Occupational Therapy for People Experiencing Illness, Injury or Impairment

For Elsevier
Senior Content Strategist: Rita Demetriou-Swanwick
Content Development Specialist: Nicola Lally
Project Manager: Kamatchi Madhavan
Designer/Design Direction: Miles Hitchen
Illustration Manager: Amy Heyden
Illustrator: Graphic World – US

Occupational Therapy for People Experiencing Illness, Injury or Impairment

PROMOTING OCCUPATION AND PARTICIPATION

Seventh Edition

EDITED BY

MICHAEL CURTIN EdD, MPhil, BOccThy

Associate Professor, Associate Head, School of Community Health, Charles Sturt University, Albury, New South Wales, Australia

MARY EGAN PhD, OT Reg. (Ont.), FCAOT

Professor, School of Rehabilitation Sciences, University of Ottawa, Ottawa, Ontario, Canada

JO ADAMS PhD, MSc, DipCOT

Professor of Musculoskeletal Health, Professional Lead for Occupational Therapy, Health Sciences, University of Southampton, Southampton, Hampshire, England

FOREWORD BY

Elizabeth Townsend, PhD, OTRegPEI, FCAOT

Professor Emerita, Dalhousie University, Halifax, Nova Scotia, Canada

ELSEVIER

Edinburgh London New York Oxford Philadelphia St Louis Sydney Toronto 2017

ELSEVIER

First edition © Longman Group Limited 1981
Second edition © Longman Group Limited 1987
Third edition © Longman Group Limited 1992
Fourth edition © Pearson Professional Group 1996
Fifth edition © Elsevier Limited 1999
Sixth edition © Elsevier Limited 2010

ISBN 978-0-7020-5446-4

Notices

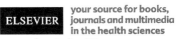

your source for books, journals and multimedia in the health sciences

www.elsevierhealth.com

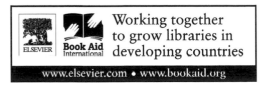

Working together to grow libraries in developing countries

www.elsevier.com • www.bookaid.org

The Publisher's policy is to use paper manufactured from sustainable forests

Printed in Great Britain
Last digit is the print number: 9   8   7

CONTENTS

PREFACE

THE RIGHT ATTITUDE

A few years ago, I (Michael Curtin) had the opportunity to work with Matthew to assist him with obtaining a new powered wheelchair and a mobile phone that he could use as an environmental control unit and as a communication device. When I met him, Matthew was in his mid-20s and was living in his own unit (apartment) in a regional town of approximately 27,000 people in northeast Victoria, Australia. I was aware, before I met Matthew, from the client notes I had read, that he had cerebral palsy – more specifically, moderately severe spastic quadriplegia. I was also aware that he required a powered wheelchair for his mobility and physical assistance with many of his personal care and daily activities.

Although I was there to assist Matthew with some of his assistive technologies, I became interested in how he came to be living by himself in his unit, a unit that he had originally rented and eventually purchased. During the course of our time together Matthew and his mother, Cathy, told me their story and also directed me to a YouTube* video they made of their story when they were asked to do a keynote presentation at a conference.

In my conversations with Matthew and Cathy I learned that he spent his childhood and adolescent years in a small rural town of approximately 280 people, which was around 20 kilometres from where he was now living. In this small rural town he lived with his parents, Cathy and Ian, and his younger sister, Abbey. Various members of the community in this town actively assisted Matthew's family with various therapies to aid Matthew's development. He attended a mainstream primary and secondary school, and after school he went to college to study for a certificate in multimedia.

I was told that when Matthew was 18 years old and studying for his certificate in multimedia, he decided he was ready to leave home. He made this decision not because he was unhappy at home but because he just 'thought it was about time'. However, it took another 3 years, until he was 21 years old, to actually make the move from the family home into a place of his own.

Cathy said that she was initially terrified at the prospect of Matthew moving out of home, as she was fearful that Matthew would be vulnerable. Despite how she initially felt, Cathy realised that if it was possible for Matthew to move out of home, there would be at least three benefits: first, Matthew would achieve his dream of being independent of the family; second, Cathy, Ian and Abbey would be able to enjoy a more spontaneous lifestyle; and third, the concerns that she and Ian had about a future in which they became too old to physically support him might be addressed.

Various options were considered, including building a flat behind the family home, purchasing a cottage away from the family home but in the same small rural town, and building three or four purpose-built units in a nearby town so that support costs could be shared between the residents of the units. However, none of these options suited Matthew's vision of living in a *regular house*, on a *regular street*. He did not want to be defined by his physical impairment, as although he used a powered wheelchair and required assistance with putting on and taking off clothes, having a shower, going to the toilet, eating a meal and having a drink, and other personal care activities, he did not see himself as disabled.

Cathy attended a series of workshops organised by Personalised Lifestyle Assistance† (PLA), where she heard stories from people who were similar to Matthew (or who had even greater support needs), who were living quite successfully in their own home in the community. She found the workshops invaluable as they laid the foundations of a new direction and renewed determination to work towards a solution for Matthew. So with the support and guidance of people from PLA she rang real estate agents looking for a wheelchair-accessible home in a good location in a nearby town. Within 6 months they came across a possible unit that was suitable. When Matthew had a look at the unit his response was immediate: 'I'll take it'! When he finally moved into his unit, he said that 'it was a GREAT day', and

---

*Interested readers can listen to Matthew and Cathy tell this story on the YouTube link: *The Story of Australian Independence with a Disability*: https://www.youtube.com/watch?v=SXEjIB8n94k

---

†Personalised Lifestyle Assistance is now called Belonging Matters. The web address for this organisation is www.belongingmatters. org. It is described as 'a small not-for-profit community education and advisory service developed by individuals and families who have a passion for social inclusion'.

indicated that even though he knew his parents were nervous, he was 'over the moon'.

Matthew chose and purchased furnishings and equipped the unit with necessary bits and pieces that he required, with the help of his parents, including a switch-operated automatic door and an accessible phone. At first he had very little money for his support needs, relying mainly on the small amount of funding he was allocated through the state government disability agency. However, he and his parents were determined to make his move work, and again with the support of PLA they developed a proposal outlining Matthew's vision for his future, including an estimation of the funding required for him to live in the unit, that they submitted to the state disability funding agency. The agency agreed to provide the funding, and with this promise of on-going support Matthew was able to really start living the life that he wanted to live.

Matthew was very comfortable living by himself and using the funding he was given to employ a team of support workers to be available at different times during the day. Support workers were recruited from a private company that was responsible for finding, interviewing, shortlisting and training prospective support workers. Matthew was then able to interview the shortlisted applicants and would make a decision about whom to appoint. The support workers provide Matthew with assistance at agreed times for his personal care and meals throughout the day.

Matthew believes that in making the decision to move out of the family home to live by himself, he became more confident when engaging with people in the community, dealing with a variety of 'different people, different personalities and, to a lesser extent, different attitudes'. These days, Matthew arranges to do the things he wants to do, the way he likes to do them. He shops, does his own banking, develops new relationships and makes his own arrangements. He is fully independent in these activities and has the control of *how* they are done and *when* they are done. From Matthew's perspective, he feels that he is able to do his 'own stuff now', is happy that he is able to buy in services as he needs them and lives life as an independent community participant.

Based on his experiences, Matthew offers the following advice: 'You just do not know the possibilities, until you try it. Whatever your disability is, whatever your fear is, whatever your abilities are […] anything is possible'. Cathy adds a caveat to Matthew's statement, explaining, 'It took a lot more than Matthew's great attitude and determination to achieve his goals. It required the support of others, both family and professionals. *He required people who shared this "can do" attitude, shared his vision, believed in him, and were willing to work with him to make his dream a reality. Anything is possible, when people have the right attitude!*'

Matthew's story of moving out of home, and his and Cathy's belief that 'anything is possible, when people have the right attitude', provides an *essential lesson* for readers of this book. Although this book has garnered the wisdom of a range of skilled and experienced occupational therapists and other professionals from around the world, and offers readers a number of approaches and strategies that can be used when working with people who have an illness, injury or impairment, all of the content is worth little if the reader does not have the 'right attitude'.

Occupational therapists who have the 'right attitude' embrace turning an individual, group, community and population's vision of possibilities into reality. Occupational therapists can do this by 'step[ping] beyond existing practices and services', and having the belief that they can do it or that they have the ability to acquire the capacity to do it (Townsend & Rappolt, 2014, p. 3, paraphrasing a Mahatma Gandhi quote). This is particularly critical when a society's invisible ableist or ageist attitudes create barriers to facilitating the right to personally valued occupation as a moral imperative for all people.

As editors of this book, we trust that readers will approach this book with 'the right attitude' and have the belief that they can acquire the capacity to 'step beyond existing practices and services' to truly meet the needs, desires, hopes and dreams of the individuals, groups, communities and populations to whom they offer client-centred, occupation-focused services.

REFERENCE

Townsend, E., & Rappolt, S. (2014). Visions of possibility: Creative occupational solutions for today's occupational challenges. *Occupational Therapy Now, 16(2)*, 3-4.

KEY FEATURES OF THE SEVENTH EDITION

Occupational Therapy and Physical Dysfunction has played a key part in preregistration occupational therapy education in the United Kingdom for more than 35 years and for the first five editions was edited by Annie Turner, Marg Foster and Sybil Johnson. The book was developed at a time when there was no book that provided a British perspective on working with people whose occupational performance was affected by physical illness, injury or impairment. It began as a collection of lecture notes on key topics and has been continually developed since the first edition was published in 1981.

Annie Turner, Marg Foster and Sybil Johnson stepped down from editing this book after the fifth edition, and the task of editing the sixth edition was taken on by Michael Curtin (Charles Sturt University, Australia), Matthew Molineux (Curtin University of Technology, Australia) and Joanne Supyk (Salford University, England). These new editors introduced significant changes to the book, which included a new subtitle of the book *(Enabling Occupation)* to reflect the primacy of occupation in occupational therapy practice; a focus on working with individuals, groups and communities; a focus on enabling skills and strategies rather than on discrete diagnostic categories; providing an international perspective to reflect the global issues that influence professional knowledge and practice; inclusion of more practice stories to illustrate the application of theory to practice; inclusion of chapter summaries and key points to provide readers with a quick overview of each chapter; and the use of person-centred and inclusive language.

When Elsevier commissioned a seventh edition of the book it was with a focus on increasing the appeal of the book within Europe and North America, as well as the Australasian region, and to appeal to occupational therapists from non-English countries. With this in mind, the editors selected for the seventh edition were Michael Curtin (Charles Sturt University, Australia), Mary Egan (University of Ottawa, Canada) and Jo Adams (University of Southampton, England).

The new editorial team for the seventh edition meant a new direction for the book, but a direction that built on the strengths of all previous editions and that would continue to contribute to preparing the next generations of occupational therapists for working in the ever-evolving world of practice. The seventh edition reflects international developments within the occupational therapy profession and the contexts of the delivery of health and social care and is built around the Canadian Practice Process Framework (CPPF), a professional reasoning process that occupational therapists may follow in practice. The following are key features of this edition of the book:

- The book is clearly aimed at preregistration occupational therapy students and early career occupational therapists. To achieve this aim we recruited an international panel of occupational therapy students who became new graduates over the course of the development of the book. This panel provided guidance on the content and the structure of the book, reviewed and provided feedback from a student/new graduate perspective on every chapter of the book, and assisted in the selection of the new book title. As editors of the book we are indebted to the exceptional contributions of each panel member and take this opportunity to publicly say thank you to Maddi Amos-Hampson, Amy Groat, Lily Ramsden, Holly Sheppard and Amanda Wangman, graduates from Charles Sturt University, Australia; Patrique Bégin, Elysia Pan and Isabelle Savage, graduates from the University of Ottawa, Canada; Anna Burroughs, Sarah Mendonca and Leah Robinson, graduates from the University of Southampton, England; and Naomi Algeo, graduate from the University of Galway.

- There has been a significant increase in the number of chapters in the book and in the number of contributors to the book. The number of chapters has increased from 33 to 50, with there now being nearly 100 contributors, with many chapters written by two or more authors. This has led to a book that more comprehensively covers the topic of working with people who have a physical illness, injury or impairment.

- Each chapter has been written to reflect the most recent research evidence that underpins occupational therapy practice.

- The inclusion of European, French Canadian and Asian occupational therapists, in a move towards having more contributors from non-English speaking countries in later editions of the book, helps better represent the global community of occupational therapists.

- In addition to occupational science, the inclusion of chapters on biomedical and social sciences showcases the sciences that underpin occupational therapy practice.

- A focus on working with groups, communities, and populations, in addition to working with individuals, reflects these growing areas of practice.

- The number of chapters on the assessment and the intervention stages of the professional reasoning process have increased.

- We've included an increased number of practice stories in chapters to provide authentic examples to illustrate the application of theory to practice. In addition, three detailed practice stories are included in the online resource for this book. The first of these practice stories focuses on Mrs Tremblay, who has experienced a cerebrovascular accident (a neurological condition); the second practice story is about Karin, a young woman diagnosed with rheumatoid arthritis (a musculoskeletal condition); and the third practice story centres on Angela, who has cancer (a medical and surgical condition) and is undergoing palliative care. These three practice stories are based on real people and provide details of the professional reasoning of the occupational therapists working with Mrs Tremblay, Karin and Angela. Reference is made at the end of each section of the book to the relevant sections of the practice stories so that readers can determine how each section of the book is practically applied to a person receiving occupational therapy.

- Each chapter includes a summary, key points and multiple choice and short-answer questions. The multiple choice questions enable readers to assess their knowledge of the content of the chapters and the short-answer questions assess application of the knowledge.

- The use of person-centred or inclusive and strengths-based language continues to be a feature in this edition of the book[‡] with some changes compared to the sixth edition. Examples include the following:
  - The term *disabled person* or *person with disability* has been used depending on the preference of the contributor. This reflects the preferred terminology of disability advocates in each contributor's country. For example, *disabled person* is the preferred term of disability advocates in the United Kingdom, as a means of politicising that disability is caused by attitudinal and environmental barriers rather than a person's impairment. In Australia and Canada disability

---

[‡]When using direct quotes, the original terminology will be retained rather than the preferred terminology for this book.

advocates prefer to use the term *people with disability* to promote people-first language. The decision to use both terms in this book depending on a contributor's preference is to reflect the global dialogue on disability. Readers will note that in many cases neither term is used as the preference was to use the phrase *a person (or people) with an illness, injury or impairment*. This choice of terminology reflects the slogan that has been used by disability organisations, 'Don't *dis* my ability'; that is what we have tried to respect in the language used in this book.

■ Where possible we have used the term *person* to refer to an individual engaged in a collaborative relationship with, and requiring the services of, an occupational therapist. The term *client* is used when referring collectively to individuals, groups, communities and populations. This means that the term *person-centred* is used when the focus is on an individual, and the term *client-centred* is used when the focus is on more than an individual.

■ The term *practice setting* continues to be used in place of *clinic* to recognise that occupational therapists provide services in a variety of workplaces.

■ *Professional reasoning*, which encompasses *occupational reasoning*, continues to be used rather than *clinical reasoning*, as the term *clinical* has medical connotations and we believe that the reasoning of occupational therapists embraces more than just the medical implications of an illness, injury or impairment on a person, group, community or population.

■ Finally, readers will note that there is a new title for the book. The term *Physical Dysfunction* was felt to be out-of-date and did not represent the contemporary strength-based and occupation-focused nature of occupational therapy practice. We feel the new title, *Occupational Therapy for People Experiencing Illness, Injury or Impairment: Promoting Occupation and Participation*, reflects this more contemporary focus of the profession. This new title, created after much consultation, acknowledges that:

  ■ occupational therapists work with people and not medical conditions and diagnoses – the term *people* here is inclusive of individuals, groups, communities and populations;

  ■ occupational therapists are interested in the lived experiences of people;

  ■ illness, injury and impairment are not the same as, and do not necessarily cause, disability (or dysfunction); and

  ■ the ultimate outcome of occupational therapy is to enable people to engage in occupations that they want, need or are expected to do, and, in the terminology used within the International Classification of Functioning, Disability and Health developed by the World Health Organization, promote the active participation of people in these occupations.

STRUCTURE OF THE SEVENTH EDITION

The chapters in this edition are set out in seven sections. These sections loosely follow the format of the CPPF, which is explained in Chapter 8, to capture the professional reasoning structure of the book.

Section 1: Introduction

Section 1: Introduction

This chapter sets the scene for occupational therapy practice by providing an overview of the evolution of the occupational therapy profession and how it has been impacted by the changing perceptions and frameworks of health care.

This section relates to the *societal and practice contexts* of the CPPF.

Section 2: Underpinning Sciences

Occupational therapy practice is underpinned by at least three broad groups of sciences. The biomedical sciences provide occupational therapists with a detailed understanding of the human body structure and function. The social sciences are important in providing a solid foundation of sociological, anthropological and psychological principles that affect the practice of occupational therapists. In many ways these two groups of sciences represent the dual heritage of the profession – the biomedical and social influences on the profession, which are identified in the first section. These sciences have been complemented by the development of occupational science, a relatively new science that aims to create an in-depth understanding of the concept of occupation, a key concept within occupational therapy practice.

This section relates to the *societal and practice contexts* of the CPPF.

Section 3: Professional Reasoning

In addition to including a chapter that provides an overview of professional reasoning and a chapter that describes the CPPF at the beginning of this section, chapters on client-centred practice and communication skills, core aspects of occupational therapy practice that are intrinsic to professional reasoning, are also included. In addition, as the practice of professional reasoning involves understanding and implementing models of practice, a number of chapters in this section provide details on key occupation-based models of practice.

This section relates to the *frame(s) of reference* component of the CPPF.

Section 4: Assessment

The assessment section includes a chapter providing an overview of the assessment process, challenging occupational therapists to remain occupation-focused. This is followed by a chapter on the Canadian Occupational Performance Measure (COPM). A series of chapters follow that present different ways of assessing a person's occupational performance, a key focus of occupational therapists when using an occupation-focused assessment approach. As occupational therapists are also interested in the environment, a chapter has been included that presents strategies to consider when assessing the environment and determining environmental factors that can facilitate and inhibit occupational performance. This section concludes with three chapters on the reasoning involved in the selection of assessments for people with neurological conditions, musculoskeletal conditions, and medical and surgical conditions.

This section relates to the *enter/initiate, set the stage, assess/evaluate, monitor/modify* and *evaluate* stages of the CPPF.

Section 5: Goals

The chapter in this section presents a structure for developing client-centred goals that have clear links to strategies and evaluation methods that address occupational engagement and performance outcomes.

This section relates to the *agree on objectives, plan* stage of the CPPF.

Section 6: Enabling Skills and Strategies

Occupational therapists use a wide range of skills and strategies when working with individuals, groups, communities and populations. This section begins with a chapter that provides an overview of these skills and strategies and then is followed by a chapter on advocacy and lobbying and one on education, as these are essential to all areas of occupational therapy practice. Then there are chapters on public health, community development and community-based rehabilitation strategies and skills that occupational therapists can use when working with communities and populations to create occupationally just societies, enabling the health and well-being of all community members. These chapters are followed by a number of chapters presenting a range of skills and strategies occupational therapists can use when working with individuals who have a physical illness, injury or impairment.

This section relates to the *implement plan* stage of the CPPF.

Section 7: Reflecting on Practice

The final chapter in this book is on *reflecting* on practice. Reflective practice is an essential skill that occupational therapists have to develop and that underpins sound professional decision-making. By developing effective reflection skills occupational therapists critically evaluate their practice, continue to evolve as practitioners, and maintain and develop their professional competencies and capacities.

This section relates to the *evaluate outcome* and *conclude/exit* stages of the CPPF.

Online Resource - Evolve Resources (evolve.elsevier.com/Curtin/OT)

This book is supported by an online resource (Evolve Resources) that includes a number of multiple choice and short-answer questions for each chapter to enable readers to assess and apply their understanding of the content within the book. In addition, three detailed practice stories are included in the online resource to clearly illustrate the application of the content of different chapters. These practice stories are referred to at the end of each section of the book.

We are grateful to the contributors from around the world who have enthusiastically given their time to share their expertise in writing the chapters for this book. We wanted to acknowledge the individuality of the each contributor, which is why there is some variance in the style of each chapter.

Working with people who are experiencing illness, injury or impairment that can affect their occupational performance and engagement is complex. Our aim for this book continues to be to provide a reference for occupational therapy students and practitioners to stimulate reflection on the knowledge, skills and attitude that inform practice, and encourage the development of occupation-focused practice.

It is an honour to be editors of this seventh edition. We trust the book will be useful to readers as they engage with working with adults who are experiencing illness, injury or impairment.

MICHAEL CURTIN

MARY EGAN

JO ADAMS

Occupational Therapy for People Experiencing Illness, Injury or Impairment:
Promoting Occupation and Participation (7th ed.)
formerly
Occupational Therapy and Physical Dysfunction

FOREWORD

O*ccupational Therapy for People Experiencing Illness, Injury or Impairment: Promoting Occupation and Participation* is a wonderfully contemporary title that jolted me to see beyond the original title, *Occupational Therapy and Physical Dysfunction,* first published in 1981. I applaud Annie Turner, Marg Foster, and Sybil Johnson, who produced the first five editions under the former title from lecture notes for occupational therapy educators, students, and practitioners within and beyond the United Kingdom. I also applaud the three international editors of the seventh edition: Michael Curtin (Australia), Mary Egan (Canada) and Jo Adams (United Kingdom). They have reconceptualised the book not only with a new title but also with contemporary theory, methods, and practice stories based on occupational therapists' current knowledge and skills for *promoting occupation and participation.*

The jolt I felt with the seventh edition's new title was followed by curiosity to read Chapter 1. Included in this opening chapter is a discussion and reflective question on *embracing the socioecological health framework* as well as the biomedical and biopsychosocial frameworks. Chapter 1 challenges occupational therapy educators, students, and practitioners to go beyond naming the environment as we do in our theoretical and practice models. To enact a socioecological framework, occupational therapists will need to engage proactively in collective, global and ecological issues that shape and are shaped by the promotion of occupation and participation in different contexts, well beyond occupational therapists' use of theoretical frameworks for understanding individual, biomedical and biopsychosocial bodies. The seventh edition also offers a critical discussion of the *International Classification of Functioning, Disability and Health* (ICF). The ICF discussion strengthens the book's concerns for promoting occupation and participation and raises questions for relying on the ICF framework in occupational therapy. A good reflective question posed here is, 'Should occupational therapists still align themselves to this [ICF] approach'?

I was delighted to see the new Chapter 2 on Occupational Science. To support practices in promoting occupation and participation, Chapter 2 builds on the introduction of the socioecological framework by emphasising 'the centrality of occupation to occupational therapy'. Here we have sections that raise 'ideas on how occupation is experienced, organised, and socially shaped', along with examples of 'how knowledge of occupation informs occupational therapy practice'. Readers may wish to consult this chapter's excellent overview of diverse definitions of occupation and the sequential arguments captured in subtitles: 'occupation as central to occupational therapy practice', 'occupational science as core to expanding knowledge about occupation', 'occupation as core to human living', and 'occupation as situated'. Chapter 2 does a marvellous job of synthesising emerging ideas from occupational science; occupation-based practice is illustrated with examples on the experience and organisation of occupation.

A valuable addition to previous editions is the inclusion of three detailed stories of occupational therapy practices that all follow the process stages of the Canadian Practice Process Framework (CPPF). The authors also attend to the enablement competencies and collaborative processes that are consistent with the Canadian Model of Client-Centred Engagement (CMCE). One story focuses on working with an individual whose occupations have been disrupted by the impacts of a stroke in the acute, inpatient rehabilitation and community rehabilitation phases of stroke recovery toward optimal home and societal participation. Another story portrays occupational therapy practice in promoting occupation and participation with an individual diagnosed with early-stage rheumatoid arthritis who is followed through on-going challenges in social participation 3 years later. The other story profiles the promotion of occupation and participation with an individual with cancer in a palliative care unit. These practice stories offer a structure for lively dialogue on the opportunities and pitfalls for occupation-based practitioners working with persons experiencing occupational changes in health contexts and in the home, employment settings and communities. The standardised stages of the CPPF used in writing these practice stories will be a useful illustration for educators, students, and practitioners of how to write their own practice stories and to critically reflect on the conditions that help and limit occupational therapists' promotion of occupation and participation associated with the CPPF process stages. The use of CMCE to guide collaborative partnerships opens the door for energetic conversations on the opportunities and pitfalls for professionals in promoting occupation and participation with individuals who encounter illness, injury and impairment in diverse contexts. Such dialogues will expand critical occupational literacy to think, talk and write about occupation with teams, clients and the public, and to advocate in health and other systems for the importance of occupation-based approaches (Townsend, 2015; Townsend & Friedland, 2016) with individuals, families, groups, communities and populations.

Finally, there is much to celebrate in the tighter cohesion and internationalisation of the seventh edition. Imagine the potential for professional cohesion in thinking about core ideas and practices in occupational therapy for promoting occupation and participation with those experiencing illness, injury and impairment around the world! One point of cohesion is the strong emphasis on reflective practice, for instance, Chapter 50 invites reflection on the self as an occupational therapist, and on practice situations. The seventh edition offers many points that can stimulate professional cohesion – on theoretical frameworks, core concerns for occupation, standard stages of the practice process and concerns for respect and power as a profession that professes to be client-centred or person-centred with individuals, families, groups, communities and populations. Reading the seventh edition, I see a contemporary, exciting vision and a growing array of practice stories for occupational therapists contributing to health, well-being and justice around the world – a vibrant profession with theories and methods that affect what people with illnesses, injuries and impairments can actually do in real life. May everyone find this seventh edition as interesting and worthwhile as I do. Here is a book that advances both a core identity and practical guidance for occupational therapists and others who may wish to see how this profession is evolving to address real life issues. Thank you for including me in such an important book by offering me the honour of writing this foreword.

Elizabeth Townsend, PhD, OT Reg PEI, FCAOT
Professor Emerita with Dalhousie University
and an Adjunct Professor with the
University of Prince Edward Island

REFERENCES

Townsend, E. A. (2015). The 2014 Ruth Zemke Lectureship in Occupational Science. Critical occupational literacy: Thinking about occupational justice, ecological sustainability, and aging in everyday life. *Journal of Occupational Science, 22,* 389–402.

Townsend, E. A., & Friedland, J. (2016). 19th & 20th century educational reforms arising in Europe, the United Kingdom and the Americas: Inspiration for occupational science? *Journal of Occupational Science.* Retrieved from. http://dx.doi.org/10.1080/14427591.2016.1232184.

CONTRIBUTORS LIST

REBECCA ALDRICH, PhD, OTR/L
Assistant Professor, Occupational Science and
Occupational Therapy, Saint Louis University,
Saint Louis, Missouri, United States of America

**SUE BAPTISTE, MHSc, OTDip, OT REG. (ONT.),
FCAOT**
Professor (tenured), School of Rehabilitation Science,
McMaster University, Hamilton, Ontario, Canada

MELANIE BERGTHORSON, MSC(OT), BMROT, BA
Faculty Lecturer, School of Physical and Occupational
Therapy, McGill University, Montreal, Quebec, Canada
Occupational Therapist, MAB-Mackay Rehabilitation
Centre, Montreal, Quebec, Canada

MATHILDA BJÖRK, PhD, BSc OT
Associate professor and Program Director
Occupational Therapy Program, Linköping
University, Linköping, Sweden

**JENNI BOURKE, SPECIALIST CERTIFICATE IN PALLIATIVE
CARE, BAPPSC(OT)**
Senior Occupational Therapist, Occupational
Therapy, Peter MacCallum Cancer Centre,
Melbourne, Victoria, Australia

**JULIA BOWMAN, PhD, MAPPSc(OT)RES, BAPPSC
(OT)DIST**
Research Operations Manager, Justice Health &
Forensic Mental Health Network, Malabar,
New South Wales, Australia

SARAH BRADLEY, MSc (HAND THERAPY), DIPCOT
Advanced Occupational Therapy Practitioner,
Hand Therapy Department, Therapy
Services Poole Hospital NHS Foundation
Trust, Occupational Therapist, BMI Harbour
Hospital, Poole, England

**CATHERINE ELIZABETH BRIDGE, PhD (ARCH),
MCOGSC, BAPPSC (OT)**
Associate Professor, Faculty of the Built Environment,
University of New South Wales, Kensington,
New South Wales, Australia

**MARTINE BROUSSEAU, PhD, MAMS, OT REG.
(ONT.)**
Professor, Department of Occupational Therapy,
Université du Québec à Trois-Rivières,
Trois-Rivières, Québec, Canada

NOÉMI CANTIN, PhD, MSc, OT
Associate Professor, Department of Occupational
Therapy, Université du Québec à Trois-Rivières,
Trois-Rivières, Québec, Canada

**GUNILLA CARLSSON, PhD, MSc(OCCTHY),
BSC(OCCTHY)**
Associate Professor, Lund University, Department of
Health Sciences, Lund, Sweden

**PHILLIPPA CARNEMOLLA, PhD, MDES(INDDES),
BDES(INDDES)**
Research Associate, Enabling Built Environment
Program, University of New South Wales, Sydney,
New South Wales, Australia

CHRIS CHAPPARO, PhD, MA, DIPOT
Discipline of Occupational Therapy, Faculty of Health
Sciences, The University of Sydney, Sydney, New
South Wales, Australia

GILL CHARD, PhD, BSc (HONS), DIPCOT
Research Director and Academic Consultant, AMPS
UK and Ireland, Lancaster, United Kingdom
Professor (retired) Occupational Science &
Occupational Therapy, University College Cork,
Cork, Ireland

PROFESSOR LESLEY CHENOWETH, PhD, MSW, BSW
ProVice Chancellor, Griffith University, Brisbane,
   Queensland, Australia

KEVIN COCKS, MSWAP, AM
Anti-Discrimination Commissioner, Anti-
   Discrimination Commission of Queensland,
   Brisbane, Queensland, Australia

LESLEY COLLIER, PhD, MSc, DipCOT
Senior Lecturer in Occupational Therapy, Faculty of
   Health Sciences University of Southampton,
   Southampton, England

**RICHARD COLLIER, PhD, MSc, PFHEA,
GRADDIPPHYS, MCSP, MMACP**
Director of Programmes: Physical & Rehabilitation
   Health, Faculty of Health Sciences University of
   Southampton, Southampton, England

**HEATHER COLQUHOUN, PHD, BScOT, OT REG.
(ONT.)**
Assistant Professor, Occupational Science and
   Occupational Therapy, University of Toronto,
   Toronto, Ontario, Canada

**CLAIRE CRAIG, PhD, MA (OXON), BSc (HONS),
BA HISTORY, FCOT**
Occupational Therapy, Sheffield Hallam University,
   Sheffield, Yorkshire, England

JANE A. DAVIS, MSc, OT REG. (ONT.)
Lecturer, Department of Occupational Science and
   Occupational Therapy, University of Toronto,
   Toronto, Ontario, Canada

**DEIRDRE R. DAWSON, PhD, MSc, BSR, OT REG.
(ONT.)**
Associate Professor, Department of Occupational
   Science & Occupational Therapy, University of
   Toronto
Senior Scientist, Rotman Research Institute, Baycrest,
   Toronto, Ontario, Canada

**MARILYN DI STEFANO, PhD, GRAD DIP
ERGONOMICS, BAppSc(OT)**
Road User Behaviour Team, VicRoads, Melbourne
Honorary Senior Lecturer, School of Allied Health La
   Trobe University, Bundoora, Australia

RACHAEL DIXEY, PhD, BSc
Emeritus Professor, Centre for Health Promotion
   Research, Leeds Beckett University, Leeds, England

**SIMONE DORSCH, PhD, MHLTHSCI, BAppSci
(PHYSIO)**
Lecturer, School of Physiotherapy, Australian Catholic
   University, Australia
StrokeEd, Sydney, New South Wales, Australia

CAROLYN DUNFORD, PhD MSc
Head of Therapy & Research, Therapy & Research,
   The Children's Trust, Tadworth, England

SALLY EAMES, PhD, BOccThy (HONS I)
Occupational Therapist, Community, Indigenous and
   Subacute Services, Metro North Hospital and
   Health Service; and Adjunct Lecturer, School of
   Health and Rehabilitation Sciences, The University
   of Queensland, Brisbane Australia

JEN GASH, KMCC, DIP CMI, BSc(HONS)OT
Coach, Occupational Therapist, Artist & Director of
   Craft Your Life Ltd., South Gloucestershire,
   England

MARIE GRANDISSON, PhD, MSc, BSc(OT)
Assistant Professor, Department of Rehabilitation,
   Laval University, Québec City, Québec, Canada

STEFANIE HAIDER, MAGPHIL, BSc
Division of Rheumatology, Department of Internal
   Medicine III, Medical University of Vienna, Austria

KAREN WHALLEY HAMMELL, PhD, MSc, DipCOT
Honorary Professor, Occupational Science &
   Occupational Therapy, University of British
   Columbia, Vancouver, British Columbia, Canada

**ALISON HAMMOND, PhD, MSc, BSc(HONS),
DipCOT**
Professor in Rheumatology Rehabilitation, Centre for
   Health Sciences Research, University of Salford,
   Salford, Greater Manchester, United Kingdom

AMY HEINZ, OTD, OTR/L, CLCP
Occupational Therapist, Fairview Health Services,
   Minnesota, United States of America

NARELLE HIGSON, BAppSc (OT)
Occupational Therapist, Sexuality Advisory Service,
    Multiple Sclerosis Society of Western Australia,
    Perth, Western Australia, Australia
Principal, Outside the Square OT Solutions, Perth,
    Western Australia, Australia

CLARE HOCKING, PhD, MHSc, ADV DIP OT,
DIP OT
Professor, Occupational Science and Therapy,
    Auckland University of Technology, Auckland,
    New Zealand

TAMMY HOFFMANN, PhD, BOccThy (HONS 1)
Professor, Centre for Research in Evidence-Based
    Practice, Bond University, Robina, Gold Coast,
    Australia

ANNE W. HUNT, PhD, MSc, BSc(OT), OT REG.
(ONT.)
Manager Student-led Concussion Clinic and
    Clinical Study Investigator, Bloorview Research
    Institute, Holland Bloorview Kids Rehabilitation
    Hospital
Assistant Professor, Department of Occupational
    Science and Occupational Therapy, University of
    Toronto, Toronto, Ontario, Canada

JEANETTE ISAACS-YOUNG, PCC, DIP TRANSPERSONAL
PSYCHOLOGY, GRAD DIP (MOVEMENT AND DANCE
EDUCATION), BAppSc(OT)
Principal, Lifestream Associates, Kiel Mountain,
    Queensland, Australia

MICHELLE JACKMAN, BOT
Occupational Therapist, John Hunter Children's
    Hospital, Newcastle, New South Wales, Australia
PhD Candidate, Cerebral Palsy Alliance Research
    Institute, The University of Sydney, Sydney, New
    South Wales, Australia

SHARON JOINES, PhD IE, MS IE, BS IE, IDSA
Associate Professor of Industrial Design,
    Graphic and Industrial Design, NC State
    University, Raleigh, North Carolina,
    United States

DOROTHY KESSLER, PhD, MSc, BMROT, OT REG.
(ONT.)
Postdoctoral Fellow, Bruyere Research Institute,
    Ottawa, Ontario, Canada

NATASHA A. LANNIN, PhD, BSc(OT),
GRADDIP
Associate Professor, School of Allied Health, La Trobe
    University, Melbourne, Australia
Associate Professor, Occupational Therapy
    Department, Alfred Health, Melbourne, Victoria,
    Australia

NATASHA A. LAYTON, PhD, MHLTSc, BAppSc
(OccTHER)
Principal, Natasha Layton & Associates, Melbourne,
    Victoria, Australia
Casual Lecturer, School of Health and Social
    Inclusion, Deakin University, Burwood, Victoria,
    Australia

ALEXANDRA LONSDALE, BHSc(OT)
Occupational Therapist, Client Services, Vision
    Australia, Bendigo, Victoria, Australia

AGNETA MALMGREN FÄNGE, PhD, DIPED,
MSc(OccTHY), BSc(OccTHY)
Associate Professor, Department of Health Sciences,
    Lund University, Lund, Sweden

CELIA MARSTON, MPALLCARE, BAppSc(OT)
Lecturer, Occupational Therapy, Faculty
    of Medicine, Nursing and Health Sciences,
    Monash University, Frankston, Victoria,
    Australia

ROSE MARTINI, PhD, OT REG (ONT)
Associate Professor, Occupational Therapy Program,
    School of Rehabilitation Sciences, Faculty of Health
    Sciences, University of Ottawa, Ottawa, Ontario,
    Canada

ANNIE McCLUSKEY, PhD, MA, DIPCOT
Honorary Senior Lecturer, Discipline of
    Occupational Therapy, Faculty of Health Sciences,
    The University of Sydney, Lidcombe, New South
    Wales, Australia
StrokeEd, Sydney, New South Wales, Australia

RACHAEL LEIGH MCDONALD, PHD, GCHE, PGDIP (BIOMECH), BAPPSC(OT)
Associate Professor, Department Chair, Department of Health and Medical Sciences, Hawthorn Victoria, Australia

SARA E. MCEWEN, PHD, MSC, BSC(PT)
Scientist, St. John's Rehab Research Program Sunnybrook Research Institute, Assistant Professor, Department of Physical Therapy, University of Toronto, Toronto, Ontario, Canada

JACQUELINE MCKENNA, MSC, PGCHEPR, NLPPRAC, BSC(HONS), DIPCOT, FHEA
Programme Leader/Senior Lecturer, Directorate of Radiography and Occupational Therapy, School of Health Sciences, University of Salford, Salford, Greater Manchester, England

SUE MESA, MSC, BSC (HONS) OT
Senior Lecturer in Occupational Therapy, School of Health Sciences, York St John University, York, England

VALERIE METCALFE, BSC (OT), OT REG. (ONT.)
Occupational Therapist, Interprofessional Rehabilitation Clinic, Ottawa, Canada

VIRGINIA MITSCH, MOT, BAPPSCI (OT)
Adult Team Leader/Occupational Therapist, South West Brain Injury Rehabilitation Service, Occupational Therapy Advisor, NSW Health-Murrumbidgee Health District, Lavington, New South Wales, Australia

LISE MOGENSEN, PHD, BAPPSC (HONS) OT
Lecturer in Medical Education (Research & Evaluation), School of Medicine, Western Sydney University, Sydney, New South Wales, Australia

HANIF FARHAN MOHD RASDI, MHSC(RES)(UKM), BOT(HONS)(UKM)
Lecturer, Occupational Therapy Programme, Centre of Rehabilitation Studies, The National University of Malaysia (Universiti Kebangsaan Malaysia), Jln. Raja Muda Abdul Aziz, Wilayah Persekutuan Kuala Lumpur, MYS

PhD Candidate, Faculty of Health Sciences, University of Southampton, Southampton, England

DEIDRE MORGAN, PHD, MCLSC, BAPPSC(OT)
Occupational Therapy, School of Health Sciences, Flinders University, Adelaide, South Australia, Australia

JANET F. MURCHISON, BSC (OT), BFA, OT REG. (ONT.)
Occupational Therapist, Brain Health Centre - Mood Clinic, - Baycrest, Lecturer, Department of Occupational Science and Occupational Therapy, University of Toronto, Toronto, Ontario, Canada

MELISSA THERESE NOTT, PHD, BAPPSC (OT)
Lecturer, School of Community Health, Faculty of Science, Charles Sturt University, Albury, New South Wales, Australia

IONA NOVAK, PHD, MSC(HONS), BAPPSC (OT)
Professor, Cerebral Palsy Alliance Research Institute, Brain Mind Research Institute, University of Sydney, Sydney, New South Wales, Australia

CHRISTINA LARISSA PARASYN, MASTER OF SOCIAL SCIENCE (INTERNATIONAL DEVELOPMENT), BAPPSC (OT)
Independent Consultant, Fairfield, New South Wales, Australia

TRACEY ELIZABETH PARNELL, PHD, MOT, BAAPPSC (OT)
Allied Health Clinical Education Coordinator, Professional Development and Research Unit, Albury Wodonga Health, Albury, New South Wales, Australia

ANDREW PAYNE, PHD, MARCH, BEDA
Department Chair and Associate Professor, Built Environment, Indiana State University, Terre Haute, Indiana, United States

WENDY PENTLAND, PCC, PHD, MED, BSC(OT), OT REG. (ONT.)
Life & Executive Coach, Kingston, Ontario, Canada

GENEVIÈVE PÉPIN, PHD, MSC, BSC (OT), GRADCERT HED
Associate Professor, Occupational Therapy Course Director and Honours Coordinator
School of Health and Social Development Deakin University, Geelong, Victoria, Australia

CYNTHIA PERLMAN, MED., BSC (OT)
Assistant Professor (Professional), School of Physical and Occupational Therapy, McGill University, Montreal, Québec, Canada

JUDITH PETTIGREW, PHD, MA, BSC (OT), DIPCOT
Senior Lecturer, Clinical Therapies, University of Limerick, Limerick, Ireland

SIMONE LUSCHIN, MA, PT
Deputy Head of Master Course, Master Course Holistic Therapy and Salutogenesis, FH CAMPUS WIEN University of Applied Science, Vienna, Austria
Lecturer of Physiotherapy, FH CAMPUS WIEN, University of Applied Science, Vienna, Austria

HELENE J. POLATAJKO, PHD, MED, BOT, OT REG. (ONT.), FCAOT, FCAHS
Professor, Department of Occupational Science and Occupational Therapy, University of Toronto, Toronto, Ontario, Canada

DR YELIZ PRIOR, PHD, PGCAP, MBPC, BSC (HONS) OT
Research Fellow and Deputy Director of PGR Studies School of Health Sciences, University of Salford, Greater Manchester, England
Advanced Clinical Specialist OT in Rheumatology, Mid-Cheshire NHS Foundation Trust, Crewe, England

LUCIA RAMSEY, BSC (HONS) OT
Lecturer, School of Life and Health Sciences, Ulster University, Jordanstown, Northern Ireland

JUDY L. RANKA, HLTHSCD, MA(EDUC&WORK), BSC (OT)
Director and Principal Occupational Therapist, Occupational Performance Network, Honorary Senior Lecturer, Discipline of Occupational Therapy, University of Sydney, Sydney, New South Wales, Australia

JACQUIE RIPAT, PHD, MSC, BMR(OT)
Associate Professor, Department of Occupational Therapy, University of Manitoba, Winnipeg, Manitoba, Canada

CARLIA RIX, BOCCSC/THY
Occupational Therapist, Vision Australia, Bendigo, Victoria, Australia

KATIE ROBINSON, PHD, MSC (DISABILITY MANAGEMENT), BSC (CUR. OCC.)
Senior Lecturer, Clinical Therapies, University of Limerick, Limerick, Ireland

KRISTY MAREE ROBSON, PHD, MHSC(ED), DIPHSC(POD)
Lecturer, School of Community Health, Faculty of Science, Charles Sturt University, Albury, New South Wales, Australia

VALMAE ROSE, BOT(HONS)
Director, Marsden Families Program, Brisbane, Queensland, Australia

DEBBIE LALIBERTE RUDMAN, PHD, MSC BSC (OT), OT REG. (ONT.)
Associate Professor, Occupational Therapy, University of Western Ontario, London, Ontario, Canada

ANICK SAUVAGEAU, M. RÉAD
Professor, Occupational Therapy, Université du Québec à Trois-Rivières, Trois-Rivières, Québec, Canada

KATRINE SAUVÉ-SHENK, MPH, BSC(OT), OT REG. (ONT.)
PhD Candidate, School of Rehabilitation Sciences, University of Ottawa, Ottawa, Ontario, Canada

KARL SCHURR, MAPPSC, BAPPSC(PHYSIO)
StrokeEd, Sydney, New South Wales, Australia

ELIZABETH R. SKIDMORE, PHD, OTR/L
Associate Professor, Department of Occupational Therapy, University of Pittsburgh, Pittsburgh, Pennsylvania, United States of America

BETH SPRUNT, MPH, BOT(HONS)
Senior Technical Adviser, Disability Inclusive
Development, Nossal Institute for Global Health,
The University of Melbourne, Carlton, Victoria,
Australia

RUTH SQUIRE, MSC, DIPCOT
Programme Manager Occupational Therapy, School
of Health Care Sciences, College of Biomedical and
Life Sciences, Cardiff University, Cardiff, Wales

**TANJA A. STAMM, PRIV DOZ, DR HUM BIOL, PHD,
MSC, MBA, MAG PHIL, OT**
Professor in Outcomes Research, chair and head of
Section for Outcomes Research, Center for Medical
Statistics, Informatics and Intelligent Systems,
Medical University of Vienna, Austria

KIRSTY STEWART, BOT
Senior Occupational Therapist, Queensland Health,
Gayndah, Queensland, Australia
Formerly, Occupational Therapist, Vision Australia,
Wagga Wagga/Albury, New South Wales, Australia

AGNES STURMA, MSC, BSC
Christian Doppler Laboratory for Restoration of
Extremity Function, Medical University of Vienna,
Master Degree Program Health Assisting
Engineering, University of Applied Sciences FH
Campus, Vienna, Austria

KIRSTY THOMPSON, PHD, BAPPSC OT (HONS)
Director, Inclusive Development, CBM Australia,
Melbourne, Victoria, Australia

INGRID THYBERG, PHD, BSC OT
Associate Professor, Rheumatology, Department of
Clinical and Experimental Medicine, Linköping
University, Linköping, Sweden

**MERRILL TURPIN, PHD, GRADDIPCOUNSEL,
BOCCTHY**
Senior Lecturer, School of Health and Rehabilitation,
The University of Queensland, St. Lucia,
Queensland, Australia

CAROLYN ANNE UNSWORTH, PHD, BAPPSC (OT)
Professor, Department of Occupational Therapy,
Central Queensland University, Melbourne,
Victoria, Australia
Adjunct Professor, School of Rehabilitation,
Jonkoping University, Jonkoping, Smaland,
Sweden
Adjunct Professor, School of Occupational Therapy
and Social Work, Curtin University, Perth, Western
Australia, Australia
Adjunct Professor, Discipline of Occupational
Therapy, La Trobe University, Melbourne, Victoria,
Australia

**HELEN VAN HUET, PHD,
GRADCERTLEARN&TEACHHIGHERED, BAPPSC
(OCCTHER)**
Lecturer, School of Community Health, Charles
Sturt University, Albury, New South Wales,
Australia

KATHY WHALLEY, BSC(HONS)(OT)
Accredited Hand Therapist, Specialist
Occupational Therapist, Hampshire Hospitals
NHS Foundation Trust, Royal Hampshire
County Hospital, Winchester, Hampshire,
England

TESS WHITEHEAD, BSC(HONS) OT
Independent Occupational Therapist, Fleet,
Hampshire, England

**BRIANA WILSON, MDVST (HUMAN RIGHTS),
BAPPSC (OCCTHER) (HONS)**
Technical Advisor Manager, Inclusive
Development Department, CBM Australia,
Melbourne, Victoria
Honorary Associate Lecturer, Faculty of
Health Sciences, The University of Sydney,
Australia

LISE ZAKUTNEY, BSC OT, OT REG. (ONT.)
Occupational Therapist, Champlain Regional Stroke
Program, The Ottawa Hospital, Ottawa, Ontario,
Canada

Section 1

INTRODUCTION

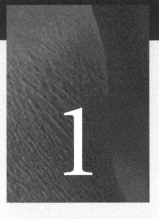

1

EVOLUTION OF OCCUPATIONAL THERAPY WITHIN THE HEALTH CARE CONTEXT

MICHAEL CURTIN ▪ JO ADAMS ▪ MARY EGAN

Abstract
The occupational therapy profession began in the early 1900s at a time when the biomedical framework of health was dominant. Although the pioneers of the profession were initially influenced by the moral treatment and arts and crafts movements, the profession became more aligned to the biomedical approach. The development of the biopsychosocial, International Classification of Functioning, Disability and Health, and socioecological health frameworks all had an impact on the evolution on the occupational therapy profession. This included a move away from the biomedical way of practice, to a stronger focus on the importance of occupation for people's health and well-being. More recently it has led to occupational therapists embracing occupation-focused strategies for working with groups, communities, populations and organisations in addition to working with individuals. The profession has moved to a stage in its evolution where it is poised to develop a secure identity, confident in its unique occupational contribution to health.

KEY POINTS

- The biomedical framework is based on the assumption that health is the absence of illness, injury or impairment in an individual.

- The biopsychosocial framework is underpinned by system theory in which a person's health is determined by the dynamic interaction of a person's body structures and functions, subjective behaviours, beliefs, thought processes, motivations and experiences, and culture, family, community and society.

- The International Classification of Functioning, Disability and Health framework integrates the biomedical and social models and recognises that health is multidimensional and affected by multiple factors.

- The socioecological framework focuses on prevention and social responsibility of illness, injury and impairment and the promotion of health and well-being, moving beyond the medical treatment of an individual and of medical conditions.

- The evolution of the occupational therapy profession has been affected by changing health perspectives influenced by which framework was more prominent.

- Contemporary occupational therapy practise embraces the profession's unique occupational focus and offers services to enhance the health and well-being and occupational engagement of individuals, groups, communities, populations and organisations.

INTRODUCTION

The concept of health is dynamic and evolving, making it difficult to define (Taylor, 2008a). The multiplicity of meanings of health are specific to the 'the unique individual, family, social and cultural context in which the term is used' (Liamputtong, Fanany, & Verrinder, 2012, p. 2). Even though health is difficult to define, the Australian Institute of Health and Welfare (AIHW) states that, 'Health, or being in good health, is important to everyone [...] [influencing] not just how we feel, but how we function and participate in the community' (Australian Institute of Health and Welfare, 2014, p. 3). Taylor (2008a, p. 4) supports this notion stating that people understand that it is important to have 'good health and access to quality health care', both of which are considered basic human rights 'in the Universal Declaration of Human Rights [...] for all people regardless of race, religion or political beliefs' (United Nations, 1948).

The nearest there is to having a universal definition of health is the one written in the Preamble to the Constitution of the World Health Organization (WHO), in which health is described as 'a state of complete physical, mental and social well-being and not merely the absence of disease or infirmity'. This definition marked a significant shift from health being the absence of illness, injury or impairment to health being each person's subjective perception of, and satisfaction with, their life whether or not they had an illness, injury or impairment (King, 2014). The WHO definition indicated that health included mental and social factors, in addition to an individual's physical factors, which eventually led to the development of the biopsychosocial view of health (Germov, 2005a) and laid the foundations for the development of health promotion as a health intervention strategy and strategies for the prevention of illness, injury and impairment (Wilcock & Hocking, 2015).

In spite of health being difficult to define, key perspectives have been identified that illustrate the evolution of understanding this concept. Taylor (2008b) proposes four key ways of understanding health, what she refers to as health frameworks: biomedical, biopsychosocial, International Classification of Functioning, Disability and Health (ICF) and socioecological. She states that these frameworks of health are 'underpinned by differing conceptualizations of core constructs like health, illness and well-being, which become translated into health policy, service delivery and professional practice' (Taylor, 2008b, p. 23-24).

Occupational therapy practice has been influenced by these frameworks. As different frameworks have become more favoured or dominant, occupational therapy practice changed and the philosophy underpinning the profession evolved. To comprehend the evolution of occupational therapy practice, from the inception of the profession in the early twentieth century to contemporary time, it helps to reflect on the development of the profession in response to the different health frameworks. Within this chapter, an overview of the four health frameworks proposed by Taylor will be described along with a broad outline of the associated evolution of the occupational therapy profession and practise.

BIOMEDICAL FRAMEWORK OF HEALTH

Overview of the Biomedical Framework of Health Care

The biomedical framework is based on the premise that health is the absence of illness, injury or impairment in an individual, and the assumption that there are two states of being: a healthy state, in which there is no illness, injury or impairment, and an ill state in which there is the presence of illness, injury or impairment (Taylor, 2008b). Germov (2005a, p. 13) states that this framework is

a traditional approach to medicine in Western societies. Illness is diagnosed and explained as a malfunction of one of the body's biological systems. [The focus within this framework is] on fixing these problems by treating individuals, particularly through surgery and drug therapy.

It is proposed that this framework emerged in the eighteenth and nineteenth centuries in line with the move towards rational and logical thinking, away from knowledge based on religious scriptures (Wilcock & Hocking, 2015). This was the period in which effective, more scientific, treatments for common diseases such as smallpox were being developed (Germov, 2005a; Wilcock & Hocking, 2015). The focus was on treating the disease, as it was believed that each disease had a single specific cause.

This was also the period in which the mind and body were considered to be separate with neither having an impact on the other (Wilcock & Hocking, 2015). This construct was known as Cartesian mind-body dualism where issues of body were the focus of medicine and issues of the mind were spiritual matters (Germov, 2005a). This led to a detailed understanding of the anatomy and physiology of the human body and the impact of pathology (Germov, 2005a). This in turn led to the creation of health experts who made clinical diagnoses based on a medical history and the use of tests and examination to identify signs of illness, injury or impairment and who prescribed drug and surgical treatments to cure disease and fix the body (Germov, 2005a; Taylor, 2008b; Wilcock & Hocking, 2015).

The biomedical framework has come under robust criticism, particularly as different perspectives of health evolved from the mid-twentieth century. According to Taylor (2008b), Germov (2005a) and Wilcock and Hocking (2015) the main criticism is that the underpinning assumptions of this framework were reductionist and did not take into account other factors that affected health and the different ways of understanding health and illness. It was evident when using this approach that the views and opinions of people experiencing the illness, injury or impairment were not sought, as the focus was on treating the condition not the person. As a result, this reductionist approach was unable to provide a sound 'explanation of who becomes ill and who stays healthy, as it does not account for the complex interplay of personal, environmental, psychological, physiological and occupational factors that impact on health' (Wilcock & Hocking, 2015, p. 67). In addition, the separation of the mind and body, a result of the reductionist approach, contributed to a number of negative outcomes, such as the objectification of people who were referred to by the name of the health condition with which they had been diagnosed or as 'patients', passive recipients of 'expert' health advice and treatment.

Even though the biomedical framework has received robust criticism, it still significantly influences current 'policies, service delivery, health-related research and professional healthcare practice' in Western countries (Taylor, 2008b). Partly this is because the scientific advances made under this framework have led to many beneficial treatments (Germov, 2005a). In spite of this, there has been a growing push for a broader approach to health, particularly since the 1970s, which led to the development of the biopsychosocial framework (Taylor, 2008b).

The Beginning of the Occupational Therapy Profession

The occupational therapy profession started in the early 1900s when the biomedical framework was the primary focus of medical intervention. In spite of the dominance of this framework the early pioneers of the profession were primarily influenced by a radically different approach. The early pioneers became focused on developing a more respectful way of working with people with mental illness, and implemented the idea of doing, or keeping busy, based on the moral treatment and the art and crafts movements, suggesting that this led to better health outcomes (Husman, 2014; Nastasi, 2014).

The moral treatment movement offered an alternative to treating people with mental health illness compared with the biomedical approach. The biomedical approach was described as subjecting people to 'terrible living conditions and horrifying treatments' based on 'the idea that people with mental illnesses

were influenced by negative supernatural forces' (Husman, 2014, p. 34). The moral movement, which began in the early 1800s, was based on a humanistic philosophy that focused on treating people with a mental illness humanely and with respect. The focus was on providing opportunities for people with mental illness to be engaged in activities such as work, art and crafts, and regular exercise, as an effective means of recovery from mental illness. Husman (2014, p. 34) stated that 'the implementation of the moral treatment paved the way for the use of occupation as a healing modality and set a course for the emerging profession of occupational therapy'.

The arts and crafts movement began in the 1800s in response to the disruption to the daily lives of people caused by the move from family farms into cities for work, mainly in factories, as a result of industrialization. Proponents of the arts and crafts movement believed that the 'reliance on machines, poor working conditions, and displacement of human skill caused a deterioration of physical health as well as the common complaint of disease, anxiety, and fatigue' (Husman, 2014, p. 34). Engaging in activities that involved making arts and crafts products by hand, in a traditional manner, was seen as a way to prevent the perceived negative effects of factory work.

Based on these movements, the early pioneers of the occupational therapy profession instigated numerous approaches to engage people in art and craft activities. The integration of the two movements was believed 'to meet the rehabilitation goals of patients with both physical and mental disabilities' (Husman, 2014, p. 34) and was considered an effective means of maintaining and improving people's health (Ward, Mitchell, & Price, 2007).

Turner (2011) proposes that at the beginning of the profession occupational therapy had a dual heritage, inheriting doctrines and practices from medicine and the moral treatment from the arts and crafts movements. She suggested that being influenced by two philosophically different heritages led to 'issues of self-esteem and identity', which was exacerbated by a directive that occupational therapy should be only 'carried out under medical direction' (Turner, 2011, p. 137). This remit to obey the medical influence led to the profession becoming dependent on medicine and, in the early years, not developing a 'sense of professional autonomy and vision' (Turner, 2011, p. 137).

Occupational Therapy Practice and the Biomedical Framework

With the advent of World War I and the increase in the number of people who developed physical and mental health illnesses, injuries and impairments, the work of the profession expanded. In addition to offering arts and crafts activities, therapists began to construct and adapt equipment, and develop alternative ways for people to do everyday activities such as washing and dressing. This led to advances in the profession and to the adoption of the biomedical framework, as it was deemed that more rigorous scientific foundations were required for the profession to develop and to fit in with other health professionals. There was a move to create a more scientific basis for using activities to facilitate recovery.

The biomedical focus of the profession continued during World War II as the rehabilitation movement developed in response to the injuries sustained by soldiers. The rehabilitation movement 'began by recognizing that, with proper care and rehabilitation, individuals with disabilities could be independent and contributing members of the community' (Husman, 2014, p. 38). Occupational therapists embraced this movement by increasing their repertoire of technical skills, becoming experts in the training and fitting of orthotics, exercises and daily living activities, and expanding their practice areas. More significantly occupational therapists became more aligned with the biomedical framework and focused primarily on treating and reducing 'deficits' and 'normalising' people who had an illness, injury or impairment (Husman, 2014).

As the rehabilitation movement expanded in the 1960s and medical knowledge became more advanced, medical fields became more specialized. Occupational therapists followed suit and became more specialized. The biomedical framework became more influential and dominant, affecting the way occupational therapy was practised (Letts, 2011). Turner (2011, p. 317) proposed that occupational therapists became 'a minority group within the medically dominated health care'. The use of arts and crafts as a therapy intervention was reduced and occupational therapists began to integrate more 'scientific' approaches into their practice, 'borrowing theory bases and specialist techniques from other profession[s]', such as medicine, psychology and sociology, as a way of enhancing credibility (Turner, 2011, p. 317).

It has been suggested that occupational therapy became more mechanistic during this period (Gillen & Greber, 2014; Hocking, 2013) as assessments and interventions were primarily focused on body structures and functions, treating illness, injury or impairment, and using quantitative measures for monitoring improvement (e.g. muscle strength increase, increased range of motion). Occupational therapy as a profession embraced the biomedical framework and neglected the original philosophy of the profession as envisaged by the founders (Hocking, 2013).

This contributed to a crisis of identity within the profession. Wilding and Whiteford (2007) proposed that this occurred because the focus on enabling occupation was not central to the profession, leading to indecision within the profession about its core values and concerns. The philosophy underpinning the occupational therapy profession became vague and poorly articulated, and the way practitioners practised varied.

THE BIOPSYCHOSOCIAL AND THE INTERNATIONAL CLASSIFICATION OF FUNCTIONING, DISABILITY AND HEALTH FRAMEWORKS OF HEALTH

Overview of Biopsychosocial Framework of Health

Germov (2005a, p. 13) wrote that the biopsychosocial framework began to gain traction in the 1970s as 'an extension of the [biomedical framework and was considered to be] a multifactorial model of illness that [took] into account biological, psychological, and social factors implicated in a [person's] condition'. A main difference between this framework and the biomedical framework is that this framework is not based on the assumption of the mind and body being separate. Rather, this framework is underpinned by system theory, which is based on the premise that health is determined by the dynamic interaction of a person's body structures and functions, subjective behaviours, beliefs, thought processes, motivations and experiences, and culture, family, community and society.

The introduction of the biopsychosocial approach led to the development of the International Classification of Impairments, Disabilities, and Handicaps (ICIDH), a manual of disease consequences issued by WHO in 1980 (Peterson, Mpofu, & Oakland, 2010; WHO, 1980). The ICIDH was developed to categorize the consequences of disease according to three dimensions: structural and functional body impairments, disabilities and handicaps (Fig. 1.1). Within the ICIDH *impairment* is defined as a problem with a person's body function and

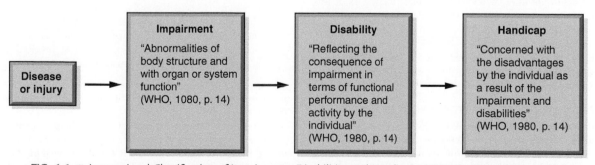

FIG. 1.1 ▪ International Classification of Impairments, Disabilities and Handicaps (ICIDH). *(From WHO, 1980.)*

structure, *disability* is defined as occurring as a result of the affected body function and structure, and *handicap* refers to the limitations experienced in the environment because of the affected body function and structure. Hence the biopsychosocial framework focuses on the individual's body function and structures being the cause of a person's disability and resulting handicap. Although some consideration is given to the impact of social and psychological factors, this framework still focuses on treatments to make a person's body structure and function as 'normal' as possible. Alford, Remedios, Webb, and Ewen (2013) state that the ICIDH 'was developed to capture the overall health status of populations but [...] focused more on disease and failed to capture the impact of the social and physical environment on functioning' (p. 2).

A positive outcome of the adoption of the biopsychosocial framework was the introduction of the concept of well-being, which Taylor (2008a) states was 'a broader concept than health as it typically involves a person's sense of overall satisfaction with [...] life' (p. 11-12). Hence, health status includes subjective experiences of quality of life (King, 2014), such that a person may have an illness, injury or impairment and feel healthy or, conversely, a person may not have an illness, injury or impairment and feel unhealthy (Liamputtong et al., 2012). Taylor (2008a, p. 12) states that 'subjective experiences of health are anchored in the complex sociocultural contexts of people's lives including their belief systems, life stage, past experiences, family context, perceived social responsibilities, cultural history and geographical locations'.

Whalley Hammell and Iwama (2012) and Wilcock and Hocking (2015) expand on the concept of well-being, considering it to be an interplay between different but interrelated factors leading to a state of contentment. These factors include a person's:

▪ physical, emotional and spiritual health and personal, economic, political and cultural safety;
▪ sense of being valued by others and belonging to social groups and communities; and
▪ ability to make choices and decisions and engage in personally valued activities.

Although the biopsychosocial framework of health was seen as a significant advance on the biomedical framework, it was eventually replaced by the International Classification of Functioning, Disability and Health, a framework that proposes that health, illness and wellness are dynamic and exist along a continuum rather than a static state fixed in time (Alford et al., 2013; Taylor, 2008b).

Overview of the ICF Framework of Health

The realization that medical conditions manifest differently across individuals and the increasing acknowledgement that the environment has a significant impact on a person's health led to the move away from the ICIDH to the International Classification of Functioning, Disability and Health, a model of health that, while still individually focused, provides recognition to internal and external factors that influence a person's health (Alford et al., 2013; Peterson et al., 2010). The ICF was developed to combine

> both biomedical and social approaches to disability and health [...] to provide a common language for disability and broader understanding of the concepts of impairment and disability by acknowledging that all people, not just those [with a medical label], have a disability, were likely to experience some impairment or disability during their life, even if only temporary (World Health Organization, 2013).
>
> *(Taylor, 2008b, p. 39)*

Taylor (2008b) sees the ICF as an extension of the biopsychosocial model, being based on the assumption that health exists along a continuum and results from dynamic interactions between the person and the person's environment. This assumption is different to the binary view of either being healthy or having an illness, injury or impairment, which underpinned the biomedical framework (Hemmingsson & Jonsson, 2005). Within the ICF impairment results from changes to a person's body functions and structures and leads to activity limitations (i.e. a person experiencing difficulty executing a task or action) and participation restrictions (i.e. the difficulty a person has doing things such as work, recreational and leisure activities, and personal care). The ICF is explained in the WHO manual as

> a framework for organising and documenting information on functioning and disability [...] It integrates the major models of disability – the medical model and the social model [and] recognises the role of environmental factors in the creation of disability, as well as the role of health conditions [and] provides a multiperspective, biopsychosocial approach which is reflected in the multidimensional model.
>
> *(World Health Organization, 2013, p. 5)*

The ICF is made up of two parts, each with two components (Peterson et al., 2010):

1. The individual: (i) a person's body functions and structures, and (ii) activities and participation; and
2. Contextual factors: (i) personal factors, and (ii) environmental factors. These contextual factors have an impact on a person's ability to participate and be involved in activity and ultimately on a person's health.

A graphic illustration of the ICF is shown in Figure 1.2 and a brief description of the components of the ICF can be found in Table 1.1.

In spite of the broad acceptance of the ICF there are a number of criticisms of this framework. Many criticisms revolve around the individual focus of the ICF and the categorization of people based on their abilities, contributing to the

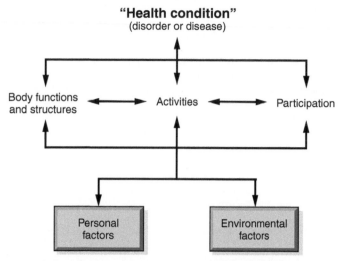

FIG. 1.2 ■ International Classification of Functioning, Disability and Health (ICF). *(From WHO, 2001.)*

TABLE 1.1
Description of Components of the ICF (Based on Definitions Provided by WHO (2001))

ICF Terms / Components	Description of Term
Health condition	This refers to a person's diagnosed disorder and/or disease. WHO defines health as 'the complete physical, mental and social functioning of a person and not merely the absence of disease' (WHO, 1948, Preamble).
Functioning	'Dynamic interaction between a person's health condition, environment factors and personal factors' (WHO, 2013, p. 5). When a person's functioning is affected this is referred to as a 'disability'. This term encompasses impairments, limitations to activities and/or restrictions to participation (Peterson et al., 2010; WHO, 2001).
Body functions and structures	*Body functions* refers to the physiological, neurological, and psychological systems that enable the body to work. *Body structures* refers to the anatomic parts of the body. When a person's body functions or body structures are affected this is referred to as an *impairment*.
Activity	The doing of a task or an action by a person. When a person has difficulty in the doing of a task or an action this is referred to as an *activity limitation*.
Participation	The involvement of a person in various occupations and life roles. When a person has difficulty or is unable to be involved in occupations and life roles this is referred to as a *participation restriction*.
Personal factors	The ICF does not provide a clear definition of personal factors because of the complex nature of social and cultural variation (Peterson et al., 2010). It is suggested that personal factors could include such things as ethnicity, gender, age, educational level, psychological assets, habits, social background and lifestyle (Wilcock & Hocking, 2015).
Environmental factors	These factors refer to the physical (natural and manufactured), social (relationships with family, friends, communities) and attitudinal (policies, services, rules and laws) environments in which people live. Environmental factors can either facilitate or inhibit an individual's functioning.

oppression, stigmatization and identification of differences of people who have an illness, injury or impairment (Conti-Becker, 2009; Hemmingsson & Jonsson, 2005; Whalley Hammell, 2004).

Conti-Becker (2009) suggests that, although the ICF was developed as an extension of the biopsychosocial model of health, it is still strongly influenced by the biomedical framework. She feels that many in the medical field use the ICF incorrectly, transposing biomedical concepts to 'fit' the ICF framework, primarily by using the ICF language but not the essence of the ICF approach. As an example, she refers to a publication by Stucki, Ewert, and Cieza (2002) in which those authors state that in rehabilitation medicine, the ICF is used to treat impaired bodies, overcome impaired functions and limitations, and prevent additional symptoms of impairment. This language is heavily based on biomedical assumptions and does not fit with the biopsychosocial philosophy that is meant to underpin the ICF.

Whalley Hammell (2004) criticizes the ICF as being based on assumptions of there being a 'normal' state, something she, and disability theorists, states does not exist. This focus on 'normality' creates hierarchical experts who make judgements on what can be considered normal and what is deviant, leading to exclusion, marginalization, and stigmatization. These experts rarely, if ever, consider the views and opinions of people with an illness, injury or impairment, and the idea that these people could be considered partners in managing their health and well-being. Hemmingsson and Jonsson (2005) also criticize the ICF because judgements about an individual's performance are made by experts, which, they suggest, does not account for the subjective experiences of people. They suggest that the participation component of the ICF is misnamed and should be renamed 'observed performance in its natural context' (Hemmingsson & Jonsson, 2005, p. 573). They further criticise the ICF for not capturing the 'complex relationship between different kinds of participation in a single life situation' (p. 573). As an example they state that the binary option of an environmental factor being either a facilitator or a barrier to participation does not account for the reality of life when a factor can be both a facilitator and a barrier at the same time. The authors use the example of a school assistant 'facilitate[ing] academic participation and at the same time be[ing] a hindrance for social participation' (p. 574).

One of the claims of the ICF is that it could be used for all people and is applicable to all cultures (Australian Institute of Health and Welfare, 2014; World Health Organization, 2001). Gilroy, Donelly, Colmar, and Parmenter (2013, p. 43) contest this assertion, stating that it does not pay 'enough attention to how the experience of colonisation influences the way that disability is conceptualised, understood and experienced in Indigenous communities'. For example, there is 'no single word equivalent to "disability" or "handicap" shared by [Australian] Indigenous communities' (p. 44). There are words for different impairments but these impairments do not necessarily equate to

people being disabled or unable to participate in community life. Although impairments are not equated to being disabled, the consequences of colonisation, the trauma and loss of lands, are felt to be disabling for Indigenous communities; yet this aspect of disability is not captured by the ICF. Hence a criticism of the ICF is that it does not capture and include Indigenous perceptions and experiences of disability; rather it imposes Western disability labels and categorisations to all cultures and societies.

Another problem with the ICF, according to Helander (2003), is that in spite of it being written with the idea of using neutral language so that the ICF could be used to express both positive and negative aspects of a person's functioning and health condition, the language in the ICF presents a negative or non–strength-based view of people who have an illness, injury or impairment. This is illustrated by words within explanations of the ICF such as 'problems', 'abnormalities', 'limitation', 'restrictions', 'losses', and 'deviations'. In addition, Helander states that the ICF does not provide a realistic understanding of the life of a person who has an illness, injury or impairment as it does not consider the impact of environmental factors such as 'poverty, lack of services, abuse and neglect in all its forms, use of alcohol and illicit drugs, [...] imprisonment, children living without parents (in institutions, on the streets and so on) and other very common problems' (Helander, 2003, p. 14). The inability to acknowledge the impact of these environmental factors means that a full understanding of the multiple determinants of health is not evident with the ICF, a framework that ultimately still focuses on the individual rather than on the social factors that affect the health of groups and populations, which is the focus of the fourth framework.

OCCUPATIONAL THERAPY PRACTICE AND THE BIOPSYCHOSOCIAL AND ICF FRAMEWORKS

Ward et al. (2007) suggest that it was during the 1960s that occupational therapists realised they were neglecting to focus on occupation.

Before this, and influenced by the biomedical framework, occupational therapists tended to be concerned with treating impairments rather than improving the occupational lives of people (Polatajko, 2014). Turner (2011) agrees, stating that at this time the profession was at odds with the dominating biomedical influence and was grappling to develop a unique identity. As a result of this growing realisation, the profession started to try to understand more fully how occupation positively affected the lives of people (Ward et al., 2007).

It was not until the 1980s that leaders in the profession pushed for a more holistic view of people who received occupational therapy services, and this led to the development of occupation-focused models of practice (Letts, 2011; Nastasi, 2014; Turner, 2011). These models assisted the occupational therapy profession to promote the concept of occupation as core to the profession internationally (Letts, 2011), leading to what Whiteford, Townsend, and Hocking (2000) refer to as the renaissance of occupation. Parnell and Wilding (2010) and Wilcock and Hocking (2015) argue that occupation, health and survival are inextricably linked and propose that any negative impact on health and well-being can only be addressed by focusing on the occupational nature of people.

Embracing of the term *occupation* was important for the occupational therapy profession (Fisher, 2013), as this started the move away from a professional identity based on a relationship with the medical profession. Wilding and Whiteford (2007) argue that many of the difficulties occupational therapists face when describing their practice stem from the clash between the philosophy underpinning medicine and that underpinning occupational therapy; they suggest that there is a clash between the two philosophies, such that aligning to the biomedical framework conflicts with occupational therapists working in an occupation-focused way.

Yerxa (cited in King, 2014) states that the renewed interest in the concept of occupation in contemporary practice led to the recognition of the importance of the relationship between being engaged in occupation and a person's health and well-being, a relationship that the early pioneers of the profession recognised (Letts, 2011; Moll, Gewurtz, Krupa, & Law, 2013; Wilding & Whiteford, 2007). However, although connections to the foundation of occupational therapy are often made, caution about the validity of these connections is advised because contemporary understandings and applications of the concept of occupation are different than the pioneers' understanding and application. Cutchin (2013) cautions that there is little evidence to indicate that the modern interpretation of the concept of occupation is similar to that proposed by the pioneers of the profession.

Whatever the connection to the pioneers' vision, the refocusing on occupation coincided with the adoption of the biopsychosocial and ICF frameworks within health. Both these frameworks, although still focused on the individual, embrace the idea that health is not just related to a person's body structure and function, but rather health involves a complex and dynamic interaction between the person and other factors, such as the social and psychological. The ICF also highlighted the impact of the environment on the health of people. Many in the occupational therapy profession were drawn to the ICF as they felt the concepts of 'activity' and 'participation' equated with the concepts of 'occupational engagement' and 'occupational performance' that were being used by occupational therapists.

Interestingly, refocusing on occupation lead the profession to be once again, as it was during the foundation years, on the periphery of mainstream medical practice. The difference this time was that the profession had matured and was becoming confident in its core foundations and philosophy, which coincided with the change in the perception of health and well-being (as evidenced by the biopsychosocial and ICF frameworks). With the move to develop its professional identity and to embrace occupation as a core concept, it also became evident, as the profession had become established in a large number of countries and was practised in a diverse range of cultural, political, economic and social contexts, that the foundation and philosophy of the profession, and much of its practice, was underpinned by middle-class Western ideas.

THE SOCIOECOLOGICAL FRAMEWORK OF HEALTH

Overview of the Socioecological Framework of Health

According to Taylor (2008b, p. 41) the socioecological framework of health maximises 'health at all levels within society, from the individual to the whole community [and promotes] health rather than simply responding to illness after it has developed'. Germov (2005a, p. 13) proposes that the ecological aspects of this framework are derived from the field of human ecology in which the 'interrelationship of human interaction, social organization, and the natural environment' are considered. In addition he states that the social aspects of this framework refer to

> *the prevention of illness through community participation and social reforms that address living and working conditions [that link] the traditional public health concerns of sanitation, hygiene, and clean air and water, with the social, cultural, behavioural and politico-economic factors that affect people's health.*
>
> *(Germov, 2005a, p. 13)*

This framework differs from the three previous frameworks because it focuses on the prevention and social responsibility of illness, injury and impairment and the promotion of health and well-being, moving beyond the medical treatment of an individual and of medical conditions. The need for medical treatment for biological and physiological aspects of illness, injury and impairment is recognised; however, it is acknowledged that this should occur within a social context.

Another term used for this framework is the *new public health approach*, as the focus is on determinants of health and the implementation of interventions at group, community, population and organisation levels (Germov, 2005a; Taylor, 2008b). Public health strategies are based on social justice principles (Hume Chambers & Walker, 2012) and focus on the health of groups, communities, populations and organisations, taking into account the interaction between the multiple social determinants of health (Moll et al., 2013). This is in keeping with the right people have to a high standard of health and health care (Taket, 2012; United Nations, 1948), not dependent on their ethnicity, religious or political beliefs or economic or social condition (Wilcock & Hocking, 2015).

The move to improve the health of populations with a focus on health promotion strategies is an outcome of the WHO (1978) Primary Health Care report of the International Conference at Alma Alta and is underpinned by the WHO Ottawa Charter of Health Promotion (1986), a charter aimed at promoting good health of groups, communities, population and organisations. This charter is underpinned by an understanding of the social determinants of health (Jirojwong & Liamputtong, 2009), which WHO (2013) consider to be the main cause of health status inequalities seen among groups of people living within a country and also between countries.

The Australian Institute of Health and Welfare (AIHW, 2014) use a diagram to illustrate the impact of determinants of health (Fig. 1.3). Within this figure it can be seen that the determinants are separated into four groups affecting a person's health and well-being over time, with the direction of determinants moving from left to right.

The AIHW (2014) use the term *social determinants* to encompass social, economic, political, cultural and environmental factors that affect health. Determinants are defined as

the conditions into which people are born, grow, live, work and age. According to this view, a person's occupation, education, material resources, social support networks and social status

can affect their health and contribute to broader health inequalities within the population. These circumstances are in turn shaped by a wider set of forces, such as economics, social policies, and politics. Some factors can be influenced by individuals and families through their pursuit of particular outcomes, while some broader forces are beyond the control of individuals. Social and economic conditions and their effects on people's lives can determine their risk of illness and the actions taken to prevent them becoming ill or treat illness when it occurs.

(Australian Institute of Health and Welfare, 2014, p. 6)

The determinants are associated with factors that facilitate good health and well-being or lead to poor health and illness (Rumbold & Dickson-Swift, 2012; Taylor, 2008a).

One of the outcomes of the focus on population health has been a growing understanding of the cultural influence on health. Black and Wells (2007, p. 5) define culture as

the sum total of a way of living, including values, beliefs, standards, linguistic expression, patterns of thinking, behavioural norms and styles of communication that influence the behaviour of a group of people that is transmitted from generation to generation.

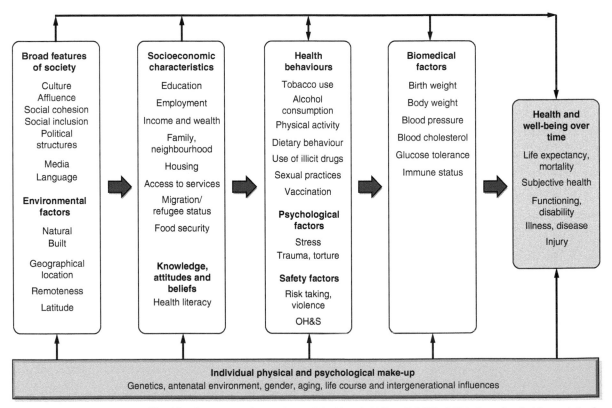

FIG. 1.3 ■ Determinants of health. *(From Australian Institute of Health and Welfare (AIHW), 2014. Reproduced with permission.)*

Whalley Hammell (2013, p. 225) concurs, stating that the term culture is used to describe 'the knowledge, beliefs, values, assumptions, perspectives, attitudes, norms, and customs that people acquire through membership in a particular society or group'.

A focus on population health, health equality and determinants of health highlights the disparity between the health of people from different cultures and also the inappropriateness of imposing a Western model of health (i.e. the biomedical, biopsychosocial and ICF frameworks) on people from non-Western backgrounds. Although culture is considered as an environmental factor in the ICF framework, a clearer understanding of culture has come from the development of population health. To illustrate this, a brief overview of the concept of health from the perspective of Aboriginal and Torres Strait Islander peoples, the Indigenous peoples of Australia, is provided. Fanany (2012, p. 235) suggests that the health experiences of Aboriginal and Torres Strait Islander peoples is characteristic of Indigenous populations in other countries who have been affected by the 'dramatic change in social structures and the living environment [that] occurred rapidly in the context of colonisation and integration into modern nation states'.

Duckett (2007, p. 32) states that the health of Aboriginal and Torres Strait Islander peoples is significantly worse than other Australians, as a result of the complex outcomes of colonisation, leading to spiritual harm caused by 'dispossession and alienation of the Aboriginal population from their land'. Land is considered fundamental to the well-being and core to the spirituality of Aboriginal and Torres Strait Islander peoples (McCalman, Tsey, Gibson, & Baird, 2009). Their health and well-being is strongly associated with their identity, which is connected to their land, and their relationship with their community. Aboriginal and Torres Strait Islander peoples' conceptualization of health is broader than that of nonindigenous people (Taylor, 2008a, 2008b).

Gee, Dudgeon, Schultz, Hart, and Kelly (2014) use the phrase 'social and emotional well-being' to capture the meaning of health for Aboriginal and Torres Strait Islander peoples. They indicate that this is a common phrase used when referring to Aboriginal and Torres Strait Islander peoples' health because it signifies 'a relatively distinct set of well-being domains and principles, and an increasingly documented set of culturally informed practices that differ in important ways with how the term is understood and used within Western health discourse' (Gee et al., 2014, p. 56-57). These authors refer to the nine guiding principles presented in the Social and Emotional Well-being Framework document (Social Health Reference Group, 2004) that shape Aboriginal and Torres Strait Islander peoples' conceptualisation of social and emotional well-being and identify core cultural values (Box 1.1).

Gee et al. (2014) build on these principles to develop a model to conceptualise social and emotional well-being from the perspective of Aboriginal and Torres Strait Islander peoples (Fig. 1.4). This conceptualisation is 'grounded within a collectivist perspective that views the self as inseparable from, and

---

BOX 1.1

NINE GUIDING PRINCIPLES THAT SHAPE ABORIGINAL AND TORRES STRAIT ISLANDER PEOPLES' CONCEPTUALISATION OF SOCIAL AND EMOTIONAL WELL-BEING AND IDENTIFY CORE CULTURAL VALUES

1. Health as holistic
2. The right to self-determination
3. The need for cultural understanding
4. The impact of history in trauma and loss
5. Recognition of human rights
6. The impact of racism and stigma
7. Recognition of the centrality of kinship
8. Recognition of cultural diversity
9. Recognition of Aboriginal strengths
   NB: Refer to the Social Health Reference Group (2004) reference for further explanation of these principles.

Modified from Gee et al., 2014.

---

embedded within, family and community' (Gee et al., 2014, p. 57). Within this illustration the social and emotional well-being of Aboriginal and Torres Strait Islander individuals, families and communities is determined by connections to seven domains: body, mind and emotions, family and kinship, community, culture, land and spirituality. The term *connection* is used to mean 'the diverse ways in which people experience and express these domains [...] throughout their lives' (Gee et al., 2014, p. 58).

Gee et al. (2014) suggest that disruption of these connections, particularly as a result of historical and political impacts of colonisation, has negatively affected the social and emotional well-being of individuals, families and communities. It has been shown that the social determinants of health are evident among Aboriginal and Torres Strait Islander communities due to the common presence of determinants such as low socioeconomic status, poverty, poor education achievement and unemployment. However, these determinants are further complicated by the historical and political determinants, and in particular unresolved issues of land rights, self-determination and cultural security. As Gee et al. (2014, p. 62) state

a community's local history of colonisation and the extent to which a cultural group is able to resist assimilation, maintain cultural continuity, and retain the right of self-determination and sovereignty will all significantly influence a community's capacity to retain their cultural values, principles, practices, and traditions. This, in turn, will differentially empower or impinge upon individual and family [social and emotional well-being].

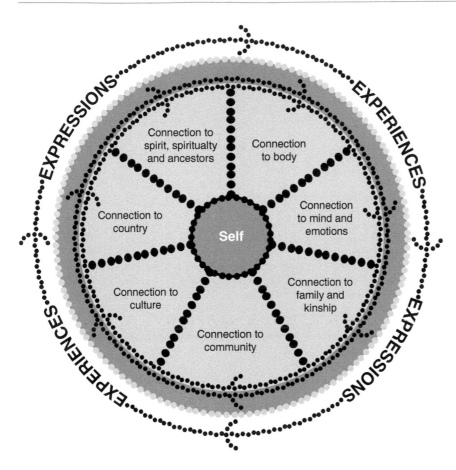

FIG. 1.4 ■ Social and emotional well-being from the perspective of Aboriginal and Torres Strait Islander peoples. *(Adapted from Gee et al., 2014, p. 57. Reproduced with permission.)*

This insight into culture, and a greater understanding and acceptance of cultural ways of knowing, identifies an ideological conflict between Western perceptions of health and the perceptions of health of Indigenous people (Foster, 2008). This has particular resonance when deciding the extent to which self-determination or assimilation should inform the guiding principles for deciding policies on Indigenous health (Foster, 2008). The continuing strong influence of the biomedical, biopsychosocial and ICF frameworks on Western health practice, and the reliance on evidence-based principles with knowledge organised according to different health disciplines, is at odds with the holistic approach to health and well-being practised by many non-Western people (Kendall, Milliken, Barnet, & Marshall, 2008).

Occupational Therapy and the Socioecological Framework of Health

In line with the socioecological framework, the occupational therapy profession began to look beyond working with individuals who had an illness, injury or impairment as the profession embraced the concept of occupation during the late 1990s and early 2000s (King, 2014). The profession began to see the potential contribution it could make to population health and wellness (Wilcock & Hocking, 2015) by developing a stronger social justice approach to practice. Hansen (2013) suggest that this is in line with the founders' vision for the profession, as it is an extrapolation of the humanistic ideals on which the profession was created. A greater understanding of the importance of occupation led to the realisation that occupation could be a health-promoting and disease-preventing force (Husman, 2014). Hence, occupational therapy as a profession expanded to address persons, groups, communities, populations and organisations, working in a variety of contexts and environments, focusing on wellness and well-being (Hocking, 2013; Nastasi, 2014; Whalley Hammell, 2009).

Occupational therapists, through multiple paradigm shifts and increased understanding of the concept of occupation, began to develop a more culturally based view of occupation (Gillen & Greber, 2014). Whalley Hammell and Iwama (2012) argue that the contemporary focus on well-being, rather than ill-health and impairment, is a focus that could be applied to people from different cultures, as the concept of well-being, although interpreted differently, is a concept that resonates with people from different cultural backgrounds. Whalley Hammell and Iwama (2012, p. 387) define well-being as:

A state of contentment – or harmony – with one's: physical/ mental health (inseparable, not dualistic concepts); emotional/ spiritual health (spiritual health is a concept defined, understood and experienced by the person); personal and economic security; self-worth (sense of being capable, and of being valued by others); sense of belonging (which includes the ability to contribute to others and to maintain valued roles and relationships, and which may include a sense of belonging and of connectedness to the land and nature); opportunities for self-determination (defined as the ability to enact choices and counteract powerlessness); opportunities to engage in meaningful and powerful occupations; and sense of hope.

A strong connection can be noted between this definition and the Aboriginal and Torres Strait Islander peoples' understanding of this concept proposed by Gee et al. (2014), as illustrated in Figure 1.4.

Contemporary Definition of Occupational Therapy

The contemporary nature of occupational therapy practice, with consideration of the socioecological framework of health, is evident in the current definition of the profession proposed by the World Federation of Occupational Therapists (WFOT). The definition is:

Occupational therapy is a client-centred health profession concerned with promoting health and well-being through occupation. The primary goal of occupational therapy is to enable people to participate in the activities of everyday life. Occupational therapists achieve this outcome by working with people and communities to enhance their ability to engage in the occupations they want to, need to, or are expected to do, or by modifying the occupation or the environment to better support their occupational engagement.

(World Federation of Occupational Therapists, 2013, p. 3)

Within this definition, phrases such as 'promoting health and well-being', 'enable people to participate' and 'working with people and communities' are consistent with the socioecological framework. In addition, this definition challenges occupational therapists to work with groups, communities, populations and organisations, rather than just individuals, and to work with ostensibly well people who have experienced occupation disruption, such as people who are homeless, refugees, or prisoners (Turner, 2011). This focus of the profession, embraced by the WFOT, is evident by the release of a number of position papers on topics such as human displacement, community-based rehabilitation, disaster management, human rights, global health, diversity and culture (see the WFOT Resource Centre at www. wfot.org/ResourceCentre.aspx).

CONCLUSION

The occupational therapy profession and the practice of occupational therapists has continually evolved since it began in the early 1900s. This evolution has been significantly influenced by the changing perception of health and health care, which has moved from the individualistic and treatment-focused biomedical, biopsychosocial and ICF frameworks, to the population- and health promotion–focused socioecological framework. It has also been influenced by a push within the profession to reconnect with the humanistic vision of the founders and by renewed interest in the importance of occupation to the health and well-being of people.

The continual evolution of the profession is seen as important to its sustainability and relevance. Hinojosa (2007) warns that the profession should not push for consistency and acceptance of one way of thinking, as this could stifle rather than enhance the evolution of the profession. He argues that

If we see the world as static, believing that occupational therapy is limited by what we currently can do, then we will act and respond consistently with those beliefs and views. But if we stretch our viewpoints and welcome change, realising interventions must be based on a client's problems or needs, we will act accordingly. We can shift our paradigms. Becoming innovators in adapting practices to meet the new realities of the world is essential to our profession's continuing development.

(Hinojosa, 2007, p. 632)

Hinojosa (2007) proposes that occupational therapists must be able to work in a volatile and changeable working climate as health services will constantly change. Perhaps the next change that the profession needs to more fully embrace is the move for health consumers to enact their rights to actively engage in planning, delivering and evaluating the services they receive (Bland & Epstein, 2008). Consumer-led health services fits with the client-centred* nature of the profession so, although this move will affect occupational therapy practice, it can be argued that its impact will not be major.

Perhaps a more significant change, and one that challenges the client-centred occupation focus of occupational therapy practice, will be the increasing rationing of health services inherent in the

---

*The terms *client-centred* and *person-centred* are often used interchangeably and are considered to have the same meaning. There has been a recent tendency for authors and therapists to prefer the use of the word *person-centred* to emphasise that individuals receiving occupational therapy services are first and foremost people, rather than clients, a term that has business connotations. The term *person-centred* is the preferred term within this book when referring to an individual. The term *client-centred* is the preferred term within this book when referring more broadly to an individual, groups, communities and populations who receive occupational therapy services. In addition, the term *client-centred* is used in the majority of historical and current research publications and hence has been retained when using direct quotes.

contemporary managerial approach to health service provision, which is strongly influenced by government and organisational policies based on budgetary and staff restraints (Germov, 2005b). This approach 'operates with a unitary purpose of work standardisation' (Germov, 2005b, p. 752) and can lead to allied health professionals losing their autonomy as their work becomes systematised and their practice constrained. Germov (2005b, p. 753) suggests that allied health professionals will need to proactively 'exercise their agency' to maintain their autonomy.

Turner (2011, p. 319) believes that the occupational therapy profession is at a stage of its evolution where it is practising 'true to its beliefs about the impact of occupation on health and wellbeing, working autonomously in a wide range of contexts in […] relationships with service users and strategic allies'. This has happened because the profession has become confident in its identity and its unique contribution to health. The profession is developing a clear vision of where it needs to go and the alliances required in order to reach this vision. The occupational therapy profession has become a profession that is in control of developing its own vision and forging these alliances so that it has the capacity to positively, constructively, dynamically and sustainably initiate and respond to inevitable future changes, developments in health frameworks and its expanding scope of practice.

 http://evolve.elsevier.com/Curtin/OT

REFERENCES

Alford, V., Remedios, L., Webb, G., & Ewen, S. (2013). The use of the international classification of functioning, disability and health (ICF) in indigenous healthcare: A systematic literature review. *International Journal for Equity in Health*, *12*(32). *Retrieved from* https://equityhealthj.biomedcentral.com/articles/10.1186/1475-9276-12-32.

Australian Institute of Health and Welfare (2014). Australia's health 2014: Australia's health series No. 14 Cat. No. AUS 178. *Australia's Health Series*, Canberra: Australian Institute of Health and Welfare.

Black, R., & Wells, S. (2007). *Culture and occupation: A model of empowerment in occupational therapy.* Bethesda, MD: American Occupational Therapy Association.

Bland, R., & Epstein, M. (2008). Encouraging principles of consumer participation and partnership: The way forward in mental health practice in Australia. In S. Taylor, M. Foster, & J. Fleming (Eds.), *Health care practice in Australia: Policy, context and innovations* (pp. 239–254). Melbourne: Oxford University Press.

Conti-Becker, A. (2009). Between the ideal and the real: Reconsidering the International Classification of Functioning, Disability and Health. *Disability and Rehabilitation*, *31*(25), 2125–2129.

Cutchin, M. (2013). The art and science of occupation: Nature, inquiry, and the aesthetics of living. *Journal of Occupational Science*, *20*(4), 286–297.

Duckett, S. (2007). *The Australian health care system* (3rd ed.). Melbourne: Oxford University Press.

Fanany, R. (2012). Language, culture and health. In P. Liamputtong, R. Fanany, & G. Verrinder (Eds.), *Health, illness and well-being* (pp. 229–241). Melbourne: Oxford University Press.

Fisher, A. (2013). Occupation-centred, occupation-based, occupation-focused: Same, same or different? *Scandinavian Journal of Occupational Therapy*, *20*(3), 162–173.

Foster, M. (2008). Fields of health service provision. In S. Taylor, M. Foster, & J. Fleming (Eds.), *Health care practice in Australia: Police, context and innovation* (pp. 74–102). Melbourne: Oxford University Press.

Gee, G., Dudgeon, P., Schultz, C., Hart, A., & Kelly, K. (2014). Aboriginal and Torres Strait Islander social and emotional wellbeing. In P. Dudgeon, H. Milroy, & R. Walker (Eds.), *Working together: Aboriginal and Torres Strait Islander mental health and wellbeing principles and practice.* Canberra: Australian Government Department of the Prime Minister and Cabinet.

Germov, J. (2005a). Imagining health problems as social issues. In J. Germov (Ed.), *Second opinion: An introduction to health sociology* (pp. 3–27). Melbourne: Oxford University Press.

Germov, J. (2005b). Managerialism in the Australian public health sector: Towards the hyper-rationalisation of professional bureaucracies. *Sociology of Health and Illness*, *27*(6), 738–758.

Gillen, A., & Greber, C. (2014). Occupation-focused practice: Challenges and choices. *British Journal of Occupational Therapy*, *77*(1), 39–41.

Gilroy, J., Donelly, M., Colmar, S., & Parmenter, T. (2013). Conceptual framework for policy and research development with Indigenous peoples with disabilities. *Australian Aboriginal Studies*, *2*, 42–58.

Hansen, A. M. W. (2013). Bridging theory and practice: Occupational justice and service learning. *Work*, *45*(1), 41–58.

Helander, E. (2003). *A critical review of the 'International Classification of Functioning, Disability and Health (ICF)'. Retrieved from* http://www.einarhelander.com/critical-review-ICF.pdf.

Hemmingsson, H., & Jonsson, H. (2005). An occupational perspective on the concept of participation in the International Classification of Functioning, Disability and Health: Some critical remarks. *American Journal of Occupational Therapy*, *59*(5), 569–576.

Hinojosa, J. (2007). Becoming innovators in an era of hyperchange [Eleanor Clarke Slagle Lecture]. *American Journal of Occupational Therapy*, *61*, 629–637.

Hocking, C. (2013). Occupation for public health. *New Zealand Journal of Occupational Therapy*, *60*(1), 33–37.

Hume Chambers, A., & Walker, R. (2012). Introduction to health promotion. In P. Liamputtong, R. Fanany, & G. Verrinder (Eds.), *Health, illness and well-being* (pp. 107–124). Melbourne: Oxford University Press.

Husman, C. B. (2014). History and philosophy. In K. Jacobs, N. MacRae, & K. Sladyk (Eds.), *Occupational therapy essentials for clinical competence* (pp. 33–42). Thorofare, NJ: Slack.

Jirojwong, S., & Liamputtong, P. (2009). Primary health care and health promotion. In S. Jirojwong, & P. Liamputtong (Eds.), *Population health, communities and health promotion* (pp. 26–42). Melbourne: Oxford University Press.

Kendall, E., Milliken, J., Barnet, L., & Marshall, C. (2008). Improving practice by respecting Indigenous knowledge and ways of knowing. In S. Taylor, M. Foster, & J. Fleming (Eds.), *Health care practice in Australia: Policy, context and innovations* (pp. 220–238). Melbourne: University of Oxford.

King, R. (2014). The experience of flow and meaningful occupation. In K. Jacobs, N. MacRae, & K. Sladyk (Eds.), *Occupational therapy essentials for clinical competence* (pp. 3–10). Thorofare, NJ: Slack.

Letts, L. (2011). Optimal positioning of occupational therapy. *Canadian Journal of Occupational Therapy, 78*(4), 209–219.

Liamputtong, P., Fanany, R., & Verrinder, G. (2012). Health, illness, and well-being: An introduction. In P. Liamputtong, R. Fanany, & G. Verrinder (Eds.), *Health, illness and well-being* (pp. 1–17). Melbourne: Oxford University Press.

McCalman, J., Tsey, K., Gibson, T., & Baird, B. (2009). Health of Indigenous Australians and health promotion. In S. Jirojwong, & P. Liamputtong (Eds.), *Population health, communities and health promotion* (pp. 69–91). Melbourne: Oxford University Press.

Moll, S., Gewurtz, R., Krupa, T., & Law, M. (2013). Promoting an occupational perspective in public health. *Canadian Journal of Occupational Therapy, 80*(2), 111–119.

Nastasi, J. (2014). Meaning and dynamic of occupation and activity. In K. Jacobs, N. MacRae, & K. Sladyk (Eds.), *Occupational therapy essentials for clinical competence* (pp. 57–70). Thorofare, NJ: Slack.

Parnell, T., & Wilding, C. (2010). Where can an occupation-focussed philosophy take occupational therapy? *Australian Occupational Therapy Journal, 57*(5), 345–348.

Peterson, D., Mpofu, E., & Oakland, T. (2010). Concepts and models in disability, functioning, and health. In E. Mpofu, & T. Oakland (Eds.), *Rehabilitation and health assessment: Applying ICF guidelines* (pp. 3–26). New York: Springer.

Polatajko, H. (2014). A call to occupationology. *Canadian Journal of Occupational Therapy, 81*(1), 4–7.

Rumbold, B., & Dickson-Swift, V. (2012). Social determinants of health: Historical developments and global implications. In P. Liamputtong, R. Fanany, & G. Verrinder (Eds.), *Health, illness and well-being* (pp. 177–196). Melbourne: Oxford University Press.

Social Health Reference Group (2004). *Social and emotion well being framework: A national strategic framework for Aboriginal and Torres Strait Islander Peoples' mental health and social and emotional well being 2004–2009*. Canberra: National Aboriginal and Torres Strait Islander Health Council and National Mental Health Working Group.

Stucki, G., Ewert, T., & Cieza, A. (2002). A value and application of the ICF in rehabilitation medicine. *Disability and Rehabilitation, 24*, 932–938.

Taket, A. (2012). Health and social justice. In P. Liamputtong, R. Fanany, & G. Verrinder (Eds.), *Health, illness and well-being* (pp. 278–301). Melbourne: Oxford University Press.

Taylor, S. (2008a). The concept of health. In S. Taylor, M. Foster, & J. Fleming (Eds.), *Health care practice in Australia: Policy, context and innovations* (pp. 3–21). Melbourne: Oxford University Press.

Taylor, S. (2008b). Contemporary frameworks of health care. In S. Taylor, M. Foster, & J. Fleming (Eds.), *Health care practice*

in Australia: Police, context and innovations (pp. 22–45). Melbourne: Oxford University Press.

Turner, A. (2011). The Elizabeth Casson Memorial Lecture 2011: Occupational therapy – A profession in adolescence? *British Journal of Occupational Therapy, 74*(7), 314–322.

United Nations (1948). *Universal declaration of human rights*. Retrieved from www.un.org/overview/rights.html.

Ward, K., Mitchell, J., & Price, P. (2007). Occupation-based practice and its relationship to social and occupational participation in adults with spinal cord injury. *OTJR: Occupation, Participation and Health, 27*(4), 149–156.

Whalley Hammell, K. (2004). Deviating from the norm: A skeptical interrogation of the classificatory practice of the ICF. *British Journal of Occupational Therapy, 67*(9), 408–411.

Whalley Hammell, K. (2009). Sacred texts: A sceptical exploration of the assumptions underpinning theories of occupation. *Canadian Journal of Occupational Therapy, 76*(1), 6–13.

Whalley Hammell, K. (2013). Occupation, well-being, and culture: Theory and cultural humility. *Canadian Journal of Occupational Therapy, 80*(4), 224–234.

Whalley Hammell, K., & Iwama, M. (2012). Well-being and occupational rights: An imperative for critical occupational therapy. *Scandinavian Journal of Occupational Therapy, 19*(5), 385–394.

Whiteford, G., Townsend, E., & Hocking, C. (2000). Reflections on a renaissance of occupation. *Canadian Journal of Occupational Therapy, 67*(1), 61–69.

Wilcock, A., & Hocking, C. (2015). *An occupational perspective of health* (3rd ed.). Thorofare, NJ: Slack.

Wilding, C., & Whiteford, G. (2007). Occupation and occupational therapy: Knowledge paradigms and everyday practice. *Australian Occupational Therapy Journal, 54*(3), 185–193.

World Federation of Occupational Therapists (2013). *Definition of occupational therapy from member organisations. (revised 2013)*. Retrieved from http://www.wfot.org/ResourceCentre.aspx.

World Health Organization (1948). *Preamble to the constitution*. Retrieved from www.who.int/hr/en.

World Health Organization (1978). *Primary health care. Report of the international conference on primary health care*. Alma Ata: World Health Organization.

World Health Organization (1980). *International classification of impairments, disabilities, and handicaps: A manual of classification relating to the consequences of disease*. Geneva: World Health Organization.

World Health Organization (2001). *International classification of functioning, disability and health (ICF)*. Geneva: World Health Organization.

World Health Organization. (2013). *Health in all policies*. Paper presented at the 8th Global Conference on Health Promotion, Helsinki.

World Health Organization, Health and Welfare Canada, & Canadian Public Health Association (1986). *Ottawa charter for health promotion*. Ottawa: World Health Organization.

Section 2

UNDERPINNING SCIENCES

SECTION OUTLINE

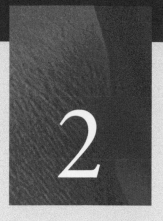

2

OCCUPATIONAL SCIENCE

DEBBIE LALIBERTE RUDMAN ■ REBECCA ALDRICH

CHAPTER OUTLINE

Abstract

Definitions and assumptions related to the concept of occupation that guide occupational therapy practice and anchor occupational science research are outlined in this chapter. Descriptions of an occupational perspective as well as occupation-based practice foreground deeper discussions of intertwined personal and environmental influences on occupational organisation and engagement. The following themes are covered: occupation as central to human living; occupation as central to occupational therapy practice; the evolution of knowledge about occupation; occupation as situated; and occupation's relation to meaning, identity and choice across the lifespan. The chapter closes with a list of resources that will help readers stay up-to-date on understandings about human occupation.

KEY POINTS

- Occupation is central to human life at individual, group, community and societal levels.

- As professionals who are concerned with how human lives are lived, occupational therapists must remain informed about developments in knowledge about human occupation.

- Occupational science generates research about human occupation that complements and enhances occupation-based occupational therapy practice.

- Assumptions about occupation must be understood relative to the sociohistorical contexts in which they emerged.

■ Understandings about occupation must account for the multiplicity of factors that influence people's occupational engagement.

■ Occupation has the potential to be a transformative force at individual and societal levels.

INTRODUCTION

No understanding of occupational therapy or occupational science is complete without a definition of occupation; however, making sense of the myriad explanations of occupation can be a daunting task. Thus the focus of this chapter is to illuminate assumptions that underpin definitions of occupation, the central construct of the occupational therapy profession, and provide an entry point into the ever-growing knowledge base regarding occupation. This chapter addresses the centrality of occupation to occupational therapy, presents ideas about how occupation is experienced, organised and socially shaped, and provides examples of how such knowledge about occupation informs occupational therapy practice. Taken together, the sections of this chapter demonstrate the ways in which occupation is fundamental to human life, occupational therapy and occupational science. A concluding list of selected resources offers readers additional opportunities for lifelong learning about occupation.

WHAT IS OCCUPATION?

Put in the simplest terms possible, occupations are the everyday pursuits that define what it means to be a human being (Yerxa et al., 1990). These pursuits can be so ordinary, such as getting dressed or completing homework (Clark et al., 1991), that people can 'do occupation all their lives, perhaps without ever knowing it' (Dickie, 2014, p. 2). Some occupations can also be extraordinary pursuits of particular significance to a person or group, such as completing a marathon or preparing a family holiday meal (Hocking, 2009; Molineux, 2010). Disruptions or barriers, such as health issues or changes in life circumstances, can unsettle the taken-for-granted nature of occupation and challenge engagement in desired and necessary occupations.

As illustrated in Table 2.1, many definitions of occupation inform research and practice around the world. Although some occupational scientists and occupational therapists are concerned by the lack of a standard definition of occupation, many authors suggest that a universal definition is neither desirable nor possible given the nature of occupation and people's diverse experiences (Galheigo, 2011; Iwama, 2003; Molineux, 2010). At the same time, it is important to articulate key assumptions about occupation and its relationships to health and well-being. Although knowledge about occupation is always developing, the following assumptions appear to guide occupational therapy practice in many contexts.

TABLE 2.1	
Example Definitions of Occupation	
Source	Definition
Yerxa et al., 1990	'Specific chunks of activity within the ongoing stream of human behaviour which are named in the lexicon of the culture' (p. 1)
Townsend & Polatajko, 2007	'Everything people do to occupy themselves, including looking after themselves (self-care), enjoying life (leisure), and contributing to the social and economic fabric of their communities' (p. 369)
American Occupational Therapy Association (AOTA) (2014)	'Occupations are various kinds of life activities in which individuals, groups, or populations engage, including activities of daily living, instrumental activities of daily living, rest and sleep, education, work, play, leisure, and social participation' (p. S19)
Frank (2013)	'Actions that rearrange and reconstruct the world in which we live' (p. 233)
Kuo (2011)	'Sociocultural practices and habits that originate from the social and express through the landscapes and places we live in' (p. 133)
International Society of Occupational Science (ISOS) (2009)	'The various everyday activities people do as individuals, in families and with communities to occupy time and bring meaning and purpose to life. Occupations include things people need to, want to and are expected to do'

A primary assumption underlying the concept of occupation is that occupation matters to individuals, groups and societies (Cutchin & Dickie, 2012). What people do, as individuals and collectives, is the core of occupational therapy practice because occupation is connected to health and well-being in a variety of ways. As well, scholars and practitioners assume that occupation is transformative; that is, engagement in occupations can evoke changes in individuals and societies (Townsend & Wilcock 2004; Watson & Swartz, 2004). Likewise, occupations are complex: they occur over time, across spaces and places, and through the context of daily experience (Christiansen & Townsend, 2010; Zemke, 2004), illustrating that people exist in relation with environments (Cutchin, Aldrich, Bailliard, & Coppola, 2008). The many meanings of everyday occupations (Hasselkus, 2011) not only illuminate the association between occupation and identity (Christiansen, 1999; Unruh, 2004), but they also show that certain ways of inhabiting everyday life are associated with individual and collective values (Laliberte Rudman, 2002). Taken together, these assumptions define occupations as what people do to live their lives as individuals and group members (Wilcock & Hocking, 2015). As Virginia Dickie (2010) suggests, occupations are not 'processes too complicated to explain' (p. 195), but they do challenge people to represent the complexity of phenomena that are often perceived as mundane.

OCCUPATION AS CORE TO OCCUPATIONAL THERAPY PRACTICE

Occupational therapy's founders argued that occupation is core to individual and collective health and well-being (Duncan, 2006; Reilly, 1962). The profession continues to be supported by research that demonstrates how occupation affects physical health, mental health, identity, social inclusion, collective functioning, well-being and group cohesion (Polatajko et al., 2007c; Polgar & Landry, 2004; Whiteford, 2004). Although the increasing influence of biomedical and mechanistic health care models between the 1940s and 1970s challenged occupational therapy's focus on occupation, the period since the 1980s has been characterised by initiatives to resituate occupation as the defining feature of occupational therapy practice (Duncan, 2006, Kielhofner, 2004). As articulated by Gustafsson, Molineux, and Bennett, (2014), the contemporary overarching paradigm informing occupational therapy practice 'is focussed sharply on occupation and recognises that humans have an occupational nature and face occupational challenges' (p. 121).

One by-product of this renaissance of occupation is the diverse use of language tying the concept to practice. Fisher (2013) noted that the terms 'occupation-centred', 'occupation-based', and 'occupation-focused' are often used interchangeably without acknowledging their distinct meanings. Fisher wrote that 'if we think of being occupation-centred as a profession-specific perspective, and occupation-based as a method of evaluation and intervention that involves engaging a person in occupation', then the practice of occupational therapy must necessarily be 'occupation focused' (p. 166). As another example, Polatajko et al. (2007a) describe occupation-based practice as centred on people as occupational beings and encompassing a range of approaches to enable occupational engagement from individual to population levels.

Occupation-focused practice entails using occupation in two primary ways: as a means and as an end (McLaughlin Gray, 1998; Polatajko et al., 2007b; Trombly Latham, 2013). The idea of occupation as a means to skill development or functional recovery implies that occupation is the therapeutic mechanism through which health and well-being are achieved. Thus 'occupation as a means' involves using occupation as a medium of change or transformation. The idea of occupation as an end suggests that occupations – especially those associated with a person's roles and identities – are the goal of any recovery or rehabilitation process. Thus 'occupation as end' shifts the focus to occupations as outcomes, or as what people want to get back to doing so they can be and become who they want to be and belong to the groups that mean most to them (Wilcock, 2006). Given this reembracing of occupation as the core of occupational therapy practice, there is an expanded need for research on occupation to provide knowledge and evidence for practice.

OCCUPATIONAL SCIENCE AS CORE TO EXPANDING KNOWLEDGE ABOUT OCCUPATION

Occupational science, a research-focused discipline committed to developing knowledge about occupation, arose in parallel with the resurgence of occupation-focused occupational therapy practice. Research in this discipline spans a range of questions: for example, questions about the nature of occupation itself, determinants of occupations, how occupation is used to organise families and societies, and the consequences of inequities in possibilities for occupation (Hocking, 2009; Molineux & Whiteford, 2011).

The development of occupational science has helped strengthen occupation as the core of occupational therapy practice. Elizabeth Yerxa (2000), one of the discipline's founders, saw occupational science as a tool for reinforcing occupational therapists' identity and expertise regarding occupation. Initial conceptualisations of occupational science also envisioned implications for a number of academic fields and professions including but not restricted to occupational therapy (Clark et al., 1991; Yerxa et al., 1990). Although the relationship between occupational science and occupational therapy has been the subject of some debate (Clark et al., 1993; Laliberte Rudman et al., 2008; Lunt, 1997; Mosey, 1992), both the discipline and the profession are committed to understanding and applying an occupational perspective as a particular way of 'looking at and thinking about human doing' (Njelesani, Tang, Jonsson, & Polatajko, 2014, p. 234). Given this perspective, occupational science has provided a powerful response to the need for knowledge that informs 'the practice terrain of occupational therapy' (Molineux & Whiteford, 2011, p. 244).

The number of authors writing about occupation has increased dramatically since the inception of occupational science, and scholars of occupation reflect increasingly diverse geographic and methodologic backgrounds (Glover, 2009; Molke, Laliberte Rudman, & Polatajko, 2004). In recognition of occupational science's importance, the World Federation of Occupational Therapists (2012) issued a position statement in support of the discipline's continued growth, noting that occupational science's 'focus on occupation is what makes occupational therapy unique among the health professions' (p. 2). The remainder of this chapter outlines key aspects of the knowledge base regarding occupation, including evolving areas of exploration in occupational science, to show links between knowledge about occupation and occupational therapy practice.

OCCUPATION AS CORE TO HUMAN LIVING

In one of the most comprehensive published accounts of occupation, Ann Wilcock (2006) linked occupation to health, survival and well-being via the nexus of human biological capacities and environmental factors. Wilcock argued that many problems in modern society stem from occupations being 'out-of-step' with people's natural needs. Accordingly, Wilcock's theory connected the doing of occupation to what a person wants to be and become and the groups to which a person might belong. Wilcock's formulation of the occupational perspective recognised that biological capacities and environmental characteristics can afford or constrain ways of doing, being or becoming (Wilcock, 1998); as such, it offered a foundation for understanding the interplay of individual and environmental characteristics that ground occupational engagement. Further scholarship built on this perspective has advanced discussions of justice and community development (Wilcock & Hocking, 2015), signalling that understandings about occupation account for both its presence and absence in people's lives.

Research within and outside an occupational perspective has addressed the centrality of what people *do* in relation to their personal identities (or, how a person views her or himself) and social identities (or, how a person wishes to be viewed and is viewed by others) (Christiansen, 1999; Laliberte Rudman, 2002). The concept of occupational identity captures the significance of the relationship (Christiansen, 2004): as defined by Kielhofner (2008), occupational identity is a 'composite sense of who one is and wishes to become as an occupational being generated from one's history of participation' (p. 106). The relationship (Christiansen, 2004) is dynamic and mutually informing because identity continuously evolves via engagement in occupations through particular contexts (Unruh, 2004). The relationship between occupation and identity is mutually informing; that is, the occupations a person does influence that person's identity, and a person's identity influences what occupations that person engages in. There is a similar relationship between occupational identity and context because engaging in identity-supporting occupations influences physical, social, and other aspects of environments, just as environmental aspects influence the types of occupations and occupational identities that are available to people (Laliberte Rudman, 2002; Phelan & Kinsella, 2009). Existing literature has also underscored that engagement in occupation can promote a sense of membership in a collective such as a family or culture (Polgar & Landry, 2004). Understanding the occupation – identity relationship sensitises occupational therapists to the challenge of occupational disruptions and losses by elucidating why particular occupations are vital to individuals and collectives. Such understandings inform how occupation can be used therapeutically to support identity management and reconstruction (Christiansen, 1999; Unruh, 2004).

Being Reflexive About Occupation-Related Assumptions

As practitioners and scholars seek evidence, they must be mindful of the perspective through which they sort and interpret occupation-related understandings. Occupational therapy and occupational science have been critiqued for adopting a middle-class, Western perspective that has constrained how occupation is studied and addressed in practice (Laliberte Rudman & Dennhardt, 2008). As one example, although research supports the long-standing assumption that occupation is connected to health and well-being, the belief that occupation is always health promoting or positive comes from particular religious and economic assumptions about the dangers of idleness and the inherent goodness of work (Kantartzis & Molineux, 2011).

Accordingly, it is important to acknowledge that occupations can have negative effects at individual and societal levels and that occupations cannot be simply categorised as positive or negative based on particular social norms (Durocher, Rappolt, & Gibson, 2014; Law, Steinwender, & LeClair, 1998; Njelesani et al., 2014; Twinley & Addidle, 2012). Existing research suggests that occupations may not promote health if an individual does not perceive having control over occupations, is not motivated to engage in occupations or finds occupations too challenging or too easy given existing skills (Law et al., 1998). Moreover, occupations can be health threatening: for instance, work-related stress has negative physical and psychological effects, and the intense training required by specific careers – such as music or athletics – can lead to physical injuries (Durocher et al., 2014).

The dominant Western view of occupation has also been critiqued for failing to acknowledge that any occupation, including those socially viewed as risky, antisocial or bad, can have both positive and negative implications for health and well-being (Kantartzis & Molineux, 2011; Kiepek, Phelan, & Magalhaes, 2014; Laliberte Rudman, 2010; Twinley & Addidle, 2012). For example, creating graffiti – which is often framed as deviant behaviour that negatively affects individual and community health – has been found to 'actually have health promoting benefits and [...] act as a potential pathway to engaging in health' (Russell, 2008, p. 95). Likewise, occupations that are ostensibly good, like automobile driving, can have detrimental environmental effects that can negatively affect human health and other occupational engagement (Hudson & Aoyama, 2008). Given the variable nature of occupation as it is expressed and experienced across circumstances, occupational therapists and occupational scientists must continue to seek evidence in relation to the assumptions that underlie occupation-focused work (Njelesani et al., 2014).

Thus within occupational therapy practice, it is important to understand how and why knowledge about occupation is sought, as well as the diverse effects occupations have on individuals, communities and the environment. It is equally important to guard against presumptions that certain occupations are negative and should be excluded from the domain of practice. Hence, scholars have argued that occupational therapists and occupational scientists should strive to be critically reflective and generate knowledge about the *situations* that promote engagement in potentially harmful occupations (Aldrich & White, 2012).

OCCUPATION AS SITUATED

Highlighting how environments influence the experience of occupation, as well as what occupations people can and do engage in, is a central part of occupational therapy practice models such as the Model of Human Occupation (Kielhofner, 2008) and the Person-Environment-Occupation model (Law et al., 1996). However, despite this incorporation of environmental aspects, occupational therapy practice and occupational science research has often taken an individualistic approach to occupation and the conditions that define people's engagement in it. In other words, occupation has often been framed as determined by individuals and as separable from environments (Dickie, Cutchin, & Humphry, 2006; Laliberte Rudman & Huot, 2013; Whiteford, 2010). In response to this trend and in line with broader moves to expand beyond individually focused models of health and well-being (Raphael, 2006), scholars have refocused their attention on the situated nature of occupation, or how occupation is continuously 'shaped and negotiated within, as well as contributing to the shaping of, social systems and structures' (Laliberte Rudman, 2014, p. 4).

The transactional perspective (Dickie et al., 2006) is one key theoretical development that has helped foster such refocusing. The development of the transactional perspective helped emphasise the situated nature of occupation by applying the work of pragmatist philosophers such as John Dewey. The transactional perspective recognises that 'people and their environments coconstitute each other' (Cutchin & Dickie, 2012, p. 27); its application represents an attempt to provide a more balanced and complex account of occupational engagement (Aldrich, 2008). Employing a transactional perspective challenges occupational scientists and occupational therapists to attend to occupation as a relational, in-process action that is a response to situations (Cutchin et al., 2008). The recognition that 'occupation occurs at the level of the situation' (Dickie, 2014, p. 6) underscores the need to think about the individual,

social, discursive, and nonhuman elements that make situations and occupations what they are. For instance, in the situation of unemployment, the lack of a work occupation cannot only be explained by a person's individual history or national economic context: it is the nexus of governmental policies, a person's demographic characteristics and experiences, and the availability of financial and social resources that shape joblessness and its effects on nonwork occupations (Aldrich & Laliberte Rudman, 2015).

Ideas about occupation have come to recognise that 'no human action is independent of the social, cultural, political and economic contexts in which it occurs' (Whiteford, Klomp & Wright-St. Clair, 2005, p. 10). Recent developments illuminate how practitioners and researchers can consider the complex intersection of individual, occupational and environmental aspects in human life. For example, occupational science research has highlighted how social constructions of gender, disability and age-based expectations can shape what occupations and identities are possible for people to take up in particular contexts (Phelan & Kinsella, 2009; Laliberte Rudman, 2010; Wicks & Whiteford, 2005). Such research demonstrates that social, physical, economic, political, cultural and geographic elements all affect whether, and in what way, people can engage in occupations. Taken-for-granted notions about gender, the physical layout of playgrounds and the structure of sports activities, for instance, are all seen as shaping the occupations and occupational identities of boys and girls (Angell, 2014). Likewise, although functional impairments can make it difficult to perform particular occupations, situated understandings of occupation reinforce that disability results from ableist assumptions and normative expectations that structure environments: a mobility impairment that reduces walking speed and a person's ability to navigate curbs only becomes problematic when traffic light durations and curb heights have been determined on the basis of assumptions about 'normal' mobility (McGrath, 2011; Polatajko et al., 2007a). Therefore it is important to always situate occupational engagement so that occupational therapy practice addresses both personal factors and environmental elements that shape occupational performance (Wicks & Whiteford, 2005).

Ideas about the situated nature of occupation have also reinforced that power influences what types of occupations various groups of people can engage in (Kronenberg & Pollard, 2006; Laliberte Rudman, 2010). Molineux and Whiteford (2011) have argued that 'when we consider occupation and its centrality not only in people's lives but in society per se, a research agenda to understand it further must necessarily address those structural issues that enable or preclude people from engaging in occupation' (p. 247). The concept of occupational justice, which was introduced in the 1990s by Elizabeth Townsend and Ann Wilcock, provides a means to understand how power affects occupation (Stadnyk, Townsend, & Wilcock, 2010). The concept of occupational justice arose from a concern that opportunities to engage in occupations are inequitably distributed across societal groups and societies (Townsend & Wilcock, 2004;

Wilcock & Townsend, 2009). The concept of occupational deprivation – one form or outcome of occupational injustice – was then developed to help practitioners and scholars attend to the ways in which external factors produce 'a state of prolonged preclusion from engagement in occupations of necessity and/or meaning' (Whiteford, 2000, p. 201).

In addition to occupational deprivation, other negative outcomes of occupational injustice include: occupational imbalance, which encompasses being overoccupied and underoccupied; occupational marginalisation, which refers to individuals or groups not having choices or opportunities to participate in valued and necessary occupations; and occupational alienation, which includes situations where individuals and groups experience everyday occupations as lacking in meaning (Nilsson & Townsend, 2010; Stadnyk et al., 2010). Illustrations of these various outcomes or forms of occupational injustice are provided in Table 2.2, using examples related to employment, underemployment and unemployment. Further work on a theory of occupational justice has enhanced knowledge of structural and social determinants, such as economic systems, social policies and transportation systems, and their impact on everyday occupations.

Aligned with the powerful premise that occupation is a human right (Galheigo, 2011; Hammell, 2008), research and practice that attend to occupational injustice seek to raise awareness of and alter situations in which 'some populations more

than others are restricted from experiencing occupational rights, responsibilities and liberties, either deliberately or through taken-for-granted social exclusion from participation' (Nilsson & Townsend, 2010, p. 58). This line of thinking about occupation also highlights the importance of collaborating with individuals and groups to enhance occupational opportunities and advocate for the reform of policies, social relations and other elements that shape occupational injustices (Townsend & Wilcock, 2004). Within the everyday context of practice, applying an occupational justice lens means that therapists work with people to understand and negotiate social and structural factors that unfairly restrict occupational engagement. Although occupational justice–focused practice may appear different from traditional occupational therapy practice, it is becoming evident that most occupational therapy practices seek to promote justice and ensure occupational rights at some level (Bailliard & Aldrich, forthcoming).

INFORMING OCCUPATION-BASED PRACTICE: EXAMPLES RELATED TO THE EXPERIENCE AND ORGANISATION OF OCCUPATION

Integrating knowledge about occupation can '[inform] therapists' understandings of the meaning, demands and context of the occupations [people] aspire to' (Hocking, 2009, p. 140). This final section provides examples of developed and emerging concepts and insights to illustrate the applicability of such knowledge to occupational therapy practice.

Experiences of Occupation: Meaning, Purposes and Categories

Many scholars have focused on creating knowledge about occupation relative to three primary points: its forms, its functions and its meanings. The form of occupation includes aspects of occupation that elicit and guide occupational performance. Knowledge about the form of occupation (Nelson, 1988) has grown as scholars have become better equipped to articulate the parameters of occupational engagement (Hocking, 2009) that exist apart from people's experience of it (Dickie, 2010). For example, understanding that learning is a central part of quilt making (Dickie, 2003a) can help a therapist move beyond focusing on a particular person's physical impairment to seeing the social or intellectual experience of quilt making as an 'end' of intervention.

Occupational science research has also endeavoured to clarify the purposes of occupation and the processes involved in its execution (Hocking, 2000). For instance, occupations related to spirituality may function as a way to connect people with a community (Beagan & Etowa, 2011), and the ways in which people engage in spiritual occupations can be understood in light of that particular purpose.

	TABLE 2.2
	Illustrations of Forms of Occupational Injustice

Form of Occupational Injustice	Example Relevant to Employment, Unemployment and/or Underemployment
Occupational deprivation	Older workers who become unemployed, who desire to return to work, and experience prolonged periods of unemployment as a result of ageist employment practices and attitudes
Occupational imbalance	Individuals who experience long-term unemployment who have to devote time and energy to resource-seeking occupations in order to survive and have few opportunities to engage in leisure or other types of occupations
Occupational marginalisation	Individuals with criminal records who are precluded from work opportunities in multiple labour market sectors
Occupational alienation	Individuals who are underemployed in work that is not commensurate with their education and skills and which they find lacking in meaning

Occupational therapists and occupational scientists have long assumed that an occupation's meaning is central to its influence on health and well-being (Christiansen, 1999). Research has shown that meaning is both individualised and socially influenced. For example, in a study examining the food-centred occupations of older women in New Zealand, researchers Chiangmai and Kentucky, found that preparing food held multiple meanings that varied across individuals, families and cultures. Participants in that study experienced cooking as meaningful when it provided a means to maintain a role in a family structure, preserve cultural teachings or create new traditions (Hocking, 2009). Such research displays the importance of understanding people's perspectives on the meanings of various occupations rather than assuming that meaning can be surmised by an outsider or inheres across similar occupations.

Researchers have also tried to understand the experience of occupation through the use of occupational categories. Although people may sometimes find it difficult to categorise their daily occupations (Aldrich et al., 2015) and the same occupation may be categorised differently by different individuals (Brooke, Desmarais, & Forwell, 2007), occupational therapists and occupational scientists often use categories to make sense of the ways in which occupation is central to human living. Such categories are often part of how occupation is defined (see Table 2.1), and they stem from foundational writings that propose work, play, rest and sleep as primary categories of occupational engagement (Hammell, 2009a). Such categories have come to be seen as exclusionary because they were derived from a Western worldview that does not encompass individual and collective experiences from around the globe (Hammell, 2009b). These critiques have led scholars to question whether or not experience-based (rather than typology-based) categories are more informative and inclusive (Jonsson, 2008), whether or not occupational categories are dichotomous (Primeau, 1995), or whether or not there is a purpose in categorising occupations at all (Aldrich et al., 2015). Developing knowledge about occupational categories has redoubled some scholars' commitment to explicating the ways in which occupations are a core feature of human life (Hammell, 2004). Thus, although the use of categories can provide an efficient way to inquire about each person's different occupations, research points to the need to use categories cautiously and to talk with people using categories or experiences that are most relevant to their occupational engagement (Aldrich et al., 2015).

Organising Occupation: Across the Lifespan, Through Routine and Habits, Transitions and Balance

Categories have also been used to conceptualise how occupations are organised across the lifespan. Human development has historically been broken down into stages using categories such as 'childhood', 'adolescence', 'adulthood' and 'older adulthood'. In looking at how occupation is organised across the lifespan (Humphry, 2002; Wiseman, Davis & Polatajko, 2005),

scholars and practitioners have helped illuminate how play occupations are central to childhood (Parham, 1996) and work occupations are central to adulthood (Dickie, 2003b; Harvey-Krefting, 1985). However, scholars have also recognised that play is culturally relative (Bazyk, Stalnaker, Llerna, Ekelman & Bayzk, 2003; Wiseman et al., 2005), that children can also work (Larson, 2004), and that adults also benefit from play and leisure (Suto, 1998). Such research illustrates that associations between categories of occupations and stages of life are not mutually exclusive; it also highlights the need to examine the diversity of occupations that comprise people's occupational repertoires at various ages. As Humphry and Wakeford (2006) articulated, research addressing the processes through which occupations are developed can inform practice that supports 'the acquisition of new occupation and transformations in occupational performance' (p. 265). That is, knowledge about how occupations develop throughout the lifespan can help occupational therapists assist people to learn or relearn occupations.

Within understandings of development, scholars have examined how habits and routines mature, persist and decline across the lifespan and how changes in habits and routines affect occupational performance (Clark, 2000). Just as with assumptions about occupational categories, emerging knowledge suggests that viewing routine as a building block of occupation may not match people's experiences in situations like unemployment (Aldrich & Dickie, 2013) or retirement (Ludwig, 1998). Therefore occupational therapists whose practices emphasise routine may have to adjust their expectations of people whose situations defy routine-based descriptions.

Scholars and practitioners have also recognised that transitioning from one developmental stage to another often brings about changes in occupations. The concept of occupational transition – or a change in the occupations that a person can, needs or wants to do – captures changes that occur for diverse reasons, such as progressive functional declines (Vrkljan & Polgar, 2006), moving out of particular age-associated roles (Wiseman & Whiteford, 2009) or the sudden onset of disability (Polatajko et al., 2007a). Occupational therapists often intervene when people are experiencing an occupational transition, and occupational therapists can thus be viewed as supporting people in negotiating transitions. Research about occupational transitions provides insights into factors that can be addressed in practice to facilitate successful transitions, such as social support, an ability to link changes to the past and future, and continued engagement in familiar occupations; (Kubina, Dubouloz, Davis, Kessler, & Egan, 2013) such research also reveals factors that can serve as barriers to the successful negotiation of transitions, such as a lack of skills to take on new occupations or having to deal with multiple transitions at the same time (Crider, Calder, Bunting, & Forwell, 2014).

Whatever developmental stage a person occupies, the notion of a person's pursuits being occupationally balanced offers a way to think about the experience and organisation of occupation. The concept of balance has had a long history in occupational therapy

(Backman, 2004; Christiansen, 1996). Broadly speaking, people can either feel that they are experiencing appropriate or inappropriate variation and duration in their daily occupations (Wagman, Hakansson, & Biorklund, 2012). The concept of occupational balance has been utilised to understand time use and qualities of experience (Jonsson & Persson, 2006) for a range of people, from those with health conditions (Bejerholm, 2010; Stamm, Wright, Mechold, Sadlo, & Smolen, 2004) to those entering new developmental stages (Pettican & Prior, 2011; Wilson & Wilcock, 2005). Drawing on this literature can benefit occupational therapists by giving them broad understandings about the types of experiences associated with health (Wilcock et al., 1997); however, as with assumptions about meaning, it is important to note that both individual and social views of balance influence the perceptions people have about their lives.

Evolving Understandings: Supporting and Challenging our Knowledge Base

This chapter has aimed to demonstrate how research has both supported and challenged assumptions about occupation. As another example, Galvaan's (2014) research, conducted with marginalised adolescents in South Africa, has challenged the pervasive view of choice as a phenomenon arising solely from individual volition, motivation, or rational decision making. Her work showed how occupational choices, such as smoking or discontinuing schooling, are constrained within particular personal, relational, historical, economic and cultural contexts, and how choices predicated on taken-for-granted assumptions can perpetuate occupational injustices. Although person-centred models of occupational therapy practice emphasise the importance of offering opportunities for choice, Galvaan's work demonstrates that understanding individual choices requires attending to past and present contexts. Similarly, her work illustrates that expanding opportunities for occupations through occupational therapy practice must account for how various contextual factors may constrain whether or not people can or will choose to take advantage of such opportunities.

CONCLUSION

This chapter has provided an overview of occupational therapy's central construct and provided examples of the knowledge that has developed since the inception of occupational science. This is an exciting time of growth for both the profession and the discipline, and the realisation of occupation-focused practice depends on increasing the number of people who use and contribute to knowledge about occupation.

FURTHER RESOURCES

In addition to exploring occupational science presentations at national and international occupational therapy conferences, the following resources will also help in that endeavour:

- *Journal of Occupational Science* (http://www.tandfonline.com/loi/rocc)
- International Society for Occupational Science (http://www.isoccsci.org/)
- Canadian Society of Occupational Scientists (https://sites.google.com/site/occupationalsciencecanada/)
- Society for the Study of Occupation: USA (https://www.sso-usa.org/cms/)
- OS4OT Facebook group (http://ot4ot.com/4-ot.html)

 http://evolve.elsevier.com/Curtin/OT

REFERENCES

Aldrich, R. M. (2008). From complexity theory to transactionalism: Moving occupational science forward in theorizing the complexities of behaviour. *Journal of Occupational Science*, *15*(3), 147–156.

Aldrich, R. M., & Dickie, V. A. (2013). 'It's hard to plan your day when you have no money': Discouraged workers' occupational possibilities and the need to reconceptualize routine. *Work, A Journal of Prevention, Assessment, and Rehabilitation, 45*, 5–15.

Aldrich, R. M., & Laliberte Rudman, D. (2015). Situational analysis: An approach to unpack the complexity of occupation. *Journal of Occupational Science.* http://dx.doi.org/10.1080/14427591.2015.1045014.

Aldrich, R. M., McCarty, C., Boyd, B., Bunch, C., & Balentine, C. (2015). Empirical lessons about occupational categorization from case studies of unemployment. *Canadian Journal of Occupational Therapy, 81*(5), 289–297.

Aldrich, R. M., & White, N. (2012). Re-considering violence: A response to Twinley and Addidle (2012) and Morris (2012). *British Journal of Occupational Therapy, 75*(11), 527–529.

American Occupational Therapy Association (AOTA). (2014). *The occupational therapy practice framework: Domain and process* (3rd ed.). Bethesda, MD: AOTA.

Angell, A. M. (2014). Occupation-centered analysis of social difference: Contributions to a socially responsive occupational science. *Journal of Occupational Science, 21*(2), 104–116.

Backman, C. L. (2004). Occupational balance: Exploring the relationships among daily occupations and their influence on well-being. *Canadian Journal of Occupational Therapy, 71*(4), 202–209.

Bailliard, A., & Aldrich, R. (forthcoming). Occupational justice in everyday occupational therapy practice. Submitted for the next edition of *Occupational Therapy without Borders.*

Bazyk, S., Stalnaker, D., Llerna, M., Ekelman, B., & Bayzk, J. (2003). Play in Mayan children. *The American Journal of Occupational Therapy, 57*(3), 273–283.

Beagan, B. L., & Etowa, J. B. (2011). The meanings and functions of occupations related to spirituality for African Nova Scotian women. *Journal of Occupational Science, 18*(3), 277–290.

Bejerholm, U. (2010). Occupational balance in people with schizophrenia. *Occupational Therapy in Mental Health, 26*(1), 1–17.

Brooke, K. E., Desmarais, C. D., & Forwell, S. J. (2007). Types and categories of personal projects: A revelatory means of understanding human occupation. *Occupational Therapy International, 14*, 281–296.

Christiansen, C. H. (1996). Three perspectives on balance in occupation. In R. Zemke & F. Clark (Eds.), *Occupational science: The evolving discipline* (pp. 431–452). Philadelphia: F.A. Davis.

Christiansen, C. H. (1999). Defining lives: Occupation as identity: An essay on competence, coherence, and the creation of meaning. *American Journal of Occupational Therapy, 53*, 547–558.

Christiansen, C. H. (2004). Occupation and identity: Becoming who we are through what we do. In C. H. Christiansen & E. A. Townsend (Eds.), *Introduction to occupation: The art and science of living* (pp. 121–139). Upper Saddle River, NJ: Prentice Hall.

Christiansen, C. H., & Townsend, E. A. (2010). An introduction to occupation. In C. H. Christiansen & E. A. Townsend (Eds.), *Introduction to occupation: The art and science of living* (2nd ed., pp. 1–34). Upper Saddle River, NJ: Prentice Hall.

Clark, F. (2000). The concepts of habit and routine: A preliminary theoretical synthesis. *Occupational Therapy Journal of Research, 20*(Suppl.), 123S–137S.

Clark, F., Parham, D., Carlson, M. E., et al. (1991). Occupational science: Academic innovation in the service of occupational therapy's future. *American Journal of Occupational Therapy, 45*(4), 300–310.

Clark, F., Zemke, R., Frank, G., et al. (1993). Dangers inherent in the partition of occupational therapy and occupational science. *American Journal of Occupational Therapy, 47*(2), 184–186.

Crider, C., Calder, C. R., Bunting, K. L., & Forwell, S. (2014). An integrative review of occupational science and theoretical literature exploring transition. *Journal of Occupational Science, 22*(3), 304–319.

Cutchin, M. P., Aldrich, R., Bailliard, A., & Coppola, S. (2008). Action theories for occupational science: The contributions of Dewey and Bourdieu. *Journal of Occupational Science, 15*(3), 157–165.

Cutchin, M. P., & Dickie, V. A. (2012). Transactionalism: Occupational science and the pragmatic attitude. In G. E. Whiteford & C. Hocking (Eds.), *Occupational science: Society, inclusion and participation* (pp. 23–37). Oxford: Wiley-Blackwell.

Dickie, V. A. (2003a). The role of learning in quilt making. *Journal of Occupational Science, 10*(3), 120–129.

Dickie, V. A. (2003b). Establishing worker identity: A study of people in craft work. *American Journal of Occupational Therapy, 57*(3), 250–261.

Dickie, V. A. (2010). Are occupations 'processes too complicated to explain'? What we can learn by trying. *Journal of Occupational Science, 17*(4), 195–203.

Dickie, V. A. (2014). What is occupation? In B. A. Boyt Schell, G. Gillen & M. E. Scaffa (Eds.), *Willard & Spackman's occupational therapy* (12th ed., pp. 2–8). Philadelphia: Lippincott Williams & Wilkins.

Dickie, V. A., Cutchin, M. P., & Humphry, R. (2006). Occupation as transactional experience: A critique of individualism in occupational science. *Journal of Occupational Science, 13*(1), 83–93.

Duncan, E. A. S. (2006). *Foundations for practice in occupational therapy* (4th ed.). London: Elsevier Churchill Livingstone.

Durocher, E., Rappolt, S., & Gibson, B. E. (2014). Occupational justice: Future directions. *Journal of Occupational Science, 21*(4), 431–442.

Fisher, A. G. (2013). Occupation-centered, occupation-based, occupation-focused: Same, or different? *Scandianavian Journal of Occupational Therapy, 20*, 162–173. http://dx.doi.org/10.3109/11038128.2014.952912.

Frank, G. (2013). Twenty-first century pragmatism and social justice: Problematic situations and occupational reconstructions in post-civil war Guatemala. In M. P. Cutchin & V. A. Dickie (Eds.), *Transactional perspectives on occupation* (pp. 229–244). New York: Springer.

Galheigo, S. M. (2011). What needs to be done? Occupational therapy responsibilities and challenges regarding human rights. *Australian Occupational Therapy Journal, 58*, 60–66.

Galvaan, R. (2014). The contextually situated nature of occupational choice: Marginalised young adolescents' experiences in South Africa. *Journal of Occupational Science, 22*(1), 39–53.

Glover, J. S. (2009). The literature of occupational science: A systematic, quantitative examination of peer-reviewed publications from 1996-2006. *Journal of Occupational Science, 16*(2), 92–103. http://dx.doi.org/10.1080/14427591.2009.9686648.

Gustafsson, L., Molineux, M., & Bennett, S. (2014). Contemporary occupational therapy practice: The challenges of being evidence based and philosophically congruent. *Australian Occupational Therapy Journal, 61*(2), 121–123.

Hammell, K. W. (2004). Dimensions of meaning in the occupations of daily life. *Canadian Journal of Occupational Therapy, 71*(5), 296–303.

Hammell, K. W. (2008). Reflections on...wellbeing and occupational rights. *Canadian Journal of Occupational Therapy, 75*(1), 61–64.

Hammell, K. W. (2009a). Self-care, productivity, and leisure, or dimensions of occupational experience? Rethinking occupational 'categories'. *Canadian Journal of Occupational Therapy, 76*, 107–114.

Hammell, K. W. (2009b). Sacred texts: A skeptical exploration of the assumptions underpinning theories of occupation. *Canadian Journal of Occupational Therapy, 76*, 6–13.

Harvey-Krefting, L. (1985). The concept of work in occupational therapy: A historical review. *American Journal of Occupational Therapy, 39*(5), 301–308.

Hasselkus, B. R. (2011). *The meaning of everyday occupation* (2nd ed.). Thorofare, NJ: Slack.

Hocking, C. (2000). Occupational science: A stock take of accumulated insights. *Journal of Occupational Science, 7*(2), 58–67.

Hocking, C. (2009). The challenge of occupation: Describing the things people do. *Journal of Occupational Science, 16*(3), 140–150.

Hudson, M. J., & Aoyama, M. (2008). Occupational therapy and the current ecological crisis. *British Journal of Occupational Therapy, 71*(12), 545–548.

Humphry, R. (2002). Young children's occupations: Explicating the dynamics of developmental processes. *American Journal of Occupational Therapy, 56*(2), 171–179.

Humphry, R., & Wakeford, L. (2006). An occupation-centered discussion of development and implications for practice. *American Journal of Occupational Therapy, 60*, 258–267. http://dx.doi.org/10.5014/ajot.60.3.258.

International Society of Occupational Science (ISOS). (2009). *ISOS has a mission*. Retrieved from http://www.isoccsci.org.

Iwama, M. (2003). Toward culturally relevant epistemologies in occupational therapy. *American Journal of Occupational Therapy, 57*(5), 582–588.

Jonsson, H. (2008). A new direction in the conceptualization and categorization of occupation. *Journal of Occupational Science, 15,* 3–8.

Jonsson, H., & Persson, D. (2006). Towards an experiential model of occupational balance: An alternative perspective on flow theory analysis. *Journal of Occupational Science, 13*(1), 62–73.

Kantartzis, S., & Molineux, M. (2011). The influence of western society's construction of a healthy daily life on the conceptualisation of occupation. *Journal of Occupational Science, 18*(1), 62–80.

Kielhofner, G. (2004). *Conceptual foundations of occupational therapy* (3rd ed.). Philadelphia: F.A. Davis.

Kielhofner, G. (2008). *Model of human occupation: Theory and application* (4th ed.). Philadelphia: Lippincott Williams & Wilkins.

Kiepek, N., Phelan, S., & Magalhaes, L. (2014). Introducing a critical analysis of the figured world of occupation. *Journal of Occupational Science, 21*(4), 403–417.

Kronenberg, F., & Pollard, N. (2006). Political dimensions of occupation and the roles of occupational therapy. *American Journal of Occupational Therapy, 60*(6), 617–626.

Kubina, L. A., Dubouloz, C. J., Davis, C. G., Kessler, D., & Egan, M. Y. (2013). The process of re-engagement in personally valued activities during the two years following stroke. *Disability and Rehabilitation, 35*(3), 236–243.

Kuo, A. (2011). A transactional view: Occupation as a means to create experiences that matter. *Journal of Occupational Science, 18*(2), 131–138.

Laliberte Rudman, D. (2002). Linking occupation and identity: Lessons learned through qualitative exploration. *Journal of Occupational Science, 9*(1), 12–19.

Laliberte Rudman, D. (2010). Occupational terminology: Occupational possibilities. *Journal of Occupational Science, 17*(1), 55–59.

Laliberte Rudman, D. (2014). Embracing and enacting an 'occupational imagination': Occupational science as transformative. *Journal of Occupational Science, 21*(4), 373–388.

Laliberte Rudman, D., & Dennhardt, S. (2008). Shaping knowledge regarding occupation: Examining the cultural underpinnings of the evolving concept of occupational identity. *Australian Occupational Therapy Journal, 55*(3), 153–162.

Laliberte Rudman, D., Dennhardt, S., Fok, D., et al. (2008). A vision for occupational science: Reflecting on our disciplinary culture. *Journal of Occupational Science, 15*(3), 136–146.

Laliberte Rudman, D., & Huot, S. (2013). Conceptual insights for expanding thinking regarding the situated nature of occupation. In M. P. Cutchin & V. A. Dickie (Eds.), *Transactional perspectives on occupation* (pp. 51–64). New York: Springer.

Larson, E. (2004). Children's work: The less considered childhood occupation. *American Journal of Occupational Therapy, 58*(4), 369–379.

Law, M., Cooper, B., Strong, S., Stewart, D., Rigby, P., & Letts, L. (1996). The Person-Environment-Occupation model: A transactive approach to occupational performance. *Canadian Journal of Occupational Therapy, 63,* 9–23.

Law, M., Steinwender, S., & LeClair, L. (1998). Occupation, health and well-being. *Canadian Journal of Occupational Therapy, 62* (2), 81–91.

Ludwig, F. M. (1998). The unpackaging of routine in older women. *American Journal of Occupational Therapy, 52*(3), 168–175.

Lunt, A. (1997). Occupational science and occupational therapy: Negotiating the boundary between a discipline and a profession. *Journal of Occupational Science, 49*(2), 56–61.

McGrath, C. (2011). Low vision and older adults: The role of occupational therapy. *Occupational Therapy Now, 13*(3).

McLaughlin Gray, J. (1998). Putting occupation into practice: Occupation as ends, occupation as means. *American Journal of Occupational Therapy, 52,* 354–364.

Molineux, M. (2010). The nature of occupation. In M. Curtin, M. Molineux & J. Supyk-Mellon (Eds.), *Occupational therapy and physical dysfunction: Enabling occupation* (6th ed., pp. 17–25). London: Churchill Livingstone.

Molineux, M., & Whiteford, G. E. (2011). Occupational science: genesis, evolution and future contribution. In E. A. S. Duncan (Ed.), *Foundations for practice in occupational therapy* (pp. 243–253). Sydney: Elsevier.

Molke, D., Laliberte Rudman, D., & Polatajko, H. J. (2004). The promise of occupational science: A developmental assessment of an emerging academic discipline. *Canadian Journal of Occupational Therapy, 71*(5), 269–280.

Mosey, A. C. (1992). Partition of occupational science and occupational therapy. *American Journal of Occupational Therapy, 46*(9), 851–853.

Nelson, D. L. (1988). Occupation: Form and performance. *American Journal of Occupational Therapy, 42*(10), 633–641.

Nilsson, I., & Townsend, I. (2010). Occupational justice – Bridging theory and practice. *Scandinavian Journal of Occupational Therapy, 17,* 57–63.

Njelesani, J., Tang, A., Jonsson, H., & Polatajko, H. (2014). Articulating an occupational perspective. *Journal of Occupational Science, 21*(2), 226–235.

Parham, L. D. (1996). Perspectives on play. In R. Zemke & F. Clark (Eds.), *Occupational science: The evolving discipline* (pp. 71–80). Philadelphia: F.A. Davis.

Pettican, A., & Prior, S. (2011). 'It's a new way of life' An exploration of the occupational transition of retirement. *British Journal of Occupational Therapy, 74*(1), 12–19.

Phelan, S., & Kinsella, E. A. (2009). Occupational identity: Engaging socio-cultural perspectives. *Journal of Occupational Science, 16*(2), 85–91.

Polatajko, H. J., Backman, C., Baptiste, S., et al. (2007a). Human occupation in context. In E. A. Townsend & H. J. Polatajko (Eds.), *Enabling occupation II: Advancing an occupational therapy vision for health, well-being, & justice through occupation* (pp. 37–61). Ottawa: Canadian Association of Occupational Therapists.

Polatajko, H. J., Cantin, N., Amoroso, B., et al. (2007b). Occupation-based enablement: A practice mosaic. In E. A. Townsend & H. J. Polatajko (Eds.), *Enabling occupation II: Advancing an occupational therapy vision for health, well-being, & justice through occupation* (pp. 177–201). Ottawa: Canadian Association of Occupational Therapists.

Polatajko, J. H., Molke, D., Baptiste, S., et al. (2007c). Occupational science: Imperatives for occupational therapy. In E. A. Townsend & H. J. Polatajko (Eds.), *Enabling occupation II: Advancing an occupational therapy vision for health, well-being, & justice through occupation* (pp. 63–82). Ottawa: Canadian Association of Occupational Therapists.

Polgar, J., & Landry, J. E. (2004). Occupations as a means for individual and group participation in life. In C. H. Christiansen & E. A. Townsend (Eds.), *Introduction to occupation: The art and science of living* (pp. 197–220). Upper Saddle River, NJ: Prentice Hall.

Primeau, L. A. (1995). Work and leisure: Transcending the dichotomy. *American Journal of Occupational Therapy, 50*(7), 569–577.

Raphael, D. (2006). Social determinants of health: present status, unanswered questions, and future directions. *International Journal of Health Services, 36*(4), 651–677.

Reilly, M. (1962). Occupational therapy can be one of the great ideas of 20th century medicine. *American Journal of Occupational Therapy, 16*, 1–9.

Russell, E. (2008). Writing on the wall: The form, function and meaning of tagging. *Journal of Occupational Science, 15*(2), 87–97.

Stadnyk, R., Townsend, E. A., & Wilcock, A. A. (2010). Occupational justice. In C. H. Christiansen & E. A. Townsend (Eds.), *Introduction to occupation: The art and science of living* (2nd ed., pp. 329–358). Upper Saddle River, NJ: Prentice Hall.

Stamm, T., Wright, J., Machold, K., Sadlo, G., & Smolen, J. (2004). Occupational balance of women with rheumatoid arthritis: A qualitative study. *Musculoskeletal Care, 2*(2), 101–112.

Suto, M. (1998). Leisure in occupational therapy. *Canadian Journal of Occupational Therapy, 65*(5), 271–278.

Townsend, E.A. & Polatajko, H.J. (2007). *Enabling occupation II.* Ottawa: CAOT.

Townsend, E., & Wilcock, A. (2004). Occupational justice. In C. Christiansen & E. Townsend (Eds.), *Introduction to occupation: The art and science of living* (pp. 243–273). Upper Saddle River, NJ: Prentice Hall.

Trombly Latham, C. A. (2013). Occupation: Philosophy and concepts. In *Occupational therapy for physical dysfunction* (6th ed., pp. 339–357). Baltimore, MD: Lippincott Williams & Wilkins.

Twinley, R., & Addidle, G. (2012). Considering violence: The dark side of occupation. *British Journal of Occupational Therapy, 75*(4), 202–204.

Unruh, A. M. (2004). Reflections on: 'So…what do you do?' Occupation and the construction of identity. *Canadian Journal of Occupational Therapy, 71*(5), 290–295.

Vrkljan, B. H., & Polgar, J. M. (2006). Linking occupational participation and occupational identity: An exploratory study of the transition from driving to driving cessation in older adulthood. *Journal of Occupational Science, 14*(1), 1–10.

Wagman, P., Hakansson, C., & Bjorklund, A. (2012). Occupational balance as used in occupational therapy: A concept analysis. *Scandinavian Journal of Occupational Therapy, 19*, 322–327.

Watson, R., & Swartz, L. (Eds.), (2004). *Transformation through occupation.* London: Whurr.

Whiteford, G. E. (2000). Occupational deprivation: Global challenge in the new millennium. *British Journal of Occupational Therapy, 63*(5), 200–204. http://dx.doi.org/10.1177/030802260006300503.

Whiteford, G. E. (2010). Occupation in context. In M. Curtin, M. Molineux & J. Supyk-Mellon (Eds.), *Occupational therapy and physical dysfunction: Enabling occupation* (6th ed., pp. 136–148). London: Churchill Livingstone.

Whiteford, G. E., Klomp, N., & Wright-St.Clair, V. (2005). Complexity theory: Understanding occupation and practice in context. In G. Whiteford & V. Wright-St.Clair (Eds.), *Occupation & practice in context* (pp. 3–15). Sydney, NSW: Churchill Livingstone.

Whiteford, G. E. (2004). When people cannot participate: Occupational deprivation. In C. Christiansen & E. Townsend (Eds.), *Introduction to occupation: The art and science of living* (pp. 221–242). New Jersey: Prentice-Hall.

Wicks, A., & Whiteford, G. E. (2005). Gender, occupation and participation. In G. Whiteford & V. Wright-St. Clair (Eds.), *Occupation & practice in context* (pp. 197–212). Sydney: Elsevier.

Wilcock, A. A. (1998). Reflections on doing, being, and becoming. *Canadian Journal of Occupational Therapy, 65*(5), 248–256.

Wilcock, A. A. (2006). *An occupational perspective of health* (2nd ed.). Thorofare, NJ: Slack.

Wilcock, A. A., Chelin, M., Hall, M., et al. (1997). The relationship between occupational balance and health: A pilot study. *Occupational Therapy International, 4*(1), 17–30.

Wilcock, A. A., & Hocking, C. (2015). *An occupational perspective of health* (3rd ed.). Thorofare, NJ: Slack.

Wilcock, A. A., & Townsend, E. A. (2009). Occupational justice. In E. B. Crepeau, E. S. Cohn & B. A. Boyt Schell (Eds.), *Willard and Spackman's occupational therapy* (11th ed., pp. 192–199). Philadelphia: Lippincott Williams & Wilkins.

Wilson, L., & Wilcock, A. (2005). Occupation balance: What tips the scales for new students? *British Journal of Occupational Therapy, 68*(7), 319–323.

Wiseman, J. O., Davis, J. A., & Polatajko, H. P. (2005). Occupational development: Towards an understanding of children's doing. *Journal of Occupational Science, 12*(1), 26–35.

Wiseman, L., & Whiteford, G. (2009). Understanding occupational transitions: A study of older rural men's retirement experiences. *Journal of Occupational Science, 16*(2), 104–109.

World Federation of Occupational Therapists. (2012). *Position statement: Occupational science (revised).* Retrieved from http://www.wfot.org/ResourceCentre.aspx.

Yerxa, E. J. (2000). Occupational science: A renaissance of service to humankind through knowledge. *Occupational Therapy International, 7*(2), 87–98.

Yerxa, E. J., Clark, F., Frank, G., et al. (1990). An introduction to occupational science, a foundation for occupational therapy in the 21st century. *Occupational Therapy in Health Care, 6*, 1–17.

Zemke, R. (2004). Time, space, and the kaleidoscopes of occupation. *American Journal of Occupational Therapy, 58*(6), 608–620.

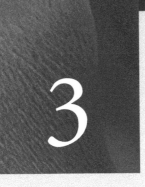

3 BIOMEDICAL SCIENCES

LESLEY COLLIER ■ RICHARD COLLIER

CHAPTER OUTLINE

Abstract
The focus of this chapter is to provide an overview of neurological, musculoskeletal, cardiovascular and respiratory anatomy and physiology. To ensure that the content is relevant to occupational therapists the anatomical and physiological information provided is related to three practice stories. These three practice stories are included to illustrate how an understanding of anatomical and physiological structures and functions can assist occupational therapists to determine the impact an illness, injury or impairment can have on a person's occupational performance.

KEY POINTS

- Understanding of anatomy and physiology underpins professional reasoning.

- The nervous system is a complex structure consisting of the brain, subcortical structures, spinal tracts and peripheral nerves.

- Perceptual and cognitive impairment may lead to discrete deficits affecting a person's occupational performance.

- The musculoskeletal system enables individuals to move around and interact with their environment.

- Understanding of the musculoskeletal system enables the understanding of how body movements may be compromised by injury.

- The respiratory and cardiovascular systems work together and so problems with one system will have a direct impact on the other.

- Emotion can have a direct impact on the cardiovascular system and so needs to be considered when working with an individual.

- A sound underpinning of anatomy and physiology assists occupational therapists in their professional reasoning and in understanding the impact an illness, injury or impairment may have on a person's occupational performance.

INTRODUCTION

An overview of key areas of anatomy and physiology that are related to neurological, musculoskeletal and medical and surgical conditions are presented in this chapter. A sound knowledge of anatomy and physiology can assist occupational therapists to understand the impact of different illnesses, injuries and impairments on a person's body structure and function, to anticipate potential occupational performance difficulties.

The chapter will use three practice stories to illustrate the importance of occupational therapists having an understanding of anatomy and physiology. The three practice stories reflect common conditions seen in practice. The first practice story focuses on Joyce and considers the anatomical and physiological structures involved in a cerebrovascular accident (CVA). The second practice story focuses on Brian and explores the anatomical and physiological structures involved in carpal tunnel syndrome. The third practice story focuses on Luc and considers the anatomical and physiological structures that are involved in a myocardial infarction.

NEUROLOGICAL ANATOMY AND PHYSIOLOGY

PRACTICE STORY: JOYCE

Joyce is a 56-year-old woman who has been admitted to an acute hospital ward with an ischaemic cerebrovascular accident (CVA) affecting the middle cerebral artery. A CVA is also known as a stroke. There are two main types of CVA: an ischaemic stroke, which is due to a lack of blood flow, and a

haemorrhagic stroke, which is due to bleeding. One of the first signs is headache followed by in inability to control one side of the body such as drooped face, inability to smile and weakness in the arm and/or leg. Risk factors for a CVA include high blood pressure, obesity and smoking.

Joyce's overall loss of function includes patterns of motor and sensory loss affecting the opposite side (contralateral) of her body to the location of the lesion. She also has perceptual problems including neglect. She has difficulty concentrating during her therapy sessions and finds her muscle spasticity increases when she becomes tired or if she tries to do a task that is too difficult.

The Brain

Brain Structure

The brain is a complex structure composed of two cerebral hemispheres. These two hemispheres have a folded surface that results in an increase in the size of the surface area (Fig. 3.1). Each raised area is known as a gyrus and each depression in between each gyrus is called a sulcus. There are a number of particularly deep sulci referred to as fissures. These two cerebral hemispheres are made up of neurones, neuroglia and capillaries that supply the high oxygen demand of nerve tissue. The cell bodies and dendrites of the neurones form the grey matter. The layer of grey matter towards the surface of the brain is referred to as the cortex, but there are also clusters of grey matter forming nuclei. These nuclei undertake specific functions; for example, the thalamus is a nuclei of grey matter that acts as a relay system to other areas of the brain. The axons of the

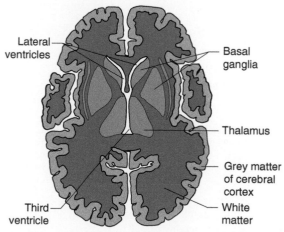

FIG. 3.1 ■ Structure of hemispheres. *(From Palastanga (2012)).*

neurones, or the tracts, lie in the white matter. The arrangement of grey and white matter can be seen in Figure 3.1.

Neuroglia are special support cells that hold the neurones in place. They also provide support and protection in the form of nutrients and oxygen and remove debris and waste.

Lobes of the Brain

The two hemispheres can be broadly mapped into a number of different areas with particular functions. Having a knowledge of the area that is damaged by a CVA or other brain injury can assist the occupational therapist in predicting the types of difficulties a person may experience. Each cerebral hemisphere can be divided into four lobes named after the skull bones that cover then. Each lobe is separated by two sulci, the central sulcus and the lateral sulcus (Fig. 3.2).

The frontal lobe lies anterior to the central sulcus and above the lateral sulcus. The posterior part of the frontal lobe, immediately in front of the central sulcus, is concerned with performance of movement and is referred to as the primary motor area. Movement is initiated from this area to the opposite side of the body and involves groups of muscles. As such, damage to this area results in loss of precision movement. In front of the primary motor area lies the premotor area. Fibres from this area descend directly to the spinal cord or indirectly via the primary motor area and are responsible for coordination and execution of learnt bilateral movements such as walking. Alongside the premotor area lies the supplementary motor area. This area is involved in the planning of movement before execution. Within the lower portion of the frontal lobe on the dominant side lies the motor speech area (Broca's area), which is involved in the production of fluent speech. The anterior part of the frontal lobe (prefrontal) connects with all the other lobes as well as other brain areas including the subcortex. This area is involved with planning of movement and behaviour in order to achieve a specific goal and to modify action according to feedback. Damage to this area affects the way a person interacts socially and how a person makes judgements based on changes to his or her environment.

The parietal lobe lies posterior to the frontal lobe. Its main function is to process sensory information from all parts of the body including the eyes and ears. This helps a person make sense of where his or her body is in space during movement and spatial awareness of the surrounding environment. The somatosensory

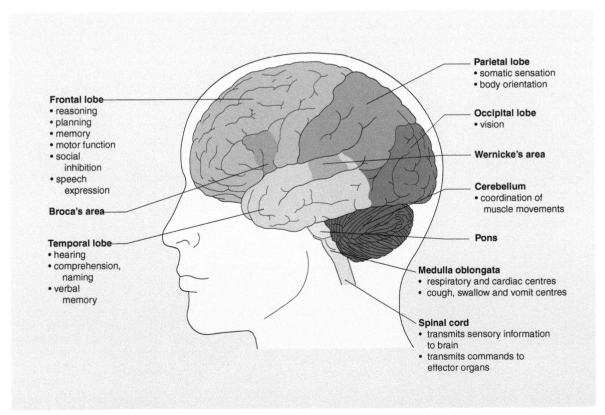

FIG. 3.2 ■ Lobes of the brain. *(From Battista, E. (2012). Crash course: Pharmacology (4th ed.). St Louis: Mosby.)*

area lies posterior to the central sulcus and receives input from muscles and joints around the body. This area allows a person to perceive danger and helps the person make sense of his or her world. Damage in this area would lead to difficulty in reading, recognising people and objects and moving around an environment.

The occipital lobe lies at the back of the brain where it receives visual information direct from the eye. Information received from the right visual field of each eye is processed in the left of the occipital lobe and vice versa. The occipital lobe links with the parietal lobe in the recognition of the written word, faces and objects. It also is involved in the processing of movement such as positioning of the hand for interaction with everyday objects. Damage to this area may lead to hemianopia, loss of sight in half of the visual field of each eye, and visual agnosia, the ability to recognise objects and faces.

The temporal lobe lies at the side of the brain and is involved in the processing in hearing and long-term memory. This area processes sound frequencies and the receptive aspects of speech and language. Lesions on the left side of the temporal lobe are associated with receptive dysphasia, and the inability to understand the spoken and written word.

APPLICATION TO JOYCE

Having a knowledge of the lobes affected by a cerebrovascular accident provides the therapist with an indication of some of the functional deficits that Joyce might experience. Involvement of the frontal lobe may lead to Joyce having difficulty in reasoning and problem solving, making it difficult for her to manage her decision making. Involvement of the parietal lobe may lead to Joyce having difficulty in telling right from left and interpreting sensation that could affect her ability to dress and perform other bilateral activities of daily living. Involvement of the temporal lobe may lead to difficulties in hearing and language that may make it difficult for Joyce to understand directions and engage in conversation. Involvement of the occipital lobe may lead to Joyce having difficulties in recognising visual objects. Involvement of the cerebellar can lead to coordination and balance problems that would make it difficult for Joyce to move around safely.

Vascular System of the Brain

The capillaries are part of the vascular system providing oxygen and removing carbon dioxide. These capillaries are supplied by a number of arteries. The carotid arteries supply the face, the scalp and the front part of the brain. Decreased blood flow to this artery can result in impairment in the frontal lobes. This can result in numbness, weakness or paralysis on the opposite side of the body to where the obstruction is. The anterior cerebral artery also supplies the frontal lobes, the parts of the brain that control logical thought, personality and voluntary movement. Decreased blood flow to this artery can result in weakness in the contralateral leg. The middle cerebral artery supplies the temporal and parietal lobes. This is the artery most often

affected in when a person has a CVA. The posterior cerebral artery supplies the temporal and occipital lobes. Decreased blood flow to this artery can lead to contralateral hemiplegia and visual field deficits (Fig. 3.3).

APPLICATION TO JOYCE

An aneurysm is a weak spot on an artery that can lead to a haemorrhagic CVA. This is where the walls of the artery have become thin because they have been stretched. Joyce may have had a haemorrhagic CVA due to high blood pressure. Aneurysms can be present from birth, but other factors including smoking, family history, using cocaine, and some medical conditions, such as autosomal dominant polycystic kidney disease, can also make them more likely to develop.

Subcortical Structures and the Brainstem
Subcortical Structures

For all the senses the final destination is the cerebral cortex, but on the way sensory signals pass through various subcortical structures. These structures allow sensory information to be modulated and modified to help make the most appropriate motor response. The thalamus is a mass of grey matter and acts as a relay station receiving sensory information from the spinal cord and sensory systems (except smell) and passing it up to the cerebral cortex and down to the brainstem. It is also thought to act as the gatekeeper of consciousness, controlling sleep and attention (Fig. 3.4).

The basal ganglia are located in the midbrain. Most of the inputs into this structure are from the motor cortex and information is sent back to the motor cortex via the thalamus. As such this structure is primarily involved in motor control. The basal ganglia select motor programmes that are most appropriate for the activity selected. They are involved in the processing of sensory stimuli for movement and the initiation of movement. Disorders of the basal ganglia result in poverty of movement (akinesia), slow movement (bradykinesia), tremor at rest, rigidity caused by increased tone in skeletal muscles, and small handwriting (micrographia).

The limbic system is made up of a number of grey matter structures linked together by white matter. These structures are sometimes referred to as the emotional brain as they process emotional and physiological responses. The amygdala is involved in processing fear, defensiveness and aggression. It contributes to deciding whether a sensory stimuli should be considered a threat or not. The hippocampus is involved establishing event memories and consolidation of short-term and long-term memory. In people with Alzheimer's disease this is one of the first structures to be affected. Also people with extensive damage to the hippocampus may experience anterograde amnesia, the inability to form and retain new memories. The hypothalamus is involved with basic homoeostasis functions such as hunger, temperature and thirst. Output from this structure is to the autonomic nervous system, which controls sweating, dilation of blood vessels and hormones from the pituitary gland.

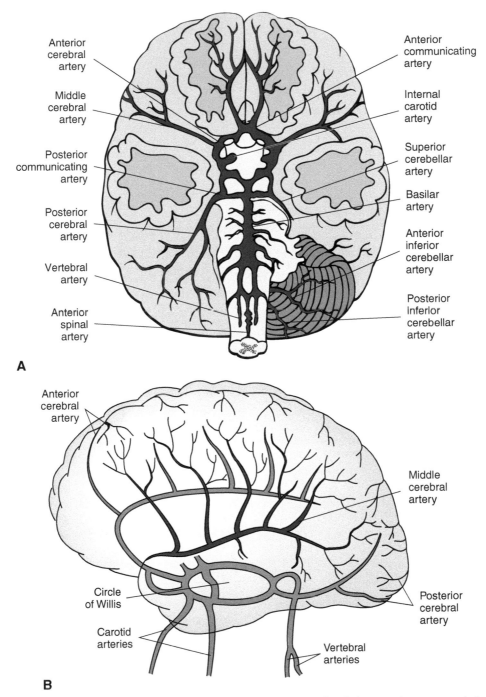

FIG. 3.3 ■ Vascular system of the brain. *(From Philips, N. (2007). Berry and Kohn's operating room technique (11th ed.). St Louis: Mosby.)*

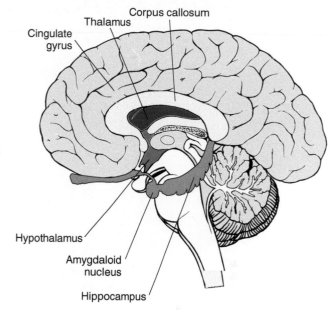

FIG. 3.4 ■ Subcortical structures. *(From Wilson, S. (2009). Health assessment for nursing practice (4th ed.). St Louis: Mosby.)*

The cerebellum is located at the back of the brain and is cauliflower-like in appearance. It controls fine movement, timing, sequencing and motor memory. Information about the position of the head is received from the vestibule of the ear, position of the rest of the body is received from the proprioceptors in muscles and joints via the spinal cord and information from the motor cortex concerning intended movement is delivered via the pons. Output is to the primary motor cortex and the brainstem. Damage to the cerebellum can result in uncoordinated, jerky movements, known as ataxia.

APPLICATION TO JOYCE

Subcortical CVA can lead to a wide range of sensorimotor and cognitive problems, including hemiparesis, paresthesias, dysarthria and dysphagia. This is different from cortical CVA, which tend to affect higher cognitive functioning.

The Brainstem

The brainstem is where the spinal cord enters the brain and controls functions such as breathing and temperature regulation. Damage to the brainstem can produce coma or death. The structures of the brainstem include the midbrain, the pons and the medulla. The reticular formation runs through these structures (Fig. 3.5).

The reticular formation is continuous through the midbrain, pons and medulla. It forms a link with the hypothalamus, the limbic system, the thalamus and the cortex and affects arousal and attention. The descending fibres affect activity in the lower motor neurones that affect the trunk and proximal muscles of our limbs. This system helps the cortex to determine which sensory information needs to be responded to and which needs to be suppressed. It also plays a role in modulating pain and respiration. It integrates autonomic functions, for example, it reduces heart rate, blood pressure and respiration when a person falls asleep and increases these systems when a person is awake so that moving from horizontal to vertical position does not cause fainting.

The midbrain is the upper part of the brainstem and contains the substantia nigra, one of the basal ganglia involved in producing parkinsonian signs after reduction in nigral cells. The pons, which lies below it, forms a relay station for fibres from the motor cortex to cross to the opposite cerebellar cortex. The medulla lies at the bottom and leads on to the spinal cord. On the ventral side of the medulla there are two triangular structures called the pyramids. These pyramids contain large (descending) motor tracts which send information down to the body. At the point the medulla joins the spinal cord most of these tracts cross to the opposite side. This crossing explains why motor areas on one side of the brain control muscular movement on the opposite side of the body. Ascending tracts containing sensory information also cross in the medulla.

APPLICATION TO JOYCE

Joyce may have difficulty in determining which environmental stimuli to respond to as a result of her CVA. Reducing sensory information in her environment may help her to focus on important sensory stimulation without being distracted.

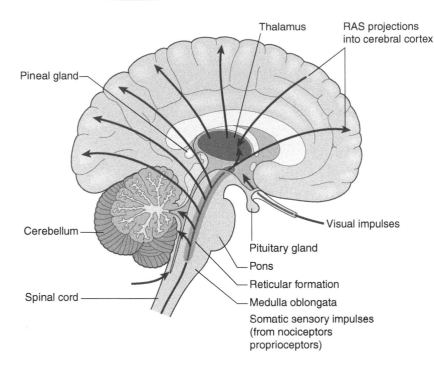

Thalamus

RAS projections
into cerebral cortex

Pineal gland

Cerebellum

Spinal cord

Visual impulses

Pituitary gland

Pons

Reticular formation

Medulla oblongata

Somatic sensory impulses
(from nociceptors
proprioceptors)

FIG. 3.5 ■ The brainstem. *(From The Worlds of David Darling, Encyclopedia of Science. Reticular formation. Retrieved from: www.daviddarling.info/encyclopedia/R/reticular_formation.html.)*

The Tracts and Sensory/Motor Feedback

Motor Pathways

Motor impulses are sent from the brain through the spinal cord via two main pathways: the pyramidal pathway and the extrapyramidal pathway. Most fibres from the pyramidal pathway originate from the motor areas of the cerebral cortex. They descend through the internal capsule of the cerebrum and cross in the medulla, terminating in the anterior grey horn of the spinal cord. These horns are part of the central core of grey matter that can be seen in a cross section of the spinal cord. This component of the descending tracts is called an upper motor neuron. A short connecting neurone completes the connection to voluntary muscles. This latter part is called a lower motor neuron. The two main tracts within this pyramidal system are the corticospinal tract and the corticobulbar tract (Fig. 3.6). The corticospinal tract links with muscles of the limbs and trunk. The corticobulbar tract links via the cranial nerves with muscles of the face.

The extrapyramidal tracts include the rubrospinal tract, which is concerned with muscle tone and body posture, the tectospinal tract, which controls movements of the head, and the vestibulospinal tract, which controls muscle tone in response to movements of the head (equilibrium) (Fig. 3.7).

APPLICATION TO JOYCE

The corticospinal tract is concerned with voluntary control of precision movement. As Joyce's CVA affected the internal capsule, the corticospinal tract was directly involved, thereby affecting her ability to perform skilled precision movements. This will affect Joyce's ability to undertake activities of daily living independently.

Sensory Pathways

Sensory information is transmitted from the periphery up the spinal cord to the sensory areas of the brain. This information travels via two general pathways, the posterior column pathway and the spinothalamic pathway (anterolateral) (Fig. 3.8). The posterior column pathway is made up of two tracts that are ipsilateral; that is, they carry sensation from the same side of the body. Fibres from the lower limbs feed in to the column to form the fasciculus gracilis. Fibres from the upper limb feed in to form the fasciculus cuneatus. This posterior column pathway transmits information via the thalamus in relation to proprioception, fine touch, two-point discrimination and vibration. This sensory information is directed to the thalamus and cortex, the conscious areas of the brain.

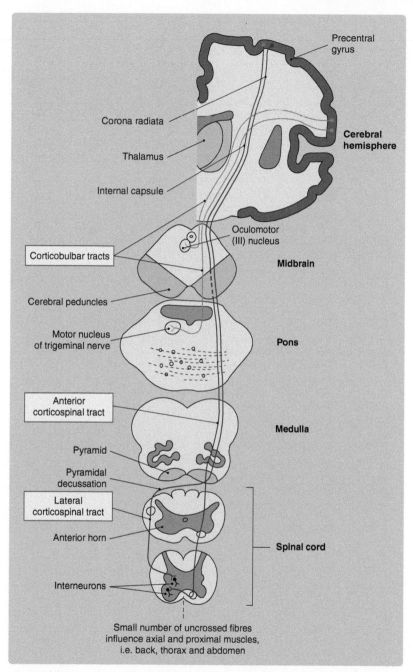

FIG. 3.6 ■ Pyramidal tract. *(From Ross, J. (2012). Crash course: Nervous system (4th ed.). St Louis: Mosby.)*

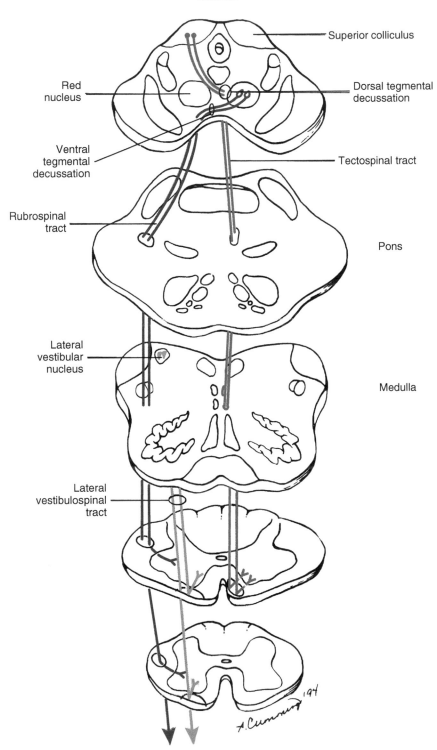

Midbrain

Superior colliculus

Red
nucleus

Dorsal tegmental
decussation

Ventral
tegmental
decussation

Tectospinal tract

Rubrospinal
tract

Pons

Lateral
vestibular
nucleus

Medulla

Lateral
vestibulospinal
tract

A. Cumming '94

FIG. 3.7 ■ Extrapyramidal tract. *(From Cramer, G., & Darby, S. (2005). Basic and clinical anatomy of the spine, spinal cord, and ANS (3rd ed.). St Louis: Mosby.)*

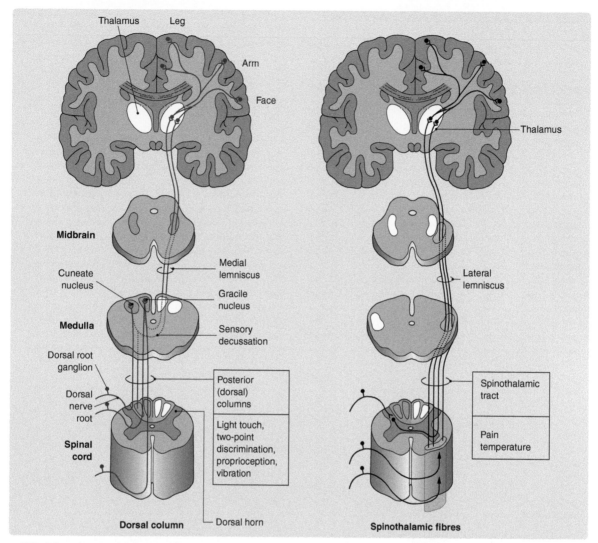

FIG. 3.8 ■ Sensory pathways. *(From Turner, C., & Gibbs, J. (2009). Crash course: Neurology (2nd ed.). St Louis: Mosby.)*

The spinothalamic pathway receives sensory information via the posterior horn of the spinal cord before crossing to the opposite side. The lateral spinothalamic pathway passes up to the thalamus via the brainstem where the conscious awareness of pain and temperature is processed. The anterior spinothalamic pathway conducts information regarding crude touch and pressure, although exact location, size and shape cannot be determined. This pathway also passes through the thalamus before reaching the cerebral cortex. As such, these two pathways send sensory signals that result in subconscious motor reactions.

APPLICATION TO JOYCE

The spinothalamic tract transmits information regarding sensation. Joyce may have difficulty in recognising different sensations such as hot and cold. This may increase her risk of burns when, for example, she is preparing a meal.

MUSCULOSKELETAL ANATOMY AND PHYSIOLOGY

Brian is a carpenter and for several months he has been experiencing an intermittent dull aching pain in the palm of his dominant right hand. Brian has been diagnosed with carpal tunnel syndrome (CTS). Carpal tunnel syndrome is a condition in which the median nerve is compressed as it passes through the carpal tunnel at the wrist. Predisposing factors may include diabetes, obesity, pregnancy and hypothyroidism. Other causes can include the use of the hand and arm in heavy manual work, using vibrating tools and performing highly repetitive tasks. The main symptom of CTS is intermittent numbness of the thumb, index, and middle fingers and the radial side of the ring finger.

Brian initially thought that the numbness was due to the fact that he was using more powerful power tools as it had been suggested by a work colleague that excessive vibration could cause the pain. More recently, he had also been experiencing numbness and a burning sensation, particularly at night. He noticed that his hand felt weak and he started

to find it difficult to use the heavier power tools. Brian feels that his hand is becoming tired more quickly and he is losing the dexterity that he once had, particularly of his thumb.

Bones and Joints of the Upper Limb

The Shoulder

The shoulder is a complex musculoskeletal region made up of a number of important joints that allow at least one hand to be placed on every part of the body and to explore the immediate space around the body (Fig. 3.9). The focus is on mobility compared with the lower limb where the focus is on stability. The glenohumeral joint is a spheroidal joint that is made up of the laterally facing shallow glenoid fossa and the partially spherical head of the humerus. Spheroidal joints are important at the root of a limb as they allow the limb to be rotated around three perpendicular axes (this is also known as 'three degrees of freedom'). This provides much greater ability to place the upper limb in numerous different positions that facilitate the use of the hand. The glenohumeral joint is part of the pectoral girdle made up of the scapular and the clavicle. These bones are connected at the acromioclavicular joint and supported by the conoid and trapezoid ligaments and the coracoclavicular ligaments. These

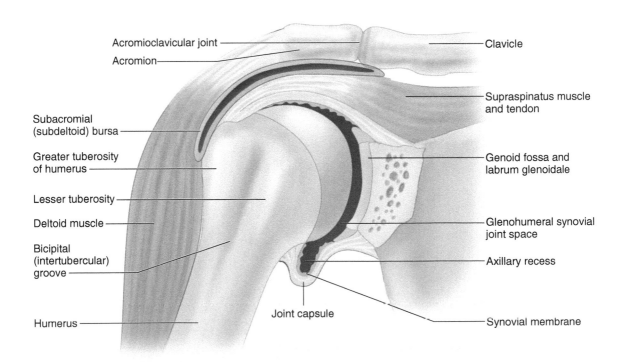

FIG. 3.9 ■ The shoulder. *(From Fam, A. (2006). Musculoskeletal examination and joint injection techniques. St Louis: Mosby.)*

strong supporting ligaments are important in providing the stability at the lateral end of the clavicle. The acromioclavicular joint is often referred to as a plane joint, which implies that the joint surfaces are flat and congruent. In reality there is considerable variation in the shape and orientation of the joint, although it is common for the orientation of the joint to be inclined in such a way that a fall onto the point of the shoulder or onto the outstretched hand drives the acromion under the lateral end of the clavicle; this is often seen in sporting injuries.

The medial end of the clavicle is much less commonly injured. The sternoclavicular joint is described as a saddle (or sellar) joint; this type of synovial joint is one of the most stable and normally consists of reciprocally concave-convex joint surfaces where joint congruency and stability are provided by the shape of the joint surfaces. This type of joint provides more flexibility than a hinge or gliding joint.

The pectoral girdle glides around the chest wall with the scapular forming a muscular joint (not a true joint) between the anterior surface of the scapular and the posterior surface of the chest. This is often referred to as the scapulothoracic joint, although it has no joint capsule or synovial membrane and so is immune from degenerative changes and inflammatory arthropathies. The function of the scapulothoracic joint is to provide stability for the glenohumeral joint; for normal movement of the upper limb to occur, the glenoid fossa is first placed in the desired starting position and the muscles stabilise the scapular. The rotator cuff muscles then stabilise the head of the humerus within the glenoid fossa. This allows the elbow, forearm and wrist joints to place the hand in the desired position.

APPLICATION TO BRIAN

When Brian first mentioned his problem to his doctor a diagnosis of rotator cuff tendonitis was considered. This condition is associated with arm movement, particularly in reaching and pain in the shoulder at night. This condition is common in active and older people.

The Elbow and Forearm

The elbow joint is a true hinge joint at which there is only one degree of freedom; it only moves about one axis and so only flexion and extension occur at this joint (Fig. 3.10). The superior radioulnar joint is a pivot joint with the superior end of the radius spinning within the annual ligament. This too only has one degree of freedom – in this case, the movement is around the longitudinal axis of the radius. This allows the radius to pronate and supinate around the ulna. The inferior radioulnar joint is also a pivot joint; the motion of pronation and supination allows the placing of the hand as required. The radiocarpal joint is an ellipsoidal joint; this type of joint has two degrees of freedom and this enables flexion and extension as well as radial and ulna deviation to occur. This type of joint is less stable than a hinge or saddle joint and consequently traumatic injuries, such as sprains and fractures of the wrist, are commonly seen in practice. The complex

movements at the radiocarpal joint can also compromise the structures that pass through the wrist and this, coupled with degenerative or traumatic pathological changes, often compromises people's wrist, forearm and hand function.

The carpal bones are situated closely together with a high degree of congruence between the bones. The joints formed between the carpal bones are normally described as plane joints which allow sliding or gliding movements. However, this is not universally the case as some of the movements that occur between carpal bones are similar to the motions seen in spheroidal joints.

APPLICATION TO BRIAN

An alternative diagnosis for Brian might be cubital tunnel syndrome, which is an ulnar nerve compression at the elbow. The signs are also numbness and tingling in the hands and fingers. Symptoms can be managed by conservative treatments such as regularly changing activities so that there is less repetition of movements.

Muscle of the Upper Limb

Muscles that control the movements that occur at the joints of the upper limb can be grouped according to function. Starting proximally, the scapular muscles can be grouped into those that protract, retract, elevate and depress the pectoral girdle (Fig. 3.11). Working in combination, muscles produce rotation of the scapular and rotation about the longitudinal axis of the clavicle; this rotation is known as conjunct rotation as is occurs largely as a result of the tension in the coracoclavicular ligaments and the shape of the joints of the clavicle. When a person lifts his or her arm above the head (i.e. elevation) the clavicle elevates as well, and this results in an increase in the distance between the coracoid process and the clavicle. This movement is limited by the coracoclavicular ligaments. As the tension in these structures increases, the posterior attachments on the clavicle of the conoid and trapezoid ligaments prevent further elevation of the back of the clavicle; this causes it to rotate backwards. This is an important adjunct movement that assists in the positioning of the glenoid fossa during elevation of the arm.

The rotator cuff muscles are the next group of muscles to consider (Fig. 3.12). These muscles effectively work as dynamic ligaments that continually work to maintain the position of the head of the humerus within the glenoid fossa. The glenohumeral joint is a relatively unstable joint; it is one of the most mobile joints of the body and has sacrificed stability for mobility. There are no ligaments of significance, only thickenings of the lax capsule, and as such they provide limited structural stability.

The rotator cuff muscles work continually to depress the head of the humerus in the glenoid fossa; this counters the biomechanical tendency for the head to roll up in the fossa to elevate the arm. The depression of the humerus in the glenoid fossa is as a result of the contraction of the rotator cuff muscles, principally supraspinatus and the long head of biceps. The other rotator cuff muscles contribute to anterior and posterior stability.

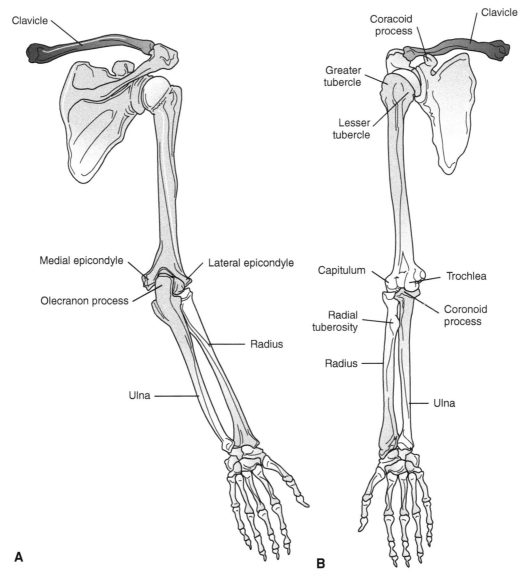

FIG. 3.10 ■ The elbow and forearm. *(From Fritz, S. (2009). Mosby's essential sciences for therapeutic massage (3rd ed.). St Louis: Mosby.)*

APPLICATION TO BRIAN

The rotator cuff muscles function as stabilisers in all movements at the glenohumeral joint. As Brian was experiencing pain and weakness in his hand he was relying more heavily on his upper limb to support the power tools he was using. This led to soreness in his shoulder.

The muscles of the forearm act on the wrist and hand and can be divided into flexor and extensor groups (Fig. 3.13).

The flexor group arises from the medial epicondyle of the humerus and passes along the medial border of the forearm. The flexor group includes flexor carpi ulnaris, flexor carpi radialis, flexor digitorum superficialis and flexor digitorum profundus. The extensor group arises from the lateral epicondyle of the humerus and passes along the lateral border of the forearm. The extensor group includes extensor carpi ulnaris, extensor carpi radialis longus, extensor carpi radialis brevis and extensor digitorum. Supinator, biceps, pronator teres and pronator quadratus produce supination and pronation of the forearm,

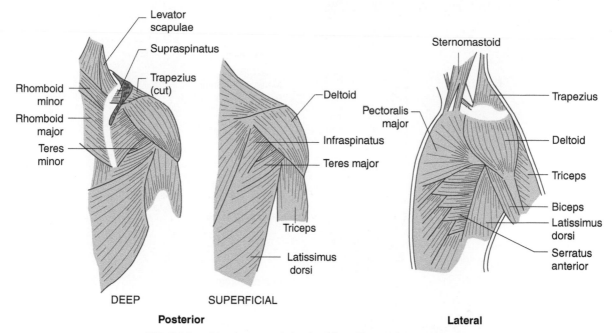

FIG. 3.11 ■ Muscles around the shoulder. *(From Palastanga (2012)).*

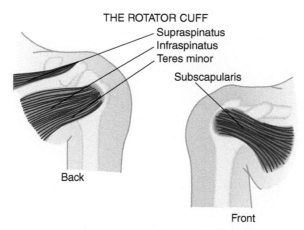

FIG. 3.12 ■ Rotator cuff muscles. *(From Miller, M. (2010). Delee & Drez's orthopaedic sports medicine: Principles and practice (3rd ed.). Philadelphia: Saunders.)*

the turning of the palm upwards or downwards. The names of these muscles refer to their action, shape and size. Their function is to position and support the hand in functional activity.

The muscles of the hand form two masses on either side of the palm. The thenar eminence is located on the thumb side of the palm and is involved in opposition of the thumb in order to facilitate grip. The hypothenar eminence is located on the side

of the little finger and has a weaker action in opposition but is instrumental in power grips. Flexor digitorum superficialis and flexor digitorum profundus, mentioned earlier, provide flexion of the fingers. These form a stronger muscle group than the extensor digitorum, hence the curled position in flexion of the relaxed hand.

APPLICATION TO BRIAN

The median nerve serves the following muscles: the muscles of the thenar eminence (abductor pollicis brevis, flexor pollicis brevis, opponens pollicis) and the first two lumbricals. As these muscles are involved with use of the thumb, CTS often results in difficulty in maintaining grip when holding an object between the thumb and other fingers. Brian may find that he drops things because of the loss of power, which will be increasingly frustrating for him. This lack of dexterity will make it difficult for him to undertake his job as a carpenter.

The Carpal Tunnel

The carpal tunnel at the wrist is an osteofibrous tunnel made up of four components: (1) the space between the flexor retinaculum, also referred to as the transverse carpal ligament or the anterior annular ligament (the roof); (2) the carpal sulcus (the floor), which is also made up of the joint capsule and the radiocarpal ligaments; (3) the hamate, triquetral and pisiform

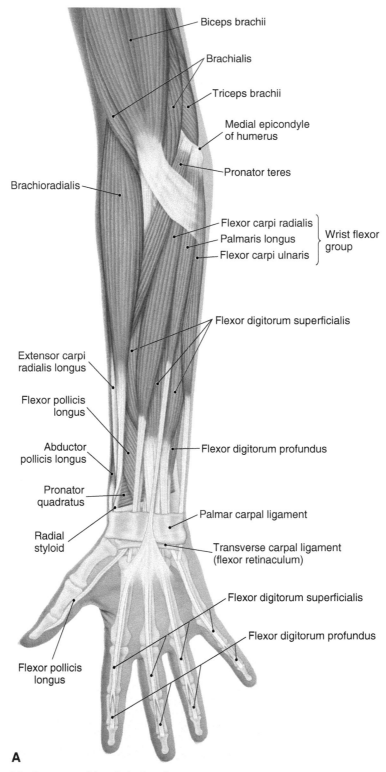

Biceps brachii

Brachialis

Triceps brachii

Medial epicondyle
of humerus

Pronator teres

Brachioradialis

Flexor carpi radialis
Palmaris longus   } Wrist flexor
Flexor carpi ulnaris   group

Flexor digitorum superficialis

Extensor carpi
radialis longus

Flexor pollicis
longus

Abductor
pollicis longus

Flexor digitorum profundus

Pronator
quadratus

Palmar carpal ligament

Radial
styloid

Transverse carpal ligament
(flexor retinaculum)

Flexor digitorum superficialis

Flexor digitorum profundus

Flexor pollicis
longus

A

FIG. 3.13 ■ Muscles of the forearm and hand. A, Anterior.

Continued

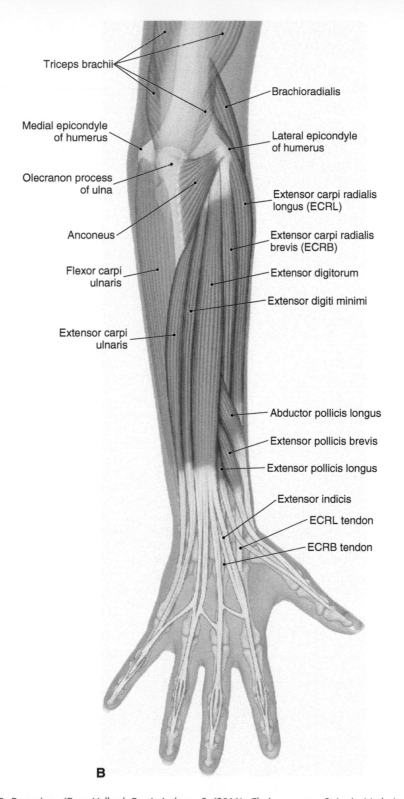

Triceps brachii

Brachioradialis

Medial epicondyle
of humerus

Lateral epicondyle
of humerus

Olecranon process
of ulna

Extensor carpi radialis
longus (ECRL)

Anconeus

Extensor carpi radialis
brevis (ECRB)

Flexor carpi
ulnaris

Extensor digitorum

Extensor digiti minimi

Extensor carpi
ulnaris

Abductor pollicis longus

Extensor pollicis brevis

Extensor pollicis longus

Extensor indicis

ECRL tendon

ECRB tendon

B

FIG. 3.13, cont'd   B, Posterior. *(From Holland, P., & Anderson S. (2011). Chair massage. St Louis: Mosby.)*

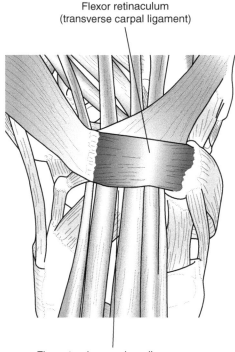

Flexor retinaculum
(transverse carpal ligament)

Flexor tendons and median nerve
travel through the carpal tunnel here

FIG. 3.14 ■ The carpal tunnel and tendons at the wrist. *From Lowe, W (2003) Orthopedic massage: Theory and technique. St Louis: Mosby.)*

bones (the ulna edge); and (4) the scaphoid, trapezoid and tendons of flexor carpi radialis (the radial edge) (Fig. 3.14). Within the carpal tunnel run the four tendons of the superficial fingers flexors, the four tendons of the deep finger flexors, the long thumb flexors and the median nerve.

APPLICATION TO BRIAN

There are anatomical variations to the contents of the carpal tunnel that may explain the variations in symptoms reported; even the ulna nerve very occasionally travels through the carpal tunnel. Tenosynovitis as a result of rheumatoid arthritis, post–Colles fracture or in individuals with osteoarthrosis of the radio-carpal or intercarpal joints can all lead to an increase in pressure of the carpal tunnel and cause symptoms. Other factors, such as the overuse or repetitive use of the hands in physical work and the use of handheld vibrating tools used in construction or heavy industry, should be considered. Brian's work involves repetitive hand actions so he should receive advice regarding taking regular breaks or interchanging activities to include a wide range of hand movements.

The Nerves of the Upper Limb

The Brachial Plexus

The brachial plexus emerges from the spinal cord from the fifth cervical vertebrae to first thoracic vertebrae. It is formed of three trunks, which are made up from two upper and two lower roots and a lateral root. Each trunk then divides into anterior and posterior divisions. The posterior divisions form nerves supplying the posterior aspect of the arm and the anterior divisions form nerves supplying the anterior aspect of the arm. These divisions form three cords (posterior, medial and lateral), which lie in the axilla (Fig. 3.15).

■ The posterior cord forms the radial and axillary nerve.
■ The medial cord forms the ulnar and medial half of the median nerve.
■ The lateral cord forms the musculocutaneous and lateral half of the median nerve.

The Axillary Nerve

The axillary nerve arises from the posterior cord and supplies the deltoid and teres minor muscles. As such, it is used in movements that involve raising the arm.

The Radial Nerve

Sensation. The radial nerve innervates the posterior surface of the upper arm, a strip of skin down the middle of the posterior aspect of the forearm and the dorsal aspect of the hand (the thumb, index finger, middle finger and medial side of the ring finger) (Fig. 3.16).

Motor. The radial nerve innervates triceps muscle, an extensor of the elbow. After the elbow, the nerve divides into two and the superficial branch continues under brachioradialis on the lateral side of the forearm. At the wrist this branch then supplies the dorsal surface of the hand on the thumb side. The second branch forms the posterior interosseous nerve and innervates the extensor muscles of the forearm.

The Musculocutaneous Nerve

The musculocutaneous nerve supplies coracobrachialis, biceps and brachialis muscles. At the elbow this nerve becomes cutaneous to supply the skin on the lateral side of the forearm.

The Ulna Nerve

Sensation. The ulna nerve is a continuation of the medial cord and passes down the medial border of the forearm (Fig. 3.17). The nerve passes on the medial aspect of the humerus and is vulnerable to knocks. A bump of the ulna nerve at this point gives a tingling sensation and is commonly referred to as hitting a person's 'funny bone'.

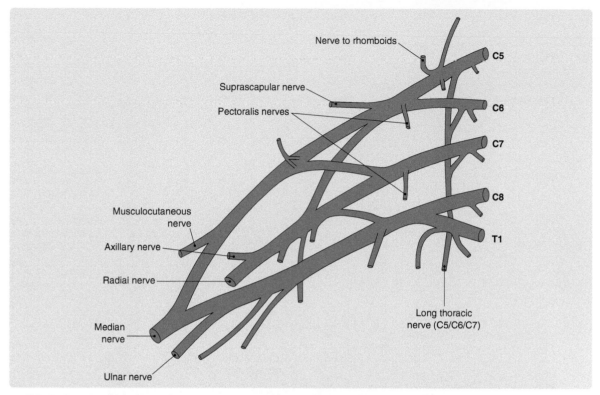

FIG. 3.15 ■ Brachial plexus. *(From Turner, C., & Gibbs, J. (2009). Crash course: Neurology (2nd ed.). St Louis: Mosby.)*

Motor. The ulna nerve innervates flexor carpi ulnaris, flexor digitorum profundus, flexor digiti mini, abductor digiti minimi, opponens digiti minimi, lumbricals, palmar and dorsal interossei and adductor pollicis. As such, this nerve is involved in the fine coordinated movements of the hand.

The Median Nerve

Sensation. The median nerve innervates the skin of the palmar surface of the thumb, index and middle finger. It also innervates the radial half of the ring finger (Fig. 3.18). There are also anatomical variations in the innervation. It is important to note that the pattern of innervation is very similar to the C7 dermatome (radial three digits), so therapists should ensure that cervical pathological conditions are excluded before concluding that compression of the median nerve is the cause of the problem.

Motor. In the forearm the median nerve innervates many of the deep and superficial flexors, including pronator teres, the flexors of the wrist and the fingers apart from flexor carpi ulnaris and the ulnar portion of flexor digitorum profundus. In the hand and at the wrist the median nerve innervates the short thumb abductors, opponens pollicis and the first two lumbrical muscles. The radial head of flexor pollicis brevis is also innervated.

APPLICATION TO BRIAN

Brian has been recommended for keyhole surgery. This involves cutting the transverse carpal ligament to create more space for the nerves and tendons in the carpal tunnel. The transverse ligament holds the flexor tendons down and forms a pulley to allow flexion of the fingers. Second, this ligament holds the carpal bones in formation. As such, this could cause postoperative complications. In addition, a scar site at the heel of the hand may cause pain when Brian returns to work as a carpenter. Alternative treatment options include steroid injections and splinting; however, the outcomes from these options are more variable.

RADIAL/AXILLARY NERVES

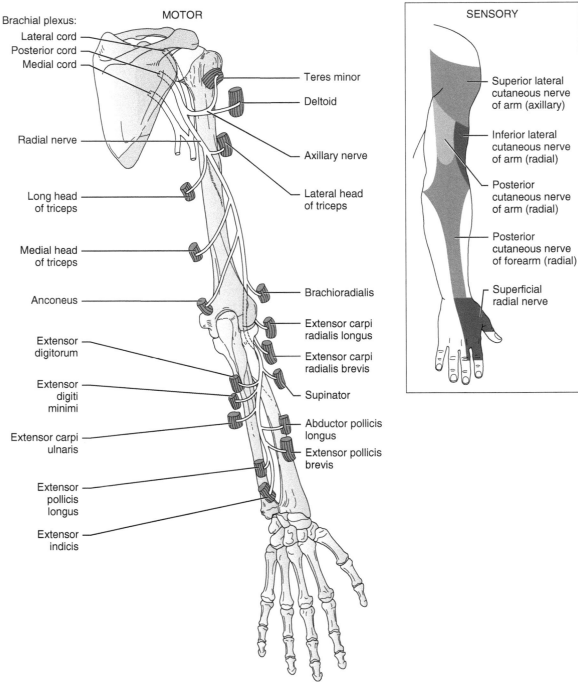

FIG. 3.16 ■ The radial nerve. *(From Jenkins, D. (2009). Hollinshead's functional anatomy of the limbs and back (9th ed.). Philadelphia: Saunders.)*

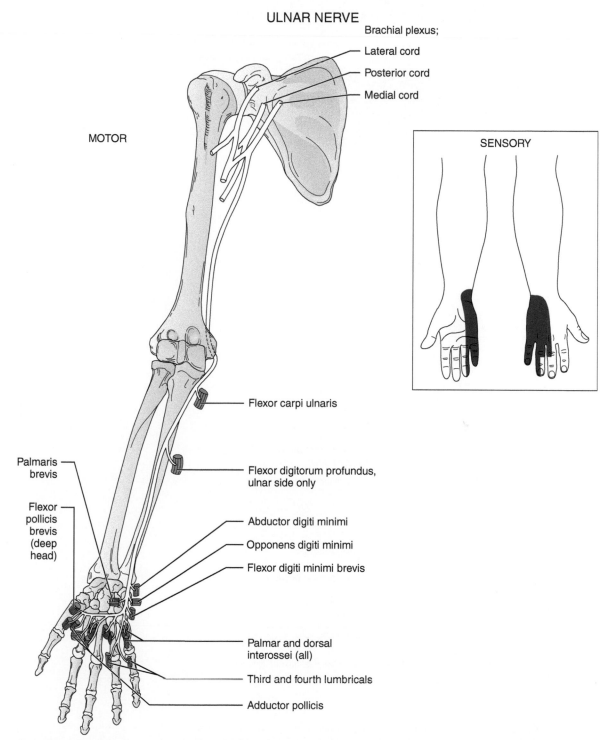

ULNAR NERVE

Brachial plexus;

Lateral cord

Posterior cord

Medial cord

MOTOR

SENSORY

Flexor carpi ulnaris

Palmaris brevis

Flexor digitorum profundus, ulnar side only

Flexor pollicis brevis (deep head)

Abductor digiti minimi

Opponens digiti minimi

Flexor digiti minimi brevis

Palmar and dorsal interossei (all)

Third and fourth lumbricals

Adductor pollicis

FIG. 3.17 ■ The ulna nerve. *(From Jenkins, D. (2009). Hollinshead's functional anatomy of the limbs and back (9th ed.). Philadelphia: Saunders.)*

MEDIAN NERVE

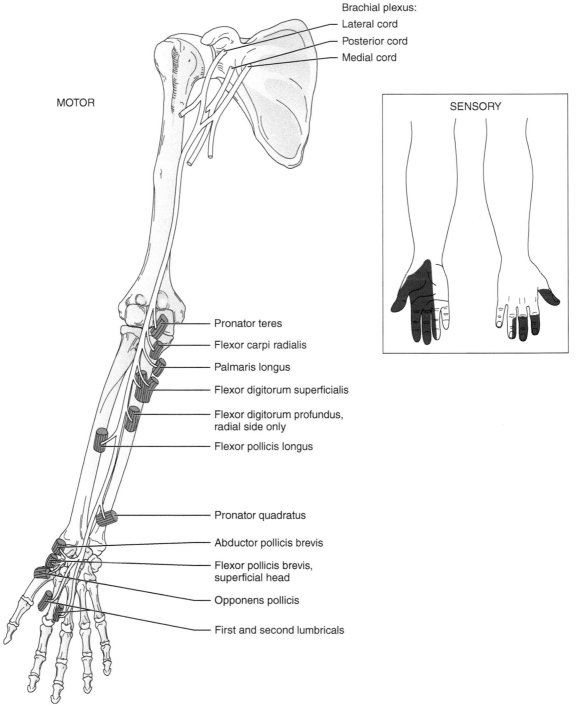

FIG. 3.18 ■ Sensation distribution of the median nerve. *(From Jenkins, D. (2009).* Hollinshead's functional anatomy of the limbs and back *(9th ed.). Philadelphia: Saunders.)*

CARDIOVASCULAR AND RESPIRATORY ANATOMY AND PHYSIOLOGY

PRACTICE STORY: LUC

Luc is a 48-year-old man who has recently experienced a myocardial infarction (MI). MI, commonly known as a heart attack, occurs when insufficient oxygen reaches cardiac muscle, leading to muscle death. A common cause of MI is coronary artery disease when the coronary arteries become blocked with atherosclerotic plaque. An MI results in symptoms of chest pain, shortness of breath and cold sweats. Risk factors of MI include smoking, diabetes and high blood pressure.

Luc was admitted into hospital complaining of chest pain, breathlessness and excessive sweating. He initially thought he was having an asthma attack because of feeling breathless as he had experienced asthma as a child. After a period in the high-dependency unit, he is now receiving cardiac rehabilitation. He finds self-care daily living tiring and finds it difficult to focus on the task in hand. He is anxious about returning to work and coping with his young family.

Respiration

The Trachea

The trachea or windpipe extends from the larynx to the point it divides into the right and left primary bronchi. The walls of this structure are made up of smooth muscle and elastic connective tissue. It is supported by a series of incomplete hyaline cartilage rings, which give support but can allow it to expand during swallowing. The lining is made from ciliated columnar cells and goblet cells that offer protection from dust and debris.

The Bronchi

The primary bronchi start where the trachea divides. The right bronchus is wider and shorter and lies in a vertical position. As it enters the lungs it divides into the three secondary bronchi. The left bronchus is narrower and enters the left lung at a more acute angle before dividing into the two secondary bronchus. As a result, any foreign object that enters the airways often becomes trapped within the bronchi. The bronchi are composed of the same tissues as the trachea. Each of these secondary bronchi then subdivide into progressively smaller structures, the bronchioles and alveoli.

The bronchioles resemble a tree trunk with branches and are commonly called the 'bronchial tree'. During an asthma attack, the smooth muscle in the bronchioles goes into spasm, and this can close off the air passages and leads to the feeling of breathlessness.

The rings of cartilage seen in the trachea and the bronchus finally disappear and are replaced with smooth muscle. These bronchioles finally lead to the alveoli, tiny structures composed of flattened epithelial cells where the interchange of gases take place.

The Lungs

The lungs are spongy balloonlike structures where gaseous exchange takes place. They are contained within pleural membrane that protects each lung. This pleural membrane forms two layers; the visceral pleura is adherent to the lung and the parietal pleura is adherent to the chest wall and the surface of the diaphragm. Between the layers of the pleura is a lubricating fluid that prevents friction and allows movement during breathing. The lungs extend from the diaphragm to just above the clavicles. Blood vessels, bronchi and nerves are held together by the pleura and form the root of the lung. The right lung is shorter and broader than the left because the diaphragm is higher on the right to accommodate the liver, which lies below it. Each lung is divided into lobes by fissures, three lobes on the right and two lobes on the left. Each lobe has its own secondary bronchus. Therefore the right lung has three secondary bronchi (superior, middle and inferior) and the left lung has two secondary bronchi (superior and inferior) (Fig. 3.19).

APPLICATION TO LUC

As Luc's heart is not pumping effectively, pressure has built up within his lungs and within the chambers of his heart. This has contributed to the sensation of breathlessness that he experiences.

Gaseous Exchange

The blood supply to the lungs is supplied via the pulmonary artery, which supplies deoxygenated blood to the lungs. These blood vessels divide down to form a dense capillary network in the walls of the alveoli. Oxygenated blood leaves the lungs via the pulmonary vein to travel to the left atrium of the heart.

Air entering the lungs has a higher concentration of oxygen than in the blood. As it passes through the respiratory airways it becomes saturated with water vapour from the moist linings of the airways, which causes the pressure to fall to 150 mm Hg. Once this air reaches the alveoli it mixes with carbon dioxide remaining as a result of diffusion from the blood to create a concentration gradient. This allows diffusion of oxygen from the alveoli into the blood in the capillaries, which then leaves the pulmonary circulation to be replaced with deoxygenated blood from the heart. The carbon dioxide in blood from the heart is about 46 mm Hg and creates a diffusion gradient between the capillaries and the alveoli. This allows the carbon dioxide in the blood to enter the alveoli, where it will be removed from the lungs during expiration.

Breathing depends on contraction and relaxation of the respiratory muscles. Inspiration is initiated by nerve impulses from the respiratory centre in the brainstem. This system is controlled by three elements. Sensors called chemoreceptors monitor changes in the blood gas composition. The central controller located in the pons and medulla integrates and coordinates this information and adjusts respiratory behaviour in

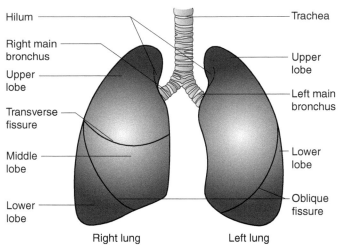

Hilum

Right main
bronchus

Upper
lobe

Transverse
fissure

Middle
lobe

Lower
lobe

Trachea

Upper
lobe

Left main
bronchus

Lower
lobe

Oblique
fissure

Right lung   Left lung

FIG. 3.19 ■ The lungs. *(From Stables, D., & Rankin, J. (2010). Physiology in childbearing (3rd ed.). Kent: Baillière Tindall.)*

response to this. The effectors are the muscles that produce changes in respiration.

APPLICATION TO LUC

Heart problems can affect the normal functioning of the lungs. Poor heart function will result in oxygen not reaching the rest of the body. Breathing will become rapid in an attempt to clear the carbon dioxide. Luc was complaining of breathlessness before his MI, which is probably partly related to the damage to his heart from coronary artery disease. At first Luc believed he was breathless because he was unfit.

The Heart and Circulatory System

Heart

The heart is at the centre of the cardiovascular system and maintains the circulation of blood through the body. It is a muscular organ that sits in the thoracic cavity lying obliquely a little to the left. It is made up of three layers of tissue: the pericardium, the myocardium and the endocardium. The pericardium is made up of two sacs: the outer sac is a tough protective membrane adherent to the diaphragm and prevents overdistension of the heart; the inner sac is adherent to the heart muscle and secretes serous fluid into the space between the layers of the pericardium. This allows for smooth movement between heartbeats. The myocardium is made up of cardiac muscle. Cardiac muscle is composed of cells and branches that connect closely with other adjacent cells. Consequently, this gives the muscle the appearance of a sheet rather than a number of individual cells. This means the cells do not need an individual nerve supply as the impulse of contraction spreads across the whole sheet. The endocardium forms a lining consisting of flattened epithelial cells continuous with the lining of blood vessels. The blood supply to the heart is

via the right and left coronary arteries, which arise from the aorta. Venous return is via the coronary sinus, which empties into the right atrium.

The heart is made up of four chambers which are divided in the middle by a muscular structure called the septum. The chambers are divided into upper and lower chambers, which are accessed by valves. The upper chambers are the left and right atrium and the lower chambers are the left and right ventricles. Oxygenated blood enters the left atrium of the heart from the pulmonary veins from the lungs. It passes through the left atrioventricular valve (bicuspid or mitral valve) into the left ventricle. From here, it then passes via the aortic valve into the aorta and from there it is pumped around the rest of the body. Deoxygenated blood returning from the body enters the right aorta of the heart via the inferior and superior vena cava. It passes into the right ventricle via the right atrioventricular valve (tricuspid valve), then through the pulmonary valve into the pulmonary artery. This artery takes the deoxygenated blood to the lungs (Fig. 3.20).

APPLICATION TO LUC

Myocardial infarct occurs as a result of faulty coronary circulation. The reduced oxygen supply leads to ischaemia of the cells, which produces pain (angina). Nitro-glycerine dilates the coronary vessels and improves the circulation and thereby reduces the pain. Luc has been given nitro-glycerine spray, which he uses before he takes part in physical activity. This helps him manage his chest pain but it can make him feel dizzy.

Cardiac Cycle

The contraction of the heart is initiated by an intrinsic system without the need of a nerve supply from the brain. Within the myocardium there are small groups of specialised cells that

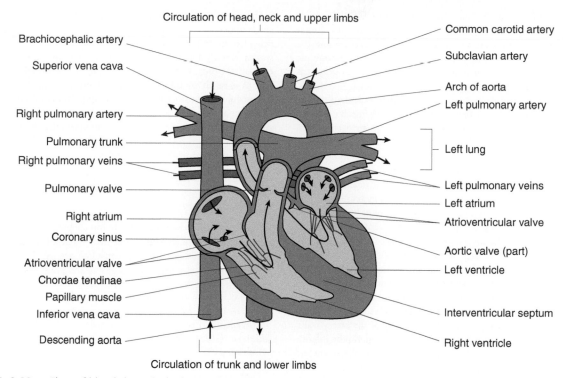

Circulation of head, neck and upper limbs

Brachiocephalic artery

Superior vena cava

Right pulmonary artery

Pulmonary trunk

Right pulmonary veins

Pulmonary valve

Right atrium

Coronary sinus

Atrioventricular valve

Chordae tendinae

Papillary muscle

Inferior vena cava

Descending aorta

Common carotid artery

Subclavian artery

Arch of aorta

Left pulmonary artery

Left lung

Left pulmonary veins

Left atrium

Atrioventricular valve

Aortic valve (part)

Left ventricle

Interventricular septum

Right ventricle

Circulation of trunk and lower limbs

FIG. 3.20 ▪ Flow of blood through the heart. *(From Watson, R. (2011). Anatomy and physiology for nurses (13th ed.). Kent: Baillière Tindall.)*

initiate and conduct a contraction of the heart muscle. This allows the two atria to contract at the same time while the ventricles relax; then, when the two ventricles contract, the two atrium relax. This is called a cardiac cycle. The sinoatrial (SA) node, located in the top right-hand corner of the heart near the opening of the superior vena cava, initiates this contraction in the myocardium. For this reason it is referred to as the 'pacemaker'. This causes the myocardium of the atrium to contract, pushing the blood down into the ventricles. The atrioventricular (AV) node located in the atrioventricular valves is stimulated by this contract from the SA node but can also initiate contraction. The atrioventricular bundle, also called the bundle of His, is located in the septum and contains fibres from the AV node. This bundle separates into two branches and travels down to each ventricle. These branches convey the contraction from the AV node to the myocardium of the ventricles, so causing them to contract to push the blood out through the pulmonary artery on the right and the aorta on the left.

The sounds that can be heard relate to the opening and closing of the values during the process described earlier. The *lubb* sound is created by the closure of the atrioventricular valves after contraction of the atrium; the second *dupp* sound is created when the aortic and pulmonary valves (semilunar valves) close after the ventricular contraction.

The heart rate can be affected by many factors. For example, strong emotions such as fear, anger, stress and anxiety can increase heart rate. Depression and grief tend to decrease heart rate.

APPLICATION TO LUC

Strong emotions such as fear, anger, stress and anxiety can increase adrenalin production, which in turn can increase heart rate. Depression and grief tend to decrease heart rate. Luc may feel anxious as a result of his heart attack. This may cause symptoms such as increased heart rate, which Luc may believe is another heart attack. Luc may also be reluctant to engage in rehabilitation as he may feel this 'works his heart too hard'. This fear may increase his heart rate and perpetuate his belief that rehabilitation is working him too hard.

Arteries and Veins

Arteries and veins make up the network that carries blood to and from the body. Arteries are thicker and stronger than veins and the pressure within arteries is always higher than the pressure in veins. Arteries have the properties of elasticity and contractibility. When the ventricles contract and force blood into the arteries, they expand; then, as the ventricles relax, the arteries recoil, forcing the blood forward. This contractibility comes from the smooth muscle that is arranged in rings around the artery. This smooth muscle is also influenced by the autonomic nervous system, so when the sympathetic nervous system is activated, the muscle constricts (vasoconstriction).

Veins have less elastic tissue and smooth muscle than arteries and as a result of this there is lower pressure in veins. Blood from a cut vein tends to flow rather than blood from an artery, which tends to spurt in rapid bursts. As the pressure in veins is low, veins also contain valves to prevent backflow of blood.

Blood pressure is the pressure that the blood exerts on the vessel in which it is contained. When the ventricle contracts it pushes blood into an already full artery, this increased pressure on the artery wall is known as systolic blood pressure. In an adult this is about 120 mm Hg. As the ventricles relax, the pressure within the artery drops. This is known as diastolic blood pressure. In the adult this is around 80 mm Hg. These figures can vary based on age, time of day and posture. Normal blood pressure is dependent on the amount of blood ejected from the heart (cardiac output), the amount of blood in circulation (blood volume), vasomotor activity on the smaller blood vessels (peripheral resistance), the elasticity of the artery walls, and the amount of blood returning to the heart via the inferior and superior vena cava. The pulse is this wave of distension and elongation felt along the artery wall.

APPLICATION TO LUC

Luc has his blood pressure taken while in hospital. His blood pressure is recorded as 138/90 mm Hg. Both the top reading (systolic) and bottom reading (diastolic) in adults between 40 and 69 years of age is important as every 20 mm Hg increase in systolic or 10 mm Hg in diastolic blood pressure doubles the risk of death from coronary artery disease.

Luc has been advised to lose weight, increase his physical activity, reduce his salt intake and moderate his alcohol intake. He has also been prescribed antihypertensive medication which he will need to take for the rest of his life.

CONCLUSION

A brief overview of neurological, musculoskeletal, cardiovascular and respiratory anatomy and physiology has been provided in this chapter. To illustrate the relevance of occupational therapists understanding anatomy and physiology, the information provided in this chapter has been related to three practice stories. Having a sound underpinning of anatomy and physiology assists occupational therapists in their professional reasoning, as a result of understanding the process and impact of illness, injury or impairment and the impact a condition may have on a person's occupational performance. Readers are encouraged to further develop this understanding by referring to texts devoted to the study of this field. A number of suitable texts are included in the bibliography.

 http://evolve.elsevier.com/Curtin/OT

BIBLIOGRAPHY

References have not been included in this chapter as a number of different texts were consulted and their inclusion would have distracted the reader. The texts consulted are listed below in the bibliography as a list of key anatomy and physiology books which will support your learning.

Cooper, C. (2013). *Fundamentals of hand therapy: Clinical reasoning and treatment guidelines for common diagnoses of the upper extremity* (2nd ed.). Philadelphia: Elsevier.

Gillen, G. (2015). *Stroke rehabilitation: A function-based approach* (4th ed.). Philadelphia: Elsevier.

Greene, D. P., & Roberts, S. L. (2016). *Kinesiology* (3rd ed.). Philadelphia: Elsevier.

Grieve, J., & Gnanasekaran, L. (2008). *Neuropsychology for occupational therapists.* Oxford: Blackwell Publishing.

McBean, D., & van Wijck, F. (2013). *Applied neurosciences for the allied health professions.* London: Churchill Livingstone.

McMillan, I., & Carin-Levy, G. (2013). *Tyldesley and Grieve's muscles, nerves and movement in human occupation.* Oxford: Wiley.

Palastanga, N., & Soames, R. W. (2012). *Anatomy and human movement* (6th ed.). Philadelphia: Elsevier.

Saladin, K. (2012). *Anatomy and physiology: The unity of form and function* (6th ed.). New York: McGraw-Hill.

Saunders, R., Astifidis, R., Burke, S. L., Higgins, J., & McClinton, M. A. (2015). *Hand and upper extremity rehabilitation* (4th ed.). Philadelphia: Elsevier.

Stone, A. J., & Stone, R. J. (2011). *Atlas of skeletal muscles* (7th ed.). New York: McGraw-Hill.

Tortora, G. J., & Derrickson, B. H. (2014). *Principles of anatomy and physiology* (14th ed.). Chichester: Wiley.

4 SOCIAL SCIENCES

JUDITH PETTIGREW ■ KATIE ROBINSON

CHAPTER OUTLINE

Abstract

The social sciences have had an enduring influence on the theory and practice of occupational therapy. The broad family of disciplines described as the social sciences include psychology, anthropology and sociology. These disciplines have had a significant impact on the development of occupational therapy theory, practice and research. In addition, two interdisciplinary fields within the social sciences, disability and gender studies, have influenced the development of the occupational therapy profession. This chapter provides an appreciation of the importance of studying, understanding and applying social science principles and concepts to occupational therapy.

KEY POINTS

- The social sciences were instrumental at the inception of the profession of occupational therapy.

- Positive psychology offers concepts to understand the experiences of people with an illness, injury or impairment who are resilient and grow and flourish in response to challenges.

- Humanistic psychology has influenced occupational therapy values and the concept of the therapeutic relationship.

- The sociology of health and illness enables occupational therapists to critically consider health, illness and the human body.

- The key anthropological concept of culture and the anthropological research method of ethnography have influenced the theory and practice of occupational therapy.

- A phenomenological way of thinking has been identified in studies on the professional reasoning of occupational therapists. Phenomenology focuses on individuals and values each individual's experience.

- Disability studies have provided useful critiques of the disabling attitudes and beliefs of health professionals, and these critical perspectives are valuable for occupational therapists to reflect on.

- Feminism refers to a range of approaches and activities that are broadly concerned with drawing attention to women's position in society. The critical perspective of feminism could enable occupational therapists to consider issues such as their gendered role in the reproduction of power relations in interactions with service users.

INTRODUCTION

The focus of this chapter is on illustrating the relevance of knowledge generated from the disciplines of sociology, psychology and anthropology. These disciplines are collectively referred to as social sciences. Although there is no standard definition of the 'social sciences', this group of sciences are a family of disciplines that began to take shape in the late nineteenth century. It is acknowledged that many terms and categorisations within the social sciences are contested and debated and to some extent the boundaries between disciplines are artificial. Approaches, methods and theories are shared across multiple disciplines. A common feature among each of the sciences in this group is a focus on dynamic and ever-changing social phenomena and relations (Calhoun, 2002).

The social sciences have been instrumental since the inception of the profession of occupational therapy. Moral treatment was an approach to working with people who had a mental illness and had been admitted to institutions that emerged at the turn of the nineteenth century based on humane psychosocial care and the provision of work and other activities (Prendiville & Pettigrew, 2015). Moral treatment was an expression of humanistic values predating the formal field of humanistic psychology (Cara & MacRae, 2012). The expression of humanistic values of the moral treatment movement marked the emergence of occupation as a treatment for people who had a mental illness (Wilcock, 2001) and ultimately created the conditions for the development of occupational therapy (Prendiville & Pettigrew, 2015).

Perspectives from the social sciences have allowed occupational therapists to respond to the many ethical and moral dilemmas experienced by the profession, drawing on critical and constructive perspectives. For example, an ongoing struggle between holism and reductionism (Kielhofner, 1997) and balancing the art and science of intervention (Schemm, 1994) are two dilemmas that have been discussed and debated using social science principles and perspectives. The depth or level of engagement with social science knowledge within the occupational therapy profession has been variable and a linear relationship certainly does not exist.

The review of the social sciences in this chapter is limited in scope, and the explanations of each of the disciplines will be brief as the focus is on providing an overview rather than a detailed explanation. The areas and topics presented have been selected based on what is relevant to occupational therapy students or practitioners in the early stages of their careers. After the explanation of the three social sciences, a further two interdisciplinary fields of study are presented: disability and gender studies. Each field is illustrated by a small number of research projects relevant to practice. This is to demonstrate the impact social science has on the profession and how principles from the different social sciences can underpin many of the research approaches that influence the continual evolution of occupational therapy. It is anticipated that by reading this chapter students will appreciate the importance of studying, understanding and applying what they learn from the different social science disciplines.

PSYCHOLOGY

Psychology has had a profound impact on occupational therapy. Psychological theories are central to the philosophical foundations of the profession and are evident in conceptual models developed for the profession. Psychology is defined as 'the study of the mind and behaviour. The discipline embraces all aspects of the human experience — from the functions of the brain to the actions of nations, from child development to care for the aged. In every conceivable setting from scientific research centres to mental healthcare services, "the understanding of behaviour" is the enterprise of psychologists' (American Psychological Association, 2015a). The field of psychology is vast with multiple subdisciplines. However, for the purposes of this chapter only the fields of humanistic psychology and positive psychology will be explored. Although the focus is on these two fields, it should be noted that there are many other psychology fields relevant to the occupational therapy profession such as cognitive, social, personality and occupational psychology.

Humanistic Psychology

Humanistic psychology emphasises the study of the whole person; humanism is central to the philosophical core of the profession of occupational therapy (Finlay, 2001). 'Humanistic psychology aims to be faithful to the full range of human experience. Its foundations include philosophical humanism, existentialism and phenomenology. In the science and profession of psychology, humanistic psychology seeks to develop systematic and rigorous methods of studying human beings, and to heal the fragmentary character of contemporary psychology through an ever more comprehensive and integrative approach. Humanistic psychologists are particularly sensitive to uniquely human dimensions, such as experiences of creativity and transcendence, and to the quality of human welfare' (American Psychological Association, 2015b).

As described earlier, the roots of occupational therapy can be traced to the philosophical movement of Moral Treatment (Barker Schwartz, 2003), which predated humanistic psychology (Cara & MacRae, 2012). The holistic and humanistic philosophy of Moral Treatment (Barker Schwartz, 2013) has had a profound influence on the philosophy and enduring values of occupational therapy. In the late 1950s and early 1960s humanistic psychology emerged as a reaction to the dominant psychological theories of the time: psychoanalysis and behaviourism. The humanistic movement championed qualitative inquiry and added a holistic dimension to psychology (Seligman & Csikszentmihalyi, 2000). Abraham Maslow (1908–70) was a key figure in the origin and evolution of this approach. Maslow's major contribution was his work on self-actualisation and needs.

Finlay (1997) described occupational therapy as imbued with humanistic understandings and approaches and identified three key areas of influence: humanistic values, the therapeutic relationship and the use of activities for healing purposes. Yerxa also described the humanistic values underpinning occupational therapy. These include optimism, holism and shared view of people as active and autonomous and having a right to life satisfaction (Yerxa, 1983). The American Occupational Therapy Association core values clearly reflect humanistic ideals of altruism, equality, freedom, justice, dignity, truth and prudence (AOTA, 1993). The following description of the core value of dignity clearly articulates a humanistic perspective: 'We view human beings holistically, respecting the unique interaction of the mind, body, and physical and social environment. We believe that dignity is nurtured and grows from the sense of competence and self-worth that is integrally linked to the person's ability to performed valued and relevant activities' (AOTA, 1993, p. 1086). Although holism is widely cited in discussions on occupational therapy philosophy, evidence suggests that therapists may struggle to enact holism in practice (Finlay, 2001). The tensions between holistic values and the often reductionist focus of the work of occupational therapists working in acute physical settings has been identified (Robertson & Finlay, 2007). A study on New Zealander occupational therapy practice in acute physical care also highlighted ambiguity between stated values of holism and actual practice (Blaga & Robertson, 2008).

Humanistic psychotherapy is described as an 'enterprise through which both therapist and client strive to marshal their differing emotional heritages in order to better connect with their common humanity' (Stern, 2014, p. xii). A range of therapeutic approaches have been developed within humanistic psychology; for example, existential psychotherapy aims to address existential anxiety that arises when people face the givens of existence – mortality, isolation, meaninglessness and freedom (Yalom, 1980). Humanistic therapies stress the importance of the service user–therapist relationship and emphasise understanding the phenomenological experience of the present moment (Waterman, 2013). These therapeutic approaches accentuate a process of meaning making in response to existential isolation and meaninglessness (Waterman, 2013). Humanistic psychology's influence is also evident in the emphasis occupational therapy places on the need for people to exercise choice, responsibility and sense of agency (Ikiugu & Ciaravino, 2007).

The humanistic therapy that has had the most profound influence on occupational therapy is client-centred therapy developed by Carl Rogers (1951). Rogerian client-centred therapy is nondirective and necessitates the development of a therapeutic relationship. In his seminal text *On Becoming a Person: A Therapist's View of Psychotherapy*, Rogers (1961) outlines significant learnings distilled from his experience as a therapist. These illustrate the central tenets of a client-centred therapeutic relationship: unconditional positive regard for the person, empathy and congruence. In communicating some of these values Rodgers stated, 'In my relationships with persons I have found that it does not help, in the long run, to act as though I were something I am not' (p. 16) and '[t]he more I am open to the realities in me and in the other person, the less do I find myself wishing to rush in to "fix things" ' (p. 21).

The therapeutic relationship has been defined as 'A trusting connection and rapport established between therapist and client through collaboration, communication, therapist empathy, and mutual respect' (Cole & McLean, 2003, p. 49). A national survey of American occupational therapists (n=568) found that, although the majority highly valued the therapeutic relationship and therapeutic use of self, they felt inadequately trained and that the field lacks sufficient knowledge in these areas (Taylor, Lee, Kielhofner, & Ketkar, 2009). A mixed methods case study of the relationship of four therapeutic dyads (i.e. therapist–person receiving therapy services) identified elements that shaped the process of relationship development, including the fostering of an interpersonal connection, a shared sense of success and a positive feedback mechanism created through successfully attaining clearly delineated person-centred therapy goals (Morrison & Smith, 2013). A study of expert occupational therapists working with people with acquired brain injury identified the importance of conscious self-awareness and use of personal characteristics as factors consistent with the concept of therapeutic use of self (Holmqvist, Holmefur, & Ivarsson, 2013). Abreu (2011), in her Eleanor Clarke Slagle lecture, discussed how affirmations of empathetic care and humanistic practice with a focus on emotion, optimism and a person's strengths are present in a range of occupational therapy literature.

Positive Psychology

Positive psychology is a branch of psychology that emerged in the late 1990s and in the intervening years has seen rapid growth and received continuing interest (Donaldson, Dollwet, & Rao, 2015). The movement has developed in response to the almost exclusive focus of psychology on human pathology. Positive psychology is defined as 'the study of the conditions and processes that contribute to the flourishing or optimal functioning of people, groups, and institutions' (Gable & Haidt, 2005, p.104).

In a seminal paper on the development of positive psychology Seligman and Csikszentmihalyi offered the following definition:

The field of positive psychology at the subjective level is about valued subjective experience: well-being, contentment, and satisfaction (past), hope and optimism (future), and flow and happiness (present). At the individual level it is about positive individual traits – the capacity for love and vocation, courage, interpersonal skill, aesthetic sensibility, perseverance, forgiveness, originality, future-mindedness, spirituality, high talent, and wisdom. At the group level it is about the civic virtues and the institutions that move individuals toward better citizenship: responsibility, nurturance, altruism, civility, moderation, tolerance, and work ethic'.

(Seligman & Csikszentmihalyi, 2000, p. 5)

Positive psychology interventions are oriented towards promoting well-being, including happiness, subjective well-being and mindfulness. Most positive psychology interventions are short-term, exercise-oriented and pragmatic, focusing on what can be done in the here and now to improve well-being (Waterman, 2013). In contrast with other branches of psychology there is not an extensive focus on the person–therapist relationship (Waterman, 2013). Typical interventions include practicing kindness, counting your blessings, gratitude exercises, hopeful thinking and strength exercises. Meta-analyses have shown that positive psychology interventions significantly enhance subjective and psychological well-being and reduce depressive symptoms (Bolier et al., 2013; Sin & Lyubomirsky, 2009). A small number of concepts developed within the field of positive psychology have had an impact on occupational therapy practice including flow theory and mindfulness (Emerson, 1998; Reid, 2011; Robinson, Kennedy, & Harmon, 2012; Wright, Sadlo, & Stew, 2007). Positive psychology constructs that have been identified as relevant to rehabilitation practitioners include optimism, hope, benefit-finding, meaning-making, posttraumatic growth and resilience (Martz & Livneh, 2015). A highly relevant area of positive psychology for occupational therapists is research concerning resilience in the face of, and positive growth after, illness, injury or impairment. A chapter by Dunn, Uswatte, and Elliott (2009) describes the experiences of people with acquired physical impairments who exhibit positive reactions to living with their impairment.

Resilience is a multidimensional construct that seeks to explain the process of positive adaptation despite adversity and has been defined as 'the potential to exhibit resourcefulness by using available internal and external recourses in response to different contextual and developmental challenges' (Pooley & Cohen, 2010, p. 30). The salience and potential of the construct of resilience to the rehabilitation of people who have faced traumatic injury has been identified and discussed (White, Driver, & Warren, 2008). A number of studies have demonstrated high rates of resilience in people with illness, injury or impairment. A study of the prevalence of resilience, recovery and distress trajectories in individuals with a severe injury during inpatient rehabilitation (n = 80) found the most common trajectory of adaptation was the resilience trajectory (54%). This trajectory was characterised by low levels of psychological distress (posttraumatic stress disorder, depression, anxiety and state negative affect) and high state positive affect (Quale & Schanke, 2010). A study of 88 adults with spinal cord injury admitted over almost 3 years into three rehabilitation units in Sydney, Australia, found almost 70% of the participants were classified as resilient at discharge, with 66% of participants classified as resilient after 6 months of living in the community (Guest, Craig, Tran, & Milddleton, 2015).

Resilience is increasingly being investigated as a protective factor that supports optimal functioning in people aging with illness, injury or impairment. A survey of a convenience sample of community-dwelling individuals with multiple sclerosis, muscular dystrophy, postpoliomyelitis syndrome or spinal cord injury (n = 1594; age range, 20–94 years) found that resilience was positively correlated with social and physical functioning ($r = .49$ and $r = .17$, respectively) (Silverman, Molton, Alschuler, Ehde, & Jensen, 2015).

Critical perspectives have brought attention to the need for care in the application of the concept of resilience and critical reflection on underlying values and assumptions. The application of the concept of resilience to understand outcomes may potentially disenfranchise the individual (Martin, 2015). A number of authors have identified that positive outcomes and success differ between groups and this may not be acknowledged in the application of the concept of resilience (Cooper & Boyden, 2007; Mohaupt, 2009). The very real risk of inadvertently blaming the victim for poor outcomes exists with unquestioned use of the concept of resilience (Masten & Obradović, 2006). Another critique centred on the lack of attention to older adults in resilience research. The focus of much resilience research has been on children and adolescents and there have been calls for greater consideration of the dynamics of resilience across the lifespan, for example, its role in healthy ageing (Windle, 2011).

Phenomenology

As a discipline, phenomenology can be defined as the study of the structures of experience, based on the premise that people can only know and understand the world on the basis of what they experience. The historical movement of phenomenology was launched in the first half of the twentieth century. Although Edmund Husserl (1859–1938) is widely regarded as the founding 'father', other key thinkers include Martin Heidegger, Maurice Merleau-Ponty and Jean-Paul Sartre who, among others, played a significant role in the development of this discipline. Phenomenology is both a disciplinary field and a movement in philosophy.

In common with other health disciplines, occupational therapy has become increasingly influenced by phenomenology, focusing as it does on individuals and valuing each person's experience. Interpretative phenomenology, which emphasises everyday life experiences, can inform how occupational therapists think about engaging in dialogue with the people they work with. According to Wright-St Clair and Smythe (2012, p. 35), '[Interpretive phenomenology] is a way of fully "listening" for that which is hidden from the outside [...] [implying that] practitioners who listen in different ways, beyond the self-evident and the taken for granted, will have richer understandings to call on when making inferences and decisions'.

As noted by Finlay (1999), the interest in phenomenology in occupational therapy was influenced by the clinical reasoning study undertaken in the United States of America by Mattingly and Fleming (1994). This study drew attention to the phenomenological way of thinking that underpinned occupational therapists' practice. Numerous occupational therapy studies drew on the phenomenological approach as a way of investigating the impact of people's experiences on practice. Hasselkus and Dickie (1994) used phenomenology to gain an understanding of the experience of doing occupational therapy. Rosa and Hasselkus (1996) examined the therapist–person relationship and demonstrated the importance of 'connecting', 'helping' and 'working together'. Finlay (1997) discussed how occupational therapists experienced the people who received their services as 'good', 'bad' and 'difficult' and demonstrated that some level of social evaluation of people was unavoidable even though therapists strove to be nonjudgemental. Eriksson and Tham (2010) identified how occupational gaps were characterised in people's lived experiences of performing everyday occupations during the first year after having a cerebrovascular accident (CVA). Laliberte Rudman, Huot, Klinger, Leipert, & Spafford (2010) used phenomenology to describe the core aspects of living with low vision in later life among older adults who had not accessed low vision rehabilitation services. The essence of the experience was identified as struggling to maintain valued and essential occupations while dealing with risk.

SOCIOLOGY

Sociology aims to understand the place of the individual within society and society's effect on the individual. A basic premise of sociology is that what an individual thinks and does is influenced by groups, organisations, cultures, societies and the world (Ritzer, 2015). Adopting a sociological perspective or 'the sociological imagination' has been described as a means to take a broad questioning view that interrogates familiar understandings and commonly accepted truths (McDonald, 2004). 'Using the sociological perspective amounts to seeing the strange in the familiar' (Macionis & Plummer, 2015, p. 5). The unique perspective of sociology has enriched occupational therapy scholarship.

The sociology of health and illness is a subdiscipline within sociology that has enabled critical consideration of health, illness and the human body. The sociology of health and illness is widely accepted as a body of knowledge that can be usefully applied by occupational therapists in practice (Jones, Sheena, & Hartery, 1998). For example, a central focus of the sociology of health and illness has been consideration and critique of the dominant paradigm of Western medicine, biomedicine, a critique that resonates with the holistic philosophy underpinning occupational therapy practice. Research within this subfield spans a range of topics that are highly relevant to occupational therapy, including the social determinants of health and illness, the experience of health and illness, health provider and health service recipient interactions and the social organisation of health care (Hyde, McDonnell, & Lohan, 2004).

The sociology of health and illness has made a major contribution to understanding the experience of illness, injury and impairment. Two major perspectives have dominated research in this area: functional and interpretative approaches. Functional approaches focus on the extent to which illness influences social roles, in particular the sick role. In contrast, interpretative approaches seek to explore how the individual makes sense of their illness (Nettleton, 2006). Parsons' 'sick role' (1951) typifies the functional approach. The 'sick role' as described by Parsons prescribes a set of obligations and responsibilities and, also, rights for a sick person. For example, a person who is sick is freed from responsibilities such as work, but is required to cooperate with medical treatment. Research on the 'sick role' has led to detailed exploration of access to and legitimation of the sick role. The 'sick role' has been problematised in terms of its application to the experience of those living with chronic illnesses where recovery and resumption of responsibilities may not occur (Varul, 2010).

Interpretative approaches within the sociology of health and illness have utilised concepts such as illness narratives, biographical disruption, stigma and coping to illuminate the experience of people who are ill. Pierret (2003) reviewed publications in the sociology of health and illness and grouped them into three thematic areas: subjectivity, coping actions and strategies for managing everyday life and the social structure. Concepts developed from the sociology of health and illness have been enthusiastically taken up and applied in occupational therapy research and theory. In a chapter on rheumatic diseases, McArthur and Goodacre (2013) provide an excellent example of how the sociology of health and illness can enable enhanced understanding of how people make sense of living with long-term conditions. The concepts of biographical disruption and narrative reconstruction are used to excellent effect to give insight into the lived experiences of people with rheumatic disease.

Individual socioeconomic status has been shown to be closely related to mortality, self-reported health and health-related behaviour (Mackenbach et al., 2008; Laaksonen et al., 2008). Sociologists have interrogated the effects of economic integration and domestic neoliberal policies on health and health inequalities (De Vogli, Schrecker, & Labonte, 2013; Navarro, 2009). Contemporary neoliberal policies have been implicated in the weakening of organisations of the working class, the redistribution of wealth and income in favour of a small minority and the dismantling of universal welfare provision (Collins, McCartney, & Garnham, 2015). Neoliberal ideology has been implicated in a shifting of responsibility for well-being onto the individual and a move away from framing public health as a public good. These changes are evident in the increasing acceptance of the view that people are personally responsible for their health through choices they make, such as decisions to smoke, drink, exercise, etc. (Brown & Baker, 2012). The sociology of health and illness encourages a critical questioning of these neoliberal policies and politics and the resultant implications for health. Rudman (2015) provides an excellent example of the application of these perspectives from the sociology of health and illness to occupational therapy practice in her critical consideration of how the imperative to govern the aging body in ways consistent with being a 'good' neoliberal citizen is negotiated by aging individuals.

ANTHROPOLOGY

Anthropology 'tries to achieve an understanding of culture, society and humanity through detailed studies of local life, supplemented by comparison' (Erikson, 2004, p. 7). The influence of anthropology on occupational therapy is considerable as both disciplines are concerned with common aspects of human experience and share an interest in the primacy of context. Frank, Block, and Zemke, (2008, p. 2) draw attention to occupational therapy's shared interests with the subdisciplines of medical anthropology and applied anthropology in promoting health and well-being through everyday activities, meaningful routines and social participation.

These authors (Frank et al., 2008, p. 3) suggest the need for a closer alignment between anthropology and occupational therapy which could benefit both professions. As occupational therapy is increasingly engaging with issue of social and occupational justice in a global context, stronger links with anthropology can deepen occupational therapy's critical perspectives. They suggest that 'Anthropologists with their training in the analysis of cultures, institutions, power structures, and social systems will understand – perhaps more clearly than professionals in occupational therapy – how a feminist or gender analysis is needed, as well as analyses of race and class'.

Additionally, critical anthropological theories could help occupational therapy to more strongly counteract forces undermining the profession such as the marginalisation of caring work, rejection of low-cost and low-tech solutions in favour of ones producing profits, domination by biomedicine, and the reproduction of entrenched forms of social stratification and exclusion (Frank et al., 2008, p. 3).

The concept of culture illustrates one impact of anthropology on occupational therapy. An awareness of the importance of culture has long been acknowledged in occupational therapy (Mosey, 1981; Hume, 1984; Krefting, 1991). Writing in the *American Journal of Occupational Therapy* in 1985, Litterst notes that the concept of culture has been brought into occupational therapy from anthropology. However, its understanding in the occupational therapy literature has often been that of a label for ethnic identification that fails to take note of change and may create static stereotypes. Krefting, writing in the early 1990s, drew similar conclusions, noting that in occupational therapy 'culture' had usually been equated with ethnicity and race or applied to immigrant health (1991). Culture was also seen as being synonymous with a geographical region such as 'rehabilitation in India'. She referred to this approach as 'windscreen' medical anthropology in which only brief contact is made with a small segment of a health care system (Krefting, 1991, p. 7). Krefting (1991) was one of the first writers to draw

attention to the importance of therapists being aware of their own cultural background and how it influenced therapy.

In the years that followed, the literature on culture in occupational therapy grew significantly, even though there was a lack of consensus on the definition of the term (Bonder, Martin, & Miracle, 2004). Bonder et al. (2004, p. 159) argued for the incorporation of the concept of 'culture as emergent in everyday interactions of individuals [which] encourages reconsideration of the main elements of culture, that it is learned, shared, patterned, evaluative, and persistent but changeable'. This approach, they argued, suggests three important characteristics that therapists could cultivate to enhance therapy encounters: careful attention, active curiosity, and self-reflection and evaluation.

In a review article on culture and diversity in occupational therapy, Beagan (2015) identified four approaches to culture within occupational therapy. The first, the cultural competence approach, centres on awareness, knowledge and skills. Echoing earlier writers, Beagan stated that, 'At their worst, cultural competence models become a kind of "laundry list" of cultural attributes that pertain to specific ethnic groups' (2015, p. 3).

The second approach, the culturally relevant model of occupational therapy, has been championed by Michael Iwama (2003, 2005, 2006) and focuses on creating space for cultural variability. Along with others such as Hammell (2009, 2011, 2013a), Laliberte Rudman and Dennhardt (2008), and Nelson (2007), Iwama further developed the idea that the profession is not culture neutral. Instead it was closely aligned with Western middle-class cultural values, beliefs, and assumptions. As Beagan (2015) points out, this perspective enabled recognition of cultural biases and assumptions within occupational therapy.

The third approach, cultural safety, is most commonly seen in the literature from New Zealand, Australia and Canada (Beagan, 2015). Cultural safety recognises that power and authority are embedded in the policies, practices and everyday procedures of heath care and emphasises the need for practitioners to critically reflect on their own values along with their personal, cultural and colonial backgrounds (Gerlach, 2012; Gray & McPherson, 2005; Thomas, Gray, & McGinty, 2011). The cultural safety approach is orientated mainly toward health equity and social justice (Jull & Giles, 2012) but provides little practical guidance for therapists (Beagan, 2015).

The fourth approach, cultural humility, was named by Tervalon and Murray-García (1998) and was first introduced into occupational therapy by Beagan and Chacala (2012) who coupled it with critical reflexivity. The concept has been championed by Hammell (2013), who writes, 'Cultural humility challenges occupational therapists to recognise the ways in which their own perspectives may differ from those of others and to acknowledge the advantages that derive from their own professional and social positions' (p. 5).

Ethnography

Ethnography is a research methodology most commonly associated with anthropology, in which the focus is on the recording and analysis of social practices inherent in a culture or society. The primary methods of gathering information when using ethnography are prolonged engagement with people within the group being researched, participant observation and interviews. As it is based in naturalistic settings it can provide detailed insights into how people construct their lives within their social contexts. 'Ethnography is particularly well suited to studying occupation focusing on everyday lived experiences and the contexts within which these are embedded' (Huot, 2015, p. 84).

Like other health care professions – especially nursing – seeking to consider experience and meaning, occupational therapy turned to qualitative research methods, including ethnography, in the early to mid-1980s. In 1985 Litterst noted that the incorporation of information from anthropology into the knowledge base of occupational therapy included fieldwork methods and culture. In 1989 Krefting coined the phrase *disability ethnography* and made a strong case for why occupational therapists should use ethnography. In 1993 Spencer et al. examined the usefulness of using ethnographic methods in assessing the functioning of people receiving occupational therapy services in the daily life domain and concluded by outlining the steps of an ethnographic assessment process. They also contrasted what they called *traditional ethnography* (a large-scale study of a designated culture most commonly carried by out by anthropologists or sociologists) with *focused ethnography* (a small-scale study concentrating on a specific area of inquiry). For example, in occupational therapy, the focus might be on a specific issue, such as the concern of mothers of children receiving intervention for obesity, or people with chronic neurological conditions who are participating in a return to work programme.

Ethnography is widely used in occupational therapy, and the results of ethnography studies have had significant effects on the profession. For example, Townsend (1996) used institutional ethnography to show how organisational context constrains the empowerment of adults with mental health illness and shaped occupational therapy practice. Through the use of ethnography Dickie (2003) identified that socially situated learning was one of the central activities of quilt makers and quilt guilds.

Inspired by institutional ethnography, Prodinger, Shaw, Rudman, and Townsend, (2012) explored the work of occupational therapists in an outpatient rheumatology setting and demonstrated that the practice of occupational therapy is ruled by a body-focused medical discourse. Huot, Laliberte Rudman, Dodson, and Magalhães, (2013) used critical ethnography to understand the integration experiences of French-speaking immigrants from visible minorities living in predominantly Anglophone Canada. An ethnographic approach allowed the experiences of women with an illness, injury or impairment living in a nursing home to be illuminated. The research highlighted that nursing homes were living situations of last resort for these women (Magasi & Hammel, 2009). Taking the emphasis on everyday occupations to anthropology, Pettigrew (2013) used ethnography to focus on the challenges to daily life activities experienced by the inhabitants of a Himalayan village in Nepal during the civil war.

Ethnographic approaches are continually developing and this has provided those who study groups and cultures with a range of new and interesting research opportunities. For example, the emergence of digital anthropology has enabled the study of the adoption of digital technologies. For occupational therapists, the methods used in ethnography provide avenues through which to explore the cultural nature of occupations and the manner in which they are embedded in social context.

Narrative Approaches

Although the narrative case history method was initially widely used in early occupational therapy to demonstrate the effectiveness of interventions, this approach became less commonly used in the 1920s when the paradigm of occupation was replaced by the scientific paradigm (Frank, 1996; Kielhofner & Burke, 1977). Case histories were subsequently short and tightly focused on a clinical problem.

With the widespread emergence in the 1980s and 1990s of narrative approaches in disciplines such as anthropology, sociology, history, counselling and psychotherapy, they once again became common in occupational therapy. Illness narratives allowed individuals to make sense of and explain their illness to others. People's stories provided significant information about what they cared about and what mattered in their lives. The work of medical anthropologists, such as Arthur Kleinman (1988), was significant in the focus on illness narratives. Research informed by a narrative approach gives occupational therapists a deeper appreciation of the meaning in people's lives as they go about their occupations in everyday life (Bonsall, 2012).

In 1986 the American Occupational Therapy Foundation initiated and funded the Boston Clinical Reasoning Study. The study was an interdisciplinary collaboration between anthropologist Cheryl Mattingly and occupational therapists Maureen Fleming, Ellen Cohn and Nedra Gillette. Using ethnographic and action research approaches they examined the clinical reasoning of occupational therapists at one hospital site over a 2-year period, resulting in seminal publications such as *Clinical Reasoning: Forms of Inquiry in a Therapeutic Practice* (Mattingly & Fleming, 1994) and *Healing Dramas and Clinical Plots* (Mattingly, 1998). Mattingly proposed the concept of therapeutic emplotment and argued that clinical encounters involved both the therapist and person receiving therapy in the creation and negotiation of a plot structure (Mattingly, 1994). In the method of therapeutic emplotment, Mattingly conceptualised the occupational therapist and the person receiving therapy as characters in an improvised action-based story that they construct together (Mattingly, 1991, 1994).

Other practice-based approaches inspired by Mattingly's work used life history approaches to investigate people's past and future worlds, such as occupational storytelling and occupational story making (Clark, 1993). In her 1993 Eleanor Clarke Slagle Lecture, Clark proposed the term *occupational storytelling* by presenting the story of her friend Penny Richardson who faced challenges when recovering from a CVA. Storytelling can both make the therapeutic process personally meaningful as well as guide therapy. Other occupational therapists who have used narrative approaches include Alsaker and Josephsson (2010), who demonstrated the narrative structure of occupations in a study of women living with chronic arthritis. Additional approaches drawing on narrative (in combination with other methods) include Frank's (2000) cultural biography approach to her work with Diane Devries, a woman who was born without arms or legs. In the book, *Venus on Wheels: Two Decades of Dialogue on Disability, Biography, and Being Female in America*, based on more than 20 years of ethnographic dialogue, Frank illuminates the experience and context of disability and gender (2000).

Autoethnographies (first used by anthropologists) are a form of self-narrative that explore the researcher's personal experiences and connects them to wider cultural, political and social meanings. For example, Neville-Jan (2003) presented a narrative of her experiences with chronic pain and subsequently problematised conceptions and reflected on how therapists could work more effectively with people with chronic pain.

DISABILITY STUDIES

Disability studies is an interdisciplinary field of study. A widely accepted description of the field was presented by the Society for Disability Studies.

> 'Disability studies recognises that disability is a key aspect of human experience, and that disability has important political, social, and economic implications for society as a whole, including both disabled and nondisabled people. Through research, artistic production, teaching and activism, disability studies seeks to augment understanding of disability in all cultures and historical periods, to promote greater awareness of the experiences of disabled people, and to advocate for social change'.
>
> *(Society for Disability Studies, n.d.)*

Disability studies can be thought of as the 'academic side' of the disability rights movement (Ferguson & Nusbaum, 2012) and parallels with various other rights movements can be identified – for example, the women's rights movement. Disability studies has reframed disability as a social phenomenon and a social construct rather than a quality or attribute of a person. 'I see disability as socially constructed in ways ranging from social conditions that straightforwardly create illnesses, injuries and poor physical functioning, to subtle cultural factors that determine standards of normality and exclude those that do not meet them from full participation in their societies' (Wendell, 1996, p. 36).

Disability studies represents a heterogeneity of perspectives, from materialist disability studies to critical and cultural disability studies, to those who seek to develop a relational understanding of disability based on a critical realist ontology (Shakespeare, 2013). The social model of disability has allowed the socially constructed nature of disability to be clearly communicated. This model conceptualises disability in terms of social oppression, and thus the locus of the problem of disability shifts away from the individual and can be located squarely within society and social organisations (Oliver, 1990). This approach has gained traction to some extent within occupational therapy and has had an identifiable influence on theory and research.

> *The social model focuses on the experience of disability [...] it considers a wide range of material and social factors and conditions, such as family circumstances, income and financial support, education, employment, housing, transport and the built environment, and more besides. At the same time, the individual and collective experience of people with disabilities is not fixed and the experience of disability therefore also demonstrates an "emergent" and temporal character. This spans the individual's experience of disability, in the context of the overall biography, social relationships and life history, the wider circumstances of disabling barriers and attitudes in society, and the impact of state policies and welfare support systems.*
>
> *(Barnes et al., 1999, p. 31)*

Disability studies have provided useful critiques of the potentially disabling attitudes and beliefs of health professionals. Abberley (1995) analysed therapists' accounts to reveal how the rhetoric of partnership and holism was employed by occupational therapists to perpetuate the notion that disability is an individual problem to which professional intervention can provide the solution, and to ascribe responsibility for any perceived failure in therapy to the person with an impairment rather than the therapist. In a study of the experiences of a small group of disabled occupational therapists, all participants faced attitudinal barriers from colleagues or managers during their training or employment (Bevan, 2014). Bevan (2014) concluded that there was further work to be done before the profession benefited fully from the inclusion of disabled therapists. Phelan (2011) applied a critically reflective lens informed by disability studies to examine notions of rehabilitation, person-centred practice, disciplinary language, independence and education in occupational therapy and revealed the ways in which occupational therapy is embedded in discourses that may reinforce negative connotations around disability. A small number of papers have described the integration of disability studies theory into occupational therapy programme curricula (Gitlow & Flecky, 2005; Block et al., 2005).

The predominant focus in occupational therapy on remediating individual deficits to enable occupational performance is at odds with disability studies theory, which emphasises the role of economic, social, political and other barriers to occupational performance (McCormack & Collins, 2010). McCormack and Collins (2010) identified five core elements of person-centred practice (power, listening and communication, partnership, choice and hope) that were linked to theoretical concepts from disability studies ('nothing about us without us', social model of disability, emancipatory research, independence and affirmation model of disability). In this manner they mapped out the contribution that disability studies made to the realisation of true person-centred practice with people with an illness, injury or impairment (McCormack & Collins, 2010).

The impact of disability studies on occupational therapy has been limited to date (Hammell, 2007); this is notable given the salience of theories and research in this field to occupational therapy practice. A seminal guest editorial on the implications of disability studies for occupational therapy was written by Kielhofner in a 2005 special issue of the *American Journal of Occupational Therapy* devoted to disability studies. Kielhofner (2005) summarised the criticisms of rehabilitation articulated by theorists in disability studies and considered in depth the potential for rehabilitation to reinforce the social oppression of people with disabilities by focusing on impairments and perpetuating the individualisation of disability (i.e. focusing on impairments as the problem rather than addressing environmental barriers, such as physical or economic barriers). Kielhofner called on the profession to integrate disability studies concepts into the profession to enable occupational therapy to be more critically self-reflective.

GENDER STUDIES

Gender studies is an interdisciplinary field in which gender identity and gendered representations are central categories of analysis (Roy, 2015). The field includes women's studies (including feminism), men's studies, and lesbian, gay, bisexual and transgender studies. The field of gender studies draws on knowledge from the social sciences, the humanities, medicine and the natural sciences. Gender research has drawn on a wide range of scholarly approaches, including empiricism, Marxism, intersectionality, postcolonial studies and body theory.

Feminism is a contested term that refers to a range of approaches and activities that are broadly concerned with drawing attention to women's position in society. 'Precisely defining feminism can be challenging, but pragmatically, a broad understanding of feminism includes women acting, speaking and writing on women's issues and rights, identifying social injustice in the status quo and bringing their own unique perspective to bear on issues' (Tandon, 2008, p. 2).

The feminist movement emerged in the late nineteenth century, and three distinct 'waves' of feminism have been identified. These waves are not entirely uniform; rather they include diverse and analytically distinct approaches to feminism. The first wave (late nineteenth to early twentieth century) was characterised by the suffrage movement. The second wave (1960s to 1980s) focused on addressing inequalities in laws and other inequalities.

The third wave (1990s to present) arose in response to perceived failures of the second wave. 'Common threads running through the diverse feminisms of the third wave are their foci on difference, deconstruction and decentering' (Mann & Huffman, 2005, p. 56). Feminists of colour and ethnicity used identity politics and intersectionality theory to criticise the 'essentialist woman' of the second wave and exposed the failure of feminism to comprehensively address the multiple simultaneous oppressions experienced by women of colour and ethnicity (Mann & Huffman, 2005). The third wave of feminism has been described as pluralistic, inclusive, nonjudgemental and respectful of self-determination (Snyder-Hall, 2010). Four major perspectives have been influential in third wave feminism: intersectionality theory, postmodernist and poststructuralist feminist approaches, feminist postcolonial theory and the agenda of younger feminists who came of adult age in the 1980s and 1990s (Mann & Huffman, 2005).

Third wave feminist scholarship contributed much to feminist disability studies; 'feminist disability studies is academic cultural work with a sharp political edge and a vigorous critical punch [...] Feminist disability studies questions the dominant premises that cast disability as a bodily problem to be addressed by normalisation procedures rather than as a socially constructed identity and a representational system similar to gender' (Garland-Thomson, 2014, pp. 1557-1559). Social constructivism has enabled disability to be considered as an identity category similar to race and gender. A large body of research and writing on disability as a social construction has used gender as a touchstone to develop these arguments. The contribution of feminism to disability studies is clear in the development of work on topics such as the politics of appearance, issues of caretaking, reproductive rights and embodiment (Garland-Thomson, 2014).

As touched on earlier, disability studies has had a limited impact on occupational therapy. The extent to which feminism has influenced scholarship in occupational therapy is far more limited. This is in contrast to other similar disciplines such as art therapy where engagement with critical viewpoints including feminism has allowed consideration of the role of art therapists in contributing to the production of meaning and reproduction of power relations in the person–therapist relationship (Hogan, 2012).

Within occupational therapy feminism had been considered to some extent in exploring the place of the profession rather than any real engagement with how feminism could inform occupational therapy theory or practice. A number of authors have drawn on feminism in discussions about occupational therapy as a predominantly female profession (Miller, 1992; Taylor, 1995). Ideas about women and what constituted appropriate work for women influenced early occupational therapy practice at the time of the emergence of the profession (Litterst, 1992). Peters' oral history work, *Powerful Occupational Therapists: A Community of Professionals 1950-80,* highlighted that there was minimal impact from the 1960s women's movement on occupational therapists with little discussion about the women's movement in workplaces or at conferences. Peters described the activities of pioneering occupational therapists at that time as 'setting up a chain of events that ultimately led to occupational therapy's professionalism, and autonomy from almost 50 years of male physician domination' (Peters, 2011, p. 381). She identified the women's movement as significant in this process as these pioneering women entered surroundings previously unfamiliar to occupational therapists, such as legislative lobbying, federal and state health care positions and academic administration. Duncan (2011) stated that the impact of the profession's gender imbalance on the development of the profession was unquestionable, and he proposed that this imbalance has affected both the value base and position of the profession in society.

Occupational scientists have paid attention on issues specific to women and engaged with gender studies/feminism to a greater extent than occupational therapy. For example, Gattuso (1996), writing on the process of self-reconstruction in aging women, considered cultural inscriptions written on women's bodies. Primeau (1992) reviewed feminist literature on the historical, political, social and personal meanings of household work and called on occupational therapists to consider the complex interactions of these meanings and to consider women's responsibility for unpaid work in the home. Primeau had also discussed the impact of gender on division of household work and identifying how parents' gender ideologies interact to create their specific gender (practices) strategies and struggles (Primeau, 2000).

Surprisingly, considering it is a female-dominated profession, feminism remains at the margins of occupational therapy and has not had a significant impact on the profession to date.

As the study of gender has expanded in recent decades so too have studies of gender issues about men and masculinities. Areas of research include the construction of masculinities, how masculinities shape and are shaped by the major institutions of modern society, the construction of masculinities in families and the intersections of war and the military with constructions of masculinity (Connell, Hearn, & Kimmel, 2004). Research on the masculine identity and the impact of disability is highly relevant to occupational therapists. Biographical research with men who have experienced spinal cord injury through playing rugby football union has illustrated the loss of specific masculine and athletic identities (Sparkes & Smith, 2002). Other highly relevant research in this field for occupational therapists includes analysis of the work–family adaptation of men (Bjørnholt, 2014).

CONCLUSION

This chapter has presented a broad overview of how theory and methods from the social sciences have influenced occupational therapy. These disciplines have permeated occupational therapy from the very origins of the profession. There is compelling evidence to suggest that the social sciences, and the critical thinking and research approaches associated with these sciences, have enriched the profession and usefully allowed critical perspectives to be taken into everyday practice. It is clear that many future opportunities for occupational therapy researchers and practitioners to use and apply the social sciences exist. The continued influence of the social sciences will deepen the profession's critical perspectives and sharpen the analysis and understanding of the interrelationship between everyday occupations, health and well-being, culture, institutions, power structures and social systems.

 http://evolve.elsevier.com/Curtin/OT

REFERENCES

Abberley, P. (1995). Disabling ideology in health and welfare-the case of occupational therapy. *Disability & Society, 10*(2), 221–232.

Abreu, B. C. (2011). Accentuate the positive: Reflections on empathic interpersonal interactions. *American Journal of Occupational Therapy, 65*(6), 623–634.

Alsaker, S., & Josephsson, S. (2010). Occupation and meaning: Narrative in everyday activities of women with chronic rheumatic conditions. *OTJR: Occupation, Participation and Health, 30*(2), 58–67.

American Occupational Therapy Association. (1993). Core values and attitudes of occupational therapy practice. *American Journal of Occupational Therapy, 47*, 1085–1086.

American Psychological Association. (2015a). *How does the APA define psychology?* Retrieved from, http://www.apa.org/support/about-apa.aspx?item=7.

American Psychological Association (2015b). *Society for humanistic psychology.* Retrieved from: http://www.apadivisions.org/division-32/about/index.aspx.

Barker Schwartz, K. (2003). History of occupation. In P. Kramer, J. Hinojosa, & C. B. Royeen (Eds.), *Perspectives in human occupation: Participation in life* (pp. 18–31). Baltimore, MD: Lippincott Williams and Wilkins.

Barker Schwartz, K. (2013). History and practice trends in physical dysfunction intervention. In H. McHugh Pendleton & W. Schultz-Krohn (Eds.), *Pedretti's occupational therapy: Practice skills for physical dysfunction* (pp. 18–27). (7th ed). St. Louis: Elsevier.

Barnes, C., Mercer, G., & Shakespeare, T. (1999). *Exploring disability: A sociological introduction.* Cambridge: Polity Press.

Beagan, B. L. (2015). Approaches to culture and diversity: A critical synthesis of occupational therapy literature. *Canadian Journal of Occupational Therapy, 82*(5), 272–282.

Beagan, B. L., & Chacala, A. (2012). Culture and diversity among occupational therapists in Ireland: When the occupational therapist is the 'diverse' one. *British Journal of Occupational Therapy, 75*, 144–151.

Bevan, J. (2014). Disabled occupational therapists – Asset, liability… or 'watering down' the profession? *Disability & Society, 29*(4), 583–596.

Bjørnholt, M. (2014). Changing men, changing times–Fathers and sons from an experimental gender equality study. *The Sociological Review, 62*(2), 295–315.

Blaga, L., & Robertson, L. (2008). The nature of occupational therapy practice in acute physical care settings. *New Zealand Journal of Occupational Therapy, 55*(2), 11–18.

Block, P., Ricafrente-Biazon, M., Russo, A. , et al. (2005). Introducing disability studies to occupational therapy students. *American Journal of Occupational Therapy, 59*(5), 554–560.

Bolier, L., Haverman, M., Westerhof, G. J., Riper, H., Smit, F., & Bohlmeijer, E. (2013). Positive psychology interventions: A meta-analysis of randomized controlled studies. *BMC Public Health, 13*(1), 119.

Bonder, B. R., Martin, L., & Miracle, A. W. (2004). Culture emergent in occupation. *American Journal of Occupational Therapy, 58*, 159–168.

Bonsall, A. (2012). An examination of the pairing between narrative and occupational science. *Scandinavian Journal of Occupational Therapy, 19*(1), 92–103.

Brown, B. J., & Baker, S. (2012). *Responsible citizens: Individuals, health, and policy under neoliberalism.* London: Anthem Press.

Calhoun, C. (2002). *Dictionary of the social sciences.* Oxford: Oxford University Press.

Cara, E., & MacRae, A. (2012). *Psychosocial occupational therapy: An evolving practice.* Boston: Cengage Learning.

Clark, F. (1993). Occupation embedded in a real life: Interweaving occupational science and occupational therapy. *American Journal of Occupational Therapy, 47*(12), 1067–1078.

Cole, M. B., & McLean, V. (2003). Therapeutic relationships redefined. *Occupational Therapy in Mental Health, 19*(2), 33–56.

Collins, C., McCartney, G., & Garnham, L. (2015). Neoliberalism and health inequalities. In K. Smith, C. Bambra, & S. Hill (Eds.), *Health inequalities: Critical perspectives* (pp. 124–137). Oxford: Oxford University Press.

Connell, R. W., Hearn, J., & Kimmel, M. S. (2004). Introduction. In M. S. Kimmel, J. Hearn, & R. W. Connell (Eds.), *Handbook of studies on men and masculinities* (pp. 1–12). Thousand Oaks, CA: Sage Publications.

Cooper, E., & Boyden, J. (2007). Questioning the Power of Resilience: Are Children Up to the Task of Disrupting the Transmission of Poverty? *Chronic Poverty Research Centre Working Paper, 73*.

De Vogli, R., Schrecker, T., & Labonte, R. (2013). Neoliberal globalisation and health inequalities. In J. Gabe & L. Monaghan (Eds.), *Key concepts in medical sociology* (pp. 32–35). (2nd ed.). Thousand Oaks, CA: Sage Publications.

Dickie, V. A. (2003). The role of learning in quilt making. *Journal of Occupational Science, 10*(3), 120–129.

Donaldson, S. I., Dollwet, M., & Rao, M. A. (2015). Happiness, excellence, and optimal human functioning revisited: Examining the peer-reviewed literature linked to positive psychology. *Journal of Positive Psychology, 10*(3), 185–195.

Duncan, E. A. (2011). *Foundations for practice in occupational therapy* (5th ed.). Edinburgh: Elsevier Health Sciences.

Dunn, D. S., Uswatte, G., & Elliott, T. R. (2009). Happiness, resilience, and positive growth following physical disability: Issues for understanding, research, and therapeutic intervention. In S. J. Lopez & C. R. Snyder (Eds.), *Oxford handbook of positive psychology* (pp. 651–664). New York: Oxford University Press.

Emerson, H. (1998). Flow and occupation: A review of the literature. *Canadian Journal of Occupational Therapy, 65*(1), 37–44.

Erikson, T. H. (2004). *Why anthropology.* London: Pluto Press.

Eriksson, G., & Tham, K. (2010). The meaning of occupational gaps in everyday life in the first year after stroke. *OTJR: Occupation, Participation and Health, 30*(4), 184–192.

Ferguson, P. M., & Nusbaum, E. (2012). Disability studies: What is it and what difference does it make? *Research and Practice for Persons with Severe Disabilities, 37*(2), 70–80.

Finlay, L. (1997). Good patients and bad patients: How occupational therapists view their patients/clients. *British Journal of Occupational Therapy, 60*(10), 440–446.

Finlay, L. (1999). Applying phenomenology in research: Problems, principles and practice. *British Journal of Occupational Therapy, 62*(7), 299–306.

Finlay, L. (2001). Holism in occupational therapy: Elusive fiction and ambivalent struggle. *American Journal of Occupational Therapy, 55*(3), 268–276.

Frank, G. (1996). Life histories in occupational therapy clinical practice. *American Journal of Occupational Therapy, 50*(4), 251–264.

Frank, G. (2000). *Venus on wheels: Two decades of dialogue on disability, biography, and being female in America.* Berkeley: University of California Press.

Frank, G., Block, P., & Zemke, R. (2008). Introduction to special theme issue anthropology, occupational therapy and disability studies: collaborations and prospects. *Practicing Anthropology, 30*(3), 2–5.

Gable, S. L., & Haidt, J. (2005). What (and why) is positive psychology? *Review of General Psychology, 9*(2), 103–110.

Garland-Thomson, R. (2014). Feminist disability studies. *Signs, 40*(1), 1557–1587.

Gattuso, S. (1996). The ageing body and the self-project in women's narratives. *Journal of Occupational Science, 3*(3), 104–109.

Gerlach, A. J. (2012). A critical reflection on the concept of cultural safety. *Canadian Journal of Occupational Therapy, 79*(3), 151–158.

Gitlow, L., & Flecky, K. (2005). Integrating disability studies concepts into occupational therapy education using service learning. *American Journal of Occupational Therapy, 59*(5), 546–553.

Gray, M., & McPherson, K. (2005). Cultural safety and professional practice in occupational therapy: A New Zealand perspective. *Australian Occupational Therapy Journal, 52*(1), 34–42.

Guest, R., Craig, A., Tran, Y., & Middleton, J. (2015). Factors predicting resilience in people with spinal cord injury during transition from inpatient rehabilitation to the community. *Spinal Cord, 53*, 682–686.

Hammell, K. W. (2007). Reflections on…a disability methodology for the client-centred practice of occupational therapy research. *Canadian Journal of Occupational Therapy, 74*(5), 365–369.

Hammell, K. W. (2009). Sacred texts: A sceptical exploration of the assumptions underpinning theories of occupation. *Canadian Journal of Occupational Therapy, 76*, 6–13.

Hammell, K. W. (2011). Resisting theoretical imperialism in the disciplines of occupational science and occupational therapy. *British Journal of Occupational Therapy, 74*, 27–33.

Hammell, K. W. (2013). Client-centred practice in occupational therapy: Critical reflections. *Scandinavian Journal of Occupational Therapy, 20*, 174–181.

Hasselkus, B., & Dickie, V. A. (1994). Doing occupational therapy: Dimensions of satisfaction and dissatisfaction. *American Journal of Occupational Therapy*, 48(2), 145–154.

Hogan, S. (2012). *Revisiting feminist approaches to art therapy.* New York: Berghahn Books.

Holmqvist, K., Holmefur, M., & Ivarsson, A. B. (2013). Therapeutic use of self as defined by Swedish occupational therapists working with clients with cognitive impairments following acquired brain injury: A Delphi study. *Australian Occupational Therapy Journal*, 60(1), 48–55.

Hume, C. A. (1984). Transcultural aspects of psychiatric rehabilitation. *British Journal of Occupational Therapy*, 47(12), 373–375.

Huot, S. (2015). Ethnography: understanding occupation through an examination of culture. In S. Nayar & M. Stanley (Eds.), *Qualitative research methodologies for occupational science and therapy.* London: Routledge.

Huot, S., Laliberte Rudman, D., Dodson, B., & Magalhães, L. (2013). Expanding policy-based conceptualizations of 'successful integration': Negotiating integration through occupation following international migration. *Journal of Occupational Science*, 20(1), 6–22.

Hyde, A., McDonnell, O., & Lohan, M. (2004). *Sociology for health professionals in Ireland.* Belfast: Institute of Public Administration.

Ikiugu, M. N., & Ciaravino, E. A. (2007). *Psychosocial conceptual practice models in occupational therapy: Building adaptive capability.* St Louis: Mosby.

Iwama, M. (2003). Toward culturally relevant epistemologies in occupational therapy. *American Journal of Occupational Therapy*, 57, 582–588.

Iwama, M. K. (2005). The Kawa (River) model. In F. Kronenberg, S. S. Algado, & N. Pollard (Eds.), *Occupational therapy without borders.* Edinburgh: Churchill Livingstone.

Iwama, M. K. (2006). *The Kawa model: Culturally relevant occupational therapy.* Edinburgh: Churchill Livingstone.

Jones, D., Sheena, E., & Hartery, T. (1998). *Sociology and occupational therapy.* London: Churchill Livingstone.

Jull, J. E., & Giles, A. R. (2012). Health equity, Aboriginal peoples and occupational therapy. *Canadian Journal of Occupational Therapy*, 79, 70–76.

Kielhofner, G. (1997). *Conceptual foundations of occupational therapy* (2nd ed.). Philadelphia F.A: Davis.

Kielhofner, G. (2005). Rethinking disability and what to do about it: Disability studies and its implications for occupational therapy. *American Journal of Occupational Therapy*, 59(5), 487–496.

Kielhofner, G., & Burke, J. P. (1977). Occupational therapy after 60 years: An account of changing identity and knowledge. *American Journal of Occupational Therapy*, 31(10), 675–689.

Kleinman, A. (1988). *The illness narratives: Suffering, healing, and the human condition.* New York: Basic Books.

Krefting, L. (1989). Reintegration into the community after head injury: The results of an ethnographic study. *OTJR: Occupation, Participation and Health*, 9(2), 67–83.

Krefting, L. (1991). The culture concept in everyday life of physical and occupational therapy. *Physical and Occupational Therapy in Paediatrics*, 11(4), 1–6.

Laaksonen, M., Talala, K., Martelin, T., et al. (2008). Health behaviours as explanations for educational level differences in cardiovascular and all-cause mortality: A follow-up of 60 000 men and women over 23 years. *European Journal of Public Health*, 18(1), 38–43.

Laliberte Rudman, D., & Dennhardt, S. (2008). Shaping knowledge regarding occupation: Examining the cultural underpinnings of the evolving concept of occupational identity. *Australian Occupational Therapy Journal*, 55, 153–162.

Laliberte Rudman, D., Huot, S., Klinger, L., Leipert, B. D., & Spafford, M. M. (2010). Struggling to maintain occupation while dealing with risk: The experiences of older adults with low vision. *OTJR: Occupation, Participation and Health*, 30(2), 87–96.

Litterst, T. A. (1985). A reappraisal of anthropological fieldwork methods and the concept of culture in occupational therapy research. *American Journal of Occupational Therapy*, 39(8), 602.

Litterst, T. A. (1992). Occupational therapy: The role of ideology in the development of a profession for women. *American Journal of Occupational Therapy*, 46(1), 20–25.

Macionis, J., & Plummer, K. (2015). *Sociology: A global introduction* (4th ed.). Essex: Pearson Education Limited.

Mackenbach, J. P., Stirbu, I., Roskam, A.-J. , et al. (2008). Socioeconomic inequalities in health in 22 European countries. *New England Journal of Medicine*, 358(23), 2468–2481.

Magasi, S., & Hammel, J. (2009). Women with disabilities' experiences in long-term care: A case for social justice. *American Journal of Occupational Therapy*, 63(1), 35–45.

Mann, S. A., & Huffman, D. J. (2005). The decentering of second wave feminism and the rise of the third wave. *Science & Society*, 56–91.

Martin, C. R. (2015). Resilience: Paradoxical insight or conceptual poverty? *Journal for Multicultural Education*, 9(3), 117–121.

Martz, E., & Livneh, H. (2015). Psychosocial adaptation to disability within the context of positive psychology: Findings from the literature. *Journal of Occupational Rehabilitation*, 1–9.

Masten, A. S., & Obradović, J. (2006). Competence and resilience in development. *Annals of the New York Academy of Sciences*, 1094 (1), 13–27.

Mattingly, C. (1991). The narrative nature of clinical reasoning. *American Journal of Occupational Therapy*, 45(11), 998–1005.

Mattingly, C. (1994). The concept of therapeutic 'emplotment'. *Social Science & Medicine*, 38(6), 811–822.

Mattingly, C. (1998). *Healing dramas and clinical plots: The narrative structure of experience.* Cambridge: Cambridge University Press.

Mattingly, C., & Fleming, M. (1994). *Clinical reasoning: Forms of inquiry in a therapeutic practice.* Philadelphia: F.A. Davis.

McArthur, M., & Goodacre, L. (2013). Living with rheumatic diseases: The theoretical perspective. In L. Goodacre, & M. McArthur (Eds.), *Rheumatology practice in occupational therapy: Promoting lifestyle management.* London: John Wiley & Sons.

McCormack, C., & Collins, B. (2010). Can disability studies contribute to client-centred occupational therapy practice? *British Journal of Occupational Therapy*, 73(7), 339–342.

McDonald, B. (2004). *An introduction to sociology in Ireland* (3rd ed.). Dublin: Gill and Macmillan.

Miller, R. J. (1992). Interwoven threads: Occupational therapy, feminism, and holistic health. *American Journal of Occupational Therapy, 46*(11), 1013–1019.

Mohaupt, S. (2009). Review article: Resilience and social exclusion. *Social Policy and Society, 8*(01), 63–71.

Morrison, T. L., & Smith, J. D. (2013). Working alliance development in occupational therapy: A cross-case analysis. *Australian Occupational Therapy Journal, 60*(5), 326–333.

Mosey, A. C. (1981). *Occupational therapy: A configuration of a profession.* New York: Raven.

Navarro, V. (2009). What we mean by social determinants of health. *International Journal of Health Services, 39*(3), 423–441.

Nelson, A. (2007). Seeing white: A critical exploration of occupational therapy with Indigenous Australian people. *Occupational Therapy International, 14*, 237–255.

Nettleton, S. (2006). *The sociology of health and illness.* Cambridge: Polity.

Neville-Jan, A. (2003). Encounters in a world of pain: An autoethnography. *American Journal of Occupational Therapy, 57*(1), 88–98.

Oliver, M. (1990). *The politics of disablement.* London: Palgrave Macmillan.

Parsons, T. (1951). *The social system.* Glencoe, IL: Free Press.

Peters, C. O. (2011). Powerful Occupational Therapists: A Community of Professionals, 1950–1980. *Occupational Therapy in Mental Health, 27*, 3–4, 199–410.

Pettigrew, J. (2013). *Maoists at the hearth: Everyday life in Nepal's civil war.* Philadelphia: University of Pennsylvania Press.

Phelan, S. K. (2011). Constructions of disability: A call for critical reflexivity in occupational therapy. *Canadian Journal of Occupational Therapy, 78*(3), 164–172.

Pierret, J. (2003). The illness experience: State of knowledge and perspectives for research. *Sociology of Health & Illness, 25*(3), 4–22.

Pooley, J. A., & Cohen, L. (2010). Resilience: A definition in context. *Australian Community Psychologist, 22*(1), 30–37.

Prendiville, C., & Pettigrew, J. (2015). Leisure occupations in the Central Criminal Lunatic Asylum 1890–1920. *Irish Journal of Occupational Therapy, 43*(1), 12–19.

Primeau, L. A. (1992). A woman's place: Unpaid work in the home. *American Journal of Occupational Therapy, 46*(11), 981–988.

Primeau, L. A. (2000). Household work: When gender ideologies and practices interact. *Journal of Occupational Science, 7*(3), 118–127.

Prodinger, B., Shaw, L., Rudman, D. L., & Townsend, E. (2012). Arthritis-related occupational therapy: Making invisible ruling relations visible using institutional ethnography. *British Journal of Occupational Therapy, 75*(10), 463–470.

Quale, A. J., & Schanke, A. K. (2010). Resilience in the face of coping with a severe physical injury: A study of trajectories of adjustment in a rehabilitation setting. *Rehabilitation Psychology, 55*(1), 12–22.

Reid, D. (2011). Mindfulness and flow in occupational engagement: Presence in doing. *Canadian Journal of Occupational Therapy, 78*(1), 50–56.

Ritzer, G. (2015). *Introduction to sociology* (3rd ed.). Thousand Oaks, CA: Sage Publications.

Robertson, C., & Finlay, L. (2007). Making a difference, teamwork and coping: The meaning of practice in acute physical settings. *British Journal of Occupational Therapy, 70*(2), 73–80.

Robinson, K., Kennedy, N., & Harmon, D. (2012). Happiness: A review of evidence relevant to occupational science. *Journal of Occupational Science, 19*(2), 150–164.

Rogers, C. R. (1951). *Client-centered therapy: Its current practice, implications and theory.* Boston: Houghton Mifflin.

Rogers, C. (1961). *A therapist's view of psychotherapy: On becoming a person.* London: Constable.

Rosa, S., & Hasselkus, B. (1996). Connecting with patients: The personal experience of professional helping. *OTJR: Occupation, Participation and Health, 16*(4), 245–260.

Roy, S. (2015). History of gender studies: A review. *Global Journal of Multidisciplinary Studies, 4*(7), 167–172.

Rudman, D. L. (2015). Embodying positive aging and neoliberal rationality: Talking about the aging body within narratives of retirement. *Journal of Aging Studies, 34*, 10–20.

Schemm, R. L. (1994). Bridging conflicting ideologies: The origins of American and British occupational therapy. *American Journal of Occupational Therapy, 48*(11), 1082–1088.

Seligman, M. E., & Csikszentmihalyi, M. (2000). Positive psychology: An introduction. *American Psychologist, 55*(1), 5–14.

Shakespeare, T. (2013). *Disability rights and wrongs revisited* (2nd ed.). Abingdon, UK: Routledge.

Silverman, A. M., Molton, I. R., Alschuler, K. N., Ehde, D. M., & Jensen, M. P. (2015). Resilience predicts functional outcomes in people aging with disability: A longitudinal investigation. *Archives of Physical Medicine and Rehabilitation, 96*(7), 1262–1268.

Sin, N. L., & Lyubomirsky, S. (2009). Enhancing well-being and alleviating depressive symptoms with positive psychology interventions: A practice-friendly meta-analysis. *Journal of Clinical Psychology, 65*(5), 467–487.

Snyder-Hall, R. C. (2010). Third-wave feminism and the defense of choice. *Perspectives on Politics, 8*(1), 255–261.

Sparkes, A. C., & Smith, B. (2002). Sport, spinal cord injury, embodied masculinities, and the dilemmas of narrative identity. *Men and Masculinities, 4*(3), 258–285.

Spencer, J., Krefting, L., & Mattingly, C. (1993). Incorporation of ethnographic methods in occupational therapy assessment. *American Journal of Occupational Therapy, 47*(4), 303–309.

Stern, E. M. (2014). Foreword to the second edition. In K. J. Schneider, J. F. Pierson, & J. F. Bugental (Eds.), *The handbook of humanistic psychology: Theory, research, and practice* (pp. xi–xii). Thousand Oaks, CA: Sage Publications.

Tandon, N. (2008). *Feminism: A paradigm shift.* New Delhi: Atlantic Publishers.

Taylor, J. (1995). A different voice in occupational therapy. *British Journal of Occupational Therapy, 58*(4), 170–174.

Taylor, R. R., Lee, S. W., Kielhofner, G., & Ketkar, M. (2009). Therapeutic use of self: A nationwide survey of practitioners' attitudes and experiences. *American Journal of Occupational Therapy, 63*(2), 198–207.

Tervalon, M., & Murray-García, J. (1998). Cultural humility versus cultural competence: A critical distinction in defining physician training outcomes in multicultural education. *Journal of Health Care for the Poor and Underserved, 9*(2), 117–125.

Thomas, Y., Gray, M., & McGinty, S. (2011). Occupational therapy at the 'cultural interface': Lessons from research with Aboriginal and

Torres Strait Islander Australians. *Australian Occupational Therapy Journal, 58*(1), 11–16.

Townsend, E. (1996). Institutional ethnography: A method for showing how the context shapes practice. *OTJR: Occupation, Participation and Health, 16*(3), 179–199.

Varul, M. Z. (2010). Talcott Parsons, the sick role and chronic illness. *Body & Society, 16*(2), 72–94.

Waterman, A. S. (2013). The humanistic psychology – Positive psychology divide: Contrasts in philosophical foundations. *American Psychologist, 68*(3), 124.

Wendell, S. (1996). *The rejected body: Feminist philosophical reflections on disability.* New York: Psychology Press.

White, B., Driver, S., & Warren, A. M. (2008). Considering resilience in the rehabilitation of people with traumatic disabilities. *Rehabilitation Psychology, 53*(1), 9.

Wilcock, A. (2001). *Occupation for health: volume 1. A journey from self health to prescription.* London: British Association and College of Occupational Therapists.

Windle, G. (2011). What is resilience? A review and concept analysis. *Reviews in Clinical Gerontology, 21*(2), 152–169.

Wright, J. J., Sadlo, G., & Stew, G. (2007). Further explorations into the conundrum of flow process. *Journal of Occupational Science, 14*(3), 136–144.

Wright-St Clair, V. A., & Smythe, E. A. (2012). Being occupied in the everyday. In M Cutchin, & V Dickie (Eds.), *Transactional perspectives on occupation* (pp. 25–37). Dordrecht: Springer.

Yalom, I. D. (1980). *Existential psychotherapy.* New York: Basic Books.

Yerxa, E. (1983). Audacious values: The energy source for occupational therapy practice. In *Health through occupation: Theory and practice in occupational therapy* (pp. 149–162).

Section 3

PROFESSIONAL REASONING

5 CLIENT-CENTREDNESS

JACQUIE RIPAT

CHAPTER OUTLINE

Abstract
Client-centredness is foundational to occupational therapy practice. Client-centredness is the spirit and attitude in which occupational therapists approach their practice and the ways in which they interact with the people receiving their services. Demonstrating respect for the inherent worth of the people receiving occupational therapy services, and enacting a commitment to redress power differences, are central to the ability of occupational therapists to provide client-centred practice. Although occupational therapists may feel challenged to implement client-centredness in practice, a number of approaches have been proposed that can assist them to enact this professional value. Beginning with engaging in a process of reflexivity, client-centred occupational therapists can work to develop their relationship-building skills such as empathy, communication and collaboration. They can explore their environments to identify opportunities to develop client-centred practice settings. Finally, building on the client-centred constructs of respect and power, occupational therapists can begin to address societal and systemic barriers that limit the occupational opportunities faced by people receiving their services.

KEY POINTS

- The occupational therapy profession has a long history of embracing client-centred practice as a core approach to the way services are provided.

- Two key constructs are foundational to client-centredness: respect for the inherent worth of the people receiving occupational therapy services and a commitment to redress power differences.

- Client-centredness is an attitude or philosophy of the occupational therapist based on internalisation of, and commitment to, the two key constructs of respect and power.

- Occupational therapists can enact client-centred approaches that reflect this spirit of client-centredness.

- Occupational therapists can influence their practice environments to reflect a commitment to client centredness.

- Occupational therapists are able to apply their client-centred thinking beyond the individual person level to address social and political barriers to occupational opportunities faced by people.

INTRODUCTION

Client-centredness* has developed as a core value of the occupational therapy profession (Aguilar, Stupans, Scutter, & King, 2013) and is foundational to the way that occupational therapists practise (Polatajko & Townsend, 2007). But what is client-centred practice, and what makes an occupational therapist client-centred? What do people who receive occupational therapy services want in terms of client-centred therapists and client-centred services? What challenges do occupational therapists face in trying to practice in a client-centred way? And what creative, innovative and forward-thinking strategies can occupational therapists draw on to enhance their ways of staying true to, and even advancing, this commitment in light of working in complex, interprofessional systems and structures? These questions are explored in this chapter. First, a brief history of client-centred practice and occupational therapy is presented. Next, two key concepts of client-centred practice, respect and power, are discussed. Finally, how internalizing client-centredness as a core value of occupational therapy can provide the foundation for implementing client-centred approaches in practice, despite implementation challenges, is outlined.

The World Federation of Occupational Therapists (WFOT, 2010) states, 'Occupational therapy is client-centred and occupation-focused' (p. 1). The notion that client-centredness is one of two key concepts defining the occupational therapy profession establishes a global commitment to incorporating

---

*The terms *client-centred* and *person-centred* are often used interchangeably and are considered to have the same meaning. There has been a recent tendency for authors and therapists to prefer the use of the word *person-centred* to emphasise that individuals receiving occupational therapy services are first and foremost people, rather than clients, a term that has business connotations. *Person-centred* is the preferred term within this book when referring to an individual. *Client-centred* is the preferred term within this book when referring more broadly to individuals, groups, communities and populations who receive occupational therapy services. In addition, *client-centred* is used in the majority of historical and current research publications and hence has been retained when using direct quotes in this chapter.

this important value into practice. If occupation is an occupational therapist's domain of interest and *what* is done in occupational therapy, then client-centredness is *how* it is done. Client-centredness is the spirit and attitude in which occupational therapists approach their practice and the ways in which they interact with the people receiving their services.

HISTORICAL ASPECTS

The occupational therapy profession can trace the roots of client-centred practice to an American psychologist, Carl Rogers. Rogers wrote about client-centred therapy in the 1940s emphasising the value of taking an approach that focused on the person. He focused his theory on the importance of the relationship between the therapist and the person, in which the therapist held an attitude of unconditional positive regard toward the person and encouraged the person through a process of self-actualisation (Bozarth, 2008). Rogers believed that a successful therapeutic process was person-led in terms of direction and pace and that this process would enable people to identify goals and autonomously solve problems (Bozarth, 2008). The *Guidelines for Client-Centred Practice of Occupational Therapy* (Canadian Association of Occupational Therapists & Department of National Health and Welfare, 1983) represented a professional adoption of some of these key ideas. More than a decade later, a seminal paper by Law, Baptiste, and Mills (1995, p. 253) took these ideas further, defining client-centred occupational therapy practice as

An approach to providing occupational therapy, which embraces a philosophy of respect for, and partnership with, people receiving services. Client-centred practice recognizes the autonomy of individuals, the need for client choice in making decisions about occupational needs, the strengths clients bring to a therapy encounter, the benefits of client-therapist partnership and the need to ensure that services are accessible and fit the context in which a client lives.

In this definition, the term *client* refers to the recipient of occupational therapy services and may include individuals, families, groups, communities, organisations, agencies, governments, corporations or populations (WFOT, 2010). Describing the people that occupational therapists work with in this way is both simple and complex. For example, working with an adult on enhancing opportunities for work the adult can be considered the client; but what about the adult's partner, family and employer? The community that the adult lives in? The funders of occupational therapy services? Should they be considered clients as well?

Mackey (2014) describes the 'triple accountability' (p. 173) that occupational therapists hold with respect to the people directly receiving occupational therapy services, to the organisations that employ occupational therapists, and to professional organisations, and how competing priorities, demands and concerns often create tension for occupational therapists. However, accountability and allegiances are not the same thing, and Hammell (2007) challenges occupational therapists to consider to whom their allegiances as client-centred therapists truly lie. Remembering that the person is the focus of therapists' professional activities in terms of identifying occupational issues, personal strengths, and desired occupational outcomes while working with the person towards those outcomes, may be a helpful way of addressing Hammell's challenge.

CLIENT-CENTRED PRACTICE IS ABOUT TWO KEY CONCEPTS: RESPECT AND POWER

Two key constructs are foundational to client-centred practice: respect and power. Therapists who practice in a client-centred way embrace a spirit of respect for the inherent dignity of people and demonstrate a caring and authentic interest in each person (Hammell, 2013). Respect is defined as 'a reflection of willingness to look past positive or negative attributes to the very core of what makes the person human' (Purtilo & Haddad, 2002, p. 4), and throughout the literature an attitude of respect has continuously emerged as central to client-centred practice. This includes respect for autonomy and choice (Law et al., 1995; Sumsion & Law, 2006; WFOT, 2010), respect for a person's values (Sumsion, 2000; Sumsion & Law, 2006), respect for prioritisation of a person's goals (Sumsion, 2000), and honouring and nurturing hope expressed by the person (Sumsion & Law, 2006; WFOT, 2010). People have consistently articulated the importance of respect and the need to have health care providers relate to them on a deep emotional level. They want therapists to honour their dignity of spirit, respond to them as individuals and experts in their own lives and recognise the broader influences of the contexts in which they live. The importance of respect emerged as central to the experience of mental health consumers and was summed up as follows: 'Client-centred care means I am a valued human being' (Corring & Cook, 1999, p. 78).

The second key construct of client-centred practice is power. In a review of the primary concepts related to client-centred occupational therapy practice, Sumsion and Law (2006) concluded that power was a foundational concept in which to consider all other concepts and was 'vital to the understanding and implementation of client-centred practice' (p. 155). *Power* refers to "the ability or right to control people or things, the possession of control, authority or influence over others, ⋯ the ability to act or produce an effect" (Merriam Webster On-line Dictionary, n.d.). It is important to spend some time teasing apart this definition as '[p]ower is neither inherently good nor bad' (Clark, 2010, p. 265). On one hand, power can be thought of in negative terms – for example, when it refers to controlling or dominating someone – an idea that does not resonate well with client-centred practitioners. However, it is important to separate the idea of dominance from other definitions of power that relate to influence or ability to create an effect. In this way, power can also be used by occupational therapists to influence and advocate on behalf of the people receiving their services (Dhillon, Wilkins, Law, Stewart, & Tremblay, 2010) or 'in the service of the public good' (Clark, 2010, p. 265).

Yet what sources of power do occupational therapists hold? Knowledge and professional status is a source of power: occupational therapists have professional status and receive income and recognition from their work (Cott, 2004; Hammell, 2015). Funders of occupational therapy services and institutions bestow therapists with power to make decisions about the present and future of the people receiving their services. Social status is also power – occupational therapists are granted societal status and privilege as they often represent the members of the predominant culture, with respect to ethnicity, socioeconomic status and ability status (Hammell, 2015). Thus an inherent power imbalance exists between people receiving services and occupational therapists by nature of the therapists' professional position and status (Falardeau & Durand, 2002; Law et al., 1995; Sumsion & Law, 2006).

Partnerships and Power

Viewing the relationship between people receiving services and the therapist as a partnership is one way of sharing power. But developing partnerships may not be as easy as it sounds – how can occupational therapists truly become partners with people when an inherent power imbalance exists? Falardeau and Durand (2002) provide a useful framework for how power-sharing between people and therapist can be conceptualised. They defined three spheres of influence related to knowledge and power, one exclusive to each of the partners and one that is mutually shared. Each person's sphere of influence is as an expert in his or her own life. This is reinforced by one consumer of health services who stated, 'The only person who is an expert on me is me' (Rebeiro, 2000, p. 12). The therapist's sphere of influence is through knowledge and expertise in enabling occupational performance and engagement and seeking and accessing resources. Falardeau and Durand (2002, p. 138) assert that 'power is shared when each partner exercises an influence over the other by respecting their respective fields of competence' and that it is in the mutually shared sphere that decision-making and collaboration over the occupational therapy process occurs. Bright, Boland, Rutherford, Kayes, and McPherson (2012) went one step further, suggesting that when therapists viewed themselves as coaches, rather than as expert practitioners, this helped move towards shared power and client-centred practice.

Power and Safety

The issue of a person's safety warrants a place in a discussion of power. An overriding concern for a person's physical and emotional safety over respect for a person's wishes and autonomy has been expressed by therapists in various studies (Durocher, Kinsella, Ells, & Hunt, 2015; Moats, 2007; Mortenson & Dyck, 2006). Protecting someone from perceived risk is an aspect that can have ethical, legal and moral implications. Client-centred occupational therapists will likely feel challenged to strike a balance between their views of what is required to maintain the physical and emotional safety of people and respect for their autonomy (Moats, 2007): how is making the decision that something is in the 'best interest' of another congruent with a practice that is client-centred? Some have begun to explore this issue, suggesting guiding frameworks that might help untangle these challenges (see, e.g., Durocher et al., 2015; Moats, 2007).

What Do the Recipients of Occupational Therapy Services Value?

The limited available literature that has explored the perspective of people receiving services supports that respect and power are central to client-centred practice. People receiving therapy services have highlighted the importance of being viewed as unique individuals who are experts in their own lives (Blank, 2004; Corring & Cook, 1999; Rebeiro, 2000) and as people who hold inherent value and are worthy of respect (Corring & Cook, 1999). Although profession-driven literature has emphasised the importance of power in a client-centred relationship, research from the perspective of service recipients have instead emphasised the nature and quality of the relationship (Corring & Cook, 1999; Crepeau & Garren, 2011; McKinnon, 2000).

Respect for each person's inherent worth is demonstrated through active listening (Blank, 2004), paying attention (Crepeau & Garren, 2011), expressing sensitivity to needs and experiences (McKinnon, 2000) and demonstrating genuine concern for and interest in their well-being (Corring & Cook, 1999; Rebeiro, 2000). People receiving services view partnerships as the creation of a climate of respect that is accepting and supportive, where there is a sense of choice and shared power and control (Blank, 2004; Corring & Cook, 1999; Rebeiro, 2000). Some have referred to an effective and positive relationship with their therapist as a friendship (Blank, 2004; Palmadottir, 2003), where a caring attitude is communicated by the therapist and the interaction is based on mutual trust and respect. It may be that what people perceive as friendship has been conceptualised as a therapeutic relationship by occupational therapists; Crepeau and Garren (2011) argue, 'What sets the therapeutic relationship apart from other friendships or partnerships is the need for competence on the part of the therapist' (p. 873). The perceived competency of the therapist and the accessibility of services has also been raised as an important aspect of service provision (Blank, 2004; McKinnon, 2000). However, examining whether people receiving services perceive therapists as client-centred, and what people want in a client-centred occupational practice, is an important area of continued research (Pizzi, 2015).

CLIENT-CENTREDNESS IN PRACTICE

Theory–Practice Divide

The gap between what occupational therapists want to do, what they believe is important and what they feel empowered to do in practice has been discussed as a challenge to putting professional values into practice (Aguilar et al., 2013; Duggan, 2005;

Mortenson & Dyck, 2006; Ripat, Wener, & Dobinson, 2013; Toal-Sullivan, 2006; Wilkins, Pollock, Rochon, & Law, 2001). In particular, goal-setting with people has emerged as one perceived barrier to implementing client-centred approach. At times there are differences between therapist and clients in the nature of goals (Richard & Knis-Matthews, 2010; Sumsion & Smyth, 2000; Wressle & Samuelsson, 2004) or a seeming discrepancy between a therapist's personal beliefs and values and client-determined goals (Krizaj & Hurst, 2012; Sumsion & Smyth, 2000). Perception of ease or extent of client involvement in goal-setting (Maitra & Erway, 2006; Sumsion & Smyth, 2000) can also be challenging for therapists. Furthermore, some have suggested that it is 'harder' to implement a client-centred approach with people who may display certain characteristics, related to age, sensory loss or motivation (Hedberg-Kristensson & Iwarsson, 2013) or when there is a perceived lack of ability to participate or lack of self-knowledge of problems (Kjellberg, Kahlin, Haglund, & Taylor, 2012). However, therapists committed to client-centred practice assert, 'We cannot say that client-centred practice only works for some clients. We must find ways for it to work with all clients' (Wilkins et al., 2001, p. 78).

As noted previously, client-centred occupational therapy involves a willingness to consider how power influences the development of collaborative partnerships with people and a commitment to redress power. The implicit nature of power and unconscious influence on the relationships therapists have with the people receiving their services is illustrated in this reflective narrative by Bright et al. (2012, p. 4): 'We unintentionally positioned ourselves as experts during interactions between ourselves and clients, resulting in a paternalistic approach to engagement. We controlled information – timing and contents of meetings and discharge reports'. A shift from profession-dominated ways of acting and thinking may be challenging for occupational therapists to accept (Wilkins et al., 2001) and instances of using what might be construed as intimidating or coercive tactics with people – for example, withholding provision of home care supports (Moats, 2007) – have been documented. Perhaps clarifying and developing general agreement on the general constructs of client-centred practice as founded on an attitude of respect and redressing the power, rather than seeing this type of practice as a prescribed set of actions, will help occupational therapy move forward as a profession. This way, occupational therapists can avoid seeing client-centred practice as an all-or-none phenomenon.

Internalising a Spirit of Client-centredness

At this juncture, there is a need to stop and make an important distinction in language (Fig. 5.1). *Client-centredness* is an attitude or philosophy based on internalisation of the two key constructs outlined earlier (i.e. respect and power). *Client-centred approaches* are the actions, behaviours and strategies that occupational therapists engage in, that reflect this spirit of client-centredness. Finally, *client-centred practice* is the way that occupational therapists can work within their contexts to reflect their commitment to client-centredness. This distinction allows

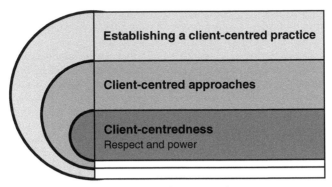

FIG. 5.1 ■ Clarifying client-centred concepts.

occupational therapists to recognise client-centred practice as a dynamic and fluid concept rather than a set of static behaviours. An occupational therapist who has embraced a spirit of client-centredness emphasises different aspects depending on the practice setting, contextual considerations and the characteristics of the clients (Hughes, Bamford, & May, 2008; Papadimitriou & Cott, 2015). Paying attention to a client's cues and preferences (Palmadottir, 2006), recognizing the diversity and heterogeneity of people and attending to each client's history and experience (Cott, 2004) is where the art of client-centred practice becomes enacted.

An internalisation of the value of client-centred practice is evident beyond the statements outlined in professional documents. Occupational therapy students quickly learn of the importance placed on client-centredness through a process of professional socialisation and identity development (Ajjawi & Higgs, 2008) throughout their preprofessional years (Ripat et al., 2013). Internalising client-centredness was also evident in a study of what occupational therapists identified as core professional values and behaviours, where many of the 61 values identified related to client-centred practice – for example, 'empowerment of the client' and 'respect for people's language, culture and views' (Aguilar et al., 2013, p. 211).

Client-centred Approaches: Client-centredness in Action

To put client-centredness 'into action', occupational therapists may find it helpful to identify strategies that they can implement (Restall & Ripat, 2008; Wilkins et al., 2001). For example, an attitude of respect can be demonstrated through the behaviours of occupational therapists. Hammell (2013) outlined a respect model of client-centred occupational therapy (p. 147) that includes active, engaged listening; critical awareness of power; cultural humility; kindness, caring and respect for people; respect for each client's right to make choices; fostering supportive relationships with people; and understanding resources, barriers and constraints to occupation and well-being. Sumsion (2006) outlined specific client-centred strategies when working

with people who may seem more difficult to engage in the occupational therapy process – for example, older adults with cognitive impairments.

Restall, Ripat, and Stern (2003) developed the client-centred strategies framework (CSF) to facilitate therapists' generation of ideas, to enhance their ability to be client-centred in practice. The CSF consists of five categories of potential strategies: personal reflection, client-centred processes, practice settings, community organising, and coalition advocacy and political action. Although not intended to be inclusive or exhaustive, the CSF provides a framework for exploring client-centredness and for thinking and acting in client-centred ways. In the next section, these strategies and ways that they can be operationalised are explored.

Personal Reflection

Cameron and McColl (2015) challenged therapists to first centre themselves in practice, stating that 'Centred client practice denotes a reminder for therapists' careful consideration of the ethics, values, beliefs, assumptions and preconceptions they bring to the relationship that may limit a truly collaborative relationship' (p. 3). To 'center' themselves, one of the most important activities therapists can engage in is a process of reflexivity. Engaging in a process of reflexivity is about uncovering the biases, assumptions and preconceived notions that may influence their thoughts, behaviours and actions.

Reflexivity is described as 'aspects of reflection [thinking about one's practice during or after an incident has occurred], in addition to the act of interrogating one's situatedness in society, history, culture, and how this may shape one's values, morals, and judgements at both individual and social levels' (Phelan, 2011, p. 165). Use of autoethnographical (Bright et al., 2012; Hoppes, Hamilton, & Robinson, 2007) or autobiographical (McCorquodale & Kinsella, 2015) methods are valuable ways for students and therapists to gain insight into their values, beliefs and tacit assumptions. Combining written reflective narratives with discussion with a trusted colleague to challenge, explore, question and bring conscious awareness to those tacit understandings has been highlighted as additionally useful (Bright et al., 2012; Duggan, 2005; McCorquodale & Kinsella, 2015; Wilkins et al., 2001). Sumsion and Law (2006, p. 159) provided a set of practice questions related to the conceptual elements of client-centred practice (i.e. power, listening and communication, partnership, choice and hope). These questions provide an important set of self-reflective questions to be used individually or in peer discussions designed to critically examine client-centredness.

Engaging in values clarification exercises is a way for therapists to explore their own biases, assumptions and preconceptions and to discover deeply held values that may influence their thoughts, behaviours and attitudes (Restall et al., 2003). Clarification of personal values and comparison with client-centred values of respect and redress of power will provide insights into how personal values shape therapy behaviours, actions and choices and, ultimately, therapists' internalisation of client-centredness. Clarification of values and comparison with a client's values may help in determining potential areas of misunderstanding. By making their values explicit, therapists sort through whether what they say they believe and how they act are congruent.

Facilitating Client-centred Approaches

In the CSF, *client-centred processes* refers to the 'clinician's active and conscious facilitation of client-centred interactions with the client' (Restall et al., 2003, p. 107). Central to facilitating client-centred processes is a focus on the relationship between the client and an occupational therapist. If therapists agree that health professionals hold power at a professional and societal level, a key to examining the role of power in client-centred practice is identifying where and how this power is exerted (McCorquodale & Kinsella, 2015). By making the implicit existence of power explicit, therapists can develop a conscious awareness of the existence and role of power in their interactions and situations, including the subtle and not so subtle expressions of control, decision-making or influence, and the effect that this power has on the other client or situation.

Development of empathy is a key client-centred strategy that helps 'the therapist to view the world through the client's eyes, walk in the client's shoes and achieve an emic or insider understanding of the disability and its effect on the client and his/her occupation' (Jamieson et al., 2006, p. 77). Learning from others who have experienced the health, educational or social system in different ways is one way of developing empathy. At a student level, one suggested strategy is to pair students with client-tutors (Cameron & McColl, 2015; Hedge, Neville, & Pickens, 2015; Jamieson et al., 2006), enhancing students' abilities to appreciate the 'humanness of people with disabilities', recognise the 'coexistence of health and disorder' and recognise the influence of the sociocultural environments in which people live (Jamieson et al., 2006, p. 83). Reading personal narratives might be another way of beginning to explore how people experience the health and social services that they receive.

Refinement of communication skills is another way of connecting on a deeper level with people. Bright et al. (2012) described how being with, rather than doing to, people by using active listening skills allowed therapists to actualise a spirit of client-centredness. Occupational therapists can draw on communication approaches described by others such as evocative empathy, a technique of communication and counselling that intended to help people to 'feel deeply understood, especially at the emotional level' (Martin, 2010, p. 4). Consistent with a client-centred approach, the therapist, using evocative empathy, views people as empowered to solve their own problems and to create their own solutions and the therapist's role is to facilitate that problem-solving. Using structured ways of checking in to find out whether or not the client felt heard, respected and understood has been found to be useful for student occupational therapists interested in adjusting their approach to the therapeutic relationship (Wener et al., 2015).

Hope and Visions of Possibility/Future

Fostering hope and visions of possibility is an important aspect of client-centred occupational therapy practice (Cott, 2004; Hammell, 2007; Sumsion & Law, 2006; WFOT, 2010). Asking key questions when initiating discussions with people, such as, 'Who is this person? What do they feel they have lost? What are their dreams for the future?' (Bright et al., 2012, p. 5) may help to appreciate their past, understand their present, and assist them to plan for and envision their future. Originating in the field of organisational change management theory, one promising method of facilitating this exploration is appreciative inquiry (AI), 'a cooperative, coevolutionary search for the best in people, their organisations, and the world around them. [⋯] AI involves the art and practice of asking unconditionally positive questions that strengthen a system's capacity to apprehend, anticipate, and heighten positive potential' (Cooperrider & Whitney, 2005). Rubin, Kerrell, and Roberts (2011) taught AI principles to occupational therapy students and found that it allowed students to focus on what a person was good at in the past, on the person's strengths, wishes and hopes for the future, and on the person's potential.

Identifying Occupational Issues and Goal-setting

Identifying issues related to performance and engagement in occupations and developing goals for intervention are key aspects of many occupational therapy process models (American Occupational Therapy Association, 2014; Fearing, Law, & Clark, 1997; Polatajko & Townsend, 2007). Although the intent is to engage in collaborative decision-making and planning, this has not consistently been the experience of therapists or people receiving their services. Bright et al. (2012) reflected, 'We now believe that we played lip service to goal setting in our previous roles. We were often setting goals for people, goals that worked with what our service could offer. Safety, length of stay and discharge took priority' (p. 3). These challenges raise several questions: Who identifies the issues and how are they identified? What goals are set? Who sets parameters on what might be considered an 'appropriate goal'?

It is important to explore the methods used for identification of issues and goal-setting as an integral aspect of the occupational therapy process.

To work with people to establish goals for occupational therapy, client-centred assessments and goal-setting tools have been developed in the profession. When selecting client-centred assessment measures, McColl and Pollock (2005) provide some useful criteria: selected assessment and measurement should be based on a client's identified goals; the client is the only 'relevant frame of reference for therapy' and thus a client-centred assessment is self-report; and the therapist's role is to create the environment and opportunities for change (p. 81). Stevens, Beurskens, Koke, and van der Weijden (2013) reviewed the feasibility of 11 instruments commonly used for goal-setting, including the Canadian Occupational Performance Measure. Although many of the ways of learning about a client's perspective, hopes, and goals are language-based (e.g. through interviews or structured assessment tools), there is opportunity to use alternate, creative ways of understanding the client's perspective. For example, Bornman and Murphy (2006) described the use of 'talking mats' as a technique for goal-setting with people with communication challenges.

Establishing a Client-centred Practice

As occupational therapists embrace and internalise a spirit of client-centredness as part of their professional identity, it is a natural extension to examine their world with this lens. If respect and a commitment to redress power imbalances are core constructs of client-centredness, examining the practice settings of occupational therapists for indicators of a practice that is client-centred and advocating for the inclusion of client-centred services, policies and mission statements helps to reconcile differences between the therapists' core values and practice experiences (Restall et al., 2003). What opportunities do therapists have that allow them to actualise respect, partnership or collaboration and redress issues of power imbalance at the practice setting level? How might therapists examine the power that is exerted through documents, policies and systems? And how might doing so help therapists to establish practice that is increasingly client-centred?

The importance of institutional, management and peer support in influencing therapists' abilities to practice in a client-centred manner must be emphasised (Sumsion & Lencucha, 2009; Sumsion & Smyth, 2000; Wressle & Samuelsson, 2004). A management philosophy and commitment to an organisation that is client-centred rather than profession-centred creates a culture where client-centred practice can evolve (Cott, 2004; Papadimitriou & Cott, 2015; Wilkins et al., 2001). However, organisational factors such as lack of time and privacy, lack of team awareness of client-centred practice, and systems factors such as the requirement for referral (Krizaj & Hurst, 2012) or competing health systems priorities (Bright et al., 2012) can create barriers. The push and pull of client-centred practice at the practice setting level was described by Durocher et al. (2015): 'While there is a systematic push to provide client-centred practice and an intrinsic pull towards it for health care professionals based on their training and ethics, systemic policies regulating the amount of time that healthcare professionals have to provide care and make discharge plans limit the potential for client-centred practice to be realized' (p. 7). This tension presents a challenge and opportunity – to take the knowledge of client-centredness and the skill of therapists in enacting client-centred approaches while working to reconcile the seeming incongruence between therapists' value of client-centredness and actualisation of client-centred practice.

Teams of professionals working together to address the complex health and social needs of people are becoming increasingly common (Gachoud, Albert, Kuper, Stroud, & Reeves, 2012), and occupational therapists are often key members of these teams. Cohesive, collaborative and effectively communicating teams are an important factor in client-centred practice (Papadimitriou & Cott, 2015; Sumsion & Lencucha, 2009). Collaborative 'patient-centred' practice is a movement focused on how health care professionals from different disciplines can come together to meet the needs of the person they centre around, with the ultimate aim of improving the client's and service provider's satisfaction and the client's outcomes (Herbert, 2005). Given increasing emphasis on interprofessional education and care provision, it is important to consider how other disciplines perceive client-centred practice. In a concept analysis of the terms *client-, family-, patient-, person-* and *relationship-centred care* over a 20-year span and in various disciplines, including occupational therapy, Hughes et al. (2008) p. 458 identified 10 common concepts. These were respect for individual values, uniqueness of the individual, therapeutic relationship, importance of social context and relationships, holistic understanding of the individual, valuing the person as expert, shared responsibility, communication, respect for autonomy, and the professional as a person. Although it appears that different professional groups are generally speaking the same language, there may be different emphasis placed on each of the concepts by members of different professions (Gachoud et al., 2012) or culture-based differences in terms of understanding and application of the concepts (Lamiani et al., 2008). It is important to engage in team discussions to ensure all members are 'speaking the same language' about client-centred practice.

The CSF strategy *influencing practice settings* refers to the creation of environments that facilitate client-centred practice where people feel empowered and respected and are provided with meaningful choice. The suggested strategies address the broader practice and organisational issues that influence the ways that therapists practice on a day-to-day basis (Restall et al., 2003). Reflecting on their practice setting as a way of examining how the institutions and systems within which occupational therapists work promote or prevent client-centred practice is one approach to increase awareness of the influence of various factors (Carrier, Freeman, Levasseur, & Desrosiers, 2015; Mortenson & Dyck, 2006). For example, Phoenix and Vanderkaay (2015) described undertaking a critical examination of the structures and systems that constrained client-centred practice in their workplace by examining two of the action points of an occupational therapy process model in the context of a practice scenario of a mother and child seeking occupational therapy services. Similarly, Carrier et al. (2015) critiqued the use of standardised referral forms on the scope and nature of community occupational therapy practice, concluding that the referral form and process were structured to meet the needs of the employer, institution and team rather than the needs of the client receiving services.

A lot can be learned from the experiences of people receiving therapy services on the nature of client-centred services. There are tools that can be used to seek this input (e.g. the Client-centred Rehabilitation Questionnaire; Cott, Teare, McGilton, & Lineker, 2006). In addition to gathering the opinion of the client receiving the services, therapists should also consider how they might advocate for the establishment and maintenance of client-centred environments by including people who receive services in positions of influence and decision making at an organisational level (Papadimitriou & Cott, 2015; Sumsion & Lencucha, 2009) and working to ensure accessibility of, and flexibility in, service delivery (Law et al., 1995; McKinnon, 2000; Sumsion & Lencucha, 2009). Finding ways to include the perspectives of people receiving services is important in actualising respect and sharing of power.

Addressing Client-centredness in the Macro Environment

There is a growing call for expanding occupational therapists' client-centred thinking and applying these ideas at macro levels to address the social determinants of health (Fleming-Castaldy, 2015; Hammell & Iwama, 2012; Pitonyak, Mroz, & Fogelberg, 2015; Restall & Ripat, 2008). Client-centred practice at the macro level addresses the duality of meeting the individual needs of people while simultaneously addressing broader determinants of health and well-being (Fleming-Castaldy, 2015). Recognising the 'constraints on client-centred practice imposed by social, economic, and political inequities and entrenched barriers to participation' (Fleming-Castaldy, 2015, p. 1) offers another opportunity for extension of the professional value of client-centredness. However, the idea of addressing client-centredness at a macro level is daunting for some, particularly if occupational therapists perceive they lack knowledge, skill and opportunity to address broader community, systems and political issues (Restall & Ripat, 2008).

Using the client-centred concepts of respect and power, therapists can think creatively about ways they might work to address client-centred practice at a macro level. Although therapists will still need to wrestle with the same issues (Who is receiving services? What are the best ways to collaborate? How are decisions made?), they can apply their understanding to address issues at the macro level (i.e. health, social, education and justice levels) that relate to communities and populations of people (Phelan, 2011). Through use of strategies such as community organising and coalition advocacy/political action (Restall et al., 2003), therapists can have widespread influence on client-centred practice. Working with a community organisation to address issues of health literacy for recent immigrants, assisting in the development of housing first initiatives for people who are homeless or advocating to decision-makers for improved playground accessibility are all examples of ways that therapists can actualise their client-centred practice ideas at a macro level.

One approach is to start at the micro (individual) level and progress to the macro (community/population/systems) level (Phelan, 2011; Wolf, Ripat, Davis, Becker, & MacSwiggan, 2010). Wolf et al. (2010) introduced a framework for doing just this by framing a client's issue in occupational justice terms focused on the 'environment and systems barriers that prevent the client from engaging in occupations that promote health and quality of life' (p. 15). Applying this framework, occupational therapists are then encouraged to consider the reasons for the occupational injustice in broader terms and their own avenues of influence and then to take action based on these considerations. Students have reported the value of addressing client-centred practice at a macro level in terms of their ability to broadly influence change, collaborate with agencies that had shared interest in addressing structural and system barriers to occupation, and practice skills of collaboration, risk-taking and advocacy (Wener et al., 2014). Through such an analysis, students learn that addressing client-centredness in macro environments is built on the same foundation as addressing client-centredness at an individual level: respect for the needs and expertise of those receiving services, engaging and using respectful communication skills to learn about these people, considering how context influences opportunity and engaging in meaningful partnerships focused on visions of possibility.

Power, Advocacy and Avenues of Influence

Advocacy is a key strategy that client-centred occupational therapists can use with a client (Dhillon et al., 2010) in a practice setting (Mortenson & Dyck, 2006) and at broader systems levels. Advocacy has been defined as a 'client-centred strategy involving a variety of actions taken by the client and therapist, directed to the client's environment to enact change for the client such that engagement in occupation is enhanced through meeting basic human rights or improving quality of life' (Dhillon et al., 2010, p. 246). At a macro level, occupational therapists are encouraged to use their advocacy skills to 'influence persons of influence' and to collaborate with, and support, communities, groups and organisations that value and uphold client-centred principles (Restall et al., 2003, p. 106).

CONCLUSION

Occupational therapists have long espoused a commitment to client-centredness and a practice that is client-centred.

Centred on key aspects of respect for people and a commitment to a consideration of power dynamics, occupational therapists have been leaders in exploring these concepts. Nevertheless, although an espoused commitment is admirable, it is not enough if therapists are unable to put their values into action in ways that address the needs of people receiving their services. Exploring their own commitment to, and understanding of, client-centredness is the first step. However, although their practice as occupational therapists often starts with the client, it expands far beyond into practice environments, community and societal settings. It is in each of these realms that therapists have both obligation and opportunity to actualise the spirit of client-centredness.

The profession is entering into a new era of client-centred practice, where the term is widely used as a central and guiding tenet of many other health care providers, systems and organizations. Occupational therapists have learned much about client-centred practice that they can share with other professions and like-minded organisations or systems interested in this concept. Occupational therapists connected within their local and global communities can seek opportunities to apply client-centred ideas beyond the individual level to also include the social and political influences that limit occupational opportunities for people. There are countless opportunities to take client-centred ideas and apply them through occupational therapy practice and processes. Occupational therapists are creative, innovative and actively focused on how they can enable occupation through a spirit of client-centredness. These are truly exciting times. A new chapter in occupational therapy's client-centred journey is about to begin.

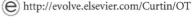 http://evolve.elsevier.com/Curtin/OT

REFERENCES

Aguilar, A., Stupans, I., Scutter, S., & King, S. (2013). Towards a definition of professionalism in Australian occupational therapy: Using the Delphi technique to obtain consensus on essential values and behaviours. *Australian Occupational Therapy Journal*, *60*(3), 206–216.

Ajjawi, R., & Higgs, J. (2008). Learning to reason: A journey of professional socialisation. *Advances in Health Sciences Education: Theory and Practice*, *13*(2), 133–150.

American Occupational Therapy Association (2014). Occupational therapy practice framework: Domain & process, 3rd edition. *American Journal of Occupational Therapy*, *68*, S1–S48.

Blank, A. (2004). Clients' experience of partnership with occupational therapists in community mental health. *British Journal of Occupational Therapy*, *67*(3), 118–124.

Bornman, J., & Murphy, J. (2006). Using the ICF in goal setting: Clinical application using Talking Mats. *Disability and Rehabilitation Assistive Technology*, *1*(3), 145–154.

Bozarth, J. D. (2008). Client centered therapy and the person-centered approach. In K. Jordan (Ed.), *The quick theory reference guide: A resource for expert and novice mental health professionals* (pp. 63–81). New York: Nova Science Publishers.

Bright, F. A., Boland, P., Rutherford, S. J., Kayes, N. M., & McPherson, K. M. (2012). Implementing a client-centred approach in rehabilitation: An autoethnography. *Disability and Rehabilitation*, *34*(12), 997–1004.

Cameron, J. J., & McColl, M. A. (2015). Learning client-centred practice short report: Experience of OT students interacting with 'expert patients'. *Scandinavian Journal of Occupational Therapy*, *22*(4), 322–324.

Canadian Association of Occupational Therapists, & Department of National Health and Welfare (1983). *Guidelines for the client-centred practice of occupational therapy H39-33/1983E*. Ottaw: Department of National Health and Welfare.

Carrier, A., Freeman, A., Levasseur, M., & Desrosiers, J. (2015). Standardized referral form: Restricting client-centered practice? *Scandinavian Journal of Occupational Therapy*, *22*(4), 283–292.

Clark, F. A. (2010). Power and confidence in professions: Lessons for occupational therapy. *Canadian Journal of Occupational Therapy*, *77*(5), 264–269.

Cooperrider, D., & Whitney, D. D. (2005). *Appreciative inquiry: A positive revolution in change*. San Francisco: Berrett-Koehler Publishers.

Corring, D. J., & Cook, J. V. (1999). Client-centred care means that I am a valued human being. *Canadian Journal of Occupational Therapy*, *66*(2), 71–82.

Cott, C. A. (2004). Client-centred rehabilitation: Client perspectives. *Disability and Rehabilitation*, *26*(24), 1411–1422.

Cott, C. A., Teare, G., McGilton, K. S., & Lineker, S. (2006). Reliability and construct validity of the client-centred rehabilitation questionnaire. *Disability and Rehabilitation*, *28*(22), 1387–1397.

Crepeau, E. B., & Garren, K. R. (2011). I looked to her as a guide: The therapeutic relationship in hand therapy. *Disability and Rehabilitation*, *33*(10), 872–881.

Dhillon, S. K., Wilkins, S., Law, M. C., Stewart, D. A., & Tremblay, M. (2010). Advocacy in occupational therapy: Exploring clinicians' reasons and experiences of advocacy. *Canadian Journal of Occupational Therapy*, *77*(4), 241–248.

Duggan, R. (2005). Reflection as a means to foster client-centred practice. *Canadian Journal of Occupational Therapy*, *72*(2), 103–112.

Durocher, E., Kinsella, E. A., Ells, C., & Hunt, M. (2015). Contradictions in client-centred discharge planning: Through the lens of relational autonomy. *Scandinavian Journal of Occupational Therapy*, *22*(4), 293–301.

Falardeau, M., & Durand, M. J. (2002). Negotiation-centred versus client-centred: Which approach should be used? *Canadian Journal of Occupational Therapy*, *69*(3), 135–142.

Fearing, V. G., Law, M., & Clark, J. (1997). An occupational performance process model: Fostering client and therapist alliances. *Canadian Journal of Occupational Therapy*, *64*(1), 7–15.

Fleming-Castaldy, R. P. (2015). A macro perspective for client-centred practice in curricula: Critique and teaching methods. *Scandinavian Journal of Occupational Therapy*, *22*(4), 267–276.

Gachoud, D., Albert, M., Kuper, A., Stroud, L., & Reeves, S. (2012). Meanings and perceptions of patient-centeredness in social work, nursing and medicine: A comparative study. *Journal of Interprofessional Care*, *26*(6), 484–490.

Hammell, K. W. (2007). Experience of rehabilitation following spinal cord injury: A meta-synthesis of qualitative findings. *Spinal Cord*, 45(4), 260–274.

Hammell, K. R. (2013). Client-centred occupational therapy in Canada: Refocusing on core values. *Canadian Journal of Occupational Therapy*, 80(3), 141–149.

Hammell, K. R. W. (2015). Client-centred occupational therapy: The importance of critical perspectives. *Scandinavian Journal of Occupational Therapy*, 22(4), 237–243.

Hammell, K. R. W., & Iwama, M. K. (2012). Well-being and occupational rights: An imperative for critical occupational therapy. *Scandinavian Journal of Occupational Therapy*, 19(5), 385–394.

Hedberg-Kristensson, E., & Iwarsson, S. (2013). Therapist attitudes and strategies to client-centred approaches in the provision of mobility devices to older clients. *Disability and Rehabilitation Assistive Technology*, 8(5), 381–386.

Hedge, N., Neville, M. A., & Pickens, N. (2015). How patient educators teach students: 'Giving a face to a story'. *The Open Journal of Occupational Therapy*, 3(1), 1–10.

Herbert, C. P. (2005). Changing the culture: Interprofessional education for collaborative patient-centred practice in Canada. *Journal of Interprofessional Care*, 19(Suppl. 1), 1–4.

Hoppes, S., Hamilton, T. B., & Robinson, C. (2007). A course in auto-ethnography: Fostering reflective practitioners in occupational therapy. *Occupational Therapy in Health Care*, 21(1–2), 133–143.

Hughes, J. C., Bamford, C., & May, C. (2008). Types of centredness in health care: Themes and concepts. *Medicine, Health Care, and Philosophy*, 11(4), 455–463.

Jamieson, M., Krupa, T., O'Riordan, A., et al. (2006). Developing empathy as a foundation of client-centred practice: Evaluation of a university curriculum initiative. *Canadian Journal of Occupational Therapy*, 73(2), 76–85.

Kjellberg, A., Kahlin, I., Haglund, L., & Taylor, R. R. (2012). The myth of participation in occupational therapy: Reconceptualizing a client-centred approach. *Scandinavian Journal of Occupational Therapy*, 19(5), 421–427.

Krizaj, T., & Hurst, J. (2012). Perceptions of a client-centred approach among Slovenian occupational therapists. *International Journal of Therapy & Rehabilitation*, 19(2), 70–78.

Lamiani, G., Meyer, E. C., Rider, E. A., et al. (2008). Assumptions and blind spots in patient-centredness: Action research between American and Italian health care professionals. *Medical Education*, 42(7), 712–720.

Law, M., Baptiste, S., & Mills, J. (1995). Client-centred practice: What does it mean and does it make a difference? *Canadian Journal of Occupational Therapy*, 62(5), 250–257.

Mackey, H. (2014). Living tensions: Reconstructing notions of professionalism in occupational therapy. *Australian Occupational Therapy Journal*, 61(3), 168–176.

Maitra, K. K., & Erway, F. (2006). Perception of client-centered practice in occupational therapists and their clients. *American Journal of Occupational Therapy*, 60(3), 298–310.

Martin, D. G. (2010). *Counselling & therapy skills* (3rd ed.). Long Grove, IL: Waveland Press.

McColl, M. A., & Pollock, N. (2005). Measuring occupational performance using a client-centred perspective. In M. Law, C. Baum, & W. Dunn (Eds.), *Measuring occupational performance: Supporting best practice in occupational therapy* (pp. 81–92). (2nd ed.). Thorofare, NJ: Slack.

McCorquodale, L., & Kinsella, E. A. (2015). Critical reflexivity in client-centred therapeutic relationships. *Scandinavian Journal of Occupational Therapy*, 22(4), 311–317.

McKinnon, A. L. (2000). Client values and satisfaction with occupational therapy. *Scandinavian Journal of Occupational Therapy*, 7(3), 99–106.

Moats, G. (2007). Discharge decision-making, enabling occupations, and client-centred practice. *Canadian Journal of Occupational Therapy*, 74(2), 91–101.

Mortenson, W. B., & Dyck, I. (2006). Power and client-centred practice: An insider exploration of occupational therapists' experiences. *Canadian Journal of Occupational Therapy*, 73(5), 261–271.

Palmadottir, G. (2003). Client perspectives on occupational therapy in rehabilitation services. *Scandinavian Journal of Occupational Therapy*, 10(4), 157–166.

Palmadottir, G. (2006). Client-therapist relationships: Experiences of occupational therapy clients in rehabilitation. *British Journal of Occupational Therapy*, 69(9), 394–401.

Papadimitriou, C., & Cott, C. (2015). Client-centred practices and work in inpatient rehabilitation teams: Results from four case studies. *Disability and Rehabilitation*, 37(13), 1–9.

Phelan, S. K. (2011). Constructions of disability: A call for critical reflexivity in occupational therapy. *Canadian Journal of Occupational Therapy*, 78(3), 164–172.

Phoenix, M., & Vanderkaay, S. (2015). Client-centred occupational therapy with children: A critical perspective. *Scandinavian Journal of Occupational Therapy*, 22(4), 318–321.

Pitonyak, J. S., Mroz, T. M., & Fogelberg, D. (2015). Expanding client-centred thinking to include social determinants: A practical scenario based on the occupation of breastfeeding. *Scandinavian Journal of Occupational Therapy*, 22(4), 277–282.

Pizzi, M. A. (2015). Promoting health and well-being at the end of life through client-centered care. *Scandinavian Journal of Occupational Therapy*, 22(6), 442–449.

Polatajko, H., & Townsend, E. (2007). *Enabling occupation II: Advancing an occupational therapy vision for health, well-being & justice through occupation*. Ottawa: CAOT Publications.

Power. (n.d.). In *Merriam-Webster On-line*. Retrieved August 3, 2016 from http://www.merriam-webster.com/dictionary/power.

Purtilo, R., & Haddad, A. (2002). *Health professional and patient interaction* (6th ed.). Philadelphia: Elsevier.

Rebeiro, K. L. (2000). Client perspectives on occupational therapy practice: Are we truly client-centred? *Canadian Journal of Occupational Therapy*, 67(1), 7–14.

Restall, G., & Ripat, J. (2008). Applicability and clinical utility of the Client-Centred Strategies Framework. *Canadian Journal of Occupational Therapy*, 75(5), 288–300.

Restall, G., Ripat, J., & Stern, M. (2003). A framework of strategies for client-centred practice. *Canadian Journal of Occupational Therapy*, 70(2), 103–112.

Richard, L., & Knis-Matthews, L. (2010). Are we really client-centered? Using the Canadian Occupational Performance

Measure to see how the client's goals connect with the goals of the occupational therapist. *Occupational Therapy in Mental Health, 26*(1), 51–66.

Ripat, J., Wener, P., & Dobinson, K. (2013). The development of client-centredness in student occupational therapists. *British Journal of Occupational Therapy, 76*(5), 217–224.

Rubin, R., Kerrell, R., & Roberts, G. (2011). Appreciative inquiry in occupational therapy education. *British Journal of Occupational Therapy, 74*(5), 233–240.

Stevens, A., Beurskens, A., Koke, A., & van der Weijden, T. (2013). The use of patient-specific measurement instruments in the process of goal-setting: A systematic review of available instruments and their feasibility. *Clinical Rehabilitation, 27*(11), 1005–1019.

Sumsion, T. (2000). A revised occupational therapy definition of client-centred practice. *British Journal of Occupational Therapy, 63*(7), 304–309.

Sumsion, T. (Ed.). (2006). *Client-centred practice in occupational therapy: A guide to implementation.* (2nd ed.). Philadelphia: Churchill Livingstone.

Sumsion, T., & Law, M. (2006). A review of evidence on the conceptual elements informing client-centred practice. *Canadian Journal of Occupational Therapy, 73*(3), 153–162.

Sumsion, T., & Lencucha, R. (2009). Therapists' perceptions of how teamwork influences client-centred practice. *British Journal of Occupational Therapy, 72*(2), 48–54.

Sumsion, T., & Smyth, G. (2000). Barriers to client-centredness and their resolution. *Canadian Journal of Occupational Therapy, 67*(1), 15–21.

Toal-Sullivan, D. (2006). New graduates' experiences of learning to practise occupational therapy. *British Journal of Occupational Therapy, 69*(11), 513–524.

Wener, P. F., Bergen, C. O., Diamond-Burchuk, L. G., Yamamoto, C. M., Hosegood, A. E., & Staley, J. D. (2015). Enhancing student occupational therapists' client-centred counselling skills. *Canadian Journal of Occupational Therapy, 82*(5), 307–315.

Wener, P., Ripat, J., Johnson, L., et al. (2014). Students as change agents in macro environments. *Occupational Therapy Now, 16*(2), 6–7.

Wilkins, S., Pollock, N., Rochon, S., & Law, M. (2001). Implementing client-centred practice: Why is it so difficult to do? *Canadian Journal of Occupational Therapy, 68*(2), 70–79.

Wolf, L., Ripat, J., Davis, E., Becker, P., & MacSwiggan, J. (2010). Theory meets practice: Applying an occupational justice framework. *Occupational Therapy Now, 12*(1), 15–18.

World Federation of Occupational Therapists (2010). *Position statement on client-centredness in occupational therapy. Retrieved from (2010).* http://www.fsa.se/Global/Om_forbundet/Internationellt/Position%20statement%20on%20Client-centredness%20in%20Occupational%20Therapy,2010.pdf.

Wressle, E., & Samuelsson, K. (2004). Barriers and bridges to client-centred occupational therapy in Sweden. *Scandinavian Journal of Occupational Therapy, 11*(1), 12–16.

6

COMMUNICATION IN OCCUPATIONAL THERAPY PRACTICE

SUE BAPTISTE

Abstract
The complex context of the interview is centrally important to excellence in person-centred occupational therapy practice. This chapter provides an overview of foundational concepts, frameworks and tools and enables an exploration of the complexities of communicating with people. The many facets of a person-centred approach to delivering occupational therapy services and the importance of enhancing self-awareness in order to enable the process to unfold naturally are presented. Understanding people's stories, hearing their descriptions of what are the central meanings and purposes of their lives, is the essence of the occupational therapy philosophy. *Fact-finding* and *interviewing* are terms that connote a clear, firm process of establishing 'true' data in an ordered and systematic fashion. Such ventures as part of the therapeutic enterprise have their place, but not perhaps at the initial interface between therapist and person. At that first point of contact, the important thing is to create a context for respectful interaction, fertile ground for a solid basis for understanding and mutual problem-solving.

KEY POINTS

■ Understanding individuals' stories, hearing their descriptions of the central meaning and purpose of their lives, is the essence of the occupational therapy philosophy.

■ Common elements of person-centred practice include: respect, partnership, collaboration, and an entrenched belief that the person is central to the endeavour of delivering the needed services.

■ The idea of practitioner personal empowerment is also one that translates well into person-centred practice, supporting the development of therapeutic partnerships with people requiring occupational therapy services and their families.

■ Communication is the basis on which health care delivery is predicated.

■ Identification of occupational performance issues is the unique perspective that is offered by engagement in a person–therapist relationship within occupational therapy.

INTRODUCTION

The profession of occupational therapy has undergone many changes over the period of its almost 100 year history, not the least of which is the most recent return to the foundational principles and pride in the occupational nature of practice. In concert with the notion of occupation being central to practice is the intention to establish a partnership between individuals and therapists. Similarly, many countries in which occupational therapists practice have embraced a regulatory model for health professions that provides protection for the public related to the services they receive from regulated professions. This trend has necessitated that individual practitioners recognise the importance of lifelong learning to ensure ongoing competence, thus engendering expectations for a conscious and aware approach to practice, acceptance of professional autonomy and accountability. The complex nature of contemporary practice is even more complicated by the contexts in which occupational therapists work. Employers and workplaces have expectations that staff will work together in interprofessional teams with common goals focusing on quality person care. At the same time, individual professionals strive to maintain their own professional mandate and philosophy. To create the context for a discussion about interviewing and information gathering, a review of foundational concepts would seem to be useful.

Through an exploration of foundational concepts, a ready appreciation can be gained regarding the complex nature of what occupational therapy practitioners do, as well as what is expected of them. Practice should be person-centred, occupation-based, acknowledge personal autonomy, and most often undertaken within a team-driven workplace or at the least within a context where communication with colleagues is essential. Thus there emerges an increased awareness of the critical importance of accurate information to enable the best care to be provided to the individuals who seek occupational therapy services.

Person-centred Practice

The origins of the central concept of client-centred practice can be traced to the ground-breaking work of Carl Rogers, which has formed a strong foundation for contemporary occupational therapy practice (Law, Baptiste, & Mills, 1995). This approach to working with people revolves around the notion of partnership, mutual regard, the art of listening and a commitment to identifying intervention priorities from the issues raised by each individual. It is from these principles that the use of *client* was chosen, perhaps a word that creates some dis-ease for many, but which does suggest a service partnership rather than a hierarchical power-based relationship of expert and patient (Law, 1998).

The emerging concept of person-centred care is similar to client-centred practice but focuses centrally on collaboration across all partners involved in the delivery of care to an individual or family. It also stresses the importance of seeing the professional as someone needing support and consideration in similar ways as the individuals receiving the service. Evidence would suggest that this multifaceted concept is showing a connection to positive health outcomes (Mead & Bower, 2000; Tinney et al., 2007) from the perspective of enhanced communication between people receiving health services and professionals as well as showing proof of the importance and relevance of education to enhance understanding of person-centred care.

Similarities between the two constructs are many; however, the additional term *patient-centred care* complicates the debate further. From an occupational therapy perspective, *client* has become the adopted term because there was a concern that *patient* tended to connote more of a passive relationship rather than a shared partnership. Conversely, concerns were also voiced that *client* painted more of a picture of a business relationship, thus creating an imbalance in power and influence that may affect the therapeutic alliance in a negative fashion because 'the client is always right'. There are common elements of client-centred care to guide us forwards, thus relinquishing the need to use the term *patient*. These common elements include: respect, partnership, collaboration and an entrenched belief that the patient or client is central to the endeavour of delivering the needed services. In the immediate context of occupational therapy practice, the term *person-centred care* does offer an alternative with similar intent for those for whom *client* is not a word that fits into the practice context or is uncomfortable for the individual practitioner.

Occupation-based Practice

The roots of occupational therapy stem from the careful attention to occupations that had meaning for those engaged in them and for the environment in which they were undertaken and performed. Somewhere over time, the way was lost and the profession struggled to define a niche in a world that was ever increasing in its reductionist stance and search for measurable 'truth'. In such a context, value and worth were best defined from observable and provable actions rather than reflective and subjective relational thought. However, since the 1980s a major practice shift has been occurring, within which a return to the original investment and belief in occupation has been realised. Component-based practice remains a viable option for care when part of an overarching occupation-based approach. Even in the most scientifically rooted practice context (such as a burns unit, hand clinic or acute care ward), there is a clear commitment to embracing person-centred practice and thus a strong inclusion of concern for links to occupation for each person and his family.

Personal Autonomy

Another element that is of key importance to communication within occupational therapy practice is the concept of personal autonomy. The central intent of personal autonomy is for an individual to possess personal rule over himself or herself while remaining free from controlling interference by others. The autonomous person acts with comfort in engaging with freely self-chosen plans and actions, the choices of which are guided by values, beliefs, knowledge and skills in the selection of those plans and actions. A person with reduced autonomy, on the other hand, can be controlled by others or feel incapable of deliberating or acting on the basis of his or her own personal choices or preferences for action. This critical concept applies to both the therapist and the person receiving occupational therapy services within the therapeutic relationship; for the optimal relational 'fit' to exist and for it to be successful in meeting the person's need, this is a desired state. It is through the detailed and rigorous process of professional regulation that occupational therapy practitioners have a clear framework against which they can measure and assess their own practice, identifying learning gaps and areas for ongoing professional development. Many of these competencies are focused upon the individual's ability to practice in a person-centred, occupation-centred manner within an interprofessional context. This idea of personal empowerment is also one that translates well into person-centred practice, supporting the development of a therapeutic partnership.

Team-based Practice

Sound communication skills in teams are essential for supporting and advocating for the needs of each individual. Most health care professionals expect to work within a team or group within their workplace. In order to be a successful and valued team participant, there is a need to articulate a ready definition of one's unique contribution to the overall enterprise. Functioning within hierarchies is becoming less obvious, and the incidence of sole representatives of individual disciplines covering a wide scope of service delivery is becoming more and more common. Therefore the ability to recognise the value and worth of other team members while firmly providing one's own piece of the puzzle is an imperative of modern practice. Sound team relationships rely heavily on the abilities and willingness of members to value mutual respect and regard, honesty and open communication, which in turn will engender trust, thus facilitating excellence in care delivery. Therefore the importance of sound information gathering through rapport building, interviewing and interpretation of information within a person-centred framework is a vital precursor to advocating well for people and their families when relating to colleagues in a team environment.

STRATEGIES TO ENABLE COMMUNICATION

Given the four foundational concepts identified in the previous section, it would appear more appropriate to begin to talk about communicating rather than simply 'interviewing' to address the intention of developing communication skills more broadly. It can be applied across all relationships within the therapeutic endeavour, from colleagues and peers to people requiring occupational therapy services, such as families, agencies, students and others.

A discussion of and reflection upon the elements that constitute communication will help to establish a framework for the development of a personal approach to obtaining information through listening to people's stories. The central strategy for enabling communication involves the use and integration of several smaller strategies and the acquisition of skill sets related to enhanced self-awareness, enriched listening and hearing skills and a conscious application of person-centred values such as respect, regard and recognition of being in a mutual partnership with the person receiving occupational therapy services (Chant, Jenkinson, Randle, Russell, & Webb, 2002; Schirmer et al., 2005).

Individuals, throughout their lives, have been 'trained' how to behave and what to expect when attending appointments with doctors and other professionals. Only in recent years has there been a move towards a consumer-based and consumer-influenced approach to health care delivery (Eysenbach & Hadad, 2001), which dictates that health professionals should work together with the person, providing care in a mutual journey towards understanding the problem and what can be done about it. In order to be able to make that transition with relative ease, it is important that health professionals become aware of their own abilities, as professionals in their own right, to listen and hear what the people receiving services are telling them. The very nature of the occupational therapy profession is a narrative one; it is second nature to want to hear what is happening in the lives of people as told from their perspectives. It is only through this process that therapists can attempt to enter and understand people's lives to enable optimal outcomes and to ensure their engagement in occupations that are meaningful.

Therapists can begin to gain a sense of the importance of understanding another person's perspective when they consider their own situation. Therapists are encouraged to think of a time when they experienced particularly effective communication between themselves and someone else; a time when they were well attuned to each other; listening, supporting and responding to each other, helping to bring out the best in each other; and resulting in a particularly good and meaningful outcome. To understand the complexity of this situation, therapists should consider the following questions:

- What made it such a good experience?
- What did the therapist bring – qualities, skills, capacities – that contributed to this positive experience?
- What did the other person contribute that made it a successful and satisfying experience?
- In what ways did the setting, context or situation contribute?
- What lessons did the therapist take from the experience?

DEVELOPING COMMUNICATION SKILLS

A discussion of and reflection on the elements that constitute communication will help in the development of a personal approach to obtaining information through listening to the stories of people who receive occupational therapy services. Communication is the basis upon which health care delivery is predicated. Currently, there is much attention being paid to the development of communication skills by many health professional groups (Chant et al., 2002; Haidet & Paterniti, 2003; Schirmer et al., 2005). This attention stems from the importance of providing services that are relevant to individuals and their families, in a caring context of skilled professionals who listen well, respond with empathy and work collaboratively to ensure the best outcomes possible in the circumstance.

The following questions need to be considered in a conscious manner when establishing comfort and developing communication skills:

- What feeling is associated with the message being delivered?
- What *is* the key message?
- How does the manner in which the person tells the story impart the essence of it?

Active listening is the desired state for anyone engaged in attending to a person's story. This is indicated by using direct eye contact as appropriate, with a welcoming, facilitative posture; facial expressions should reflect a state of attentiveness while remaining open and nonjudgemental. Tone and volume of voice should be moderate, suggesting an understanding of the feelings and information being shared.

Perhaps one of the main difficulties in gaining awareness of personal practice skill levels relative to communication and relationship building is internalising the ability to reflect and act on the insights gained. This is particularly hard in the area of communication because of the complexity of the process and the number of potential influences on outcomes. Building any relationship is a process fraught with potential pitfalls; building a

therapeutic partnership is no exception, necessitating enhanced levels of self-awareness to provide individuals with quality input and an investment in the partnership (Chant et al., 2002).

Empathy and Sympathy

Empathy and sympathy are similar constructs that can be confusing. Empathy is the process of developing rapport through the ability to be intuitive to another person's feelings and to be cognisant of nonverbal cues. Sympathy, on the other hand, results in a person feeling sorry for another person. Many people respond negatively to sympathy and to sensing a feeling of being pitied. When working within a person-centred context, the ability to have an empathic stance is essential to the maintenance of partnership. Although empathy and sympathy are used interchangeably in the context of practitioner–client relationships, there are subtle differences.

Barriers to Communication

There can be many barriers to communication and they can reside in the environment within which the conversation or information-finding process is taking place. It is important to pay attention to the setting in which the interaction will take place, the manner in which the furniture is arranged and the comfort of the available seating. In addition, a positive communication environment is one within which there is a low noise level and more subtle lighting. The key to appreciating the impact of the immediate environment upon a conversation with a person is to be constantly aware and to check in with the person to ensure that comfort levels are such that the process can move forward in a positive fashion. It is also critical that language used to explore ideas with individuals is such that the use of forms, professional jargon or medical terminology is kept at a minimum while guarding against sounding pedantic or patronising.

Assumptions

Assumptions can be made, and often are, based on past experiences, perceptions, and observations thus influencing the manner in which a relationship unfolds. It is critical that practitioners develop an awareness of their personal values and beliefs, anything in their personal pasts that could have created certain biases, fears or a sense of dis-ease that might impinge upon their ability to listen respectfully and process new information. Similarly, working from an expert-centred framework, not a person-centred one, may influence the manner in which a person shares the information and how openly and naturally the story will evolve. Experiences are common where the person is asked what seem like interminable questions throughout which the person begins to feel more of an automaton than a human being, a repository of data rather than an individual with rich life stories to tell.

SPECIFIC AREAS OF COMMUNICATION REQUIRING EMERGENT SKILL SETS

As systems have become more and more sophisticated and technology has gained serious traction in society overall, it is essential for health professionals to redirect many communication efforts towards and through technological platforms. Along with this radical shift comes a necessity to gain totally new skills in many different domains including: keyboard, understanding software programs, negotiating the Internet and navigating the complexities of multiple social media options.

Additionally, while society is gaining in the use of everyday technology, the growth of multicultural environments is burgeoning. As the world becomes more and more accessible, with people moving across borders and boundaries either as voluntary immigrants or in response to unsafe, even dangerous conditions and seeking safe haven. Both of these conditions (advancing technology and growing multicultural contexts) bring certain communication imperatives that need to be addressed and integrated into existing person-centred health care environments in the role of a regulated health professional. Key elements will be identified as being valuable additions to the occupational therapy communication toolbox.

Virtual Communication

There are several different types of virtual communication. Consequently, there are differing protocols to be learned that support the core values and principles of person-centredness as well as ethical, boundaried professional practice.

Texting and Email

It is critical to keep a consistently professional tone within online messages. When emails are to become part of a person's file they need to be printed, scanned, and saved electronically. Any online documentation and communication must be undertaken through and saved on a secure system; email is not considered ideal so if necessary should consist of only the most essential information. Encryption and password protection are also required, with a person's information anonymized by applying a coding system. Personal details such as personal email addresses, cell phone and other contact numbers should not be shared with people receiving services and their families. The sharing of email addresses can be very convenient in relation to staying connected to people; therefore having one specific email for this type of communication can be a viable and sensible option. Nevertheless, the content of emails is considered to be part of the person's record and can be used as evidence in chart audits, court proceedings and so forth. It is essential that practitioners are in the habit of seeing everything said, written or done for people receiving their services as professional communication that be undertaken with that in mind.

There are many resources that outline best practice 'netiquette'; one that is simple and informative can be obtained from http://www.albion.com/netiquette/corerules.html. This particular resource is based on extrapolated information from a text by Shea (1994) and outlines the core skill set for online communication. If there are alternate ways of corresponding with colleagues regarding a person receiving services and other confidential information (face-to-face, telephone), then they remain an acceptable and often preferable method in professional practice.

Social Media

There are three central areas requiring vigilance pertaining to the use of social media.

Maintaining Professionalism. There should be no difference between the therapeutic partnerships that are established face-to-face and those that are played out online. It is also essential that decisions about posting are predicated on information that the health professional is comfortable making public. If there is a sense of uncertainty, then the advice is to be conservative rather than take a risk.

Ensuring Personal Privacy and Confidentiality. Decisions made related to the area of privacy and confidentiality need to be informed by the policies and protocols of the associated facility as well as the regulations articulated by any relevant professional college. Every social medium platform has privacy settings that should be read and applied at the very least. In addition, informed consent must be obtained from the person receiving services before anything is posted.

Communication. Any language used online should be clear, simply expressed and devoid of short forms and colloquialisms. An interesting point that has been raised is to suggest strongly that once a maximum of three interactions has been reached, one is best advised to move the conversation to the telephone or face-to-face.

Tele-health. The term *tele-health* refers to the group of communication methods that enable health care consultations, interviews and some examinations to be completed through technological means. This can be facilitative to therapists when they are working with people who live in remote locations. When reassessments are required or a judgement requested about readiness for discharge, and if distances are far, then using technological methods (e.g. Skype, telephone conference) can be sound alternatives. There are differing schools of thought about the use of distance communication methods when working with people particularly within the health care system. A decrease in personal contact can potentially increase a sense of isolation and being disconnected. Managing an empathic conversation with no visual connection can be extremely difficult; what is said can often be misconstrued based on tone of voice, sound level of delivery and the use of language. Nevertheless, using distance technology can be timely when a quick response is required and there are no limits on distance to consider with technologies that know no global boundaries.

CULTURAL COMMUNICATION

Tomas and Inkson (2003) wrote about the construct of cultural intelligence that has assisted in heightening understanding and sensitivity to the complexities of communicating with people from other regions and countries. As they stated, 'Most people operate interpersonally in a condition of "cruise control", in which their experiences are interpreted from the standpoint of their own culture' (p. 21). This is not the place in which to engage in a discussion of what is culture, however fascinating it may be; but it is essential that, as health professionals working with people at their most vulnerable, occupational therapists become aware of the need to practise with respect, knowledge and sensitivity to people's cultural contexts. When speaking of culture, the meaning of *culture* is not limited to ethnicity or race, but rather refers to the following insight offered by Tomas and Inkson (2003): 'Culture is not just a set of surface behaviours, it is deeply imbedded in all of us. The surface features of our social behaviour – for example, our mannerisms, our ways of speaking to each other, the way we dress – are often manifestations of deep culturally based values and principles' (p. 22).

Culture is an important element of daily life, but it can be difficult to raise cultural issues during a conversation. Within groups and between seemingly similar groups there are cultural differences that can be unrecognised or at least not understood. These statements have direct relevance to working within health care environments where professionals from different disciplines, possibly from different countries or ethnic groups, with differing values, have external expectations that they will apply best practices in delivering quality care to clients. For this to become an established reality, there is an important skill set that these team members would do well to develop; that is, the sensitivity and awareness of cultural difference, the ability to respect and value diversity and to integrate this cultural intelligence into their communication and relationship-building with colleagues, clients and families. Communication is a complex vehicle but one that is fundamentally essential; it is not difficult to appreciate then how cultural differences (of all kinds) can and do lead to misunderstanding. The following examples of nodes of difficulty will help to add clarity to this discussion.

Individualism versus Collectivism

In countries and groups with cultures that are termed *individualistic*, the focus of concern is the self, the immediate sphere of influence of the person. Conversely, those environments that are considered *collectivistic* are founded upon values of the community or at least of the group. Canada tends to be more individualistic, whereas India and the Philippines are examples of collectivistic cultures. This difference can have a marked impact on the manner in which communication can take place in the partnership between a person and a health professional.

Power Distance

Power distance refers to the perceived distance between those at the top of the hierarchy and others at different levels of the pyramid. Overall, there tends to be less attention paid to hierarchies in Canada and the United States of America – in fact, in Western countries overall. Deference between a department head, a new staff member and a student rarely is observable. It is more a matter of perceived respect as one would have hopefully for anyone who is new to one's contacts or from whom a person hopes to learn. However, many lands that were colonised still retain certain behaviours from that period of colonisation, one of which is serious attention being paid to position and title. It is not unusual to receive letters or messages sent by individuals from India or Malaysia, for example, with long salutations and sounding somewhat obsequious. These communication patterns can leave a faulty impression with the recipient of the message of which the sender is totally oblivious.

Uncertainty Avoidance

The more structure that exists within an organisation or a system, the less chance there is perceived to be of mistakes being made or oversights happening. Form and expectations are valued by those coming from cultures of more orderliness and lines of authority than those where flexibility, proactiveness and responsiveness is expected and appreciated. There are often examples cited where new immigrants are seen to be nonassertive or reticent, with little 'get up and go'. In reality, they are being what they believe is respectful and awaiting directions about what comes next.

Masculinity/Femininity

The concept of *masculinity/femininity* refers to the societal balance that exists between male and female traditional roles. This can be illustrated through the notions of ambition and achievement being valued in men, whereas nurturance and the maintenance of relational harmony is deemed to be desirable attributes for women.

DIMENSIONS OF COMMUNICATION

There are many key domains of day-to-day communications that can be the source of much misunderstanding in relationship building. Consideration of these can inform and clarify and thus avoid misunderstandings and unfortunate interpretations or reactions. As these terms are presented here, consider personal experiences that could be linked to these concepts and for which understanding has remained a mystery.

Time

Some cultures and societies expect timeliness, often becoming uncomfortable when an interviewee, for example, is even 5 minutes late. On the other hand, other cultures value more flexibility in scheduling. People may find it very important to have the opportunity to spend the amount of time felt necessary for interactions.

Handshake

For hundreds of years, a handshake has been seen as a behaviour suggesting respect and a positive approach to meeting the other. Of late, the handshake has undergone much scrutiny as a social expectation because of global virulent diseases and a wish to protect oneself. Also, there have been increases in cultural and religious groups travelling more widely where preferred ways of relating in public are markedly different from those within the host country; these ways of being include strict rules of interaction that do not include men touching women, or often women communicating with men at all. Upon meeting initially it is a universal hope that each individual will be respectful to the individuals other as the minimal acceptable behaviour. However, discovering what 'respect' means in a particular context is a critical element of building successful relationships across borders.

Personal Space

Personal space can be a very difficult communication element to assess. Too close and a person tends to feel somewhat threatened or challenged by the other, stepping backwards to regain more distance; too far away and one runs the risk of being seen as superior or unapproachable. It is often best to consider the other person in this transaction, watching his or her behaviour and taking a lead from there.

Gestures and Body Language

The domain of body language can be riddled with potholes and chances for social misunderstandings. Many simple gestures can invite vastly different interpretations in different cultures; a raised thumb, for instance, a frown or looking into the distance. It is by far best to avoid making these potential social faux pas and containing enthusiasm or passion for the topic of conversation. Smiling at someone is generally construed as a friendly sign in North America and Europe; however, elsewhere globally it is often a sign of embarrassment. Conversely, not smiling can suggest aloofness. Eye contact is measured as a sign of confidence and trustworthiness, but lack of eye contact can suggest the reverse. Also, maintaining eye contact for lengthy periods is often construed as challenging. Head nodding means different things in different places, so it is best to clarify meaning if uncomfortable feelings or reactions are experienced.

FRAMEWORKS TO GUIDE THE SEARCH FOR UNDERSTANDING AND ESTABLISHING RELATIONSHIPS

For the purposes of the discussion here, the focus will be on two tools that represent structures and processes to guide the understanding of a person's circumstance and provide a framework for developing foci for intervention. These frameworks are the Calgary Cambridge Model of History Taking (CCMHT) (http://skillscascade.com 2007) and the Canadian Occupational Performance Measure (COPM) (Law et al., 1990).

The Calgary Cambridge Model of History Taking

The CCMHT (Table 6.1) is a framework designed to clarify the steps and stages along the process of history taking in medicine (Haidet & Paterniti, 2003; Kurtz, Silverman, & Draper, 2005). Although occupational therapists focus on building a story rather than taking a history, a brief overview of the defined steps can assist in understanding the core elements of the basic process.

This approach has been embraced widely by medical practice in many countries with some gratifying resulting trends. The literature indicates that better physician communication skills result in heightened satisfaction of, and outcomes for, the person receiving services and that such skills can be taught (Kurtz et al., 2005; Susuki Laidlaw, MacLeod, Kaufman, Langille, & Sargeant, 2002).

The kinds of information that are of importance to occupational therapists are different from the core information needs of physicians, although there are some areas of commonality. Commonalities exist as both professions have similar needs to uncover what has caused the individual to seek help, to identify clear goals for intervention, to articulate a synopsis of the conversation with first steps in planning what will happen next. The main difference lies in the approach to gaining an understanding of the person's circumstances in order to guide the encounter. The physician is often focused, by perceived necessity and purpose, on understanding symptoms and starting immediately to frame a differential diagnostic picture in order to cure or care. The occupational therapist, again by necessity when guided by the central professional construct of 'occupation', is most interested in establishing a relationship that will enable conversations informed by the purpose and meaning of each person's life. From this understanding a mutually agreed upon determination of priority issues of occupational performance and engagement to be addressed during the period of intervention will evolve.

The first essential task is to attend to the location chosen for the interaction as well as the comfort and setup in which the conversation will unfold. Details concerning furniture type and placement, lighting, space, sound and light levels must be

TABLE 6.1	
Five Stages of the Calgary Cambridge Model of History Taking (CCMHT)	
Stage 1: Initiating the session	Make preparations for engaging in the session to ensure a comfortable environment, establishing initial rapport and clarifying the reason for being there.
Stage 2: Gathering information	Exploring the person's problems from an occupational perspective, against a backdrop of the person's environments, personal resources, strengths and areas requiring attention.
Stage 3: Providing structure	Make clear to the person the path being followed to paint a picture of the problem, while making sure that the conversation flows in a logical and comfortable manner.
Stage 4: Building the relationship	Pay attention to the moment and ensure that appropriate nonverbal behaviour and cues are utilised, involving the person in an open and honest manner and thus developing a deeper rapport. The explanation of the conversation and making plans for next steps incorporates the person's health and illness perspective, the provision of needed information and explanations. This important part of the process ensures a shared understanding that will culminate in shared decision-making.
Stage 5: Closing the session	It is essential that the conversation ends in a timely and respectful fashion, incorporating a clear path for any further assessment as needed and plans for potential intervention as appropriate.

considered. Setting the context also involves ensuring that the person understands who is there with them, why, what they can expect from participating in this conversation and what the therapist is hoping to gain from the interaction. The person is then asked to give consent for the conversation and the relationship to continue.

The clearer these issues are at the outset, the more successful the outcome. However, there is also a need to be flexible and not to adhere totally to the expected conversational outline. If the person takes matters in a totally different direction, then this is where enhanced skills in listening and hearing are critical, as throwing away the plan might be the most valuable and appropriate response.

The body of the interview will differ depending on the purpose, the timing and the place of it within the person–therapist relationship. It is very important to be clear about the purpose of the interaction: is it to inform selection of a theoretical approach or an assessment tool, to develop an intervention plan, or to evaluate work completed and decide whether or not discharge is appropriate? Having clarity of purpose will help both partners in making the most of the time spent together.

Identification of occupational performance issues is the unique perspective that is offered by engagement in a person–therapist relationship within occupational therapy. This is the specific philosophical focus of the discipline and, as such, requires the use of a framework that supports the articulation by individuals of occupational performance issues of importance and meaning to them. It is here, within the body of the interview, that occupational performance issues can be identified and rapport consolidated, thus enabling a rich partnership to be forged. Most recently, an additional concept has been articulated as being a central piece of occupational therapy's unique contribution and that concept is occupational engagement. Townsend and Polatajko (2007) have proffered this construct as an addition to the original Canadian Model of Occupational Performance. They posit that the central construct of occupational therapy goes beyond occupational performance and embraces the essential notion of engagement. Occupational engagement suggests the broadest view of occupation that is recognised and addressed by occupational therapists (Townsend & Polatajko, 2007).

Ending an interview/conversation within a framework of person-centred practice demands that there is a mutual agreement regarding what is hoped for in the interchanges, what was achieved and what will be the next steps. This approach supports a process that is fluid and flexible and yet is contained within goals, targeted outcomes and overarching mutually determined expectations.

The Canadian Occupational Performance Measure

The Canadian Occupational Performance Measure (COPM) is an outcome measure that was developed in response to the need for a measure that would support the practice process of Canadian occupational therapists. Since its debut, the COPM has been the subject of much research, resulting in an emerging picture of a tool that is reliable, valid, responsive and has clinical utility (Carswell et al., 2004; Law et al., 2014; McColl et al., 2006) and is now used around the world.

The COPM uses a person-centred process to identify an individual's occupational performance issues that are of the highest priority from his perspective. This process also builds upon an occupation-centred expectation, thus illustrating a clear and transparent process of guiding occupational therapy assessment and intervention. This process does not replace specific assessment tools or approaches that are used by practitioners already and address particular areas such as neurological, sensory, cognitive, physical rehabilitative, socioadaptive and environmental. Rather, the COPM frames the identification of priorities for an intervention plan, based upon stated personal need and priority. This tool also offers the person and therapist the opportunity to use it as a focus for grounding partnerships rather than relying upon home-grown data collection options. Specific details related to the COPM can be found in another chapter in this text.

CONCLUSION

Practice is becoming progressively more complex, with many emerging trends making the need for enhanced communication and information-seeking skills ever more critical. Organisational changes, from hierarchical to programme-based systems, have placed a very clear responsibility on the shoulders of individual practitioners to practice with a clear and readily identifiable mandate that easily illustrates each discipline's unique contribution. By engaging in a person-centred process of addressing occupational performance issues, occupational therapists are well placed to deliver this kind of service. Again, approaching the establishment of person–therapist partnerships from the perspective of learning about someone's story instead of developing a personal case database helps those with whom occupational therapists work to have a very clear understanding of the reasons for occupational therapy and the steps in the intervention process. Time is at a premium in systems that still claim to be sadly underresourced; thus there is less time readily available in which to create supportive intervention environments – therefore, another reinforcement of the need to streamline rapport-building skills. A needed congruence between practice style and person-centred principles has emerged from the consumer movement, a societal expectation that is increasingly reinforced. Perhaps most critically, there is a deeply rooted need for occupational therapists to practice in a manner that is respectful and sensitive to cultural differences.

If occupational therapists embrace an approach to finding out about the occupational performance issues of the people who require their services that was enriched by individual's stories, notions of 'taking a history' or 'completing an interview' could be relinquished in favour of allowing those stories to unfold, thus shaping the nature of occupational therapy assessments and interventions. This would become then a truly person-centred approach to practice. Guidelines to assist occupational therapists to develop excellent communication skills are provided in Box 6.1.

BOX 6.1
EXCELLENCE IN PERSON-CENTRED COMMUNICATION

The following information aims to assist occupational therapists to develop person-centred listening and learning styles.

A. CONTEXTUAL CONSIDERATIONS

Setting: it is imperative that the space in which the conversation is taking place be large enough to accommodate the participants with comfort, that the furniture and lighting are appropriate and that there are as few distractions as possible.

Professional presentation: At all times, it is very important to appear professional in dress and manner and to be punctual and unhurried in approaching the person. Dress codes differ depending on the type of practice setting but, regardless of the degree of formality or informality, tidiness and cleanliness are not negotiable!

Background knowledge and skill: Reviewing the information available about the person is important before meeting in order to feel as prepared as possible. This will allow for the optimal use of possibly limited time, which also shows respect for the person's time and priorities. It is also critical that a therapist feels prepared to understand and respond professionally to expectations for the conversation that may stem from the person's cultural background or other elements of why he is there and who he is.

Recording: It is important to advise the person at the beginning of the conversation if the preference is to take notes in order to remember the details of what occurred. Also, when completing the notes, report or letter to the referral source, the content should be organised using a person-centred, occupation-based framework that includes an honest and authentic representation of what the person said, followed by a clear accounting of the professional reasoning that led to the assessment and enabling strategies.

Confidentiality: All notes and personal information should be kept in a secure location. All practitioners must be aware of any ethical responsibilities around confidentiality that are expected by a regulatory college or any government legislation.

Individual, family or group interview: When there are several people or one person plus family and others, there are very different expectations of the therapist. It is more complex to manage an interview environment when there are many potential agendas and therefore it is important to be aware of personal skill levels in handling such a situation. If someone else being present would enhance the outcomes, then asking for another team member perhaps to join the conversation is an

Continued on following page

BOX 6.1
EXCELLENCE IN PERSON-CENTRED COMMUNICATION (Continued)

excellent strategy. In any case, it is essential that the existence and awareness of who is the primary person be maintained.

B. NONVERBAL COMMUNICATION

The importance of nonverbal communication can never be underestimated.

Facial expression: Facial expressions can telegraph a great deal of information, so it is important to be conscious of personal impact and to respond to feedback from others about impressions made. Projecting an authentic interest in the person can make a profound difference when establishing new relationships and reconfiguring existing ones. If you feel confused or uncertain, it is important to talk about it rather than simply raise eyebrows or frown in a quizzical manner.

Eye contact: Direct eye contact can project a sincere interest in and engagement with the conversation; however, it is important to ensure that such a direct gaze is not confrontational. In addition, eye contact can be culturally inappropriate, so it is imperative that cultural sensitivity and awareness are applied at all times.

Posture: Offering an open and welcoming stance either when seated or standing provides a positive beginning to any interaction. Mirroring the position of the other participant in the conversation can be seen as a message of comfort and engagement.

Movement/gestures: Awareness of personal use of gestures and movement during conversations is an important skill to develop. Similarly, comfort with individuals who tend to be demonstrative is a valuable skill to include in your practice tool kit.

C. VERBAL COMMUNICATION

Tone and inflections: Sounding confident is desirable, whereas verging on arrogant is not. Keeping the voice at a conversational level, controlling the speed with which the conversation unfolds and ensuring the tone is pleasantly heard are critical pieces of developing a helpful and productive interviewing style.

Reflecting understanding: An open and appreciative style of communicating will give the person a clear sense of what to expect and an appreciation of the therapist's authenticity.

Messages: At all times the language used should reflect empathy, positive engagement and authenticity. Being oneself is crucial to productive engagement with individuals.

D. THERAPEUTIC CONVERSATIONS (INTERVIEWS)

Introductions and clarification of purpose: When doing an introduction the therapist must ensure that the person becomes familiar with the therapist's name and the therapist's perception of why the conversation is taking place. It is also essential that the role of an occupational therapist is made clear, with particular emphasis being placed on the role in the context of the person's particular circumstances.

Building a history/story: It is essential to create a context within which the person will feel comfortable in telling his story on his own, letting the story unfold at its own pace, providing words of assurance and interest to move the process along.

Identifying occupational performance issues from the perspective of the person: In the case of a true partnership, power and control are shared, with attention being paid to when the person's experiences and life knowledge are central to the conversation or when the therapist's skills and expertise take precedence. In fact, the person is the expert when addressing his life circumstances and identifying what is meaningful and a priority occupational performance issue.

E. SILENCE

Silence can be a powerful tool in reinforcing a partnership between therapist and person. Three to four seconds is a natural pause in a conversation but may appear longer and rather threatening early on in the establishment of a relationship. A silence lasting up to 10 seconds is reasonable and to be expected when someone is trying to share a story that is complex, disturbing and rich with personal meaning. However, gaining comfort with short silences is also a skill to be developed, together with a built-in ability to recognise when some interjection is required or deemed appropriate. At times, it can be a good strategy to share such discomfort with the person and therefore resolve it together.

 http://evolve.elsevier.com/Curtin/OT

REFERENCES

Carswell, A., McColl, M. A., Baptiste, S., Law, M., Polatajko, H., & Pollock, N. (2004). The Canadian Occupational Performance Measure: A research and clinical literature review. *Canadian Journal of Occupational Therapy, 71*(4), 210–222.

Chant, S., Jenkinson, T., Randle, J., Russell, G., & Webb, C. (2002). Communication skills training in health care; a review of the literature. *Nurse Education Today, 22,* 189–202.

Eysenbach, G., & Hadad, A. (2001). Evidence-based patient choice and consumer health informatics in the internet age. *Journal of Medical Internet Research, 3*(2).

Haidet, P., & Paterniti, D. A. (2003). 'Building' a history rather than 'taking' one. *Academic Medicine, 16*(3), 1134–1140.

Kurtz, S. M., Silverman, J., & Draper, J. (2005). *Teaching and learning communication skills in medicine.* Oxford: Radcliffe.

Law, M. (1998). *Client-centred occupational therapy.* Thorofare, NJ: Slack.

Law, M., Baptiste, S., & Mills, J. (1995). Client-centred practice: What does it mean and does it make a difference? *Canadian Journal of Occupational Therapy, 62*(5), 298–301.

Law, M., Baptiste, S., McColl, M. A., Opzoomer, A., Polatajko, H., & Pollock, N. (1990). The Canadian occupational performance measure for occupational therapy. *Canadian Journal of Occupational Therapy, 57*(2), 82–87.

Law, M., Polatajko, H., Pollock, N., McColl, M. A., Carswell, A., & Baptiste, S. (1994). Pilot testing of the canadian occupational performance measure: Clinical and measurement issues. *Canadian Journal of Occupational Therapy, 61*(4), 191–197.

Law, M., Polatajko, H., Pollock, N., McColl, M. A., Carswell, A., & Baptiste, S. (2014). *COPM: Canadian Occupational Performance Measure* (5th ed.). Ottawa: Canadian Association of Occupational Therapists/ACE.

McColl, M. A., Carswell, A., Law, M., Baptiste, S., Pollock, N., & Polatajkp, H. (2006). *Research on the COPM: An annotated resource.* Ottawa: Canadian Association of Occupational Therapists.

Mead, N., & Bower, P. (2000). Patient-centredness: A conceptual framework and review of the empirical literature. *Social Science and Medicine, 51*(7), 1087–1110.

Schirmer, J. M., Mauksch, L., Lang, F, et al. (2005). Assessing communication competence: A review of current tools. *Family Medicine, 37*, 184–192.

Shea, V. (1994). Netiquette. San Francisco, CA: Albion Books.

Susuki Laidlaw, T., MacLeod, H., Kaufman, D. M., Langille, D. B., & Sargeant, J. (2002). Implementing a communication skills programme in medical school: Needs assessment and programme change. *Medical Education, 36*(2), 115–124.

Tinney, J., Fearn, M., Hill, K., Dow, B., Haralambous, B., & Bremner, F. (2007). *Best practice in person-centred health care for older victorians: Report of phase 1. report to sub-acute and transitional care services.* Washington, D.C: Department of Human Services, National Ageing Research Institute.

Tomas, D. C., & Inkson, K. (2003). *Cultural intelligence.* San Francisco: Berrett-Koehler.

Townsend, L., & Polatajko, H. (2007). *Enabling occupation II: Advancing an occupational therapy vision for health, well-being and justice through occupation.* Ottawa: Canadian Association of Occupational Therapists.

7

PROFESSIONAL REASONING IN OCCUPATIONAL THERAPY PRACTICE

CAROLYN ANNE UNSWORTH

CHAPTER OUTLINE

Abstract
Professional reasoning is the thinking processes of an occupational therapist when engaging in practice. Learning about professional reasoning, and promoting a language to share this reasoning stimulates best practice and facilitates students and novice therapists to develop their practice. Several types of professional reasoning have been documented, and these are described in the chapter. These types of reasoning are illustrated through the use of a practice story of a therapist working with a person recovering from a traumatic brain injury. A recent review of the literature provides insights to the amount and nature of professional reasoning research, and this is summarised in a figure that also provides ideas on where research attention might best be directed in the future. Given that students and novice therapists are required to attain expertise as quickly as possible, an exploration of novice and expert differences and the features of expert practice, which includes professional reasoning, is outlined. As professional reasoning may also be viewed as growing into a theory that supports practice, information on how theories evolve and the professional reasoning models currently under development are provided.

KEY POINTS

- *Professional reasoning* is a term used to describe thinking processes of occupational therapy professionals when undertaking practice.

- Professional reasoning relies on both cognitive skills and embodied knowledge and enables occupational therapists to work from both phenomenological 'lived experience' as well as medical model perspectives.

- Researchers and writers have described a number of types of professional reasoning, and this language has helped occupational therapists to understand, describe and educate students about professional reasoning.

- Research suggests that professional reasoning skills and expertise are linked, so that as students and novice therapists enhance and develop their reasoning skills, they will move towards expert status.
- From 1982 to 2014, 140 journal articles were written on professional reasoning in occupational therapy, and this mounting evidence contributes to the development of a theory of professional reasoning.

WHAT IS PROFESSIONAL REASONING?

To examine what professional reasoning is in occupational therapy, how this construct came to the occupational therapy profession has to be considered. In 1983 Donald Schön published *The Reflective Practitioner: How Professionals Think in Action*. At around the same time, occupational therapy researchers were inspired to ask questions about how therapists think and how occupational therapy educators could facilitate students and practitioners to 'think smarter'. Rogers and Masagatani published the first study on clinical reasoning in occupational therapy in 1982, and the following year Rogers (1983) delivered an Eleanor Clarke Slagle lecture that focused on this topic. The collective interest of the profession sparked as the potential of this construct to help understand and articulate occupational therapy practice was recognised. The American Occupational Therapy Association Commission on Education recommended that the American Occupational Therapy Research Foundation set up the Clinical Reasoning Study. This ethnographic action research study on clinical reasoning was conducted in Boston between 1986 and 1990 by Mattingly (an anthropologist), Fleming, Gillette and Cohen (occupational therapists) and was greatly influenced by Schön as the project's consultant. Key findings from the study were reported in a special issue on clinical reasoning of the *American Journal of Occupational Therapy*, in November 1991, and in the text *Clinical Reasoning: Forms of Inquiry in a Therapeutic Practice* (Mattingly & Fleming, 1994), which laid a solid foundation for the current understanding of the construct.

Clinical reasoning was aptly named at this point as the profession's focus was centred around clinical environments, despite Mattingly and Fleming (1994) articulating that occupational therapy practice was not limited to a medical (clinical) model. However, over the ensuing years the occupational therapy practice culture has changed, with the focus of the profession now more clearly centred on the concepts of occupation, health and well-being. In addition, the places where occupational therapy is currently practiced vary widely. Therefore rather than using the term *clinical reasoning*, terms such as *therapeutic*, *occupational* or *professional* reasoning are being embraced. The term *professional reasoning* is adopted throughout this chapter and this book, as this term is inclusive of practice that occurs in all settings, such as in the community or schools, at people's place of work, in homes or in clinical environments.

Professional reasoning may be defined as the thinking processes of occupational therapy professionals when undertaking practice. Professional reasoning involves the therapists' thinking when planning and reflecting on therapy, as well as the whole body experience of engaging in therapy.

The Whole Body Process of Professional Reasoning

The professional reasoning an occupational therapist engages in when determining what standardised assessment to administer can appear to be relatively straightforward; however, it is complex as it involves more than just the therapist's cognitive skills. When meeting a young woman for an initial assessment as an outpatient after rehabilitation for upper limb burns in a work accident, the occupational therapist may choose to conduct an initial assessment and establish goals, assess range of motion and examine skin condition, and then conduct a standardised upper limb assessment. However, during administration of these assessments, the reasoning processes the therapist uses are both cognitive/perceptual and sensory. The therapist needs to feel the range of movement during the assessment and determine where the contractures are forming or have formed. The therapist also feels for muscle disuse and weakness. Similarly, the therapist views and feels the condition of the skin and also uses smell to determine where wounds are not healing or there might be hygiene problems with a thermoplastic splint. In other words the therapist is using all senses when working with the person. That means that the professional reasoning of an occupational therapist is not only cognitive, it is a whole body process.

Cognitive Processes That Underpin Professional Reasoning

An understanding of professional reasoning for occupational therapists is underpinned by information processing theory and the related field of memory (Carr & Shotwell 2008; Ericsson & Simon 1993). The information gathered through the therapist's senses, cognitive reasoning (thinking), theoretical knowledge and intuition (Chaffey, Unsworth, & Fossey, 2010) is 'chunked'; logically connected material is put together and incorporated into 'scripts' or 'frames' that are mentally stored and used repeatedly with people who participate in occupational therapy. Although there are no set definitions for these terms, it is generally understood that straightforward, linear-style information about a particular issue or problem is stored in memory as a script. Frames are similar in that they are also a method of gathering information to be stored in a therapist's long-term memory; however, they are generally perceived as more structured and complex (Carr & Shotwell, 2008). Frames are an approach for storing rich and complex knowledge in which there are many possible pathways with many possible outcomes. Expert occupational therapists are able to rapidly (sometimes simultaneously) draw upon stored scripts or frames and use them to interact at the 'just right' level with each person.

Although there are differing theories as to how professionals such as occupational therapists organise information in memory systems and access it when appropriate, the three most widely used are frame theory (Barsalou, 1992), the adaptive control of thought – rational (ACT-R) model (Anderson, 1983) and dual coding theory (Paivio, 1971). Each of these theories proposes a way to understand how people process, organise and code information and store it for later use (Carr & Shotwell, 2008). Frame theory focuses on how people organise and connect information when multiple possibilities for relationships between this information exists. For example, frame theory helps provide an understanding of how a therapist might choose a particular intervention from an available selection. The ACT-R model describes both a person's memory for concepts and facts (declarative) and procedures of how to do things (procedural). To do something with a person, a therapist needs to bring both procedural and declarative memories into the working memory and then generate the frame to engage in therapy. Finally, dual coding theory posits that knowledge is represented in memory using sensory-based coding (e.g. from sight, sound, touch, etc.). People are believed to have both verbal and nonverbal systems for encoding and storing information, and these systems interact to allow them to understand and respond (Carr & Shotwell, 2008). What all three theories have in common is that the key to recognising patterns and being able to construct and access scripts and frames is organisation of knowledge. An important role for educators is to facilitate students to organise their knowledge, as this will aid them to construct more complete scripts and frames that can be accessed more quickly when needed. This will aid novices on their journey to expert status.

ENHANCING PROFESSIONAL REASONING SKILLS AND BECOMING AN EXPERT

As described earlier, occupational therapists gather information and incorporate this into scripts or frames that are stored and accessed to use and adapt with different people seen in therapy (Carr & Shotwell, 2008). Professional reasoning supports the creation of these scripts and frames and subsequently enables frames to be appropriately enacted. However, the speed with which therapists access and adapt these scripts and frames, the range of scripts and frames available, and the depth and complexity of information they contain depend on the level of expertise of the therapist. An expert is someone who has special skill or knowledge because of what they have been taught or derived from training or experience (Merriam-Webster.com, 2016) and through intuition (Benner, 1984). A detailed literature review conducted by King et al. (2008) identified the six main attributes of expertise as being: superior outcomes, reputation, experience, skills and attributes, personal characteristics and qualities and knowledge. These terms are described in Table 7.1. Furthermore, King et al. identified that three main

variables are generally associated with the development of expertise; motivation, openness to experience (including critical thinking, truth-seeking, cognitive maturity and open-mindedness), and features of their clinical caseload over time (such as range of services and people worked with).

TABLE 7.1

Six Attributes of Expert Practice Among Occupational Therapists

Feature	Description
Superior outcomes	Achieving outcomes above peers. These outcomes may be at service, team or individual person levels.
Reputation	Peers and colleagues describe the occupational therapist as being an expert, based on the contributions to practice and outcomes achieved over time.
Experience	Time practicing in the health environment. High experience is generally defined as 10 years of professional practice. Experience is generally viewed as necessary for the attainment of expertise, but not sufficient. Expert status can be achieved by occupational therapists who may only have limited experience. Additionally, experience in one area of practice may contribute to expertise in that area, whereas the same practitioner may be viewed as a novice in other specialist areas of practice (such as hand therapy or cognitive behavioural therapy).
Skills and abilities	Technical, interpersonal, self-regulation, cognitive, and metacognitive skills that the occupational therapist brings to the professional encounter.
Personal characteristics and qualities	These consist of personal attitudes, values and traits. These are unique to the individual and need to be consciously recognised so their role/influence in the therapeutic encounter can be understood and changed if desired by the therapist.
Knowledge	Content, propositional knowledge (knowing facts) and nonpropositional knowledge (knowing how), as well as self-knowledge (insight to what you know and where gaps in knowledge are).

Modified from King et al., 2008.

Most of the literature in occupational therapy on expertise has been constructed from Dreyfus and Dreyfus' (1980) model of skill acquisition, which was adapted to nursing by Benner (1984). The Dreyfus and Dreyfus model posits that from novice to expert status there are five levels: novice, advanced beginner, competent, proficient and expert. In this model, novice therapists are described as having very few experiences of the situations in which they are involved. Although novice therapists know some of the rules, principles and theories, they are often rigidly applied. Advanced beginner therapists begin to recognise recurring themes and patterns and begins to create scripts for practice. Advance beginner therapists are still remembering theoretical information and as a result have limited flexibility in the application of theory. Competent therapists are said to be consciously aware of the outcome of their actions; however, they lack the speed and flexibility of the proficient therapist. Therapists who are thought to be at the proficient level of expertise have a rapid and clear picture of a person's whole situation and recognise the recurring patterns in the people who present for therapy. In the final level, an expert therapist uses multiple frames to engage in a flexible and reflexive practice. Experts need less information when working on a problem, and make better judgements, as they seem to have an intuitive grasp of the therapy situation (Benner, 1984; Dreyfus & Dreyfus, 1986; Unsworth, 2011).

Drawing on the Dreyfus and Dreyfus model, there have been several studies on differences between novice and expert occupational therapists (Gibson et al., 2000; Hallin & Svidán, 1995; Mitchell & Unsworth, 2005; Robertson, 1996; Strong, Gilbert, Cassidy, & Bennett, 1995; Unsworth, 2001a). These studies have also included excellent strategies, centred on reflection, that novices can use to help them improve their reasoning. However, the research has not been able to tease out differences beyond the novice–expert dichotomy. Further, occupational therapy writers have recently argued that the Dreyfus and Dreyfus model may not be the best basis for understanding expertise given that this work was developed with pilots where a strong relationship exists between hours of flying and expertise (Robertson, Warrender, & Barnard, 2015). Indeed, occupational therapy research consistently supports the idea that the passage of time or experience does not automatically equate with expertise (Hallin & Svidán, 1995; Mitchell & Unsworth, 2005; Robertson, 1996; Strong et al., 1995; Unsworth, 2001a).

Instead, Robertson and colleagues suggest that the 'critical occupational therapy practitioner' model could be used, which is based on Barnett's (1997) three forms of criticality. Three elements are encompassed in this model: the therapist is professionally engaged, informed by evidence, and critically self-reflective. However, it remains difficult to determine whether a therapist is achieving these ideals and practicing at this level. Therefore a multimodal approach may be better to objectively identify expert practice. For example, in research by King et al. (2008) these authors attempted to determine variables associated with expertise in paediatric allied health practitioners. They identified a range of measures such as the California Critical Thinking Disposition Inventory (CCTDI) (Facione, Facions, & Giancarlo, 1996) and Clinical Behaviours of Paediatric Therapists – Multidimensional Peer Rating (Gilpin et al., 2005), among others, to help measure and subsequently determine expert status. As the number and level of sophistication of scales that can be used to help measure thinking and practice skills grows, so too does the opportunity to determine expertise. Although being able to quantify or determine level of expertise continues to challenge researchers, the fact remains that expertise and professional reasoning capacity remain inextricably linked.

THE TWO-BODIED PRACTICE

The occupational therapy profession focuses on the relationships among occupation, health and well-being. 'Occupation' is everything people do in their lives, is at the core of practice and provides the therapeutic means as well as the focus for the therapy. When Mattingly and Fleming and their colleagues examined how occupational therapists reasoned in their practice, they found that the way occupational therapists think about the 'health' and 'well-being' components and their arrangement in this triangular relationship was different from other health professionals. The 'health' component of occupational therapy is based on a biomedical framework. A biomedical framework provides opportunity to explore people's medical issues and the assessments, technologies and interventions that surround their health care. This approach views the body as a machine (Mattingly, 1994). In contrast, people's well-being is concerned with their psychological, social and cultural attributes, their experience of their health issues and the meanings attached to this experience. The focus on well-being is phenomenological in nature as it is about the 'lived body'.

Professionals who work in health care usually associate more strongly with either a biomedical or phenomenological approach. Hence, although nurses and physiotherapists might align themselves with a biomedical perspective, medical social workers might approach people from a more social/psychological/cultural perspective. However, occupational therapists consider both the biomedical and phenomenological understanding of people as important, described by Mattingly as a 'two-bodied' practice. Moreover, Mattingly noted that occupational therapists seemed to be able to shift easily between these two perspectives. To achieve this, occupational therapists have two quite distinct language processes, which Mattingly labelled as 'chart talk' and 'narrative reasoning'.

Chart Talk and Narrative Reasoning

When a therapist is thinking about a person's health condition and medical issues, the therapist communicates using 'chart talk'. This is a shared language among allied health and medical professionals where a person's situation is summarised and reduced to essential information on history, current status and future concerns. This information can be presented orally during team meetings or documented in formal or informal records.

In contrast, when the therapist is thinking about the person and taking a more phenomenological view, the therapist uses narrative reasoning. Hence, if the therapist is having a conversation with another team member, the therapist may describe more details about how the person is coping, what the person's mood is like, and what strategies might help the person to move forward. Narrative reasoning is aptly named as these conversations appear to be like stories. These stories are co-created, adapted and rewritten with the person in therapy and with other team members. Within the construct of professional reasoning, narrative reasoning is one of the strands of thinking that has been identified, but because of its pervasive and foundation nature, it's important that students and new graduates understand what it is and the central role it plays in the process (Mattingly & Fleming, 1994).

TYPES OF PROFESSIONAL REASONING

To access knowledge and convey it to students and new graduates, there needs to be a way of communicating it. This is particularly important, as without this language, a great deal of an expert's knowledge remains tacit, or unspoken, and therefore not able to be accessed by novices. One of the major outcomes of the foundational clinical reasoning study (Mattingly & Fleming, 1994) was the identification of different types of reasoning: narrative, procedural, interactive and conditional reasoning. It was also noted that these types of reasoning could be used in isolation, sequentially or concurrently. The term *types of reasoning* is adopted throughout this chapter; however, it should be noted that other writers in this area also use the interchangeable terms *tracks* or *facets*.

Following on from the foundational clinical reasoning study, and drawing on the earlier work of Rogers and Masagatani (1982), many different types of reasoning have now been identified, including scientific, diagnostic, ethical, generalisation, pragmatic, collaborative and even occupational reasoning. These types of reasoning are defined in Table 7.2. However, in addition to these terms, there are other constructs that help contextualise these types of reasoning: worldview, reflection, embodiment and intuition. These constructs are presented in Table 7.3 along with an explanation of how each construct relates to the professional reasoning of the therapist and the person receiving occupational therapy services.

	TABLE 7.2
	Types of Professional Reasoning
Mode of reasoning	**Description**
Narrative reasoning	When the therapist makes sense of a person's circumstances though his or her story. The emphasis is on the meaning of the person's health experience (Mattingly & Fleming, 1994). Narrative reasoning forms a platform for the other forms of reasoning.
Scientific reasoning	A systematic approach to reasoning that includes hypothetico-deductive reasoning. This is centred around hypothesis generation and testing (Rogers & Holm, 1991).
Diagnostic reasoning	The process of identifying the person's occupational performance issues, or needs (Rogers & Holm, 1991; Schell & Schell, 2008).
Procedural reasoning	The reasoning processes associated with the evaluations and interventions to be used with a person. This reasoning refers to all the 'procedures' of therapy. Mattingly and Fleming suggested that procedural reasoning includes systematic data collection, hypothesis formation and testing and the reasoning that underpins interventions (Mattingly & Fleming, 1994).
Interactive reasoning	This is the type of reasoning that therapists used when communicating with a person, both verbally and nonverbally. Mattingly and Fleming referred to this as the underground practice because therapists easily describe what they have done with the person but do not articulate their interactions so easily. Therapists use interactive reasoning to engage a person in therapy, consider the best approach to communicate with a person, to understand the person, understand the person's problems from the person's point of view, individualise therapy, convey a sense of acceptance/trust/hope to the person break tension through the use of humour, build a shared language of actions and meanings, and monitor how the treatment session is going (Mattingly & Fleming, 1994). More recently, Taylor (2008) has explored this type of reasoning through understanding the 'intentional relationship' between therapists and the people they work with.

TABLE 7.2	
Types of Professional Reasoning (Continued)	
Mode of reasoning	**Description**
Conditional reasoning	Conditional reasoning is one of the more complex to understand and has several components. A therapist is reasoning conditionally when thinking about the person's condition and how change is conditional upon participation in the therapeutic process. But more than this, the therapist is reasoning conditionally when thinking temporally about the person's past, present and future in order to understand what the person's life was like before the therapy encounter, what it is like now, and what it could be in the future. Hence, this type of reasoning is used when trying to understand what is meaningful to each person in their social and cultural world (Mattingly & Fleming, 1994).
Ethical reasoning	Reasoning about a moral conflict, where one moral stand or action conflicts with another (Barnitt & Partridge, 1997; Rogers, 1983).
Pragmatic reasoning/ management reasoning	The therapist's thinking related to personal, organisational, political and economic contexts. Hence, this thinking is about how therapy can operate given resources and reimbursement issues. Personal context includes the reasoning surrounding therapists' own motivations, negotiation skills, repertoire of therapy skills and what Törnebohm (1991) described as life knowledge and assumptions (Barris, 1987; Lyons & Crepeau, 2001; Schell & Cervero, 1993).
Generalisation reasoning	Within the forms of procedural, interactive, conditional and pragmatic reasoning, therapists use generalisation reasoning when drawing on past experience or knowledge to assist in making sense of a current situation or client circumstance. This kind of reasoning occurs within procedural, interactive, conditional and pragmatic reasoning as the therapist thinks about a particular person, then reflects on general experiences or knowledge (i.e. making generalisations) related to the situation, and then refocuses back on the person (Unsworth, 2005).

TABLE 7.3	
Constructs That Coexist with Professional Reasoning	
Construct	**Description**
Embodiment	As a therapist works with a person, the therapist gathers information not only from what the person says (i.e. aurally) but also from the therapist's other senses. A therapist will look at the person's body language and how the person's body is positioned. A person's smell may inform the therapist about the person's hygiene and, for example, how well a wound may be healing. Therapists use sensation often, for example, to feel is a person's muscles are moving as expected, or whether there is flaccidity or hypertonicity. Professional reasoning may be described as 'embodied' because therapists reason with their whole bodies.
Intuition	Intuition may be defined as 'knowledge of a fact or truth, as a whole; immediate possession of knowledge; and knowledge independent of the linear reasoning process' (Rew, 1986, p. 23). Sometimes intuition is described as a 'gut' feeling or instinct. Intuition means not consciously thinking about something, and therefore knowing something intuitively is quite different from consciously thinking about something and analysing it. Therefore, if a therapist's thinking could be placed on a continuum, it would stretch from intuition to analysis.
Reflection	This is the activity of turning experiences into learning. There are several types of reflection including reflection about past experiences (reflection on action), reflecting in the present (reflection in action) and looking forward or anticipatory reflection (reflection for action).
Worldview	Wolters (1989) defined worldview as a person's global outlook on life and the world. This construct was first explored in occupational therapy by Hooper (1997) through the thinking of an expert clinician. Since that time, very little has been written or researched about an occupational therapist's worldview. However, it has been found (Unsworth, 2004) that worldview is distinct from pragmatic reasoning (as described by Schell & Cervero (1993)), which had been previously described as incorporating practical as well as personal views of the therapist. As proposed by Unsworth, worldview describes the influence of the therapist's personal context on professional reasoning but is not a form of reasoning itself.

USING DIFFERENT TYPES OF PROFESSIONAL REASONING ACROSS THE OCCUPATIONAL THERAPY PROCESS

Practice Story 7.1 provides the background to a therapy session between Jess, an occupational therapist, and James who has had a traumatic brain injury. Jess's professional reasoning is explored in detail in Table 7.4 using the eight action points of the Canadian Practice Process Framework (CPPF) (Townsend & Polatajko, 2013) from the Canadian Model of Occupational Performance and Engagement (CMOP-E) (Townsend & Polatajko, 2013) illustrate the different types of professional reasoning than have been mentioned earlier. The practice story is based on previously published research (Unsworth 2001a; 2004). The research used head-mounted video camera technology (Unsworth, 2001b) in which a therapist records a therapy session, then watches the footage immediately after the session and provides an account of their reasoning processes as the session unfolds. This professional reasoning soundtrack is then recorded together with the original footage and forms the data that are then transcribed and analysed.

PRACTICE STORY 7.1

The Story of James and His Occupational Therapist, Jessica

Jess has worked in a brain injury unit for 8 years and works with people who are recovering from moderate to severe brain injury. James had his injury 6 months ago. He was in a coma for 3 weeks and spent more than a month in intensive care before being transferred to the specialist brain injury rehabilitation unit where he began to work with Jess. In the following quotes, Jess introduces James and begins to reveal her professional reasoning as she watches the video of the session, filmed from her perspective (i.e. from a head-mounted video camera). At the end of this excerpt, Jess talks briefly about the influence of James' occupational hopes and dreams on the narrative of therapy. This is also beautifully illustrated by Smith's (2006) writings on how stories co-create change in therapy.

Jess: So this is a young gentleman who is aged 20 and has been involved in a motor vehicle accident. We're about to do an upper limb functional assessment. We're always assessing as we're treating at the same time with someone like this. At the start here, just before we started these computer game activities, I gave James the choice of what he wanted to do. I always give him lots of choices, and a variety of occupations or activities, but they are always working towards the same goals that we have been working on from the start. But I give him the choice of what he wants to do and when, because there might be something he doesn't want to do and we always need to make sure that he is empowered in the sessions as well.

At the minute we're doing some simple basic exercises that are like a warm-up so we need to warm him up so we can complete the assessment and then the computer-based activities he wants to do next, and this is set out for him so he can see its coming and he knows it's part of what we are doing now. So I'm supporting his torso there so that he doesn't substitute movement patterns. So what we are encouraging James to do there is forward shoulder flexion and elbow extension and he likes to move his trunk forward at the same time. He's got some associated tonal patterns there. My prompt on the shoulder is just controlling that trunk involvement there so we get the right movement coming back. So getting proximal stabilisation and maximising his left upper limb, so, that's what our session involves, facilitating return of the movement that he's got, building strength and endurance, so then he can manage the computer activity next.

So you can see James' mother and younger sister [in the video], they are very, very involved in his rehab and very committed to his rehab programme as well. They're invited to come to every therapy session whenever they want as are all of our family members. James responds really well to them and they like to be involved in the process, they're here almost every day, so we encourage them to be involved in sessions whenever possible. Also it helps out of therapy, because they understand the rationale and reasons why we're doing what we're doing and the goals we all want to achieve. They can facilitate those out of therapy sessions and they're actually doing that, they're a great family. They have a good understanding of James' injury and what he wants and needs to work on. And if I ask them to do something after therapy, they do, and that's really nice to see. And they are a good motivating factor for James too. He always wants to perform well in front of his family.

I guess I've talked a lot about what we are doing in this session, but I haven't really put this into the bigger picture of what are James' hopes and dreams for the future. There is no easy way to describe the devastation for the person and their family when a brain injury happens. And it's just so sudden. One minute everything is fine and the next its chaos, intensive care and then it's a whole journey of recovery. And I guess I haven't talked much about that in what I've just described, so I guess it's important to add that this therapy session fits into a whole shared story that James and I are making. I want to add that we are working towards his goals and dreams of returning home, and getting a girlfriend and working again, and hanging out with mates playing his video games.

TABLE 7.4	
The Eight Action Points of the Occupational Performance Process Framework (Townsend & Polatajko, 2013) and Associated Professional Reasoning	
Action points	**Examples of Associated Professional Reasoning from the Case of Jess and James— Jess Reflects on her Work with James as She Watches the Video of One of Their Initial Therapy Sessions**
Enter/initiate Set the stage	Generalisation reasoning (with interactive and conditional reasoning as Jess thinks about how she will work with James, and what the future holds):
	James was in a coma following his car accident for over 2 weeks and his Glasgow Coma Score was 5, and so I know that when I see him, he has a very severe brain injury and I can expect that he is going to have the full range of physical, cognitive, sensory and behavioural problems and that it's a long road to get him to be able to live at home with his family again. The underlying issues around independence and getting as much functional return are the same for all my clients, but what's different for each is their personal stories and personalities, what will motivates them in therapy and what's really important to them to achieve. Clients I work with who have similar injuries can have such different outcomes, based on these things. Yeah, so I've read the medical file notes on James and I know that we will start to work on self-care independence, and the underlying issues of seating, posture balance, and the notes also suggest that there are lots of issues with his right upper limb, so we're going to need to do some work there so he can do fun stuff he want[s] to do. I'm guessing that he's 20 and he might be motivated by computer games and so if that's the case then I can work with him on building upper limb skills through computer games.
	Pragmatic and conditional reasoning:
	I know that James has compensation [insurance] through the state scheme so he's going to be able to stay in this facility for about 5 to 9 months and I know I'm really going to see lots of changes and be able to get him back home [...] but just how far we are going to get [is] too early to say, so I'm always really keen to get started and meet the client and start to make some plans for the best future we can.
	Throughout the eight action points, the therapist is choosing and using theoretical approaches to guide practice.
	Procedural reasoning:
	I don't really think about the occupational therapy models that I will use any more as they are so ingrained, and I'm using the same models all the time. So I usually work within the CMOP-E. I find it a great way to organise my thinking around the person I'm working with and what the issues are. And then for practice models I'm mostly using the Biomechanical Model, Motor Relearning Approach, and then Noomie Katz' Retraining Approach for working on cognitive and perceptual problems. The CPPF from the CMOP-E, and using the eight action points, is how I organise my practice. I know this session is not as occupation focussed as I want it to be... but we are working towards the computer games James wants to play.
	Worldview:
	I guess when I do stop and think about the theory I use, that despite my best efforts to keep everything occupation-focussed, sometimes I find this hard to do. It's a real challenge to be able to get client participation and power-sharing when our clients have such severe brain trauma. So we try to empower clients as much as possible through simply daily choices, and also getting family fully involved and sharing in the decisions and choices. In our staff journal club we are reviewing articles on goal setting with clients following acquired brain injury and this is sparking lots of heated debates about whether occupation is truly central in our practice, and whether we are truly client centred... which has been really interesting, but really challenging!
Assess/evaluate	Procedural reasoning:
	The assessments I'm using fit within those models I've just listed which are the CMOP-E, Motor Relearning, Retraining. Therefore I'm using COPM (Canadian Occupational Performance Measure), DASH (Disabilities of Arm, Shoulder, Hand), ARAT (Action Research Arm Test), and LOTCA (Lowenstein Occupational Therapy Cognitive Assessment). Sometimes I will also use the AMPS (Assessment of Motor and Process Skills). It depends on where we are up to in the client's recovery. My team is now measuring all clients on a global outcome measure, AusTOMS-OT, and this really helps to identify client outcomes over a long period and is based on the goals we are working on at the time. So at the moment I'm working on self-care, transfers, and upper limb function, so I've scored James on scales 3 (Upper Limb Function), 5 (Transfers), and 7 (Self-care). We've only been using this outcome measure for about 18 months and we've been able to show how much clients have improved and used it with management to argue for more hours in OT activities for our clients by employing another part time OT assistant.
	Pragmatic and interactive reasoning (with generalisation at the end):
	But you know, we're always assessing as we're treating at the same time with someone like this. So in that way, it's not like we assess for 3 weeks and then move to intervention as we have to start straight away working on core treatments.

Continued on following page

	TABLE 7.4
	The Eight Action Points of the Occupational Performance Process Framework (Townsend & Polatajko, 2013) and Associated Professional Reasoning (Continued)
Action points	**Examples of Associated Professional Reasoning from the Case of Jess and James—Jess Reflects on her Work with James as She Watches the Video of One of Their Initial Therapy Sessions**
	So in the next session, I'm going to get James to do some hand activities there on the table. He's still on the warm-ups. He's doing a bit of wrist extension here, and what I'm doing, I'm actually modelling and demonstrating to James what is going on there at his wrist and then he's copying my actions so he can get the right movement patterns. Verbally, he has quite good comprehension for simple phrases and commands, but if I just said 'James, can you bend your wrist up', he could bend it in the wrong pattern or the wrong way. So I know I'm going to get the best understanding from him if I say it, and show him and then he really gets what I want to do understanding of what to do. And I find that with a lot of my clients, I really need to find multiple ways of communicating through gestures, and demonstrations and small amounts of plain language and consistent communication patterns... so no small talk and chatter as that takes my clients so much energy to process and to try and understand. So instead I'm using simple phrases, that I say over and over, and lots of smiles and encouragement with that.
	If he can get these wrist movements, then he can really participate in the occupations he wants to do, like playing computer games.
Agree on objectives and plan	Procedural reasoning (with interactive reasoning):
	With James, his strengths are really around his motivation and willingness to give 100% in his therapy. In terms of impairments and activity limitations, we have lots of motor, sensory, behavioural and cognitive problems that we need to work on through engaging in daily occupations and so together (and through using the COPM) we have agreed that we will work on getting on and off the toilet from the wheelchair, showering and getting dressed, and then being able to play his computer games.
	And of course his family are a major strength as well. They are coming to as many therapy sessions as they can and are really invested in getting him to be able to come home. It's a really long road ahead of them, but they are a fantastic support and he will be able to return home with them. Of course we may [need] to make some adaptions to the house, but it's just way too early to tell what these might be, and when he starts going on weekend leave, then we can put some temporary equipment in place for what he needs at the time.
	As I mentioned earlier, I'm working with James on getting on and off the toilet from the wheelchair, showering and getting dressed, and then being able to play his computer games, which is also about getting better control over his right upper limb. So at the moment in this session, we are working on playing a computer game and I'm doing some upper limb work to get him started so he has better control in the game and less frustration. I find if he can't get enough control over the adapted joystick, he gets really frustrated and demoralised and then it's no fun anymore, so I think I can get the best from James, and he can have the most fun, if we work beforehand [before going on the computer game] to get a bit of control. The behavioural objective for the session is:
	Who: James
	Given what: a precursor upper limb wrist and finger control activity (using elbow stabilisation techniques, cones, and Thera-putty), adapted joystick and gradable computer game.
	Does what: engage in the basic level of a computer game of his choice.
	How well: so that he is challenged but can manage to manoeuvre the controls with sufficient success to be able to play the game continuously for 10 minutes at a time, before needing to restart.
	By when: by the end of a 60 minute therapy session.
	Pragmatic reasoning:
	I need to consult with my OT colleague, Sophie, as I think James really needs to have a resting splint overnight for his right hand and wrist, and splinting actually isn't my strength at all. But I really want to learn more splinting techniques and improve my skills so I am going to see if Sophie has some time later in the week to have a look at James with me and then I might get her to supervise me making the splint.
Implement the plan	Procedural and interactive reasoning (shared language of meaning):
	So I'm working with him on interventions to improve his right upper limb function. So, I am watching his arm to make sure he doesn't have any associated reactions, and I just want to see movements from his wrist, rather than associated reactions, and I'm using lots of layman's terms, because if I said we were going to do ulnar and radial wrist movements, it's just meaningless. I do have nick names I have made up with James already, and I say to him 'do some of that side to side wrist stuff', and I explain it to him and he then forgets it of course because he does have problems with his memory but he thinks it's funny and likes all the terms as well as our nicknames.

	TABLE 7.4

The Eight Action Points of the Occupational Performance Process Framework (Townsend & Polatajko, 2013) and Associated Professional Reasoning *(Continued)*

Action points	Examples of Associated Professional Reasoning from the Case of Jess and James— Jess Reflects on her Work with James as She Watches the Video of One of Their Initial Therapy Sessions
	And now I want to work on his control of deltoid as [he has] had some substitution patterns happening in his arm while he was trying to turn his shoulder — he was externally rotating his shoulder and bringing his elbow in whilst he was trying to move his trunk there. So I stabilised his forearm and shoulder and brought his attention to it so we were just concentrating on the isolated movement patterns we wanted to see there. *I'm also being very careful about how I touch him and where, and preparing him that I am going to stabilise his arm. He's a young man who a few days ago, whenever I touched his hand, he'd [⋯] get a bit excited and be a bit inappropriate and say 'Jess's holding my hand!' and think that it's because I like him as a boyfriend, so I have to be careful about how I'm touching James, and really explain it to him.* *And we have the computer joystick and the hardware sitting over there, so after I do these activities with James, we can really link the improvements he is making to the occupation he wants to do which is play computer games. But it's just been too frustrating to launch in and play a game as he just doesn't have the control he wants. So he knows that these activities are helping him to get better control to play the computer. Our next task is to upgrade from these table-top tasks to an adapted joystick, which isn't so sensitive as the one he was using in the past. The therapy joystick allows for more tremor and doesn't need the fine control that most of the commercial games need. The downside of our joystick is that it links to computer programs that are a bit child-like, so I'm just trying to balance all these issues of the occupation James wants to do, managing his upper limb, and what we are going to do in therapy together to enable him to play on the computer games he wants to.*
Monitor and modify Evaluate outcome Conclude/ exit	Procedural (evaluating the session), interactive (James' response to the session) and conditional (what will the next session involve) reasoning: *So this session went pretty well. I'm really happy that James had a good time and enjoyed the game. And of course he really is making gains with his wrist and finger control and I can see that he is also beginning to understand that if he stabilises his elbow on the table then he does much better in the activity, so he is doing it automatically himself. His mum and sister were also in the session and they are also seeing some small progress and so it's great for them as well as we are just at the very beginning with many, many months ahead of us together, working as a team.* *In the next session I think we can increase the level of the game so its little harder as I can really see that he is making progress, but I'm going to check with James before we do this, as its OK if he really wants to have some fun and master this level as its all good in terms of continuing to work on his wrist and also in terms of being able to improve his cognitive skills like concentration and attention and problem solving and so on.* *And then I am also thinking about his outcome measures scores that we are scoring for the start of these goals, on AusTOMs-OT (see the website for manual and scoring at www.austoms.com), so for Scale 3, Upper Limb Function, he is scoring 3 for Impairment Domain, 2 for Activity Limitation Domain, and then for the global scores for the Participation Domain he is 2, and then a 3 for Well-being—Distress.* *I guess we will continue to work on this goal for quite a few months and make sure that James really gets as good skill as possible on both the computer games he really likes but also on his upper limb control.*

WHAT EVIDENCE SUPPORTS THERAPIST'S UNDERSTANDING OF PROFESSIONAL REASONING IN OCCUPATIONAL THERAPY?

A recent systematic review on professional reasoning (Unsworth & Baker, 2016) revealed a total of 140 peer-reviewed articles over 33 years (1982 to 2014) written about the reasoning of occupational therapists or occupational therapy students. Although 43 of these articles were discussion or theoretical pieces that contained no data, 97 were research studies that included more than 3000 participants. These articles appeared in 25 different journals, as documented in Table 7.5.

A topic analysis was conducted to determine what these articles covered, and six topic areas were developed: what is professional reasoning?; ethics and moral reasoning; methods of studying professional reasoning; novice–expert differences; professional reasoning of assistants; and advancing specific fields of practice using professional reasoning. These topics, and how many papers were written on each, are presented on the left side in Figure 7.1. Since some articles covered more than one topic, there are 157 topics represented across the 140 articles. On the right side of Figure 7.1 ideas for further research are presented. To facilitate this research, time should be spent on developing methods and techniques to access therapist thinking and collect professional reasoning data. Research conducted to date uses very simple techniques to access therapist thinking, such as written case studies, and very little attention has been paid to

TABLE 7.5

Number of Articles on Professional Reasoning of Occupational Therapists or Students Published in Indexed Journals (1982–2014)

Journal	Number	Journal	Number
American Journal of Occupational Therapy	41	Medical Anthropology Quarterly	2
British Journal of Occupational Therapy	26	Medical Journal of the Islamic Republic of Iran	1
Occupational Therapy in Health Care	18	Assessment and Evaluation in Higher Education	1
Australian Occupational Therapy Journal	11	Computer Methods and Programs in Biomedicine	1
Scandinavian Journal of Occupational Therapy	6	Health and Social Care in the Community	1
Occupational Therapy Journal of Research	5	Journal of Physical Therapy Education	1
Journal of Allied Health	4	Medical Teacher	1
Occupational Therapy International	4	Physiotherapy Research International	1
Canadian Journal of Occupational Therapy	3	Reflective Practice	1
Physical and Occupational Therapy in Geriatrics	3	Technology and Disability	1
Disability and Rehabilitation	2	Journal of Interprofessional Care	1
Occupational Therapy in Mental Health	2	Work	1
International Journal of Therapy and Rehabilitation	2	**Total**	**140**

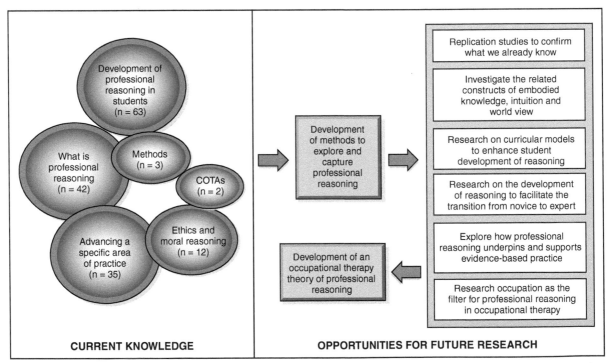

FIG. 7.1 ■ Conceptualisation of current knowledge (scope and size) of occupational therapy research and writing on professional reasoning and opportunities for future research.

adopting more innovative data collection methods (such as video capture and analysis) or using protocol analysis (as has been described by Ericsson & Simon, 1993).

The largest field of professional reasoning research is 'development of professional reasoning in students' and includes journal articles written about classroom experiences, fieldwork,

novice–expert differences and scales to measure student acquisition of reasoning. This last subtopic is of particular interest given research on capturing and 'measuring' reasoning is useful to educators wanting to determine whether their courses are promoting development of professional reasoning skills. However, this information is also very important to researchers in the

TABLE 7.6
Scales Used to Measure Professional Reasoning Skills (1982–2014)

Scale Name	Research Using the Scale	Source
The Structured Oral Self-directed Learning Examination (SOSLE)	Chapman (1993)	Included as an appendix in Chapman (1993)
California Critical Thinking Skills Test (CCTST)	Coker (2010), Velde (2006)	Available from Insight Assessment (www.insightassessment.com)
California Critical Thinking Dispositions Inventory (CCTDI)	Lederer (2007), Velde (2006)	Available from Insight Assessment (www.insightassessment.com) Facione (1996)
The Questionnaire for Reflective Thinking (QRT)	Kember (2000), Dunn (2011)	Included as an appendix in Kember (2000)
Watson-Glaser Critical Thinking Assessment (WGCTA)	Mitchell (2009), Mitchell (2011)	Watson and Glaser (1980)
The Self-Assessment of Clinical Reflection and Reasoning (SACRR)	Scaffa (2004a), Scaffa (2004b), Coker (2010)	Included in Table 1 in Scaffa (2004a)
Critical Thinking Survey (adapted from the work of Paul and Elder)	Schaber (2012)	Included in Table 2 in Schaber (2012)
The Professional Reasoning Case Analysis Test (CRCAT)	Sladyk (2000)	Created by Sladyk (2000) for the study, no example provided
Interactive Video Client Evaluation Simulation	Tomlin (2005)	Included as an appendix in Tomlin (2005)
The Sociomoral Reflection Measure-Short Form (SRM-SF)	Gibbs (1982)	Included in Gibbs (1992)

Note. Only the first author of each article has been included in the table for ease of reading.

field as a way of accessing and measuring therapist mastery and reasoning skills in general. Therefore Table 7.6 provides a summary of scales that can be used to measure the acquisition of professional reasoning skills, together with supporting literature and where the scales can be obtained. Finally, from Figure 7.1 it can be seen that the collective writing on professional reasoning in occupational therapy is contributing to the development of a theory of professional reasoning.

PROFESSIONAL REASONING IS MORE THAN THE LINK BETWEEN THEORY AND PRACTICE: DEVELOPING A THEORY OF PROFESSIONAL REASONING

Theories are connected sets of ideas that form the basis for action. Theories are generally developed away from that action and are referred to as 'espoused', which means held as true. Occupational therapy models such as the Model of Human Occupation (MOHO) (Kielhofner, 2008), or the CMOP-E (Townsend & Polatajko, 2013) are espoused theories. However, some researchers suggest that theory can arise from practice (Creek & Ormston, 1996). Argyris and Schön (1974) refer to this approach as building 'theories in use', and Kielhofner (2005) describes a similar process as building a 'scholarship of practice'.

When the foundational clinical reasoning study was developed, the research team wanted to discover the practical theories that occupational therapists used, and build a language to describe these. Therefore the clinical reasoning study was more than a way of gathering insights to how occupational therapists think in practice, because it also laid the foundation for building a theory of clinical, or professional, reasoning. All the descriptive and empirical research conducted over the past 33 years and published in the 140 articles referred to earlier has been slowly building a theory of professional reasoning. More structure around this theory is required, as is a process to test and prove the theory.

A summary of four models of professional reasoning that have been articulated or are under development have been presented previously (Schell, Unsworth, & Schell, 2008) and include Dewey's Linear Model of Clinical Reasoning, Higgs and Jones' Spiral Model of Clinical Reasoning, Schell's Ecological Model of Professional Reasoning and Unsworth's hierarchical model (Schell et al., 2008). Unsworth's Hierarchical Model of Professional Reasoning is presented as an example in Figure 7.2 and depicts the combined reasoning of both the therapist and the person as they interact during a therapeutic encounter. For both therapists and the people they work with, three levels of reasoning are articulated. Both the person and the occupational therapist have their own worldview, which overarches all forms of thinking. Worldview is described as encompassing an individual's personal-cultural-historical context and produces the individual's global view on life (Wolters, 1989). Occupational therapy research investigating the worldview of therapists (Unsworth, 2004) suggests that worldview incorporates values, beliefs, faith and spirituality, as well as ability to read the practice culture, interest in the profession, repertoire of therapy

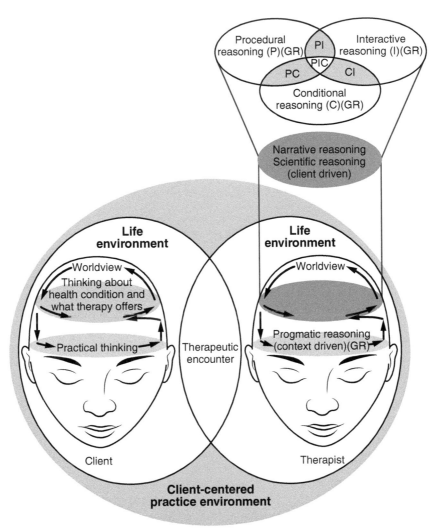

FIG. 7.2 ■ Current conceptualisation of professional reasoning in occupational therapy. Note: GR = Generalisation reasoning. *(Modified from Fig. 16.1 in Unsworth, 2011a; Unsworth, 2004.)*

skills and motivation. Unsworth proposed that *worldview* describes the influence of the therapist's personal context on professional reasoning but is not a form of reasoning itself. Occupational therapists cannot divorce the therapy they provide from the individuals they are. Therefore worldview will influence everything the therapist does. However, the extent of this influence will be modified by the therapist's willingness to reflect and insightfulness concerning how worldview may be affecting therapy in a positive or potentially negative way (see also Table 7.3).

The 'middle' level of reasoning that the person engages in is concerned with thinking about his or her health condition and

what the therapy offers, whereas for the occupational therapist this middle level depicts the interactions of all the types of professional reasoning (as described in Table 7.2). Finally, for the therapist, the most basic level of thinking involves pragmatic reasoning, which is concerned with what can be done given finite resources, and how the therapist negotiates with the person, their family and the therapy services as well as funders and the health care environment to deliver services (Unsworth, 2004). For the person, this reasoning involves the practical thinking around resources such as funding therapy, allocating the time to therapy tasks required and getting to and from the service.

CONCLUSION

An overview of professional reasoning in occupational therapy has been provided in this chapter, including an introduction to a framework to understand what professional reasoning is, and a language to enable students and experts to better articulate what is happening in practice so that it can be more clearly voiced and shared. Using a framework and a common language is vital if novices are to learn and experts are to gain access to their often tacit knowledge. The story of James and his occupational therapist was told to illustrate Jess' professional reasoning. The excerpts from the narrative illustrate many of the modes of reasoning, as they relate to the eight action phases of therapy as described by the CPPF. These excerpts also highlight the need to ensure the client's occupational hopes and dreams are at the centre of the co-created narrative. A brief summary of research into professional reasoning over the past three decades provides insights into where further research is needed, and it is suggested that this body of work is laying the foundation for the development of a theory of professional reasoning in occupational therapy.

Acknowledgment

Many thanks to Dr. Anne Baker who through her work as a research assistant, helped source the clinical/professional reasoning literature presented in this Chapter.

 http://evolve.elsevier.com/Curtin/OT

REFERENCES

Anderson, J. R. (1983). *The architecture of cognition.* Cambridge, MA: Harvard University Press.

Argyris, C., & Schön, D. A. (1974). *Theory in practice: Increasing professional effectiveness.* San Francisco: Jossey-Bass.

Barnett, R. (1997). *Higher education: A critical business.* Buckingham: The Society for Research into Higher Education and Open University Press.

Barnitt, R., & Partridge, C. (1997). Ethical reasoning in physical therapy and occupational therapy. *Physiotherapy Research International, 2*(3), 178–194.

Barris, R. (1987). Clinical reasoning in psychosocial occupational therapy: The evaluation process. *Occupational Therapy Journal of Research, 7*(3), 147–162.

Barsalou, L. W. (1992). Frames, concepts and conceptual fields. In A. Lehrer, & E. F. Kittay (Eds.), *Frames, fields and contrasts: New essays in semantic and lexical organisation* (pp. 21–74). Hillsdale, NJ: Erlbaum.

Benner, P. (1984). *From novice to expert. Excellence and power in clinical nursing practice.* Menlo Park, CA: Addison-Wesley.

Carr, M., & Shotwell, M. (2008). Information processing theory and professional reasoning. In B. B. Schell, & J. W. Schell (Eds.), *Clinical and professional reasoning in occupational therapy* (pp. 36–67). Baltimore: Lippincott Williams & Wilkins.

Chaffey, L., Unsworth, C. A., & Fossey, E. (2010). A grounded theory of intuition among occupational therapists in mental health practice. *British Journal of Occupational Therapy, 73*(7), 300–308.

Chapman, J. A., Westmorland, M. G., Norman, G. R., Durrell, K., & Hall, A. (1993). The structured oral self-directed learning evaluation: One method of evaluating the clinical reasoning skills of occupational therapy and physiotherapy students. *Medical Teacher, 15*(2-3), 223–236.

Coker, P. (2010). Effects of an experiential learning program on the clinical reasoning and critical thinking skills of occupational therapy students. *Journal of Allied Health, 39*(4), 280–286.

Creek, J., & Ormston, C. (1996). The essential elements of professional motivation. *British Journal of Occupational Therapy, 59*, 7–10.

Dreyfus, H. L., & Dreyfus, S. E. (1986). *Mind over machine: The power of human intuition and expertise in the era of the computer.* New York: Free Press.

Dunn, L., & Musolino, G. M. (2011). Assessing reflective thinking and approaches to learning. *Journal of Allied Health, 40*(3), 128–136.

Ericsson, K. A., & Simon, H. A. (1993). *Protocol analysis: Verbal reports as data.* Boston: MIT Press.

Facione, P. A., Facione, N. C., & Giancarlo, C. A. F. (1996). *The California critical thinking disposition inventory: Test manual.* Millbrae, CA: The California Academic Press.

Fearing, V. G., Law, M., & Clark, J. (1997). An occupational performance process model: Fostering client and therapist alliances. *Canadian Journal of Occupational Therapy, 64*(1), 7–15.

Gibbs, J. C., Basinger, K. S., & Fuller, D. (1992). *Moral Maturity: Measuring the Development of Sociomoral Reflection.* Hillsdale, NJ: Lawrence Erlbaum.

Gibbs, J. C., & Widaman, K. F. (1982). *Social intelligence: Measuring the development of sociomoral reflection.* Englewood Cliffs, NJ: Prentice Hall.

Gibson, D., Velde, B., Hoff, T., Kvashay, D., Manross, P. L., & Moreau, V. (2000). Clinical reasoning of a novice versus an experienced occupational therapist: A qualitative study. *Occupational Therapy in Health Care, 12*(4), 15–31.

Gilpin, M., King, G., Currie, M., et al.(2005). The multidimensional peer rating of the clinical behaviours of pediatric therapists (MPR). *Focus On, 5*(4).

Hallin, M., & Svidán, G. (1995). On expert occupational therapists' reflection on practice. *Scandinavian Journal of Occupational Therapy, 2*(2), 69–75.

Hooper, B. (1997). The relationship between pretheoretical assumptions and clinical reasoning. *The American Journal of Occupational Therapy, 51*(5), 328–338.

Kember, D., Leung, D. Y. P., Jones, A., et al.(2000). Development of a questionnaire to measure the level of reflective thinking. *Assessment and Evaluation in Higher Education, 25*(4), 381–395.

Kielhofner, G. (2005). A scholarship of practice: Creating discourse between therapy, research, and practice. *Occupational Therapy in Health Care, 19*, 7–16.

Kielhofner, G. (2008). *Model of human occupation: Theory and application* (4th ed.). Baltimore: Lippincott Williams & Wilkins.

King, G., Currie, M., Bartlett, D. J., Strachan, E., Tucker, M. A., & Willoughby, C. (2008). The development of expertise in paediatric rehabilitation therapists: The roles of motivation, openness to experience, and types of caseload experience. *Australian Occupational Therapy Journal, 55*(2), 108–122.

Lederer, J. M. (2007). Disposition toward critical thinking among occupational therapy students. *American Journal of Occupational Therapy*, 61(5), 519–526.

Lyons, K. D., & Crepeau, E. B. (2001). The clinical reasoning of an occupational therapy assistant. *American Journal of Occupational Therapy*, 55(5), 577–581.

Mattingly, C. (1994). Occupational therapy as a two-body practice: The body as Machine. (pp. 37-63). In C. Mattingly, & M. H. Fleming (Eds.), *Clinical reasoning: Forms of inquiry in a therapeutic practice*. Philadelphia: F.A. Davis.

Mattingly, C., & Fleming, M. H. (1994). *Clinical reasoning: Forms of inquiry in a therapeutic practice*. Philadelphia: F.A. Davis.

Merriam-Webster.com. (2016). Retrieved from www.merriam-webster.com

Mitchell, A. W., & Batorski, R. E. (2009). A study of critical reasoning in online learning: Application of the Occupational Performance Process Model. *Occupational Therapy International*, 16(2), 134–153.

Mitchell, R., & Unsworth, C. A. (2005). Clinical reasoning during community health home visits: Expert and novice differences. *British Journal of Occupational Therapy*, 68(5), 215–223.

Mitchell, A. W., & Xu, Y. J. (2011). Critical reasoning scores of entering bachelor's and master's students in an occupational therapy program. *American Journal of Occupational Therapy*, 65(6), e86–e94.

Paivio, A. (1971). *Imagery and visual processes*. New York: Holt, Rinehart & Winston.

Rew, L. (1986). Intuition: concept analysis of a group phenomenon. *Advances in Nursing Science*, 8(2), 21–28.

Robertson, L. J. (1996). Clinical reasoning, Part 2: Novice/expert differences. *British Journal of Occupational Therapy*, 59(5), 212–216.

Robertson, D., Warrender, F., & Barnard, S. (2015). The critical occupational therapy practitioner: How to define expertise? *Australian Occupational Therapy Journal*, 62, 68–71.

Rogers, J. C. (1983). Clinical reasoning: The ethics, science, and art. *American Journal of Occupational Therapy*, 37, 601–616.

Rogers, J. C., & Holm, M. B. (1991). Occupational therapy diagnostic reasoning: A component of clinical reasoning. *American Journal of Occupational Therapy*, 45, 1045–1053.

Rogers, J. C., & Masagatani, G. (1982). Clinical reasoning of occupational therapists during initial assessment of physically disabled patients. *Occupational Therapy Journal of Research*, 2, 195–219.

Scaffa, M. E., & Smith, T. M. (2004a). Effects of Level II fieldwork on clinical reasoning in occupational therapy. *Occupational Therapy in Health Care*, 18(1/2), 31–38.

Scaffa, M. E., & Wooster, D. M. (2004b). Effects of problem-based learning on clinical reasoning in occupational therapy. *American Journal of Occupational Therapy*, 58(3), 333–336.

Schaber, P., & Shanedling, J. (2012). Online course design for teaching critical thinking. *Journal of Allied Health*, 41(1), e9–e14.

Schell, B. B., & Cervero, R. M. (1993). Clinical reasoning in occupational therapy: An integrative review. *American Journal of Occupational Therapy*, 47, 605–610.

Schell, B. B., & Schell, J. W. (Eds.), (2008). *Clinical and professional reasoning in occupational therapy*. Philadelphia: Lippincott Williams & Wilkins.

Schell, B. B., Unsworth, C. A., & Schell, J. W. (2008). Theory and practice: New directions for research in professional reasoning.

In B. B. Schell & J. W. Schell (Eds.), *Clinical and professional reasoning in occupational therapy* (pp. 401–431). Philadelphia: Lippincott, Williams & Wilkins.

Schön, D. A. (1983). *The reflective practitioner: How professionals think in action*. New York: Basic Books.

Sladyk, K., & Sheckley, B. (2000). Clinical reasoning and reflective practice: Implications of fieldwork activities. *Occupational Therapy in Health Care*, 13(1), 11–22.

Smith, G. (2006). The Casson Memorial Lecture 2006: Telling Tales—How Stories and Narratives Co-Create Change. *The British Journal of Occupational Therapy*, 69(7), 304–311.

Strong, J., Gilbert, J., Cassidy, S., & Bennett, S. (1995). Expert clinicians' and students' views on clinical reasoning in occupational therapy. *British Journal of Occupational Therapy*, 58(3), 119–123.

Taylor, R. (2008). *The intentional relationship. Occupational therapy and use of self*. Philadelphia: FA Davis.

Tomlin, G. S. (2005). The use of interactive video client simulation scores for the prediction of clinical performance of occupational therapy students. *American Journal of Occupational Therapy*, 59(1), 50–56.

Townsend, E. A., & Polatajko, H. J. (2013). *Enabling occupation II: Advancing an occupational therapy vision for health, well-being, and justice through occupation* (3rd ed.). Ottawa: Canadian Association of Occupational Therapists.

Unsworth, C. A. (2001a). The clinical reasoning of novice and expert occupational therapists. *Scandinavian Journal of Occupational Therapy*, 8(4), 163–173.

Unsworth, C. A. (2001b). Using a head-mounted video camera to study clinical reasoning. *American Journal of Occupational Therapy*, 55, 582–588.

Unsworth, C. A. (2004). Clinical Reasoning: How do worldview, pragmatic reasoning and client-centredness fit? *British Journal of Occupational Therapy*, 67(1), 10–19.

Unsworth, C. A. (2005). Using a head-mounted video camera to explore current conceptualizations of clinical reasoning in occupational therapy. *American Journal of Occupational Therapy*, 59, 31–40.

Unsworth, C. A. (2011a). The evolving theory of clinical reasoning. In E. A. S. Duncan (Ed.), *Foundations for Practice in Occupational Therapy* (pp. 209–231). (5th ed.). Edinburgh: Elsevier.

Unsworth, C. A. (2011b). How therapists think: Exploring therapists' reasoning when working with patients who have cognitive and perceptual problems following stroke. In G. Gillen, & A. Burkhardt (Eds.), *Stroke rehabilitation: A function-based approach* (pp. 438–455). (3rd ed.). St. Louis: Mosby.

Unsworth, C. A., & Baker, A. (2016). A systematic review of professional reasoning literature in occupational therapy. *British Journal of Occupational Therapy*, 79(1), 5–16.

Velde, B. P., Wittman, P. P., & Vos, P. (2006). Development of critical thinking in occupational therapy students. *Occupational Therapy International*, 13(1), 49–60.

Watson, G., & Glaser, E. M. (1980). *Watson-Glaser Critical Thinking Appraisal Manual*. San Antonio, TX: The Psychological Corporation – Harcourt Brace & Co.

Wolters, A. M. (1989). On the idea of worldview and its relationship to philosophy (pp. 14–26). In P. A. Marshall, S. Griffioen, & R. Mouw (Eds.), *Stained glass: Worldviews and social science*. New York: University Press of America.

8

CANADIAN PRACTICE PROCESS FRAMEWORK

NOÉMI CANTIN ■ MARTINE BROUSSEAU

CHAPTER OUTLINE

Abstract
The Canadian Practice Process Framework (CPPF) (Polatajko, Craik, Davis, & Townsend, 2007a) is introduced as a tool designed to guide occupational therapists as they enable the individual, group, community or population to engage in and perform occupations, placing these people at the centre of the occupational therapy process. The CPPF represents the progression of a partnership between an occupational therapist and the people receiving occupational therapy services that enables the move from an occupational challenge to successful occupational performance, within a given societal and practice context. In this chapter, the practice stories of three individuals are used to guide occupational therapy students, as well as novice and experienced occupational therapists, as they reflect on the practical use of the CPPF.

KEY POINTS

- The Canadian Practice Process Framework (Polatajko et al., 2007a) is a generic framework that ensures occupational therapists position an individual, group, community or population at the centre of the occupational therapy process.

- The CPPF graphically represents the occupational therapy practice process through eight action points.

- The eight action points are contained within the frame(s) of reference element of the CPPF to illustrate that theories, models of occupational therapy practice and interdisciplinary frames of reference influence everything that an occupational therapist does.

- The CPPF represents the occupational therapy process across the different contexts within which occupational therapy can take place, while also highlighting the influence of the societal context.

- The CPPF emphasises the necessity for occupational therapists to become expert reflective practitioners throughout the practice process.

INTRODUCTION

Exemplary occupational therapy is based on the fundamental concepts of the profession, focuses on enabling an individual, group, community or population to engage in and perform occupations, places these people at the centre of the process, is research informed, and is congruent with the services offered within the practice context. In this chapter, the Canadian Practice Process Framework (CPPF) (Polatajko et al., 2007a) is introduced as a tool designed to guide occupational therapists as they carry out such practice. First, the elements of CPPF are briefly introduced. Then, each of the action points of the process framework are described and illustrated using practice stories.

THE CANADIAN PRACTICE PROCESS FRAMEWORK

In general, occupational therapy practice models graphically depict beliefs regarding the interaction of concepts critical to the production of occupational performance or engagement. The CPPF (Polatajko et al., 2007a) belongs to a different category of models. The CPPF is a generic framework that graphically represents the occupational therapy practice process. It represents this process across the different contexts within which occupational therapy can take place when working with an individual, group, community or population (Craik, Davis, & Polatajko, 2013). The CPPF represents the progression of a partnership between an occupational therapist and an individual, group, community or population receiving occupational therapy services that enables the move from an occupational challenge to successful occupational performance within a given societal and practice context.

Four specific elements are illustrated in the CPPF (Fig. 8.1): the societal context (outer box), the practice context (inner box), the frames of reference (large circle) and the action points (small circles) (Craik et al., 2013). Each element will be briefly described here and illustrated in the practice stories.

Societal Context

The societal context is included in the framework to highlight the influence of cultural, institutional, physical and social elements of the environment on all occupational therapy practice processes. Occupational therapists from around the world can use the CPPF to frame their actions and reflect on how their particular societal context influences what they do. Examples of influential elements could be health care funding policies, cultural expectations or societal values.

Practice Context

The practice context is embedded within this societal context, which is why the line separating the two in Figure 8.1 is dotted. It also includes cultural, institutional, physical and social elements of the environment, but this time it is specific to an occupational therapist's practice environment. This might include physical characteristics of the spaces where interventions are carried out, the presence of other team members, an institution's culture, or the prevailing model of service delivery. The practice context also includes personal elements related to the therapist and the client's "knowledge, abilities,

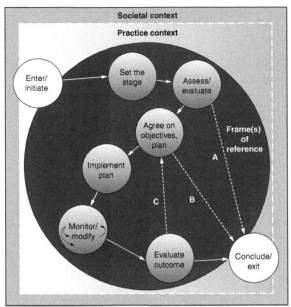

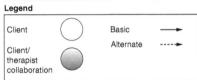

FIG. 8.1 ■ Canadian Practice Process Framework (CPPF) *(From Polatajko, H. J., Craik, J., Davis, J., & Townsend, E. A. (2007). Canadian Practice Process Framework. In E. A. Townsend & H. J. Polatajko,* Enabling occupation II: Advancing an occupational therapy vision for health, well-being, & justice through occupation *(p. 233). Ottawa: CAOT Publications ACE.)*

skills, habits, values, beliefs and attitudes" (Craik et al., 2013, p. 236). As illustrated by the graded shading in Figure 8.1, the practice context is where the therapeutic relationship between the occupational therapist and the individual, group, community or population begins.

Frames of Reference

The circle representing frames of reference is embedded within the practice context. The frames of reference hold the eight action points in the practice process. This illustrates that theories, models of occupational therapy practice and interdisciplinary frames of reference influence everything that an occupational therapist does (Craik et al., 2013). In occupational therapy, a frame of reference is understood to be based on a set of theories and assumptions that influence and constrain an occupational therapist's perception and understanding of occupational challenges, ultimately guiding professional reasoning during the occupational therapy process (Mosey, 1986; Townsend & Polatajko, 2013). In the CPFF, this element is defined broadly to include paradigms, theories, occupational therapy practice models and specific interdisciplinary frames of reference (Craik et al., 2013).

Despite numerous studies proposing that using theory intentionally and explicitly throughout the occupational therapy process is important, this remains a challenge for many therapists (Boniface et al., 2008; Leclair et al., 2013; Melton, Forsyth, & Freeth, 2010; Wimpenny, Forsyth, Jones, Matheson, & Colley, 2010). Indeed, the integration of theory into practice requires considerable commitment. When models of practice and frames of reference are mastered, their application results in solid professional reasoning. However, when understanding is superficial, or when the use of theory in practice is not valued, professional reasoning is weak and application of a theory's tools is haphazard and often ineffective (Boniface et al., 2008; Leclair et al., 2013). The CPPF highlights the importance of frames of reference and theories by depicting that the action points for intervention are based within these frames of reference that guide professional reasoning.

Action Points

The eight action points represent actions to be completed by occupational therapists to ensure their practice is centred on the individual, group, community or population, research informed, and occupation based. As such, the CPPF does not depict professional reasoning itself. Instead, it depicts the key action points where professional reasoning and reflection occur. The shading of the circles represents that both the individual, group, community or population and the therapist are actively engaged in each action step. Recognising that therapists work within varied societal and practice contexts, the process is meant to be flexible, allowing therapists to skip or repeat an action while still ensuring that they are following best practices. The dotted arrows in Figure 8.1 illustrate this flexible practice process. Furthermore, although each action point is represented separately, it is important to note that, sometimes, certain action points can be carried out simultaneously. For the purposes of illustrating the action points, the practice stories of three individuals will be used; it should be noted that these same action points can be used when working with groups, communities and populations.

Enter, Initiate

Victoria is a 40 year-old sole parent of two teenagers. She works at a local automobile manufacturing plant. She was referred to an outpatient chronic pain programme because of chronic back, shoulder and neck pain. Today, during the weekly team meeting, her file was presented by the nurse responsible for admissions. Victoria's pain was described in terms of its location, duration, frequency and intensity, and the nurse expressed her concerns about Victoria's mental health. As was

typical in this programme, an appointment was scheduled for a psychologist to conduct an initial assessment and provide an introduction to cognitive behavioural therapy. Victoria's initial meeting with the occupational therapist was scheduled for 2 weeks after the MDT meeting.

In this practice story, the occupational therapist's first point of contact with Victoria occurs when her file is presented during a weekly team meeting. This meeting marks the beginning of the occupational therapy process. At this action point, it is important to develop a clear understanding of the reason for referral. Such an understanding is essential to assess whether conflicts of interest could impede the therapist's ability to work with Victoria. Knowing the reason for referral helps the therapist evaluate whether the issue falls within the therapist's scope of practice and expertise. In a perfect world, referral sources would always understand that the goal of occupational therapy is to enable people to perform and engage in occupations that are important and meaningful to them (Polatajko, Davis, Cantin, Dubouloz, & Trentham, 2013b). However, in some practice contexts, occupational therapists report that they have to reframe the reason for referral so that it reflects what they actually do (Brousseau, 2004; Ordre des Ergothérapeutes du Québec (OEQ), 2010). In such cases, occupational therapists may need to educate and advocate to ensure that referral sources understand their expertise and scope of practice.

Even though Victoria was not physically present at the Enter/Initiate stage, this first action point forms the foundation of the therapeutic process. By identifying this as the initial action point, the CPPF highlights the importance of placing Victoria at the centre of the process and ensuring that occupations are the starting point of the interaction. To this end, before meeting Victoria, the therapist should read her file. During this reading, the therapist reviews information from the referral source and begins to form an image of Victoria. At the same time, the therapist reflects on her own thoughts, feelings and first impressions of Victoria, and reflects on the possible influence of previous experiences on the upcoming interaction with Victoria.

Reid (2009) proposes that occupational therapists can enhance their practice by intentionally setting the expectation that they will practice mindfully throughout the therapeutic process. Mindfulness has been discussed by many authors and disciplines. Reid chooses to define it as 'a means of paying attention in a particular way, on purpose, in the present moment, and in a nonjudgemental way' (Kabat-Zinn, 1994, p. 4)

The occupational therapist sat in her office, going over Victoria's file and reading the psychologist's report in preparation for her initial meeting with Victoria. She allowed herself to critically reflect on her typical practice, hoping to interrupt her usual ways of thinking and acting so that she could approach Victoria with an open mind, with creativity and an appreciation for Victoria's unique occupational experiences.

The therapist noted that the information currently in Victoria's file offered a very biomedical perspective of her pain. The occupational therapist really wanted to know Victoria as an occupational being, to learn more about her occupational roles, routines and habits and understand her perspective on her current occupational performance and engagement. The occupational therapist reflected on what she learnt and reflected on this through the lens of the occupational therapy practice model used to frame her practice. The therapist's knowledge of the research and previous experience with people with chronic pain suggested to her that Victoria's pain was likely to have an impact on her occupational roles and identity. The therapist expected that, to a certain extent, Victoria had adapted to her condition, had developed coping strategies, and had probably discovered that being engaged in some occupations helped distract her momentarily from the pain.

The occupational therapist met Victoria in the waiting room and invited her into the assessment room for their initial meeting.

Setting the Stage

It is during the Setting the Stage action point that the strengths and resources of people referred for occupational therapy are identified, as well as the occupational challenges that will be the focus of the occupational therapy process. At this action point the reason for referral might need to be reframed with, and centred on, the individual, group, community or population to ensure that the stage is set for a therapeutic process focused on significant occupations (Brousseau, 2004; Cup, Scholte Op Reimer, Thijssen, & Van Kuyk-Minis, 2003, OEQ, 2010). Indeed, since the importance and meaning of occupations is unique to each individual performing them, these can only be understood and explained by the people engaged in their performance (Polatajko et al., 2013a). Accordingly, the person receiving the occupational therapy services must be the ones who identify their occupational challenges.

The practice context will have a certain influence on an occupational therapist's scope of practice and the occupational challenges that can be addressed throughout the therapeutic process. The influence of the practice context on the therapeutic process should be discussed with the individual, group, community or population. It is nevertheless important for occupational therapists to remember that, despite their practice context, their scope of practice is occupational enablement and, accordingly, therapists should strive to enable people to not only see 'what is' but also consider 'what could be' (Townsend et al., 2013, p. 121) with regards to their occupational performance and engagement. Here again, the occupational therapist may need to educate and advocate to ensure managers and third party payers understand the health-promoting benefits of engagement in a broad range of occupations.

Engaging people in sharing their occupational narratives – that is, offering them the opportunity to tell their stories by organising past events, perceptions and experiences into meaningful wholes (Bonsall, 2012) – enables them to share the meanings they ascribe to their occupational performance and engagement, occupational roles and identities (Bonsall, 2012; Goldstein, Kielhofner, & Paul-Ward, 2004). The use of narratives early in the practice process also motivates them to be invested in their rehabilitation as it positions occupational therapy within the context of their life stories (Cup et al., 2003; Mattingly, 1998). Furthermore, narratives allow therapists to gain a greater understanding of the cultural meaning of occupations, which is critical to a culturally sensitive occupational therapy practice (Awaad, 2003).

The overarching occupational model of practice used by a therapist should have an influence on the structure of this initial therapeutic encounter and the information sought. For example, a therapist who ascribes to the Canadian Model of Occupational Performance and Engagement (CMOP-E) (Polatajko, Townsend, & Craik, 2007b) might consider using the Canadian Measure of Occupational Performance (Law et al., 2014) to guide the narratives of the individual, group, community or population and prioritise occupational challenges needing to be addressed. As therapists move on to the next action point, they would be interested in understanding how the dynamic interaction between factors related to people, their environments and occupations results in the current occupational performance and engagement issues.

Assess, Evaluate

Matthew's practice story will be used to illustrate the next two action points of the CPPF.

Matthew is a 36-year-old high school teacher. He had a spinal cord injury 4 years ago when he was involved in a motor vehicle accident. He was quite frustrated with his current wheelchair and asked to be seen at the seating clinic where an occupational therapist responsible for wheelchairs and adaptive seating systems procurement works.

During the initial meeting, the occupational therapist inquired about Matthew's current occupational engagement and performance to identify the occupational challenges that would be the focus of assessment. He explained that he felt quite limited by his current wheelchair. To him, it looked too medical, it seemed very slow and he felt that it limited the upper body movements he needed for many of the tasks and activities he had to do at work. Furthermore, his current wheelchair was not adequate for him to participate in most recreational activities he wished to engage in. Before his accident, Matthew was involved in many activities with his friends such as floor hockey, ultimate Frisbee and soccer. He wanted to get involved in adapted sports. The occupational challenges he identified were: (1) performing work activities requiring upper body mobility, and (2) engaging in adapted sports.

After gathering this information, the occupational therapist was ready to proceed with her evaluation to better understand why Matthew was experiencing these occupational challenges.

It is important to highlight here the many influences on this action point. Receiving a referral for occupational therapy does not always imply the need to perform an in-depth assessment of an individual, group, community or population's overall occupational performance. Sometimes, professional reasoning might suggest that only a screening assessment is needed; at other times the in-depth assessment of a single occupation might be most appropriate. The societal and practice contexts, and identified occupational challenges, as well as the chosen model of practice and relevant frames of reference will all contribute important elements to the professional reasoning leading to this decision.

Recognising the influence of the societal and practice contexts on this action point is essential. Sometimes, the practice context might determine the assessment tools that are available, the ones that must be routinely performed for reimbursement purposes or the ones for which the therapist has expertise to perform.

As well, given occupational therapists' understanding that occupational performance is the result of a dynamic interplay between a person, the person's environment and the occupation being performed, this action point is ideally carried out in the environment where occupational challenges are experienced. When the practice context prevents this from happening, the expertise of the individual, group, community or population should be relied upon for additional information. Reflecting on the likely influence of the environment on an individual, group, community or population's occupational challenges involves placing them at the centre of the assessment process and evaluating in the environments where these activities actually take place. Again, the therapist is called on to educate and advocate when managers or funders have difficulty supporting best practices in occupational therapy evaluation.

The occupational therapy model of practice guiding the therapeutic process will also influence the assessment process by drawing the focus of evaluation to specific elements of the model. Indeed, although each occupational therapy model has similarities, each model also uniquely presents its assertions with regards to the dynamic interaction of components of the person, the environment or the occupation that lead to occupational performance (Polatajko et al., 2013b). In an attempt to explore plausible explanations for the occupational challenges identified by an individual, group, community or population, frames of reference and related theories guide a therapist to explore specific components of the person, the environment or the occupation. Research-informed best practices and professional experiences will also come into play.

The occupational therapist commenced her evaluation of Matthew's occupational challenges. She explained her assessment plan and obtained his consent to proceed. She wanted to start her assessment by observing Matthew at his workplace; however, her current practice context limited her ability to leave

the seating clinic. Accordingly, she attempted to reproduce similar environmental conditions in the clinic and choose to rely on Matthew's assessment of his own work environment to explore the role it could play in explaining his current occupational challenges. Then, drawing from a biomechanical frame of reference, the occupational therapist proceeded to assess the fit of the chair and Matthew's postural alignment. Biomechanical theories further guided her professional reasoning and her decision about which measures to focus on. Finally, because of her practice experience, she decided to perform muscle testing to compare it with Matthew's previous assessment on file, wondering whether his current occupational challenge at work was related to a decrease in his strength.

Matthew had researched the different adapted sports available to him and had decided that he would like to join a local wheelchair hockey team. The occupational therapist had ordered adapted wheelchairs for that sport before and proceeded to take the necessary measurements.

Once the assessment is completed, this action point ends by putting all of the information gathered together to elaborate an analysis of an individual, group, community or population's current occupational challenges. This analysis represents an occupational therapist's interpretation of assessment findings and professional reasoning as to why an individual, group, community or population is experiencing such challenges (OEQ, 2010). This analysis provides the transition point between the assessment and evaluation of occupational challenges, the elaboration of occupational objectives, and a related intervention plan. This analysis is discussed with the individual, group, community or population before moving on to the next action point.

Matthew's satisfaction and performance of significant occupations was moderately altered. Specifically, his performance of tasks and activities related to his teaching had been affected by mobility restrictions secondary to the wheelchair's high back. Related reduced efficiency had also resulted in deconditioning of his postural muscles. His wheelchair offered too much postural support. Furthermore, his actual wheelchair was inadequate for playing wheelchair hockey.

The occupational therapist was ready to discuss potential objectives and develop an intervention plan with Matthew to enable him to resolve his occupational challenges.

Agree on Objectives and Plan

The specifics of an occupational therapist's practice context will influence the therapist's professional decision making while collaborating with an individual, group, community or population to establish objectives and plan the occupational therapy intervention. Available resources will vary by culture, values and beliefs, such as the value placed on universal accessibility to activities. Each practice context comes with its own set of factors that will influence a therapist's professional decision making at this action point, and it is important to actively consider if such factors will be facilitators to be exploited or obstacles to be overcome while forming objectives and the intervention plan.

At this action point, situating people at the centre of the process requires that they be actively engaged in setting the objectives and elaborating the intervention plan. Engaging them signifies more than simply asking for agreement with the objectives established by the therapist; it involves enabling them to see what is possible, to express their wants and needs, and to make informed choices (Ripat & Colatruglio, 2016). In a study exploring the wheelchair procurement process from the perspectives of therapists and people who use wheelchairs, Mortenson and Miller (2008) discovered that not all people who used wheelchairs were actively engaged in the process of setting objectives or elaborating the intervention plan. Some authors have suggested that this lack of involvement could explain the high levels of wheelchair abandonment reported in the literature (Kittel, Di, & Stewart, 2002). In fact, when the wants and needs of an individual who uses a wheelchair are not at the centre of the process, a wheelchair, which is supposed to offer great benefits such as improved comfort, increased autonomy in mobility and community participation (Mortenson & Miller, 2008), can lead to disability by, for example, limiting the individual's mobility or engagement in recreational activities (Kittel et al., 2002; Ripat, Brown, & Ethans, 2015).

After identifying the objectives, the occupational therapist developed a detailed intervention plan comprised of enabling skills, actions, and strategies in collaboration with Matthew that could be implemented to assist him to reach those specific objectives. The plan included answers to the what, when, where, who and how of the intervention. As the therapist elaborated the intervention plan, Matthew's unique experiences and expertise, as well as the therapist's previous professional experiences, research evidence from the literature, selected occupational model of practice, specific frames of reference and related theories, guided the therapist's professional reasoning.

Implement the Plan

Mrs Chin's practice story will be used to illustrate the remaining CPPF action points.

Mrs Chin was a 61-year-old widow, mother of four grown children and grandmother of two grandchildren. She experienced a stroke and was transferred to the inpatient rehabilitation unit. More than anything, Mrs Chin wanted to return home. Living alone and without access to support services, Mrs Chin felt she had to regain her autonomy in self-care occupations if she was to feel at ease at home. The occupational challenges she identified and prioritised when completing the Canadian Occupational Performance Measure

(COPM) (Law et al., 2014) during her initial meeting with an occupational therapist were showering, getting dressed and preparing a nutritious meal.

With these priorities in mind, at the next session her occupational therapist began an initial assessment of Mrs Chin's performance of those occupations. Once the evaluation was complete, the occupational therapist's analysis suggested that Mrs Chin was not able to complete these tasks as problems with bilateral coordination and dexterity, limited mobility of her right upper extremity, and mild attention deficits affected her function.

The occupational therapist determined that a cognitive-based approach to intervention, the Cognitive Orientation to daily Occupational Performance Approach (CO-OPApproach™) (Polatajko & Mandich, 2004), was likely to help Mrs Chin return to her chosen occupations. The occupational therapist's decision to use CO-OPApproach™ was research informed and based on her positive practice experience with the approach.

In collaboration with Mrs Chin, the occupational therapist proceeded to set the following specific occupational therapy objectives: Mrs Chin (1) will shower herself independently within 3 weeks, (2) will dress herself independently within 3 weeks, and (3) will prepare a nutritious lunch independently within 4 weeks. The occupational therapist developed an intervention plan with Mrs Chin, framed within the CO-OPApproach™. Mrs Chin agreed that this approach fitted with her general objective of regaining her autonomy before returning home.

When implementing the intervention plan elaborated with Mrs Chin, the specifics of the societal context and context of practice come into play. For example, stroke rehabilitation programs vary between regions and countries. Understandably, elements of the societal context will ultimately influence which intervention plans can be implemented. For example, for Mrs Chin, health care funding mechanisms and available health and social services resources within her community could have an impact on the type of intervention plan that would be possible.

Similarly, the context of practice on inpatient rehabilitation units also varies greatly. Some occupational therapists work within interprofessional teams where multiple professionals collaborate to achieve person-driven goals; others work on occupational therapy units where the scope of practice of each health care professional is dictated by their programme director or prescriptive treatment pathways. With Mrs Chin, the context of practice would likely influence the frequency and length of occupational therapy sessions and the duration of her stay on the rehabilitation unit. Once again, the therapist is called on to educate and advocate when managers or funders are not yet supporting best practices for occupational therapy intervention.

The occupational model of practice and frames of reference selected at the previous action point will guide the implementation of the intervention plan. For example, in this practice story, the protocol for the CO-OPApproach™ suggests that the first session be focused on establishing baseline performance of the chosen occupations and on teaching the global cognitive strategy. The CO-OPApproach™ protocol, adapted for adults who have experienced stroke, proposes that the approach be implemented over approximately 10 sessions, on a weekly basis or twice a week (McEwen, Polatajko, Huijbregts, & Ryan, 2009). However, it is important to note here that this protocol was initially tested with community-dwelling participants experiencing a more chronic phase of stroke. Professional reasoning may lead a therapist to increase the frequency of sessions to three times a week or daily for Mrs Chin. Evidence-based practice integrates research evidence, person expertise and professional expertise to inform professional reasoning and decision making (Kristensen, Person, Nygren, Boll, & Matzen, 2011; Sackett, Rosenberg, Gray, Haynes, & Richardson, 1996). In this case, when developing the intervention plan, the occupational therapist considered the fit between her previous experience using the approach on the rehabilitation unit, the research evidence and Mrs Chin's current condition.

Additionally, when implementing an intervention plan, occupational therapists must be acutely aware of the intervention burden imposed on people and ensure that it is minimised (Gallacher et al., 2013). Positioning people at the centre of the therapeutic process and weaving interventions within their daily lives is one of the ways in which the burden of an intervention plan can be reduced (Gallacher et al., 2013; Shippee et al., 2012). This begins with open dialogue between the therapist and the individual, group, community or population to identify potential issues and strategies to resolve them. It also requires a constant dialogue with the rest of the health care team to ensure coordination of everyone's efforts.

As the occupational therapist implemented the plan, she closely monitored Mrs Chin's progress toward her occupational goals to ensure that the intervention plan was helping her move towards her objectives.

Monitor and Modify

Positioning people at the centre of the therapeutic process also ensures that interventions are not futile, that they make sense to those receiving the interventions and that they lead to positive outcomes. However, to ensure that positive outcomes are reached, progress towards occupational objectives must be monitored and intervention plans must be modified and adapted to respond to the changing needs of people. Sometimes, this may even involve going back to 'assess/evaluate' and redrafting occupational objectives and developing a new intervention plan.

To be flexible and open to modifying an intervention plan, a therapist must necessarily be engaged in critical self-reflection throughout the therapeutic process; this reflection must necessarily involve the individual, group, community or population. By definition, the word *reflection* suggests thinking back about something that has happened (Yanow & Tsoukas, 2009), reflective practice being 'the practice of stepping back to ponder the meaning [of] what has recently transpired' (Raelin, 2001, p. 11). The term *reflection-on-action* describes reflection that takes place after the event has happened, whereas the term *reflection-in-action* has been coined to describe reflection that takes place in the moment, while the event is happening (Schön, 1987; Yanow & Tsoukas, 2009).

At the simplest level, therapists monitor progress to ensure that the intervention plan is truly helping people move towards their goals. As well, it is important to monitor whether progress appears to be sufficiently rapid that people's goals are likely to be met before discharge. If not, the intervention plan should be modified or a plan should be put in place to ensure people receiving occupational therapy services will be able to continue working towards these goals after discharge.

On a somewhat more abstract level, it is important that occupational therapists periodically review the plan to ensure that their understanding of the individual, group, community or population's goals aligns with their understanding. For example, if autonomy is a goal, is the occupational therapist's definition of autonomy consistent with the individual, group, community or population's definition? It is important to recognise that how autonomy is defined and what it means for different people, within a particular societal context, will be highly variable. Positioning people, with their wants, needs and specific contexts, at the centre of the therapeutic process will ensure that the occupational therapist is working in collaboration with them to reach the same goal.

Evaluate Outcome

Mrs Chin worked towards her occupational objectives for 3 weeks. As was determined when the objectives were set, it was time to evaluate the outcome of the intervention plan implemented. To gain Mrs Chin's perspective on her current performance in showering, dressing and preparing lunch, the occupational therapist readministered the COPM. Mrs Chin rated her performance and her satisfaction with her performance as significantly improved for all three objectives. The occupational therapist observed her performing the occupations and noted that the original breakdowns in performance have all been resolved. However, despite her progress, Mrs Chin was still anxious at the idea of being discharged back to her home. She felt that there was much to do to maintain her home and was unsure that she would be able to manage it all.

The focus of the summative evaluation was to determine the outcome of the implemented intervention plan in relation to the occupational challenges identified at the outset of the therapeutic process, the occupational objectives agreed upon after the initial evaluation, and the model of practice and frames of reference selected to guide the intervention. When people are positioned at the centre of the therapeutic process, outcome evaluation necessarily relies on their perceptions of goal attainment, as well as their satisfaction. What is most important is that, once an intervention plan has been implemented, people receiving occupational therapy services can perform and engage in the occupations they need and want to do, to their satisfaction. Sometimes, when the context of practice permits, outcome evaluation marks the transition to the identification of new occupational goals and beginning of a new therapeutic process. Other times, outcome evaluation marks the transition to concluding the occupational therapy process.

Beyond the importance of outcome evaluation for the individual, group, community or population, this action point is an important part of an occupational therapist's reflective practice. Professional expertise was mentioned earlier when briefly discussing evidence-based practice. Professional expertise can be thought of as the judgement and competencies that therapists acquire through experience and practice (Sackett, Rosenberg, Gray, Haynes, & Richardson, 1996). It is often this expertise that guides a therapist's professional reasoning when deciding how to integrate research-based evidence in an intervention plan. To build expertise, therapists must critically evaluate the outcome of each intervention plan implemented. Evaluating outcomes allows occupational therapists to accumulate a repertoire of personal practice stories, documenting on a very small scale the efficiency of their interventions. However, studies have demonstrated that with increased experience, professional decisions sometimes become intuitive and based on habitual patterns of practice (Boudrieu, 1990; Jarvis, 1999). Occupational therapists should be careful not to fall into this trap; instead, they must continuously question usual ways of doing through self-reflection while remaining open to the integration of research evidence into practice.

Conclude/Exit

The occupational therapist agreed that, although Mrs Chin had reached her occupational goals, further important occupational issues remained. However, unit policy required that Mrs Chin be discharged. In preparation for her imminent discharge from the unit, the occupational therapist engaged Mrs Chin in a discussion of her hopes with regards to her future occupational engagement and identified new occupational challenges. With Mrs Chin and the rest of the team, the occupational therapist arranged for follow-up services to help Mrs Chin meet these new occupational goals.

At the end of the therapeutic process, once intervention objectives have been met, the last action point remaining is to conclude the therapeutic relationship. Sometimes, and for many different reasons, the individual, group, community or population and therapist might decide to end the therapeutic relationship earlier in the process. Regardless, it is important that this action point be planned as carefully as the others. For example, for Mrs Chin, recognising that stroke recovery is a long-term and complex process, concluding the therapeutic relationship would necessarily involve coordinating with the community-based occupational therapist and other community agencies and services to ensure continuity of care beyond the inpatient rehabilitation unit.

It is important to remember that, although the conclusion of the therapeutic process does represent an end in itself, it also represents an important transition for people. Indeed, while on the rehabilitation unit, people like Mrs Chin are actively engaged in creating new meanings and order in their lives while attempting to keep a certain continuity in their sense of self (Dubouloz 2014; Mezirow, 2000; Purves & Suto, 2004). It could be said that they are in a transitional process between their previous selves and their future selves. In this sense, the conclusion of the therapeutic relationship would actually mark the continuation of this transitional process, with new challenges to face and new contexts to adapt to. When people are positioned at the centre of the therapeutic process, they are included in planning the conclusion.

CONCLUSION

In this chapter, the Canadian Practice Process Framework (Polatajko, 2007) was introduced and each element of the model was presented. The impact of societal and practice contexts on the occupational therapy practice process was highlighted throughout the chapter. The eight action points of the framework were depicted using three practice stories to offer varied exemplars of how the CPPF can be used to frame an occupational therapist's practice process and professional reasoning, keeping the individual, group, community or population and their occupations at the centre of the process. Finally, the influence and importance of models of practice and frames of reference in professional reasoning and practice was emphasised.

In many ways, although the CPFF may at first appear to represent a simple process to be followed, there is a complexity to this process, which clearly emphasises the necessity for occupational therapists to keep abreast of advances within the profession and their area of practice, integrate research evidence within their professional reasoning and strive to become expert reflective practitioners.

 http://evolve.elsevier.com/Curtin/OT

REFERENCES

Awaad, J. (2003). Culture, cultural competency and occupational therapy: A review of the literature. *British Journal of Occupational Therapy, 66*, 356–362.

Boniface, G., Fedden, T., Hurst, H., et al. (2008). Using theory to underpin an integrated occupational therapy service through the Canadian model of occupational performance. *British Journal of Occupational Therapy, 71*, 531–539.

Bonsall, A. (2012). An examination of the pairing between narrative and occupational science. *Scandinavian Journal of Occupational Therapy, 19,* 92–103.

Boudrieu, P. (1990). *The logic of practice.* Cambridge, UK: Polity Press.

Brousseau, M. (2004). *La tenue de dossiers en ergothérapie. Habiletés de rédaction.* Montréal: Ordre des Ergothérapeutes du Québec.

Craik, J., Davis, J., & Polatajko, H. J. (2013). Presenting the canadian practice process framework. In E. A. Townsend, & H. J. Polatajko (Eds.), *Enabling occupation II: Advancing an occupational therapy vision for health, well-being & justice through occupation.* (2nd ed.). Ottawa: CAOT Publications ACE.

Cup, E. H. C., Scholte Op Reimer, W. J. M., Thijssen, M. C. E., & Van Kuyk-Minis, M. A. H. (2003). Reliability and validity of the Canadian Occupational Performance Measure in stroke patients. *Clinical Rehabilitation, 17,* 402–409.

Dubouloz, C.-J. (2014). Transformative occupational therapy: We are wired to be transformers. *Canadian Journal of Occupational Therapy, 81,* 204–212.

Gallacher, K., Morrison, D., Jani, B., et al. (2013). Uncovering treatment burden as a key concept for stroke care: A systematic review of qualitative research. *PLoS Medicine, 10,* e1001473.

Goldstein, K., Kielhofner, G., & Paul-Ward, A. (2004). Occupational narratives and the therapeutic process. *Australian Occupational Therapy Journal, 51,* 119–124.

Jarvis, P. (1999). The way forward for practice education. *Nurse Education Today, 19,* 269–273.

Kabat Zinn, J. (1994). *Wherever you go you are there.* New York: Hyperion.

Kittel, A., Di, M. A., & Stewart, H. (2002). Factors influencing the decision to abandon manual wheelchairs for three individuals with a spinal cord injury. *Disability and Rehabilitation, 24,* 106–114.

Kristensen, H. K., Persson, D., Nygren, C., Boll, M., & Matzen, P. (2011). Evaluation of evidence within occupational therapy in stroke rehabilitation. *Scandinavian Journal of Occupational Therapy, 18,* 11–25.

Law, M., Baptiste, S., Carswell, A., Mccoll, M. A., Polatajko, H., & Pollock, N. (2014). *Canadian measure of occupational performance* (5th ed.). Ottawa: CAOT Publications ACE.

Leclair, L. L., Ripat, J. D., Wener, P. F., et al. (2013). Advancing the use of theory in occupational therapy: A collaborative process. *Canadian Journal of Occupational Therapy, 80,* 181–193.

Mattingly, C. (1998). In search of the good: Narrative reasoning in clinical practice. *Medical Anthropology Quarterly, 12,* 273–297.

McEwen, S. E., Polatajko, H. J., Huijbregts, M. P., & Ryan, J. D. (2009). Exploring a cognitive-based treatment approach to improve motor-based skill performance in chronic stroke: Results of three single case experiments. *Brain Injury, 23,* 1041–1053.

Melton, J. J., Forsyth, K., & Freeth, D. (2010). A practice development programme to promote the use of the Model of Human Occupation: Contexts, influential mechanisms and levels of engagement amongst occupational therapists. *British Journal of Occupational Therapy, 73,* 549–558.

Mezirow, J. (2000). *Learning as transformation: Critical perspectives on a theory in progress.* San Francisco: Jossey-Bass.

Mortenson, W. B., & Miller, W. C. (2008). The wheelchair procurement process: Perspectives of clients and prescribers. *Canadian Journal of Occupational Therapy, 75,* 167–175.

Mosey, A. C. (1986). *Psychosocial components of occupational therapy.* New York: Raven Press.

Ordre des Ergothérapeutes du Québec (2010). *Référentiel de compétences lié à l'exercice de la profession d'ergothérapeute au Québec.* Montréal: Ordre des Ergothérapeutes du Québec.

Polatajko, H. J., & Mandich, A. (2004). *Enabling occupation in children: The cognitive orientation to daily occupational performance (CO-OP) approach.* Ottawa: ON, CAOT Publications ACE.

Polatajko, H. J., Craik, J., Davis, J., & Townsend, E. A. (2007a). Canadian practice process framework (CPPF). In E. A. Townsend, & H. J. Polatajko (Eds.), *Enabling occupation II: Advancing an occupational therapy vision of health, well-being, & justice through occupation.* Ottawa: CAOT Publications ACE.

Polatajko, H. J., Townsend, E. A., & Craik, J. (2007b). Canadian model of occupational performance and engagement (CMOP-E). In E. A. Townsend, & H. J. Polatajko (Eds.), *Enabling occupation II: Advancing an occupational therapy vision of health, well-being, & justice through occupation.* Ottawa: CAOT Publications ACE.

Polatajko, H. J., Backman, C., Baptiste, S., et al. (2013a). Human occupation in context. In E. A. Townsend, & H. J. Polatajko (Eds.), *Enabling occupation II: Advancing an occupational therapy vision for health, well-being, & justice through occupation.* (2nd ed.). Ottawa: CAOT Publications ACE.

Polatajko, H. J., Davis, J., Cantin, N., Dubouloz, C. J., & Trentham, B. (2013b). Occupation-based practice: The essential elements. In E. A. Townsend, & H. J. Polatajko (Eds.), *Enabling Occupation II: Advancing an occupational therapy vision for health, well-being, & justice through occupation.* (2nd ed.). Ottawa: CAOT Publications ACE.

Purves, B., & Suto, M. (2004). In limbo: Creating continuity of identity in a discharge planning unit. *Canadian Journal of Occupational Therapy, 71,* 173–181.

Raelin, J. (2001). Public reflection as the basis of learning. *Management Learning, 29,* 11–30.

Reid, D. (2009). Capturing presence moments: The art of mindful practice in occupational therapy. *Canadian Journal of Occupational Therapy, 76,* 180–188.

Ripat, J., & Colatruglio, A. (2016). Exploring winter community participation among wheelchair users: An online focus group. *Occupational Therapy in Health Care, 30,* 95–106.

Ripat, J. D., Brown, C. L., & Ethans, K. D. (2015). Barriers to wheelchair use in the winter. *Archives of Physical Medicine and Rehabilitation, 96,* 1117–1122.

Sackett, D. L., Rosenberg, W. M., Gray, J. A., Haynes, R. B., & Richardson, W. S. (1996). Evidence based medicine: What it is and what it isn't. *British Medical Journal, 312,* 71–72.

Schön, D. A. (1987). *Educating the reflective practitioner: Toward a new design for teaching and learning in the professions.* San Francisco: Jossey-Bass.

Shippee, N. D., Mullan, R. J., Nabhan, M., et al. (2012). Adherence to preventive recommendations: Experience of a cohort presenting for executive health care. *Population Health Management, 15,* 65–70.

Townsend, E. A., Beagan, B., Kumas-Tan, Z., et al. (2013). Enabling: Occupational therapy's core competency. In E. A. Townsend, & H. J. Polatajko (Eds.), *Enabling occupation II: Advancing an occupational therapy vision for health, well-being, & justice through occupation*. (2nd ed.). Ottawa: CAOT Publications ACE.

Townsend, E. A., & Polatajko, H. J. (Eds.). (2013). *Enabling occupation II: Advancing an occupational therapy vision for health, well-being & justice through occupation*. (2nd ed.). Ottawa: CAOT Publications ACE.

Wimpenny, K., Forsyth, K., Jones, C., Matheson, L., & Colley, J. (2010). Implementing the model of human occupation across a mental health occupational therapy service: Communities of practice and a participatory change process. *British Journal of Occupational Therapy, 73*, 507–516.

Yanow, D., & Tsoukas, H. (2009). What is reflection-in-action? A phenomenological account. *Journal of Management Studies, 46*, 1339–1364.

9

OCCUPATIONAL THERAPY PRACTICE MODELS

MERRILL TURPIN

CHAPTER OUTLINE

Abstract

In occupational therapy, there has been substantial development of models of practice. In this chapter five occupational therapy models of practice are reviewed: Model of Human Occupation (MOHO), Person-Environment-Occupation Model (PEO), Occupational Performance Model (Australia) (OPM(A)), Canadian Model of Occupational Performance and Engagement (CMOP-E), and Kawa Model. Each model is described and the notion of occupation, conceptualisation of the occupational therapy scope of practice and recommendations for use in practice are made explicit. These five models of practice demonstrate different conceptualisations of occupation and therefore occupational therapy. MOHO emphasises the intertwined nature of the action of people in their environments and contributes a substantial bank of assessment tools to occupational therapy practice. PEO takes an ecological view, in which the congruence among person, environment and occupation in an event underpins occupational performance. OPM(A) presents occupation as a process through which people enact occupational performance roles. CMOP-E presents occupation as the bridge between person and environment. Kawa highlights the importance of creating a culturally relevant approach to occupation.

KEY POINTS

■ Occupational therapy has substantial development of models of practice.

■ MOHO highlights how occupation is selected, organised and undertaken within particular environments. It also contributes a substantial bank of assessment tools to occupational therapy practice.

■ PEO emphasises the importance of the congruence among person, environment and occupation (PEO fit) to occupational performance within an event.

■ OPM(A) provides a framework for guiding occupational analysis, which is used to understand and facilitate occupational role performance.

■ CMOP-E conceptualises occupation as the bridge through which individuals can affect the environment.

■ Kawa highlights the importance of maintaining a culturally relevant approach to occupation and uses the collectivist nature of the Japanese culture to highlight the Western-centric notions that are often uncritically accepted in occupational therapy.

INTRODUCTION

In occupational therapy there has been substantial development of models of practice. The term *model of practice* refers to frameworks that aim to 'assist therapists by providing a conceptual framework for thinking about, planning and interpreting action (both their own and that of their clients)' (Turpin & Iwama, 2011, p. 22). Thus occupational therapy models of practice are important to consider when using the Canadian Practice Process Framework (CPPF), because they link theory to action. Models of practice aim to guide practice by providing a basis for both the *thinking in action* in which occupational therapists engage (Mattingly & Fleming, 1994) and planning for action.

Decision making in relation to action is central to professional practice. Occupational therapists have to make decisions about the following:

■ What information to collect
■ How to collect it
■ How best to organise it
■ How to interpret it
■ What to do (e.g. plan intervention)
■ Whether the chosen action adequately addresses the identified occupational issues and consequent goals for occupational therapy
■ What, if any, modifications need to be made to the current plan of action

Models of practice support the complex decision making that is required of occupational therapists in practice.

Turpin and Iwama (2011) outlined five ways that models of practice can guide practice. They are as follows: (1) make explicit occupational therapy assumptions regarding human occupation; (2) assist in defining the scope of practice; (3) facilitate the systematic and comprehensive collection of information that contributes to a holistic understanding of occupational issues of the people receiving occupational therapy; (4) assist occupational therapists to think about what *ideally* could be done, rather than being constrained in their thinking by a particular practice context (although occupational therapists need to be practical and consider the actual context in which they are working, they can become blind to other possibilities regarding what *could* be done, and using models of practice can assist in overcoming this); and (5) enhance professionalism, in that, by making explicit the theoretical assumptions of the profession and how it organises concepts, models contribute to demonstrating the profession's body of knowledge, opening it to critical review (internal and external).

This chapter outlines five occupational therapy models of practice. These are: Model of Human Occupation (MOHO), Person-Environment-Occupation Model of Occupational Performance (PEO), Occupational Performance Model (Australia) (OPM(A)), Canadian Model of Occupational Performance and Engagement (CMOP-E) and Kawa Model. Although occupational therapy has a well-developed suite of models of practice (see Turpin & Iwama, 2011 for a detailed review of nine occupational therapy models of practice), these five provide an overview of some of the different ways that concepts have been organised in order to guide occupational therapy practice. For each, the notion of occupation, the scope of occupational therapy and any guidelines provided for using the model in practice are presented (see Table 9.1 for a summary).

MODEL OF HUMAN OCCUPATION

MOHO was the first published of the models of practice to be reviewed in this chapter, and its development has continued over the greatest span of time. Publications commenced in the early 1980s and MOHO grew out of the tradition of occupational behaviour established by Mary Reilly at the University of Southern California (Madigan & Parent, 1985). The model has been published in four editions, in the years 1985, 1995, 2002 and 2008, and has undergone substantial change over that extended time (see Turpin & Iwama, 2011 for a further historical perspective on the model).

Right from its inception, exploring and making explicit the influences on human occupation has been the central concern of MOHO. Human occupation (i.e. doing or action) is conceptualised as always occurring in a context. Thus MOHO provides a framework (Fig. 9.1) that details the following:

1. Components within a person that contribute to occupation
2. Environmental context in which a person's occupation occurs
3. Three dimensions of doing

TABLE 9.1
Comparison of Models

	MOHO	PEO	OPM(A)	CMOP-E	Kawa
Major concepts	Provides a framework for how people select, organise and carry out occupation through volition, habituation, and performance capacity and the lived body, respectively	Ecological model: Transactive (not interactive) relationship among person, environment and occupation. Event as the unit of analysis and P, E and O fit as the purpose of analysis	Occupational performance in context (person-environment-performance). Uses concepts from OP models (performance areas, performance components) but emphasises occupational performance in context	Occupational engagement includes performing and having occupations	River metaphor: Offers a cultural critique of occupational therapy assumptions and presents a collectivist understanding
Concept of occupation	Three dimensions of doing – participation, performance, skill – lead over time to occupational adaptation (which comprises occupational identity and competence)	One of three components (P, E and O) which, when in a congruent relationship, enhance occupational performance. Performed by particular people in particular places at particular times	A process rather than an entity. The process of purposeful and meaningful engagement, rather than the things in which people engage	All the tasks and activities in which a person engages in everyday life that are both culturally and personally meaningful. They are performed with regularity and consistency. Occupation is the bridge between person and environment	In a collectivist culture, occupation (doing) is a consequence of belonging and being. Harmony with the environment and context determines the meaning and purpose of occupation
Scope of practice	Occupational therapy practice should be occupation focused, client centred and evidence based	Facilitate occupational performance by analysing events in terms of person, environment and occupation and their combinations	Occupational therapy should address occupation roles. Interventions this may target any aspects of the internal or external environments	Occupation is the core domain of concern for occupational therapy, and enablement is the core competency	Occupation is life flow and occupational therapists are enablers of people's life flow
Use in practice	Extensive theoretical reasoning table. Six steps: 1. Generate questions to guide information gathering 2. Gather information on or with the person	Goal: to promote occupational performance by enhancing the person-environment-occupation fit. Three-stage process 1. Identify occupational strengths and problems in occupational performance in collaboration with person	Goal: to facilitate performance of occupational roles. Seven questions regarding the following: 1. Occupational roles 2. Routines, tasks and subtasks from the occupational areas	Six enablement foundations: 1. Choice, risk and responsibility – requires negotiation and awareness of the person's value and interests and considers legal responsibilities	Creative ways of using the model should be explored. Six steps: 1. Determine the appropriateness of the model and who should draw the river

Continued on following page

TABLE 9.1

Comparison of Models (*Continued*)

MOHO	PEO	OPM(A)	CMOP-E	Kawa
3. Include strengths and challenges in conceptualisation of the person 4. Identify therapeutic goals and plans 5. Implement and review intervention 6. Assess outcomes	2. Assess performance components, environmental conditions and occupations contributing to occupational performance problems 3. Combine information in a transactional framework to plan intervention and evaluate outcomes	3. Performance components or environmental factors 4. Core element functions 5. Time and space fit 6. Therapist's preferred approach to intervention 7. Use of techniques within the context of a task or relevant performance environment PRPP system of task analysis	2. Client participation 3. Visions of possibility (help clients form visions of what might be possible) 4. Change – to enable occupational patterns and balance and negotiate occupational transitions 5. Justice – recognising systematic injustice and advocating for people 6. Power sharing	2. Clarify the context of life flow by exploring elements in the drawing 3. Prioritise issues according to the person's perspective and exploring possibilities for facilitating life flow 4. Assess using formal, informal and qualitative assessments 5. Intervention 6. Evaluation

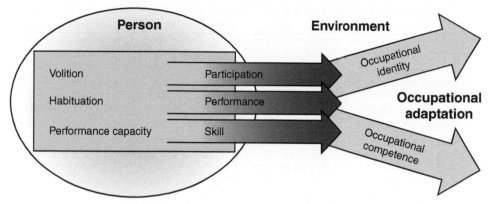

FIG. 9.1 ■ The process of occupational adaptation. *(Adapted from Kielhofner, 2008f, p.108.)*

These three aspects in combination result in occupational adaptation, which is defined as 'the construction of a positive occupational identity and achieving occupational competence over time in the context of one's environment' (Kielhofner, 2008f, p. 107). Each component is discussed next.

Components within the Person

MOHO provides a framework for conceptualising how people 'select, organise and undertake their occupations' (Kielhofner, 2008b, p. 12). The internal components of humans are vehicles through which these are achieved. These are volition, habituation, and performance capacity, and the lived body.

Volition

Humans are perceived as having an intense and pervasive need to act; that is, an impetus towards action. Motivation for action is addressed through the first component of the model, *volition*, which is defined as 'a pattern of thoughts and feelings about oneself as an actor in one's world which occurs as one anticipates, chooses, experiences, and interprets what one does' (Kielhofner, 2008b, p. 16). A volitional process of anticipating, choosing, experiencing and interpreting that courses through each of the three subcomponents of volition – personal causation, values and interests.

Personal causation refers to an individual's sense of his or her ability to act purposefully in the world and achieve outcomes. This is often referred to as a sense of agency (Germov, 2014). At the level of volition, it is not that people need to have the capacity to carry out the required tasks themselves, but rather they must have a sense that they can achieve the result they seek (perhaps by being able to prevail upon someone else). Previous experiences contribute to personal causation, so that depending on past experiences of self-efficacy and personal capacity, past successful outcomes might prompt people to persist in some areas of their lives while avoiding others.

Values is the second subcomponent of volition. These are 'beliefs and commitments about what is good, right, and important to do' (Kielhofner, 2008c, p. 39) that people acquire over their lives. They develop in the broader cultural contexts in which people grow, develop and belong and shape people's expectations about behaviour, the relative importance of various phenomena and happenings and their dreams and goals. They influence personal convictions, including beliefs, worldviews and perspectives and sense of obligation. 'Values bind people to action' (p. 41). When people choose to and are able to act in ways that are consistent with their values, they gain a sense of belonging to and value within their cultural group. When their actions contravene their values, they can experience guilt and shame.

The third subcomponent of volition is *interests*. These are defined as 'what one finds enjoyable or satisfying to do' (Kielhofner, 2008c, p. 42). Enjoyment can derive from the activity itself (e.g. simple routine activities or those a person undertakes with intense passion) or the context (e.g. being with friends). Enjoyment could arise from factors (and their combinations) such as: bodily pleasure, the handling of particular objects and materials, intellectual engagement, aesthetic satisfaction, successfully meeting challenges, creating a pleasing product and communing with others (Kielhofner). Each person develops a unique constellation of preferred activities. As with personal causation, interests can be influenced by past experiences, and their enjoyment often requires congruence between a person's capabilities and the demands of the activity (except, of course, when the enjoyment derives from overcoming a challenge or succeeding at a demanding activity).

Habituation

Whereas volition deals with the choices that people make about occupation, *habituation* outlines the way occupation is organised. People develop consistent patterns in their behaviour appropriate to the temporal, physical and social environments in which they occur. Habituation comprises habits and roles. Each is discussed.

When environmental conditions are sufficiently stable, people are able to respond in automatic ways. They form *habits* that help them adapt to and locate themselves within familiar environments. Habits allow people to act while reducing the cognitive load associated with decision making. For example, when in familiar environments, people can use routine ways of performing familiar activities, such as bathing and dressing. A clear sign that an activity has become habitual is when people perform it without conscious awareness. When in unfamiliar environments, activities that ordinarily would be routine might take longer and require more conscious effort. Kielhofner (2008d) emphasised the importance of the environment to habituation when stating that 'a large component of any habitual action will be strategies for incorporating the things, people, and events around us into what we do' (p. 54).

Habits have advantages for both individuals and society. Although habits can reduce cognitive load and allow individuals to do several things at once, they also serve the society. They can promote the transmission of culture and convey the customs of a society. They embody the values and expectations of the culture (whether society, group or organisation) and promote a sense of 'this is how we do things here'.

Another aspect of habituation, important to participation in society comprises internalised roles. Although roles carry social expectations, they are also internalised and individualised by the people adopting them. Society shapes roles by determining what roles are expected of people in particular situations and which roles are available or denied to particular people. However, people also shape the roles they carry out and internalise them. As Kielhofner (2008d) explained, the process of internalising roles 'means taking on an identity, an outlook, and actions that belong to that role. Consequently, an internalised role is the incorporation of a socially and/or personally defined status and a related cluster of attitudes and actions' (p. 59).

Performance Capacity and the Lived Body

Whereas the components of volition and habituation deal with how occupation is selected and organised, the third component deals with how occupation is undertaken. Kielhofner, Tham, Baz, & Hutson, (2008) explained that doing requires people to 'sense and interpret the world, move their bodies in space, manipulate objects, plan actions, and communicate and interact with others' (p. 68). In MOHO, the ability to undertake such action is called *performance capacity,* which has both objective and subjective components. The objective components are physical and mental abilities such as range of motion or cognitive processing. They are often observable. The subjective components of performance capacity are addressed using the concept of the lived body (i.e. the body as it is lived), which comes from phenomenology (a tradition in philosophy). Kielhofner et al. defined the lived body as 'the experience of being and knowing the world through a particular body' (p. 70). They explained that, at times, people are aware of their bodies, which can be the focus of their attention (e.g. a person might look at and think about his or her hand). At other times,

people experience the world *through* their bodies; their conscious attention is directed to something outside of themselves and their body becomes the invisible means through which they perceive and make a connection with it (e.g. a person reaches for a glass, a person looks at something). In everyday life, people take their bodies for granted, the unnoticed background to their conscious awareness, and only become conscious of them when something changes (e.g. they feel pain, their body does not work as it normally does). Although people may find it relatively easy to think about how their bodies contribute to the way they *do* things, it is often more difficult to think about how fundamental their bodies are to their *being* and *knowing.* Their bodies are central to both their sense of self and their perception of the world.

Environment

MOHO emphasises that occupation always occurs within contexts that can enable occupation by providing opportunities and resources or constrain it. The environment is seen as having four dimensions – spaces, objects, occupational forms or tasks and social groups – as well as its culture and economic and social conditions. *Spaces* are the physical contexts in which human occupation occurs and which shape it. *Objects* are the things with which people interact. They could be fabricated or naturally occurring and their properties influence how people interact with them. *Occupational form* refers to what is done and the cultural expectations regarding how it is done, which imbue an occupation with meaning and purpose. When performing occupation, an occupational form is enacted. *Social groups* refers to the social context in which occupation is undertaken. These social groups have norms that shape values, interests and the behaviours in which people engage when undertaking occupation.

These four dimensions of the environment occur within the broader cultural context, which is complex and has considerable variation within subcultures. Kielhofner (2008e) defined culture as 'the beliefs and perceptions, values and norms, customs and behaviours that are shaped by a group or society and are passed from one generation to the next through both formal and informal education' (p. 95). Culture also creates political and economic conditions that influence occupation by providing opportunities or constraining it. For example, conditions might enhance or diminish people's access to employment and education. In summarising the importance of the environment to occupation, Kielhofner stated, 'if we want to understand human occupation, we must also understand the environment in which it takes place. Occupation is, after all, action that occupies a particular social and physical space' (p. 97).

Concept of Occupation: Three Dimensions of Doing

In MOHO, human occupation is understood as shaped by both factors internal to people and the physical and social environments in which they live. Doing or action is conceptualised as having three dimensions: occupational participation, occupational performance and occupational skill. These three dimensions are described as embedded levels, whereby occupational skill is embedded within occupational performance, which is embedded within occupational participation. *Occupational participation* refers to engaging in occupations within a person's sociocultural context that are 'desired and/or necessary to one's well-being' (Kielhofner, 2008f, p. 101) and have personal and social significance. It is broader than simply performing occupation, as it includes subjective experience. The notion of *occupational performance* is informed by Nelson's (1988) distinction between occupational form (what is being done) and occupational performance (doing it). Consequently, 'occupational performance refers to doing an occupational form' (Kielhofner, p. 103). *Occupational skill* refers to the purposeful actions that contribute to occupational performance. Three types of skills are identified in MOHO: motor skills, process skills and communication and interaction skills.

Over time, occupational participation results in occupational adaptation. As Kielhofner (2008f) stated:

Occupational adaptation is the consequence of one's history of participation in life occupations. From the time we learn our first occupational forms and begin to participate in the world around us by doing things, we shape our own volition, habituation, and performance capacity. Throughout this process, we are in constant interaction with the physical and social environment that shapes the development of our volition, habituation, and performance capacity. These personal characteristics, in interaction with the environment, influence our occupational participation. (p. 107)

Occupational adaptation has two components, occupational identity and competence. Occupational identity is the subjective sense a person has of who he or she is that is developed over time through participation in the world. It includes who the person has been as well as a sense of who the person might become in the future. Occupational competence is 'the degree to which one sustains a pattern of occupational participation' (p. 107) over time. It is the action aspect of occupational adaptation.

Scope of Occupational Therapy

Kielhofner (2008a) stated, 'The vision for MOHO has been to support practice throughout the world that is occupation-focussed, client-centred, evidence-based, and complementary to practice based on other occupational therapy models and interdisciplinary theories' (p. 1). As MOHO centres on human occupation, rather than occupational therapy per se, the text does not specifically outline a scope for occupational therapy, apart from stating that human occupation is central to it. However, it bases the history of the model's development firmly in occupational therapy. Consequently, it proposes that occupational therapy should be occupation focused, client centred and evidence based.

Using MOHO in Practice

Kielhofner and Forsyth (2008) outlined six steps to guide the therapeutic reasoning required for practice and provided an extensive 'theoretical reasoning table' (p. 205) to guide these steps. The steps are as follows:

Step 1: Generating questions to guide information gathering. MOHO emphasises the narrative aspects of life and how occupational participation is developed and changes over the lifespan. Consequently, the purpose of this questioning is to understand people and their circumstances in terms of the various aspects of the model. Therefore questions can be devised around each MOHO concept. Seven questions, one for each aspect of MOHO, are provided by the authors to guide this step.

Step 2: Gathering information on or with the person receiving occupational therapy. Structured assessments and unstructured approaches can be used. MOHO has an extensive battery of structured assessments (e.g. Occupational Performance History Interview II, Worker Role Interview, MOHO Screening Tool, Assessment of Communication/ Interaction Skills).

Step 3: Creating a conceptualisation of the person that includes strengths and challenges. The MOHO framework forms the basis for this holistic understanding through the questions asked and information gathered. This provides the foundation for planning action for change.

Step 4: Identifying goals and plans for engagement of the person and therapeutic strategies. The MOHO framework guides the generation of goals and interventions. For example, intervention might target a component of the three aspects of the person and/or the environment.

Step 5: Implementing and reviewing therapy. Kielhofner and Forsyth emphasised 'being vigilant to monitor how therapy is unfolding' (p. 151). Therapists should expect some outcomes to be unanticipated and there should be a constant process of working through the earlier steps again.

Step 6: Collecting information to assess outcomes. The outcomes of therapy should be documented, including goal achievement and readministration of structured assessments.

PERSON-ENVIRONMENT-OCCUPATION MODEL OF OCCUPATIONAL PERFORMANCE

The Person-Environment-Occupation Model of Occupational Performance (Law, Cooper, & Strong, 1996) presents an understanding of occupation that is based on human ecology, an area of study concerned with the relationships between people and their environments. The PEO model was published in 1996 and has been very influential in occupational therapy since that time. It is currently being reviewed (including reviewing the occupational therapy literature regarding its use) and updated. Given that the model was published approximately 20 years ago, many of the concepts in the original publication, particularly regarding occupation and the terms used for different aspects of human action, might appear dated in the light of current occupational therapy literature.

Although there are three major components of the model – person, environment and occupation – they are conceptualised as richly interconnected, with their level of *fit* affecting occupational performance (Fig. 9.2). Law et al. (1996) described the PEO model as taking a 'transactive' perspective (p. 9) and distinguished this from an interactive approach in which the person and environment are considered as separate and independent entities that interact. In an interactive approach, where the components are considered independent, they can be studied separately. In contrast, an *event* is the unit of interest in a transactive perspective, because the components are interconnected and are not considered separately.

Law et al. (1996) described each component of the model and their assumptions. Their interconnectedness is evident when each is discussed. The *person* is seen holistically as a unique being that is a composite of mind, body and spiritual qualities, has skills and abilities that are learned or innate, and has attributes and life experiences that are brought into interaction with the environment. Attributes and life experiences include 'self-concept, personality style, cultural background, and personal competencies. This last factor incorporates abilities related to motor performance, sensory capabilities, cognitive aptitude

and general health' (p. 16). Some personal attributes are amenable to change, whereas others, such as cultural values, are likely to remain stable. In describing the person component, Law et al. (1996) emphasised that people are constantly interacting with the environment and fulfil multiple roles at once. These roles vary in importance, duration and personal significance.

The *environment* is considered dynamic and is defined broadly as having five domains. These are cultural, socioeconomic, institutional, physical and social. The rich complexity of the environment is evident as each environmental domain is considered 'from the unique perspective of the person, household, neighbourhood and community' (Law et al., 1996, p. 16). For example, it is important to consider the shared values and expectations of the community and their influence on an individual. The five environmental domains will influence and be influenced by the roles people have and the activities they undertake. For example, a particular place (physical environment) might have different purposes at different times (e.g. a church hall might be used for worship at one time and a community dance at another) because of the different roles that might be undertaken there. Law et al. (1996) proposed that the environment is generally more amenable to change than the person.

The concepts of activity, task and occupation are considered to be 'nested within each other' (Law et al., 1996, p. 16). The way these three concepts were defined in the 1996 publication, with activity being the 'basic unit of a task' (p. 16), would be at odds with many of the current hierarchies, which place task at a more fundamental level and often do not use the term *activity* at all. Occupations are regarded as meeting people's needs for self-maintenance, expression and fulfilment within the context of their life circumstances and roles. They are purposeful, pluralistic and complex. Emphasizing the transactive nature of the components, Law et al. (1996) stated that occupations are 'carried out within the context of individual roles and multiple environments' (p. 16).

Occupational performance is the result of the transaction among person, environment and occupation. The complexity of creating occupational performance is evident when considering that the meanings and purposes individuals ascribe to their actions are shaped by their worldview, goals, responsibilities and desires, as well as by the demands of the context in which they live and the occupations they are undertaking. The influence is multidirectional, in that the way people think about themselves and the actions in which they engage also affects their environments. Similarly, the experience of and need for particular occupations, as well as the way they are carried out, depend on the nature of both the individual and his or her environment. Therefore occupational performance is understood as a person-, occupation- and context-specific process, in which particular people take particular actions at particular times and in particular places.

The notion of the 'person-environment-occupation fit' (Law et al., 1996, p. 17) (PEO fit) is central to the model. This term encapsulates the assumption that the 'three major components (person, environment, occupation) interact continually across

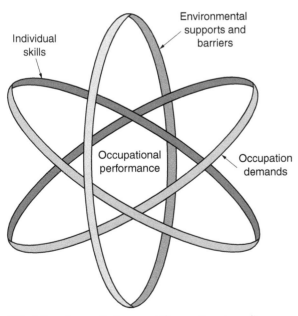

FIG. 9.2 ■ Person-Environment-Occupation atom diagram. *(From Law et al., 1996, p. 15.)*

time and space in ways that increase or decrease their congruence' (p. 17). The more congruence, or the better the fit, the more occupational performance will be increased. Conversely, the poorer the fit among the components, the poorer the outcome in occupational performance. The congruence between the three elements changes with time and space. These changes might be the consequence of the typical changes that occur across the lifespan or of unexpected disruptions.

Across the lifespan, changes are likely in a person's skills and abilities, the occupations expected of, or engaged in by, people at different times will differ, and there is often a great variety in the contexts in which these occupations are undertaken. For example, a person might attend university and undertake the occupations relevant to the role of university student at one time in his or her life and be in or out of work at another time. This will bring changes in the occupations and environments in which the person engages and the level of congruence with that person's skills. Within a shorter temporal period such as in daily life, people move between occupations and environments, creating a constant flux in the congruence of the three at any moment.

Concept of Occupation

Occupation is considered one of three components that contribute through their congruence to occupational performance. Occupation is performed by particular people in particular places at particular times. It cannot be understood outside of the context of persons and environments in which it occurs. Drawing upon the work of Csikszentmihalyi and Csikszentmihalyi (1988), Law et al. (1996) stated, 'When the challenges presented by an activity being carried out within an environment are in harmony with a person's skills, satisfaction with the experience of that activity is greater' (p. 13). It is the PEO fit in any particular event, rather than occupation per se, that is the central concern of this model.

Scope of Occupational Therapy

Law et al. (1996) stated that 'the model can be used to enrich and expand the clinical approach of occupational therapy' (p. 19). By focusing on an event, rather than the three components separately, occupational therapists aim to enhance the congruence of components in order to facilitate occupational performance in a particular circumstance. The repertoire of intervention options is quite broad, because it encompasses person, environment and occupation and their combinations. It provides for 'multiple avenues for eliciting change' (p. 18) and emphasises intervening in context.

Rich complexity in the concepts of person and environment creates expanded options for intervention. For example, viewing an individual as part of a family and community means that intervention might not be limited to centring on the individual. Similarly, considering all five domains of the environment

develops a much more complex understanding of the environments in which people perform occupations. Law et al. (1996) encouraged the profession to attend to the environments in which people live their lives.

Use in Practice

The goal of occupational therapy is to promote occupational performance by enhancing the person-environment-occupation fit. The PEO model outlines a three-stage process to follow when using it in practice. The first is identification of occupational strengths and problems in occupational performance. This is done in collaboration with the person receiving occupational therapy services and by using informal interviews, semistructured interviews such as the Canadian Occupational Performance Measure and standardised measures such as the Occupational Performance History Interview (Law et al., 1996). The second stage is the assessment of personal performance components, environmental conditions and occupations that might be contributing to occupational performance problems. Finally, all of this information is brought together 'in a transactional framework' (p. 19) to plan intervention, and then outcomes are evaluated.

OCCUPATIONAL PERFORMANCE MODEL (AUSTRALIA)

The name Occupational Performance Model (Australia) denotes the country from which this model originated. It was developed in 1986 at the University of Sydney, Australia. It was published as a monograph in 1997 (Chapparo & Ranka, 1997) and has a website that was launched in 2001, restructured in 2005 and relaunched in 2014 (http://www.occupationalperformance.com).

OPM(A) is based on the occupational performance models, the dominant models of practice in occupational therapy from the 1970s. These occupational therapy models focused on the component capacities (called performance components) that a person requires for occupational performance. These include biomechanical, sensory, perceptual, cognitive, psychological and social performance components. By the 1990s, occupational therapy models centred on a broader and deeply contextualised notion of occupational performance. Both of these historical trends are evident on OPM(A). Consistent with other occupational performance models, OPM(A) uses the structure of performance areas and performance components. However, like the models of the 1990s, it emphasises the interconnectedness of person and environment. This interconnectedness is particularly evident through the labels *internal* and *external environment* (which, in other models, would be called *person* and *environment*).

The internal environment encompasses four levels – occupational performance roles, performance areas, performance components, and the core elements of mind, body and spirit. The external environment provides the context for occupational performance. The central concern of OPM(A) is the performance of occupational roles (Fig. 9.3).

Occupational performance roles are defined as "patterns of occupational behaviour composed of configurations of self-maintenance, productivity, leisure, and rest occupations. Occupational performance roles are determined by individual person-environment-performance relationships. They are established through need and/or choice and are modified with age, ability, experience, circumstance and time" (Chapparo and Ranka, 2011, p. 6). In OPM(A), occupational performance roles are of primary importance, with the model advocating that all occupational therapists should aim to facilitate them, even when interventions target other aspects of the internal environment such as performance components.

The primacy of occupational performance roles indicates a contextualised notion of occupational performance. Occupational performance roles are influenced by both the person performing them and social expectations regarding their performance. Individuals uniquely configure their occupational performance roles according to their own goals, interests and preferences, their perceived abilities, and the expectations and values they have internalised. However, social expectations (those of society and of significant others) greatly influence occupational performance roles. They have socially agreed upon functions and an accepted code of norms (Chapparo & Ranka, 1997) and the broader context determines the need for and shapes a person's choice to engage in occupational performance roles. They change over time and with changing circumstances, abilities, and expectations.

The next two aspects of the internal environment, performance areas and performance components (traditional components of

occupational performance models), guide understanding and facilitation of occupational role performance (Chapparo & Ranka, 1997). Performance areas and components guide the classification and analysis of occupation, respectively.

Performance areas provide a framework for classifying occupation. In OPM(A), the occupational performance areas are self-maintenance, productivity, leisure, and rest. Because of the idiosyncratic nature of occupation, its classification into these performance areas should be undertaken by the performer (e.g. an occupation might be productivity for one person and leisure for another). Classification of occupation by a particular person can change over time and with age, circumstance and ability.

Performance components and the notions of structure and time guide the analysis of occupation. OPM(A) identifies five performance components: biomechanical, sensory-motor, cognitive, intrapersonal and interpersonal. Whereas occupational performance models traditionally present performance components as abilities of the performer, OPM(A) presents performance components as 'forming both the component attributes of the performer as well as the components of the occupational tasks' (Chapparo & Ranka, 1997, p. 10), which mirror and prompt the operations in the performer. For example, the biomechanical performance component is defined as the operation of and interaction between physical structures of the body such as range of motion, prompted by the biomechanical attributes of the task such as size and weight.

In OPM(A), three levels of complexity in occupation – subtasks, tasks and routines – are analysed in terms of structure and time. Regarding *structure*, tasks can be broken down into subtasks and grouped into routines. For example, the task of drinking

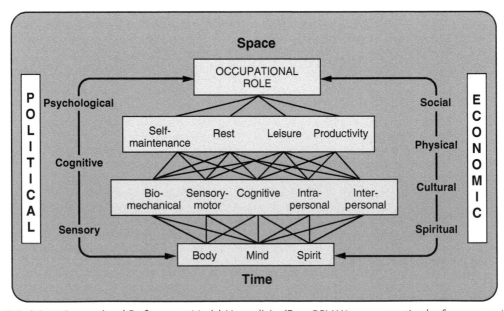

FIG. 9.3 ■ Occupational Performance Model (Australia). *(From OPM(A), www.occupationalperformance.com.)*

has subtasks such as reaching for the glass, grasping it and lifting it. Additionally, drinking could be part of a routine. Routines are sequences of tasks and can be prompted by internal or external cues. They create patterns of tasks that can be fixed or flexible. Many self-maintenance routines comprise fixed task patterns, because there is generally a defined set of tasks to be performed. Chapparo and Ranka (1997) emphasised that sociocultural expectations shape these fixed routines. Flexible routines can be undertaken in many different ways and can contain a varied range of tasks, provided they are acceptable to the performer.

In terms of *time*, routines can be regular or intermittent. Regular routines are performed on a daily basis and are usually critical to a person's functioning in a particular environment. Regular routines often become habitual through repetition, whereby they can be performed without conscious attention. For example, a person could shower or undertake a daily commute while thinking about something else. This may leave him or her with a sense of time having flown and little recollection of performing the task. Intermittent routines do not have to be carried out daily but may still be critical to the performance of occupation in a particular environment. In the longer term, the temporal dimension of occupational performance also applies to the lifespan, whereby routines, tasks and subtasks vary with age, circumstance and ability.

The *core elements* of occupational performance constitute the final aspect of the internal environment, comprising body, mind and spirit. The performer is considered holistically, whereby all three elements combine to influence what a person does, how it is done and how it is experienced. The body element refers to 'all of the tangible physical elements of human structure', mind is defined as 'the core of our conscious and unconscious intellect which forms the basis of our ability to understand and reason', and the spiritual element is 'defined loosely as that aspect of humans which seeks a sense of harmony within self and between self and nature, others and in some cases an ultimate other; seeks an existing mystery to life; inner conviction; hope and meaning' (Chapparo & Ranka, 1997, pp. 12-13). These core elements translate to the doing, knowing, and being dimensions of occupational performance, respectively.

The *external environment,* illustrated in the most recent diagram (Ranka & Chapparo, 2011), has six dimensions – sensory, physical, cultural, social, psychological and cognitive. Only the first four, which appeared in the 1997 publication, are discussed in descriptions of OPM(A). However, the inclusion of these last two are part of a larger conceptual shift to consider context (rather than environment) and the contextualising of occupation. In the 2001 diagram, the context also has political and economic dimensions. All dimensions of the context combine to shape what action is taken and how, as well as how it is experienced.

The first four dimensions of the external environment are as follows: the physical environment is 'the natural and constructed surroundings of a person' (Chapparo & Ranka, 1997, p. 15). The sensory environment 'provides the natural cues that direct occupational performance' (p. 15) and is most closely linked to the sensory and cognitive performance components.

The social environment results from people's relationships and contributes to expectations regarding behaviour. The cultural environment 'is composed of subsystems of values, beliefs, ideals, and customs which are learned and communicated to contribute to the behavioural boundaries of a person or groups of people' (p. 15). Cultural expectations influence occupational roles and the related tasks, subtasks and routines performed, as well as how they are performed, the standards expected and how people think and feel about themselves (self-identity).

The constructs of space and time are aspects of the external environment that pervade occupational performance. Both space and time have physical and felt dimensions, referring to how they manifest and how they are experienced, respectively. *Physical space* includes 'our understanding about body structures, body systems, objects with which people interact and the wider physical world within which people exist and function' (Chapparo & Ranka, 1997, p. 16). *Felt space* is the subjective experience of space and includes the way people use space, their interactions within it and its meaning to them. Space pervades all aspects of occupational performance. For example, performance components will be activated by the demands of performing occupation in a particular place and the experience will be created through interpretation by the body-mind-spirit core elements. In turn, this experience will influence the performance of occupation and occupational roles.

Similarly, time has both physical and felt dimensions. *Physical time* (chronological time) can be measured. Physical time is required when recording muscle response times and forms the basis of schedules and deadlines. *Felt time* is 'a person's understanding of time based on the meaning that is attributed to it' (Chapparo & Ranka, 1997, p. 18) and constantly changes through experience. Felt time underpins a person's sense of how much time is available for an occupation and whether it could be completed in that time, as well as whether it is the 'right' time to do something.

Concept of Occupation

The central construct of the model is occupational performance (consistent with occupational therapy models in the 1990s and in contrast to more recent editions of models that include participation), which is defined as 'the ability to perceive, desire, recall, plan and carry out roles, routines, tasks and subtasks for the purpose of self-maintenance, productivity, leisure and rest in response to demands of the internal and/or external environment' (Chapparo & Ranka, 1997, p. 4). The requirements for both occupation and its performance are evident in this definition. Occupation serves a purpose in a person's life through occupational roles and the performance areas, all of which stimulate perceiving and desiring. Performing occupation requires recalling, planning and carrying out.

In OPM(A), occupation is presented as a *process*, rather than an entity. It is the process of purposeful and meaningful engagement, rather than the things in which people engage (i.e. tasks and subtasks within routines and roles). People are engaged in the process of occupation when they undertake routines, tasks and subtasks for the purpose of fulfilling occupational roles in the areas of self-maintenance, productivity, leisure and rest. It is through occupation that people create their occupational being or identity. Occupational being 'is expressed through occupational performance and ultimately defined by people's occupational roles' (Chapparo & Ranka, 1997, p. 4). Occupational roles are shaped by the demands and expectations of the external environment as well as the capacities and interests of the person. Therefore occupation is presented as the conduit between the person and the environment (internal and external environments). It is through occupation that people and environments interact.

Scope of Occupational Therapy

The occupational nature of humans is the fundamental concern of occupational therapy. The profession is understood in terms of four principles. These are as follows: (1) Occupational therapists address the occupational needs of the people receiving occupational therapy. (2) Occupational therapists aim for these people to be satisfied with their occupational existence. (3) Occupational therapists use strategies to enhance people's occupational performance. (4) Occupational performance is the ability to perform (including 'doing', 'knowing' and 'being' dimensions) the occupations (roles, activities and tasks) a person wants to do, needs to do and is capable of doing (Ranka & Chapparo, 1997).

The centrality of occupational role performance is encapsulated in the statement, '[T]herapy provided which is not related to occupational role performance is NOT occupational therapy' (Ranka & Chapparo, 1997). However, OPM(A) assumes that, providing that the ultimate aim is addressing occupational need and facilitating occupational role performance, the methods used in occupational therapy could target any level of the internal and external environments. For example, interventions could address performance components, performance areas, or aspects of the external environment.

Use in Practice

OPM(A) provides a framework for guiding occupational therapists to address people's occupational needs. Occupational therapists should provide 'opportunities for choice and participation in role (Occupational Performance Role), routine, and task performance (Occupational Performance Areas)' (Ranka & Chapparo, 1997) and through goal-directed tasks. Programmes can be designed to alter or compensate for underlying components of occupational performance and address their relationship with the three core elements of body, mind, and spirit, as well as address barriers to occupational performance posed by the external environment.

Occupational analysis provides the foundation for practice using OPM(A). Occupational analysis is a holistic process. Identifying occupational role demands – that is, what people desire or need to do – is the primary purpose of the analysis. Relevant to these, analysis of the other components of the

model is undertaken. The following questions are provided to guide occupational therapists in using the model (Ranka & Chapparo, 1997):

- What occupational roles are desired or needed? (What does the person need or want to 'do'? What does the person's family, partner or other significant people require them to 'do'? What is the person capable of 'doing'?)
- What occupational routines, tasks and subtasks from the occupational areas are required to enable role performance (e.g. brushing teeth; conducting a meeting – 'doing'; instructing others to transfer – 'knowing'; being comfortably seated and positioned – 'being')?
- What performance components or environmental factors are causing difficulty in task performance (e.g. weakness, lack of confidence, inadequate knowledge, inaccessible bathroom, absence of cultural tools, socially shunned, room is too dark and hot, lack of finances)?
- Are core element functions damaged, at risk or healthy (e.g. fractures, systemic illness, mental processing, will to live and sense of hope)?
- What is this person's time and space fit? Are things 'in place' to support occupational performance (e.g. environmental supports, personal preparedness)?
- What is the therapist's preferred approach to intervention (e.g. biomechanical, neurodevelopmental, sensory integrative, behavioural, psychodynamic or interpersonal techniques)?
- How can the therapist apply preferred techniques to enhance a person's role, routine, task or subtask accomplishment (e.g. use techniques within the context of a task or relevant performance environment)?

The main practice resource available is the Perceive, Recall, Plan and Perform (PRPP) system of task analysis. It is an assessment and intervention model and addresses the cognitive dimension of performance. The PRPP model has four interconnected quadrants to categorise cognitive processing strategies used for task performance. These are: 'sensory perception (Perceive), memory (Recall), response planning and evaluation (Plan) and performance monitoring (Perform)' (Nott, Chapparo, & Heard, 2009, p. 308) and three information processing strategies are identified for each quadrant. The PRPP assessment is described as a 'standardised, client-centred, criterion referenced, ecological occupational therapy assessment of occupational performance' (Ranka, 2014). The PRPP system uses a two-stage analysis process. Stage one uses a standard behavioural task analysis and stage two adopts a cognitive task analysis.

CANADIAN MODEL OF OCCUPATIONAL PERFORMANCE AND ENGAGEMENT

In the book *Enabling Occupation II: Advancing an Occupational Therapy Vision for Health, Well-being, & Justice Through*

Occupation (Townsend & Polatako, 2007), the Canadian Model of Occupational Performance and Engagement is outlined, along with the CPPF and the Canadian Model of Client-Centred Enablement (CMCE). The CMOP-E is the revised edition of the Canadian Model of Occupation, which was published in the first edition of *Enabling Occupation* (CAOT, 1997). The CMOP-E has three main components – person, occupation and environment. These are represented in a three-dimensional diagram (Fig. 9.4) with the person in the centre (affective, cognitive and physical performance components and a core of spirituality) embedded within an environmental context (physical, institutional, cultural and social). In between these two is occupation, conceptualised as a bridge that connects the person and his or her environment and having three occupational purposes: self-care, productivity and leisure. Occupation is presented as the core domain of occupational therapy,

In CMOP-E, a distinction is made between *performing* occupations and *having* them, thus broadening the scope of the model from occupational performance. Although people can only perform one occupation at a time, they have many. Therefore performance is only one aspect of a person's potential engagement in occupation and there are many other 'modes of occupational interaction' (p. 24), including occupational competence, development and history. Consequently, *occupational engagement* is used to represent the breadth of modes of occupational interaction.

Concept of Occupation

Enabling Occupation II provided the definition of occupation used in *Enabling Occupation*, as follows:

> *Occupation refers to groups of activities and tasks of everyday life, named, organised, and given value and meaning by individuals and a culture. Occupation is everything people do to occupy themselves, including looking after themselves (self-care), enjoying life (leisure), and contributing to the social and economic fabric of their communities (productivity).*
> *(Polatajko et al., 2007b, p. 17)*

Polatajko, Backman, Baptiste, (2007a) explained that occupation is difficult to define, because: (1) it is 'a broad class [of phenomena that] is composed of all the tasks and activities in which a person engages in every-day life that are both culturally and personally meaningful' (p. 39), (2) it is a performed event and is not observable until a person engages in it, and (3) it has subjective and personal meaning and therefore cannot be understood by observation alone.

In explaining occupation, Polatajko et al. (2007b, p. 19) used the revised Taxonomic Code of Occupational Performance (TCOP) to place it in the context of other concepts relating to people's 'doing'. The TCOP outlines a hierarchy of five levels of occupational performance, with occupation at the top. These

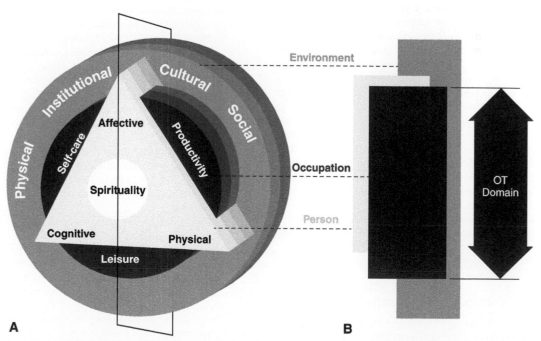

FIG. 9.4 ■ The Canadian Model of Occupational Performance and Engagement (CMOP-E). A, Referred to as the CMOP in *Enabling Occupation* (1997a, 2002) and CMOP-E as of this edition. B, Transsectional view. *(From Townsend & Polatajko, 2007, p. 23.)*

are (in ascending complexity): (1) voluntary movement or mental processes, defined as 'a simple voluntary muscle or mental activation' (e.g. flexion, extension, blinking, memory, scanning); (2) action, which is 'a set of voluntary movements or mental processes that form a recognisable and purposeful pattern (e.g. holding, standing, walking, remembering, smiling, chewing); (3) task, 'a set of actions having an end point or a specific outcome'; (4) activity, defined as 'a set of tasks with a specific end point or outcome that is greater than that of any constituent task'; and (5) occupation, 'an activity or set of activities that is performed with some consistency and regularity, that brings structure, and is given value and meaning by individuals and a culture'.

The model assumes that 'humans are occupational beings with a basic need for occupation' (Polatajko et al., 2007b, p. 15). Four further assumptions are as follows:

1. Occupation affects health and well-being.
2. Occupation organises time and brings structure to living.
3. Occupation brings meaning to life.
4. Occupations are idiosyncratic.

As these four basic assumptions show, the importance of occupation is not limited to health. As the authors stated, 'Occupation has value in its own right as a resource for everyday life' (p. 15). CMOP-E uses the framework of 'who, what, when, where, how and why' (Polatajko et al., 2007a, p. 40) to discuss the essential characteristics of human occupation:

- *Who:* Occupation is dependent on people to perform it; therefore who is performing is central. People are considered occupational beings who develop 'occupational repertoires' (p. 40) and patterns of occupation over the course of their lives. As these patterns usually involve connection to others, *who* is categorised in six ways: individuals, families, groups, communities, organisations and populations.
- *What:* This refers to *what* people do in their daily lives that has meaning for them.
- *When:* Occupation has a temporal dimension. People form 'occupational patterns' (p. 44) in which they organise their occupations over days, weeks, years and their lives. The model proposes that, unique to each individual, there is an ideal balance ('occupational balance' p. 46), which will contribute to health and well-being.
- *Where:* Occupations are performed in physical, social, cultural, and institutional environments.
- *How:* How people engage in and undertake their occupations develops and changes over time.
- *Why:* The purpose of engaging in occupation is health, well-being and justice.

Scope of Occupational Therapy

CMOP-E presents occupation as the core domain of concern for occupational therapy, and enablement as the core competency. *Enabling Occupation II* makes it clear that issues that do not pertain to occupation in its broader sense of culturally and individually meaningful tasks and activities of everyday life are beyond the occupational therapy scope of practice. The following definition of occupational therapy shows the connection between occupation and enablement:

Occupational therapy is the art and science of enabling engagement in everyday living, through occupation; of enabling people to perform the occupations that foster health and well-being; and of enabling a just and inclusive society so that all people may participate in their potential in the daily occupations of life.

(Townsend, Beagan, Kumas-Tan, 2007, p. 89)

The following example was used to illustrate that occupational therapy, at its best, should use occupation as its main strategy to enable people in their daily lives. A filmmaker who had a debilitating brainstem stroke while making a film was determined to complete the film and (guiltily) prioritised this over other aspects of rehabilitation. When she reflected on this time, she said of working on and finishing the film, 'I realized myself that this was my occupational therapy (as occupational therapy was meant to be)' (Polatajko et al., 2007b, p. 14).

Using CMOP-E in Practice

Guiding occupational therapy practice are six enablement foundations:

1. *Choice, risk, and responsibility:* The process of ensuring this requires negotiation and close attention to the perspectives, interests and safety of the people receiving occupational therapy services as well as the professional and legal responsibilities of professionals. As Townsend et al. stated, 'The aim in occupational therapy is to enable safe engagement in just-right risk-taking' (p. 101).
2. *Client participation:* The notion of 'occupational citizenship' (p. 101) is used to emphasise that a person's participation in everyday occupation in the context of being able to participate fully in society is key to occupational enablement.
3. *Visions of possibility:* Both occupational therapists and the people they work with need to form visions of what might be possible. A role in occupational therapy is to support people to imagine a life (that sometimes might not be in their vision).
4. *Change:* Occupational therapy is conceptualised as going beyond being 'guided to develop, maintain or restore occupational performance, or to prevent problems in occupational performance' (p. 103) and includes facilitating change that enables people to develop (or further develop) occupational patterns and balance and negotiate occupational transitions.
5. *Justice:* Rather than assuming that people who have body impairments should be made to function more normally, taking a justice perspective to enablement would involve recognising systematic injustices that affect people,

accepting people as they are and assisting others to do the same, and assuming that all people should have a place in society and advocating for that.

6. *Power sharing:* Person-centred practice requires a high level of power sharing characterised by mutual respect and acknowledgement of and regard for values, interests and skills.

Central to the enablement foundations is the assumption that occupational therapists also need to promote enablement at the level of society. Townsend et al. (2007) emphasised the importance of taking 'a critical social perspective' (p. 91) in which attention is given to the social construction of power.

CMOP-E also combines with the CPPF (with its 6 steps between Enter/Initiate and Conclude/Exit) and the CMCE (with its 10 enablement skills, presented in alphabetical order: Adapt, Advocate, Coach, Collaborate, Consult, Coordinate, Design/ Build, Educate, Engage, Specialise) to provide systematic guidance for practice.

KAWA MODEL

The final model reviewed in this chapter is the Kawa Model. This model was developed by Michael Iwama, a Japanese-Canadian occupational therapist and social scientist, along with a group of Japanese occupational therapists. The book *The Kawa Model: Culturally Relevant Occupational Therapy* was published in 2006 (Iwama, 2006). The word *Kawa* is Japanese for river, and the model uses the metaphor of a river to map the course of a person's life from birth to death (Fig. 9.5). Any particular time in a person's life can be represented using a transection of the river at that point (Fig. 9.6).

The life course is represented by the river flowing from the source in the mountains (birth) to the ocean (end of life). Just as the course of a particular river is shaped by the landscape through which it flows, the context in which a person lives shapes his or her life. A river might be calm and flat when wide and largely unimpeded or quite turbulent when flowing over shallow rocks or descending waterfalls. So, too, a person's life might appear to be proceeding calmly at times and have other periods in which obstacles have to be overcome or 'lived through'.

The central concern of the Kawa Model is 'life energy' or 'life flow' (Iwama, 2006, p. 142), represented by water. At various times in a person's life, the elements of the river (the river walls and floor, driftwood and rocks) might combine to impede or facilitate the flow of water. The river metaphor is used for identifying these elements in a person's 'river' and understanding their effect on the flow of water.

The first element in the model is *water* (*mizu* in Japanese). Water is a fluid and, as such, can both be shaped by and shape the context surrounding it. For example, water will conform to the contours of its receptacle. However, these also can be changed by the erosion caused by water flowing over or through them. Iwama explained that, in the same way, people's lives will be shaped 'by their surroundings, people and circumstances' (p. 144), as well as shaping them. The emphasis in this

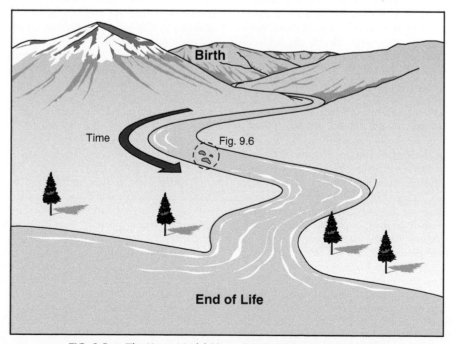

FIG. 9.5 ■ The Kawa Model River. *(Iwama, 2006, Fig. 7.1, p. 143.)*

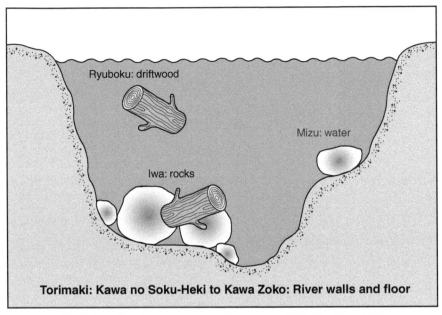

Ryuboku: driftwood

Mizu: water

Iwa: rocks

Torimaki: Kawa no Soku-Heki to Kawa Zoko: River walls and floor

FIG. 9.6 ■ The river cross-section. *(From Iwama, 2006, Fig. 7.2, p. 144.)*

description of the context shaping the individual is indicative of the collectivist culture in which the model was developed. It might be challenging for people from individualist cultures to appreciate fully that, for people from collectivist cultures, allowing the social context to shape them might be of a higher value than acting upon the context to change it. Individuals expressing their agency in working to change their situation, represented by the image of river water shaping the landscape through which it flows, might be an image that arises more naturally for some people than others.

The second element is the *river walls and floor,* which in Japanese is *kawa no soku-heki* and *kawa no zoko,* respectively. In a river, the walls and floor could be wide and deep, and water might flow unobstructed. Where the river winds, narrows or shallows, the flow of the water will be altered. In the Kawa Model, the river walls and floor refer to the contexts that surround people, such as their social and physical environments. Iwama (2006) emphasised the significance of context in collectivist cultures when stating that 'these are perhaps the most important determinants in a person's life flow in a collectivist social context because of the primacy afforded to the environmental context in determining the experiences of self and subsequent meanings of personal action' (p. 146). Regardless of whether a culture is primarily collectivist or individualist, the meaning given by an individual to his or her action will be shaped to varying degrees by shared understandings.

The third element of the Kawa model is *rocks.* The word *iwa* in Japanese refers to large rocks or crags. Rocks are used to refer to obstacles in a person's life that impede his or her *life flow.* Just

as some rocks in a river do not disrupt the flow of water, because their shape and positioning allow the water to flow freely under, over or around them, a person's 'impairments' may or may not be obstacles. As Iwama stated, 'If you reflect on your own life as a river, you may see a variety of rocks (of different shapes and sizes) in your river. Some of these rocks remain unremarkable until they butt up against certain aspects of the social and physical environment' (p. 147).

The fourth element in the model is *driftwood,* or *ryuboku.* Driftwood represents the personal attributes and resources that can affect circumstances and life flow either positively or negatively. These include values, character, personality, special skill, material and immaterial assets (e.g. wealth and relationships, respectively) and living situation. Just as driftwood in a river can block water flow, have no impact or enhance it by dislodging obstacles, these factors in a person's life can be obstructive, neutral or facilitatory.

Since the model's original publication, Orange Tang fish and sparkles have been added. These denote those aspects of a person's life that are going well. This addition facilitates a strengths approach in which situations of stronger life flow can be identified and built upon.

The concept of harmony is central to the Kawa Model. Harmony is a state in which a balance exists between a subject (whether an individual or community) and its context; the elements of the river are in balance. The need for synergy between the elements of the river, creating an integrated whole, is fundamental to the Kawa Model. Harmony is central to the notion of *life flow.*

Concept of Occupation: Transforming the Occupational Therapy Body of Knowledge by Reconceptualising the Notion of Occupation

In presenting the Kawa Model and the need for it, Iwama (2006) made a distinction between East Asian and Western worldviews. Understanding this distinction is important, because it highlights how occupation is conceptualised and the cultural critique of occupational therapy inherent in this model.

The subtitle of the Kawa Model book, *Culturally Relevant Occupational Therapy,* signals the emphasis in the model. Iwama (2006) stated, 'the meanings of people's actions vary according to *culture,* that is, according to shared spheres of common experience, situated in a particular place and time' (p. 159, italics in original). Thus culture is an important construct and is understood in its broader sense of 'shared spheres of meaning' (p. 160). In particular, the Kawa Model highlights the differences between the collective cultures characterising East Asian countries and the individualist cultures that are prevalent in Western countries. He used the example of differing conceptions of the *self* to illustrate this. He proposed that occupational therapy models are dominated by a Western notion of the self. This is characterised by a 'centrally situated *self,* separated from a surrounding, discrete environment that one "occupies" through rational, purposeful, action or "doing"'. Consequently, 'independence, autonomy, egalitarianism, and self-determinism' are highly valued ideals that are embedded in 'mainstream occupational therapy ideology' (p. 161). In this perspective, a privileged self exerts control over the environment. In contrast, in collectivist cultures, there is not the same sharp distinction between a centrally situated self, environment and context; rather, they are seen as 'integrated parts of a whole frame' (p. 161). That is, the self is not privileged over other parts, but one with them and part of them.

This fundamental view of the interconnectedness of all things shapes how meaning is ascribed by people within collectivist cultures regarding their actions and place in the world. This interconnectedness is central to an understanding of occupation. Iwama (2006) emphasised that 'the claim that we occupy our environs through occupation [and] self-deterministic notions of unilaterally controlling life circumstances through occupation are lost on people who ascribe to more naturalistic viewpoints of reality and who are oriented towards a harmonious existence with nature and its circumstances' (p. 53). In an East Asian collectivist culture, then, rather than acting on the environment, being at one with, belonging to, taking one's place within and fulfilling one's role in the environment, gives meaning to one's action or occupation. Belonging precedes being, and doing comes last in the sequence, as it results from the others.

Iwama cautioned that taking accepted occupational therapy assumptions and transplanting them into other cultures without critical review 'will ensure that occupational therapy will fall far short of its mandate to enable people through meaningful action' (p. 54). Thus underlying the Kawa Model is the call for a transformation in occupational therapy's body of knowledge through the acknowledgement and analysis of the cultural constructions that underpin its assumptions, generally, and notion of occupation in particular.

Scope and Purpose of Occupational Therapy

Within the Kawa Model, the scope of occupational therapy is quite broad. The purpose of occupational therapy is to facilitate the life flow of the subject (whether an individual or collective) through a balanced synergy between the elements of the river. As Iwama stated, 'Occupation is life flow and occupational therapists are enablers of people's life flow' (p. 154). Any elements in the river and their combinations can be used to achieve this.

Use in Practice

The Kawa Model outlines six steps for its use in practice settings. As Iwama (2006) stated, 'In keeping with the relational qualities and the philosophical bases of the Kawa Model, occupational therapists should explore various and creative ways for utilizing the Kawa Model' (p. 164). The six steps are as follows:

1. Determine the appropriateness of the model, who is receiving occupational therapy services, and who should draw the river diagram. The river metaphor needs to have meaning for both the person and the therapist and its appropriateness for a particular situation needs to be determined. Who or what the client is needs to be clearly identified. Is the client an individual or collective, an organisation, a community, or a process such as a rehabilitation team mandate? Once this is determined, then a decision can be made as to who should draw the river diagram. The diagram is then used as a basis for discussion. Iwama emphasised that the way the model is used will (and should) change over time to ensure that it remains relevant to the occupational therapist's practice. The drawings can serve as a record of progress over time.

2. Clarify the context. Through discussion with the client who did the drawing, the therapist gains an understanding of the context being represented in the Kawa Model drawing. The therapist can ask questions about the elements in the river, such as why the client has made a rock so big or what is represented by the particular shape of the river walls and floor.

3. Prioritise issues according to the person's perspective. This step centres on identifying possibilities for occupational therapy intervention. Using a strengths-based approach, the Kawa Model particularly focuses on the 'potential courses and channels through which a person's [or organization's etc.] life continues to flow' (p. 168). As well as identifying current channels of flow, an occupational therapist using this model looks for potential ways that life flow could be expanded, by intervening to change the relationships between the various elements in the river.

4. Assess focal points of occupational therapy intervention. The occupational therapist engages the person in a process of 'quantifying the magnitude and ascertaining the quality of the various structures involved [elements of the river]' (p. 169). This can be done by utilising formal and informal assessments and through qualitative methods.

5. Implement the intervention. This step involves the planning and implementation of intervention. The interrelatedness of the elements of the river is emphasised in the conceptualisation of intervention in this model. As Iwama stated, 'When change is introduced in any point in the context, all other parts of the whole are affected and also subject to change' (p. 171).

6. Evaluate the intervention. Person-centred criteria are used for evaluation of the effectiveness of intervention. One way this could be undertaken is by comparing the river drawings that the relevant person has made at different times throughout the process of occupational therapy. The aim of evaluation is to determine how well occupational therapy has met the person's goals.

CONCLUSION

Occupational therapy has made substantial development to models of practice. These assist the profession in articulating its assumptions and body of knowledge. The five models reviewed in this chapter each present a particular view of occupation, which is generally accepted to be the central concern of occupational therapy. They all assume that the environment or context in which people live influences their action or occupation. However, each model makes it explicit how the relationship between people and their environment is conceptualised.

 http://evolve.elsevier.com/Curtin/OT

REFERENCES

Canadian Association Occupational Therapy (CAOT) (1997). *Enabling occupation: An occupational therapy perspective.* Ottawa: CAOT Publications ACE.

Chapparo, C., & Ranka, J. (1997). *Occupational performance model (Australia): Monograph 1.* Castle Hill, NSW: Occupational Performance Network.

Csikszentmihalyi, M., & Csikszentmihalyi, I. S. (1988). *Optimal experience: Psychological studies in flow in consciousness.* Cambridge, MA: Cambridge University Press.

Germov, J. (2014). Imagining health problems as social issues. In J. Germov (Ed.), *Second opinion: An introduction to health sociology* (pp. 5–22). (5th. ed.). Melbourne: Oxford University Press.

Iwama, M. K. (2006). *The Kawa model: Culturally relevant occupational therapy.* Edinburgh: Churchill Livingstone Elsevier.

Kielhofner, G. (2008a). Introduction to the model of occupational performance. In G. Kielhofner (Ed.), *Model of human occupation: Theory and application* (pp. 1–7). (4th ed). Baltimore, MD: Lippincott Williams & Wilkins.

Kielhofner, G. (2008b). The basic concepts of human occupation. In G. Kielhofner (Ed.), *Model of human occupation: Theory and application* (pp. 11–23). (4th ed.). Baltimore, MD: Lippincott Williams & Wilkins.

Kielhofner, G. (2008c). Volition. In G. Kielhofner (Ed.), *Model of human occupation: Theory and application* (pp. 32–50). (4th ed.). Baltimore, MD: Lippincott Williams & Wilkins.

Kielhofner, G. (2008d). Habituation: Patterns of daily occupation. In G. Kielhofner (Ed.), *Model of human occupation: Theory and application* (pp. 51–67). (4th ed.). Baltimore, MD: Lippincott Williams & Wilkins.

Kielhofner, G. (2008e). The environment and human occupation. In G. Kielhofner (Ed.), *Model of human occupation: Theory and application* (pp. 85–100). (4th ed.). Baltimore, MD: Lippincott Williams & Wilkins.

Kielhofner, G. (2008f). Dimensions of doing. In G. Kielhofner (Ed.), *Model of human occupation: Theory and application* (pp. 101–109). (4th ed.). Baltimore, MD: Lippincott Williams & Wilkins.

Kielhofner, G., & Forsyth, K. (2008). Therapeutic reasoning: Planning. implementing, and evaluating the outcomes of therapy. In G. Kielhofner (Ed.), *Model of human occupation: Theory and application* (pp. 143–154). (4th ed.). Baltimore, MD: Lippincott Williams & Wilkins.

Kielhofner, G., Tham, K., Baz, T., & Hutson, J. (2008). Performance capacity and the lived body. In G. Kielhofner (Ed.), *Model of human occupation: Theory and application* (pp. 68–84). (4th ed.). Baltimore, MD: Lippincott Williams & Wilkins.

Law, M., Cooper, B., & Strong, S. (1996). The person-environment-occupation model: A transactive approach to occupational performance. *Canadian Journal of Occupational Therapy, 63*(1), 9–23.

Madigan, M. J., & Parent, L. H. (1985). Preface. In G. Kielhofner (Ed.), *A model of human occupation: Theory and application.* Baltimore, MD: Williams & Wilkins.

Mattingly, C., & Fleming, M. H. (1994). *Clinical reasoning: Forms of inquiry in a therapeutic practice.* Philadelphia: FA Davis.

Nelson, D. (1988). Occupation: Form and performance. *American Journal of Occupational Therapy, 42*, 633.

Nott, M. T., Chapparo, C., & Heard, R. (2009). Reliability of the perceive, recall, plan and perform system of task analysis: A criterion-referenced assessment. *Australian Occupational Therapy Journal, 56*, 307–314.

Polatajko, H. J., Backman, C., Baptiste, S., et al. (2007a). Human occupation in context. In E. Townsend, & H. Polatajko (Eds.), *Enabling occupation II: Advancing an occupational therapy vision for health, well-being and justice through occupation* (pp. 13–36). Ottawa: CAOT Publications ACE.

Polatajko, H. J., Davis, J., Stewart, D., Cantin, N., Purdie, L., & Zimmerman, D. (2007b). Specifying the domain of concern: Occupation as core. In E. Townsend, & H. Polatajko (Eds.), *Enabling occupation II: Advancing an occupational therapy vision for health, well-being and justice through occupation* (pp. 13–36). Ottawa: CAOT Publications ACE.

Ranka, J., & Chapparo, C. (1997). Occupational performance: A practice model for occupational therapy. Retrieved from, In C. Chapparo, & J. Ranka (Eds.), *Occupational performance model (Australia): Monograph 1* (pp. 45–57). Occupational Performance Network: Sydney.

Ranka, J., & Chapparo, C. (2011). *Draft illustration of the 2011 illustration of the occupational performance model (Australia). Retrieved from,* www.occupationalperformance.com/model-illustration.

Ranka, J. (2014). *Description of OPM(A) assessments. Retrieved from,* www.occupationalperformance.com/assessments.

Townsend, E. A., Beagan, B., Kumas-Tan, Z., et al. (2007). Enabling: Occupational therapy's core competency. In E. Townsend, & H. Polatajko (Eds.), *Enabling occupation II: Advancing an occupational therapy vision for health, well-being and justice through occupation* (pp. 87–171). Ottawa: CAOT Publications ACE.

Townsend, E. A., & Polatajko, H. J. (2007). *Enabling occupation II: Advancing an occupational therapy vision for health, well-being and Justice through occupation.* Ottawa: CAOT Publications ACE.

Turpin, M., & Iwama, M. (2011). *Using occupational therapy models in practice: A fieldguide.* Edinburgh: Churchill Livingstone Elsevier.

10

OCCUPATIONAL PERFORMANCE MODEL (AUSTRALIA): A DESCRIPTION OF CONSTRUCTS, STRUCTURE AND PROPOSITIONS

CHRIS CHAPPARO ■ JUDY L. RANKA ■ MELISSA THERESE NOTT

Abstract

This chapter describes how the Occupation Performance Model (Australia) (OPM(A)) is structured around eight interacting constructs: occupational performance (the central construct) and its conceptual elements, which include occupational roles, occupational performance areas, occupational performance capacities, core elements of occupational performance, context, space, and time. The constructs outlined in this chapter can be applied to people and groups. Practice stories of people who have a physical impairment are included in the chapter to illustrated how reduced physical capacity or impairment may affect all constructs of the OPM(A). Considerations for identifying performance strengths and evaluating the impact of physical impairments on occupational performance are provided.

KEY POINTS

- The OPM(A) is a conceptual framework that simultaneously explains occupational performance and scope of occupational therapy practice.

- The focus of the OPM(A) is the relationship between people and their contexts relative to performance of occupations throughout life.

- The OPM(A) is a self-organising, interactive system comprising eight major constructs: *occupational performance, occupational roles, occupational performance areas, occupational performance capacities, core elements of occupational performance, context, space* and *time.*

- *Performance,* as defined in this model, extends the usual notions from that of motor action only to include antecedent and subsequent physical, cognitive, sensory, mental and emotional processes relevant to the task performed.

- The relationship between constructs is strategic in nature. Tasks and routines are configured strategically by people to comply with their occupational role performance needs. People use their performance capacities strategically to support performance of relevant tasks and routines.

- The external context can afford or inhibit performance.

- Personal interpretations of time and space are embedded in the performance of all occupations throughout life.

- Notions of 'normal' and 'typical' are rejected in favour of the 'specific' and 'particular'.

- The constructs can be applied to individuals and groups.

- People with reduced physical capacity can experience difficulty engaging in occupational performance within any construct.

INTRODUCTION

Models of occupation and therapy are used by researchers and practitioners in a variety of ways so it is not surprising that one single model has been unable to meet the range of theoretical, practice and explanatory demands of the profession. This chapter describes how one model, the Occupational Performance Model (Australia) (OPM(A)) (Chapparo & Ranka, 1997; Jurkowitsch & Ranka, 2009) conceptualises both elements of occupation and the performance of occupations and can be used in practice to

explain, delineate and make decisions about the scope and focus of occupational therapy for individuals and groups.

A conceptual model must be developed in such a way as to provide an easily understood interpretation for the model users. A conceptual model, when implemented properly, should satisfy the following four fundamental objectives (Gemino & Wand, 2004):

1. Enhance a person's understanding of the representative system. In this instance the OPM(A) contributes to students', therapists' and others' understanding of occupational performance and occupational therapy.
2. Facilitate communication of elements of the system between relevant people. The OPM(A) provides a common, well-defined and easy-to-use language system that can assist with communication of occupation-centred issues among all people in the system where it is used (e.g. therapists, people who receive occupational therapy services, researchers and other stakeholders).
3. Provide a point of reference for system designers to extract system specifications. This means that constructs and propositions within the OPM(A) can be used by occupational therapists and students to develop and explain the nature and focus of practices used.
4. Document the system for future reference and provide a means for collaboration. Publication of the constructs within the OPM(A) (such as the information contained in this chapter) and propositions about how they may be related provides a vehicle for further research and development within the profession.

Discussion of the OPM(A) in this chapter is limited to outlining (1) the structure of the model by defining the major constructs, (2) propositions about the relationship between constructs and (3) examples of how the constructs and propositions can be used by practitioners. Although some aspects of the constructs are not unique to the OPM(A) and reflect a synthesis of decades of ideas about the nature of human occupations (e.g. Christensen, Bass, & Baum, 2015; Kielhofner, 2002, 2009; Meyer, 1922), those emphasised in this chapter form a configuration of occupational performance that differs from other performance-focused models and reflects concepts in the OPM(A) outlined originally by Chapparo & Ranka (1997).

OPM(A): PHILOSOPHICAL BASIS AND ASSUMPTIONS

The OPM(A) is considered a conceptual framework that simultaneously explains occupational performance and scope of occupational therapy practice. The overarching philosophy that informs its structure and use is *pragmatism,* a defining philosophy of practice underpinning early and contemporary occupational therapy (Meyer, 1922; Morgan, 2007). The focus of pragmatism is on addressing issues that are relevant to people and that result in action (Glasgow & Steiner, 2012). Pragmatists believed that knowledge is generated by personal experience through 'knowing' and 'doing' (Hooper & Wood, 2002). Early pragmatists emphasised the following two perspectives that are aligned with the assumptions, focus and use of the OPM(A):

1. People construct visions of desired futures and direct their everyday activity towards realising those futures. The focus of occupational therapy for people who experience reduced physical capacity is on their needs and the practical, active ways those needs can be met.

2. The daily activity of people is inextricably interwoven with their biology and their physical and social environments, and each of these may pose possible barriers or enablers to desired activity in unique ways (Dewey, 1930). Mirroring Meyer's (1922) original ideas about the focus and methods used in occupational therapy, the OPM(A) proposes that people harness their physical, mental and psychological capacities strategically to carry out their daily occupations. Occupational therapy is not solely interested in people's physical, cognitive or psychosocial capacity per se, but rather how people can develop and use their capacities in a way that is demanded by the occupations they do and in the contexts where they live.

Although the OPM(A) uses *general terms* to describe its constructs and processes, its application to each situation by therapists *is specific and unique* to each person or group. Notions of 'typical' and 'normal' are rejected in favour of the 'specific' and 'particular'. To this end, the OPM(A) provides a template that can be used to assist practitioners and researchers discover the experiences of people (unique particularities) when they engage in activities (occupations) that may pose difficulty (problems of moving, sensing, thinking, feeling and communicating) and the ways that these can be addressed (through the use of personal and other resources) in their own contexts. Key features of pragmatism in occupational therapy practice that uses the OPM(A) as a guiding framework include the following:

■ The perspectives, practices and outcomes of therapy are those that are *important to the person or group receiving occupational therapy.*
■ The focus of therapy practice is on *real-world events* rather than artificial or manipulated scenarios.

OCCUPATIONAL PERFORMANCE: CONSTRUCTS AND STRUCTURE

Consistent with other existing and evolving models in occupational therapy, the primary focus of the OPM(A) is the lifelong person–context relationship and its activation through occupation. Eight major constructs form the theoretical structure of this model. These are *occupational performance, occupational roles, occupational performance areas, occupational performance capacities, core elements of occupational performance, context, space* and *time.* Each of these constructs incorporates many interrelating elements.

In addressing a person–context–performance relationship, the structural framework of the model considers the interactions between two contexts relative to people and occupation: the *internal* context and the *external* context (Fig. 10.1).

The internal context is the central core of the model and reflects both the person or people (the performer) and the

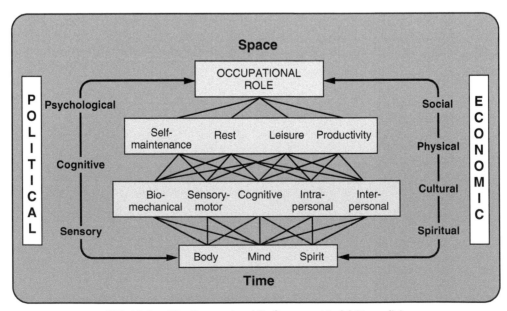

FIG. 10.1 ■ The Occupational Performance Model (Australia).

occupation being performed. The OPM(A) does not separate person and occupation constructs, emphasising the assumption that occupation does not exist as a separate entity, but is only actualised through engagement of the performer (the performance). The internal context comprises four layers that reflect the increasing complexity of occupations and their performance: the core elements of occupational performance, occupational performance capacities, occupational performance areas and occupational roles. The external context is composed of structures, conditions and influences that are outside of the person within which occupations are performed. The external context has several layers consisting of sensory, physical, cognitive, social, cultural, spiritual, economic and political dimensions. Functions of the internal and external contexts operate in time and space (see Fig. 10.1).

In the OPM(A), use of the word *context* rather than *environment* is proposed for conceptual and semantic reasons. Participation in any life task requires that people assign meaning to the contexts in which they perform occupations. Although concrete aspects of the environment are common to all, individuals create their own view of it. As a part of every daily task people do, they make interpretations of what they are *able to do* (internal context), what they *want to do* (internal context) and what they see are the *affordances or limitations* that surround them (external context). The OPM(A) refers to this process as *contextualising*, bringing the external context into the mind. People's internal and external contexts become fused to form an understanding of their own performance and its place in the world around them. Context is both a *place* and a *process* in occupational performance.

CONSTRUCT 1: OCCUPATIONAL PERFORMANCE

The major construct around which the Occupational Performance Model (Australia) is conceptualised is occupational performance. The central proposition in this model is that all goal-oriented behaviour related to daily living is occupational in nature. *Performance*, as defined in this model, extends the usual notions from that of motor action only to include antecedent and subsequent physical, cognitive, sensory, mental and emotional processes relevant to the task performed. *Performance* is the ability to *perceive, desire, recall, plan* and *carry out occupations* in response to *demands* of the internal and/or external contexts, and is characterised by changes that can be *physical, cognitive* or *psychosocial*. *Occupation* refers to meaningful *roles, routines, tasks and subtasks* performed for the purpose of *self-maintenance, productivity, leisure* (Reed, 2005) and *rest* (Meyer, 1922).

> **Occupational performance** is the ability to perceive, desire, recall, plan and carry out roles, routines, tasks and subtasks for the purpose of self-maintenance, productivity, leisure and rest in response to demands of the internal and/or external context (Chapparo & Ranka, 1997).

CONSTRUCT 2: OCCUPATIONAL ROLES

> **Occupational roles** are *patterns of occupational behaviour* composed of configurations of *self-maintenance, productivity, leisure/play* and *rest* occupations. Occupational roles are determined by each unique *person–context–performance relationships*. They are *established* through *need* and/or *choice* and are *modified* with *age, ability, experience, circumstance* and *time* (Chapparo & Ranka, 1997).

Humans are active in the process of creating their occupational being or identity through active participation in tasks and with others. Active participation can be intrinsically driven by choice or need or externally imposed by contextual factors. This occupational identity is expressed through a person's occupational performance and defined by peoples' occupational roles. *Occupational roles* comprise patterns of occupational performance that are determined by a person's unique daily routines of self-maintenance, productivity, leisure and rest within that person's particular contexts (Chapparo & Ranka, 1997; Hillman & Chapparo, 2008; Kielhofner, 2002).

Occupational role behaviour is complex, probably because roles are content specific and tied to the context in which they are embedded. People adopt a number of roles that become functionally interlocked. For example, people are expected to be workers at work. However, they simultaneously behave in the roles of 'friend' when talking to others with whom they have a close relationship, 'worker' when working on tasks that are directed by the job, 'learner' when learning new work skills, 'player' when socialising during breaks and out-of-work hours, 'self-carer' when eating lunch and looking after themselves while going to and from work, and 'community member' when engaging in activities that support the particular work institution that employs them and when helping others. Premium value may be assigned to any of these roles. For example, a person might value the role of friend over other interlocking roles at work. Assessment of role performance of people with reduced physical capacity should therefore pay attention to all interlocking roles and identify those that are most important to the person or group.

Each role has its own repertoire of behaviours that support it. Roles are lost, gained and changed throughout the lifespan in a process of transition (Chapparo & Ranka, 1997; Forsberg-Wärleby & Möller, 1996; Hillman & Chapparo, 2008). Challenges occur when people experience life and health events that disrupt their ability to carry out their roles in a manner that is expected or desired. Role change that is imposed rather than chosen may be accompanied by stress. People who sustain reduced physical capacity may experience permanent or temporary *role loss* (e.g. inability to engage in self-care activities after a stroke). They may have difficulty *with resuming or acquiring new roles* (e.g. resuming work in a different capacity after back or hand injury; becoming a carer for a spouse with significant physical impairment), or they may have difficulty identifying which role is the most appropriate in a specific situation and making the *transition* between different roles. For example, people who have significantly reduced physical capacity because of a fluctuating disorder such as rheumatoid arthritis or chronic fatigue syndrome may have difficulty making the transition from a self-maintainer role (managing physical fatigue and joint pain at work) to a worker role when returning to the work station after resting during lunch break.

Roles appear to be governed by a complex relationship between demands placed upon people in their contexts and their own personal choices (Hillman & Chapparo, 2008; Landis, 1995). Over time, people learn to balance their roles between what others *expect* them to do and what they *want* to do. Sudden onset of reduced physical capacity results in a period of role change during which people learn to understand and balance personal and expected roles in light of their physical capacity and the resources available to them.

Although personal choice is thought to motivate adoption of roles throughout life, the OPM(A) also recognises that, as both a construct and a personal/social system of values, individual choice is alien to a number of social groups whose sociocultural identity is collectivistic (Manstead & Hewstone, 1995). Occupational role performance can therefore be determined by the individual, the social group or combinations of both.

Consistent with the pragmatist view outlined earlier, the OPM(A) conceptualises occupational roles as having *three dimensions*. One is *knowing*. Knowing is having an intuitive or concrete understanding of roles people want to enact and what roles are expected by their physical-sensory-sociocultural context. The second involves a process of *doing* and usually entails action. The third dimension addresses the interpersonal and socioemotional aspects of role identity and acknowledges the notion of *being* as a fulfilment or satisfaction component of occupational performance roles (Rowles, 2009). It is possible that this dimension is linked to personal meaning, which contributes to valuing one's occupational roles (Hillman & Chapparo, 2008).

People participate fully or partially in the performance of occupational roles. For example, full participation in the occupational role of homemaker (work role) produces occupational behaviour involving physical activity during the performance of many tasks and routines (doing). This may be carried out with family members requiring interpersonal interaction (social context) and knowledge of their needs (knowing). The role carries with it aspects of satisfaction and fulfilment that are linked both to personal notions of competence in the performance of the role and personal perceptions of its sociocultural worth (being).

Alternatively, a man who is elderly, and who requires considerable physical assistance may be deemed to have no occupational role as a self-maintainer because he can no longer 'do' self-maintenance routines or tasks (for example, getting dressed). However, he does 'know' what he wants done and how he wants it done, thereby participating in the 'knowing' dimensions of role performance. He can also experience satisfaction when the self-maintenance routines are carried out to his directions and experience the 'being' dimensions of role function in terms of fulfilment.

Someone with severe and multiple physical impairments may not be able to contribute to the 'doing' or 'knowing' aspects of an occupational role such as self-maintainer. Personal and family expectation may be related to 'being' cared for in a safe, comfortable situation that provides satisfaction and contentment to the level needed by that person. In this instance a person who lacks the ability to organise the 'doing' or 'knowing' aspects of occupational roles has the right to 'being' cared for in a way that supports the person's role as a family member whose existence is valued.

The OPM(A) is thought to function as a self-organising, interactive system, in which occupational role is the central organising construct (Chapparo & Ranka, 1997). Roles influence and are influenced by other parts of the system, a relationship that is depicted by the recursive arrows in Fig. 10.1. For example, a person's occupational role as a worker determines the balance of time and activity allotted to self-maintenance, productivity, leisure and rest areas of occupational performance. These, in turn, determine the personal capacities necessary for engagement in work. Alternatively, when circumstance allows a person to choose an occupational role, the choice may be based on the presence or absence of particular capacities they have, such as the outstanding motor coordination of an athlete or the cognitive creativity of an artist. When illness strikes core elements of a person (e.g. a stroke affecting the body and mind function), relationships throughout the system are disturbed, affecting role function.

Analysis of Occupational Role Performance

Given the doing, knowing, being, view of occupational roles, the OPM(A) asserts that identification of important roles should not be limited simply to interpretation of observable actions (what the person does) or by an external source (such as a predetermined role checklist) (see, e.g., Crepeau & Schell, 2009 for summary). The unique construction of occupational roles assumes that there is not just one meaning (shared by everyone) for a named role (such as 'gardener', or 'churchgoer'). Theorists warn against imposing normative interpretations or expectations while obtaining information about occupational role performance during assessment (Jackson, 1998). Any analysis of occupational role performance relative to the OPM(A) definition of occupational roles would include examples of questions such as those listed in Box 10.1.

CONSTRUCT 3: OCCUPATIONAL PERFORMANCE AREAS

Occupational performance areas comprise self-maintenance, work, play and rest, and their relationship to other constructs in the OPM(A) is illustrated by arrows in Fig. 10.1. Occupational therapy has traditionally categorise performance of daily occupations to three areas: self-maintenance occupations, productivity/school occupations and leisure/play occupations. The OPM(A) proposes a fourth area: rest occupations (Chapparo & Ranka, 1997). Others, including early pragmatists, have also recognised its importance as a dimension of occupational performance (American Occupational Therapy Association [AOTA], 2008; Meyer, 1922).

Rest occupations refer to the *purposeful pursuit* of *nonactivity*. This can include time devoted to *sleep* as well as routines, tasks, subtasks and rituals undertaken in order to *relax* (Chapparo & Ranka, 1997).

Inclusion of this category as separate from self-maintenance occupations acknowledges that there are sociocultural, daily and lifespan reasons for the degree to which people are, or wish to be, passive and contemplative rather than active and productive. People who experience reduced physical capacity find that planned periods of rest become important to sustaining occupational performance in other areas (Matuska & Barrett, 2014).

Self-maintenance occupations are routines, tasks and subtasks done to *preserve* a person's *health* and *well-being* in the environment (Reed, 2005). These routines, tasks and subtasks can be in the form of habitual routines (dressing, eating) or occasional nonhabitual tasks (taking medication) that are demanded by circumstance (Chapparo & Ranka, 1997).

Productivity/school occupations are routines, tasks and subtasks which are done to enable a person to engage in *learning*, *provide support* for *self*, *family* or *community* through the production of *goods* or provision of *services* (Chapparo & Ranka, 1997) (Reed, 2005).

Leisure/play occupations are those routines, tasks and subtasks that are done for purposes of *entertainment*, *creativity* and *celebration* (Chapparo & Ranka, 1997).

Occupational Performance Areas: Subtask, Tasks and Routine Units of Performance

Although *activity* has been a term traditionally used in occupational therapy to denote purposeful action (Christiansen, 1991; Cynkin, 1979; Fidler & Fidler, 1978; Meyer, 1922; Mosey, 1981), meanings attributed to the term have become so broad and flexible that it has lost its power to describe elements of occupations and performance at varying levels (Nelson, 1988). In the OPM (A), occupations in each occupational performance area have been classified into subtask, task and routine units according to their size and complexity (Fig. 10.2).

Subtasks consist of steps or single units of the total task and are stated in terms of observable behaviour (e.g. putting an arm in a sleeve) (Romiszowski, 1984). *Tasks* are a sequence of subtasks that are ordered from the first step performed to the last performed to accomplish a specific purpose (e.g. putting on a jacket). Tasks can be carried out in action (doing) or thought (planned) and have definite beginning and end points. For example, drinking can be divided into subtasks such as locating the glass, reaching for the glass, grasping the glass, lifting the glass and taking a mouthful of liquid. All of these subtasks, when put together in an orderly sequence, result in execution of the total task: drinking. *Routines* are larger 'chunks' of occupation that are made up of a number of tasks that are sequenced to achieve a specific function (Brown, 1987). For example, drinking is one of the tasks involved in the routines of preparing and eating a meal.

Patterns of performance can be fixed or flexible. Many routines are fixed, determined by the prevailing sociocultural or physical context (such as using an escalator or lift, using the entry gates at a train station). A flexible routine is one that can be accomplished in many different ways, as long as it is

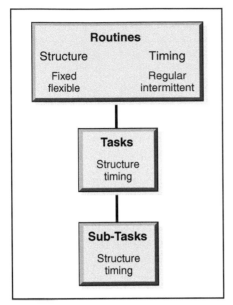

FIG. 10.2 ■ Occupational performance areas: routines, tasks and subtasks.

accomplished in a way that is acceptable to the performer and others. For example, there are many ways to complete morning routines. When someone sustains physical injury, one of the functions of occupational therapy is to explore alternative or more flexible patterns for task performance that may be quite different from those previously used by the person.

The classification of subtasks, tasks and routines can also be described according to their temporal patterns. Routines can be regular or intermittent. Regular routines occur on a daily basis and are usually critical to a person's function relative to the demands of his or her context. Intermittent routines do not have to be accomplished every day but may still be crucial to independent or satisfying function in life. For example, sudden illness prompts a person to engage in the routine of going to the doctor. Other intermittent routines have a qualitative impact on a person's life. For example, going to the movies is not a critical routine for most people but may be perceived by people as life enriching.

The extent to which people participate in performance of subtasks, tasks and routines is dependent on age, circumstance and ability. People with reduced physical capacity because of injury or illness are often unable to complete routines without assistance from others. Many may never be able to master the performance of daily routines. However, having the opportunity to choose to participate in part of the routine (a task or a subtask) contributes to establishing an occupational identity that is linked to an occupational role. For example, a young man who uses a wheelchair, has reduced upper limb physical capacity, and who is unable to complete the whole routine of shopping need not be excluded from family shopping excursions. His participation in those tasks and subtasks of the shopping routine which he is able to master, such as selecting items, transporting them on his lap and paying for them, confirms his occupational identity by participating in the occupational role performance of shopper and family member.

Classification of Occupational Performance Areas: An Idiosyncratic Process

Naming a task as either self-maintenance or work is an idiosyncratic function that can only be done by the performer, and the way a person classifies any one occupation as work, leisure, rest or self-maintenance may change day to day relative to its purpose. For example, reading may be classified by a person at one time as self-maintenance (to read medication instructions), or work (to read a computer screen), or leisure (to read a book for enjoyment), or rest (reading to get to sleep). Moreover, classification of occupations varies among sociocultural groups. Similarly, the pattern of time spent or value afforded each of the occupational performance areas are individually determined relative to desired or expected occupational role performance. Contrived notions of the balance of occupational performance cannot be externally imposed. The absence of lines separating the occupational performance areas of self-maintenance, rest, leisure and productivity in Fig. 10.1 illustrate that in the OPM(A), any division that is externally imposed is artificial.

Analysis of Occupational Performance Areas

Occupations at this level can be analysed and described using standard task analysis methods. Elements of the routine, task or subtask to be performed can be examined using a *task demands analysis*. The performance can be measured using *behavioural task analysis*. For example, cooking a meal can be described as a routine that requires performance of the tasks and subtasks of cutting, reading, stirring, tasting and grasping objects in such a way that a meal is produced within a specific time frame (task demands analysis). The performance of the person producing the meal can be analysed according to how successful the performance of each step of these routines, tasks and subtasks is relative to goals (behavioural task analysis). Errors in performance usually fall into one or more of four categories: errors of accuracy (does the wrong thing: for example, putting the wrong ingredients in a cake mix), errors of omission (leaves part of the performance out: such as forgetting to turn on the oven when cooking), errors of repetition (perseverates on steps: such as repeating steps in cooking that have already been completed) and errors of timing (too slow or quick such that performance is affected: for example, not cooking ingredients for long enough).

Questions listed in Box 10.2 represent examples of analysis and intervention that would be addressed in occupational performance areas.

CONSTRUCT 4: OCCUPATIONAL PERFORMANCE CAPACITIES

Accomplishment of routines and tasks in the occupational performance areas is predicated on the ability to use a variety of personal capacities or attributes in a way that is determined by the occupation and the performance context. This aspect of the model is conceptualised as being comprised of the capacities of the performer as well as the capacity requirements of occupations. There are motor, sensory, cognitive and psychosocial dimensions to any task performed that prompt a person to use motor, sensory, cognitive, interpersonal and intrapersonal capacities in a particular or *strategic* manner. Observation and analysis of occupational performance capacities focuses on task demands, the performance capacities of the person, and the relationship between them. For example, if a person with reduced motor capacity in the upper limbs had to dress, a task demands analysis would identify the specific range, strength, coordination and control needed for dressing in that person's context. Observation of the person's performance would be used to assess whether the person's motor capacities (range, strength, coordination and control) were sufficient for successful performance or whether there was poor 'fit' between the physical demands of the task and the physical capacity of the person. This approach differs from using standard methods of assessing physical capacity per se. The OPM(A) categorises occupational performance capacities into five areas: motor, sensory, cognitive, intrapersonal and interpersonal (see Fig. 10.1).

Motor capacity (move): From the perspective of the *performer* this component refers to the operation and

interaction of and between *physical structures* of the body during task performance. This can include range of motion, muscle strength, grasp, muscular and cardiovascular endurance, circulation, elimination of body waste, regulation of muscle activity, generation of motor responses and coordination. From the perspective of the *task* being done this component refers to the *physical attributes* of the task, such as size, load, dimension and location of objects (Chapparo & Ranka, 1997).

Sensory capacity (sense): From the perspective of the *performer* this component refers to the registration of sensory stimuli and discrimination required by the task. From the perspective of the *task* this component refers to the *sensory aspects* of the task, such as colour, texture, temperature, weight, movement, sound, smell and taste (Chapparo & Ranka, 1997).

Cognitive capacity (think): From the perspective of the *performer* this component refers to the operation and interaction of and between *mental processes* used during task performance. This can include thinking, perceiving, recognising, remembering, judging, learning, knowing, attending and problem solving. From the perspective of the *task* this component refers to the *cognitive dimensions* of the task. These are usually determined by the symbolic and operational complexity of the task (Chapparo & Ranka, 1997).

Intrapersonal capacity (feel): From the perspective of the *performer* this component refers to the operation and interaction between *internal psychological processes* used during task performance. This can include feelings, emotions, self-esteem, mood, affect, rationality and defence mechanisms. From the perspective of the *task* this component refers to the *intrapersonal attributes* that can be stimulated by the task and are required for effective task performance such as valuing, satisfaction and motivation (Chapparo & Ranka, 1997).

Interpersonal capacity (communicate): From the perspective of the *performer* this component refers to the continuing and changing *interaction between* a *person* and *others* during task performance. This can include interaction among individuals in relationships such as partnerships, families, communities and organisations both formal and informal. Interactive examples include sharing, cooperation, empathy, verbal and nonverbal communication. From the perspective of the *task* this component refers to the nature and degree of *interpersonal interaction* required for effective task performance (Chapparo & Ranka, 1997).

There is a complex network of interactions between the capacities and other constructs within the model. Influence of one capacity on another is illustrated by the absence of lines between capacities within this level of the model (Fig. 10.1). The interaction between the capacities and other levels of the model is illustrated by the arrows between levels in the Model (Fig. 10.1).

Analysis of Occupational Performance: Occupational Performance Capacities

Occupational therapists use many human capacity assessments that are independent from the tasks and contexts where they are used. For example, goniometry can be used to analyse restrictions in joint range of motion; the Mini Mental State Examination (Folstein, Folstein, & McHugh, 1975) can be used to analyse short- and long-term memory operations; measures of social interaction can be used to analyse interpersonal operations; and loneliness or depression inventories have been used as measures of intrapersonal operations (Borg & Bruce, 1991). The OPM(A) assumes each capacity is only functional if the person can apply existing capacities strategically. For example, people with back injuries may demonstrate strength that is within normal limits and good memory on formal tests of those capacities, but they may not use their motor and cognitive capacity in a strategic way when lifting and handling heavy objects (think then move), resulting in further injury. An elderly woman who has sustained a stroke may score poorly on formal measures of memory but may demonstrate adequate memory for everyday function in her own home environment when assessed using task analysis in her context. Analysis at the capacity level of the OPM(A) requires a criterion-referenced approach, similar to that described earlier. In other words, performance is determined as successful or not depending on how the capacity has to be used for particular tasks, in particular contexts with particular supports.

Successful strategy use implies salience or use of known motor, sensory, cognitive, interpersonal and intrapersonal capacities in the 'here and now'. It is the *ability to choose and apply the 'best' strategy* to fit a particular situation. Effective strategy use is dependent on having a large repertoire of strategies – in other words, many alternatives from which to choose when faced with a problem of function – and efficiency in the use of strategies (Torbeyns, Verschaffel, & Ghesquiére, 2004). This level of the OPM(A) lends support for three intervention approaches relative to improving occupational performance: *capacity building* (increasing the number and strength of strategies that are needed for tasks and routines), *capacity application* (learning how to apply newly learned strategies or residual strategies in different ways), and *grading* the capacities demanded by occupations to be performed.

Questions listed in Box 10.3 represent considerations to be made during assessment and intervention at this level of occupational performance.

CONSTRUCT 5: CORE ELEMENTS OF OCCUPATIONAL PERFORMANCE

Construct 5 acknowledges the body–mind–spirit interactionist paradigm that has long been recognised as key to physical and mental health and well-being (Townsend, Brintnell, & Staisey, 1990) and is illustrated at the bottom of the internal construct

---

---

in Fig. 10.1. Although each of the three aspects of this construct is described separately in this section, they cannot be functionally separated, reduced or understood as independent elements. This is not a new concept in occupational therapy and reflects pragmatist views of an integrated being whose mind, body and soul seek harmony (Meyer, 1922). In the OPM(A), body, mind and spirit are viewed as core elements reflecting the essential 'makeup' of humans from a corporeal (physical and tangible) and incorporeal (intangible and without material existence) perspective (Chapparo & Ranka, 1997).

Body element is defined as all of the tangible *physical* elements of human structure (Chapparo & Ranka, 1997).

Acknowledging the core element of the physical body affirms that within the boundaries of human understanding, aspects of performance can be described in terms of their smallest known structure such as cells, molecules and tissues. The interaction within and between the physical structures of the body may either contribute to occupational performance by providing the intrinsic physical elements required for occupational performance or inhibit desired occupational performance if affected by ill health, injury or disease (such as degenerative joint disease, musculoskeletal trauma and amputation).

Mind element is defined as the core of a person's conscious and unconscious intellect that forms the basis of the person's ability to understand and reason (Chapparo & Ranka, 1997).

The concept of the mind is understood in many different ways by many different cultures. Neurobiological approaches, for example, take a physicalist view of the mind and describe mind–brain relationships on the basis of neurotransmitters, neuronal circuitry and cell function. It is generally agreed that the mind is that which enables a person to have consciousness and the capacity for thought that, in turn, produces individual paradigms of reality from which people plan their daily routines, tasks and subtasks and construct their beliefs. Disorders of the mind (such as acquired brain impairment and schizophrenia) may affect occupational performance at all levels in the OPM(A).

Spirit element is defined loosely as that aspect of humans that *seeks* a sense of *harmony* within self and between self, nature, others and in some cases an ultimate other; *seeks* an *existing mystery* to life; *inner conviction; hope* and *meaning* (Chapparo & Ranka, 1997).

Spirituality is a broad concept with room for many perspectives. In general, it includes a sense of connection to something bigger than oneself. This view mirrors earlier interpretations of spirituality in occupation as expressed by Meyer (1922), who observed that as people live their life through daily occupations, they concern themselves not only with the performance of occupations but with deriving meaning from them. In the OPM(A), spirituality, as distinct from religiosity, is not viewed as separate from everyday occupations, but as a part of every level of occupational performance.

Although many idiosyncratic definitions of spirituality have been derived in health literature, three concepts are recurrent and relate to notions of 'meaning', 'hope', and a sense of 'interconnectedness'. The link between human occupations and meaning is at the heart of 'purposefulness' of life. Particularly for Aboriginal and Torres Strait Islander peoples of Australia, spirituality is a dynamic, evolving, contemporary expression of indigineity connecting past, present and future (Poroch et al., 2009). For all people, a strong sense of 'spirit' is considered an important determinant of health.

The OPM(A) does not view spirituality as one human subsystem, but a fundamental core element that is embedded in all aspects of occupational existence. At the level of occupational performance routines, tasks and subtasks it contributes to the person's sense of purposefulness when creating, thinking about and doing desired and needed occupations. At the capacity level in the OPM(A), spirituality, when defined as meaning and hope, contributes to using cognitive strategies that involve imagination, decision making and the ability to reflect. Intrapersonal aspects of meaning and hope relate to notions of a personal locus of control, intention, will, motivation. Interconnectedness is fundamental to the desire for and the development of interpersonal strategies that satisfy a personal need to 'fit' with the external social world.

BOX 10.4
CORE ELEMENTS CONSIDERATIONS IN ASSESSING OCCUPATIONAL PERFORMANCE

What specific *body* system disorder might interfere with occupational performance such as swelling, soft tissue shortening, inflammation, compromised cardiovascular system compromised respiratory system and other pathologies of body systems?

What specific disorder of the *mind* arising from compromised central nervous system function might interfere with occupational performance such as disordered neuronal transmission, brain damage and disordered neurochemistry that result from development, injury or chemical, drug and alcohol use?

What specific disorder of *spirit* might interfere with occupational performance such as loss of hope, loss of resolve, loss of 'connectedness', loss of purpose?

Relative to occupational performance, the body–mind–spirit core element of this model translates into the 'doing–knowing–being' dimensions at all levels of performance. The influence between the core elements and other levels of the model is reflected by the arrows which link the core elements to the occupational performance capacities (see Fig. 10.1).

Analysis of Occupational Performance: Core Elements of Performance

Aspects of core elements of performance that may be considered during assessment and intervention for occupational performance are listed in Box 10.4.

CONSTRUCT 6: EXTERNAL CONTEXT

People participate in occupations that occur in specific contexts. The ecology of their task performance is a critical element of successful participation reinforcing the notion that context-based *performance* (what a person actually does in his or her own context) may be quite different from clinic-based *capacity* (a person's ability to perform a task at the highest level of functioning in a test situation). For this reason an ecological approach to assessment with a focus on the discordance between person/people and context, as well as factors within the person, or people is needed.

In the OPM(A) the external context is an interactive world which has physical, sensory, cognitive, psychological, social, cultural, spiritual, and political-economic elements (Chapparo & Ranka, 1997). Aspects of the external context are labelled and defined briefly here. Their position around the internal context in Fig. 10.1 reflects the scope of ongoing press and affordance they exert on daily performance. An *affordance* is when the performance context enables opportunities for optimum performance. For example, a handle affords pulling, a quiet room affords reading, and a slippery surface affords balance reactions. *Press* has to do with the level of demand placed on performance and presents barriers, risks and restrictions to performance. Although all people at various times experience contextual demand that is beyond their capacity to cope, it is usually temporary. People with reduced physical capacity experience greater demand (press) from the external context as their physical capacity changes. It also cannot be assumed which of the contextual elements asserts greatest press. The cumulative effects of all contextual elements affecting performance may be greater than a single element. For example, some people who experience difficulties with the cognitive dimensions of planning movement find the cumulative cognitive load of thinking about how to do the task (cognition) and controlling actions in situ (physical) contributes to reduced physical skills. Each of the contextual elements in Fig. 10.1 assume prominence relative to salient performance demands. For example, the physical context assumes importance when climbing stairs at a railway station, sensory and cognitive contexts assume importance when cooking a meal from a complicated recipe. Their relationship to roles, tasks, capacities and core elements changes constantly.

Physical Context

The physical, tangible elements of situations in which people perform or participate, the location and arrangement of objects in the physical world and the physical characteristics of tools, objects, equipment, materials, supplies, food and liquids used (e.g. size, dimension, position, weight, viscosity). This includes naturally occurring characteristics and those that are built, engineered, manufactured or assembled.

Sensory Context

The sensory characteristics of tools, objects, equipment, materials, supplies, food and liquids used. It also includes sensory aspects of a wider performance context including temperature, texture, sound, light, odour, taste, humidity, movement and vibration.

Cognitive Context

The cognitive and perceptual complexity of situations where people do their everyday occupations, the clarity of information presented and the ease with which information presented can be interpreted in order to know what things are, what to do and how to use items, including tools, objects, equipment, materials, supplies, food and liquids. A virtual context exists when along with displacement of time and place, an alternate reality is contextualised for performance.

Psychological Context

The characteristics of situations that support or challenge a person's psyche. This includes dimensions that may invoke high levels of arousal, strong emotions, stress responses or have a calming effect.

Social Context

The characteristics of situations that require interactions with others and the expectations and supportiveness of people in those interactions. They include a range of social interactions from solitary, dyad, triad and small group to large group membership that may be closed or open.

Cultural Context

The characteristics of situations that reflect the traditions and ways of 'doing' that are passed down through generations and are unique to social groups. These include cultural symbols, arrangement of space, tools and materials used, modes of dress, modes of interaction, place for rituals, customs and ceremonies.

Spiritual Context

The characteristics of situations that support people's spiritual beliefs – for example, places of worship and sacred sites or places to be meditative, tools, materials, clothing and food associated with sacred rites and rituals.

Political Context

The explicit and implicit laws, policies and rules that govern and regulate performance and participation. Disability discrimination legislation, for example, is an aspect of the political context which mandates opportunities for equal participation for people with reduced physical capacity in all performance contexts.

Economic Context

The explicit and implicit financial systems and structures that fund and reward performance and participation. The costs of goods and services, taxation and health insurance, are important to all people, but assume greater importance where the cost of equipment, access and ongoing intervention is required for people with reduced physical capacity.

Analysis of Occupational Performance: External Context

Examples of the focus of analysis and intervention for occupational performance at this level of the OPM(A) include those listed in Box 10.5.

BOX 10.5
CONSIDERATION OF THE EXTERNAL CONTEXT IN ASSESSING OCCUPATIONAL PERFORMANCE

What are the barriers, risks and/or restrictions (press) in present and future physical, sensory, cognitive, social, psychological, cultural, spiritual, political and economic contexts that affect occupational performance?

What affordances (opportunities, support and resources) exist in present and future performance environments?

What affordance or press is required (modifications) in the physical, sensory, cognitive, social, psychological, cultural, spiritual, political and economic contexts for optimal occupational role performance?

CONSTRUCT 7: SPACE

Space refers to compositions of *physical matter* (physical space) as well as a person's view of *experience of space* (felt space) (Chapparo & Ranka, 1997).

Space is defined as an expanse that extends in all directions, in which all material objects or forms are located. The OPM(A) extends these notions of surrounding space to incorporate both internal and external components (see Fig. 10.1). External space surrounds people and contains objects in space, but people themselves contain internal space that is filled with objects in the form of body structures. Human understanding of internal and external space is conceptualised in this model as *physical space* and *felt space*. *Physical space* is derived from the technical construct of space as viewed by physics and from this is derived, in part, people's understanding about body structures, body systems, objects with which they interact and the wider physical world within which they function.

Of more importance to occupational performance is the notion of *felt space*. Although people are surrounded by physical space, the meaning they attribute to it, the way they use it and their interactions within it are largely determined by how they interpret it. Felt space is a personal, dynamic view of physical space as experienced by individuals. The meaning that is attributed to physical space during occupational performance has representation within all the constructs. For example, external objects and space impinge on people's various sensory receptors at the level of core elements of occupational performance. This information results in an understanding of the form and space elements of the context through a complicated process of interpretation. Motor, cognitive, sensory, interpersonal and intrapersonal perspectives of form and space are integrated to generate a highly individualised personal schema (body scheme), an account of form and space components of every step of every occupational task that is perceived, remembered, planned or carried out in life. People who experience reduced physical capacity work hard to reorder their personal schema.

CONSTRUCT 8: TIME

Time refers to a temporal ordering of physical and other events (physical time) as well as a person's understanding of time based on the meaning attributed to it (felt time) (Chapparo & Ranka, 1997).

Time is the final construct of the OPM(A) and has been defined as a system of relating one successive event to another. Just as with descriptions of the spatial construct outlined previously, time is conceptualised in this model as *physical time* and *felt time* (see Fig. 10.1).

Physical time is also derived from laws of physics which attempt to explain the temporal aspects of physical changes seen during occupational performance. This is usually expressed in terms of sequential or simultaneously occurring events.

Felt time is a person's understanding of time based on the meaning that is attributed to it. As with felt space, felt time involves highly personal abstractions of time that have representation at all levels of the model. It is an experiential abstraction that is being constantly changed and modified by experience. At the core elements, it is essential to muscle contraction, neuronal transmission and a spiritual feeling of the 'right' time. At the capacities level, it is the application of strategies when required by the tasks being performed. At the level of the occupational performance areas, timed ordering of steps in performance is essential to forming sequential routines. At the occupational role performance level, timing of performance links people to their social and environmental circumstances and enables feelings of being in the 'right place' at the 'right time'. As with the concept of felt space, notions of felt time vary from person to person and from one culture to another. Before using this model to explain abstractions of time relative to other cultures, therapists would need to investigate the prevailing abstraction of time within that culture and revise its relationship to other constructs within the model.

Analysis of Occupational Performance: Space and Time

As described, elements of space and time are embedded in occupational performance at every level of the model. The implication for analysis of occupational performance is to consider space and time dimensions within all the constructs of occupational performance.

CONCLUSION

This chapter describes how the OPM(A) is structured around eight constructs: occupational performance (the central construct) and its conceptual elements, which include occupational roles, occupational performance areas, occupational performance capacities, core elements of occupational performance, context, space and time. The proposed interaction between the constructs has been illustrated in Fig. 10.1 by arrows between these constructs. The arrows conceptualise a particular relationship between constructs that is strategic in nature and reflects a self-organising occupational performance system. Tasks and routines are configured strategically by people to comply with their occupational role performance needs. People apply their occupational performance capacities strategically to support relevant tasks and routines to be performed. Core elements comprising human composition are used strategically to develop and maintain performance capacities. These arrows not only link constructs conceptually but propose a place for occupational therapy intervention that centres on how people can gain or regain the most strategic use of self for occupational performance and the place for external affordance. Notions of 'normal' and 'typical' are rejected in favour of the 'specific' and 'particular'. The constructs outlined in this chapter can be applied to people and groups. The OPM(A) can be used as a means of identifying performance strengths and evaluating the impact of impairments on occupational roles, occupational performance areas and occupational performance capacities.

 http://evolve.elsevier.com/Curtin/OT

REFERENCES

American Occupational Therapy Association (2008). Occupational therapy practice framework: Domain and process (2nd ed.). *American Journal of Occupational Therapy, 62,* 625–683.

Borg, B., & Bruce, M. A. (1991). Assessing psychological performance factors. In C. Christiansen, & C. Baum (Eds.), *Occupational therapy: Overcoming human performance deficits* (pp. 539–590). Thorofare, NJ: Slack.

Brown, F. (1987). Meaningful assessment of people with severe and profound handicaps. In M. E. Snell (Ed.), *Systematic instruction of persons with severe handicaps* (3rd ed.) (pp. 29–63). Columbus, OH: Charles e. Merrill Publishing Company.

Chapparo, C., & Ranka, J. (1997). *Occupational performance model (Australia), monograph 1.* Sydney: Total Print Control.

Christiansen, C. (1991). Occupational therapy: Intervention for life performance. In C. Christiansen, & C. M. Baum (Eds.), *Occupational performance: Overcoming human performance deficits* (pp. 3–44). Thorofare, NJ: Slack, Inc.

Christiansen, C., Bass, J. D., & Baum, C. M. (Eds.). (2015). *Occupational therapy: Performance, participations, and well-being.* (4th ed.) Thorofare, NJ: Slack, Inc.

Crepeau, E. B., & Schell, B. A. B. (2009). Analysing occupation and activity. In H. Willard, E. B. Crepeau, E. S. Cohn, & B. A. B. Schell (Eds.), *Willard & Spackman's occupational therapy* (p. 165). Philadelphia: Wolters Kluwer Health/Lippincott Williams & Wilkins.

Cynkin, S. (1979). *Occupational therapy: Toward health through activities.* Boston: Little, Brown.

Dewey, J. (1930). *Human nature and conduct: An introduction to social thought.* New York: Modern Library.

Fidler, G., & Fidler, J. (1978). Doing and becoming: purposeful action and self actualization. *American Journal of Occupational Therapy, 32*(5), 305–310.

Folstein, M. F., Folstein, S. E., & McHugh, P. R. (1975). Mini-mental state: A practical method for grading the cognitive state of patients for the clinician. *Journal of Psychiatric Research, 12,* 189–198.

Forsberg-Wärleby, G., & Möller, A. (1996). Models of adaptation – An adaptation process after stroke analysed from different theoretical perspectives of adaptation. *Scandinavian Journal of Occupational Therapy, 3,* 114–122.

Gemino, A., & Wand, Y. (2004). A framework for empirical evaluation of conceptual modeling techniques. *Requirements Engineering, 9*(4), 248–260.

Glasgow, R. E., & Steiner, J. F. (2012). Comparative effectiveness research to accelerate translations: recommendations for an emerging field of science. In R. C. Brownson, G. A. Colditz, & E. K. Proctor (Eds.), *Dissemination and implementation research in health: Translating science to practice* (pp. 498–508). New York: Oxford University Press.

Hillman, A., & Chapparo, C. (2008). *Living a meaningful life with chronic illness.* Germany: VDM Verlag.

Hooper, B., & Wood, W. (2002). Pragmatism and structuralism in occupational therapy: The long conversation. *American Journal of Occupational Therapy, 56,* 40–50.

Jackson, J. (1998). Contemporary criticisms of role theory. *Journal of Occupational Science, 5*(2), 49–55.

Jurkowitsch, A., & Ranka, J. (2009). Occupational Performance Model of Australia (OPMA). In C. Habermann, & F. Kolster (Eds.), *Ergotherapie im arbeitsfeld neurologie* (pp. 90–106). Stuttgart: Thieme.

Kielhofner, G. (2002). *A model of human occupation: Theory and application.* Philadelphia: Lippincott Williams & Wilkins.

Kielhofner, G. (2009). *Conceptual foundations of occupational therapy practice* (4th ed.). Bethesda, MD: AOTA.

Landis, J. R. (Ed.). (1995). *Sociology: Concepts and characteristics.* Belmont: Wadsworth.

Manstead, A. S. R., & Hewstone, M. (Eds.). (1995). *The Blackwell encyclopedia of social psychology.* Boston: Blackwell Reference.

Matuska, K., & Barrett, K. (2014). Patterns of occupation. In B. A. B. Schell, G. Gillen, & M. E. Scaffa (Eds.), *Willard and Spackman occupational therapy* (12th ed.) (pp. 163–172). Philadelphia: Lippincott William & Wilkins.

Meyer, A. (1922). The philosophy of occupational therapy. *Archives of Occupational Therapy, 1,* 1–10.

Morgan, D. (2007). Paradigms lost and pragmatism regained. Methodological implications of combining qualitative and quantitative methods. *Journal of Mixed Methods Research, 1*(1), 48–76.

Mosey, A. C. (1981). *Occupational therapy: Configuration of a profession.* New York: Ravens Press.

Nelson, D. (1988). Occupation: Form and performance. *American Journal of Occupational Therapy, 42*(10), 633–641.

Poroch, N., Arabena, R., Tongs, J., Larkin, S., Fisher, J., & Henderson, G. (2009). *Spirituality and aboriginal people's social and emotional wellbeing: A review.* Cooperative Research Centre for Aboriginal Health Discussion Paper Series: No. 11.

Reed, K. L. (2005). An annotated history of the concepts used in occupational therapy. In C. H. Christiansen, M. C. Baum, & J. Bass-Haugen (Eds.), *Occupational therapy: Performance, participation, and well-being* (pp. 567–626). Thorofare, NJ: Slack.

Romiszowski, A. (1984). *Designing instructional systems.* London: Kogan Page.

Rowles, G. D. (2009). Meaning of place. In H. Willard, E. B. Crepeau, E. S. Cohn, & B. A. B. Schell (Eds.), *Willard & Spackman's occupational therapy* (11th ed.) (pp. 80–92). Philadelphia: Wolters Kluwer Health/Lippincott, Williams & Wilkins.

Torbeyns, J., Verschaffel, L., & Ghesquiére, P. (2004). Strategy development in children with mathematical disabilities: Insights from the choice/no choice method and the chronological-age/ability-level match design. *Journal of Learning Disabilities, 37,* 119–131.

Townsend, E., Brintnell, S., & Staisey, N. (1990). Developing guidelines for client-centred occupational therapy practice. *Canadian Journal of Occupational Therapy, 37*(2), 69–76.

11

THE CANADIAN MODEL OF OCCUPATIONAL PERFORMANCE AND ENGAGEMENT (CMOP-E)

JANE A. DAVIS

CHAPTER OUTLINE

Abstract
Conceptual models of practice are important tools for occupational therapy practitioners to facilitate organisation of information, identify assessment needs, and support occupational therapy reasoning and practice processes. The Canadian Model of Occupational Performance and Engagement (CMOP-E) is a widely used occupational therapy conceptual model. In this chapter, the history of the development of the model is described and its key elements are defined. An example is provided of how the CMOP-E can be used in practice, in combination with other models, to guide occupational therapy practitioners as they work to enable occupational performance and engagement.

KEY POINTS

- The Occupational Performance Model (OPM) was developed based on the Human Occupations Model by Reed and Sanderson. The ideas presented in the OPM have remained foundational to and continue to play significant roles in the articulations of occupational therapy theory, practice and research.

- The Canadian Model of Occupational Performance (CMOP) replaced the OPM and emphasised the dynamic nature of the interaction of person, occupation and environment, the three core dimensions of interest for the occupational therapy profession.

- The Canadian Model of Occupational Performance and Engagement (CMOP-E) replaced the CMOP in 2007 with the publication of *Enabling Occupation II*. In that publication, client-centred enablement is identified as the core purpose, client-centredness as a core philosophy, occupation as the core domain, and enablement as the core competency of the occupational therapy profession.

- The Taxonomic Code of Occupational Performance (TCOP) focuses on *doing* or observable performance aspects of occupation and not on other areas such as purpose, meaning or engagement.

- The Fit Chart offers a practical way to think about enabling occupation and applying the dimensions of the CMOP-E in more detail.

HISTORICAL DEVELOPMENTS OF THE CANADIAN MODEL OF OCCUPATIONAL PERFORMANCE AND ENGAGEMENT

The OPM

During the 1980s, an influential group of occupational therapy thinkers, along with colleagues from medicine and medical sociology, engaged in a multi-year project focused on articulating the conceptual foundations, processes, and outcomes of occupational therapy in Canada. Their work, in collaboration with a federal guidelines programme for health professions and published by the Canadian Association of Occupational Therapists (CAOT), resulted in three documents: *Guidelines for the Client-centred Practice of Occupational Therapy, Intervention Guidelines for the Client-centred Practice of Occupational Therapy,* and *Toward Outcome Measures in Occupational Therapy* (Department of National Health and Welfare (DNHW) & CAOT, 1983, 1986, 1987, respectively). Within these documents the first iteration of the Occupational Performance Model (OPM) was elaborated based on the Human Occupations Model by Reed and Sanderson (1980). The OPM was depicted by a simple black-and-white line drawing of three concentric circles (Fig. 11.1; DNHW & CAOT, 1983, 1986; CAOT, 1991*). The inner circle, representing the individual,[†] contained four performance components—the physical, mental, sociocultural and spiritual. The individual was situated within the physical, social and cultural environments—the outer circle—with the occupation dimension of self-care, productivity and leisure acting as the bridge between the individual and the environment, resulting in occupational performance.

As one of the earliest conceptual models, the ideas presented in the OPM have remained foundational to and continue to play significant roles in the articulations of occupational therapy theory, practice and research. The reconceptualisation of the OPM into the Canadian Model of Occupational Performance (CMOP) allowed for a clearer understanding of the relationship of the dimensions of person, occupation and environment as well as a more complex evolution of their features.

The Canadian Model of Occupational Performance

In 1997, the publication of *Enabling Occupation: An Occupational Therapy Perspective,* the sixth Canadian practice guidelines,[‡]

presented a new version of the OPM, the CMOP (CAOT, 1997[§]). The new three-dimensional image of a triangle with a small centre circle and two larger concentric circles (Fig. 11.2A) emphasises the dynamic nature of the interaction of person, occupation and environment, the three core dimensions of interest for the profession of occupational therapy. The three points of the triangle (person) extend over the inner circle (occupation) to highlight that the person and environment interact in other ways independent of 'occupation' as well as that occupations (in form and structure) exist within the environment even if they are not being performed. Thus occupational performance is represented by the 'dynamic, interwoven relationship' of all three dimensions (CAOT, 2002), where occupation remains the bridge between person and environment; that is, people interact with their environment through doing. As such, occupational performance, as an embedded part of the CMOP graphic illustration, is conceptualised in a different and more simplified manner than in most other occupation-informed conceptual models that often depict their occupational outcome of interest as an end point of a fairly detailed process that moves through the person, occupation, and/or environment dimensions. Although the person, occupation and environment dimensions and most of their features—first conceptualised within the OPM—were retained in the CMOP, important features were added or amended (CAOT, 2002). These changes are highlighted here along with the original features of the OPM that were retained as part of the CMOP.

Person

The changes made to the performance components of the person dimension of the Canadian model in its evolution from the OPM to the CMOP were (a) partitioning out spirituality, (b) renaming the 'mental' performance component as cognitive and affective, and (c) removing the sociocultural performance component. These are described below along with brief descriptions of the CMOP performance components.

Partitioning Out Spirituality. In addition to the new graphic, significant changes were made in the representation of the 'spirit', now situated at the core of the entire model as 'spirituality'. The placement of spirituality or 'essence of the self' (CAOT, 2002, p. 43) at the core of the CMOP reinforced its long-standing importance within Canadian occupational therapy (Friedland, 2011; Urbanowski & Vargo, 1994). Spirituality is

---

*The 1991 version of the CAOT guidelines was an amalgam of the three original documents. It included the OPM and the content was left essentially unchanged.

[†]The term *individual* was used in the OPM; this was changed to *person* in the Canadian Model of Occupational Performance.

[‡]In keeping with the original tripartite focus—foundations, process, and outcomes—of the 1980s practice guidelines, the sixth guidelines not only moved forward the evolution of the OPM to the CMOP, it also presented a new practice process framework, the

Occupational Performance Process Model (OPPM; CAOT, 1997; Fearing et al., 1997), to complement the Canadian Occupational Performance Measure (COPM), which was created in keeping with the philosophies and dimensions of the OPM and first published in 1991 (see Law et al., 2014, for the current [fifth] edition of the COPM), as a tool for guiding practitioners in exploring their clients' occupational lives to understanding the occupational issues deemed important by each client.

[§]The 2002 edition of *Enabling Occupation: An Occupational Therapy Perspective* is considered the 7th guidelines as it was updated with a new preface.

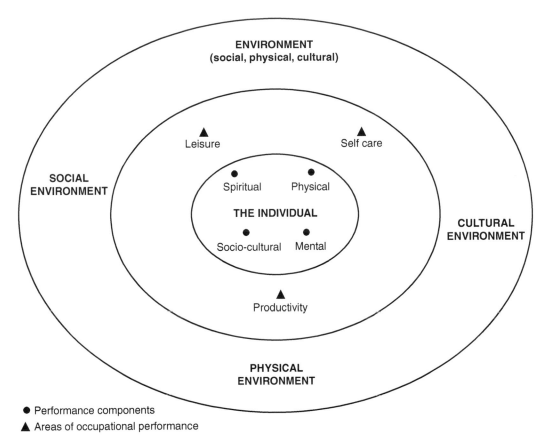

FIG. 11.1 ■ Occupational Performance Model (OPM), adapted from Reed and Sanderson, 1980. *(Reproduced with permission from Department of National Health and Welfare and the Canadian Association of Occupational Therapists. (1983). Guidelines for the client-centred practice of occupational therapy (H39-33/1983E) (p. 9). Ottawa: Department of National Health and Welfare.)*

viewed as infused through the person, occupation and environment, in that not only are people regarded as spiritual beings, but occupations and environments are viewed as containing spiritual elements that are experienced by people as they interact in doing within contexts (CAOT, 1997). The CAOT (1997) characterises spirituality as 'a pervasive life force, manifestation of a higher self, source of will and self-determination, and a sense of meaning, purpose and connectedness that people experience within the context of their environment' (p. 182). A person's truest *self* is expressed through his or her actions and shared through his or her occupational narratives (Kirsh, 2011). These occupations include religious and spiritual practices (Brémault-Phillips & Chirovsky, 2011; Smith & Suto, 2012), spiritual occupations (Kang, 2003), activities of spirit (Christiansen, 1997) and everyday activities that sustain and enhance life and support health and well-being (Kang, 2003; McColl, 2011; Wilding, May, & Muir-Cochrane, 2005). For further discussion and debate on spirituality and occupational therapy, see McColl, 2011.

Renaming Mental as Cognitive and Affective. The term *mental* was viewed as too narrow to represent both cognitive and affective

features as it did in the OPM. Thus mental was divided into two components, cognitive and affective, to ensure that both these components of performance were considered throughout the practice process. Depicting the cognitive and affective components in this way accentuates their essential nature alongside the physical and the breadth of occupational therapy practice.

Removing Sociocultural. When looking back at the OPM and its conceptualisation of the sociocultural performance component and the social and cultural environments, the overlap and conflicting understandings of where the 'sociocultural' was situated becomes apparent. The removal of the sociocultural as a performance component from the CMOP asserted a new Canadian perspective of the *social* and *cultural* as inherent aspects of the environment that interact with and shape the person. This perspective captured the shift from viewing involvement in community, relationships with family and friends and the effect of illness or injury on those relationships as features of the sociocultural performance component. Instead, these features were incorporated into the existing environment dimensions and expressed in the things that we do with others as

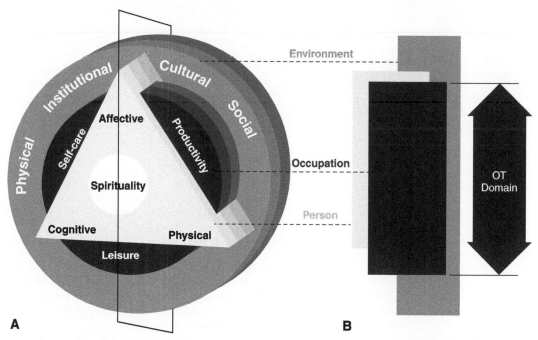

FIG. 11.2 ■ The CMOP-E: Specifying occupational therapists' domain of concern. A, This was referred to as the CMOP in *Enabling Occupation* (1997, 2002) and CMOP-E in *Enabling Occupation II* (2007, 2013). B, The transsectional view of the CMOP-E. *(Reprinted with permission. Copyright by CAOT Publications ACE. From Polatajko, H. J., Townsend, E. A., & Craik, J. (2013). Canadian Model of Occupational Performance and Engagement (CMOP-E). In E. A. Townsend & H. J. Polatajko (Eds.), Enabling occupation II: Advancing an occupational therapy vision of health, well-being, & justice through occupation (p. 23). Ottawa: CAOT Publications ACE.)*

shaped by society and culture. Conceptually, this shift affords occupational therapy practitioners a new understanding about the possibilities for advocacy and effective occupational enablement through environmental change as well as a more nuanced understanding of the essential features of occupational performance.

CMOP Performance Components. Although some might argue that spirituality is a performance component of the person, it is depicted in the CMOP as the core to the entire model, and thus distinct from the CMOP's three performance components: cognitive, affective and physical (known as CAP).

COGNITIVE. The cognitive performance component comprises aspects such as memory, orientation, concentration, intellect, insight, judgement and general knowledge. It covers how people think and remember and what they know.

AFFECTIVE. The affective performance component involves aspects that describe emotions, mood, affect, volition, body image, coping skills and reaction and adaptation to illness or injury.

PHYSICAL. The physical performance component pertains to aspects of movement, strength, coordination, balance, endurance, sensation, pain, appearance and physical illness and/or injury of body systems and/or structures.

Occupation

The original definition of occupation used in the OPM was that used by Reed and Sanderson (1980): 'activities or tasks which engage a person's resources of time and energy' (p. 243). This definition has evolved within the Canadian guidelines over time from one focused solely on 'activities and tasks' that involve a person's 'time and energy' to one that captures the complexities of occupation, including its meaning and significance in people's lives and how it is shaped by society and culture (CAOT, 1997, p. 34). Known as the areas of occupational performance in the OPM, the three categories of occupation or purposes—self-care*, leisure and productivity—have remained a part of the model since its inception in 1983; however, this more recent definition of occupation holds that how an occupation is understood and named is defined, and hence decided, by the individual and culture.

Self-care. Self-care is viewed in the CMOP as aspects of personal care, such as grooming, dressing, bathing, feeding and toileting. Some people may also argue that self-care includes aspects such as exercise, meditation and sleep, whereas others may view these aspects as leisure. Unlike the categories of

---

*Reed and Sanderson used *self-maintenance, productivity,* and *leisure. Self-maintenance* was changed to *self-care* in the OPM.

occupation often used in the United States of America and other countries, the CMOP does not have a separate category for sleep.

Leisure. The leisure category is meant to capture occupations that are performed as hobbies, games and collecting, sports and recreation, to fill free time, to fulfil cultural and creative interests, within clubs and groups and in nature. If the notion of play is defined as filling time with a self-chosen occupation, then it could be placed here as well.

Productivity. Productivity is understood within the CMOP as occupations that provide remuneration such as paid employment, as well as occupations that give back to the community or society, such as volunteering, homemaking, and schooling. An ongoing debate in occupational therapy remains with respect to the categorisation of the play of children. The notion that 'play is the "work" of children' has long been argued, whereas others assert that children play and children work, and the nature of children's play[††] and work differs.

Classifying Occupation. The typological categories for occupation used within the CMOP illustrate one way of classifying occupations—that is, by purpose. This type of classification has been critiqued by theorists as biased toward Western assumptions that give work the dominant position in the classification (Aldrich, McCarty, Boyd, Bunch, & Balentine, 2014; Hammell, 2009). Many other classifications systems have been proposed as a way of understanding 'types' of occupations (e.g. work, rest, play; self-care, productivity, leisure) and 'experiences' of occupation (e.g. social connectedness, control, purpose and continuity [Aldrich et al., 2014]; restorative, as ways to connect and contribute, as ways of engagement in doing, and as ways to connect the past and present to a hopeful future [Hammell, 2009]; calming, exacting, flowing [Jonsson & Persson, 2006]). The CMOP definitions for self-care, productivity and leisure do convey some experiential aspects; however, they do not dominate the classification. As typological classifications have a more concrete structure, they may be a useful way of starting off conversations about what people do, providing the practitioner with clues to occupational aspects that need further clarification (Aldrich et al., 2014). The use of different classification systems for occupations offers diverse avenues for understanding why people do and the different ways that people experience their occupations.

Environment

The environment as depicted in the CMOP was expanded from the three environmental aspects described in the OPM to four aspects: physical, social, cultural and institutional. The first three have remained relatively stable in how they have been

conceptualised across the evolution of the Canadian guidelines, whereas the institutional environment was a new addition to the CMOP.

Physical Environment. The physical environment is viewed as encompassing all built and natural aspects of the environment from the micro, such as the type of door knobs, to the macro, such as how a society is built to provide accessible spaces. It includes indoor features of a house or building to natural features, such as paths and roads.

Social Environment. The social environment pertains to the people in the environment, our relationships with them, the networks we can leverage when requiring assistance and the general availability of assistance to support living. Social environments can vary depending on the institutional environments as described later.

Cultural Environment. The cultural environment extends from the micro, such as person or family rituals, to the macro, such as expectations and attitudes of the broader culture. The extent to which a person 'takes up' a culture will shape his or her behaviours, rituals and practices.

Institutional Environment. This fourth environmental aspect, institutional environment, was added to the three existing environments in the CMOP. Although typically viewed as part of the social environment, the institutional environment was created as distinct from the existing social environment described in the OPM to reinforce the critical importance of understanding how structural and systemic elements comprising the broad-level social environment can enable or obstruct occupational performance. This broad-level understanding was missing from the description of the social environment in the OPM. The institutional environment is viewed as not only comprising governmental and organisational structures, policies and practices, but also often hidden or underconsidered social determinants of health (Mikkonen & Raphael, 2012),[‡‡] such as income, education, unemployment, aboriginal status, race, gender and disability as well as stigmatising, fear-mongering and bullying systemic practices. For occupational therapy practitioners, these institutional elements can be viewed as social determinants of occupational engagement, therefore demanding their consideration when working with individuals, groups, communities and population to enable occupation.

[‡‡]The *Social Determinants of Health: The Canadian Facts* (Mikkonen & Raphael, 2012) considers 14 social determinants of health: (1) Income and Income Distribution; (2) Education; (3) Unemployment and Job Security; (4) Employment and Working Conditions; (5) Early Childhood Development; (6) Food Insecurity; (7) Housing; (8) Social Exclusion; (9) Social Safety Network; (10) Health Services; (11) Aboriginal Status; (12) Gender; (13) Race; (14) Disability.

[††]The notion of playfulness is beyond this categorisation as it implies the way one performs and not the type or purpose of the occupation.

The changes made to the CMOP illustrate the complexities involved in understanding the dynamic relationship of the person, occupation and environment dimensions. However, during the reconceptualisation of the CMOP, its outcome of occupational performance was left unchallenged even though the original guidelines described the 'essence' of occupational therapy practice as 'the engagement of clients in purposeful activities' (DNHW & CAOT, 1983, p. 1), whereas occupational performance was simply defined as 'activities carried out' (p. xv). So although the concept of engagement has been part of the lexicon of occupational therapy for decades, it took until 2007 for the concept of 'occupational engagement' to be included in a conceptual model of practice, when the CMOP became the CMOP-E. The CMOP-E shines a light on key occupational concepts that have moved us forward in our thinking as a profession.

THE CANADIAN MODEL OF OCCUPATIONAL PERFORMANCE AND ENGAGEMENT

The Canadian Model of Occupational Performance and Engagement (CMOP-E; Polatajko, Townsend, & Craik, 2013b) is the most recent version of the Canadian model. It was first published in the eighth Canadian practice guidelines in 2007, *Enabling Occupation II: Advancing an Occupational Therapy Vision for Health, Well-Being, & Justice Through Occupation* (Townsend & Polatajko, 2007, 2013) based on input from a national advisory panel made up of occupational therapists and stakeholders from across Canada. The CMOP-E is depicted in two ways, as the original CMOP with the addition of a new transsectional view (see Fig. 11.2A and B, respectively). Since the 2007 publication, client-centred occupational enablement has become established as the core purpose of occupational therapy, with client-centredness as a core philosophy, occupation as the core domain of concern of the profession and enablement as its core professional competency.

With the addition of the transsectional view of the CMOP-E (see Fig. 11.2B), occupation is clarified decisively as the core domain of concern of occupational therapy (Polatajko et al., 2013a), where occupational therapists are concerned primarily with the collective interaction of the person, occupation and environment. However, where the CMOP focused only on this collective interaction of the three dimensions—person, occupation and environment—the CMOP-E clarifies that the concern of occupational therapists can extend to situations where occupation and person interact (e.g. an activity analysis) or occupation and environment interact (e.g. policy creation to afford availability/accessibility of occupations). Foregrounding occupation in the CMOP-E has heightened the need for further refinement and development of occupational concepts that are important for clearer articulation of the profession's core purpose. Three of these concepts central to the CMOP-E are discussed next: occupational repertoire, occupational performance and occupational engagement.

Occupational Repertoire

The occupation dimension within the CMOP-E is presented as a bridge between the environment and the person (community/group). This dimension captures all the occupations that compose a person's occupational repertoire. As with a repertoire of music, which is understood as what a musician knows or is prepared to perform, an occupational repertoire is viewed as the constellation of occupations that a person performs or has the capacity to perform at one point in time (Davis & Polatajko, 2006, 2010). Understanding the extent of a person's occupational repertoire offers practitioners a clear illustration of an occupational life and how occupations form patterns and trajectories that support performance and engagement. It also accentuates the occupational transitions that may reveal occupational issues. Although occupational therapy has been focused predominantly on a person's performance of one occupation, the concept of occupational repertoire as depicted in the occupation dimension of the CMOP-E broadens the scope of practice for occupational therapists to issues of 'repertoire', such as occupational balance/imbalance, marginalisation, and deprivation.

Occupational Performance

The concept of occupational performance is one of the longest standing and most commonly used occupational terms in the profession's lexicon. Occupational performance captures what an individual *can* do or has the *capacity, skills, and knowledge to* do. Thus it pertains to observable aspects of doing or how an occupation is carried out. It was defined in the CMOP as the 'result of a dynamic, interwoven relationship between persons, environment, and occupation over a person's lifespan; the ability to choose, organise, and satisfactorily perform meaningful occupations that are culturally defined and age appropriate for looking after oneself, enjoying life, and contributing to the social and economic fabric of a community' (CAOT, 1997, p. 181). This definition has been retained within the CMOP-E, which continues to view occupational performance as embedded in the model where occupation bridges person and environment.

Taxonomic Code of Occupational Performance

A number of hierarchies of occupational performance have been proposed, and these differ from the classifications of occupation described earlier. The hierarchies of occupational performance capture how occupations that are performed can be broken down into smaller aspects of doing. Once such hierarchy is the *Taxonomic Code of Occupational Performance* (TCOP; Table 11.1), which evolved from the work of an occupation interest group that began in 1999 at the University of Western Ontario (now Western University), in London, Ontario, Canada, and involved academics, master's students and practitioners. The purpose of the group was to attempt

TABLE 11.1		
The Taxonomic Code of Occupational Performance (TCOP)		
Level of complexity	Definition	Example
Occupation	An activity or set of activities that is performed with some consistency and regularity, that brings structure, and is given value and meaning by individuals and a culture	Accountancy
Activity	A set of tasks with a specific end point or outcome that is greater than that of any constituent task	Financial report writing
Task	A set of actions having an end point or a specific outcome	Printing the report
Action	A set of voluntary movements or mental processes that form a recognisable and purposeful pattern (such as grasping, holding, pulling, pushing, turning, kneeling, standing, walking, thinking, remembering, smiling, chewing, winking, etc.)	Folding, remembering the meaning of numbers
Voluntary movement or mental processes	A simple voluntary muscle or mental activation (such as flexion, extension, adduction, abduction, rotation, supination, pronation, blinking, memory, attention, focusing, scanning, etc.)	Flexing, attending

All levels of performance are subserved by cognitive, physical, and affective performance components. Spirituality pervades.

Reprinted with permission. Copyright by CAOT Publications ACE. From Polatajko, H. J., Davis, J., Stewart, D., Cantin, N., Amoroso, B., Purdie, L., & Zimmerman, D. (2013). Specifying the domain of concern: Occupation as core. In E. A. Townsend & H. J. Polatajko (Eds.), *Enabling occupation II: Advancing an occupational therapy vision for health, well-being, and justice through occupation* (pp. 13-36). Ottawa: CAOT Publications ACE. p. 19.

to clarify aspects of occupation-based practice that often led to confusion. In the first few meetings, it was recognised that the profession's definitions and understandings of the terms *occupation, activity,* and *task* differed greatly, acting as a barrier to the clear articulation of the core concern of our profession. Thus terms and definitions used within the occupational therapy literature were uncovered to capture occupation and the aspects that it subsumes, as well as relevant terms and definitions within other disciplines and professions. An affinity analysis process was used to construct the initial 'Taxonomic Code', which was published in 2004 (Polatajko, Davis, Hobson, et al., 2004), and face validity testing was carried out in 2006 (Zimmerman, Purdie, Davis, & Polatajko, 2006). The version of the TCOP published in the *Enabling Occupation II* guidelines offers a way of understanding the occupational levels of occupational performance and highlights how breakdowns at different levels in the hierarchical TCOP structure may result in occupational performance challenges. The focus of the TCOP was specifically on the *doing* or observable performance aspects of occupation and not on other areas such as purpose, meaning or engagement. This tool was viewed as a way of supporting practitioners and students in articulating where their practice is focused, or at what level, in relation to the outcome of occupational performance specifically. This tool can help

practitioners to articulate the target for change in relation to an occupational performance issue.

For example, if Becca, a 24-year-old student, had a tendon repaired in her hand resulting in decreased range of motion, the TCOP would help to illustrate how the breakdown for using her hand in performing occupations occurs at the *physical* foundational level. As Becca increases her range of motion, she may then find that she is now able to hold a fork but not able to use it to stab food because of her poor grip strength. Using the TCOP, the occupational therapist could demonstrate how there is a breakdown at the action level due to her poor grip strength. The therapist would then work with the individual to determine the next steps toward enabling her occupational performance in eating, whether to modify the occupation and/or environment or continue to work on building grip strength (a physical foundational component) to support her actions and ultimately her occupational performance of that one occupation.

The TCOP is not meant to be a definitive hierarchical structure for occupational performance, but instead a tool to help clarify where breakdowns in occupational performance may be occurring. Although definitions and examples are provided for each level, what one practitioner may consider an activity may be viewed as an occupation or even a task by another. The point of the tool is to clarify the different possible levels of focus regarding an occupational performance issues to enhance decision making and bring light to the evidence required to support the decisions made about targets for changing performance.

Occupational Engagement: Beyond Performance

The term *engagement* is often used in the occupational therapy literature interchangeably with *performance, participation* and *involvement*. Because of this lack of specificity in use, the concept of occupational engagement has not been well described, defined or critiqued. The conceptual modification from CMOP to CMOP-E added occupational engagement as a distinct outcome of importance for occupational therapy. The addition of occupational engagement to the CMOP-E highlights the complexities in discussing and understanding the profession's core concern of occupation. Conceptualising occupational engagement as *beyond* performance substantially broadens the breadth or scope of the profession's core purpose to not only enable individuals to *do* occupation, but also to be engaged as a performer in or a director of that doing. The literature that describes occupational engagement often conveys a strong cognitive/affective dimension and argues that the doing of an occupation is not enough to conclude engagement and in fact may not be required for engagement (Xavier, Ferreira, Davis, & Polatajko, 2012). This perspective adds an experiential aspect to doing, highlighting the level of subjective involvement in the doing of the occupation. This involvement in doing has been discussed in the literature in various ways—for example, *being, becoming,* and *belonging* (see Hammell, 2004; Rebeiro, 2001; Wilcock, 1998)—and through debates about categorisations of meaning (see Hammell, 2009) and the existential nature of occupation (see Pierce, 2001). Thus engagement in occupation must be subjectively experienced (Xavier et al., 2012) and typically involves some form of intrinsicality (Hammell, 2001). A just-right occupational challenge is essential to achieving occupational engagement, along with receiving a positive outcome or feedback and being in an environment that can support and sustain engagement through accessibility, resources, time, opportunities and social support (Kennedy, Davis, & Polatajko, 2010).

Although much debate has centred around the proliferation of professional jargon and use of occupational concepts in occupational therapy—for example, how their use produces a separation in interprofessional understanding—the concept of occupational engagement offers an important new lens for examining occupational therapy practice. In their research with persons living with severe and persistent mental illness, Sutton, Hocking, & Smythe, (2012) contend that occupational engagement exists along a continuum from disengagement to full engagement. They argue that disengagement may be an essential nature of being for some people who need to disengage so that they can be fully engaged at other times. More intense or frequent occupational engagement may not always be supportive

of health (Egan, Kubina, Lidstone, Macdougall, & Raudoy, 2010), and people may pull back from more intense engagement for various reasons. Although such pulling back is commonly perceived as 'unhealthy' within the occupational therapy profession, a reconceptualisation of diversity in the needs for engagement is an important idea to consider as well as the significance of health, quality of life and meaning in relation to occupational engagement outcomes (Stewart, Fischer, Hirji, & Davis, 2016). Traditionally, occupational therapy practitioners have focused on occupational performance as their outcome, ensuring that the people they work with are able to 'do' or carry out the occupation. Consideration of the concept of occupational engagement within practice reveals how a focus on occupational performance is just not enough, as if a person is not interested in or motivated to 'do' an occupation or does not find meaning in that doing, then he or she is less likely to continue performing that occupation. Or, if he or she does perform that occupation out of necessity, his or her involvement in it will be constrained. The concept of occupational engagement also broadens the scope of occupational therapy practice to help characterise people's social participation in occupation regardless of their capacity to perform an occupation; for example, Rick Hoyt's participation in 1108 endurance races as of April 2014 (72 marathons, 32 Boston Marathons, and 6 Ironman triathlons) with his father, Dick, in spite of not being able to swim, run or bike, let alone walk. Although many would consider that Rick is not performing the occupation, no one could say that he was not occupationally engaged in that occupation when watching him race or listening to him speak about racing. As Dave McGillivray, Race Director of the Boston Marathon, clearly illustrated, "He [Rick] is dealing with all the elements too. It takes a lot of strength to say "dad, I want to continue, I want to participate." ... I realized how much of an incredible athlete Rick is." (Driscoll & Thyer, 2010).

Using the CMOP-E as a Conceptual Tool

The CMOP-E provides occupational therapy practitioners with a strong conceptual tool for understanding, collecting and organising informal and formal knowledge about the person, group, community or population with whom they are working, bringing to the forefront elements and outcomes of occupational concern. The CMOP-E framework (see Box 11.1) supports professional reasoning and enhances decision making and documentation by highlighting what is known and what still needs to be known about a person's occupational life. This framework can include past, present and future aspects of a person's occupational life to help monitor the progress of a person's situation. For example, consider the recent life events of Mr. Jackson Pernell, a 53 year old divorced man, who works as a produce manager for a large grocery chain within a small rural community located 6 hours from the closest urban centre. He is well known in the community as he has lived there since he started working at the grocery store when it was first built 24 years ago.

BOX 11.1

Organisational Framework based on the Canadian Model of Occupational Performance and Engagement. The information below provides examples of Mr. Jackson Pernell's occupational life analysis. [Two Days Post Discharge from Hospital]

Spirituality (essence of the self)
- Sense of self is strongly routed in being a good father and provider of a safe and secure home for his children
- Feels his job is vital to his sense of well-being and connectedness to his rural community

Person (performance components)

Cognitive	- Has good memory and attention
	- Exceptional insight into current situation
Affective	- Is upset about the possibility of not continuing in his current job
	- Before hospitalisation, was experiencing high levels of anxiety and distress trying to manage day-to-day when working full time
Physical	- 53 year old man
	- Has lived with ulcerative colitis (UC) for 26 years; it has become more severe over the past 6 years
	- Maintains a special diet of mostly raw foods; no dairy, wheat, processed foods or seeds
	- Has lived with moderate to severe fatigue over the past 3 years; has B12 injections and iron infusions to help manage fatigue
	- Has lived with abdominal pain, gastro-intestinal issues, and diarrhea for many years; it occurs sporadically and often without warning.
	- Has been hospitalised 4 times (for 3 months in total) over the past 3 years
	- Has been in the hospital in a large urban area for 4 weeks due to exacerbation of his UC; lost 5.5 kg the week before he was hospitalised and had severe dehydration.
	- Is currently taking Remicade for his UC
	- Is experiencing general weakness due to his most recent hospitalization

Occupation (areas of occupation composing repertoire)

Self-care	- Cooks all meals
	- Dresses, grooms, bathes
	- Drives
	- Meditation
Productivity	- Cleans home: dishes, vacuums, laundry
	- Mows lawn and cares for garden and general tasks around his property
	- Works full-time as produce manager in local grocery store
	- Volunteers at his children's schools
	- Coaches Jack Jr.'s hockey team
Leisure	- Played hockey in local intermural league (two nights per week11pm-12midnight) until about 18 months ago
	- Sails with friends in the summer
	- Reads fiction books and sports magazines

Environment (areas of environment)

Physical	- Lives in a two-storey home in a small rural town 6 hours outside a large urban area
	- Town has a community centre and a few local restaurants and shops
	- His work is a 10 minute walk from his home
Social	- Has three children; Michael 16 years, Jack Jr. 12 years, and Celia 10 years
	- Shares custody of his children with his ex-wife, Madeleine

BOX 11.1
Organisational Framework based on the CMOP-E. *(Continued)*

- His children stay with him on the weekends and for two months in the summer.
- Madeleine lives three blocks away
- His parents and his brother's family live in the next town
- The store supervisor feels that he should take long-term disability from the company as he is not able to work full time
- Two close friends/hockey teammates live across the street from him and are supportive
- Most of his other friends have stopped calling over the past year
- His father does not understand why he has not been able to work full time

Cultural
- Workplace culture of large grocery store chain; currently on short term disability benefits
- Small town culture with close community ties
- He has experienced some stigma about his illness from local town's people and some friends who do not understand
- He has a Scottish background

Institutional
- Employed by a grocery store with certain policies and procedures related to work and return to work
- Has a mortgage on his home
- Management positions in the grocery chain are only full time; no part-time positions available
- Governmental policies on accessibility rights and work
- Disability benefits offered by the grocery chain and required by law

Occupational Performance and Engagement Strengths and Issues
- Is managing his cooking, dressing, and grooming
- Has good memory and attention skills
- Has not started driving again
- Has good support from two close friends and family
- Is experiencing stigma from people who do not understand his illness and fatigue issues
- Worried that without his employment income he will not be able to afford to keep his home and his children will not have a room when they come to stay with him
- His store supervisor thinks he should take long-term disability benefits because he has missed a lot of work due to his illness and has not been able to work full time over the past year
- Wants to return to his job as produce manager but is concerned about returning to long-term, full time employment

He and his ex-wife, Madeleine, who divorced 4 years ago, have shared custody of their three children. Jackson has lived with ulcerative colitis for the past 26 years and recently returned home after spending 4 weeks in a large urban hospital due to a severe relapse of his illness. Box 11.1 demonstrates how the CMOP-E framework facilitates the organisation of knowledge and the identification of gaps in what is known about Mr. Pernell that require clarification through informal or formal assessments of person, occupation and/or environment dimensions. Once all the gaps in knowledge have been filled and occupational performance/engagement strengths and issues identified, the information organised within the CMOP-E framework can be used along with the Canadian Occupational Performance Measure (COPM; refer to Chapter 13) to identify potential occupational performance and/or engagement goals and choose the specific goal(s) to be enabled through the therapeutic relationship following the eight action points of the Canadian Practice Process Framework (CPPF; refer to Chapter 8).

The Fit Chart

Although the CMOP-E provides occupational therapy practitioners with an initial framework and a visual representation of the interaction of the person, occupation and environment dimensions of occupational performance and engagement that firmly articulates occupation as the core domain of concern, it does not offer any insight into how this interaction occurs. The Fit Chart (Polatajko, 2013; Figure 11.3) provides an expanded visual of the CMOP-E, facilitating initial theorising about how the dimensions interact and what factors may mediate this interaction pertaining to the identified

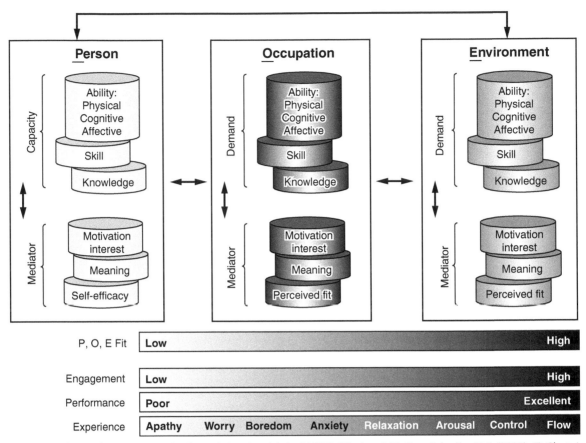

FIG. 11.3 ■ The Fit Chart. *(Reprinted with permission. Copyright by CAOT Publications ACE. From Polatajko, H. J. (2013). Fit Chart. In E. A. Townsend & H. J. Polatajko (Eds.),* Enabling occupation II: Advancing an occupational therapy vision for health, well-being, and justice through occupation *(p. 213). Ottawa: CAOT Publications ACE.)*

occupational goal. Once occupational issues are identified and goals are selected using the CMOP-E and COPM, the Fit Chart can be used by practitioners to ascertain plausible explanations for the issue pertaining to the selected goal, as well as possible solutions for enabling successful achievement of the goal (a list of questions that can be asked to collect and organise information is presented in Table 11.2A and 11.2B). The solutions that are generated through the Fit Chart analysis will involve the identification of targets for change in relation to person-, occupation- and/or environment-focused interventions.

Returning to Mr. Pernell's story, he clearly identifies his occupational performance/engagement issue as concern about maintaining long-term, full time attendance at his current job and his goal as wanting to return to his job as produce manager at the local grocery store. Mr. Pernell's abilities, skills and knowledge pertaining to his work as a produce manager as well as the mediators of his occupational engagement, that is, his motivation/interest, meaning and self-efficacy and perceived fit with the occupation (produce manager) and environment (local grocery store in small community) of concern are captured in Box 11.2. Now that the possible targets for change have been identified in relation to Mr. Pernell's goal, the practitioner will work with him to make decisions about his next steps in the practice process and potential enablement strategies that will facilitate his successful return to work, fulfilling his desire to be a good father and provider of a safe and secure home for his children.

TABLE 11.2A

Reasoning for Understanding Potential for Occupational Performance and Possible Solutions to Identified Occupational Performance-based Issues

		Analysis of Personal Capacity	Analysis of Occupational Demands/Supports	Analysis of Environmental Demands/Supports (for All Relevant Environments)	Analyses Of Goodness of Fit For Performance (Plausible Explanations)	Target(s) for Change (Possible Solutions)
ABILITIES	*Cognitive*	What cognitive strengths and difficulties does the person have related to the occupational issue?	What are the general cognitive demands/ requirements and supports of the specific occupation?	What are the general cognitive demands/ requirements and supports of the relevant environments?	Discuss FIT among the personal capacity (cognitive), the cognitive demands/supports of the occupation, and the cognitive demands/supports of the environment in which the occupation takes place. State whether the FIT is **HIGH, MODERATE, or LOW.**	Based on FIT analysis, state the possible target(s) for change (personal capacity, occupational demand/support, and/or environmental demand/support) and state recommended intervention/ enablement strategy.
	Affective	What affective strengths and difficulties does the person have related to the occupational issue?	What are the general affective demands/ requirements and supports of the specific occupation?	What are the general affective demands/ requirements and supports of the relevant environments?	Discuss FIT among the personal capacity (affective), the affective demands/supports of the occupation, and the affective demands/supports of the environment in which the occupation takes place. State whether the FIT is **HIGH, MODERATE, or LOW.**	Based on FIT analysis, state the possible target(s) for change (personal capacity, occupational demand/ support, and/or environmental demand/support) and state recommended intervention/ enablement strategy.
	Physical	What physical strengths and difficulties does the person have related to the occupational issue?	What are the general physical demands/ requirements and supports of the specific occupation?	What are the general physical demands/ requirements and supports of the relevant environments?	Discuss FIT among the personal capacity (physical), the physical demands/supports of the occupation, and the physical demands/supports of the environment in which the occupation takes place. State whether the FIT is **HIGH, MODERATE, or LOW.**	Based on FIT analysis, state the possible target(s) for change (personal capacity, occupational demand/support, and/or environmental demand/support) and state recommended intervention/ enablement strategy.
SKILLS		What skills does the person have related to occupational issue? [Consider if the person has a history of skilled performance of this occupation?]	What are the skill demands/ requirements and supports of the specific occupation?	What are the skill demands/ requirements and supports of the relevant environments?	Discuss FIT among the person's skills, the skill demands of the occupation, and the skill demands/ supports of the environment in which the occupation takes place. State whether the FIT is **HIGH, MODERATE, or LOW.**	Based on FIT analysis, state the possible target(s) for change (personal capacity, occupational demand/support, and/or environmental demand/support) and state recommended intervention/ enablement strategy.

Continued on following page

TABLE 11.2A

Reasoning for Understanding Potential for Occupational Performance and Possible Solutions to Identified Occupational Performance-based Issues (*Continued*)

	Analysis of Personal Capacity	Analysis of Occupational Demands/Supports	Analysis of Environmental Demands/Supports (for All Relevant Environments)	Analyses Of Goodness of Fit For Performance (Plausible Explanations)	Target(s) for Change (Possible Solutions)
KNOWLEDGE	What knowledge does the person have related to occupational issue? [Consider if the person has a history of knowledgeable performance of this occupation?]	What are the knowledge demands/requirements and supports of the specific occupation? [What does the person need to know to perform this occupation?]	What are the knowledge demands/requirements and supports of the relevant environments? [What does the person need to know about the environments?]	Discuss FIT among the person's knowledge, the knowledge demands/supports of the occupation, and the knowledge demands/supports of the environment in which the occupation takes place. State whether the FIT is **HIGH, MODERATE, or LOW.**	Based on FIT analysis, state the possible target(s) for change (personal capacity, occupational demand/support, and/or environmental demand/support) and state recommended intervention/enablement strategy.

Copyright Jane A. Davis and Helene J. Polatajko.

TABLE 11.2B

Reasoning for Understanding Potential for Occupational Engagement and Possible Solutions to Identified Occupational Engagement-based Issues

	Analysis of Personal Mediators	Analysis of Occupational Mediators	Analysis of Environmental Mediators	Analyses of Potential for Engagement (Plausible Explanations)	Target(s) for Change (Possible Solutions)
MOTIVATION/INTEREST	What motivations/interests does the person have to support engagement in the occupation?	What motivations/interests may be derived from the specific occupation?	What motivations/interests may exist within the relevant environments?	Discuss FIT among the person's motivation and interest, and those that exist within the occupation and environment in which the occupation takes place. State whether the FIT is **HIGH, MODERATE, or LOW.**	Based on FIT analysis, state the possible target(s) for change (personal, occupational, and/or environmental mediators) and state recommended intervention/enablement strategy.
MEANING	What meaning does the person hold in relation to this occupation to support engagement in it?	What meaning may be derived from the specific occupation?	What meaning may exists within the relevant environments?	Discuss FIT among the personal meaning, and those that exist within the occupation and environment in which the occupation takes place. State whether the FIT is **HIGH, MODERATE, or LOW.**	Based on FIT analysis, state the possible target(s) for change (personal, occupational, and/or environmental mediators) and state recommended intervention/enablement strategy.
SELF – EFFICACY/PERCEIVED FIT	What is the person's self-efficacy in relation to this general occupation to support engagement in it?	What is the person's perceived fit with this specific occupation?	What is the person's perceived fit with the relevant environments?	Discuss the FIT among the person's self-efficacy and their perceived fit with the specific occupation and environment in which the occupation takes place. State whether the FIT is **HIGH, MODERATE, or LOW.**	Based on FIT analysis, state the possible target(s) for change (personal, occupational, and/or environmental mediators) and state recommended intervention/enablement strategy.

BOX 11.2

Organisation Framework based on the Fit Chart to facilitate an occupational performance and engagement analysis. The information below provides examples of Mr. Jackson Pernell's occupational analysis, plausible explanations and possible targets and solutions to enable change.

Occupational Performance/Engagement Issue: Return to Work as Produce Manager at Local Grocery Store

PERFORMANCE CAPACITY

	Analysis of Personal Capacity	Analysis of Occupational Demands/Supports	Analysis of Environmental Demands/Supports (for All Relevant Environments)	Analyses Of Goodness of Fit For Performance (Plausible Explanations)	Target(s) for Change (Possible Solutions)
Cognitive	- Exceptional insight into current strengths and limitations - Has good memory and attention	- Managing produce ordering and delivery - Creating schedules for workers - Multitasking: Attending to tasks, possibly many at one time.	- Social environment of the grocery store in this small community may require the performance of many activities at once including speaking to shoppers - Large floor space of grocery store; produce section is only 1/6th of store. - Small town grocer so everyone knows him and speaks to him	**HIGH** - He has the cognitive abilities to perform his work tasks and activities and has a 24 year history of working in grocery produce and meeting the cognitive demands of the environment. He has good insight into how to manage his limitations.	NONE
Affective	- Experiences high levels of anxiety and distress trying to manage day-to-day when working full time	- Working on the store floor requires a positive social disposition for interaction with shoppers - Managing workers requires stable affect and capacity to manage stress	- Social environment of the grocery store requires employees to have a positive and engaging disposition when interacting with the shoppers - Managing stigma/community members views of hidden illness	**MODERATE-LOW** - He is concerned about returning to work and not being able to manage his full time job. This concern elevates his level of distress and anxiety which affects the symptoms of his illness and makes it difficult for him to engage fully in his work environment.	**PERSONAL CAPACITY (Affective)** The occupational and environmental demands of a positive and engaging disposition lack fit with his current personal capacity to manage his anxiety and distress. - *Consideration of possible solutions for decreasing his anxiety and distress is recommended.*
Physical	- Ulcerative colitis symptoms of abdominal pain and gastrointestinal issues	- Lifting boxes of produce - Breaking down boxes - Wheeling carts of produce	- Company requires that he manage a full time position - Store supervisor not supportive of return to work gradually	**LOW** - His current decreased physical strength, increased fatigue, and pain do not match the occupational demands of his job.	**PERSONAL CAPACITY (Physical)** His personal capacity (strength, pain, fatigue) does not fit with the occupational and environmental demands of this job.

BOX 11.2

Organisation Framework based on the Fit Chart. *(Continued)*

- Experiencing moderate to severe fatigue
- Is experiencing general weakness

- Standing for long periods fixing displays
- Managing stigma/community members views of hidden illness

- Parttime or flexible alternatives for his employment are not supported by the company or the store supervisor.

- *Consideration of possible solutions for increasing his general strength and management of pain and fatigue is recommended.*

OCCUPATIONAL DEMANDS

The occupational demands are too great for his current physical capacity.

- *Consideration of possible solutions for decreasing the physical occupational demands of the job is recommended.*

ENVIRONMENTAL DEMANDS

The current environment of his employment does not support parttime options or his gradual return to work.

- *Consideration of possible solutions for managing stigma around his 'hidden' illness and for changing the employer's views on parttime and gradual return to work, his capacity, and making the company/employer aware of disability, accessibility, and return to work legislation is recommended.*

Continued on following page

BOX 11.2

Organisation Framework based on the Fit Chart. *(Continued)*

SKILL	- Has been in current job for 24 years and has a high level of skill in the performance of the tasks and activities it requires.	- A moderate level of skill is required for the competent performance of the numerous tasks and activities required for this job.	- Social environment demands a moderate level of skill to navigate the interactions with shoppers, employer, and fellow employees.	**HIGH** - He has a high skill level which fits with the skill level demanded by the occupation and environment. **NONE**
KNOWLEDGE	- Has been in current job for 24 years and has a high level of knowledge related to the performance of the tasks and activities it requires.	- A moderate level of specific knowledge is required for the completion of the numerous tasks and activities required for this job.	- The environment demands a moderate level of knowledge pertaining to the social, institutional, and cultural environments of her workplace.	**HIGH** - He has a high knowledge level due to 24 years of experience in his current workplace, which fits with the skill level demanded by the occupation and environment. **NONE**

MEDIATORS OF ENGAGEMENT

	Analysis of Personal Mediators	Analysis of Occupational Mediators	Analysis of Environmental Mediators	Analyses of Potential for Engagement (Plausible Explanations)	Target(s) for Change (Possible Solutions)
MOTIVATION / INTEREST	- To maintain his financial independence and manage mortgage payments on his home - Provide a safe home for his children - To maintain socialisation with his community in which he has worked for 24 years - Worried about possible having to go on long term disability	- Engaging in paid work can be motivating in different ways, including the provision of income and a venue for continued learning.	- Working in this community grocery store maintains his socialisation and links to one's community. - The company and employer feel that managers should work full time and do not support gradual return to work.	**MODERATE-LOW** - He is very motivated to return to his job. However, he is very worried about being forced to go on long term disability benefits because of his company/employer's policy on full time employment for managers. He sees this as a potential barrier to his continued employment as the produce manager.	**ENVIRONMENTAL MOTIVATORS** The current environment in which he is working holds decreased motivation due to his employer's attitudes about parttime and gradual return to work. This lack of fit may act to limit his continued occupational engagement in his current job. - *Consideration of possible solutions for changing the employer's views on part-time and gradual return to work, his capacity, and making the company/employer aware of disability, accessibility, and return to work legislation is recommended.*

BOX 11.2

Organisation Framework based on the Fit Chart. *(Continued)*

MEANING

- His sense of self is strongly rooted in being a good father and provider of a safe and secure home for his children
- Feels his job is vital to his sense of well-being and connectedness to his rural community
- His job maintains his occupational engagement and identity.

- Engaging in work may provide individuals with a sense of contributing to society.
- This grocery store and job has been a part of his life for 24 yrs.
- Company/employer conveys that only full time workers are useful contributors.

HIGH-MODERATE

- Great meaning and significance is attached to his work as a produce manager. Although his company/employer have attached a negative meaning to part-time and gradual return to work, much personal and occupational meaning exists for him with this job.

NONE

Although the inherent meaning of his job has been altered slightly by some negative environmental mediators, his potential for engagement remains fairly high. Therefore the negative environmental meaning is not seen as a sufficient to be a target for change at this time. In addition, since motivation and meaning are closely linked, the current negative environmental meaning will most likely be altered through targeting the negative environmental motivators. (See above in motivation / interest).

SELF-EFFICACY/PERCEIVED FIT

- Believes that he has the skills and knowledge to complete his job.
- Feels he is a good worker.
- Is concerned that his UC will impact his attendance at work over the long term and that he will not have the energy to work full time.

- Perceives that his knowledge and skills fit with the demands of his current job.
- However, currently perceives reduced fit between his physical capacity and the demands of his job.

LOW

- Perceives that his knowledge and skills fit with the demands of his current job.
- However, his employer feels that he should go on long-term disability benefits instead of returning to his job. Because he does not feel he is physically able to return to his job full time, which his employer is enforcing, he perceives reduced fit with the demands of his workplace environment.

SELF-EFFICACY

His personal capacity (strength, pair, fatigue) does not fit with the occupational and environmental demands of this job, thus decreasing his self-efficacy.

- *Consideration of possible solutions for increasing his general strength and management of pain and fatigue is recommended.*

LOW

- He believes he is a skillful and knowledgeable worker. Realistically, however, he is aware that he cannot return to full time employment due to his fatigue and ongoing health issues.
- He perceives decreased fit with his occupational environment because his employer has a negative view of part-time and gradual return to work and thus is not supportive of having him continue in his current position as a produce manager.

PERCEIVED FIT / OCCUPATIONAL DEMANDS

His perceives decreased fit between his personal capacity and the occupational demands.

Continued on following page

BOX 11.2
Organisation Framework based on the Fit Chart. *(Continued)*

- *Consideration of possible solutions for altering the physical occupational demands of the job is recommended.*

PERCEIVED FIT / ENVIRONMENTAL DEMANDS

The current environment of his employment does not support part-time options or his gradual return to work.

- *Consideration of possible solutions for managing stigma around his hidden illness and for changing the employer's views on part-time and gradual return to work, his capacity, and making the company/employer aware of disability, accessibility, and return to work legislation is recommended.*

CONCLUSION

The CMOP-E provides a strong conceptual tool for understanding many aspects of occupation. It can be used as a framework for professional reasoning, decision making, and documentation allowing significant features of our occupational perspective and occupation-based practice to be highlighted. The CMOP-E and such tools as the TCOP and the Fit Chart offer occupational therapy practitioners additional resources to support the work that they do, clarifying what they do for other health care professionals and laypeople.

 http://evolve.elsevier.com/Curtin/OT

REFERENCES

Aldrich, R. M., McCarty, C. H., Boyd, B. A., Bunch, C. E., & Balentine, C. B. (2014). Empirical lessons about occupational categorization from case studies of unemployment. *Canadian Journal of Occupational Therapy, 81*, 289–297.

Brémault-Phillips, S., & Chirovsky, A. (2011). Spiritual practices. In M. A. McColl (Ed.), *Spirituality and occupational therapy* (2nd ed., pp. 183–192). Ottawa: CAOT Publications ACE.

Canadian Association of Occupational Therapists (1991). *Occupational therapy guidelines for client-centred practice.* Toronto, ON: CAOT Publications ACE.

Canadian Association of Occupational Therapists (1997). *Enabling occupation: An occupational therapy perspective.* Ottawa: CAOT Publications ACE.

Canadian Association of Occupational Therapists (2002). *Enabling occupation: An occupational therapy perspective* (2nd ed.). Ottawa: CAOT Publications ACE.

Christiansen, C. (1997). Acknowledging a spiritual dimension in occupational therapy practice. *American Journal of Occupational Therapy, 51*, 169–172.

Davis, J., & Polatajko, H. (2006). The occupational development of children. In S. Rodger, & J. Ziviani (Eds.), *Occupational therapy with children: Understanding children's occupations and enabling participation* (pp. 136–157). Oxford, UK: Blackwell Science.

Davis, J. A., & Polatajko, H. J. (2010). Don't forget the repertoire: The meta occupational issue. *OT Now, 12*(3), 20–22.

Department of National Health and Welfare and the Canadian Association of Occupational Therapists (1983). *Guidelines for the client-centred practice of occupational therapy (H39-33/1983E).* Ottawa: Department of National Health and Welfare.

Department of National Health and Welfare and the Canadian Association of Occupational Therapists. (1986). *Intervention guidelines for the client-centred practice of occupational therapy (H39-100/1986E).* Ottawa: Department of National Health and Welfare.

Department of National Health and Welfare and the Canadian Association of Occupational Therapists. (1987). *Toward outcome measures in occupational therapy (H39-114/1987E).* Ottawa: Department of National Health and Welfare.

Driscoll, T., & Thyer, J. (Eds.). (2010, Nov. 23). Labor of love. [Television series episode]. In: J. Perskie & L Gaffney (Producers), *Real Sports with Bryant Gumbel.* New York, NY: HBO.

Egan, M. Y., Kubina, L. A., Lidstone, R. I., Macdougall, G. H., & Raudoy, A. E. (2010). A critical reflection on occupational therapy within one assertive community treatment team. *Canadian Journal of Occupational Therapy, 77*, 70–79.

Friedland, J. (2011). *Restoring the spirit: The beginnings of occupational therapy in Canada, 1890–1930.* Montreal: McGill-Queen's University Press.

Fearing, G., Law, M., & Clark, J. (1997). An Occupational Performance Process Model: Fostering client and therapist alliances. *Canadian Journal of Occupational Therapy, 64*, 7–15.

Hammell, K. W. (2001). Intrinsicality: Reconsidering spirituality, meaning(s) and mandates. *Canadian Journal of Occupational Therapy, 68*, 186–194.

Hammell, K. W. (2004). Dimension of meaning in the occupations of daily life. *Canadian Journal of Occupational Therapy, 71*, 296–305.

Hammell, K. W. (2009). Self-care, productivity, and leisure, or dimensions of occupational experience? Rethinking occupational 'categories'. *Canadian Journal of Occupational Therapy, 76*, 107–114.

Jonsson, H., & Persson, D. (2006). Towards an experiential model of occupational balance: An alternative perspective on Flow Theory analysis. *Journal of Occupational Science, 13*, 62–73.

Kang, C. (2003). A psychospiritual integration frame of reference for occupational therapy. Part 1: Conceptual foundations. *Australian Occupational Therapy Journal, 50*, 92–103.

Kennedy, J., Davis, J., & Polatajko, H. (27 May 2010). Clarifying occupational engagement: A first step in measurement development. In: *Paper presented at the Canadian Association of Occupational Therapists Conference*, Nova Scotia: Halifax.

Kirsh, B. (2011). What makes narratives spiritual and how can we use them in OT. In M. A. McColl (Ed.), *Spirituality and occupational therapy* (2nd ed., pp. 201–208). Ottawa: CAOT Publications ACE.

Law, M., Baptiste, S., Carswell, A., McColl, M. A., Polatajko, H., & Pollock, N. (2014). *The Canadian Occupational Performance Measure* (5th ed.). Ottawa: CAOT Publications ACE.

McColl, M. A. (Ed.). (2011). *Spirituality and occupational therapy* (2nd ed.). Ottawa: CAOT Publications ACE.

Mikkonen, J., & Raphael, D. (2012). *Social determinants of health: The Canadian facts.* Toronto: York University School of Health Policy and Management. Retrieved from, (2012). *http://www.thecanadianfacts.org/The_Canadian_Facts.pdf.*

Pierce, D. (2001). Untangling occupation and activity. *American Journal of Occupational Therapy, 55*, 138–146.

Polatajko, H. J. (2013). Fit Chart. In E. A. Townsend, & H. J. Polatajko (Eds.), *Enabling occupation II: Advancing an occupational therapy vision for health, well-being, and justice through occupation* (p. 213). Ottawa: CAOT Publications ACE.

Polatajko, H. J., Davis, J. A., Hobson, S., et al. (2004). Nationally speaking: Meeting the responsibility that comes with the privilege: Introducing a taxonomic code for understanding occupation. *Canadian Journal of Occupational Therapy, 71*, 261–268.

Polatajko, H. J., Davis, J., Stewart, D., et al. (2013a). Specifying the domain of concern: Occupation as core. In E. A. Townsend, & H. J. Polatajko (Eds.), *Enabling occupation II: Advancing an occupational therapy vision for health, well-being, and justice through occupation* (pp. 13–36). Ottawa, ON: CAOT Publications ACE.

Polatajko, H. J., Townsend, E. A., & Craik, J. (2013b). Canadian Model of Occupational Performance and Engagement (CMOP-E). In E. A. Townsend, & H. J. Polatajko (Eds.), *Enabling occupation II:*

Advancing an occupational therapy vision of health, well-being, & justice through occupation (p. 23). Ottawa: CAOT Publications ACE.

Rebeiro, K. (2001). Enabling occupation: The importance of an affirming environment. *Canadian Journal of Occupational Therapy, 68,* 80–89.

Reed, K. L., & Sanderson, S. R. (1980). *Concepts of occupational therapy.* Baltimore, MD: Williams & Wilkins.

Smith, S., & Suto, M. J. (2012). Religious and/or spiritual practices: Extending spiritual freedom to people with schizophrenia. *Canadian Journal of Occupational Therapy, 79,* 77–85.

Stewart, K., Fischer, T., Hirji, R., & Davis, J. A. (2016). Toward the reconceptualization of the relationship between occupation and health and well-being. *Canadian Journal of Occupational Therapy, 83,* 249–259.

Sutton, D. J., Hocking, C. S., & Smythe, L. A. (2012). A phenomenological study of occupational engagement in recovery from mental illness. *Canadian Journal of Occupational Therapy, 79,* 142–150.

Townsend, E. A., & Polatajko, H. J. (2007). *Enabling occupation II: Advancing an occupational therapy vision of health, well-being, and justice through occupation.* Ottawa: CAOT Publications ACE.

Townsend, E. A., & Polatajko, H. J. (2013). *Enabling occupation II: Advancing an occupational therapy vision of health, well-being, & justice through occupation* (Rev. ed.). Ottawa: CAOT Publications ACE.

Urbanowski, R., & Vargo, J. (1994). Spirituality, daily practice, and the occupational performance model. *Canadian Journal of Occupational Therapy, 61,* 88–94.

Wilcock, A. A. (1998). Reflections on doing, being and becoming. *Canadian Journal of Occupational Therapy, 65,* 248–256.

Wilding, C., May, E., & Muir-Cochrane, E. (2005). Experience of spirituality, mental illness and occupation: A life-sustaining phenomenon. *Australian Occupational Therapy Journal, 52,* 2–9.

Xavier, S., Ferreira, J., Davis, J., & Polatajko, H. (6 June 2012). Beyond performance: Clarifying the construct of occupational engagement. In: *Paper presentation at the Canadian Association of Occupational Therapists Conference. Quebec City, QC.*

Zimmerman, D., Purdie, L., Davis, J. A., & Polatajko, H. J. (5 May 2006). A classification of occupational performance: Testing face validity. In: *Paper presented at the 3rd Canadian Society of Occupational Scientists Conference, Vancouver.*

PROFESSIONAL REASONING - EXCERPTS FROM BONUS PRACTICE STORIES

ⓔ [Read the full practice stories on Evolve at http://evolve.elsevier.com/Curtin/OT]

MRS TREMBLAY: A PRACTICE STORY OF A PERSON EXPERIENCING REHABILITATION FOLLOWING A STROKE - PROFESSIONAL REASONING

DOROTHY KESSLER, KATRINE SAUVÉ-SHENK, & VALERIE METCALFE

Part 1: Acute Care

Social/Practice Context. I am an occupational therapist working at a Canadian regional acute care hospital, located in a large urban centre. The hospital has over 1000 beds, and the neurosciences unit on which I work has 60 beds. The neurosciences unit admits a variety of people with neurological issues and the length of stay is on average seven days. All services are covered by the government health insurance plan …

ⓔ **To read the full Practice Story and complete a reflective exercise please visit Evolve at http://evolve.elsevier.com/ Curtin/OT**

KARIN: A PRACTICE STORY OF A PERSON EXPERIENCING RHEUMATOID ARTHRITIS - PROFESSIONAL REASONING

MATHILDA BJÖRK & INGRID THYBERG

Part 1: Initial Diagnosis

Social/Practice Context. In Sweden, when people have symptoms of joint pain, stiffness and fatigue they will visit their general practitioners. If their symptoms are indicative of a rheumatic inflammatory disease they will be referred to a physician who works at a hospital clinic that specialises in rheumatology. The most common rheumatic diagnoses that people have when presenting to a rheumatology clinics are rheumatoid arthritis (RA), ankylosing spondylitis and psoriatic arthritis …

ⓔ **To read the full Practice Story and complete a reflective exercise please visit Evolve at http://evolve.elsevier.com/ Curtin/OT**

ⓔ

ANGELA: A PRACTICE STORY OF A PERSON EXPERIENCING PALLIATIVE CARE - PROFESSIONAL REASONING

DEIDRE MORGAN & CELIA MARSTON

Social/Practice Context. The World Health Organisation (WHO) defines palliative care as an approach that addresses the physical, psychosocial and spiritual issues faced by person with a life limiting illness. Palliative care also extends to family and other caregivers over the course of the illness and also during bereavement …

ⓔ **To read the full Practice Story and complete a reflective exercise please visit Evolve at http://evolve.elsevier.com/ Curtin/OT**

Section 4

ASSESSMENT

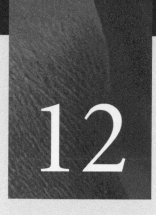

12 PROCESS OF ASSESSMENT

CLARE HOCKING ■ KAREN WHALLEY HAMMELL

Abstract

Occupational therapy assessments are undertaken to assemble information about people and the occupations in which they choose to engage. This process focuses on occupations (rather than impairments); on the abilities, skills, knowledge, roles and resources of the person, family, group or community; and on dimensions of people's environments, which may support or prohibit occupational opportunities. Congruent with an understanding of the social determinants of health, assessment identifies qualities of the broader context – social, political, policy, economic – that determine the opportunities available to disabled people collectively. Assessment provides the knowledge necessary to act appropriately to address people's occupational needs. This entails collecting, synthesising and interpreting information in collaboration with recipients of occupational therapy, screening to ensure the suitability of intervention, planning strategies for action, monitoring progress and evaluating outcomes. Professional and ethical considerations include consent processes, documentation and reporting, using evidence to select and evaluate culturally appropriate assessment tools and ongoing review of assessment strategies.

KEY POINTS

■ Assessment is a considered and collaborative process of collecting, synthesising and interpreting information that provides occupational therapists with the knowledge necessary to take appropriate actions to address people's occupational needs.

■ Parallel with the profession's evolving conceptual shifts, occupational therapy assessments have shifted focus, from measuring impairments and dysfunctions, to exploring the nature of occupational disruptions and to identifying abilities, skills and resources – of individuals and, whenever appropriate, of couples, families, groups and communities.

■ The occupational focus of assessment may pertain to orchestration (the organisation and balance of occupations within everyday life) or to analysis of people's performance of and engagement in specific occupations. These assessments address participation in the occupations that matter to those being assessed.

- Congruent with an understanding of the social determinants of health and with the profession's commitment to human rights, assessments explore the opportunities available to people to exercise their abilities and engage in the occupations they need, want or are required to do.

- The assessment process encompasses screening, assessing contextual and person-related factors, monitoring progress and evaluation of outcomes and continues throughout the occupational therapy process.

- Assessment responds to people rather than their 'conditions'. This implies that those assessments focused on understanding people's abilities, skills and resources should be appropriate to their age, gender roles and cultural background, a requirement that demands attention to cultural safety.

- Standardised assessments may be employed: where there is evidence of their validity with people of the same age group, demographic profile, cultural background and language as those whose abilities and priorities are to be assessed; in situations where the assessment will not be distressing or unreasonably arduous; and where these forms of assessment are able to explore people's abilities and opportunities to engage in those occupations they have reason to value. Other forms of assessment are available and in some situations are more appropriate.

- Occupational therapists are responsible for ensuring assessment processes are conducted professionally and ethically, with particular attention to transparency in obtaining informed consent.

INTRODUCTION

The social construction of a problem shapes our social and institutional responses to its resolution.

(Priestley, 2005)

The 'problem' addressed by this book is how to best respond to the occupational needs of people with physical impairments. The type of response depends on prevailing societal beliefs about the nature of disability and disfigurement and the risk of contagion. In different times and cultures, people with impairments have been constructed as merely unfortunate, attracting assistance and pity, godless creatures deserving the deepest loathing and fear (Wilcock & Hocking, 2015), or bearing the consequences of previous lives badly lived.

With the rise of Western medicine, impairments associated with medical conditions came to be viewed as amenable to preventive or rehabilitative efforts. Because of occupational therapists' early association with rehabilitation, the profession became embedded in institutional responses to disability and

continues to carry that legacy into our work within schools, institutions and workplaces, and, more recently, within agencies tackling homelessness, poverty, disaster relief and the ill effects of colonisation, displacement, torture, human trafficking and war.

This chapter addresses one aspect of assisting people to engage in occupation despite physical impairments: the process of assessing the problem and evaluating intervention outcomes. Like societal views of disability, occupational therapists' efforts to assess and resolve people's daily living problems have reflected profound shifts in thinking over the decades. It is important to understand those conceptual shifts because traces of earlier assumptions live on, continuing to shape practice despite espoused commitment to newer ways of thinking and working. In the following section, three distinct paradigms that have characterised occupational therapy's worldview are outlined, from the perspective of the assessment and evaluation process.

THE SHIFTING FOCUS OF ASSESSMENT

In the mechanistic era that gained favour in the 1950s and 1960s (Kielhofner, 2004), assessment efforts focused on identifying and precisely measuring the extent and impact of body impairments and dysfunctions. From the late 1980s, the renaissance of occupation (Whiteford, Townsend, & Hocking, 2000) that spawned occupational science and changed the face of occupational therapy practice brought discussions of 'top-down' assessment, in which occupational therapists were encouraged to initiate assessments by enquiring into the occupations people need, want or are required to do, delving into impairments only if necessary to clarify the nature of occupational disruption (Fisher, 2009). That radical shift, from the assessment and remediation of body impairments to directly observing and intervening with occupation, can be understood in its societal context; it parallels the World Health Organization's scrapping of the International Classification of Impairments, Disabilities and Handicaps (ICIDH) (World Health Organization, 1980) in favour of the International Classification of Functioning, Disability and Health (ICF) (World Health Organization, 2001). That was an important change. The ICIDH assumed that impairments were the root cause of disability and handicap, which implied that alleviating them would automatically reduce disability. In contrast, the ICF positions participation as the ultimate concern of all health practitioners and no longer privileges body impairments as the logical starting point for health assessments and interventions. Importantly, it also recognises the role of environments in creating impairments and in exacerbating disabilities.

Some of the legacy of occupational therapy's mechanistic era persists in the continued use of assessment tools that measure the status of various physical, cognitive and perceptual functions. Think, for instance, of using a goniometer to assess range of movement or the Occupational Therapy Adult Perceptual

Screening Test (OT-APST), which screens adults who have experienced a stroke or traumatic brain injury for agnosia, apraxia, acalculia and impairments in constructional and visuospatial skills (Cooke, McKenna, & Fleming, 2005). Assessing those components of body structure and function, which might or might not explain difficulty with occupation, with the intention of treating them would be out of step with occupational therapists' espoused commitment to occupation-focused practice.

Another example is the Barthel Index, which generates a score out of 100 to represent people's level of dependence in various tasks of daily living (Mahoney & Barthel, 1965). Calculating dependence levels does not reveal what people want to do or can do or the skills and strategies they employ as they try. Nor does it acknowledge that independence may be possible in some environments but not in others. Moreover, the scoring system reflects a specific value judgement that privileges physical independence in activities of daily living as though that were central to living. This erases people's priorities and denies the legitimacy of needing help, preferring to be helped or choosing to accept help to save time and energy for more meaningful or productive occupations. No wonder many people view independence as synonymous with quality of life and say they would rather die before they lose the ability to bath, dress and toilet themselves (Bush, 2009). Regrettably, through our assessment choices, the occupational therapy profession has colluded with the promotion of this destructive ideology.

The next paradigm shift has been signalled by the World Health Organization (WHO) and the United Nations (UN), along with economists, philosophers, scholars and human rights activists: from health as participation to health as a human right. For instance, the World Report on Disability (World Health Organization and World Bank, 2011) asserts that 'disability is increasingly understood as a human rights concern' (p. xxi). Indeed, there is increasing recognition that improvements in human health can only occur with improvements in human rights (Siegert & Ward, 2010). Aligning with occupational therapy assessments that focus on what people can and might be able to do, what's important to them, and the barriers in their immediate context, the Report on Disability directs attention to the 'everyday life activities' of disabled people (p. xxi). However, its concern is not what individuals need and want to do; rather it is on the fact that disabled people 'do not have equal access to health care, education, and employment opportunities [...] and experience exclusion from everyday life activities' (p. xxi). That concern directs attention to important issues that occupational therapists have not traditionally included in their assessments; it points to societal influences on the things people do. Among those influences are inequitable distribution of access and opportunity for occupation, which result in some people accruing benefits they were not due while others shoulder more than their share of the burden and risk (Wilcock & Hocking, 2015).

Importantly, the discussion of health as a human right extends well beyond health services. As one example among many, The Right to Health, a fact sheet jointly published by the United Nations High Commissioner for Human Rights and the WHO (2008), identifies relationships between health, poverty and discrimination. It urges governments to give priority to improving the health of vulnerable and marginalised groups through efforts that directly address the social determinants of health. Although disabled people are identified as just one group among many that experience disadvantage, discrimination and disempowerment, it is acknowledged that even in resource-rich countries they are among the most poor, excluded and disenfranchised populations (Stienstra, 2012).

A human rights discourse thus brings the social determinants of health into sharp focus. For instance, providing substance to claims that low educational attainment, limited employment options, substandard housing and discriminatory exclusion from valued occupations are determinants of poor health and disability, direct associations between childhood socioeconomic status and noncommunicable physical health disorders such as arthritis have been established (Baldassari, Cleveland, & Callahan, 2013; Bowen & González, 2010). Poverty, in itself, is both a cause and a consequence of impairment and disability (Canadian Medical Association (CMA), 2013). It is known to negatively affect children's neurological development and is a significant contributor to stress, substance abuse, anxiety, depression and other forms of mental illness (CMA, 2013). This implies that growing up in or living in relative deprivation is a significant risk factor for physical impairment, which is a human rights issue when societies could act to lift vulnerable groups out of poverty but fail to do so (Wilcock & Hocking, 2015). Clearly then, assessments undertaken to inform health interventions must identify vulnerable groups and appraise the social conditions that create vulnerabilities and reduce opportunities.

The occupational therapy profession is experiencing the same shift in consciousness. Internationally the World Federation of Occupational Therapists' position statement on human rights (WFOT, 2006) unequivocally asserts the profession's concern with occupational justice, declaring that the human right to occupation should be ensured by equitable access to participation, regardless of difference. In the British occupational therapy literature, for example, discussions of human rights have identified the inequities in communities' access to being and doing arising from sociopolitical, economic and environmental factors (Pollard & Sakellariou, 2007); have noted the risks to human rights inherent in systems that classify people according to their impairments (Hammell, 2004a); and have addressed the complex balance that must be negotiated between disabled people's right to participate in occupations in the community (citing shopping, horse riding, swimming) and the possible risk to carers' rights to safety (Mandelstam, 2003). Although the implications of these discussions are yet to be fully realised, it is clear that considering human rights will require occupational therapists to pay much greater attention to the broad societal factors that create inequities in participation and well-being. Given that 'our assessments establish the boundaries of our vision, within which we shall only find what we are looking for' (Hammell, 2015a), occupational therapy assessments of structural barriers to health and well-being must become the 'new normal', an accepted component of the assessment and evaluation process.

OPENING UP THE ASSESSMENT PROCESS

Occupational therapists have long recognised that, broadly speaking, practice proceeds through a series of stages, each influencing the next. The process gives order and predictability, keeping practice on track, and, once integrated, is experienced as the natural way of proceeding. At three points in the process, screening, assessment and evaluation, attention is given to gathering information to inform the next step. Simply put, assessment is designed to generate an accurate understanding of what is going on, what outcomes are sought, and appropriate ways of achieving those outcomes. But assessment is complex because there will be multiple perspectives on what is happening, important and acceptable. Occupational therapists' commitment to person-centred practice directs attention to the people with the occupational need as a critical source of that information, because they have experiential evidence of the quality, circumstances and outcomes of their occupations. They also make judgements about what would be better, have expectations about the way intervention decisions will be made and have opinions about which courses of action are acceptable and preferable. The profession's knowledge of evidence-based practice brings another strand, informing choices about the best means of gathering the information needed, what might be possible to achieve, and how effective different courses of action are likely to be.

A human rights perspective further opens up thinking about the assessment process. Hammell (2015a) reminded occupational therapists of the substantial evidence indicating that environmental barriers and social inequities, rather than physical impairments, account for much of the diminished quality of life experienced by disabled people. Acknowledging this fact implies that, contrary to established practice, assessments need to draw in information about the ways social, economic and political barriers impede people's ability to pursue occupations 'that give expression to their being' (Duncan & Creek, 2014, p. 464). The assessment results might signal the need for actions outside the sphere of people's day-to-day performance contexts, directing attention to structural factors such as social attitudes and policies that oppress and exclude them. Thus occupational therapists must acknowledge that people need more than skills, knowledge, the right genes and a measure of good luck to be healthy and to participate in their society; they need opportunities to gain and apply skills and knowledge. It is this combination of abilities and opportunities that Amartya Sen refers to as capabilities (Hammell, 2015b; Pereira, 2012; Whiteford & Pereira, 2012), recognising that a vicious cycle works against marginalised people such that lack of opportunity removes the possibility of acquiring skills, knowledge and experience. This leaves people ill equipped to exercise their abilities and capitalise on their opportunities.

Viewed from a capabilities perspective, disability is recognised to be the denial of choices and opportunities to be and to do. Like occupation, disability is understood to be the result of interactions of people's personal characteristics, such as their gender, age and impairments; the resources available to them (e.g. assets, income); and the social, economic, political and cultural environment (Mitra, 2006). Taking this perspective into the assessment process shifts attention from a singular focus on impairments, inabilities and problems, to abilities (skills, knowledge, experience), resources and strengths (e.g. supportive relationships, adequate finances). Thus informed, issues of health and occupational justice can be considered in light of the opportunities afforded or denied by the environment, irrespective of whether the occupational need sits with an individual, family, selected community members and the agencies that serve them or an entire community (Pizzi, Reitz, & Scaffa, 2010). Making this shift in the scope of assessments is important because occupational therapists treat what they measure. When they concentrate on assessing the minutiae of impairments and inabilities, they generate partial understandings, at best, and therefore apply partial, inadequate interventions. Additionally, by focusing so much attention on all that has been lost, the assessment process can be distressing and demoralising. To assess specific deficits in ability alongside strengths, skills, assets and opportunities provides a more nuanced, more hopeful and more complete picture. Moreover, following the lead of disability researchers such as Peter Evans (2002), the capability approach can be harnessed to assess the collective capabilities of marginalised groups and communities, such as self-help networks or the self-determination expertise of indigenous peoples. This way of thinking opens up possibilities for less individualistic and more culturally inclusive modes of assessment and intervention.

CRITICALLY INFORMED ASSESSMENT PROCESSES

As the discussion earlier reveals, commitment to human rights demands critical reflection on the assessment process, encompassing what information is needed, where to get it, and the appropriate focus for action. For example, knowledge of the association between socioeconomic status and arthritis alerts us to the value of attending to the social determinants of health (e.g. poverty, discrimination) as indicators of the differential health risk and prognosis of rich and poor people and majority and minority groups. In this way, the assessment process becomes somewhat less person-centred, because that information is about groups, not individuals, and is available as demographic rather than diagnostic data. Equally, however, the assessment of health determinants might not need to be repeated until new data or evidence are available. Moreover, the insights gained might usefully be shared across therapists. The results of such an assessment, in our view, must be weighed against data generated by assessing specific people's occupational needs, to determine which referrals to accept, how therapists' time is apportioned across different people, and the balance of interventions targeting change in the sociopolitical environment, the social and economic resources available to support participation, and people's skills, knowledge and impairments.

To illustrate those ideas, stimulating change in the sociopolitical environment might incorporate lobbying for legislative changes to enforce access to sports clubs for disabled people, to bring their activity levels up to those of other people and ensure equality of opportunity for community participation, as is their human right. Another example might be legislation to enforce reasonable workplace accommodations for people with enduring mental illness, on a par with environmental modifications for people with physical impairments. Although these examples are limited, in both being disability focused, their achievement would be supported by occupational therapists assessing and documenting discrepancies between health-promoting occupations people and communities want and are able to do versus what they can gain access to (their opportunities to do). A resource-focused intervention might be promoting the provision of comfortable seating in shopping malls to encourage older adults to socialise and be physically active in a relatively safe environment. Such initiatives would be supported by asking about and documenting the community-based exercise opportunities preferred by older adults, alongside evidence of managerial efforts to displace them in favour of a more fashion-conscious consumer demographic with more disposable income (Hart & Heatwole Shank, 2015).

The capabilities of disabled people to function might most usefully be understood by assessing their practical opportunities rather than their personal attributes. Consider the following account, reported by the Canadian Broadcasting Corporation (CBC, 2015). A nine-storey building in Vancouver's most economically deprived neighbourhood houses some of the city's most marginalised citizens. In the spring of 2015, the only elevator in the building broke down. More than a week later it had still not been repaired, leaving 'John', a man with a spinal cord injury, stranded on an upper floor. This had repercussions for his occupational opportunities: he was unable to shower because the only wheelchair-accessible shower was on the ground floor, he lost money because he couldn't get to his job and he was unable to get outside to enjoy the sunshine. John will have discovered that his options, and his abilities to accomplish self-care, to work and to participate in the life of his community, are of little use without opportunity. Clearly, his capabilities – options and opportunities – are constrained due to socially structured barriers to his full participation in society.

Adopting a mode of assessment that permits consideration of both abilities and opportunities will reveal appropriate targets for intervention. For example, an assessment of workers with diabetes, HIV infection, dyslexia or other invisible impairments, who experience excessively demanding work requirements and fear the consequences of revealing their condition, might expose a need to equip employers with strategies for creating inclusive and accessible workplaces. This is a human right, as described in the United Nations Convention on the Rights of Persons with Disabilities (2006), which asserts the right to equality of opportunity and to full and effective participation and inclusion in society and access to facilities and services on an equal basis with others. Regrettably, these rights to equality of opportunity are violated, even in resource-rich countries such as Canada, where it is reported that almost 90% of employers have no provisions in place for people with such challenges (Reeve & Gottselig, 2011). Although time spent accessing and assessing demographic data, documenting and reporting barriers to health-giving occupations, educating others and lobbying will inevitably take time from interventions targeting people's impairments and immediate context, the societal impact would be more far reaching. Further, therapists would be freed from the self-perpetuating cycle of solving the same problem over and over again with each person individually (Hocking, Townsend, Galheigo, Erlandsson, & de Mesquita Chagas, 2014).

A critical rethinking of assessment practices also brings into question the profession's commitment to seeking people's perspectives without paying attention to 'individual conceptions of well-being, and to their interplay with political, social and cultural settings, thus, ultimately, with conditions that may influence choice and reasoning' (Terzi, 2005, p. 206). As epidemiologists have long emphasised, the choices people make are dependent on the choices available to them. Indeed, structural barriers may constrain the choices of entire vulnerable communities, effectively limiting their life options and opportunities (Quesada, Hart, & Bourgois, 2011). These insights can also be found in the occupational science literature – for example, Laliberte Rudman's (2012) work with governmentality theory, exposing how older adults are shaped by contemporary social discourses of 'ageing well' to be active consumers; Galvaan's (2012) work with disadvantaged youths in South Africa whose occupational choices are constrained by the legacy of the apartheid era; and Beagan and Etowa's (2011) revelation that older Afro-Canadian women accept the daily racism they encounter as a test of their faith. These findings all point to ways that people's experience of wanting, needing and being expected to do certain things is influenced by political, social and cultural factors and are not solely expressions of personal volition. This fact further highlights the importance of assessing and addressing 'the socially structured and inequitable shaping of choice' (Frohlich & Abel, 2014, p. 210) that affects the health and well-being of individuals, families and entire communities and suggests that there are situations wherein it is more useful to reinforce the collective capabilities (opportunities) of a family or community than to target assessments and interventions at the capabilities of an individual disabled person (Dubois & Trani, 2009).

AN OCCUPATIONAL FOCUS

Having argued the need for assessment processes infused with an occupational justice perspective, we now turn to other occupational and professional issues, and considerations for the selection and design of assessment strategies. Primary among these is having an occupational focus, which means assessing people's and communities' level of participation in preferred and necessary occupations, the quality or ease of performing occupations that matter to them, plus the barriers encountered and their effect. An occupational focus makes both the relevance and intended outcome of occupational therapy evident (Hocking, 2001; Molineux, 2004), revealing problems such as not knowing how to do something (Polatajko, Mandich, & Martini, 1999), not wanting to do it (Fisher, 1992) or not having opportunities to engage in the occupations of concern. Two broad approaches to analysing occupation have been proposed: analysing how occupations are orchestrated, or brought together into a pattern or lifestyle, and occupational analysis, which drills down to people's actual engagement in occupation (Crepeau, Boy Schell, Gillen, & Scaffa, 2014). These approaches carry through to the assessment process and, depending on the issues identified, assessments might focus on one or both of these. When orchestration of occupations is the concern, attention is given to how people manage multiple occupations, which might include coordinating occupations with others, managing competing role demands and time use. Systemic barriers to occupation, such as the absence of fresh food outlets in lower socioeconomic neighbourhoods (American Nutrition Association, 2010), discriminatory practices of employers and sporting organisations or appointments with health services that impinge on the working day (Jakobsen, 2004) might become apparent as impediments to orchestration.

Occupational analysis examines the way people actually carry out an occupation. Consistent with the idea that engagement in occupation is a transactional process, people's performance is viewed as an interaction with the demands of the occupation in which they are engaged, the performance environment and the sociopolitical and cultural context (Cutchin & Dickie, 2012). The focus is on how experienced people are and how skilfully they perform, as demonstrated by how the occupation proceeds and the barriers to effective performance that become apparent. Two commonly cited categorisations of performance skills are motor and process skills and social interaction skills, which direct attention to actions such as manipulating objects, coordinating the movement of different body parts, restoring tools to their usual position, noticing and responding to things in the environment, turning towards people during interaction and expressing emotion in socially acceptable ways (Fisher & Griswold, 2014). Assessment of occupational performance can be highly personalised, revealing much about people as occupational beings (Crepeau et al., 2014). We emphasise, however, that being personalised does not necessarily equate to honing in on an individual. That individualistic view of occupation is challenged by

researchers who explored the occupations of an older couple after one of them sustained a stroke. They found that the timing, balance, choice and orchestration of the couple's occupations had become a co-occupational endeavour, demonstrating the possible interdependency of everyday occupations (Van Nes, Runge, & Jonsson, 2009). This reinforces the legitimacy and importance of assessments that seek input from all those engaged in cooperative or communal occupations.

It is now taken as given that body impairments do not preclude skilful occupational performance (Fisher & Griswold, 2014), and evidence to support focusing on performance skills rather than deficits in motor, cognitive or perceptual skills and emotional regulation is found in research. For instance, a comparison of almost 4000 people with either left or right hemispheric strokes, and thus different patterns of impairments, exhibited no significant differences in the 36 motor and process skills that were evaluated (Bartels, Duffy, & Beland, 2011). If impairments are hampering performance, that should become evident through observational assessments (Payne & Howell, 2005). Direct assessment of impairments might sometimes be necessary to inform the diagnosis (Missiuna, Gaines, & Soucie, 2006), clarify which intervention approach to use, such as remedial or compensatory, or ascertain people's capacity to take up new skills (Copley & Ziviani, 2005). Nonetheless, the goals negotiated to direct intervention should address enhanced participation in occupations that matter to people (e.g. quality, quantity or ease of performance) or inclusion (e.g. removal of societal barriers). To support such outcomes, rather than evaluating the performance of people with impairments, assessments might more profitably focus on the ways community members or work colleagues could support others' participation. Research to identify the skills people use to include others in shared occupations holds promise in this regard but is yet to be tested among adults (Jones & Hocking, in press).

ENACTING ASSESSMENT PROCESSES

Although there is general agreement about what the assessment process includes, terminology such as needs analysis, capacity assessment and environmental scanning are more typical when working with institutional clients or in public health settings, where the process might include establishing a formal contract. What actually happens also varies because assessments occur within specific societal and practice contexts that frame the organisational policies and procedures and the attitudes, values, beliefs and actions of both therapists and the people with whom they work (Craik, Davis, & Polatajko, 2013). To fulfil occupational therapy's commitment to occupational rights (WFOT, 2006), responsiveness to the social determinants of health must become a primary concern, as discussed earlier. Culturally safe practice, which requires health professionals to ensure they are safe to practice with people of other cultures, is also imperative. That includes respecting and actively responding to diverse occupations, languages and health beliefs, working inclusively, and confronting institutional and personal racism (WFOT, 2009).

The assessment process is usually depicted as beginning with an initial screening, to decide whether input from an occupational therapist is indicated and beneficial outcomes likely. This is followed by more detailed assessment to inform decisions about what to do, and then evaluation of the outcomes to determine whether the intentions were achieved. On the basis of that evaluation, the process is concluded or further goals or the need to refer to other services are identified. In community development contexts, which might involve engagement with diverse individuals and issues, the initial steps in the process are more elaborated. For example, the Ontario Healthy Communities Coalition (n.d.) specifies the following stepwise process: learning about the community; listening to community members; bringing people together to develop a shared vision; assessing community assets, resources, needs and issues; helping community members to recognise and articulate areas of concern and what causes them; and reaching agreement on the 'vehicle for change'.

Although assessment is described as occurring at specific points in the occupational therapy process, it is in effect an ongoing process to monitor the implementation of planned actions and appraise progress towards anticipated outcomes. Judgements about what information to gather and how, who will do that, and when there is sufficient information to agree on a course of action are also ongoing (Table 12.1). Recognising that assessment continues throughout occupational therapy interventions suggests that this is a dynamic process, with therapists exploring aspects of participation in occupation 'as they become relevant and meaningful during the course of the assessment' (Wilby, 2005, p. 41). One lamentable failure of ongoing review of assessment results concerns a woman who told her therapists that she wanted to walk after sustaining a stroke but later worried whether 'my arm got neglected' (Brown et al., 2014, p. 1023). If assessment had been dynamic and ongoing throughout the rehabilitation process, the importance of engaging in everyday occupations requiring use of her arm might have been identified. A final point is that, in addition to informing intervention, assessments may also be undertaken to determine eligibility for services on the basis of symptom severity (Corr & Siddons, 2005) or to monitor change in occupational status.

Screening

The purpose of screening is to gain a sense of people's aspirations, current occupational status, context, issues and potential and to look for indicators that occupational therapy intervention is likely to prove beneficial (Mozley et al., 2007). Contrary to much existing practice, we assert the necessity of taking a capabilities approach to screening that attends to people in context (Fig. 12.1). A strengths-based approach that acknowledges people as experts in their own occupations (Craik et al., 2013) and circumstances is also essential (and congruent with occupational therapy's espoused person-centred philosophy). Careful screening avoids wasting the time and resources of both service

TABLE 12.1	
Questions Addressed By Assessment Findings at Each Step of the Occupational Therapy Process	
Step in the Occupational Therapy Process	**Questions Assessment Findings Address**
Screening	Does occupational therapy have anything to offer?
	Is what occupational therapy has to offer welcome?
	Is intervention likely to be beneficial? (evidence)
Assessing	What is the occupational issue?
	What is the context? (social determinants, cultural and physical context)
	What is their perspective? How might that perspective be shaped/restricted by the context?
	What might help?
	What abilities, resources and opportunities do people have? Are there additional collective capabilities?
	What is the nature of the problem? (if this needs to be clarified to determine how to intervene)
Identifying needs	What occupational needs are apparent?
	Do they warrant intervention?
	Is this the best service to address those needs?
	Is referral to another service warranted?
Negotiating goals	What does the community/group/family/person want?
	What do others want?
	What has priority?
	Should the focus for change be the people, the physical or social environment, at an institutional or policy level (or a combination of these)?
	Can the goals be legally and ethically supported?
Planning and implementing intervention	Are things progressing as expected?
	Are observations consistent with previous understandings?
	If not, why not?
Evaluating outcomes	What was achieved?
	Was that enough?
Renegotiating goals or discharge	Are further needs apparent?
	If so, can occupational therapy address them?

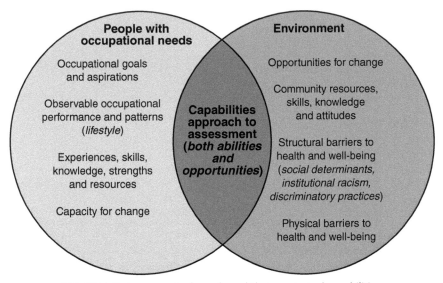

People with occupational needs

Occupational goals and aspirations

Observable occupational performance and patterns (*lifestyle*)

Experiences, skills, knowledge, strengths and resources

Capacity for change

Capabilities approach to assessment (*both abilities and opportunities*)

Environment

Opportunities for change

Community resources, skills, knowledge and attitudes

Structural barriers to health and well-being (*social determinants, institutional racism, discriminatory practices*)

Physical barriers to health and well-being

FIG. 12.1 ▪ Assessment of people and their contextual capabilities.

recipients and providers. It is the first step in negotiating the parameters for further assessment and the broad goals of intervention (Copley & Ziviani, 2005), and as such it provides a sense of what occupational therapy can realistically offer. Put another way, this is the consultation and contracting phase of the occupational therapy process, where therapists and people referred to them identify whether occupational therapy has anything to offer and thus whether to continue. It is also an opportunity to start to get to know people and establish a professional alliance.

In medical or rehabilitation contexts, screening is often about prioritising therapists' caseload and, as discussed earlier, that judgement should include consideration of occupational justice issues in relation to disadvantaged groups. In determining how to proceed with individuals, occupational therapists consider a range of factors including their health status, cognitive and communication abilities, the practicalities of observing them participating in the occupations of concern and the availability of suitable standardised screening tools.

Assessing

Having determined that occupational therapy is indicated, a more extensive process of inquiry begins. Assessment of the context to identify possibilities for and barriers to occupation may involve exploration and interpretation of the determinants of health, collection of demographic data and becoming familiar with the human and nonhuman environment. Environmental scanning includes identifying services that are already in place, both because replicating existing services is inefficient and, in the case of community development initiatives, because diverting resources or income away from existing services can inadvertently jeopardise the livelihood of the local people (Thibeault, 2013).

Considerations in relation to the intended recipients of occupational therapy include the nature of the assessment itself – what it would be like to 'be assessed' (Hocking, 2001). Is it a supportive experience of cooperative discovery and problem solving or a 'scientific' exercise where the assessor strives to achieve a detached and objective stance? Does it involve self-chosen, familiar occupations in a familiar context or simulated activities and unfamiliar tasks in an unfamiliar context? Are the assessment activities and the way they are administered consistent with people's background, status and worldviews or foreign and irrelevant? To address cultural safety, assessment tasks and materials should reflect people's culture by incorporating their language and familiar occupations, concepts and images, because failure to do so risks subtly (or blatantly) conveying disrespect and undermining their performance. This requirement largely eliminates the use of standardised assessments developed on a different population or in a different time and place. Consistent with cultural practices, thought must also be given to welcoming support people, or indeed including them as active participants where they have a socially sanctioned role in providing assistance with whatever is being assessed, or in speaking for or making decisions on behalf of family members. Again, administering assessments in a group or family context challenges the use of standardised assessments, most of which are designed to be administered one-on-one in a controlled environment. Implicit assumptions that discussion of the results will immediately lead into decisions about intervention, without time, for example, for recipients of occupational therapy to reflect, consult and pray, are also challenged.

More technical considerations include whether the same assessment can be used as a reassessment once intervention is completed and where this assessment should be conducted. There is some evidence, for example, indicating that people with cognitive deficits perform better in their own home (Bottari et al., 2006). The picture gained of the people being assessed, the context and occupational concern sets the stage for relevant goals addressing valued occupational outcomes. In turn, occupation-focused goals support the development of intervention strategies that are perceived to address the issue and to be achievable and tolerable. As the intervention proceeds, initial assumptions and findings may come into question and further assessment following new lines of inquiry may be necessary.

Evaluating

To evaluate something means to appraise it, and often, to find out how much of it there is. In this context, 'it' refers to the outcomes of intervention and the extent to which they were achieved. People value this information because it provides feedback on what has been accomplished, helping them both to realise how far they have progressed and feel satisfied with their efforts. This motivational boost can help people sustain the changes they have made. Evaluation results also assist therapists and others to determine whether intervention is complete, and if not, whether new goals or different ways of intervening need to be explored.

There are a number of additional reasons for ascertaining what was accomplished. The recording of evaluation results completes the written record, showing the progression from presenting issues to outcomes. Occupational therapists also report evaluation results to others: such as referral sources and health insurer, services that people are referred on to, a community that will decide whether occupational therapy input helps move things forward and so on. Whatever the audience, therapists must carefully consider how to present evaluation findings. In some cases, specific observations of improved performance skills and more favourable outcomes or reporting the removal of risk factors and barriers will suffice. Equally, therapists may seek subjective accounts of the outcomes or report objective measures of change that can be compared with research reporting outcomes using similar intervention strategies with the same population.

ASSESSMENT STRATEGIES

Occupational therapists have a range of assessment strategies available to them. Information about the social determinants of health or systemic barriers to occupation may be gleaned from health statistics, demographic data and reports. More nuanced information about the presence and impact of human rights issues will be available through engagement with indigenous peoples, minority groups, disability rights activists and cultural advisors. Strategies employed to gather information directly from people include observation, evaluation, dialogue – more formally referred to as interviews – and self-rating

(Corr & Siddons, 2005). Assessments can be standardised or nonstandardised. This section of the discussion addresses the relative strengths and weaknesses of each.

Selecting and Using Standardised Assessments

Standardised assessments generally require people to respond to set questions, be interviewed about set topics, rate their experiences on a set scale, or engage in a set task, sometimes within a set time frame. Assessors are required to administer the assessment and record and score the findings in a prescribed way. The objects used and how they are arranged may be specified. There may or may not be normative data, which enable people's results to be compared with the population representative of the context in which the assessment was developed.

There are many reasons to opt for standardised assessments. They provide consistency across therapists and practice settings and generate a baseline against which people's performance can be later compared (Fisher & Griswold, 2014). Many also have a conceptual framework that guides interpretation of findings and some identify cut-off scores – that is, scores that indicate a possible problem or a severe problem warranting intervention. The developers of standardised assessments attend to their validity, meaning that the assessment does assess what it was intended to assess, and face validity, which means that the assessment tasks or items are perceived as relevant to whatever is being assessed. Test developers also attend to reliability, ensuring that the result would be much the same if the assessment was administered at another time (test-retest reliability) or by another person (interrater reliability), unless an actual change has occurred. In turn, therapists are responsible for preserving the integrity of standardised assessments and carefully documenting minor deviations from the administration protocol and their possible impact on validity and reliability.

The relative strength of an assessment's psychometric properties is an important consideration in adopting it into practice. Therapists looking for assistance in identifying or choosing between standardised assessments might usefully consider published reviews or, if none are available, evidence-based approaches to critically evaluating assessment tools are available to guide therapists through a rigorous process of evaluation. Another important consideration is whether assessments were developed or adapted for use with people of the same age, demographic profile, cultural background, and language as those to be assessed. For example, standardised life satisfaction scales developed for elderly people (who are predominantly female) have been used to assess the perspectives of people with recent spinal cord injuries, who are primarily young and predominantly male (Hammell, 2004b). If questions appropriate to the people concerned are not asked, it is unlikely that meaningful results will be attained. In some cases there are published reports that substantiate the use of the chosen assessment with a relevant population. In other cases, therapists must make a judgement based on the developer's claims and information about participants in the studies undertaken to develop the assessment or generate validity, reliability or normative data. If the available standardised assessments do not capture information concerning engagement in occupations that are valued, or how occupational engagement enables the enactment of meaningful roles, they are inadequate to inform or appraise occupation-based practices.

The renewed focus on occupation has stimulated both the development of occupationally focused standardised assessments (Diamantis, 2006) and evaluation of the extent to which previously developed assessments align with the ICF. Where no existing tools adequately address the participation outcomes of concern, therapists might justifiably conduct a nonstandardised assessment. Of the standardised occupation-focused assessments available, those that encompass 'occupations related to all aspects of daily life' (Lexell, Iwarsson, & Lexell, 2006, p. 241), such as the Canadian Occupational Performance Measure, are more suited to an approach to practice that acknowledges the complexities of occupation than assessments that evaluate a predetermined selection of skills and occupations. As mentioned previously, cultural safety must also be considered. That often means making judgements about people's language capability and the relevance of assessment items that assume normative life experiences such as 'fingerpainting, walking barefoot or standing in line' (Brown & Brown, 2006, p. 242). Such judgements are important because, as critical race theorists contend, standardised assessments are premised on the assumption that specific skills – valued by the designers of the assessment – are universal, rather than culturally specific. Using them with people from other cultural contexts risks conveying a misleadingly negative portrayal of the abilities of members of minority groups, who may have cultivated a different skill set. Ensuring the cultural safety of all recipients of occupational therapy is one consideration in resisting the blanket adoption of particular assessments, even at the cost of generating a standard data set across the population served.

Safety concerns, for both the therapist and the person being assessed, may constitute a further reason to opt for a standardised rather than unstandardised assessments, such as choosing a virtual driving assessment over an on-road test (Lee, 2006). Local practice is also influential. Surveys in the United States of America and Canada (Korner-Bitensky et al., 2006) and Sweden (Larsson et al., 2006), for example, revealed wide variations between countries in the assessment tools therapists prefer. An additional pragmatic consideration is whether therapeutic application of an assessment has been reported or whether its use is confined to research. Having incorporated a standardised assessment into practice, therapists must remain open to reviewing that decision as new assessments become available and occupational therapy theory and broader assessment practices change.

Selecting and Using Nonstandardised Assessments

Nonstandardised assessments include locally developed checklists, report formats, 'standard' interview questions, self-care and kitchen tasks that therapists use repeatedly and hand on to each other, as well as one-off interviews and observations. Whatever the format, therapists opt for nonstandardised assessments because they fit the situation or the population or because no standardised assessment suits the purpose. Their advantages include enormous flexibility, both in being able to be modified to the particular person or context and in being able to intermingle assessment with problem solving and trialling of solutions. Dynamic performance analysis, initially developed by Polatajko et al. (1999) and further developed in this text, is a prime example of this.

Reasons cited for using nonstandardised assessments include the sometimes prohibitive cost of acquiring standardised assessments, lack of knowledge about how to administer them, lack of time to evaluate which are most suitable (Blenkiron, 2005) and managers who do not actively support changes in practice (Chard, 2006). Opting for nonstandardised assessments also seems to be driven by therapists' discomfort with administration protocols that require them to suspend efforts to engage with and encourage people, to wait and watch while they struggle with tasks and fail, and to resist intuitions about ways to modify tasks, instructions or questions to elicit a more adaptive response (Managh & Cook, 1993). From an occupational perspective, nonstandardised assessments might be more likely to use actual occupational performance as a point of comparison – typically, what the person concerned could previously do.

Using nonstandardised methods to gather information means that the findings are entirely dependent on the therapist's expertise (Wilby, 2005), and the repeatability of the assessment depends on detailed documentation of the assessment process. Their limitations include the frequent lack of rationale for what is included and what is left out and the reliance on therapists to update assessment practices to keep pace with emerging professional concerns and new evidence, including the things disabled people and carers are concerned about (Welch & Lowes, 2005). Compared with standardised assessments, locally developed assessment processes do not generate strong evidence of therapy outcomes and the overall efficacy of services provided, and it is difficult to relate the results of efficacy studies to local practice because the similarities and differences are unknown (Bowman, 2006). To be fair, however, standardised assessments do not always provide a clear rationale for their content and, equally, may not be revised in a timely fashion to reflect shifts in the profession's philosophy or available evidence.

Although it is important for occupational therapists to be able to demonstrate both the effectiveness of their interventions and accountability to employing institutions, it is equally important to consider whether standardised assessments are being used primarily – or solely – to benefit the profession (through ensuring 'market share') while usurping the time and efforts of people receiving occupational therapy. If standardised assessments do not enable the assessment of outcomes that are valued by them and are not undertaken to further their interests, those assessments do not fit within a mode of practice that aspires to be named person-centred. Such measurements as range of motion or functional independence are inadequate surrogates for what occupational therapists surely ought to assess: the effect of occupational therapy interventions on people's abilities and opportunities to engage in occupations they have reason to value. From a human rights perspective, it has been suggested that outcome measures used to gauge the effectiveness of occupational therapy services should assess the degree to which disabled people are able to transcend a marginalised status and assume the occupational rights and opportunities accorded other citizens (Hammell, 2006). This might be accomplished through assessments of capabilities (abilities and opportunities) and of community participation. This will require new forms of assessment.

PROFESSIONAL AND ETHICAL COMMITMENTS

Skills in conducting assessments, synthesising information from multiple sources and engaging in professional reasoning are vital to the assessment process (Wilby, 2005), affecting the accuracy of information gained and the meanings and interpretations that therapists and therapy recipients derive from and attribute to this information. Occupational therapy's commitment to person-centredness demands skilfully working in partnership with people, tailoring the assessment process to their needs. It also means recognising that people may have extensive or lifelong experience of the issue and its context, such as people who have lived with an impairment for many years, or at the other extreme, very limited knowledge of it, such as a group facing a situation they have not previously encountered or a person with a newly acquired impairment. Therapists must vary their approach accordingly, acknowledging some people as experts and guiding others in their role as 'coinvestigators' of issues that they may be only vaguely aware of. Additionally, regardless of how careful or comprehensive the assessment process has been, therapists must not conflate having sufficient information to make an informed judgement with understanding people's life experience (Duncan & Creek, 2014).

The relationships established with people affect whether they feel inclined to share information, concerns and aspirations. Occupational therapists rely on people divulging sensitive information, such as feeling that carers sometimes help too much, explaining that the person available to assist is a same sex partner or disclosing abuses of power within a community or institution. The sensitivity therapists employ in gathering information will, in turn, influence people's preparedness to coach the therapist through cultural practices. This may include how occupations are carried out, decisions made and agreement or disagreement conveyed and how the therapist ought to behave as a visitor, convey respect for high-status individuals, negotiate gender boundaries and so on.

Therapists' professional responsibilities include ensuring that 'every client [has] a clearly recorded assessment of need' (College of Occupational Therapists, 2005, p. 529) and that assessment methods and findings are reported in full (College of Occupational Therapists, 2005; Gibson, Sykes, & Young, 2004). That includes representing the views of therapy recipients (Gibson et al., 2004) and providing an interpretation of results, so that others can understand what they mean (Corr & Siddons, 2005). Careful consideration must also be given to who has a right to know the assessment results and the recommendations arising from them and how best to convey that information (Welch & Lowes, 2005).

The assessment process incorporates multiple ethical demands. Primary among those is the issue of informed consent, which means recognising that people have a legitimate choice about engaging in assessment, having been given sufficient information about its purpose, what it will involve and how the information generated is likely to be used. Despite its importance, little attention has been given to the complexities of eliciting consent from people whose capacity to give consent is compromised or who might be disadvantaged by the outcome. One small-scale study in New Zealand revealed that therapists in both mental and physical health services used various strategies to entice people with cognitive impairments into cooperating with assessments, including being friendly, providing rewards (such as cooking tasks), eliciting their help with providing information 'the doctors' want, skimping on information about what the assessment would involve or how the results would be used, selecting informal occupational-based assessments over formal assessments and modifying standardised assessments if they anticipated that people would resist completing some assessment tasks. That is, they prioritised fulfilling their role by gathering information to inform rehabilitation decisions and preserving harmonious relationships with the person to be assessed over their right to give or withhold consent (White, Hocking, & Reid, 2014). Aside from the other issues, modifying a standardised assessment nullifies its psychometric properties, rendering the results useless. Moreover, exerting professional dominance through such strategies as persuasion and coercion (Moats, 2007) is incompatible with person-centred practices.

Ethical considerations also include the responsibility to 'obtain relevant information to enable [people] to determine the appropriateness of the referral' (College of Occupational Therapists, 2005, p. 529) and only gather relevant information that will be used to inform occupational therapy interventions. In relation to using standardised assessments, therapists must recognise the limitations of their knowledge and expertise (College of Occupational Therapists, 2005), including their proficiency in administering an assessment, which affects its reliability, and whether they administer it in the same way as other therapists, which is the basis of interrater reliability. A final consideration is not overstating the significance or trustworthiness of findings, given that they potentially inform life-changing decisions such as discharge destination or the focus for community development.

CONCLUSION

Occupational therapy assessments are conducted in a professional context that increasingly demands responsiveness to human rights and occupational justice, occupation and evidence-focused practice, person-centredness and cultural safety. Their purpose is to generate information about what occupations mean to people, the functions those occupations serve in their lives, what is happening when participation is disrupted or dysfunctional and the impact of opportunities on the ability to participate in occupation – opportunities that are not equally distributed across a society. Assessment processes are complex. They span the most intimate to the most public occupations, the mundane requirements of everyday living to spiritual expression, and every occupational setting people might create or enter, alone or in cooperation with others. Running through this diversity is a consistent demand for high levels of ethical and professional behaviour, which requires constant updating of therapists' knowledge and skill in evaluating and administering relevant standardised assessment tools and devising trustworthy nonstandardised assessment processes. The imperative for the best possible assessment practices lies in the consequences for people and communities with an occupational concern as well as the societal messages occupational therapists reinforce about human rights, the value of occupation and the meaning of living if occupational performance is compromised.

 http://evolve.elsevier.com/Curtin/OT

REFERENCES

American Nutrition Association. (2010). USDA defines food deserts. *Nutrition Digest, 37*(2) Retrieved from http://americannutrition association.org/.

Baldassari, A. R., Cleveland, R. J., & Callahan , L. F. (2013). Independent influences of current and childhood socioeconomic status on health outcomes in a North Carolina family-practice sample of arthritis patients. *Arthritis Care Research, 65*(8), 1334–1342.

Bartels, M. N., Duffy, C. A., & Beland, H. E. (2011). Pathophysiology, medical management, and acute rehabilitation of stroke survivors. In G. Gillen (Ed.), *Stroke rehabilitation: A function-based approach* (3rd ed., pp. 1–48). St Louis: Mosby Elsevier.

Beagan, B. L., & Etowa, J. B. (2011). The meanings and functions of occupations related to spirituality for African Nova Scotian women. *Journal of Occupational Science, 18*(3), 277–290.

Blenkiron, E. L. (2005). Uptake for standardised hand assessments in rheumatology: Why is it so low? *British Journal of Occupational Therapy, 68*(4), 148–157.

Bottari, C., Dutil, É., Dassa, C., et al. (2006). Choosing the most appropriate environment to evaluate independence in everyday activities: Home or clinic? *Australian Occupational Therapy Journal, 53,* 98–106.

Bowen, M. E., & González, H. M. (2010). Childhood socioeconomic position and disability later in life: Results of the health and retirement study. *American Journal of Public Health, 100*(S1), S197–S203.

Bowman, J. (2006). Challenges to measuring outcomes in occupational therapy: A qualitative focus group study. *British Journal of Occupational Therapy, 69*(10), 464–472.

Brown, G. T., & Brown, A. (2006). A review and critique of the touch inventory for elementary school-aged children (TIE). *British Journal of Occupational Therapy, 69*(5), 234–243.

Brown, M., Levack, W., McPherson, K. M., et al. (2014). Survival, momentum, and things that make me 'me': Patients' perceptions of goal setting after stroke. *Disability and Rehabilitation, 36*(12), 1020–1026.

Bush, S. S. (Ed.). (2009). Questionnaire of surrogate values. In *Geriatric mental health ethics: A casebook.* New York: Springer.

Canadian Broadcasting Corporation, (2015). *Disabled Portland Hotel residents left stranded without elevator.* Retrieved from http://www.cbc.ca/news/canada/british-columbia/disabled-portland-hotel-residents-left-stranded.

Canadian Medical Association. (2013). *Health care in Canada. What makes us sick?* Ottawa: CMA. Retrieved from *https://www.cma.ca/ Assets/assets-library/.../What-makes-us-sick_en.pdf.*

Chard, G. (2006). Adopting the assessment of motor and process skills into practice: Therapists voices. *British Journal of Occupational Therapy, 69*(2), 50–57.

College of Occupational Therapists. (2005). College of Occupational Therapists: Code of ethics and professional conduct. *British Journal of Occupational Therapy, 68*(11), 527–532.

Cooke, D. M., McKenna, K., & Fleming, J. (2005). Development of a standardised occupational therapy screening tool for visual perception in adults. *Scandinavian Journal of Occupational Therapy, 12,* 59–71.

Copley, J., & Ziviani, J. (2005). Assistive technology assessment and planning for children with multiple disabilities in educational settings. *British Journal of Occupational Therapy, 68*(12), 559–566.

Corr, S., & Siddons, L. (2005). An introduction to the selection of outcome measures. *British Journal of Occupational Therapy, 68* (5), 202–206.

Craik, J., Davis, J., & Polatajko, H. J. (2013). Introducing the Canadian Practice Process Framework (CPPF): Amplifying the context. In E. A. Townsend, & H. J. Polatajko (Eds.), *Enabling occupation II: Advancing an occupational therapy vision for health, well-being, & justice through occupation* (2nd ed., pp. 229–246). Ottawa: CAOT Publications ACE.

Crepeau, E. B., Boyt Schell, B. A., Gillen, G., & Scaffa, M. E. (2014). Analyzing occupations and activity. In B. A. Boyt Schell, G. Gillen, & M. E. Scaffa (Eds.), *Willard and Spackman's occupational therapy* (12th ed., pp. 234–248). Philadelphia: Wolters Kluwer Lippincott Williams & Wilkins.

Cutchin, M. P., & Dickie, V. A. (Eds.). (2012). *Transactional perspectives on occupation.* New York: Springer.

Diamantis, A. D. (2006). Use of standardised tests in paediatrics: The practice of private occupational therapists working in the United Kingdom. *British Journal of Occupational Therapy, 69*(6), 281–287.

Dubois, J.-L., & Trani, J.-F. (2009). Extending the capability paradigm to address the complexity of disability. *ALTER: European Journal of Disability Research, 3,* 192–218.

Duncan, E. M., & Creek, J. (2014). Working on the margins: Occupational therapy and social inclusion. In W. Bryant, J. Fieldhouse, & K. Bannigan (Eds.), *Creek's occupational therapy and mental health* (5th ed., pp. 457–473). London: Churchill Livingstone.

Evans, P. (2002). Collective capabilities, culture, and Amartya Sen's development as freedom. *Studies in Comparative International Development, 37*(2), 54–60.

Fisher, A. (1992). Functional measures, Part 2: Selecting the right test, minimizing the limitations. *American Journal of Occupational Therapy, 46,* 278–281.

Fisher, A. G. (2009). *Occupational therapy intervention process model: A model for planning and implementing top-down, client-centred, and occupation-based interventions.* Fort Collins, CO: Three Star Press.

Fisher, A. G., & Griswold, L. A. (2014). Performance skills. In B. A. Boyt Schell, G. Gillen, & M. E. Scaffa (Eds.), *Willard and Spackman's occupational therapy* (12th ed., pp. 249–264). Philadelphia: Wolters Kluwer Lippincott Williams & Wilkins.

Frohlich, K. L., & Abel, T. (2014). Environmental justice and health practices: Understanding how health inequities arise at the local level. *Sociology of Health and Illness, 36,* 199–212.

Galvaan, R. (2012). Occupational choice: The significance of socio-economic and political factors. In G. E. Whiteford, & C. Hocking (Eds.), *Occupational science: Society, inclusion and participation* (pp. 152–162). Oxford: Wiley-Blackwell.

Gibson, F., Sykes, M., & Young, S. (2004). Record keeping in occupational therapy: Are we meeting the standards set by the College of Occupational Therapists? *British Journal of Occupational Therapy, 67*(12), 547–550.

Hammell, K. W. (2004a). Deviating from the norm: A sceptical interrogation of the classificatory practices of the ICF. *British Journal of Occupational Therapy, 67*(9), 408–411.

Hammell, K. W. (2004b). Exploring quality of life following high spinal cord injury: A review and critique. *Spinal Cord, 42*(9), 491–502.

Hammell, K. W. (2006). *Perspectives on disability and rehabilitation: Contesting assumptions; Challenging practice.* Edinburgh: Churchill Livingstone Elsevier.

Hammell, K. W. (2015a). Occupational rights and critical occupational therapy: Rising to the challenge. Early Online: *Australian Occupational Therapy Journal.*

Hammell, K. W. (2015b). Quality of life, participation and occupational rights: A capabilities perspective. *Australian Occupational Therapy Journal, 62*(2), 78–85.

Hart, E. C., & Heatwole Shank, K. (2015). Participating at the mall: Possibilities and tensions that shape older adults' occupations. *Journal of Occupational Science, 22*(3), 1–15.

Hocking, C. (2001). The issue is: Implementing occupation based assessment. *American Journal of Occupational Therapy, 55*(4), 463–469.

Hocking, C., Townsend, E., Galheigo, S. M., Erlandsson, L.-K., & de Mesquita Chagas, J. N. (2014). Driving societal change: Occupational therapy, health and human rights. In *16th international congress of the World Federation of Occupational Therapists: Sharing traditions, creating futures.* Yokohama, Japan.

Jakobsen, K. (2004). If work doesn't work: How to enable occupational justice. *Journal of Occupational Science, 11*(3), 125–134.

Jones, M., & Hocking, C. (in press). Crossing the practice border: Participation skills for communities. In N. Pollard & D. Sakellariou (Eds.), *Occupational therapies without borders: Integrating justice with practice* (2nd ed.). St. Louis, MO: Elsevier.

Kielhofner, G. (2004). *Conceptual foundations of occupational therapy* (3rd ed.). Philadelphia: FA Davis.

Korner-Bitensky, N., Bitensky, J., Sofer, M., et al. (2006). Driving evaluation practices of clinicians working in the United States and Canada. *American Journal of Occupational Therapy, 60*(4), 428–434.

Laliberte Rudman, D. (2012). Governing through occupation: Shaping expectations and possibilities. In G. E. Whiteford, & C. Hocking (Eds.), *Occupational science: Society, inclusion and participation* (pp. 100–116). Oxford: Wiley-Blackwell.

Larsson, H., Lundberg, C., Falkmer, T., et al. (2006). A Swedish survey of occupational therapists' involvement and performance in driving assessments. *Scandinavian Journal of Occupational Therapy, 14*(4), 215–220.

Lee, H. C. (2006). Virtual driving tests for older adult drivers? *British Journal of Occupational Therapy, 69*(3), 138–141.

Lexell, E. M., Iwarsson, S., & Lexell, J. (2006). The complexity of daily occupations in multiple sclerosis. *Scandinavian Journal of Occupational Therapy, 13,* 241–248.

Mahoney, F. I., & Barthel, D. (1965). Functional evaluation: The Barthel Index. *Maryland State Medical Journal, 14,* 56–61.

Managh, M. F., & Cook, J. V. (1993). The use of standardised assessment in occupational therapy: The BAFPE-R. *American Journal of Occupational Therapy, 47*(10), 877–884.

Mandelstam, M. (2003). Disabled people, manual handling, and human rights. *British Journal of Occupational Therapy, 66*(11), 528–530.

Missiuna, C., Gaines, R., & Soucie, H. (2006). Why every office needs a tennis ball: A new approach to assessing the clumsy child. *Canadian Medical Association Journal, 175*(5), 471–473.

Mitra, S. (2006). The capability approach and disability. *Journal of Disability Policy Studies, 16,* 236–247.

Moats, G. (2007). Discharge decision-making, enabling occupations and client-centered practice. *Canadian Journal of Occupational Therapy, 74,* 91–101.

Molineux, M. (2004). Occupation in occupational therapy: A labour in vain? In M. Molineux (Ed.), *Occupation for occupational therapists* (pp. 1–14). Oxford: Blackwell.

Mozley, C. G., Schneider, J., Cordingley, L., et al. (2007). The care home activity project: Does introducing an occupational therapy programme reduce depression in care homes? *Aging & Mental Health, 11*(1), 99–107.

Ontario Healthy Communities Coalition. (n.d.). *Ten steps to community development.* Retrieved from http://www.ohcc-ccso.ca/en/courses/community-development-for-health-promoters/module-two-process-strategies-and-roles/ten-steps.

Payne, S., & Howell, C. (2005). An evaluation of the clinical use of the Assessment of Motor and Process Skills with children. *British Journal of Occupational Therapy, 68*(6), 277–280.

Pereira, R. B. (2012). Viewpoint: The potential of occupational therapy services for students with disabilities within tertiary education settings. *Australian Occupational Therapy Journal, 59,* 393–396.

Pizzi, M. A., Reitz, M., & Scaffa, M. E. (2010). Assessments for health promotion practice. In M. E. Scaffa, S. M. Reitz, & M. A. Pizzi (Eds.), *Occupational therapy in the promotion of health and wellness* (pp. 173–194). Philadelphia: FA Davis.

Polatajko, H., Mandich, A., & Martini, R. (1999). Dynamic performance analysis: A framework for understanding occupational performance. *American Journal of Occupational Therapy*, 54, 65–72.

Pollard, N., & Sakellariou, D. (2007). Occupation, education and community-based rehabilitation. *British Journal of Occupational Therapy*, 70(4), 171–174.

Priestley, M. (2005). Disability and social inequalities. In M. Romero, & E. Margolis (Eds.), *The Blackwell companion to social inequalities*. http://dx.doi.org/10.1111/b.9780631231547.2005.00021.x (Chapter 16). Blackwell Reference Online.

Quesada, J., Hart, L. K., & Bourgois, P. (2011). Structural vulnerability and health: Latino migrant laborers in the United States. *Medical Anthropology*, 30, 339–362.

Reeve, T., & Gottselig, N. (2011). *Investigating workplace accommodation for people with invisible disabilities*. Vancouver: BC Coalition of People with Disabilities. Retrieved from *http://www. disabilityalliancebc.org/docs/employmentinvisibledis.pdf*.

Siegert, R. J., & Ward, T. (2010). Dignity, rights and capabilities in clinical rehabilitation. *Disability and Rehabilitation*, 32, 2138–2146.

Stienstra, D. (2012). *About Canada: Disability rights*. Halifax, NS: Fernwood.

Terzi, L. (2005). A capability perspective on impairment, disability and special needs: Towards social justice in education. *Theory and Research in Education*, 3, 197–223.

Thibeault, R. (2013). Occupational justice's intents and impacts: From personal choices to community consequences. In M. P. Cutchin, & V. A. Dickie (Eds.), *Transactional perspectives on occupation* (pp. 245–256). Dordrecht: Springer.

United Nations. (2006). *Convention on the rights of persons with disabilities*. Vienna: United Nations.

United Nations High Commissioner for Human Rights and World Health Organization. (2008). *The right to health. Fact sheet No. 31*. Geneva: United Nations. Retrieved from *http://www.ohchr.org/ Documents/Publications/Factsheet31.pdf*.

Van Nes, F., Runge, U., & Jonsson, H. (2009). One body, three hands and two minds: A case study of the intertwined occupations of an older couple after a stroke. *Journal of Occupational Science*, 16, 194–202.

Welch, A., & Lowes, S. (2005). Home assessment visits within the acute setting: A discussion and literature review. *British Journal of Occupational Therapy*, 68(4), 158–164.

White, A., Hocking, C., & Reid, H. (2014). How occupational therapists engage adults with cognitive impairments in assessments. *British Journal of Occupational Therapy*, 77(1), 2–9.

Whiteford, G. E., & Pereira, R. B. (2012). Occupation, inclusion and participation. In G. E. Whiteford, & C. Hocking (Eds.), *Occupational science: Society, inclusion and participation* (pp. 187–207). Oxford: Wiley-Blackwell.

Whiteford, G., Townsend, E., & Hocking, C. (2000). Reflections on a renaissance of occupation. *Canadian Journal of Occupational Therapy*, 67(1), 61–69.

Wilby, H. J. (2005). A description of a functional screening assessment developed for the acute physical setting. *British Journal of Occupational Therapy*, 68(1), 39–44.

Wilcock, A. A., & Hocking, C. (2015). *An occupational perspective of health* (3rd ed.). Thorofare, NJ: Slack.

World Federation of Occupational Therapists. (2006). *Position statement: Human rights*. Retrieved from http://www.wfot.org/ ResourceCentre.aspx.

World Federation of Occupational Therapists. (2009). *Diversity matters: Guiding principles on diversity and culture*. Retrieved from http://www.wfot.org/ResourceCentre/tabid/132/did/306/Default. aspx.

World Health Organization. (1980). *International classification of impairments, disabilities and handicaps*. Geneva: WHO. Retrieved from *http://apps.who.int/iris/bitstream/10665/41003/1/ 9241541261_eng.pdf?ua = 1*.

World Health Organization. (2001). *International classification of functioning, disability and health*. Geneva: WHO. Retrieved from *http://www.who.int/classifications/icf/en/*.

World Health Organization and World Bank. (2011). *World report on disability*. Geneva: WHO Press. Retrieved from *http://www.who. int/disabilities/world_report/2011/report.pdf*.

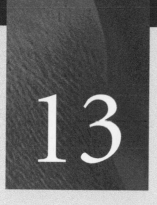

13 CANADIAN OCCUPATIONAL PERFORMANCE MEASURE

HEATHER COLQUHOUN ■ ANNE W. HUNT ■ JANET F. MURCHISON

Abstract

This chapter describes the Canadian Occupational Performance Measure and how it is used to determine a person's self-identified occupational performance issues and measure improvements in these issues over the course of occupational therapy intervention. The chapter will provide a historical review of the Canadian Occupational Performance Measure and describe current resources for incorporating the Canadian Occupational Performance Measure into practice. A review of the key characteristics of the Canadian Occupational Performance Measure, including theoretical considerations, will be addressed, as will key issues related to the administration of the Canadian Occupational Performance Measure. Focus is placed on common communication pitfalls that hinder occupational performance issue identification and professional considerations or 'tips' for each of the steps undertaken to administer the tool. A general overview of the tool's psychometric characteristics is provided.

KEY POINTS

- The Canadian Occupational Performance Measure (COPM) is a standardised assessment for identifying occupational performance issues and measuring individuals' perceptions of change in occupational performance and satisfaction.

- The COPM encourages practice that is evidence-based, person-centred and occupation-focused.

- The COPM consists of a semistructured interview to identify occupational performance issues, followed by a rating of these issues for importance and current performance and satisfaction regarding this performance.

- Common COPM pitfalls include a disconnection between what an individual said and what an occupational therapist heard or judged important, questions that include too many occupational performance issues, and moving too quickly from one issue to another.

- The COPM is reliable and valid with good clinical utility.

INTRODUCTION

The Canadian Occupational Performance Measure (COPM) is a standardised assessment designed specifically to be used by occupational therapists (Law et al., 2014). Considered a gold standard for identifying occupational performance issues and measuring individuals' perceptions of change in the performance and satisfaction of occupations (McColl et al., 2005; Parker & Sykes, 2006; Wressle, Eeg-Oldofsson, Marcusson, & Henriksson, 2002), the COPM encourages practice that is evidence-based, person-centred and occupation-focused. It is applicable for use with people who have a wide range of diagnoses and within a broad range of practice settings.

The COPM is valuable both as an individual assessment and as a tool for demonstrating the effectiveness of occupational therapy practice. Individual results of the COPM demonstrate the extent to which individuals feel they have improved over the course of occupational therapy in valued occupations that they identified as ones they had difficulty performing. Aggregated results of the COPM – that is, results averaged across numerous people who have been assessed using the COPM – demonstrate the level of change experienced by people who receive occupational therapy within a caseload or service.

After a brief word about the history of the COPM, the tool is described. Throughout this description, advice is provided and some potential barriers are discussed regarding the administration of the tool. A general overview of the tool's psychometric characteristic is provided.

THE CANADIAN OCCUPATIONAL PERFORMANCE MEASURE

The COPM was developed by Canadian occupational therapy leaders Mary Law, Sue Baptiste, Anne Carswell, Mary Ann McColl, Helene Polatajko and Nancy Pollock and first published in 1990 (Law et al., 1990). It is now in its fifth edition (Law et al., 2014). In addition to complete administration and scoring instructions, the latest COPM administration manual provides an excellent summary of research related to the COPM to date. The COPM has been used in practice with diverse range of people and age spans. It has been translated into 36 languages. In addition, an aphasia-friendly version has recently been developed (Coates, Irvine, & Sutherland, 2015).

The COPM is a standardised instrument designed to aid in the selection of relevant and meaningful occupational performance issues and measures an individual's perception of change in performance and satisfaction with those issues over time (Law et al., 2014). The COPM is an individualised outcome measure in that the occupational performance issues to be addressed and measured are unique to the individual (Donnelly & Carswell, 2002). It is also person-centred, because the individual plays an essential role in identifying these issues. This is consistent with a core principle of the profession: that the individual is a partner and key decision maker in occupational therapy (Townsend & Polatajko, 2007).

Theoretical Considerations

The COPM was developed for use in practice guided by the Canadian Model of Occupational Performance (Law, Polatajko, Baptiste, & Townsend, 1997), and by extension, the Canadian Model of Occupational Performance and Engagement (Townsend & Polatajko, 2007). Person-centred application of these models requires an approach that views people both as experts regarding their occupations and partners in their own care. The COPM enables people to participate meaningfully in their occupational therapy by identifying occupational performance problems and evaluating performance and satisfaction in these problem areas (Law, Baum, & Dunn, 2005). Use of the COPM is also consistent with person-centred applications of other occupational therapy models, including the Person Environment Occupation model (Law et al., 1996) and the Occupational Performance Model (Australia) (Chapparo & Ranka, 1997). Additionally, the COPM is in keeping with a core aspect of evidence-based practice – the inclusion of the perspective of people receiving occupational therapy services (Law et al., 2005). The COPM's format as a self-report measure is in keeping with this commitment to the inclusion of the individual's perspective in all steps of the therapy process, from identification of priorities to evaluation of outcomes.

THE COPM PROCESS

The COPM is carried out using a semistructured interview in which the person is guided to identify occupational performance issues in self-care, productivity and leisure. This is followed by a rating of the importance of these issues and a discussion leading to the selection of up to five key issues that the person wishes to address in therapy. Then, the person rates his or her current performance and satisfaction regarding this performance on these prioritised occupational performance issues. The COPM manual provides detailed instructions for this process. Scoring sheets allow for efficient recording of the person's responses, as well as performance and satisfaction scores during initial administration and reevaluation. The manual and scoring sheets are necessary for administering the COPM.

The COPM is considered a standardised assessment, as there are specific steps that need to be included in the process and specific results that are gathered. However, there is no one script for the semistructured interview. Each interview is unique. Exactly what will be said during the interview depends on a combination of the style of the therapist and of the individual characteristics of the person being interviewed.

It is common to complete the COPM as part of an initial assessment. The COPM interview is an opportunity to facilitate the development of the therapeutic relationship and to set an initial standard of individual engagement in the therapeutic process. However, for people who have difficulty working in such collaboration, it may be beneficial to develop the therapeutic relationships in other ways before introducing the COPM.

Once a therapist is experienced with the process, administering the COPM takes approximately 20 to 40 minutes. People who are familiar with occupational therapy services and their own occupational performance and engagement priorities may complete the process relatively quickly. Those who are less knowledgeable regarding occupational therapy, or who have little experience working in a collaborative relationship with a health care provider, may require more time. In addition, if there are communication challenges between the occupational therapist and the individual, as for example when the therapist does not speak the individual's first language or when the individual has expressive or receptive language problems, additional administration time may be needed.

Care should be taken to ensure that the person understands what occupational therapy is and why the COPM is being used. That is, the person should appreciate that the COPM results will guide which occupations will be the focus for occupational therapy. Additionally, care must be taken to allow for the interaction necessary to develop the therapeutic relationship while carrying out this assessment.

Implementing the COPM in practice may be challenging for a number of reasons. It can be difficult to listen to and acknowledge an individual's occupational performance issues, knowing that these may be quite different from what the therapist thinks should be the focus of therapy. Also it does take time, something that always seems to be in short supply in a busy practice (McColl et al., 2005). However, the overall therapeutic experience is enhanced when time is taken at the outset of therapy to identify meaningful occupational performance issues using the COPM.

There are five steps to administering the COPM. Each is briefly described next. Suggestions that may be helpful in administration are given and recommendations for potentially challenging situations are made. Each step concludes with a boxed set of key professional considerations. For specific instructions regarding COPM administration, readers are asked to refer to the most recent COPM manual (Law et al., 2014) or the COPM website (www.thecopm.ca).

Step 1: Identify Occupational Performance Issues

The COPM begins with the identification of the occupational performance issues the individual is experiencing. The individual is prompted to identify problems in self-care, productivity and leisure. The therapist may ask individuals specifically what they need to do, want to do and are expected to do in their daily lives. Therapists may ask individuals to describe a typical day or prompt individuals with examples of occupations that are often identified by others with similar health or developmental issues.

The therapist records all of the occupational performance issues that the individual identifies so no important problems are missed.

Identification of occupational performance issues that are of importance to the individual is the key to both accurate identification of priority occupational performance problems and the initiation of effective, person-centred occupational therapy. Key facilitators of this process include reflective listening, acknowledgement and affirmation and open-ended questioning. Reflective listening means providing each individual with the time he or she need to respond, listening carefully to what has been said, and responding in a way that promotes additional information and clarification.

Simple acknowledgements (such as, 'Okay' or 'hmm') and affirmations (such as, 'That seems really important for you') have been shown to facilitate occupational performance issue identification (Hunt, Le Dorze, Polatajko, Bottari, & Dawson, 2015). In interviews, these types of statements are typically followed by a natural pause in conversation. These pauses provide people with opportunities to talk more about their specific concerns and priorities. This in turn facilitates the identification of key occupational performance issues.

Open-ended questions are used to learn more about occupational performance issues in general. They may also be used to prompt people to talk about issues that they may not have considered. For example, 'How are you managing your grocery shopping?' may prompt a person who is having difficulty getting around the community to consider this occupation as a potential occupational performance issue. Such prompts may be particularly helpful for people experiencing cognitive impairment.

A number of common communication pitfalls that hinder occupational performance issue identification have been highlighted (Hunt et al., 2015). These problems tend to reflect a disconnection between what an individual has said and what the occupational therapist has heard or judged important. This can happen when therapists do not obtain enough detail about an occupational issue to properly define it. This can also occur when therapists prematurely form a picture in their minds of the issue or dismiss some occupations as not achievable and therefore not worthy of discussion.

Posing a question that includes multiple occupational performance issues can also inhibit the identification of important occupational performance issues. For many people, a question that includes a list of multiple occupational performance issues may be confusing. People experiencing cognitive or communication difficulties may still be processing the first occupational performance issue raised after the occupational therapist has moved on to other occupational performance areas. Specific questions that encourage a person to reflect on everyday occupations may be more useful than a long list of items. For example, rather than saying, 'Tell me about your self-care: your showering, dressing and meal preparation', the therapist could say, 'Tell me about your morning routine'.

BOX 13.1
KEY PROFESSIONAL CONSIDERATIONS FOR STEP 1

SET THE STAGE FOR USING THE COPM:

Ensure the person understands that the therapist wants to engage in a collaborative therapeutic relationship in which the person's needs and wants are of critical importance. Situate the COPM within the overall assessment process. For example, the therapist should explain that the COPM is one of the assessments that will be conducted to gain an overview of the difficulties the person is experiencing in daily life. The person should be informed that the COPM will help determine the focus of therapy.

BE READY TO HELP THE INDIVIDUAL SPEAK IN TERMS OF OCCUPATIONAL PERFORMANCE ISSUES:

If instead of occupational performance issues the person identifies issues relating to performance components (such as strength or pain), the therapist should assist the person to identify how these problems are affecting what the person needs to do and wants to do. For example, 'What does your fatigue mean for your morning routine?'

PHRASE THE ISSUE IN A WAY THAT IS SHORT BUT CLEAR:

Ensure that the wording clearly reflects the performance issue. For example, 'swimming' could be more clearly stated as 'knowing how to swim' or 'going swimming regularly' depending on the person's concern.

AVOID CENSORING THE PERSON'S OCCUPATIONAL PERFORMANCE CONCERNS:

Therapists need to be aware of their own thoughts about the feasibility of a particularly occupation, the potential to work on the occupation within the practice setting or other issues related to their feelings about the occupation, as these can cause the therapist to consciously or unconsciously dismiss particular concerns raised by the person. Write down all of the person's concerns to ensure that this does not happen.

Moving abruptly from one occupational performance issue to another is also a common cause of inadequate therapist understanding of occupational performance issues. Sudden changes of topic may signal to the person that his or her responses are not important or are to be kept short. This not only limits the amount of information the person is able to provide; it may also make the person reluctant to share important concerns. In addition to listening carefully, leaving space for details and confirming that the therapist's understanding of the issue is accurate, it is suggested that therapists make a concluding statement or question before moving on to the next section – for example, 'Before we finish with our discussion of self-care, is there anything else you would like to discuss?'

Key professional considerations for Step 1 are listed in Box 13.1.

Step 2: Rate and Choose the Five Occupational Performance Issues That Are Most Important to the Person

Stage 2 involves the therapist working together with the person to choose up to five most important occupational performance issues. This begins with a numeric rating of all of the occupational performance issues identified earlier. For some people this is easy; for others it is not. It is acceptable and even encouraged to try different approaches to rating importance; there is no 'one way' to complete this task. The COPM manual contains a visual rating scale that can be used to facilitate this rating of importance.

Once the rating is done, the therapist confirms with the person that the five most highly rated issues are those that the person wishes to work on in occupational therapy. This is done by reviewing these issues in light of the other highly rated issues and asking the person to confirm that these are in fact the issues he or she wants to focus on. Five key occupational performance issues are generally considered the maximum number of issues that can be worked on at one time (Law et al., 2014). A person may choose fewer issues. If there are additional issues, these can be considered later.

Key professional considerations for Step 2 are listed in Box 13.2.

Step 3: Score Performance and Satisfaction with Performance

For each identified occupational performance issue that will be the focus of occupational therapy, each individual rates: (1) his or her perception of his or her current performance and (2) how satisfied he or she is with the current performance. Again a visual rating scale is provided in the COPM manual to facilitate this task. The order for conducting this scoring is flexible; however, generally people will find it easier to first consider how well they feel they perform an occupational performance issue and then think about how satisfied they are with this performance. That is, it is usually easiest for the person to rate performance and satisfaction of each issue in turn.

Key professional considerations for Step 3 are listed in Box 13.3.

BOX 13.2
KEY PROFESSIONAL CONSIDERATIONS FOR STEP 2

USE THE VISUAL RATING SCALE AS NEEDED:

The visual rating scale may be helpful for people who might benefit from the use of a prompt (such as people experiencing cognitive impairments).

CONSIDER ADAPTING RATING SCALES:

Some people have difficulty making decisions and feel anxious committing to a number. Feel free to use descriptors instead of numbers if this seems to be the case (e.g. very important, somewhat important, not that important, very unimportant).

HELP THE PERSON TO PRIORITISE AREAS OF EQUAL IMPORTANCE:

If the person rates more than five areas of equal importance, ask, 'Which is more important to you, this problem or that problem?' or 'Which issues are most important for you to work on in therapy?' or 'Which issues are the ones that you would like to start working on today, knowing that if we have time, we could go back to some of the other ones?

EXPLAIN HOW OCCUPATIONAL PERFORMANCE ISSUES WILL BE USED:

Ensure that the person understands that the occupational performance issues identified as most important will form the basis of goals that will be addressed in occupational therapy.

REMEMBER THAT IDENTIFYING OCCUPATIONAL PERFORMANCE ISSUES IS NOT GOAL SETTING:

Although the priority occupational performance issues will indicate what the person wants to work on in therapy, typically it will not provide an indication of the goal (i.e. what the person wants the performance to look like after intervention). Working with the person to develop a clear description of the goal for each occupational performance issue is an important step that must take place after completion of the COPM and before intervention begins.

BOX 13.3
KEY PROFESSIONAL CONSIDERATIONS FOR STEP 3

COMPLETE BOTH RATINGS FOR AN OCCUPATIONAL PERFORMANCE ISSUE AT THE SAME TIME:

Have the person complete the performance and satisfaction ratings for each problem before rating the next occupational performance issue.

USE THE VISUAL RATING SCALE AS NEEDED:

The visual rating scale may be helpful for people who benefit from the use of a prompt (such as those experiencing cognitive impairment).

PROVIDE EXAMPLES:

Use examples of numeric rating systems that may be familiar to the person (e.g. rating an Olympic performance).

OFFER REASSURANCE:

For people who are anxious about committing to a number, emphasise that their rating is only a general way of gaining an understanding of how they feel about their performance at this time. That there is no right or wrong answer.

MODIFY THE LANGUAGE USED:

Experiment with different ways of simply explaining performance and satisfaction.

Step 4: Reassessment

The COPM is used to reassess the person's performance and satisfaction with performance at the end of therapy or at any other time when an indication of progress may be helpful. Reassessment consists simply of returning to Step 3 and having the person rate his or her current performance and satisfaction with occupational performance issues.

Key professional considerations for Step 4 are listed in Box 13.4.

PSYCHOMETRIC PROPERTIES OF THE COPM

The COPM can be used as a descriptive measure to simply identify priority occupational performance issues and related current performance and satisfaction. However, it was primarily designed for use as an evaluative measure. Specifically, it was designed to measure changes in occupational performance and satisfaction after occupational therapy.

BOX 13.4
KEY PROFESSIONAL CONSIDERATIONS FOR STEP 4

INTERPRETATION OF RESULTS SHOULD INCLUDE THE PERSON:

Therapists should work in partnership with the person to appropriately interpret the person's scores.

APPRECIATE THAT EACH INDIVIDUAL'S CONCERNS AND STANDARDS MAY SHIFT:

Sometimes, people rate their performance and satisfaction differently as they progress in therapy. During the course of therapy people may become knowledgeable about their occupational performance. They may find that they are having more difficulty than they thought they would with a particular occupation, or that they are able to carry out this occupation more easily than they had imagined. Either situation may lead them to alter the way they approach their performance or satisfaction ratings. It may also lead them to alter their goals. Such changes may lead to smaller change scores than the therapist had anticipated based on the changes the therapist observed in the person's performance.

REMEMBER THAT THE COPM IS NOT A GOAL ATTAINMENT SCALE:

COPM scores may not always reflect the degree to which goals have been met, but rather reflect each individual's perspective on how well they currently perform the occupational performance issues and their satisfaction with that performance. In addition to COPM change scores, occupational therapy reports should include an indication of the attainment of goals that were set at the beginning of therapy.

There have been many studies of the COPM's psychometric properties. Summaries of these can be found in an annotated bibliography (CAOT, 2006) and the COPM manual (Law et al., 2014). Brief highlights of these studies are discussed below.

Clinical Utility

The clinical utility (i.e. ease of administration and usefulness) (Law, 1987) of an instrument is critical to its value in practice. The COPM is easily accessible to therapists and may be purchased online through the Canadian Occupational Performance Measure website (www.thecopm.ca/). The materials required to conduct the COPM are a manual and the assessment form. No specific qualifications are required to conduct the COPM; however, using the COPM requires that the therapist be comfortable with a person-centred and occupation-based approach to both assessment and intervention (Law et al., 2014).

Therapists have indicated that the COPM is useful in the occupational therapy process. Studies suggest that using the COPM assists with goal setting and intervention planning, provides useful feedback on the performance improvements of people receiving occupational therapy and facilitates communication (Wressle et al., 2002). Use of the COPM has been found to increase the person-centred nature of practice (Colquhoun, Letts, Law, Macdermid, & Missiuna, 2012; Donnelly & Carswell, 2002; McColl et al., 2005), to improve goal setting (Chen, Rodger, & Polatajko, 2002), and to assist in defining the work of occupational therapy (Fedden, Green, & Hill, 1999). Therapists state that using the COPM allows them to work more holistically with people and assists with developing realistic and person-centred goals (Chen et al., 2002). Using the COPM as a routine part of practice improved the quality of occupational therapy service on eight important dimensions of practice, such as

therapist knowledge of the person's perspective, professional decision-making and documentation (Colquhoun et al., 2012). Therapists indicate that their priorities are often different from the priorities of people receiving occupational therapy (Law et al., 1990), suggesting that the COPM provides an important window on these people's perspectives.

Reliability

Test-retest reliability is important when tools are used to measure change as a result of occupational therapy intervention. *Test-retest reliability* refers to the degree scores are consistent across two administrations of the tool over a period when scores would not be expected to change. Test-retest reliability has been found to be between $r = .65$ and $r = .85$ (Law et al., 2014), meaning that the COPM demonstrates moderate to high reliability (Portney & Watkins, 2000).

Validity

A valid tool measures what it is supposed to measure (Portney & Watkins, 2000). Overall, the COPM demonstrates good validity across multiple studies and validity types. Content validity is generally viewed as good, as the COPM has strong conceptual grounding in the CMOP and it explicitly addresses the three core dimensions of occupation: self-care, productivity and leisure.

The COPM has been shown to have good convergent and divergent validity. That is, its scores correlate with scores of related measures rather than with scores of measures to which its results should be unrelated. For example, the COPM correlates well with other self-report measures of occupation such as the Return to Normal Living Index (Chen et al., 2002) but tends to correlate poorly with measures of functional status and performance components, such as the Functional Independence Measure

(Chan & Lee, 1997), the Disability of the Arm, Shouler and Hand scale and the Michigan Hand Outcomes Questionnaire (van de Ven-Stevens, Graff, Peters, Van Der Linde, & Geurts, 2015).

The COPM appears to be responsive to change in an individual's performance and satisfaction (Carpenter, Baker, & Tyldesley, 2001; Eyssen et al., 2011). A two-point change in performance and satisfaction is generally considered clinically significant (Law et al., 2014).

CONCLUSION

The COPM is an individualised outcome measure that provides the occupational therapist and the person receiving occupational therapy with prioritised occupational performance issues and pre- and postintervention measures of the person's performance and satisfaction with this performance. It is applicable for use with a very broad range of people receiving occupational therapy and is available in many languages. In addition to providing an excellent indication of how well therapy has addressed an individual's issues, it can also be used to demonstrate the overall effectiveness of occupational therapy within a caseload or service.

 http://evolve.elsevier.com/Curtin/OT

REFERENCES

Canadian Association of Occupational Therapists (2006). *Research on the Canadian occupational performance measure: An annotated resource*. Ottawa: CAOT Publications ACE.

Carpenter, L., Baker, G. A., & Tyldesley, B. (2001). The use of the Canadian occupational performance measure as an outcome of a pain management program. *Canadian Journal of Occupational Therapy, 68*, 16–22.

Chan, C. C., & Lee, T. (1997). Validity of the Canadian occupational performance measure. *Occupational Therapy International, 4*, 231–249.

Chapparo, C., & Ranka, J. (1997). *OPM: Occupational performance model (Australia): Monograph 1*. Occupational Performance Network.

Chen, Y. H., Rodger, S., & Polatajko, H. (2002). Experiences with the COPM and client-centred practice in adult neurorehabilitation in Taiwan. *Occupational Therapy International, 9*, 167–184.

Coates, R., Irvine, C., & Sutherland, C. (2015). Development of an aphasia-friendly Canadian occupational performance measure. *British Journal of Occupational Therapy, 78*, 196–199.

Colquhoun, H. L., Letts, L. J., Law, M. C., Macdermid, J. C., & Missiuna, C. A. (2012). Administration of the Canadian occupational performance measure: Effect on practice. *Canadian Journal of Occupational Therapy, 79*, 120–128.

Donnelly, C., & Carswell, A. (2002). Individualized outcome measures: A review of the literature. *Canadian Journal of Occupational Therapy, 69*, 84–94.

Eyssen, I., Steultjens, M., Oud, T., Bolt, E. M., Maasdam, A., & Dekker, J. (2011). Responsiveness of the Canadian occupational performance measure. *Journal of Rehabilitation Research & Development, 48*, 517–528.

Fedden, T., Green, A., & Hill, T. (1999). Out of the woods: The Canadian occupational performance measure, from the manual into practice. *British Journal of Occupational Therapy, 62*, 318–320.

Hunt, A. W., Le Dorze, G., Polatajko, H., Bottari, C., & Dawson, D. R. (2015). Communication during goal-setting in brain injury rehabilitation: What helps and what hinders? *British Journal of Occupational Therapy, 78*, 488–498.

Law, M. (1987). Measurement in occupational therapy: Scientific criteria for evaluation. *Canadian Journal of Occupational Therapy, 54*, 133–138.

Law, M., Baptiste, S., Carswell, A., Mccoll, M., Polatajko, H., & Pollock, N. (2014). *Canadian occupational performance measure* (5th ed.). Ottawa: CAOT Publications ACE.

Law, M., Baptiste, S., Mccoll, M., Opzoomer, A., Polatajko, H., & Pollock, N. (1990). The Canadian occupational performance measure: An outcome measure for occupational therapy. *Canadian Journal of Occupational Therapy, 57*, 82–87.

Law, M. C., Baum, C. M., & Dunn, W. (2005). *Measuring occupational performance: Supporting best practice in occupational therapy*. Thorofare, NJ: Slack.

Law, M., Cooper, B., Strong, S., Stewart, D., Rigby, P., & Letts, L. (1996). The person-environment-occupation model: A transactive approach to occupational performance. *Canadian Journal of Occupational Therapy, 63*, 9–23.

Law, M., Polatajko, H., Baptiste, S., & Townsend, E. (1997). Core concepts of occupational therapy. In E. Townsend, S. Stanton, & M. Law, et al. (Eds.), *Enabling occupation: An occupational therapy perspective* (pp. 29–56). Ottawa: CAOT Publications.

McColl, M. A., Law, M., Baptiste, S., Pollock, N., Carswell, A., & Polatajko, H. J. (2005). Targeted applications of the Canadian occupational performance measure. *Canadian Journal of Occupational Therapy, 72*, 298–300.

Parker, D. M., & Sykes, C. H. (2006). A systematic review of the Canadian occupational performance measure: A clinical practice perspective. *British Journal of Occupational Therapy, 69*, 150–160.

Portney, L. G., & Watkins, M. P. (2000). *Foundations of clinical research: Applications to practice*. Upper Saddle River, NJ: Prentice Hall.

Townsend, E. A., & Polatajko, H. J. (2007). *Advancing an occupational therapy vision for health, well-being, and justice through occupation*. Ottawa: CAOT Publications.

van de Ven-Stevens, L. A., Graff, M. J., Peters, M. A., Van Der Linde, H., & Geurts, A. C. (2015). Construct validity of the Canadian occupational performance measure in participants with tendon injury and Dupuytren disease. *Physical Therapy, 95*, 750–757.

Wressle, E., Eeg-Olofsson, A.-M., Marcusson, J., & Henriksson, C. (2002). Improved client participation in the rehabilitation process using a client-centred goal formulation structure. *Journal of Rehabilitation Medicine, 34*, 5–11.

14

TASK, ACTIVITY AND OCCUPATIONAL ANALYSIS

CYNTHIA PERLMAN ■ MELANIE BERGTHORSON

CHAPTER OUTLINE

Abstract
Occupational analysis, a perspective unique to the profession of occupational therapy, is explored as a continuum beginning with task analysis, followed by activity analysis and culminating in occupational analysis itself. The analysis process begins with understanding the sequential components of and inherent skills needed for specific activities, and then builds towards meaningful person-specific, goal-directed occupations. An activity becomes an occupation when it is personally meaningful and when participation is reinforced through the process of grading and adapting. The chapter highlights the conceptual frameworks and models needed for a successful occupational analysis, including the Person-Environment-Occupation (PEO) Model, the Canadian Model of Occupational Performance and Engagement (CMOP-E) and the Model of Human Occupation (MOHO).

Examples of each type of analysis and the subsequent grading and adapting of the activity/occupation, including discussion of the environmental contexts (physical, social, cultural, institutional), are provided through a practice story in which grocery shopping is analysed.

KEY POINTS

- The analysis process is viewed as a continuum beginning from a task analysis, to an activity analysis, leading to an occupational analysis.

- An activity becomes an occupation when its personal meaning is acknowledged and pursued, the goals are personally set, the required skills to perform are considered and the environmental context is acknowledged.

- Occupational analysis is a perspective unique to the profession of occupational therapy enabling the therapist to evaluate and validate the meaning of the occupation for a specific person when performing it within a chosen environmental context.

- Occupational analysis is supported by the philosophical influences of the value of purposeful, meaningful occupation on health and well-being.

- The Person-Environment-Occupation Model (Law et al., 1996), an open systems theory-based approach, can be used as a foundational support and preanalysis tool for occupational analysis, to further build upon the value of purposeful, meaningful occupations, as well as to promote further understanding of the occupation-based contexts.

- Using the results of an occupational analysis, occupational therapists can grade or adapt the activity/occupation to lead to optimal participation, engagement and autonomy for their people receiving occupational therapy.

THE MEANING OF OCCUPATION FOR ANALYSIS OF ACTIVITIES AND OCCUPATIONS

A historical shift in the paradigm of occupational therapy occurred in the 1970s when there was a transition from a mechanistic/reductionist perspective to an occupation-based perspective, which allowed the development of occupation-based intervention (Aiken, Fourt, Cheng, & Polatajko, 2011; Bauerschmidt & Nelson, 2011; Kielhofner, 2008; Wilding & Whiteford, 2007). This shift addressed the personal values and meaning attributed to occupations by an individual, group or community performing the occupation. Meaning is individually constructed and interpreted, thereby acknowledging the human experience – performing in a unique person-specific manner (Blesedell Crepeau, Gillen, & Scaffa, 2013; Kielhofner, 2008; Peloquin, 2005). Occupations are personalised activities chosen and performed by individuals because they hold personal meaning and purpose to that individual (Reed, Hocking, & Smythe, 2011; Thomas, 2012; Townsend & Polatajko, 2013). These chosen occupations occur within the unique context of the person and the environment. Occupational therapists understand the impact of activities and occupations on participation and engagement, through fundamental analysis frameworks that analyse an activity or occupation as a whole considering its inherent component parts, including the environmental contexts (physical, social, cultural, institutional).

The focus of this chapter is on the concepts of task analysis, activity analysis and occupational analysis as a continuum of an analysis process from understanding sequential component parts and inherent skills associated with tasks and activities to more person-specific, goal-directed occupations in which the personal meaning of doing is identified. Through occupation-based activity analysis, and subsequent grading and adapting, the activity's or occupation's therapeutic potential is identified (Thomas, 2015).

To understand this continuum, it is first important to differentiate the terms *task, activity* and *occupation,* as described in Table 14.1.

When Does an Activity Become an Occupation?

Therapeutic and meaningful activities and occupations remain core professional concepts that are valued as both a *means and an end* or outcome from the intervention process. An activity becomes an occupation when the personal meaning of it is acknowledged and pursued, the goals are personally set, the required skills to perform it are considered and the environmental context is acknowledged. Hinojosa, Sabari, and Pedretti (1993) described the attributes of purposeful and meaningful therapeutic activity in occupational therapy. These are presented in Box 14.1.

The Influence of Meaningful Occupation on Practice

An *occupation-focused* practice founded on a belief that humans are occupational in nature underpins occupational therapy practice. Nelson (1997) reiterated that pride and professional

TABLE 14.1	
Differentiating Among Task, Activity and Occupation	
A task	A conventional sequence and timing of actions or list of steps required to complete an activity (Thomas, 2015).
An activity	The actual concrete doing or completion, without a context, of the list of actions or steps that involve skills, materials and interaction with the environment. Activities comprise components and parts that can be analysed (Mosey, 1986).
An occupation	The contextual, meaningful, goal-directed everyday activities that people choose to do to occupy themselves, including caring for oneself (self-care), enjoying and participating in life outside of work (leisure) and contributing to society (productivity/work) (CAOT, 2002). Occupations are shaped by culture and evolve through the lifespan as they are reflective of personal goals, skills, roles, habits and values (Kielhofner, 2008; Thomas, 2015).

> **BOX 14.1**
> **EIGHT CHARACTERISTICS OF A PURPOSE-FUL AND MEANINGFUL THERAPEUTIC ACTIVITY**
>
> 1. Goal directed and goal driven
> 2. Reflects life experiences
> 3. Unique to the individual
> 4. Requires active participation within occupational context of productivity/self-care/leisure
> 5. Requires the use of body structures and functions
> 6. Dependent on environmental context
> 7. Is used therapeutically to evaluate, facilitate and restore or maintain functional abilities
> 8. Gradable or adaptable to ensure participation
>
> From Hinojosa et al., 1993.

confidence result from full identification and adoption of the term *occupation,* a definitive domain of occupational therapy. Fisher (2013) posited that a worldview and appreciation of occupation to guide professional reasoning is termed *occupation-centred.* The actual therapeutic process of engaging a person in meaningful occupations that foster choice-making, satisfaction and restoration is termed *occupation-based* (Fisher, 2013; Polatajko & Davis, 2012). Emphasis should be placed on the value and meaning personally attributed to the particular occupation. 'Occupation-based means that practice must enable the performance of, or engagement in, an occupation that a person wants to, needs to, or is expected to do' (Polatajko & Davis, 2012, p. 259).

When occupational therapists are grounded by the occupation-based paradigm, they acknowledge their expertise in enabling occupation and in maintaining the occupational perspective throughout the therapeutic process (Aiken et al., 2011; Gray, 1998; Letts, 2011). Aiken et al. (2011) revealed the significance of embracing occupation-based practices and placing interventions in the context of meaningful occupation. They found that occupational therapists can gain personal and professional meaning through occupation-based practices using a conscious connection between their actions and the future occupational performance and engagement of people receiving occupational therapy services. Townsend and Polatajko (2013) identified occupation as the following:

■ Basic human drive to do and participate
■ Source of meaning and purpose as it reflects personal interests, values and pursuits

■ Source of control over one's life through intentional choice making
■ Source of self-expression leading to self-identity and a trueness of oneself across the lifespan
■ Source of satisfaction and self-fulfilment through purposeful doing
■ Means for interaction with the environment (physical, social, cultural, institutional)
■ Means of organising time, behaviour, space and materials to foster efficiency
■ Means of skill development and competence

CONTINUUM OF ANALYSES: TASK, ACTIVITY AND OCCUPATION

An extensive search of the literature reveals minimal consensus on definitions of, and how to properly differentiate among, the terms *task analysis, activity analysis* and *occupational analysis.* This is especially true for the terms *task analysis* and *activity analysis,* because delineations between activity and occupational analyses are more evident when based on occupation-based philosophy and terminology. Blesedell Crepeau et al. (2013) advocated for using both activity and occupational analyses to gain a deeper understanding of how people relate to their occupations. 'Practitioners must be able to analyse both the general idea of how an activity occurs within culture as well as the actual occupations as they are performed by the particular individuals' (Blesedell Crepeau et al., 2013, p. 237). Extrapolating from the American Occupational Therapy Association position paper on purposeful activity (Hinojosa et al., 1993), the continuum is defined in Figure 14.1.

The continuum of the analysis process begins with the task analysis, with an appreciation of the sequence and timing of actions or list of steps comprising an activity or typical procedure (Allen, 1982; Thomas, 2015). Activity analysis, the next step in the continuum, then examines the skills and context of the activity. This step acknowledges the context in which the activity is being performed, how it is normally done and the required body structures or functions (but not specific to an individual's potential) (Polatajko, Mandich, & Martini, 2000). Hersch, Lamport, and Coffey (2005) stated that an activity analysis involves a step-by-step dissection of an activity and determining the skills required to perform the activity in order to discover its therapeutic characteristics. The third step in the continuum is the occupational analysis, the perspective most unique to the profession of occupational therapy. This perspective validates the meaning of the activity to the individual. This analysis is person specific and combines the two previous analyses with a focus on the person's specific challenges, interests and lifestyle, as well as the environmental contexts (Pierce, 2001). To demonstrate this continuum, the occupation of grocery shopping will be explored from the perspective of a young mother, Bernice (Practice Story 14.1).

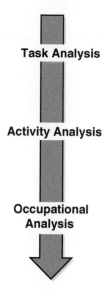

Task Analysis

The activity is examined to identify its component parts to determine which skills and abilities are necessary to complete the task.

Activity Analysis

The activity is examined in terms of the skills and context in which it will be performed to enable participation and engagement.

Occupational Analysis

In determining the meaningfulness of the activity for the individual, the practitioner considers the person's age, occupational roles, cultural background, gender, interests and preferences.

FIG. 14.1 ■ The task analysis–activity analysis–occupational analysis continuum based on the American Occupational Therapy Association position paper on purposeful activity (Hinojosa et al., 1993).

PRACTICE STORY 14.1

Bernice

Bernice was a 34-year-old woman with a recent diagnosis of multiple sclerosis. Bernice was referred to occupational therapy to address her symptoms of decreased upper extremity strength, fatigue and decreased endurance. She lived with her husband of 6 years and her 18-month-old son in a two-bedroom apartment. Bernice recently returned to work part time (3 days a week) as a librarian at her community library after an extended maternity leave.

An initial evaluation using the Canadian Occupational Performance Measure (Law et al., 2014) was implemented. Bernice identified the following occupations as challenging: work-related activities that required endurance (sorting, cataloguing both manually and electronically using the computer) and self-care activities of grocery shopping and house cleaning. Bernice expressed significant satisfaction with her roles as wife, mother and homemaker and stated that she hoped to maintain her capacity to fulfil these roles. She expressed strong, foundational family values as experienced from her Italian heritage. She looked forward to her weekly trips to the grocery store with her son as it enabled her to stimulate her child with the sights, smells and tastes while grocery shopping and to participate in an activity within the community. She often asked her mother to join them for the activity and they usually followed up this activity with a light lunch at a local Italian bistro.

The environmental context comprised a large general grocery store with outdoor parking situated within her local suburban neighbourhood. She drove to the grocery store.

Task Analysis of Grocery Shopping

Bernice's grocery shopping activity can be broken down into the following component parts or tasks to determine the required skills and abilities. The task analysis simply breaks down grocery shopping into a sequence of steps that could be completed by anyone in any generic store.

1. Retrieve cart and enter store.
2. Walk through aisles to targeted destination while pushing cart; start and stop.
3. Item One – Apples:
   a. Retrieve small plastic produce bag.
   b. Select and grasp apple.
   c. Release apple in bag; repeat for desired number of apples.
   d. Twist or tighten bag to close.
   e. Release bag of apples into cart.
4. Walk through aisles to targeted destination while pushing cart; start and stop.
5. Item Two – Bread:
   a. Select and grasp bread from shelf.
   b. Read label on bag for freshness date.
   c. Release bread into cart.
6. Walk through aisles for targeted destination while pushing cart; start and stop.
7. Repeat previous steps for additional items:
   a. Reach, hold, and release 2 L carton of orange juice.
   b. Reach and grasp aluminium foil package and release into cart.
8. At checkout, bend, reach, grasp, lift and place each item onto conveyor belt.
9. Retrieve wallet and take out required amount of money or credit card for purchase.

10. Hand money or credit card to cashier and obtain receipt.
11. Shopping items are bagged and placed into cart by cashier.
12. Push cart out of store to car.
13. Open trunk of car, lift and release each bag into trunk of car.
14. Replace cart.

Activity Analysis of Grocery Shopping

'Activity analysis is a clinical practice tool which must be learned and applied by all occupational therapy students in order to meet and fulfil the occupational performance needs of their clients, at any point within the lifespan' (Perlman, Weston, & Gisel, 2005, p. 154). As a result of an activity analysis, the inherent skills and abilities needed to perform the activity are identified; however, they are not specific to a particular individual. The environmental and activity demands are examined in preparation for optimal participation. With regards to Bernice's grocery shopping, the occupational therapist may anticipate the following expected demands of the activity:

- Position of the person in relation to the activity as well as the position of the activity in relation to environmental space
- Tools/utensils/objects/materials used to participate in the activity
- Environmental opportunities, demands and/or constraints of the large grocery store (physical, social, cultural, institutional)
- Contextual opportunities and demands to enable meaning of activity for the client (space; objects; tools; equipment, including virtual or electronic forms; sequence and temporal patterns; social interactions)
- Requisite performance skills and abilities needed for successful completion of the activity (motor, sensory-perceptual, cognitive, emotional, social/communicative)

To illustrate, an activity analysis description of the sensory performance skill domain as well as the environmental domain for the activity component of selecting apples are provided in Tables 14.2 and 14.3. Separating each activity component and determining the expected outcomes for success for each component is strongly suggested for an activity analysis (Thomas, 2015).

Examples of subcomponents or domains, particularly the sensory and environmental domains that can be analysed for an activity analysis, are provided in Table 14.2 and 14.3, respectively. In Table 14.4, the task of retrieving apples from a fruit bin in the grocery store is analysed through the sensory domain. The expected skill actions within this domain are described. Success for this task would be defined as physically collecting a set number of fresh, unblemished red apples from the bin and placing them in a plastic bag.

In Table 14.5, the task of retrieving apples from a fruit bin in the grocery store is analysed through the domains of the

TABLE 14.2
Activity Analysis of Selecting Apples: Sensory Performance Skill Domain

Visual	Visually scanning the environment to locate the plastic bags and to determine where apples are located and which specific type is desired. Visual awareness of potential obstacles or people in path. Visual assessment of apple to ensure it is blemish free, lacking bruises or holes. Visually checking the price above the apple bin.
Auditory	Tuning out/habituating to background noise of store (other shoppers, music playing, announcements, etc.)
Gustatory	Not utilised at this time unless samples are offered; possible activation of salivary glands when thinking about taste of apple.
Olfactory	Smelling apples to help determine freshness. Tuning out other odours in the store (odours of meat, fish, other vegetables, etc.)
Tactile	Tactile discrimination is utilised through handling of each apple to verify the appropriate firmness, smooth texture and lack of any spots. Temperature of apple is noted, as well as overall weight. Secured grasp may be adapted according to size and weight of an apple.
Vestibular	Maintaining balance while retrieving apples and visually scanning the environment.
Proprioceptive	Awareness of position in space relative to the apple display, location of bag in hand and the distance to other shoppers or store displays.

environmental context: physical, social, cultural and institutional. These subdomains reflect the environmental domains expressed within the Canadian Model of Occupational Performance and Engagement (CMOP-E) (Canadian Association of Occupational Therapists (CAOT), 2002; Townsend & Polatajko, 2013). The expected opportunities and demands or expected behaviours within the domain are described. Success for this task would be defined as easily accessing the apple bins and choosing preferred produce.

OCCUPATIONAL ANALYSIS: A CORNERSTONE OF OCCUPATIONAL THERAPY PRACTICE

Philosophical Influences on Occupational Analysis

An appreciation of the influence of occupation and purposeful doing on health and self-efficacy promotes a thorough occupational analysis that identifies the meaning and purpose of

TABLE 14.3
Environmental Context for Selecting Apples

Domain	Opportunities	Demands (Expected Behaviours)

Physical setting:
  Natural/built
  Space
  Objects
	■ Choice making
	■ Sensorial experience with food items (taste, touch, smell, visual)
		■ Access to area and equipment
		■ Location of objects
		■ Availability of fresh items
		■ Ease of navigation, way-finding

Social:
  Groups
  Roles
	■ Interact with staff, other shoppers, accompanying participants
	■ Fulfil roles (i.e. homemaker)
		■ Respect of others
		■ Social and conversational skills
		■ Social pragmatics (i.e. turn taking)

Cultural
  Temporal
    concepts
  Values
  Life situations
  Experiences
	■ Choice making for health promotion
	■ Choice making of culturally preferred apples
	■ Support meal planning
		■ Temporal availabilities (store hours)
		■ Budget constraints (organic versus nonorganic, local versus imported)
		■ Availability of apple variety

Institutional:
  Physical spaces
  Policies and
  procedures
  Rules and
  regulations
	■ Variety of apple selection to choose from
	■ Purchasing power for discounted items at large commercial institution
	■ Ease of navigation in larger stores
		■ Access to scale to weigh produce
		■ Self-serve policies
		■ Provisions for taste testing

chosen occupations for the person. Two philosophical influences that support current practices of occupational analysis are an occupational perspective on health and values-based medicine.

The influence of an occupation perspective on health (promotion) leading to well-being supports the opportunity to do, to be true to oneself and to strive to become (Wilcock, 2006). Engagement in occupation is strongly linked to health maintenance systems and the drive to meet not only survival needs but also progression of dignity, self-identity and competence (Kielhofner, 2008; Peloquin, 2005). The outcome is health and well-being through choice, meaning, balance, satisfaction, opportunity and self-actualisation (Wilcock, 1998). Doing, being and becoming (Fidler & Fidler, 1978; Wilcock, 1998) and belonging (Hitch, Pepin, & Stagnitti, 2014; Wilcock, 2007) lead to outcomes of improved health. Doing is living and participating in meaningful occupations. Doing is synonymous with function and occupation. Being is a philosophical state: being true to oneself while engaging in meaningful occupations (spirituality). Becoming is a process leading to self-actualisation, augmenting one's full potential, in constant development (Wilcock, 1998). Belonging is a socially driven connection to others, connecting within a social network. The social context may be collaborative or competitive, acknowledging the existing diversity of interactions, expectations and role scripts (Hitch et al., 2014). This philosophical perspective highlights the significance of occupational engagement for health, well-being and development.

Values-based medicine, as a theory of philosophical values, promotes the integration of person-centred practice in professional skills development. Fulford (2004) postulated that person-perspective values are at the top of a values hierarchy, signifying the importance of the person's narrative in collaborative decision making. Embracing differences and diversity in values, beliefs and decisions certainly supports ethical reasoning in daily occupational therapy practice. Values and beliefs are significantly correlated to sense of being (or spirituality) through the occupational experience. In addition, scientific and evidence-based practices are linked with values-based philosophies. 'Scientific progress increasingly opens up choices and with choices goes values' (Fulford, 2004, p. 59). When the people receiving occupational therapy services are given volitional power to enable choice making, their values and interests are acknowledged and integrated. The recognition and transparency of values and choices inherent in practice-based decision making facilitates ethical reasoning in occupational therapy practice (Clair & Newcombe, 2014). These value-based philosophies are evident within the Model of Human Occupation (MOHO) (Kielhofner, 2008). For example, personal causation drives the volitional process for choice making and motivation, which are reflective of the human experience and human behaviour in which human values are particularly diverse and personal.

Both philosophies support the occupation-based practice in which occupation remains proximal to health and well-being. Through occupational analysis, the details of the occupations a person chooses to engage in and the benchmarks for personal

TABLE 14.4
Preanalysis Step to Set the Context of the Activity Leading to Occupational Analysis (Perlman & Gisel, 2000)

Activity: _____

OCCUPATION: Identify area(s)

☐ productivity	☐ leisure	☐ self-care

PERSON: Identify predominant skill components:

☐ motor	☐ sensory	☐ cognitive
☐ perceptual	☐ social	☐ affective/emotional

ENVIRONMENT:

☐ physical	☐ social	☐ cultural

Preanalysis, person

Physical:	☐ trunk stability	☐ balance	☐ U/E strength (including hands)
	☐ L/E strength	☐ coordination	
	☐ mobility	☐ endurance ☐ hand dexterity	

Identify characteristics:

Sensory processing:	☐ visual	☐ tactile	☐ vestibular
	☐ auditory	☐ proprioceptive	☐ kinesthetic

Affective:	☐ satisfied	☐ optimistic	☐ pessimistic
	☐ introverted	☐ extroverted	
Cognitive:	☐ memory for this activity	☐ oriented to time and place	
	☐ concentration for this activity	☐ attention span for this activity	
	☐ problem solving skills		
	☐ activity is meaningful to the individual		

Spiritual:	☐ values quality of life	☐ expresses choices	
	☐ is motivated to perform this activity	☐ positive attitude towards autonomy	

Physical	Setting:	☐ natural	☐ built
	Objects/items:	☐ required	☐ not necessary

Preanalysis, environment
Identify characteristics:

Rules of physical accessibility	Orientation and wayfinding:	☐ observe safety	☐ general accessibility

Social	Group size:	☐ small	☐ large	☐ N/A
	Individual:	☐ in isolation	☐ alone but within a social milieu	☐ N/A
	Roles:	☐ leader	☐ follower ☐ participant	☐ N/A
	Task:	☐ serious	☐ playful	☐ competitive
		☐ collaborative	☐ educational	

Cultural:	☐ ethnicity	☐ age	☐ religion
	☐ gender	☐ life situations and experiences	
Rules of social conduct:	☐ code of conduct in this environment	☐ observe safety	☐ respect for others

TABLE 14.5		
Generic Subdomains Listed Under the Domains of the Person, Environment and Occupation for Occupational Analysis		
Person	**Environment**	**Occupation**
■ Motor ■ Sensory/perceptual ■ Cognitive ■ Affective ■ Social communication ■ Spiritual	**Physical** ■ Natural or built setting ■ Objects and tools ■ Space management ■ Accessibility	**Productivity** ■ Work ■ Play ■ Volunteer work ■ Retirement preparation or adjustment
	Social ■ Social groups ■ Socially constructed tasks	**Leisure** ■ Sports ■ Social participation ■ Community participation ■ Play
	Culture ■ Values and beliefs ■ Generational transmission of knowledge ■ Rituals; customs; rite of passage ■ Temporal significance	**Self-care** Activities of daily living: ■ Rest and sleep ■ Dressing ■ Bathing ■ Feeding ■ Toileting ■ Transfers
	Institutional ■ Policies and procedures ■ Rules and regulations ■ Accessibility ■ Integration	Instrumental activities of daily living: ■ Community mobility ■ Health management ■ Banking ■ Meal preparation ■ Grocery shopping

success are examined to determine their therapeutic benefit. Ensuring that the chosen occupations are tailored to address a person's occupational performance goals, skills and values can promote health and well-being.

Theoretical Influences on Occupational Analysis

Occupational therapy embraces a dynamic systems approach to the interaction among person, environment and occupation. This is described as an open system in which there is constant interplay among these domains. A change in one domain will affect change in the other two domains and change necessitates adaptation for performance, participation and even survival. For example, a change in a person's motor capacity (e.g. proximal humeral fracture) will affect the way the person performs or engages in occupations (e.g. washing hair), thereby affecting the environmental demands (e.g. assistance from a family member). Environmental demands will influence the need for

adaptation or adaptive aids, for social support or for possibly institutional advocacy.

Occupational performance is an outcome from the dynamic interaction of the person, environment and occupation that continues to evolve throughout a person's life; as a result occupational performance is flexible and variable. Occupational performance comprises interpretations and experiences by the individual so that the personal meaning of the occupation is acknowledged. It can shape self-identity and adaptability to changing priorities (Law et al., 1996). It enables choice making, occupational organisation and satisfaction from performing and engaging in meaningful occupations (CAOT, 2002).

Occupational engagement fundamentally underlies the notion of enablement, in that people can have the capacity to identify their own needs, to solve their own problems and to generally know what is best for them (Townsend & Polatajko, 2013). To become engaged requires involving oneself through participation in an occupation that has value, thereby fostering meaning. Meaning in occupations is derived from dynamic interactions and personal experiences and therefore is critical to self-identity, self-development and well-being.

The Person-Environment-Occupation Model as a Foundational Framework for Occupational Analysis

The Person-Environment-Occupation (PEO) Model (Law et al., 1996) supports occupation-based intervention and the application of occupational analyses, particularly when applying other models of human occupation. The PEO Model may be seen as a foundational conceptual framework for occupational analyses as it facilitates an understanding of how an individual, group or community may choose meaningful occupations. It also facilitates communication within and outside the profession through a common language of occupation-based domains (Strong et al., 1999). The model assumes that the three major domains (person, environment, occupation) continually interact across time and space in ways that increase or decrease their support for occupational performance. Law et al. (1996) posited that a person is active, determined and perpetual in building skills and

attributes, across the lifespan, while interacting with various occupations and environments (Fig. 14.2). If the interaction and overlap of domains is greater, it is assumed that the occupational performance is better supported and therefore more satisfying and meaningful for the person (Law et al., 1996). In a meaningful occupation, the human skills and capacities (of the person) are acknowledged and the environmental context is explored and accounted for through person-centred approaches to intervention. When the interaction between domains is optimal, the person will pursue occupational choices that are meaningful and satisfying.

In-depth understanding of the person–environment–occupation dynamic supports the occupational analysis as it recognises what is required for full participation (person: skills, attributes, roles, habits, spiritual capacity) and how and where the activity/occupation is performed (environments: physical, social, cultural, economic, political). In addition, the personal meaning behind the chosen occupations (tasks and activities comprising necessary functions of daily life) is acknowledged and pursued in order to maintain participation and engagement.

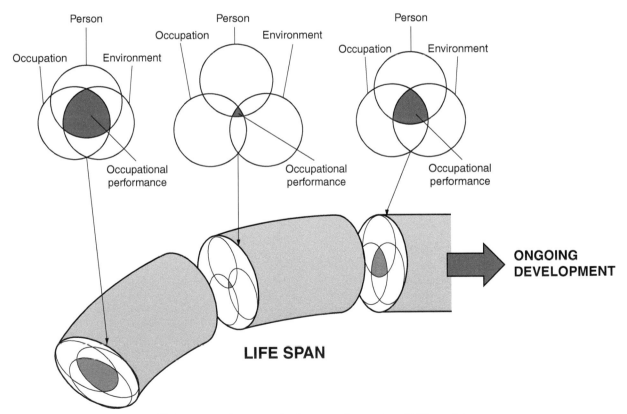

FIG. 14.2 ■ The Person-Environment-Occupation (PEO) model.

A thorough analysis of the environmental contexts must also be implemented to fully enable participation and engagement at the micro, macro and community levels (Leclair, 2010).

Environmental contexts can accommodate or constrain adaptation as they are never static. These contexts function as a feedback loop – for example, the context can affect behaviour, but in turn, behaviour influences the environmental context. Intervention planning comprises activity and occupational analyses, thereby supporting the inclusion of the PEO Model as an appropriate theoretical framework to guide occupational therapy practice applications (Strong et al., 1999). The occupational therapist enables this pursuit and supports meaningful choice through occupational analysis.

The Person-Environment-Occupation Model for Preanalysis

The PEO Model as a framework (Law et al., 1996) may be chosen to support a *preanalysis* step to set the context of the activity leading to occupational analysis. A preanalysis builds on values of purposeful, meaningful activity and occupation-based frameworks and promotes an understanding of the person-based and occupation-based contexts (Perlman, Weston, & Gisel, 2010; Perlman & Gisel, 2000). By first reflecting on the domains of the PEO Model, the occupational therapist gains an appreciation and understanding for the specific contexts of the person, environment and occupation, so that the occupational analysis remains aligned with the tenets of occupation-based and values-based perspectives. The preanalysis (Perlman & Gisel, 2000) format presented in Table 14.4 allows the therapist to do the following:

■ Build on prior knowledge of occupation-based models and meaningful activities through the sequence of steps
■ Review the domains of occupation-based models and appreciate the dynamic relationship between each domain and the impact on performance and participation
■ Recognise the components of two models of occupation: CMOP-E (Townsend & Polatajko, 2013) and MOHO (Kielhofner, 2008); these two models provide a comprehensive framework for an occupational analysis
■ Analyse more complex situations and occupations and focus on salient issues for enablement of occupation relevant to specific clients

Essential Domains for Occupational Analysis

Embracing the PEO framework provides a scaffold for an occupational analysis comprising the specific subdomains that should be included in the analysis. A generic list of subdomains or characteristics under each domain of the person, environment and occupation that should be included in an occupational analysis are listed in Table 14.5. This framework aligns well with the two evidence-based models of occupation: CMOP-E (Townsend & Polatajko, 2013) and MOHO (Kielhofner, 2008). These two

models focus on domains reflective of human occupation (performance skills and choice making), the person's attributes and skills and his or her dynamic interactions with the physical, social, cultural and institutional environments. The CMOP-E (Townsend & Polatajko, 2013) comprises the domains of the person (motor, cognitive, affective and spiritual), the occupation (productivity, leisure and self-care) and the environment (physical, social, cultural and institutional). It embraces person-centred enablement of occupation across the lifespan and supports a vision for health, well-being and occupational justice. The model postulates that engagement in meaningful occupations leads to occupational development, competence and identity, which are linked to spirituality (a source of self-determination and personal control through occupational choices).

The MOHO (Kielhofner, 2008) advances an understanding that human occupation is chosen (volition), organised and patterned through habits and roles (habituation) and performed (performance capacity) within an environmental context (physical, temporal, sociocultural). Occupation is described through a person's participation, occupational performance and skills (motor, process, social and communication skills) while doing (subjective experience through the lived body) within an environmental context (Kielhofner, 2008). Each environmental context affords opportunities, resources, demands and constraints, thereby dynamically influencing the person and occupation. This model also embraces person-centred enablement of occupation (person's unique attributes and values) across the lifespan and supports occupational competence and self-identity through purposeful, meaningful doing.

The assumptions to support each model's proximity to occupation-based practice through person-centred enablement and its influence on health and well-being are presented in Table 14.8. In addition, a comparison of the domains of the CMOP-E (Townsend & Polatajko, 2013) and the MOHO (Kielhofner, 2008) with the PEO domains to highlight their association with occupation-based concepts that support an occupational analysis is also presented in Table 14.6.

Application of an Occupational Analysis: Examples Using the CMOP-E and MOHO

An example of the occupational analysis of environment domain of the CMOP-E (Townsend & Polatajko, 2013) as Bernice participates in the occupation of grocery shopping is provided in Table 14.7. The analysis remains specific to the environmental context of the large community-based grocery store. The subdomains of the environment are identified as physical (settings natural or built; objects and space), social (social groups and interactions at the micro [personal], meso [families or work groups] and macro [societal] levels), cultural (values, beliefs, life experiences) and institutional (economic, political, legal and societal influences). These environmental domains may offer facilitators or barriers to participation, engagement and performance.

TABLE 14.6			
Comparison of Domains of Two Models of Occupation, the CMOP-E and the MOHO, with the Domains of the PEO Model			
Model	**PEO (Law et al., 1996)**	**CMOP-E (Townsend & Polatajko, 2013)**	**MOHO (Kielhofner, 2008)**
Assumption	Explains person-centred enablement through the dynamic relationship of the person, environment and occupation. Changes in one domain will influence the others and will affect occupational performance and satisfaction	Explains person-centred occupational therapy enablement of occupation to ensure occupational engagement, participation and adaptation. The model envisions health, well-being and justice as attainable through occupation and embraces the dynamic relationship among the person, environment and occupation	Explains how human occupations are motivated (volition), patterned through doing (habituation – habits and roles), and performed (performance capacity) within everyday environmental contexts. These occupations influence the capacity for occupational identity, competence and adaptation through the dynamic relationship among the person, environment and occupation
Domains	Person	Person ■ Physical ■ Cognitive ■ Affective ■ Spiritual	Person ■ Volition ■ Habituation ■ Performance capacity
	Environment	Environment ■ Physical ■ Social ■ Cultural ■ Institutional	Environment ■ Physical ■ Temporal ■ Sociocultural
	Occupation	Occupation ■ Productivity ■ Leisure ■ Self-care	Occupation/doing ■ Participation ■ Performance ■ Skills

CMOP-E, Canadian Model of Occupational Performance and Engagement; *MOHO,* Model of Human Occupation; *PEO,* Person-Environment-Occupation Model.

TABLE 14.7			
Application of CMOP-E for Grocery Shopping: Domain of Environment			
Physical	**Social**	**Cultural**	**Institutional**
■ Built space ■ Objects and equipment required (cart, bags, money, credit cards, purse) ■ Aisles to navigate ■ Obstacles to navigate ■ Food items ■ Nonfood items	■ Interaction with staff to request items or ask for assistance ■ Interaction with child and/or family member ■ Interaction with cashier	■ Value activity as a leisure occupation (mother/child outing) ■ Value the productivity role as homemaker, wife, mother ■ Choose culturally specific, meaningful food items ■ Perform activity at own pace, be respectful of personal preferences	■ Follow rules and regulations of public space including not eating food without paying ■ Respect other shoppers ■ Pay for all items ■ Bring recyclable shopping bags ■ Expectation to load bags into car and to return cart

CMOP-E, Canadian Model of Occupational Performance and Engagement

An example of the occupational analysis of the domain of volition of the MOHO (Kielhofner, 2008) as Bernice participates in the occupation of grocery shopping is provided in Table 14.8. The analysis remains specific to Bernice's skills, attributes, roles, habits and spiritual capacity as she performs the activity within the environmental context of the large community-based grocery store. The subdomains of volition are identified as *personal causation* (knowledge of skill capacity and self-efficacy), *values* (personal values/beliefs, sense of obligation) and *interests* (attraction and preferences of a given activity). The volitional domain can be used to explain how Bernice anticipates, chooses, experiences and interprets the grocery shopping activity in its entirety, thereby influencing her occupational engagement. Success in engagement will be determined by her thoughts and feelings about her own capacity for mastery, her values and her enjoyment and satisfaction attributed to the tasks of grocery shopping.

THERAPEUTIC APPLICATION OF ACTIVITY AND OCCUPATIONAL ANALYSES

Grading and Adapting an Occupation

Once an occupational analysis is complete and the intrinsic values of the activity and environment are described, the occupational therapist will then grade or adapt the activity components or environmental factors to understand its meaning and value to an individual. Both grading and adapting foster change and adaptation that potentially leads to greater participation and engagement, as well as increased independence.

Grading is a modification of the occupational challenge (either increased or decreased) for a person as that person performs the activity (Thomas, 2012). Hersch et al. (2005) suggested that this is done by using the results of the occupational analysis and then working backwards to find a way to change the task to allow successful completion. This can be achieved by progressively changing the task complexity, the steps, the physical assistance, the social interaction or the environmental demands. In addition, the demands of the sequence of steps and temporal variables should be considered, including timing or scheduling of the activity during specific times of the day, week or month and the duration of the whole activity. To grade the occupation for success, consider the most challenging activity demands for the person and the impact of these demands on performance and satisfaction.

Examples of grading an occupation include the following:

- Reducing steps or repetitions of movements to promote completion
- Providing preprepared materials to eliminate task components

---

TABLE 14.8

Application of the MOHO Occupational Analysis for Grocery Shopping: Domain of Volition

PERSONAL CAUSATION		VALUES		INTERESTS	
Knowledge of Capacity	**Sense of Efficacy**	**Personal Convictions**	**Sense of Obligation**	**Attraction**	**Interests**
■ Organisational skills for planned outing: shopping list, materials, child and transportation by car ■ Drive car to grocery store ■ Choose food and nonfood items according to list ■ Restriction of navigation of whole store due to fatigue and decreased endurance ■ May choose lighter items	■ Appropriate control of organisational and choice-making skills ■ Decreased control of physical endurance and strength to complete activity and carry heavy bags — may affect choice of items on a given day	■ Values activity to fulfil roles as homemaker, wife, mother and daughter ■ Values choice making and selection of culturally preferred items ■ Values activity for social participation in her community ■ Values choice making for health promotion	■ To fulfil roles as homemaker, wife, mother and daughter ■ To complete this instrumental activity of daily living with success, leading to food preparation for family	■ Social participation and social outing in community ■ Fulfilment of roles as wife, mother, daughter and homemaker	■ Grocery shopping as a weekly pleasurable activity ■ Social outing with child and mother ■ Choice making of culturally preferred food items

MOHO, Model of Human Occupation.

- Providing lighter weight materials to facilitate grasp or increase endurance
- Pairing up two individuals to complete one activity
- Positioning all materials on the functional side for easy access

Adapting is explained as modifying or changing an aspect of the occupation or environment with the goal of allowing participation or increased independence (Thomas, 2012). Although adapting shares similarities to grading, the objective is not to increase or decrease the demands of the activity on the person. An occupational therapist can creatively adapt the task or the environment to improve the individual's ability to perform and succeed at the chosen activity (Hinjosa & Kramer, 1997). This can involve changing components of the environment such as physical space, tools and equipment, lighting and sensory input or may involve the provision of adaptive technologies. Technologies are comprised of technical aids, adaptive supports and virtual or simulated environments that enable participation. Technology in its simple (low) or complex (high) forms supports an adaptive intervention approach that promotes acquisition or restoration of compensatory skills, habits and routines and is often integrated when grading and adapting activities or occupations. An example of a simple low-technology adaptation is the application of a built-up handle of a spoon to facilitate self-feeding. An example of more complex, high-technology grading application is the use of motion capture sensors through a virtual program, such as *Jintronix*, to stimulate range of motion of the upper extremity and provide biofeedback to the person who will use the technology.

Examples of adapting an occupation include the following:

- Providing a tool that allows for a modified grasp (i.e. replace a conventional computer mouse with a joystick mouse for easier grasp and manipulation)
- Providing prompting or personal assistance with the activity (i.e. verbal prompting to guide actions to complete a puzzle; hand-over-hand support to brush teeth)
- Providing online support to ensure participation (i.e. online shopping with home delivery)
- Choosing a time of day when a location is likely to be less occupied and overstimulating (i.e. playing in a park early in the morning rather than midmorning)
- Reading a book with an enlarged font (for visual impairments) or with a condensed story line (for attention difficulties)
- Engaging in a simplified version of a board game to promote successful participation

A number of possible ways that the occupation of grocery shopping can be graded or adapted for Bernice are presented in Table 14.9. The activity demands are reflective of Bernice's challenges with decreased upper extremity strength, fatigue and decreased endurance.

CONCLUSION

An overview of the concepts of task analysis, activity analysis and occupational analysis within occupation-based frameworks has been provided in this chapter. These analyses are recognised to form a continuum of the analysis process and are appreciated from an occupation-based perspective, in which meaningful occupation is proximal and essential to occupational therapy

TABLE 14.9		
Grading and Adapting of Grocery Shopping for Bernice		
Activity Demands (challenges)	**Grade**	**Adapt**
Complete navigation of circumference of grocery store	■ Preplan route to minimise backtracking ■ Decrease the time allowance per shopping trip by scheduling a second trip to grocery store within the week, to complete shopping list	■ Use a scooter provided by store to reduce walking and to conserve energy ■ Use an online shopping/delivery service
Manoeuvre cart through stops and starts	■ Reduce selection of number of weighted items to reduce cart weight ■ Minimise starts and stops of cart by reducing items for purchase on a given visit	■ Use smallest cart available to reduce weight ■ Ensure chosen cart is easy to manoeuver
Reach and grasp objects from shelf or produce bin	■ Use bilateral grasp for heavier objects ■ Select items within reach on shelf ■ Ensure cart is within close proximity to minimise distance object is carried	■ Ask for assistance from her mother (or staff) for items that are too high or too heavy
Hold objects and release into grocery cart	■ Use bilateral grasp for heavier objects and hold closer to body ■ Limit number of items in bags to decrease weight	■ Ask for assistance from mother (or staff) for heavier items

TABLE 14.9
Grading and Adapting of Grocery Shopping for Bernice *(Continued)*

Activity Demands (challenges)	Grade	Adapt
	■ Ensure cart is within close proximity to minimise length of time object is grasped and released	■ Use online services for heavier items and personally shop for lighter, more manageable items
Release apples in bag and twisting bag to close	■ Secure placement of plastic bag on top of apples or in cart to minimise weight of bag as apples are released ■ Buy preselected bag of apples	■ Use plastic reusable clips to close bag rather than twisting or knotting
Attend to active child in child seat of cart	■ Actively engage child in shopping experience (provide pictures of items to be purchased; play 'I Spy' game). ■ Reduce time of shopping trips to habituate child to the routine of grocery shopping	■ Find childcare for child ■ Ask her mother to assist in keeping child safely seated in cart while she shops ■ Ask her mother gather items while she engages her child in other shopping experiences
Complete grocery shopping activity within 45 minute time frame	■ Shop for items only itemised on shopping list ■ Set watch or phone timer to monitor time frame ■ Follow preplanned route	■ Shop during early morning or evening hours when store is less occupied ■ Wear comfortable shoes and clothing to facilitate efficiency of movements

intervention. The continuum of the analysis process begins with a task analysis describing the sequence and timing of actions or list of steps within an activity. An activity analysis then examines the skills and context of the activity in the environment. Finally, an occupational analysis, the perspective most unique to the profession of occupational therapy, validates the meaning of the activity for the specific person performing it within a chosen environmental context. An activity becomes an occupation when it becomes meaningful to the person performing it.

Theoretical practice models are useful to occupational therapists as a tool to enable analysis of occupations to help guide their interventions. The PEO Model (Law et al., 1996) provides foundational support for occupation-based application of activity/occupational analyses and highlights the dynamic and influential relationship among the person, environment and occupation. The outcome of this dynamic relationship is occupational performance, comprised of interpretations and experiences of the person so that meaning of the occupation is personally expressed. The CMOP-E (Townsend & Polatajko, 2013) and the MOHO (Kielhofner, 2008), two occupation-based models of practice aligned with the concepts and philosophy of the PEO Model (Law et al., 1996), are applied to the occupational analyses. They each focus on domains reflective of human occupation (performance skills and choice making), the person's attributes and skills, and his or her interactions with the physical, social, cultural and institutional environments.

Occupational therapists have the expertise to assess the environment, inherent sequence and timing of occupations, as well as the required skills and capacities needed for participation in an activity or occupation, to achieve a therapeutic outcome. By grading and adapting activities or occupations, personal meaning is reinforced, potentially leading to greater participation, engagement and independence. This outcome further fosters health, well-being and quality of life for people receiving occupational therapy services.

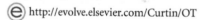 http://evolve.elsevier.com/Curtin/OT

REFERENCES

Aiken, F. E., Fourt, A. M., Cheng, I. K. S., & Polatajko, H. J. (2011). The meaning gap in occupational therapy: Finding meaning in our own occupation. *Canadian Journal of Occupational Therapy, 78*(5), 294–302.

Allen, C. K. (1982). Independence through activity: The practice of occupational therapy (psychiatry). *American Journal of Occupational Therapy, 36*(11), 731–739.

Bauerschmidt, B., & Nelson, D. L. (2011). The terms occupation and activity over the history of official occupational therapy publications. *American Journal of Occupational Therapy, 65*(3), 338–345.

Blesedell Crepeau, E., Gillen, G., & Scaffa, M. E. (2013). Analyzing occupations and activity. In B. A. Schell, G. Gillen, M. E. Scaffa, & E. S. Cohn (Eds.), *Willard and Spackman's occupational therapy* (12th ed., pp. 234–248). Baltimore, MD: Lippincott Williams & Wilkins.

Canadian Association of Occupational Therapists (2002). *Enabling occupation: An occupational therapy perspective.* Ottawa: CAOT Publications ACE.

Clair, V. A., & Newcombe, D. B. (2014). Values and ethics in practice-based decision making. *Canadian Journal of Occupational Therapy, 81*(3), 154–162.

Fidler, G. S., & Fidler, J. W. (1978). Doing and becoming: Purposeful action and self-actualization. *American Journal of Occupational Therapy, 32*(5), 305–310.

Fisher, A. G. (2013). Occupation-centred, occupation-based, occupation-focused: Same, same or different? *Scandinavian Journal of Occupational Therapy, 20*(3), 162–173.

Fulford, K. L. M. (2004). Ten principles of values-based medicine (VBM). In T. Schramme, & J. Thome (Eds.), *Philosophy and psychiatry* (pp. 50–82). Berlin: Walter de Gruyter.

Gray, J. M. (1998). Putting occupation into practice: Occupation as ends, occupation as means'. *American Journal of Occupational Therapy, 52*(5), 354–364.

Hersch, G. I., Lamport, N. K., & Coffey, M. S. (2005). *Activity analysis: Application to occupation* (5th ed.). Thorofare, NJ: Slack.

Hinjosa, J., & Kramer, P. (1997). Statement – Fundamental concepts of occupational therapy: Occupation, purposeful activity, and function. *American Journal of Occupational Therapy, 51*(10), 864–866.

Hinojosa, J., Sabari, J., & Pedretti, L. (1993). Position paper: Purposeful activity. *American Journal of Occupational Therapy, 47*(12), 1081–1082.

Hitch, D., Pepin, G., & Stagnitti, K. (2014). In the footsteps of Wilcock, Part One: The evolution of doing, being, becoming, and belonging. *Occupational Therapy in Health Care, 28*(3), 231–246.

Kielhofner, G. (2008). *Model of human occupation: Theory and application* (4th ed.). Baltimore, MD: Lippincott Williams & Wilkins.

Law, M., Baptiste, S., Carswell, A., McColl, M. A., Polatajko, H. J., & Pollock, N. (2014). *Canadian occupational performance measure* (5th ed.). Ottawa: CAOT Publications ACE.

Law, M., Cooper, B., Strong, S., Stewart, D., Rigby, P., & Letts, L. (1996). The person-environment-occupation model: A transactive approach to occupational performance. *Canadian Journal of Occupational Therapy, 63*(1), 9–23.

Leclair, L. L. (2010). Re-examining concepts of occupation and occupation-based models: Occupational therapy and community development. *Canadian Journal of Occupational Therapy, 77*(1), 15–21.

Letts, L. J. (2011). Muriel Driver Memorial Lecture 2011: Optimal positioning of occupational therapy. *Canadian Journal of Occupational Therapy, 78*(4), 209–217.

Mosey, A. C. (1986). *Psychological components of occupational therapy.* New York: Raven Press.

Nelson, D. L. (1997). The 1997 Eleanor Clarke Slagle Lecture: Why the profession of occupational therapy will flourish in the 21st century. *American Journal of Occupational Therapy, 51*(1), 11–24.

Peloquin, S. M. (2005). The 2005 Eleanor Clarke Slagle Lecture: Embracing our ethos, reclaiming our heart. *American Journal of Occupational Therapy, 59*(6), 611–625.

Perlman, C., & Gisel, E. (2000). *Pre-analysis: Web-based tutorial for activity analysis. OCC1 550-002 Enabling Human Occupation (MYcourses).* Montreal, Canada: McGill University.

Perlman, C., Weston, C., & Gisel, E. (2005). A web-based tutorial to enhance student learning of activity analysis. *Canadian Journal of Occupational Therapy, 72*(3), 153–163.

Perlman, C., Weston, C., & Gisel, E. (2010). Enabling meaningful learning through web-based instruction with occupational therapy students. *Educational Technology Research & Development, 58*(2), 191–210.

Pierce, D. (2001). Untangling occupation and activity. *American Journal of Occupational Therapy, 55*(2), 138–146.

Polatajko, H. J., & Davis, J. A. (2012). Advancing occupation-based practice: Interpreting the rhetoric. *Canadian Journal of Occupational Therapy, 79*(5), 259–263.

Polatajko, H. J., Mandich, A., & Martini, R. (2000). Dynamic performance analysis: A framework for understanding occupational performance. *American Journal of Occupational Therapy, 54*(1), 65–72.

Reed, K. D., Hocking, C. S., & Smythe, L. A. (2011). Exploring the meaning of occupation: The case for phenomenology. *Canadian Journal of Occupational Therapy, 78*(5), 303–309.

Strong, S., Rigby, P., Stewart, D., Law, M., Letts, L., & Cooper, B. (1999). Application of the person-environment-occupation model: A practical tool. *Canadian Journal of Occupational Therapy, 65*(3), 122–133.

Thomas, H. (2012). *Occupation-based activity analysis.* Thorofare, NJ: Slack.

Thomas, H. (2015). *Occupation-based activity analysis* (2nd ed.). Thorofare, NJ: Slack.

Townsend, E. A., & Polatajko, H. J. (2013). *Enabling occupation II: Advancing an occupational therapy vision for health, well-being & justice through occupation* (2nd ed.). Ottawa: CAOT Publications ACE.

Wilcock, A. A. (1998). International perspective: Reflections on doing, being and becoming. *Canadian Journal of Occupational Therapy, 65*(5), 248–256.

Wilcock, A. A. (2006). *An occupational perspective of health* (2nd ed.). Thorofare, NJ: Slack.

Wilcock, A. A. (2007). Occupation and health: Are they one and the same? *Journal of Occupational Science, 14*(1), 3–8.

Wilding, C., & Whiteford, G. (2007). Occupation and occupational therapy: Knowledge paradigms and everyday practice. *Australian Occupational Therapy Journal, 54*(3), 185–193.

15

DYNAMIC PERFORMANCE ANALYSIS

ROSE MARTINI ■ DOROTHY KESSLER

Abstract

Dynamic performance analysis (DPA) is a task-oriented, performance-based approach to occupational performance analysis that is centred on the person's actual performance of an occupation or activity. The purpose of DPA is to identify a person's performance problems or breakdowns. The analysis process focuses on the dynamic transaction of the activity, person and environment relative to the person's performance of the activity and not on the components necessary for that performance. The DPA process (depicted by a decision tree) begins by observing the person perform the activity and identifying whether performance is competent or not, taking note of the errors or breakdowns. For each performance breakdown, an iterative analysis process is undertaken that considers the person, the activity and the environmental context. Two practice stories, with illustrated decision trees, are presented to guide the reader through this iterative analysis process.

KEY POINTS

■ Dynamic performance analysis (DPA) is an analysis process that focuses on the actual performance of an occupation or activity so as to be able to identify performance problems or breakdowns (Polatajko, Mandich, & Martini, 2000).

■ Although activity analysis is usually done without a particular person in mind, DPA requires the observation of the person performing the activity.

■ DPA is a nonstandarised performance analysis process that can be used with any activity and anyone receiving occupational therapy.

■ DPA is a task-oriented assessment process that is continuous and iterative and can be applied not only at the beginning and end of the intervention but continuously throughout the intervention sessions.

■ In addition to being a tool for therapists to use, DPA may be considered an ability that can be developed by people receiving occupational therapy services, which may be key for improving skill performance and intertask transfer.

INTRODUCTION

Activity analysis is useful to identify potential activity demands and required performance skills. However, activity analysis does not generally allow for consideration of the individualised, interactive and dynamic components of real-time task performance by a specific individual. Dynamic Performance Analysis (DPA) was developed to meet this need. DPA is a performance-based approach to occupational performance analysis. The analysis process focuses on the actual performance of an occupation or activity and the identification of performance problems or breakdowns (Polatajko et al., 2000). DPA evolved in the context of the development of a person-centred, top-down intervention approach called Cognitive Orientation to daily Occupational Performance CO-OP Approach™ (Polatajko et al., 2000). The CO-OP Approach™ is a metacognitive problem-solving approach in which a therapist guides individuals to identify their task performance breakdowns and discover strategies that will enable them to overcome or solve the issues identified (Polatajko & Mandich, 2004). To be able to guide a person through this metacognitive problem-solving process, the therapist needs to first identify where during task performance the performance breaks down. Such analysis requires the observation of actual task performance.

PERFORMANCE ANALYSIS

When occupational therapists talk about *performance,* they tend to refer to an accomplishment or an execution of an occupation, activity, task or action. For each of these levels, a person's performance proficiency is the result of a dynamic interaction among the activity, person and environment. The ability to examine and analyse activities is a fundamental skill for occupational therapists to develop and provides the therapist with an understanding of what is needed to perform an activity. Whereas the activity analysis processes recognises the interaction among person, occupation and environment factors, the focus of the analyses remains targeted on the underlying components from each of these dimensions. When an occupational therapist carries out an activity analysis, the activity is analysed as it is typically done, without a particular person in mind (Thomas, 2012). To understand the intricacies of a particular person's performance breakdown, activity analysis is not enough; a performance analysis must be done.

Performance analysis is embedded in a top-down, task-oriented framework and based on the direct observation of a person performing a desired, needed, or expected occupation or activity (Fisher, 1997, 2013; Fisher & Griswold, 2014; Polatajko et al., 2000). The focus is on the quality of the dynamic transaction among the elements (of activity or occupation, person, and environment) with respect to the person's performance of the activity or task, rather than the components necessary for performance (Fisher, 2013; Fisher & Griswold, 2014). In this type of analysis, the units of observations are the skills required for accomplishing the activity or occupation. For example, the skills required for the activity of putting on socks are: grasping sock, orienting sock to foot, pulling sock onto foot. Each skill itself is a result of a goal-directed transaction among the person, the occupation and the environment (Fisher & Griswold, 2014).

Standardised performance analysis procedures exist, such as the Assessment of Motor and Process Skills (Fisher, 1997), a standardised, observational assessment that is used to assess the quality of a person's performance in real-life tasks, and the Activities of Daily Living Profile (Dutil, Bottari, Vanier, & Gaudreault, 2005), developed to assess everyday activities of people with traumatic brain injury (TBI). Fisher and Griswold (2014) describe several advantages of using a standardised performance analysis it allows objectivity of analysis, consistency in evaluation practices, and facilitated interpretation of results by virtue of established criterion measures and normative values. On the other hand, these authors also identify: (a) the formal training needed to be able to administer these assessments as a disadvantage of these standardised analysis instruments; (b) the lack of flexibility these instruments provide with respect to the tasks and activities encompassed; and (c) lack of generalisability to other populations.

A significant advantage of a nonstandardised performance analysis process, such as DPA, is that it does not require costly therapist training, it affords unlimited flexibility with respect to the activities and tasks that can be analysed, and it can be conducted with people experiencing a broad range of difficulties. Furthermore, this dynamic assessment process permits a continuous and iterative assessment process, not only at the beginning and end of the intervention, but throughout the intervention sessions.

DYNAMIC PERFORMANCE ANALYSIS

DPA is a top-down, task-oriented framework for analysing occupational performance applicable to all occupations, activities and tasks. Although its development began with the analysis of task performance of children with developmental coordination disorder, it is not limited to use with people of any particular age or diagnosis. Unlike activity analysis, in DPA the reference point is not the typical way a task is done. Rather, the occupational therapist bases his or her analysis on the *person's* way of doing the task, taking into consideration the person's characteristics, the occupation and the environment, all in interaction with each other (Polatajko et al., 2000).

The Hierarchy of Occupational Performance

Occupational performance can be understood as having different levels of complexity (Polatajko et al., 2012), and in DPA it is important to understand the hierarchical structure of occupational performance (Polatajko, Davis, Stewart, et al., 2007) whereby the occupation is composed of a set of activities and activities are composed of a set of tasks, which are composted of a set of actions. These actions, in turn, are composed of voluntary movements or mental processes (Polatajko et al., 2007). It is important to note that each higher level of this hierarchical structure subsumes the characteristics of those below it, permitting a therapist to focus on a particular level of performance at a time (Polatajko et al., 2000). For instance, when considering the occupation of *self-care* (Fig. 15.1) the activities may include *dressing, bathing, toileting,* and so on. Each of these activities are composed

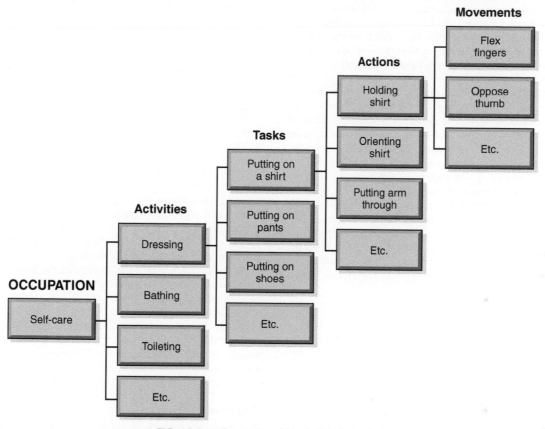

FIG. 15.1 ■ Occupational hierarchy of dressing.

of different tasks; *dressing,* for example, can involve *putting on a shirt, putting on pants, putting on shoes,* and so on. Similarly, each of these tasks will consist of actions; *putting on a shirt,* for example, may require *holding the shirt, orienting the shirt, raising the arm,* and so on. Finally, each of these actions are composed of individual voluntary movements or mental processes; when *holding a shirt,* for example, one needs to *flex fingers, oppose thumb,* and so on. When undertaking a DPA, it is helpful to keep this hierarchical nature of occupational performance in mind.

Other than the occupational performance, which is the central aspect of the DPA, two other elements need to be considered before going ahead with the dynamic analysis: the therapist and the person doing the occupation, activity, task, action or movement (the performer).

Therapist Prerequisites

To successfully carry out a DPA, it is helpful if the therapist enters the process with the following four prerequisites.

1. It is important for the therapist to begin the process with a *task-orientation or top-down mind set.* The focus in DPA is on the activity and sublevels of activity, rather than on the person's weakness impairment (e.g. strength, coordination, balance, etc.) in relation to the activity demands and performance skills (as is the case in activity analysis). When the focus is on the person's impairment and activity demands, the tendency is to identify problems with respect to how a person would typically do a task, rather than pay attention to the fit between the occupation and environment and the person's abilities, skills and actions (Polatajko & Mandich, 2004). The aim with DPA is to identify at what point in the activity (task or action), a person's performance breaks down. Only after the activity performance breakdown is identified can the therapist then examine the person–occupation–environment interaction to determine how to overcome this breakdown.

2. The therapist needs to *have a certain level of knowledge with respect to the occupation or activity at hand.* It is difficult to identify where a performance is breaking down if the therapist does not know or understand the activity.

3. The therapist appreciates that *there is more than one way to do things*. Unlike activity analysis, where a specific manner of doing an activity forms the template for the analysis, DPA recognises that there is more than one way to achieve a task or action. For the activity of dressing, for instance, the task of putting on a pair of pants requires putting both legs into the pant legs. This can be done by: (a) standing and putting one leg into a pant leg at a time, (b) sitting on a chair and putting one leg into a pant leg at a time, or (c) sitting on a chair and putting both legs into both pant legs at the same time. Any one of these three methods will accomplish the task of putting both legs into the pant legs (other methods may also exist). Although one method may be the more 'typical' method or the more 'preferred' by the therapist, this may or may not be the method used or selected by the person to whom the therapist is providing services.

4. To undertake a DPA, the therapist needs to actually observe the person doing the activity or task, to identify where the performance breakdown occurs. This is because the actions or methods to achieve a task or activity are contingent on the person.

Performer Prerequisites

From the person's perspective, two prerequisites are required to engage in the occupational performance: *motivation* and *task knowledge* (Polatajko et al., 2000).

1. Motivation is what provides the impetus to do. It not only predicts learning (Pintrich, 2003), but also a person's readiness to learn (Shonkoff & Phillips, 2000). Motivation is necessary for the acquisition and performance of occupations and subsumed activities, tasks and actions. Researchers have shown that motivation is an important factor in the ability to use existing knowledge and skills, as well as to persist when a task becomes extremely challenging (Anshel, Weinberg, & Jackson, 1992; Deci & Ryan, 1992; Dweck, 1986; Miller, Ziviani, Ware, & Boyd, 2014). For an occupation or activity to be initiated, a person must have a minimum level of motivation for that occupation or activity (Polatajko et al., 2000). As such, before embarking on a DPA, the therapist needs to determine whether the person is motivated or willing to perform the activity, task or action being considered. If the person is not motivated or willing to perform the activity or its sublevels, it will not be possible to do a proper DPA.

2. *Task knowledge* refers to the level of understanding the person has about the activity being performed (Polatajko & Mandich, 2004). At least a minimum or basic level of knowledge about the activity is necessary for performance. For instance, to put on a pair of pants, one must have an idea of what pants are and that the two legs go into the pant legs individually. Without basic task knowledge, it will not be possible for the person to initiate task performance and so not possible to undertake a DPA.

DPA Decision Tree

The DPA process is guided by the DPA decision tree (Fig. 15.2). This decision tree provides the therapist with a framework for structuring observations. There are two sets of questions that the therapist will ask himself or herself: *performer prerequisites* and *performance requisites*.

Performer Prerequisites

As described earlier, the purpose of the first set of questions is to determine whether the person has the prerequisites for engaging in the occupational performance. If the person is not motivated or willing to perform the activity,* then the DPA process stops here. The therapist exits the decision tree and explores the person's motivational issues with respect to the activity. Once motivation is addressed, the person is asked to try the activity, and the therapist then determines the person's general level of task knowledge. The therapist does this by questioning or observing the person attempt the activity. If the person does not demonstrate a rudimentary level of task knowledge, the therapist cannot proceed with the DPA. The therapist needs to exit the decision tree and provide the person with information on the activity or demonstrate the task. If the person has basic task knowledge, then she or he can attempt the activity and enter the performance requisites part of the decision tree. As mentioned, DPA is an interactive process. The therapist repeats this line of questioning considering each level of the occupational performance (i.e. occupation, activity, task, action).

Performance Requisites

Once it has been determined that the person possesses the necessary motivation and general task knowledge, the therapist can begin analysing the actual performance. At this point, the person is asked to perform the activity as the therapist observes. The therapists uses task knowledge and observation skills to identify whether the performance is competent or not, taking note of errors or breakdowns. Once the therapist identifies a breakdown, the next series of questions in the decision tree are asked to ascertain the possible source(s) of the difficulties.

For each breakdown, the (a) knowledge, (b) motivation, and (c) competence are verified (depicting the embedded, iterative process of DPA). The person's competence is explored by considering his or her (1) abilities relative to the (2) occupational and (3) environmental demands and supports. Once the sources of the person–occupation–environment imbalance are identified, the therapist can then begin intervention to address these imbalances. This process is undertaken for each identified breakdown as depicted in Figures 15.3 and 15.4.

---

*For the purpose of simplicity, the *activity* level of the occupational hierarchy is being used; however, please note that this can be replaced by any other level (e.g. occupation, task or action).

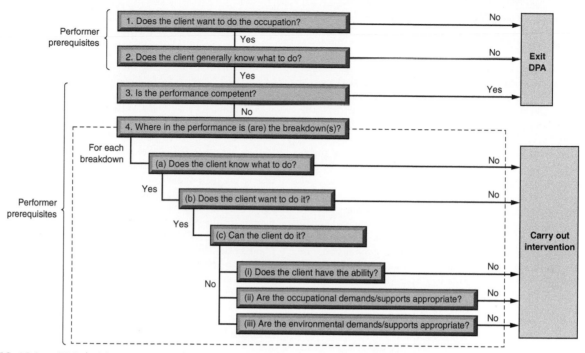

FIG. 15.2 ■ DPA decision tree. *(Reproduced with permission from Polatajko, H. J., Mandich, A., & Martini, R. (2000). Dynamic performance analysis: A framework for understanding occupational performance.* American Journal of Occupational Therapy, 54, 65-72.)

It should be noted that there is a certain hierarchy of break-downs. In some instances, a breakdown can be identified that does not impede the client from continuing with the activity (Practice Story 15.1 and Fig. 15.3). In an such instance, subsequent breakdowns in performance can be identified, resulting in a series of breakdowns that can be addressed. However, there are times when a breakdown does not permit the ongoing performance of the activity (Practice Story 15.2 and Fig. 15.4). In such cases, the therapist needs to address this breakdown before the DPA process can continue for the rest of the activity. In this way intervention can be closely tied to the DPA process. DPA does not just occur before intervention; it is a process that continues throughout the intervention process. Once the breakdown is addressed, the person will be able to continue the activity performance and further breakdowns can be identified if that is the case.

PRACTICE STORY 15.1

Making Tea

Marie was referred to community occupational therapy because her family reported that her memory was decreasing and they were concerned about her ability to cook safely. They had found a stove burner left turned on a few times when visiting her.

The occupational therapist visited Marie in her home and began by interviewing Marie. When talking about her cooking habits, Marie reported that she did not make big meals, just simple meals like soup, a sandwich and tea. She also reported that her children had arranged for one meal a day to be delivered to her and this was usually enough food for the whole day. Marie acknowledged that her children had noticed a stove burner left on when visiting and had made quite a fuss about it. With a bit of probing, Marie admitted that this was a concern for her as well. She did not want to start a fire but wanted to remain in her apartment.

The occupational therapist asked if she could observe Marie making tea to see how she managed and determine whether there was anything that could be done to address her and her family's concerns. Marie agreed, stating that she enjoyed having a quiet cup of tea and had been making tea since she was a young girl. To make tea she had always used a kettle that was boiled on the stove (Steps 1 and 2, Fig. 15.3).

Continued

PRACTICE STORY 15.1

Making Tea (Continued)

While observing Marie making tea Beth noted two areas of performance breakdown. First, when Marie poured the water into the cup, she poured more water on the table than in the teacup. Second, Marie left the stove burner on after the kettle had boiled and replaced the kettle on the burner (Steps 3 and 4, Fig. 15.3).

In analysing the first breakdown, the occupational therapist determined that Marie knew what to do – that is, that water should be poured into the cup instead of on the table (Step 4 Breakdown i-a, Fig. 15.3) and that she did not want to pour the water onto the table and make a mess (Step 4 Breakdown i-b, Fig. 15.3). However, although Marie was physically able to fill the kettle, the kettle shook in her hand when pouring it. On further analysis the occupational therapist determined that Marie was not able to hold the full kettle still with one hand while pouring (Step 4 Breakdown i-c-i, Fig. 15.3) and that the occupational demands were not appropriate because the kettle was too heavy (Step 4 Breakdown i-c-ii, Fig. 15.3). Keeping this analysis in mind, the occupational therapist considered intervention options.

Similarly, when analysing the second breakdown, during which Marie left the stove burner on after the kettle had boiled and replaced the kettle on the burner, the occupational therapist determined that Marie knew that she should turn the stove burner off when she was finished with it and that Marie wanted to remember to turn it off, recognising the fire risk. Despite her physical ability to turn off the burner, during the task Marie did not realise that she had left the burner on. During the performance analysis the occupational therapist determined that (a) Marie did not appear to have the memory ability to consistently remember to turn off the stove burner; (b) the occupational demands or supports were not adequate – that is, the task provided insufficient cues to help Marie notice that the stove burner was still on; and (c) the environmental demands or supports were not appropriate to facilitate competent task completion that is, there were not enough cues in the environment to help Marie notice that the burner is still on. The occupational therapist considered all of these factors when determining an intervention with Marie to enable her make tea in a safe manner.

PRACTICE STORY 15.2

Putting on a Buttoned Shirt

Mr Smith experienced a right hemispheric cerebrovascular accident (CVA) 1 week ago and was recently admitted to an inpatient stroke rehabilitation programme. As a result of the CVA, he had left hemiparesis with a flaccid left upper extremity. He was beginning to have some movement in this arm (e.g. minimal movement at his shoulder and slight finger flexion).

During the initial interview with the occupational therapist Mr Smith commented that he was not able to get dressed by himself and that he was tired of wearing a hospital gown. On further inquiry, the occupational therapist learned that Mr Smith worked in a bank and always wore a buttoned dress shirt. When it was suggested that they could explore ways for Mr Smith to put a buttoned shirt on by himself, Mr Smith sat up straighter and immediately agreed. The occupational therapist arranged to see Mr Smith the following morning.

The occupational therapist had determined that Mr Smith had the performance prerequisites (Steps 1 and 2, Fig. 15.4) of wanting to be able to put on a buttoned shirt and knowing what was involved in putting one on. During the assessment,

he examined whether Mr Smith's performance was competent (Step 3, Fig. 15.4). The occupational therapist noted that Mr Smith began dressing by putting his right arm into the shirt sleeve. After he had his right arm in the sleeve and the shirt pulled around to his left side, he could not get his left arm into the sleeve. At this point, the occupational therapist knew that Mr Smith's performance was not competent and that he had to address this performance breakdown before continuing with the DPA. In analysing this performance breakdown (Step 4, Fig. 15.4) where Mr Smith was not able to reach with his left arm to find the sleeve and push his arm through the sleeve, the occupational therapist determined that Mr Smith knew that both arms needed to go into the shirt sleeves (Step 4 Breakdown i-a, Fig. 15.4) and that he wanted to be able to get both arms into the sleeves (Step 4 Breakdown i-b, Fig. 15.4). However, Mr Smith was not capable of lifting his left arm to position his hand to go into the sleeve (Step 4 Breakdown i-c-i, Fig. 15.4). In addition, the demands of the task based on Mr Smith's usual sequence of putting his right arm into the sleeve first did not allow successful performance (Step 4

Putting on a Buttoned Shirt (Continued)

Breakdown i-c-ii, Fig. 15.4). The occupational therapist implemented an intervention to enable Mr Smith to put both arms into the shirt sleeves and continued with the DPA.

The occupational therapist observed that after putting both arms into the sleeves, Mr Smith straightened his shirt and aligned the buttons. He started to do up the buttons starting with the top button. Mr Smith was able to grasp the button but was not able to get it completely through the buttonhole (Step 4 Breakdown ii, Fig. 15.4). In examining Mr Smith's performance, the occupational therapist determined that Mr Smith knew what was required to fasten a button and that he wanted to be able to do it (Steps 4 Breakdown ii-a & b, Fig. 15.4). He observed that Mr Smith was able to hold the

button of the shirt but was not holding the buttonhole part of the shirt in a way that enabled him to manipulate the button through the hole so that he could grasp it and pull it all the way through (Step 4 Breakdown ii-c, Fig. 15.4). Mr Smith did not have the motor ability in his left hand to assist his right hand by either stabilising the shirt or manipulating the button (Steps 4 Breakdown ii-c-i, Fig. 15.4). In addition, the shirt that Mr Smith had was smooth and a bit slippery and the buttons were small, making the demands of the task more challenging (Step 4 Breakdown ii-c-ii, Fig. 15.4). The occupational therapist discussed intervention options with Mr Smith and together they decided on an intervention approach to enable Mr Smith to be able to do up his buttons.

Collaborative DPA. One of the prerequisites for DPA is that the therapist be able to observe the person participate in the activity. However, there are times that the nature of the activity undertaken makes it impractical for observation. Elements such as (a) the time the activity occurs (e.g. getting ready for bed at night), (b) the duration of the activity (e.g. preparing Christmas dinner), (c) the location of the activity (e.g. at a work site), or (d) the social construct of the activity (e.g. a job interview) render it impossible for a therapist to be present to observe the person in action. At such times, other techniques can be used to initiate DPA, such as talking the person through the task, as used with adults after a traumatic brain injury by Dawson et al. (2009), or talking through and roleplaying, as used with children diagnosed with high functioning autism spectrum disorder by Rodger, Ireland, and Vun (2008); Rodger and Vishram (2010). Through these strategies, the therapist seeks to obtain as much information as possible about how a person does an activity so as to understand how it is actually performed by the person. To ensure proper detailed understanding of the person's performance, a therapist may ask questions to obtain more details or to clarify the information already obtained.

A SKILL FOR DEVELOPMENT

Besides being a tool for therapists to identify occupation performance issues, DPA may also be considered as a skill to develop in the people receiving occupational therapy services. Martini, Wall, and Shore (2004) showed that during their attempt to evaluate their performance, children recognised that something in their performance was not working. Hyland and Polatajko (2012). Unlike their non-DCD peers, the evaluation of children with DCD is inappropriate or inaccurate, leading to ineffective strategy selection. reviewed videos and examined statements of children who received a CO-OP Approach™ intervention and those who did not receive CO-OP Approach™. They found that

children who received CO-OP Approach™ demonstrated a greater number and quality of statements that reflected a DPA and they were able to spontaneously apply DPA to the performance of another child. This finding indicated that DPA may be considered as an ability that can be improved.

Furthermore, Polatajko, McEwen, Ryan, and Baum (2012) suggest that the process of learning DPA plays a role in enabling transfer of strategies and skills to new situations. Indeed, in their multiple-baseline, single-subject investigation (across three participants) on the effectiveness of the CO-OP Approach™ with adults who had experienced cerebrovascular accident, McEwen, Polatajko, Huijbregts, and Ryan (2010) found significant improvement in the skill performance of trained skills as well as transfer to untrained skills. These positive findings are thought to be due to the combination of learning DPA and problem-solving strategies within the context of meaningful skill acquisition (Polatajko et al., 2012).

CONCLUSION

DPA is a performance-based, top-down, task-oriented approach to occupational performance analysis. This analysis process takes into consideration the dynamic interaction between a person's characteristics, the occupation, and the environment. As such, unlike activity analysis, where the analysis is based on the typical way a task is done, in DPA the analysis is based on the *person's* way of doing the task. Its focus is on the actual performance of an occupation or activity and identifying performance problems or breakdowns (Polatajko et al., 2000). DPA is a flexible analysis process that can be applied with any and at all levels of the hierarchical structure of occupational performance as well as any and all client populations. Finally, although DPA was developed as a tool for therapists to use, there are early indications that DPA may be considered an ability that can be developed and that it may be key for improving skill performance and intertask transfer.

Performer prerequisites

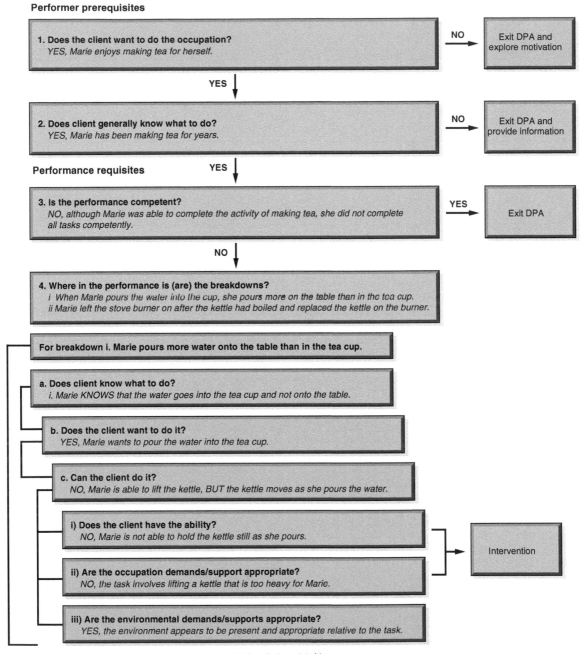

1. **Does the client want to do the occupation?**
   YES, Marie enjoys making tea for herself.

   NO → Exit DPA and explore motivation

   YES ↓

2. **Does client generally know what to do?**
   YES, Marie has been making tea for years.

   NO → Exit DPA and provide information

Performance requisites   YES ↓

3. **Is the performance competent?**
   NO, although Marie was able to complete the activity of making tea, she did not complete all tasks competently.

   YES → Exit DPA

   NO ↓

4. **Where in the performance is (are) the breakdowns?**
   i When Marie pours the water into the cup, she pours more on the table than in the tea cup.
   ii Marie left the stove burner on after the kettle had boiled and replaced the kettle on the burner.

For breakdown i. Marie pours more water onto the table than in the tea cup.

a. Does client know what to do?
   i. Marie KNOWS that the water goes into the tea cup and not onto the table.

b. Does the client want to do it?
   YES, Marie wants to pour the water into the tea cup.

c. Can the client do it?
   NO, Marie is able to lift the kettle, BUT the kettle moves as she pours the water.

i) Does the client have the ability?
   NO, Marie is not able to hold the kettle still as she pours.

ii) Are the occupation demands/support appropriate?
   NO, the task involves lifting a kettle that is too heavy for Marie.

Intervention

iii) Are the environmental demands/supports appropriate?
   YES, the environment appears to be present and appropriate relative to the task.

FIG. 15.3 ■ Making tea.

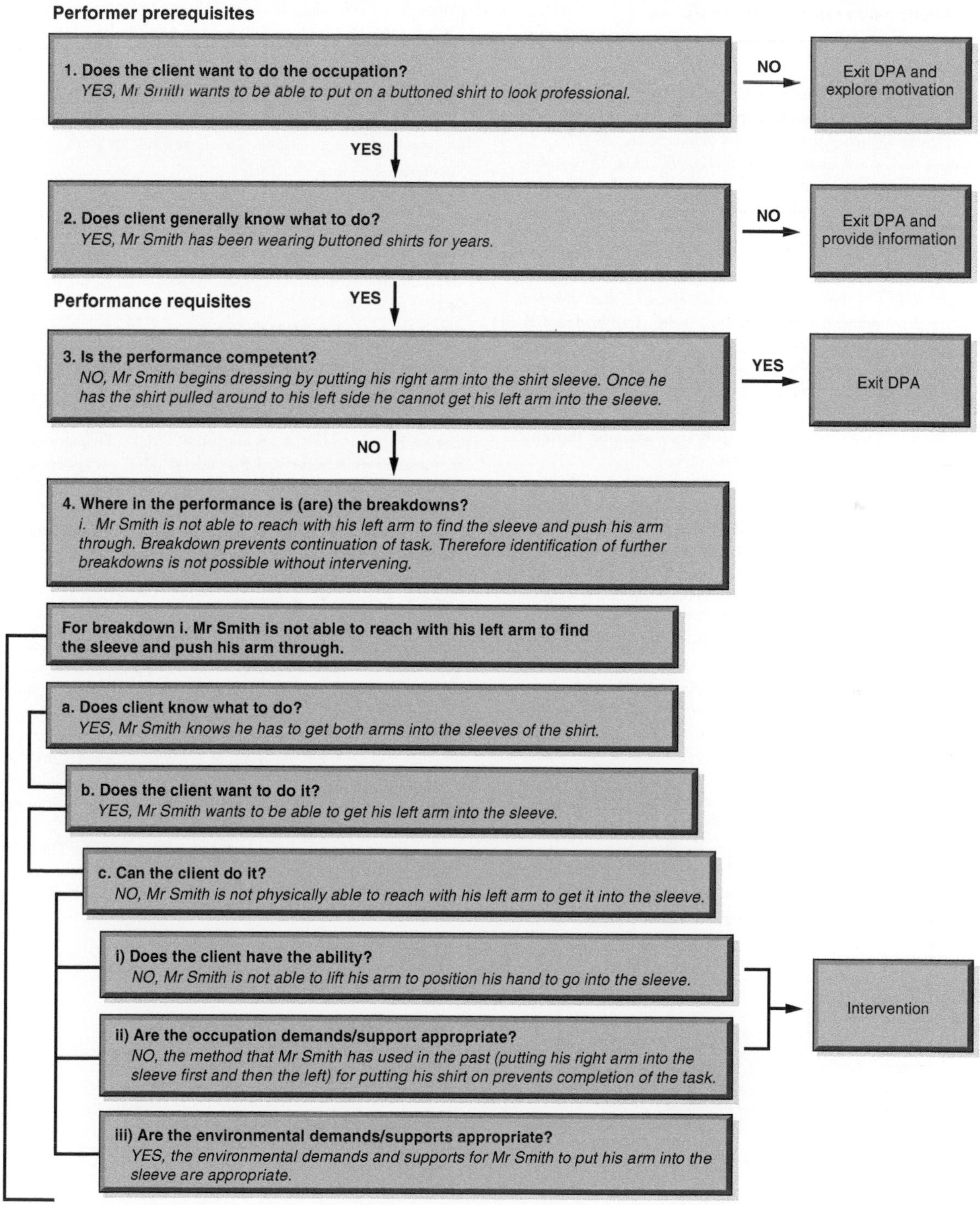

Performer prerequisites

1. Does the client want to do the occupation?
YES, Mr Smith wants to be able to put on a buttoned shirt to look professional.

NO → Exit DPA and explore motivation

YES ↓

2. Does client generally know what to do?
YES, Mr Smith has been wearing buttoned shirts for years.

NO → Exit DPA and provide information

Performance requisites   YES ↓

3. Is the performance competent?
NO, Mr Smith begins dressing by putting his right arm into the shirt sleeve. Once he has the shirt pulled around to his left side he cannot get his left arm into the sleeve.

YES → Exit DPA

NO ↓

4. Where in the performance is (are) the breakdowns?
i. Mr Smith is not able to reach with his left arm to find the sleeve and push his arm through. Breakdown prevents continuation of task. Therefore identification of further breakdowns is not possible without intervening.

For breakdown i. Mr Smith is not able to reach with his left arm to find the sleeve and push his arm through.

a. Does client know what to do?
YES, Mr Smith knows he has to get both arms into the sleeves of the shirt.

b. Does the client want to do it?
YES, Mr Smith wants to be able to get his left arm into the sleeve.

c. Can the client do it?
NO, Mr Smith is not physically able to reach with his left arm to get it into the sleeve.

i) Does the client have the ability?
NO, Mr Smith is not able to lift his arm to position his hand to go into the sleeve.

ii) Are the occupation demands/support appropriate?
NO, the method that Mr Smith has used in the past (putting his right arm into the sleeve first and then the left) for putting his shirt on prevents completion of the task.

iii) Are the environmental demands/supports appropriate?
YES, the environmental demands and supports for Mr Smith to put his arm into the sleeve are appropriate.

Intervention

FIG. 15.4 ■ Putting on a buttoned shirt.

http://evolve.elsevier.com/Curtin/OT

REFERENCES

Anshel, M. H., Weinberg, R., & Jackson, A. (1992). The effects of goal difficulty and task complexity on intrinsic motivation and motor performance. *Journal of Sport Behavior, 15*, 159–176.

Dawson, D. R., Gaya, A., Hunt, A. , et al. (2009). Using the cognitive orientation to occupational performance with adults with traumatic brain injury. *Canadian Journal of Occupational Therapy, 76*, 115–127.

Deci, E. L., & Ryan, R. M. (1992). The initiation and regulation of intrinsically motivated learning and achievement. In A. K. Boggiano, & T. S. Pittman (Eds.), *Achievement and motivation: A social-developmental perspective* (pp. 9–36). Cambridge, UK: Cambridge University Press.

Dutil, E., Bottari, C., Vanier, M., & Gaudreault, C. (2005). *ADL profile: Description of the instrument* (H. Scott & C. Bottari, Trans. 4th ed., vol. 1). Montreal: Les Éditions Émersion.

Dweck, C. S. (1986). Motivational processes affecting learning. *American Psychologist, 41*, 1040–1048.

Fisher, A. G. (1997). Multifaceted measurement of daily life task performance: Conceptualizing a test of instrumental ADL and validating the addition of personal ADL tasks. *Physical Medicine and Rehabilitation: State of the Art Reviews, 11*, 289–303.

Fisher, A. G. (2013). Occupation-centred, occupation-based, occupation-focused: Same, same or different? *Scandinavian Journal of Occupational Therapy, 20*, 162–173.

Fisher, A. G., & Griswold, L. A. (2014). Performance skills: Implementing performance analyses to evaluate quality of occupational performance. In B. A. B. Schell, G. Gillen, M. E. Scaffa, & E. S. Cohn (Eds.), *Willard & Spackman's occupational therapy* (pp. 249–264). (12th ed.). Philadelphia: Wolters Kluwer Lippincott Williams & Wilkins.

Hyland, M., & Polatajko, H. J. (2012). Enabling children with developmental coordination disorder to self-regulate through the use of Dynamic Performance Analysis: Evidence from the CO-OP approach. *Human Movement Science, 31*, 987–998.

Martini, R., Wall, A. E., & Shore, B. M. (2004). Metacognitive processes underlying psychomotor performance in children with differing psychomotor abilities. *Adapted Physical Activity Quarterly, 21*, 248–268.

McEwen, S. E., Polatajko, H. J., Huijbregts, M. P. J., & Ryan, J. D. (2010). Inter-task transfer following a cognitive based treatment: Results of three multiple baseline design experiments in chronic stroke. *Neuropsychological Rehabilitation, 20*, 541–561.

Miller, L., Ziviani, J., Ware, R., & Boyd, R. N. (2014). Mastery motivation in children with congenital hemiplegia: individual and environmental associations. *Developmental Medicine & Child Neurology, 56*, 267–274.

Pintrich, P. R. (2003). A motivational science perspective on the role of student motivation in learning and teaching contexts. *Journal of Educational Psychology, 95*, 667–686.

Polatajko, H., Davis, J., Stewart, D. , et al. (2007). Specifying the domain of concern: Occupation as core. In E. A. Townsend, & H. J. Polatajko (Eds.), *Enabling occupation II: Advancing an occupational therapy vision for health, well-being, & justice through occupation* (pp. 9–36). Ottawa: CAOT Publications ACE.

Polatajko, H. J., & Mandich, A. (2004). *Enabling occupation in children: The Cognitive Orientation to Daily Occupational Performance (CO-OP) approach.* Ottawa: CAOT Publications ACE.

Polatajko, H. J., Mandich, A., & Martini, R. (2000). Dynamic performance analysis: A framework for understanding occupational performance. *American Journal of Occupational Therapy, 54*, 65–72.

Polatajko, H. J., McEwen, S. E., Ryan, J. D., & Baum, C. M. (2012). Brief report – Pilot randomized controlled trial investigating cognitive strategy use to improve goal performance after stroke. *American Journal of Occupational Therapy, 66*, 104–109.

Rodger, S., Ireland, S., & Vun, M. (2008). Can cognitive orientation to daily occupational performance (CO-OP) help children with Asperger's syndrome to master social and organizational goals? *British Journal of Occupational Therapy, 71*(1), 23–32.

Rodger, S., & Vishram, A. (2010). Mastering social and organizational goals: Strategy use by two children with Asperger's syndrome during cognitive orientation to daily occupational performance. *Physical and Occupational Therapy in Pediatrics, 30*(4), 264–276.

Shonkoff, J. P., & Phillips, A. J. (2000). *From Neurons to neighbourhoods: The science of early childhood development.* Washington, DC: The National Academies Press.

Thomas, H. (2012). *Occupation-based activity analysis.* Thorofare, NJ: Slack.

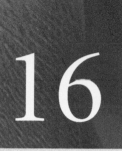

16

ANALYSIS OF OCCUPATIONAL PERFORMANCE: MOTOR, PROCESS AND SOCIAL INTERACTION SKILLS

GILL CHARD ■ SUE MESA

CHAPTER OUTLINE

Abstract

This chapter focuses on occupational performance analysis and provides guidance on how to perform this core skill. Occupational performance analysis is defined and described in the context of the *doing* of a task. A distinction is made between task analysis, activity analysis and occupational performance analysis. Individual performance skills (motor, process and social interaction) are defined and described. A rationale for the use of occupational performance analysis is provided and the Occupational Therapy Practice Framework (American Occupational Therapy Association (AOTA), 2014) is used to define and apply occupation terminology. Occupation is explored from five broad perspectives: occupations, client factors, performance skills, performance patterns, and contexts and environments. Occupational performance analysis is described and applied within a top-down (person-focused) approach. The Assessment of Motor and Process Skills (AMPS) and the Evaluation of Social Interaction (ESI) are used in the context of a practice story as the basis for the application of occupational performance analysis for people with disabilities. Occupational performance analysis is explored through the process of assessment in the practice story. How information from this assessment process is used for intervention planning and re-evaluation is also discussed.

KEY POINTS

- *Occupational performance analysis* is a structured assessment process that uses observation of an individual doing an occupation to identify and define factors that support or hinder occupational performance and prevent that person from being a full participant in life.

- Occupational performance analysis should always be placed in the context of the occupations that people want and need to engage in or *do*. *Occupation* refers to the doing of meaningful and purposeful tasks. Occupational performance analysis is the observation of the smallest parts of the task, referred to as *performance skills.*

- Performance skills include motor skills, process skills and social interaction skills. These are influenced by the dynamic interaction among the person (client factors), the environment (environments and contexts) and the occupations (the tasks performed).

- Occupational performance analysis is the unique skill of occupational therapists. It enables them to identify strengths and limitations of occupational performance and draw conclusions about the needs of individuals with body structure limitations and activity or participation restrictions.

- Detailed information about strengths and limitations of occupational performance can be used in collaboration with the person and the person's family to clarify the cause of the problem and identify solutions to enable or enhance occupational performance.

INTRODUCTION

It is no accident that the early founders gave the profession the name *occupational* therapy. They saw the need for individuals to be busy, or *occupied* with the ordinary and the necessary, the occupations and roles that were their everyday lives. The early founders were quick to note that when individuals were deprived of occupation, their lives lacked purpose and meaning. By observing and analysing the skills required, occupations provided a therapeutic medium, either as 'therapy' or treatment in itself, or as a means to enable individuals to achieve independence to participate in home and community life by adapting or changing the way that occupations were performed. As the profession developed over the decades, analysis of everyday occupations has remained but the focus has shifted towards achieving or maintaining health and well-being and enhancing full participation in life.

This chapter defines and describes occupational performance analysis and explores how to apply it within occupational therapy practice. The domain and process of occupational therapy practice, as defined and described in the practice framework of the American Occupational Therapy Association (AOTA, 2014), is the underpinning theoretical framework and language used throughout this chapter. The Assessment of Motor and Process Skills (AMPS) (Fisher & Jones, 2012, 2014) is used to demonstrate the application of occupational performance analysis in an individual performance context, and the Evaluation of Social Interaction (ESI) (Fisher & Griswold, 2015) is used to demonstrate the application of occupational performance analysis in a social context or during social occupations.

The AOTA practice framework describes what individuals *do* as occupations: activities of daily living (ADL), sleep/rest, education, work, play, leisure and social participation (AOTA, 2014). The Canadian Association of Occupational Therapists (CAOT) describes occupation as everything that people do in the course of everyday life (CAOT, 2012). Moreover, CAOT goes on to state that occupations describe who individuals are and how individuals feel about themselves (2012). Whereas *occupation* refers to the *doing* of everyday activities, occupational performance analysis is the detailed observation of the smallest units (or performance skills) of the task being undertaken in environments and contexts (physical, social and cultural) relevant to the person. *Performance skills* are goal-directed actions that are observable in daily life occupations and include motor skills, process skills and social interaction skills (Fisher, 2009).

The AOTA practice framework (AOTA, 2014) and occupation terminology used in this chapter forms the basis of occupational performance analysis and how it is applied in occupational therapy practice. According to the AOTA practice framework (2014), the way that the person carries out occupations is referred to as *performance patterns* and include habits, routines, roles and rituals. The spaces or environment in which individuals carry out their occupations are referred to as *performance contexts and environments* and include cultural, personal, physical, social, temporal and virtual. The doing of occupations is influenced by the person themselves, or *client factors* (a person's body functions and body structures, values, beliefs and spirituality).

DEFINITION OF TERMS

In this chapter specific terms are used to help define occupational performance analysis. It is recognised that some of these terms are used in occupational therapy literature to mean subtly different things and that the same terms are also used differently internationally. To assist the reader in understanding the content and meaning of this chapter, the main terms used in this chapter are defined next.

Occupation, Activity and Task

Occupation, activity and *task* are used interchangeably in some literature to refer to the same thing, whereas some authors argue that they are different concepts (Christiansen & Townsend,

2004; Pierce, 2001; Polatajko et al., 2004; Reed, 2005). In this chapter *occupation* refers to:

> *The everyday activities that people do as individuals, in families and with communities to occupy time and bring meaning and purpose to life. Occupations include things people need to, want to and are expected to do.*
> *(World Federation of Occupational Therapists, 2012)*

In this chapter both the terms *activity* and *task* are used and mean the same thing. That is, both terms are a way of describing a general idea about a group of human actions that are not personal or experienced by a specific person and therefore are not observable (Pierce, 2001). For example, within a given culture there are shared understandings of what it means to *make tea*. The outcome of the activity (or task of making tea) is the same but the way of doing or presenting the tea may vary with personal, cultural and social expectations. A key perspective for differentiating between occupation and activity is that activity is a shared concept about 'what' is done. It becomes an occupation when a person does the activity (it is observable) and it has individual meaning and purpose to the person.

Occupational Performance Analysis and Activity or Task Analysis

Activity analysis outlines the typical process (steps of) and demands of a particular activity on any given person. It does not consider a particular person or the environment or context in which the activity will be done (O'Toole, 2011). Generally, it outlines the typical sequence of the activity, the skills required to safely complete it and typical equipment used (O'Toole, 2011). Activity analysis has long been part of the occupational therapy curriculum in order to outline the requirements for successful completion of an activity and its therapeutic potential (O'Toole, 2011). This is essential to assist the occupational therapist to select activities that are the right challenge and for which the necessary equipment is available to use in assessment and treatment. It assists students and practitioners to understand the complexity of activities, and for novice practitioners it can be a lengthy paper-based exercise. In professional practice this process is often not replicated in the same way. It is a process learned at university but not visible to students on practice placement. For the more advanced practitioner this knowledge is almost automatic and therefore *tacit* as it becomes embedded within occupational performance analyses.

Occupational performance analysis extends the activity analysis process, examining a *person* doing an activity, which has meaning and purpose to them, within a specific environment and context. Although it is recognised that activity analysis is important, in this chapter the focus is on occupational performance analysis, the analysis of an observed event of a person doing an occupation.

Performance Skills

Skills are goal-directed, practiced abilities that develop over time showing deftness and dexterity (Connelly & Dalgleish, 1989). They are learned, observable and relate directly to occupational performance (Fisher, 2009). They are not a person's body functions nor do they relate to underlying body impairments. Performance skills include motor skills, process skills and social interaction skills and are always observable. Performance skills are the smallest units of occupational performance that, when linked together one after another, are observed in an ongoing stream of action (performance) or social interaction. Sometimes performance skills are referred to as actions – for example, motor actions. The motor skill *grips* is an action, or the process skill *navigates* is an action or the social interaction skill *turns towards* is an action; this relates to the concept that skills are observable and relate to 'doing', not an abstract concept like remembering or thinking.

Top-down and Bottom-up

Bottom-up practice, sometimes referred to in the literature as *deficit focused,* is closely aligned with the medical model and primarily focuses on a person's underlying ability at the body function and structure level of the International Classification of Functioning Disability and Health (ICF) (Brown & Chien, 2010; WHO, 2001). The theoretical assumption is that remediating impairments – for example, in cognition, muscle strength or perception – will result in successful changes in performance in activities of daily living (Weinstock-Zlotnick & Hinojosa, 2004).

A top-down approach, often referred to as *occupation-centred* or *occupation-focused,* is advocated by several occupational therapy theorists (Cantin & Polatajko, 2013; Diamantis, 2010; Fisher, 2013; Hocking, 2001; Rodger, 2010; Trombly, 1993). With a top-down approach the focus is on the person's role competence and participation in occupations and can be considered at the activity and participation level of the ICF (World Health Organization (WHO), 2001). Underlying abilities are only considered, if this is necessary, after assessing the occupational performance of the person first. This approach is described and advocated in the AOTA practice framework (AOTA, 2014) as well as discussed and supported in occupational therapy models such as the Person-Environment-Occupation Model (Law et al., 1996), Canadian Model of Occupational Performance and Engagement (Townsend & Polatajko, 2007), Model of Human Occupation (Kielhofner, 2008) and Occupational Therapy Intervention Process Model (Fisher, 2009).

Assessment Versus Evaluation, Outcome Measurement Versus Reevaluation

In this chapter the term *assessment* is used to refer to gathering detailed information to form a snapshot of a person's abilities and needs at a given time (College of Occupational Therapy

(COT), 2012). This usually consists of gathering information about the person through an interview with and observation of the person, which may or may not include the use of formal standardised assessment tools. In some of the literature this process is referred to as *evaluation,* but the term *assessment* is used in this chapter to refer to the initial process of gathering information.

Outcome measurement is the term used to refer to the process of reassessing (or reevaluating) a person, group or community to establish if any change has occurred after intervention (COT, 2012). In other literature this may be referred to as *reevaluation.*

WHAT IS OCCUPATIONAL PERFORMANCE ANALYSIS?

Fisher (1998, 2009, 2013) defines occupation as *the action of seizing or taking possession of, or occupying space or time. Also as the holding of positions – as in one's role.* In fact, occupation is everything that people do: it is the way people spend their time productively, in leisure pursuits and taking care of themselves. Occupation is a process that unfolds over time; the doing of something meaningful, towards a purpose – for example, dressing oneself for work or walking the dog. It implies action or, as Fisher (2009) points out, the carrying out of actions – the *doing* of something and not what is done. Fisher describes *what* is done as the task (to get dressed), whereas occupation implies action, either the global action of *dressing* oneself or the more specific actions of *grasping* the shirt and *manipulating* the button. Actions then are verbs: *doing* words, denoted by their *ing* ending – grasp*ing*, reach*ing*, ask*ing*. This is an important concept in understanding the breaking down of or analysis of an occupation into smaller performance units (or skills).

Activity or task analysis, therefore, is analysis of *what is done* – to get dressed or to make a drink or to share information with a colleague, in other words the demands of the *task* (biopsychosocial and environmental) rather than the performance of skills by the person. Tasks consist of *shared concepts:* the making of a cup of tea is a concept understood by people from different communities, cultures and countries. The process, tools and materials may vary with culture, age and ability, but the task will result in the same end product (water that is heated, flavoured with leaves, with or without additions). All persons who engage in this task will need to select and gather culturally specific tools and materials, move themselves and task objects from place to place and make changes in their environment in order to proceed with and complete the task. The task (what is done) is composed of a number of steps, and each step is composed of a number of smaller units or actions. Each step is dependent on the development of skilled actions that have been practised on many occasions over time.

Occupational performance analysis extends the activity analysis process (O'Toole, 2011) and places the person in the foreground (Crepeau, 2013). It assists with understanding the person: what individuals do, why individuals do what they do, how individuals do what they do; the places where individuals conduct their occupations: home, workplace, school or community; and how phenomena such as health, physical, social, societal, economic or political restrictions can disrupt an individual's roles and way of life. Occupational performance analysis is a structured, observational process used by occupational therapists to identify and define *actions* that support or limit a person's occupational performance and factors that prevent the person from being a full participant in home and community life.

Occupational performance analysis can be used to assess the quality and effectiveness of these small, discrete steps and actions (the *process*) of performance rather than the outcome. The purpose is not just to see if the person can do the task but to determine how competent the person is in performing each action and step: are there signs of increased physical effort or difficulty or clumsiness, or performance being slow or delayed, either by inefficient use of time (it takes a long time to complete an action) or inefficient use of spaces (the steps or actions are organised in such a way that the person has to constantly move from one space to another to complete the steps)?

Polatajko, Mandich, and Martini (2000) discuss two further performer prerequisites for optimal occupational performance: motivation and task knowledge. Motivation is an important factor that is known to influence a person's willingness to participate in and continue to the completion of tasks, especially under challenging conditions. There must be a desire or need on the part of a person or an expectation by the person (or the person's cultural group) that the tasks should be performed. Nelson and Thomas (2003) identify that motivation, or human purpose may be intrinsic or extrinsic. Intrinsic purpose involves doing something for its own sake, for the pleasure of it, whereas extrinsic purpose involves doing something for a reason. Second, Fisher (2009) and Fisher and Jones (2012) point out that task knowledge, or having had experience, at least at some basic level, of what is done is also an important consideration. Mastery is only achieved after much practice until knowledge of the task has become implicit.

Occupational performance analysis is a top-down process, as the focus is on the person's skills while doing an occupation of importance and not on underlying capacities – capacities are underlying body functions (musculoskeletal, neurological, cardiovascular, etc.). When using a top-down therapy approach, underlying capacities are only considered, along with environmental factors and the demands of the activity, *after* occupational performance analysis has been completed. By observing the person's occupational performance first, the occupational therapist is better able to interpret the causes for the person's difficulties and make informed judgements about why a person is having problems.

WHY IS OCCUPATIONAL PERFORMANCE ANALYSIS IMPORTANT?

Over time people become adept and skilful through repetition and practice, so that by adulthood performance patterns form part of their habits and routines, often to the extent that they are not even aware of what they do or how they do it. Getting dressed in the morning is a good example of this. When working with individuals whose occupations have been disrupted – for example, by age, illness, injury or impairment – occupational therapists can see the impact of body structure impairments on occupational performance. The frail elderly person who falls and fractures a hip is no longer able to use the same dextrous movement patterns in standing and sitting, in reaching and bending; the person who has had a stroke must adapt performance skills and patterns in response to increased muscle tone or muscle weakness in one side of the trunk and the upper and/or lower limb of the same side; and the person with a dementia is no longer able to remember where items are kept in the kitchen cupboards and either needs help to find them or to keep them visible on the countertop.

Occupational therapists conduct occupational performance analysis to assess the extent to which the doing of occupations has been disrupted and to identify skills that are still intact and skills that inhibit competent occupational performance. Such detailed information about strengths and limitations of performance can be used in collaboration with individuals and their families to clarify the cause of the problem and identify solutions (an intervention plan) to enhance occupational performance. This ensures the intervention is targeted at the problem (AOTA, 2014). Fisher (2013) noted that the use of occupation as a tool for assessment and intervention provides a unique focus for occupational therapists. Using occupation as an assessment and therapeutic (intervention) medium underpins occupational therapy practice (AOTA, 2014; COT, 2015; Fisher, 2013). The ability to analyse and understand the demands of different kinds of occupations to use them as a medium for assessment and/or intervention is also the unique skill of occupational therapists.

Fisher (2013) states that if occupational therapists are occupation-centred in the way they work with people (i.e. putting occupation at the centre of everything they do), they become grounded in occupation and demonstrate to others that occupation is the unique focus of the profession. This means using occupation as methods for assessments (including standardised assessment tools) and interventions. Thus occupational performance analysis should be occupation-based (Fisher, 2013) – that is, using occupation as the *method* of assessment. This method enables the occupational therapist to gather information on the ability of the *person* to perform occupations competently and with satisfaction in the person's spaces or naturalistic environments. Beginning with a focus on the person and the person's needs (rather than the underlying capacities or impairments) constitutes a top-down approach (Fisher, 2009; Ideishi, 2003). Ideishi also recommends a top-down approach as occupations are then chosen by the person for their intrinsic meaning and purpose and their perceived importance to life roles or social expectations of the culture.

AMPS AND ESI AS STANDARDISED, OBSERVATIONAL OCCUPATIONAL PERFORMANCE ANALYSIS TOOLS

In this chapter two standardised occupational therapy assessment tools are used to illustrate how motor, process and social interaction skills are used to identify strengths and limitations of performance in an occupational performance analysis. The same tools can be used at baseline and after intervention to measure and demonstrate the outcomes of therapy. These two standardised assessment tools help to conceptualise how what is observed during the performance of a task is translated into an occupational performance analysis with a person. This is a key process to grasp and is often a difficult process for the novice initially as occupational performance analysis is complex to learn and requires practice and skill to implement. These two assessment tools are the Assessment of Motor and Process Skills (AMPS) and the Evaluation of Social Interaction (ESI). The AMPS and the ESI focus specifically on performance skills that are observable, which is essential in the context of occupational performance analysis.

Assessment of Motor and Process Skills

The Assessment of Motor and Process Skills, or AMPS, is an observational assessment designed to be used by occupational therapists to assess the quality of a person's performance of activities of daily living in natural, task-relevant environments (Fisher & Jones, 2012, p. 1-1). It is a standardised ADL performance analysis. Motor skills are defined as 'the observable, goal directed actions a person performs in order to move him or herself or task objects while interacting with the task objects and environment as he or she performs an ADL task' (Fisher & Jones, 2012, p. 2-5). Process skills are defined as 'the observable, goal directed actions a person performs as he or she (a) selects, interacts with, and uses task tools and materials; (b) logically carries out individual actions or steps of an ADL task; and (c) modifies his or her performance when problems occur' (Fisher & Jones, 2012, p. 2-5). There are 16 motor skills and 20 process skills, each scale (motor and process) forming a universal skill taxonomy. During any occupational performance, every skill will be observed, and this is why each scale is called a universal taxonomy. The list of motor and process skills can be found in Table 16.1.

TABLE 16.1
Performance Skills: Motor and Process

Motor Skills

Body Positions

Stabilises	Maintains an upright sitting or standing position while moving through the task environment or interacting with task objects such that there is no evidence of momentary propping or loss of balance that affects performance
Aligns	Sustains an upright sitting or standing position, as required during the task performance, such that there is no evidence of persistent propping, leaning or loss of balance that affects the ongoing task performance
Positions	Positions body, arms or wheelchair in relation to task objects (i.e. not too close or far away) as required for efficient arm movements during task performance

Obtaining and Holding Objects

Reaches	Extends the arm, and when appropriate bends the trunk, to effectively grasp or place objects that are out of reach; includes skilfully using a reacher to obtain task objects
Bends	Actively flexes, rotates or twists the trunk in a manner and direction appropriate to the task, as when bending to pick up a task object from the floor or to sit down in a chair
Grips	Pinches or grasps task objects such that the task object does not slip, e.g. from between the person's fingers, from between the teeth
Manipulates	Uses dextrous grasp and release patterns, isolated finger movements, and coordinated in-hand manipulation patterns when interacting with small task objects, e.g. difficulty manipulating buttons when buttoning, difficulty manipulating a pencil when writing
Coordinates	Uses two or more body parts together to stablise and manipulate task objects during bilateral motor tasks such as when holding a jar with one hand (or between the knees) and removing the lid with the other hand

Moving self and Objects

Moves	Pushes or pulls task objects along a supporting surface, pulls to open or pushes to close doors and drawers, or pushes on wheels to propel a wheelchair
Lifts	Raises or lifts task objects, including lifting an object from one place to another, but without ambulating or moving from one place to another
Walks	Ambulates on level surfaces and changes direction while walking without shuffling the feet, lurching, instability, propping or using assistive devices (cane, walker, wheelchair) during the task performance
Transports	Carries task objects from one place to another while walking, seated in a wheelchair or using a walker
Calibrates	Regulates or grades the force, speed and extent of movement when interacting with task objects, e.g. not too much and not too little, pushing a door with enough force to close it but not too much that it bounces open
Flows	Uses smooth and fluid arm and wrist movements when interacting with task objects

Energy

Endures	Persists and completes the task without obvious evidence of physical fatigue, pausing to rest, or stopping to catch one's breath
Paces	Maintains a consistent and effective rate or tempo of performance throughout the performance of actions and steps of the entire task

Process Skills

Sustaining Performance

Paces[a]	Maintains a consistent and effective rate or tempo of performance throughout the performance of actions and steps of the entire task
Attends	Maintains focus on the task performance such that the person does not look away from what he or she is doing, thus interrupting the ongoing task progression
Heeds	Uses goal-directed task actions that are focused towards carrying out and completing a specified task, e.g., the outcome originally agreed on, e.g. to make a cup of hot instant coffee for one person

Applying Task Knowledge

Chooses	Selects necessary and appropriate type and number of tools and materials for the task, includes choosing the tools and materials that the person said they would choose before initiating the task

TABLE 16.1	
Performance Skills: Motor and Process *(Continued)*	

Uses	Employs tools and materials as they are intended, e.g. uses a knife to cut and spread but not to stir food; and in a reasonable (including hygienic) fashion
Handles	Supports, stabilises and holds tools and materials in an appropriate manner, protecting them from damage, slipping, moving or falling
Inquires	Seeks needed verbal or written information by asking questions or reading directions or labels; does not ask for information where the person has a prior awareness of the answer

Temporal Organisation

Initiates	Starts or begins the next action or step without hesitation
Continues	Performs single, sustained actions or action sequences without unnecessary interruptions or pauses so that once the action has started, e.g. filling the cup with water, the person continues on until the action or step is completed (the cup is filled)
Sequences	Performs steps in an effective or logical order for efficient use of time or energy and with an absence of randomness or lack of logic in the ordering of steps, or inappropriate repetition of steps (washing the same cup twice when it is already clean)
Terminates	Brings to completion single actions or single steps without inappropriate persistence (continuing to sweep the same piece of floor long after all the dirt has been swept up) or premature cessation (stopping sweeping the floor before all the dirt has been swept up)

Space and Objects

Searches/ locates	Looks for and locates tools and materials in a logical manner, both within and beyond the immediate environment, including not asking where task objects are located before looking for them (provided the person was aware before beginning the task where tools and materials are located)
Gathers	Collects together needed or misplaced tools and materials in a logical manner including: collecting related tools and materials into the same workspace; collecting and replacing materials that have spilled, fallen or been misplaced
Organises	Logically positions or spatially arranges tools and materials in an orderly fashion including: in a single workspace; between multiple appropriate workspaces, in order to facilitate ease of task performance, e.g. the workspace is not too crowded or too spread out
Restores	Puts away tools and materials in appropriate places; closes or seals containers and covering where appropriate; restores immediate workspace(s) to original condition (including wiping up any spills or saving work on a computer before closing the program)
Navigates	Modifies the movement pattern of the arm, body or wheelchair to manoeuvre around obstacles that are encountered in the course of moving through space such that undesirable contact with obstacles (knocking over, bumping into) is avoided

Adapting Performance

Notices/ responds	Responds appropriately to: (i) nonverbal task related cues (task object rolling or falling, liquid dripping, appliances heating) that provide feedback regarding task progression; (ii) the spatial arrangement of objects one to another (alignment of objects during stacking, edges of laundry during folding); (iii) notices and responds to cupboard doors and drawers that have been left open during task performance
Adjusts	Changes working environments in anticipation of, or in response to, problems that arise; anticipates or responds to problems effectively by making some change: between workspaces by moving to a new workspace or bringing in or removing tools and materials from the present workspace; or in an environmental condition (turning a tap on or off or a temperature up or down)
Accommodates	Modifies actions or the location of objects within the workspace, in anticipation of, or response to problems that might arise; anticipates or responds to problems effectively by changing the method with which one is performing an action sequence; changing the manner in which one interacts with or handles tools and materials already in the workspace; asking for assistance when appropriate or needed
Benefits	Anticipates and prevents undesirable circumstances or problems from recurring or persisting; includes responding appropriately to verbal cues intended to lead to correction of errors.

[a]Paces is both a motor skill and a process skill, but it is only scored once based on the person's overall rate or tempo of performance.
Reproduced with permission from Fisher & Jones, 2014.

There are more than 120 ADL tasks in the AMPS task list, each with specific guidelines for standardisation with flexible task options to allow for cross-cultural application (Fisher & Jones, 2014). Two tasks are observed by the occupational therapist, in a naturalistic context (never contrived) and are selected based on occupations that the person (and/or the person's caregiver) has identified as meaningful and needed for everyday living. The rating on a 4-point scale of each of the 36 skills allows the occupational therapist to assess the quality of the person's ADL performance in terms of increased effort, decreased efficiency, level of safety and need for assistance while simultaneously completing an occupational performance analysis. As the AMPS focuses on observable skills that are seen in every task (and not on underlying body functions or impairments), it is free from cross-cultural bias and can be used with any person of any age with any type of diagnosis, including well people. It can also be used with those who have not yet received a formal diagnosis but who may be at risk of functional decline (Fisher & Jones, 2012).

Evaluation of Social Interaction

The Evaluation of Social Interaction (ESI) is a standardised, observation-based assessment of the quality of a person's social interaction (Fisher & Griswold, 2015, p. 1). When the ESI is used, the person engages in *real* social interactions, with specific intended purposes relevant to the person and with social partners with whom the person would typically interact (Fisher & Griswold, 2015). Social interaction skills are defined as 'the individual actions or units of social interaction that are observable within the ongoing stream of a social exchange' (Fisher & Griswold, 2015, p. 11). There are 27 social interaction skills and, like motor and process skills, they form a universal skill taxonomy as all the social interaction skills will be observed during every social exchange. The list of social interaction skills can be found in Table 16.2. As the ESI focuses on observable skills (and not on underlying body functions or impairments), it is also free from cross-cultural bias and can be used with any person of any age older than 2 years with any type of diagnosis, including well people and those who have not yet received a formal diagnosis but who may be demonstrating diminished quality of social interaction (Fisher & Griswold, 2015; Simmons, Griswold, & Berg, 2010).

The intended purpose of each social exchange is identified by the person, and the exchanges are similar to typical social interactions that would take place in the home, workplace and leisure or play environments (Fisher & Griswold, 2015), such as

TABLE 16.2
Performance Skills: Social Interaction

Social Interaction Skills

Initiating and Terminating Social Interaction

Approaches/starts	Use strategies appropriate to the social context to approach and/or initiate interaction with social partner; includes catching the attention of social partner through (a) asking a question or (b) sending a greeting or introductory phrase to initiate social interaction; also includes responding to the arrival or greeting from a social partner
Concludes/disengages	Terminate the conversation or social interaction using customary termination statements, brings to closure the topic under discussion, and disengages or says goodbye using appropriate phrases and ceremonies, as appropriate to the context and degree of familiarity with the social partner; includes the ability to send verbal and nonverbal messages that termination is desired, and then using appropriate strategies to carry the termination of conversation or social interaction through to an appropriate end

Producing Social Interaction

Produces speech	Produce spoken, signed or augmentative (i.e. computer-generated) messages with literal meaning; includes producing clearly articulated speech that is audible and expresses meaning, given the social context
Gesticulates	Use socially appropriate gestures to communicate or support a message (e.g. shaking one's head, frowning, smiling, waving one's hand) to send signals to the social partner
Speaks fluently	Speak in a fluent and continuous manner with an even flow (not too fast, not too slow); includes speaking without pauses or delays during spoken, signed, or augmentative (i.e. computer-generated) message

Physically Supporting Social Interaction

Turns towards	Actively position or turn the body and the face toward the social partner or the person who is speaking
Looks	Make eye contact with the social partner in a manner that is relaxed; includes adjusting the frequency and duration of eye contact to match that of the social partner

TABLE 16.2
Performance Skills: Social Interaction *(Continued)*

Places self	Place oneself at an appropriate distance from the social partner during the social interaction and as appropriate, given the social context and degree of familiarity with the social partner; implies acting according to the social partner's cues about personal space, and adjusting one's distance to the type of social interaction and degree of familiarity with the social partner
Touches	Respond to and use touch or bodily contact with the social partner in a manner that it socially appropriate
Regulates	Control impulses and behaviours that are not part of communication and not appropriate to the social situation; includes assuming body positions that are appropriate to the type of social interaction and degree of familiarity with the social partner

Shaping Content of Social Interaction

Questions	Ask questions that support the intended purpose of the social interaction (e.g. requesting relevant facts or information; asking questions in order to seek socially relevant information about the social partner's opinions, interests, or needs; asking questions needed to manage a task)
Replies	Keep conversation going by replying to questions and comments that are appropriate to the social context; includes providing information or opinions when asked for them; also includes giving a relevant reply to an apology or feedback expressed by the social partner or elaborating on the ideas being discussed
Discloses	Reveal opinions, feelings, and private information about oneself or others in a manner that is appropriate, given the social context and degree of familiarity with the social partner
Expresses emotion	Display affect and emotions in a way that is socially acceptable, and appropriate to the context and the level of familiarity with the social partner; includes expressing emotion through one's facial expression or tone of voice in a manner that matches the message sent; also includes expressing emotion both as a listener and as a speaker
Disagrees	Express differences of opinion in a socially appropriate manner and as appropriate in the social context and degree of familiarity with the social partner
Thanks	Use appropriate words, phrases, gestures, and ceremonies to confirm receipt of services, offers, gifts, and/or compliments; includes expressing gratitude for the generosity or kindness shown by the social partner or showing conventional courtesy in the context of economical transactions involving goods and services

Maintaining Flow of Social Interaction

Transitions	Smoothly transition the conversation to a closely related topic, and/or change the topic without disrupting the conversation
Times response	Reply to social messages without delay or hesitation, or without interrupting social partner
Times duration	Speak for reasonable time periods that are appropriate, given the social partner and the context; includes adjusting the length of one's turn, depending on the situation and the complexity of the message
Takes turns	Take one's turn and give the social partner the freedom to take his/her turn; includes sending cues or messages that signal whose turn it is to send a message; also includes not allowing oneself to be dominated by others

Verbally Supporting Social Interaction

Matches language	Use a tone of voice, dialect, and level of language that is appropriate to the situation and the social partner's abilities and level of understanding; implies varying one's level of language according to (a) the type of social interaction (e.g. formal speech versus casual conversation), (b) the level of language used by the social partner (e.g. that of a child versus that of an adult; use of dialect or jargon), and (c) the intended purpose of the social interaction and degree of familiarity with the social partner
Clarifies	Ensure, in a manner appropriate to the social context and the degree of familiarity with the social partner, that the social partner is *following* the conversation of social interaction; includes recognising when the social partner does not comprehend or understand a message and then responding appropriately by clarifying or giving an explanation

Continued on following page

TABLE 16.2	
Performance Skills: Social Interaction *(Continued)*	
Acknowledges/encourages	Acknowledge receipt of messages and/or encourage the social partner to continue interaction by nodding, using facial expressions (e.g. smiling), gesturing or verbalising encouraging statements (e.g. uh-huh, good point); includes sending messages to encourage all social partners to participate in social interaction
Empathises	Express a supportive attitude towards the social partner by agreeing with, empathising with, or expressing understanding of the social partner's feelings and experiences; includes using gestures of concern (e.g. hugging, patting the social partner on the back) as appropriate, given the social context and degree of familiarity with the social partner
Adapting Social Interaction	
Heeds	Use goal-directed social interactions that are focused towards carrying out and completing the intended purpose of the social interaction
Accommodates	Modify his/her social interactions in anticipation of, or response to problems that might arise; includes apologising or excusing oneself, when socially indicated. The person anticipates or responds to the problems effectively by (a) changing the method with which he/she is interacting, or (b) asking for assistance when appropriate or needed
Benefits	Anticipate and prevent undesirable circumstances or problems in the social interaction from recurring or persisting; includes responding appropriately to verbal cues intended to lead to correction of appropriate social interaction

Reproduced with permission from Fisher & Griswold, 2015.

interacting with co-workers to seek information, giving instructions, making decisions, collaborating with others, engaging in small talk over a coffee break or purchasing goods and services. Intended purposes of social interactions can be found in Table 16.3.

Two social exchanges are observed by the occupational therapist in a naturalistic context (never contrived) and are selected based on what the person (and/or the person's caregiver) sees as limiting the quality of social interaction. The types of behaviours that may limit effective social interactions include shouting, staring (or avoiding eye contact), inappropriate touching of others, not replying to a social partner or not taking a turn in the conversation, interrupting others, replying or disagreeing in a disrespectful or impolite way, whining, swearing or hitting one's social partner in the course of the ongoing conversation. Such behaviours have a significant negative impact on the quality of social interaction and the person's social relationships with family, work colleagues and friends. If problems have been identified during social occupations, then these need to be captured during an occupational performance analysis. The rating of each of the 27 social interaction skills, also on 4-point scale, allows the occupational therapist to assess the quality of the person's social interaction in terms of polite, respectful, well-timed, relevant and mature social interactions, while simultaneously completing an occupational performance analysis.

DOMAINS OF OCCUPATIONAL THERAPY

The AOTA Occupational Therapy Practice Framework is a useful guide for practice as it provides a common understanding of the central tenets of occupational therapy and it purveys, through occupation terminology, first that there is a positive relationship between occupation and health, and second, that people are viewed as occupational beings (AOTA, 2014). The framework is divided into two major sections: *Domains*, which outlines the scope, range and intentions of occupational therapy theory and practice; and *Process*, which describes what occupational therapists do in providing occupational therapy services (occupational therapy process). In this chapter, the main focus is on the five domains of practice: Occupations, Client Factors, Performance Skills, Performance Patterns and Contexts and Environments.

Occupations

The first domain is *Occupations* and includes occupations that individuals *do* such as caring for self (personal and domestic/instrumental activities of daily living), education, productive work, play, leisure activities and social participation (AOTA, 2014). This also includes occupations such as rest, meditation, sleep that focus on *being* (rather than doing). When the

TABLE 16.3
Intended Purposes of Social Interaction

Gathering Information (GI)

Social interactions with a *preplanned* purpose related to the person asking for and/or gathering information from someone who knows the answer; can be related to information that involves demonstration using tangible objects. An expectation is that the person *must ask one or more questions focused on gathering relevant information.*

GI-1   Interacting with someone to gather *facts or information about experiences, people, places, or services,* but *not* about tangible objects or in the context of an interview, lecture, or providing assistance to others (e.g. gathering information from someone to get directions to a restaurant, inquiring about what types of services are available from a telephone provider, gathering information from a friend about a favourite recipe, asking a student questions about a required reading assignment, asking for clarification or expectations or scope of a specific task, gathering information about recommendations for what to order at a restaurant)

Note. Tangible objects may be used during the social exchange, but they are not the focus on the information provided (e.g. a map may be used when getting directions, a pencil and paper may be used to write down the recipe)

GI-2   Interacting with someone to gather information *about a tangible object* that is present during the social exchange, but with *no demonstration* of how the object is operated or used (e.g. gathering information about the features included in a mobile telephone, gathering information about the ingredients included in a dish that has been served at a restaurant)

GI-3   Interacting with someone to gather information *about how to use or operate a tangible object – with demonstration* (e.g. learning how to use the calendar function included in a mobile telephone, learning how an electronic appliance works)

GI-4   Interacting with someone to gather information *during an interview or lecture* (e.g. gathering information about the client during an occupational therapy interview, gathering information about a social partner's prior work experience during a job interview, gathering information about how to manage fatigue during a workshop offered for people with chronic fatigue)

Sharing Information (SI)

Social interactions with a *preplanned* purpose related to giving information to someone; can be related to information that involves demonstration using tangible objects. Depending on the social context, there *may be no expectation that the person ask questions.*

SI-1   Interacting with someone to share *facts or information about experiences, people, places, or services,* but *not* about tangible objects or in the context of an interview, lecture, or providing assistance to others (e.g. giving someone directions to a restaurant, explaining what types of services are available from a telephone provider, sharing a favourite recipe, sharing information about a recent trip or book one has read, answering questions posed by a teacher, clarifying the expectations or scope of a specific task, giving recommendations for what to order at a restaurant)

Note. Tangible objects may be used during the social exchange, but they are not the focus on the information provided (e.g. a map may be used when giving directions, a pencil and paper may be used to write down the recipe)

SI-2   Interacting with someone to give that social partner information *about a tangible object* that is present during the social exchange, but *not with demonstration* of how the object is operated or used (e.g. sharing information about the features included in a mobile telephone, sharing information about the ingredients included in a dish that has been served at a restaurant, sharing information about a piece of artwork)

SI-3   Interacting with someone to teach that social partner about *how to use or operate a tangible object – with demonstration* (e.g. teaching a social partner how to use the calendar function included in a mobile telephone, demonstrating how an electronic appliance works, teaching a social partner how to position a wheelchair and lock the wheelchair brakes)

SI-4   Interacting with someone to share information *during an interview or lecture* (e.g. sharing information about occupational therapy during a patient interview, sharing information about one's prior work experience during a job interview, providing an in-service lecture to colleagues)

SI-5   Interacting with someone to share *opinions or perspectives* but *not* to come to an agreement about a shared viewpoint (e.g. debating political viewpoints or candidates, sharing opinions about a movie or book, discussing perspectives on a recent event

Problem Solving/Decision Making (PD)

Social interactions with a *preplanned* purpose related to making decisions, discussing options, or *debating differences of opinion,* but without tangible objects as the focus of the interaction. The use of tools and materials (e.g. pen, paper, computer) to record ideas and decisions may be used. An expectation is that the person *must ask one or more problem-solving/decision-making questions.*

PD-1   Interacting with someone to *discuss and agree upon a shared viewpoint* (e.g. coming to an agreement on the rules of a game, coming to an agreement on a joint perspective to share with others)

PD-2   Interacting with someone to *plan a social event, a project, a trip,* but not who will do what tasks (e.g. planning a party, planning an awards ceremony, planning how to remodel a bathroom)

Continued on following page

TABLE 16.3
Intended Purposes of Social Interaction *(Continued)*

PD-3   Interacting with someone to *plan who will do what tasks* when implementing an event or project together (e.g. planning who will prepare which parts of a meal, planning who will complete which parts of an art project, planning who will act which parts in a play)

PD-4   Interacting with someone to *plan a time and/or place* for an appointment, a meeting, or getting together for dinner

PD-5   Interacting with someone to *decide which option to choose* (e.g. deciding which movie to go and see, deciding which game to play, choosing which task to do)

Collaborating/Producing (CP)

Social interactions with a *preplanned* purpose focused on collaborative interaction with tangible objects. An expectation is that the person *must ask one or more collaboration questions.*

CP-1   Interacting with someone in the context of and in relation to *cooking a meal together*

CP-2   Interacting with someone in the context of and in relation to *completing a shared/joint arts and crafts project* (e.g. making a collage or mural, making a quilt)

CP-3   Interacting with someone in the context of and in relation to *playing a collaborative team game or playing collaboratively with tangible objects,* but *not* in the context of using a computer, tablet, or mobile telephone (e.g. playing volleyball; playing *dress-up,* but without pretending to be another person; playing with trains)

CP-4   Interacting with someone in the context of and in relation to *jointly doing a work or school project/assignment,* but *not* in the context of using a computer, tablet, or mobile telephone (e.g. creating a poster, filling in a worksheet, writing a story, drawing a floor plan for a new house)

CP-5   Interacting with someone in the context of and in relation to *jointly learning how to use and/or using a computer, tablet, or mobile telephone* (e.g. working together to learn how to use a new calendar app, using a computer to collaboratively complete a joint assignment or create a poster, playing a collaborative game on the same computer)

CP-6   Interacting with someone in the context of and in relation to *jointly constructing, building, or repairing a tangible object* (e.g. tiling a floor, building a bird house, planting a garden, building with blocks)

Acquiring Goods and Services (AG)

Social interactions with a *preplanned* purpose of requesting, ordering, and/or purchasing goods or services; does not include social interactions related to gathering or sharing information about a product a social partner is selling or in the process of deciding what to order or purchase. Depending on the social context, there *may be no expectation that the person ask questions.*

AG-1   Interacting with a salesperson in the context of *ordering goods or services*

AG-2   Interacting with a salesperson or cashier in the context of *paying for goods or services*

AG-3   Interacting with personnel in the context of *making bank or postal transactions*

AG-4   Interacting with a librarian or clerk when *checking out books and/or other media from a library*

AG-5   Interacting with someone at a ticket counter in the context of *purchasing tickets* (e.g. train, bus, movie)

AG-6   Interacting with a service provider in the context of *requesting assistance or support* (e.g. requesting help with personal ADL tasks, requesting help with a schoolwork assignment)

Note: Gathering information *about* a product a social partner is selling in the process of deciding what to order or purchase is a social interaction related to *Gathering information.* Similarly, sharing information about a product is a social interaction related to *Sharing information.*

Providing/Serving Goods and Services (PG)

Social interactions with a *preplanned* purpose of responding to requests for assistance, taking orders, and/or serving goods or services; does *not* include social interactions related to gathering or sharing information about a product a social partner is buying or in the process of a social partner deciding what to order or purchase. An expectation is that the person *must ask one or more questions related to providing services.*

PG-1   Interacting with a customer in the context of *taking an order for goods or services* (e.g. taking an order for meat at a meat counter, taking an order for coffee at a coffee shop, taking an order for a meal at a restaurant)

PG-2   Interacting with a customer in the context of *serving goods or services* (e.g. serving coffee at a coffee shop, serving a meal at a restaurant)

PG-3   Interacting with a customer in the context of *accepting payment for goods or services*

PG-4   Interacting with a customer in the context of *providing bank or postal transaction services*

PG-5   Interacting with a customer when *providing services to check out books and/or other media from a library*

PG-6   Interacting with a customer at a ticket counter in the context of *selling tickets* to a customer (e.g. train, bus, movie)

PG-7   Interacting with someone) in the context of *providing assistance to that person* (e.g. assisting a social partner with personal ADL tasks, helping a student with a schoolwork assignment)

TABLE 16.3
Intended Purposes of Social Interaction *(Continued)*

Note.   Sharing information with a social partner about a product in the process of the social partner's deciding what to order or purchase is a social interaction related to *Sharing information.* Similarly, gathering information about a product is a social interaction related to *Gathering information.*

Conversing Socially/Small Talk (CS)

Social interactions without an explicit or *preplanned* focus and that are determined by the participants during the interaction. The intended purpose of this type of social interaction may be intrinsic (e.g. to *socialise* and enjoy being with friends) or extrinsic (e.g. to take a break from work, to eat a meal, to get one's haircut, to have a massage), and may vary for each participant. An expectation, however, is that all participants involved in the social interaction take on a variety of social roles. The person, therefore, *must ask (and respond to) questions.*

CS-1   Engaging in a casual conversation with friends or colleagues *while eating a meal together*

CS-2   Engaging in *small talk* with friends or colleagues at work *during a coffee break*

CS-3   Engaging in a casual conversation *while just sitting or standing beside another person* (e.g. sitting on a park bench, sitting on a bus, standing in a queue and waiting one's turn, sitting in a theater waiting for a concert to start)

CS-4   Engaging in *small talk* with others *while playing together or while engaged in a leisure or sport activity* (e.g. playing a card game, playing golf, bowling, swimming)

CS-5   *Engaging in small talk with customers or service providers* while providing or receiving services at a spa, hair salon, or clinic

CS-6   Engaging in *small talk* with others *while preparing a meal or performing some other productive task* (e.g. building a bird house)

Note.   A critical feature of *small talk* is that it pertains to social interactions that start with *no preplanned focus.* Rather, they most often begin spontaneously and in the context of "just being together" in the same location with others. Even when such a social interaction (i.e. one that started with no *preplanned* focus) ends up focusing on a specific purpose that matches another type of social interaction, it is still coded under *Conversing socially/Small talk.*

ADL, Activities of daily living.
Reproduced with permission from Fisher & Griswold, 2015.

occupational therapist gathers information from the person in order to carry out an occupational performance analysis, all occupations that are important to the person are considered. When using a top-down approach, occupational performance is observed first and the analysis of this helps describe not just *what* the person does, but *how* they do what they do. The focus here is specifically on occupations, described in terms of *actions* or the *doing* of something (dress*ing,* shopp*ing,* play*ing*), rather than as a list of tasks (personal hygiene, household chores, care of pets). Occupational performance analysis is about observing an individual's active engagement in something. If nothing is being done or engaged in, it is not possible for the occupational therapist to observe any actions; hence *personal hygiene* has little meaning in terms of occupational performance analysis (there is no performance to observe or analyse), whereas comb*ing* one's hair, or clean*ing* one's teeth implies actions that can be observed and analysed.

Client Factors*

Client factors are specific factors, characteristics and beliefs that reside within the person (the client) who is in receipt of occupational therapy services (AOTA, 2014). Client factors can

*The term *client factors* is used here rather than *person factors,* the preferred term for this book, as this is the terminology used in the Occupational Therapy Practice Framework (AOTA, 2014).

include factors pertaining to an individual, at a group level or at the level of a population. Client factors incorporate values, beliefs and spirituality and may be influenced by the presence or absence of illness, injury or impairment (body functions and body structures) and by the person's life experiences (AOTA, 2014). Although beliefs relate to cognitive content, values are principles, standards or qualities considered important by the person (AOTA, 2014) and might include personal integrity and commitment to the family, for example. Spirituality includes a person's search for and expression of purpose or meaning in life and as such guides that person's actions towards a greater purpose beyond the personal. Values, beliefs and spirituality can influence what occupations are important to the person and the way in which these are carried out. Beliefs can be so embedded in the fabric of the person's identity that they are not even aware that they exist, and a simple intervention may result in a disruption to the person's way of life that is so great that it is not possible for the person to change.

When considering the ICF (WHO, 2001) in the context of occupational therapy practice domains, Occupations are loosely seen as 'Activity Limitations & Participation Restrictions'. Client Factors are partly covered by 'Impairments of Body Functions and Body Structures', and Contexts & Environments are listed under 'Environmental Factors'. Occupational therapy domains of Performance Skills and Performance Patterns are not covered by the ICF checklist. The ICF categorisation can be found in Table 16.4.

TABLE 16.4
Structure of the International Classification of Functioning, Disability and Health as it relates to the Domains of Occupational Therapy Practice (AOTA 2014)

ICF Part 2: ACTIVITY LIMITATIONS & PARTICIPATION RESTRICTIONS (OCCUPATIONS)	ICF Part 1: IMPAIRMENTS OF BODY FUNCTIONS & BODY STRUCTURES (CLIENT FACTORS)		ICF Part 3: ENVIRONMENTAL FACTORS (CONTEXTS & ENVIRONMENTS)
Learning/applying knowledge	Mental functions	Brain & nervous systems	Products and technology
General tasks and demands	Sensory functions & pain	Eyes, ears, tongue, nasal, sensation	Natural & man-made environments
Communication	Voice and speech functions	Lips/tongue, pharynx/larynx	Support & relationships
Mobility	Cardiovascular/haematological	Heart/cardiovascular, blood	Attitudes (personal/social/societal)
Self-care	Respiratory functions	Lungs & related structures	Service policies (including:):
Domestic life	Digestive/metabolic/endocrine	Digestive tract & related structures	Housing
Interpersonal/relationships	Genito-urinary/reproductive	Urinary/reproductive structures	Transport
Education/employment	Neuro-musculoskeletal	Central/peripheral nervous systems	Health
Community/social/civic life (including leisure)	Movement	Joints, muscles-power/tone	Education
	Skin & related functions	Skin, hair nails	Employment Financial Social

Retrieved from: www.who.int/classification/icf

Body functions are the physiological functions of the body systems and include mental, sensory; neuromusculoskeletal; cardiovascular, immunological, respiratory; voice/speech; digestive, endocrine; genitourinary; and skin functions. Body structures include the anatomical parts of the body such as organs, limbs and their components that support body functions (WHO, 2001) (Table 16.5).

Although occupational performance analysis does not focus on or measure a person's body function, this domain can assist the occupational therapist to interpret the reasons the person has problems with performance skills. Client factors will also influence the intervention offered.

Performance Skills

Performance skills are the universal, goal-directed, observable actions, linked together one after another, that unfold over time as the person engages in a daily life task performance (Fisher & Jones, 2012) or constructs a social exchange (Fisher & Griswold, 2015). They are called skills as each one is learned and developed over time in order to complete a specific task or social interaction. If they are not observable, they may relate to underlying body structure impairment such as cognition (remembering) or praxis (motor planning). Occupational performance analysis involves observing the person perform these small units of the

task, noting the quality of each and the context in which it takes place as it unfolds over time. Performance skills therefore must be observable. They are divided into three taxonomies (aspects): motor skills, process skills and social interaction skills (AOTA, 2014). Motor and process skills are derived from the AMPS, (Fisher & Jones, 2014). Social interaction skills are derived from the ESI (Fisher & Griswold, 2015). These skills are listed in Table 16.1 (motor and process skills) and Table 16.2 (social interaction skills).

Motor skills, process skills and social interaction skills in the context of occupational performance analysis are considered in this domain. Motor skills are the observable, goal-directed actions that a person performs in order to move himself or herself or the task objects while interacting with the task objects and environment as he or she performs a task (Fisher & Jones, 2012, p. 2-5). These skills pertain to positioning, stabilising and aligning the body in relation to the task; obtaining and holding task objects using one or more body parts in a way that supports task performance; moving the entire body or body part in space or when interacting with task objects; and sustaining effort throughout the task performance. The motor skills, observed in context when Sarah is brushing her hair, are identified in Box 16.1 (the motor skills are written in italics and are listed in Table 16.1).

TABLE 16.5

International Classification of Functioning, Disability & Health: Body Functions

Mental Functions (Including Affective, Cognitive and Perceptual)

Consciousness	Level of consciousness, arousal
Orientation	To person, place, time, self and others
Intellectual	Retardation, dementia
Energy and drive functions	Motivation, impulse control, interests, values
Sleep	Quality, quantity, sleep patterns
Attention	Sustained and divided
Memory	Retrospective, prospective
Emotional functions	Appropriate range and regulation of emotions, self-control
Perceptual functions	Visuospatial, body schema, sensory interpretation
Higher cognitive functions	Executive functions of judgement, concept formation, time management, problem solving, decision-making
Psychomotor functions	Experience of self, regulation of motor response to psychological events, motor planning
Language functions	Receive and express self through spoken/written/sign language
Calculation functions	Ability to calculate (add and subtract, etc.)

Sensory Functions and Pain

Seeing functions	Visual acuity, visual field
Hearing functions	Responding to sounds, pitch and volume
Vestibular functions	Balance
Gustatory functions	Taste including smell
Touch functions	Sensitivity to touch, ability to discriminate
Proprioceptive functions	Kinaesthesia, joint position sense
Pain functions	Pain sensation – dull/stabbing/ache

Voice and Speech Functions

Voice functions	Articulate and produce sounds, words and communication

Functions of the Cardiovascular, Haematological, Immunological, Respiratory Systems

Heart	Pulse rate, physical endurance, stamina, fatigue
Blood pressure	Hypotension, hypertension, postural hypotension
Haematological	Blood
Immunological	Allergies, hypersensitivity
Respiration	Breathing, rate, rhythm, depth

Functions of the Digestive, Metabolic and Endocrine Systems

Digestive/defecation	Food intake/output
Weight maintenance	Diet, obesity
Endocrine glands	Hormonal changes

Genitourinary and Reproductive Functions

Urination functions	Fluid intake/output, micturition
Sexual functions	Libido, pregnancy, birth

Neuromusculoskeletal and Movement Related Functions

Mobility of joint	Range of motion, postural alignment, joint stability/mobility
Muscle power	Strength, endurance
Muscle tone	Degree of tone, spasticity, flaccidity
Movement functions	Hand–eye/foot coordination, bilateral integration, walking patterns and gait
Involuntary movements	Motor reflexes, righting reactions
Tics, tremors, motor perseveration	

Functions of the Skin and Related Structures

Skin functions	Presence/absence of wounds, cuts, abrasions; healing
Hair and nail functions	Protective, appearance

From World Health Organization, 2001. Retrieved from www.who.int/classification/icf.

Similarly, process skills are described as the observable, goal-directed actions a person performs when (a) selecting, interacting with and using task tools and materials; (b) logically carrying out individual actions and steps of an ADL task; and (c) modifying the performance when problems occur (Fisher & Jones, 2012, p. 2-5). Process skills pertain to maintaining attention on the task throughout the performance; seeking and using task-related knowledge; beginning, continuing, logically ordering and completing actions and steps in a timely way; organising task spaces and objects; and anticipating problems and adapting performance as problems are encountered. The process skills, observed in context when Andrew is cleaning his car, are identified in Box 16.2 (the process skills are written in italics and are listed in Table 16.1).

Social interaction is an exchange of verbal and nonverbal messages and social behaviours, in a back and forth manner, that occurs between two or more individuals (Fisher & Griswold, 2015, p. 11). Fisher and Griswold define social interaction skills as 'observable actions of social behaviour' that occur within the ongoing stream of performance that occurs within the context of engagement in an occupation that involves social interaction (i.e. a social exchange). Social interaction skills pertain to initiating and terminating interactions; producing speech and speaking fluently; physically supporting social interactions by turning towards, looking at and touching one's partner appropriately and controlling repetitive behaviours; shaping the content of a social interaction by questioning, replying, disagreeing, thanking and expressing emotions politely and respectfully; maintaining the timing and flow of social interaction, verbally supporting the interaction using appropriate language, tone of voice and empathy; and adapting social interactions as problems occur. The social interaction skills, observed in context when Sarah is purchasing a camera, are identified in Box 16.3 (the social interaction skills are written in italics and are listed in Table 16.2).

Fisher and Griswold (2015) point out that social interaction skills (like motor and process skills) should be observed and evaluated in the appropriate context (social interaction as it occurs during a meaningful social occupation) and with real social partners. They stress that role play or contrived social interactions are not acceptable as they are not 'real'. As with Sarah buying the camera, the occupational therapist would go to the store with Sarah and observe (from nearby) as she interacts with the sales person (real social partner) in the store where she purchases the camera (naturalistic context). In this way interactions that are difficult or problematic for the person will be observed in the real context – that is, with a noise level and typical distractions of other people and events and interruptions that might occur. Fisher and Griswold also assert that this is what differentiates an occupational therapist's assessment from that of other professionals – the ability to observe the quality of the smallest units of performance (skills) that unfold over time in real contexts. If social interaction (and other) skill are assessed in contrived or 'test' situations using checklists of isolated components, then it is underlying body functions or person factors (articulation or vocalisation of sounds) that are recorded rather than social interaction *skills* during engagement in a social occupation.

The unfolding of social interactions can be observed in a similar way to the unfolding of actions over time during the doing of a task. Fisher (2009) suggests a comparison of skills (motor, process, social interaction) with the ICF terminology and codes in the context of a communication exchange. In Sarah's interaction the links with the temporal organisation process skills – initiating, continuing, sequencing and terminating the social interaction as a natural flow of steps or events – can be noted:

- She initiates interactions using a range of appropriate strategies: eye contact, gestures, placing herself and speaking. Similarly, she is able to terminate or conclude the social interaction by thanking her social partner and leaving in a timely manner.
- She is able to produce words and speech fluently and uses appropriate gestures to support the social interaction.
- She supports the social interactions physically by turning towards and looking at her social partner and placing herself appropriate to the social context (not too close and not too far). In this interaction there was no need for touch and it was observed that overall she regulated repetitive behaviours except when tapping her foot.
- She shapes the content of the interaction by asking questions, providing replies when others ask, expressing emotion such as smiling, disagreeing politely and thanking her social partner when appropriate. There is no need to and she does not disclose information inappropriately.
- She maintains the flow of social interactions and sustains the conversations by taking turns, changing topics, responding to her social partner without hesitations and in a timely way and completing messages appropriately.

- She verbally supports the social interaction by clarifying or explaining messages, acknowledging and encouraging her social partner to continue by nodding and smiling and matching language appropriate to camera terminology. There is no need for her to empathise with her social partner in this context.
- Finally, she adapts her social interactions appropriately by heeding or undertaking the social exchange that she agreed to, by accommodating or changing her method of interacting when needed (changing the questions that she asks or asking for help).

Skills and Capacities

When carrying out occupational performance analysis it is important to distinguish between performance skills (motor, process and social interaction skills) and underlying body functions (musculoskeletal, neurological, cardiovascular and cognitive) and body structures (muscles, joints, skin, eyes, voice, etc.). Performance skills focus on what the person is doing, whereas body functions (capacities) focus on what the person's body is doing. When conducting an occupational performance analysis, occupational therapists are able to observe motor skills (skills pertaining to moving oneself and tasks objects), process skills (skills pertaining to organising and sequencing events over time and preventing/overcoming problems as they occur during the task performance), and social interaction skills when verbally interacting in a social context. When an occupational therapist observes Sarah interacting with a salesperson, the therapist can see her asking questions, tapping her foot as she waits, disagreeing with a point of view and asking for clarification. The occupational therapist cannot see that she does not understand about camera features, only that she is asking for clarification (more information), or know that she is bored, only that she is tapping her foot. The occupational therapist does not *know* that she is bored or does not understand as these are capacities (understanding, boredom) and cannot be *seen*. Only the manifestations as enacted during the task or social exchange (the performance skills) can be seen, so this is what should be observed and later measured.

This distinction is a very important one for occupational therapists. An occupation-focused approach places the person and the person's chosen occupations at the centre of the analysis process. By observing individuals actually carrying out occupations (including social occupations) of their choice, performance skills (motor, process and social interaction) are directly observed. Moreover, when the person is observed performing occupations in a preferred environment/context (physical, social and cultural), the interaction of person, environment and occupation can readily be seen. The person is central to the assessment process and the focus is on the doing of tasks. When occupational performance analysis is based on actual performance in context, there is rarely a need to assess the underlying body function capacities. The occupational therapist is able to observe the quality of performance as well as challenges presented by physical, social, cultural or other environments/contexts and impact of the people in that environment. There is no need to make inferences (or guesses) about the person's strengths or limitations as these can be seen in context. Further, occupational performance analysis (as opposed to activity analysis) does not rely on the identification of underlying capacities and deficits as it is focused on what is done. Most available assessment tools begin by focusing on body functions and body structures, including assessment of memory, behaviours, hand function or perception, and are conducted by appropriately trained professionals using specific standardised tests of impairment and incorporate a bottom-up approach. By conducting occupational performance analysis first in the context of what a person wants and needs to do, results that focus on performance issues can be used to plan and implement appropriate occupation-based interventions (occupation used as method).

Performance Patterns

Having considered client factors and performance skills, it is important to consider how performance patterns might influence the doing of occupations. Performance patterns include the habits, routines, roles and rituals that support or limit occupational performance (AOTA, 2014). What a person does and why that person does it is dependent on the person's personal habits, routines and rituals, as well as social and societal roles and expectations.

Habits, Routines and Rituals

Habits involve learned ways of doing occupations or specific behaviours that have developed through repeated experience and unfold automatically (Kielhofner, 2008). Dunn (2000) maintains that habits can be useful, dominating or impoverished and as such can either support or limit occupational performance. Routines are established sequences of occupations that provide a structure for daily life (AOTA, 2014). Routines are *what* a person does, whereas habits are the *way* a person does them. Habits and routines are observable behaviours repeated at predicable intervals such as eating dinner, going to bed and getting up. They are often organised by physical context such as day and night, sleep and wake, and provide stability in a person's life – for example, the morning dressing routines or the route taken to drive to and from work each day.

Kielhofner (2008) believes that habits guide behaviour through repeated experience of them over time and within a context (or environment). Rituals are symbolic actions with spiritual, cultural or social meaning that shape the identity of an individual and reinforce their values and beliefs (AOTA, 2014). Segal (2004) described routines as patterned behaviours that have instrumental goals and rituals as a form of symbolic communication. She describes routines as giving life order and rituals giving it meaning; for example, mealtime rituals are not just about providing nourishment but provide opportunities for socialisation, conflict resolution and determination of power relationships.

This is also important when working with people as habits and routines may have been disrupted by illness, injury or impairment and are often the first kinds of occupations that individuals want to reestablish (e.g. the morning routine of washing and dressing). Engaging people in familiar and regular occupations means connecting them with socially recognisable routines.

Roles

A role is defined as a set of behaviours expected by society and shaped by culture and context and can refer to a person, group or population (AOTA, 2014), such as, in a group context, the formal role of a chairperson on a committee, or the informal role of a parent within a family unit. Individuals participate in many different roles – student, worker, parent, homemaker, and so on – and behave in different ways according to whom they are interacting with (behaviours with a friend are usually different to behaviours with an employer) as well as societal and cultural expectations. Thus particular roles may be internalised and associated with behaviours expected by cultures or societies.

The roles that people assume say much about who they are and how they see themselves; it is usual for people only to assume roles that they want and need to do and those that would be expected by the society and culture in which they live. These are important considerations when working with people as a person's role gives occupations meaning. For example, the purpose of preparing a meal is to provide physical sustenance. However, the meaning of meal preparation (and cooking) will vary depending on the role: a working parent providing a meal for the family, a single person cooking for himself or herself, or a host or hostess preparing food for a celebration dinner for friends. Although the outcome will be similar (a meal on the table), the intrinsic meaning (and enjoyment) of the occupation will vary depending on the role.

Context and Environment

The importance of the interaction between persons and contexts/environments has long been recognised by occupational therapists. For example, the Person-Environment-Occupation Model (Law et al., 1996), Occupational Therapy Intervention Process Model (Fisher, 2009), Person-Environment-Occupation-Performance Model (Christiansen & Baum, 2005), Canadian Model of Occupational Performance and Engagement (Townsend & Polatajko, 2007) and Model of Human Occupation (Kielhofner, 2008) all outline the influence of this dynamic interaction on occupational performance.

The AOTA (2014) defines contexts and environment as different and separate concepts. *Context* refers to interrelated but different conditions, which are within and surround individuals and their families or carers and includes cultural, personal, temporal and virtual aspects. Environments are defined as the physical and social spaces within which the individual performs needed occupations and may potentially support or limit performance (AOTA, 2014).

Contexts

Cultural context includes customs, beliefs, activity patterns and behavioural standards expected by the society in which a person lives (AOTA, 2014). The cultural context influences who the person is (identity) and what activities are performed. This might include societal traditions and cultural celebrations such as specific religious festivals or customs. These are especially important where occupations include social interactions or understanding what should or should not be said or done in the home, education, employment or social circumstances.

Personal contexts include age, gender, educational and socioeconomic status (AOTA, 2014). These values and traditions are especially important where occupations include social interactions; for example, children or teenagers may interact differently in more formal school or work settings than when meeting with each other. Differences in personal contexts may include norms such as shaking hands when being introduced or understanding what should or should not be said in different social circumstances, including how different age groups meet and greet each other.

Temporal contexts place the occupation in a time frame (e.g. lifetime, year, day), a sense of history through past, present and future, and include the rhythm of activity. Occupations unfold over time and can provide temporal barriers or resources; the key feature here is to note how the temporal context changes during the course of an occupation rather than what changes for the *person*.

Virtual contexts refers to interactions that occur in simulated, real-time or near-time situations absent of physical contact (AOTA, 2014). These contexts usually require an ability to use technology such as mobile devices, smart phones, tablets, computers, video-game consoles in order to carry out their occupations or daily routines. Communication by virtual means may include the Internet, wireless or satellite communications, email, texts and social media such as blogs, Facebook and Twitter. Such environments can support performance, as in a home teleworker using Skype or Facetime on a computer, tablet or mobile device to conduct business, or inhibit performance, as in the case of an older adult with dementia who can no longer grasp the concept of a wireless alarm and thus refuses to carry the call device.

Environment

Physical environment refers to the natural environment and built surroundings in which daily life occupations take place (AOTA, 2014). The built environment not only includes the spaces but also the tools, devices and materials that are normally found in that context. For example, a kitchen would normally include a sink with running water, cupboard units, appliances such as cooker and refrigerator and tools and devices needed to prepare,

cook and serve food and clean up afterwards. This is important as occupations should occur in appropriate contexts.

The physical environment can either support or limit participation in occupations. For example, a kitchen can be designed with enough space to enable a wheelchair user to work, socialise and interact with task objects, people and the operation of devices in that space. In the same way, the familiarity of a kitchen may support or limit how well an older person with memory loss is able to search for and locate needed items, sequence steps logically over time or even be able to complete the task. In general, it is assumed that individuals perform occupations better in a familiar environment. However, this may not always be the case and so it is important not to make assumptions about the settings in which assessment of occupational performance takes place, but to be aware that context can and does have an impact. Observing and assessing individuals in their environment is the best way to determine whether the physical environment supports or limits occupational performance and, if there are limitations, what these are and how they may be overcome.

Task objects can also support or limit occupational performance. When making a hot drink or a snack in an unfamiliar kitchen, a person's performance would probably be less efficient as it would take longer to search for and find task objects and materials, and there may be some difficulty using unfamiliar electrical equipment (devices) such as the kettle, toaster or microwave. This is an important point to remember when working with people in an environment that they are unfamiliar with. The physical spaces, tools and materials that support performance are often referred to as 'naturalistic'. According to Fisher (2009), occupations should occur in naturalistic or an *ecologically relevant* environment. This usually means that it is the person's usual environment using tools and materials that the person would typically use and be familiar with. However, a naturalistic environment does not automatically support performance. Increasing age, frailty or physical, sensory, mental or cognitive decline may also negatively increase the demands of familiar activities even in a naturalistic environment.

It is important to remember that *context* refers to elements within and surrounding a person that can be less tangible than physical objects and spaces (AOTA, 2014). This is especially relevant when thinking about what is done in different cultural contexts and how performance rituals may affect (positively or negatively) aspects of occupational performance. A person's identity and which activities are chosen to be done are influenced by the person's culture, beliefs and customs. The roles expected of men and women; the people expected to be present, including chaperones for women in some cultures; and norms expected when eating are good examples of this. The way that spaces are used and the kinds of tools and materials in the environment are also affected by the culture of the person and the society where the person lives. For example, different tools and utensils would be found in a Western or European kitchen compared with an Asian or African kitchen as the kinds of foods that are prepared and the cooking methods are different.

The social environment consists of relationships and expectations of those with whom a person has regular contact. Fisher and Griswold (2015) refer to the 'client constellation' that includes others who live with, work with or are otherwise closely connected to the person. This may include (but is not limited to) family members, friends and caregivers. Environments will differ according to their purpose (work, family, church, leisure) and social expectations (such as dress, behaviours and rules). If specific rules or obligations apply, then the context may have to accommodate these; a sports centre would have changing rooms with gender-specific facilities, a church would have spaces, objects and symbols necessary and appropriate for religious acts, and so on. The presence or absence of individuals significant to the person is also important. Cavallin (2011) examined the impact of the environment on social interaction and concluded that the social environment had a stronger impact on the quality of a person's social interaction than does the physical environment. Fisher and Griswold (2015) examined aspects of the social environment on social interaction. Using the ESI they concluded that, overall, the quality of the social partner's social interaction has the greatest (observable) impact on the client's quality of social interaction.

THE APPLICATION OF OCCUPATIONAL PERFORMANCE ANALYSIS WITHIN THE OCCUPATIONAL THERAPY PROCESS

Occupational performance analysis can be completed during the assessment phase and reassessment or outcome measurement phase of the occupational therapy process.

The AOTA (2014) outlines the assessment phase as consisting of an occupational profile followed by an occupational performance analysis. The occupational profile is established through initial and ongoing interviews with the individual and significant others and establishes information pertaining to the domains already outlined. The occupational therapist will use the information from the occupational profile to begin to generate working hypotheses regarding possible reasons for the identified problems and concerns (AOTA, 2014). This information will therefore directly influence which occupational performance or performances will subsequently be observed and analysed. Nelson and Thomas (2003) highlight that observing a person doing a task is essential as what a person or significant others report can often differ from what the therapist sees. The focus here is on occupational performance skills and the *doing* of the occupations and not the limitations of body functions or body structures. This observation can be a nonstandardised observation or a standardised assessment tool such as the AMPS (Fisher & Jones, 2014) or the ESI (Fisher & Griswold, 2015). Performance skills and patterns are observed and the occupational therapist draws on professional knowledge and experience to analyse occupation (performance analysis). An overview of the performance skills is provided in Tables 16.1 and 16.2.

After an occupational performance analysis has been completed, the occupational therapist, using his or her professional reasoning skills, considers and interprets the impact of client factors (body functions and structures), the context and the environment in order to more specifically identify all the factors that are supporting or hindering the performance or the doing of occupations. Crepeau (2013) states that practitioners analyse occupations using both theoretical and practical knowledge and perspectives. Occupational performance analysis is a highly skilled and dynamic process that cannot be separated from the observation of the performance, the person who performed it or his or her needs in a specific context. Highlighting strengths and limitations of performance skills and patterns, contexts and task demands are all integral to this process. Keeping an occupation focus ensures that methods chosen for intervention will also be occupation-based (Fisher, 2013).

As strengths and limitations in performance skills, patterns, contexts, task demands and client factors are identified, goals and outcomes can be discussed and developed with the person. This in turn leads to the development of an intervention plan which is implemented. After intervention, the person is reassessed, again using an occupational performance analysis tool (such as the AMPS or the ESI). A comparison can then be made between this reassessment score and the initial baseline score in order to measure the outcomes of the intervention.

In Practice Story 16.1 Mary (an occupational therapist) is implementing a top-down process with David, a newly referred user of the community occupational therapy stroke service.

CONCLUSION

The purpose of this chapter has been to define and describe occupational performance analysis and discuss factors that affect how it is applied in occupational therapy practice. *Occupational performance analysis* refers to the analysis of performance skills, not body functions, and as such the difference between performance skills (motor, process and social interaction) and body functions (as described in the ICF) has been emphasised. After the implementation of occupational performance analysis and assessment of performance skills, task analysis is used to evaluate the impact of body functions and activity demands. A top-down approach has been emphasised as this focuses first on the needs of the person and the person's performance skills. Once a full occupational performance analysis has been completed, the range of person factors, contexts and environment that affect performance can be considered.

Occupation is the core of the occupational therapy profession and occupational therapists are experts in applying occupation as assessment and as intervention. Learning to analyse occupational performance takes time; it is a complex and skilled process in itself and should not be expect to be mastered overnight. Practice and application to meaningful daily activities will allow skills to develop and occupation terminology to become second nature.

David

OCCUPATIONAL PROFILE

Mary, an occupational therapist, interviewed David at home with his wife (Ellen); their daughter (Kate) who lives nearby was also present. David was 66 years old and 6 weeks before Mary's visit he had a right hemisphere cerebrovascular accident (CVA). After 4 weeks of rehabilitation in the local stroke unit he returned home to the two-bedroom bungalow in which he and Ellen had lived for the past 8 years. He was able to carry out most personal care tasks independently and safely but needed supervision with showering. He was not able to go outside unassisted.

Before his CVA David helped with heavier household chores, enjoyed do-it-yourself (DIY) projects and gardening, and kept the bungalow and garden in good order. Since returning home he had not yet attempted any domestic or meal preparation tasks, but he wanted to be able to make his own breakfast and other simple snacks, wash the dishes and help with laundry tasks so as not to be a burden on Ellen. Mary noted that Ellen appeared very anxious and protective of David and reluctant to let him do anything on his own. After some discussion, it was clear that Ellen's anxiety, manifested by a somewhat fussy and overbearing demeanour, was preventing David from progressing any further in his rehabilitation since returning home. After the initial interview, Mary agreed with David and Ellen that she would observe David in his home environment doing some domestic activities of daily living.

OCCUPATIONAL PERFORMANCE ANALYSIS: MOTOR AND PROCESS SKILLS

Assessment of Motor and Process Skills (AMPS)*

Mary observed David perform two AMPS tasks: preparing a bowl of cereal and a glass of juice (a typical breakfast for David) and hand washing the dishes. She used the AMPS as her standardised assessment tool and, in addition, was able to use information collected during the two AMPS observations to conduct an occupational performance analysis. As Mary was setting up the kitchen for the first task with David (cereal and juice), Ellen came into the kitchen to 'help'. Mary explained to David and Ellen that this was an assessment and therefore she wanted to observe David on his own first (without help) so that she could see what David could and could not do on his own. David and Ellen understood this and both readily agreed.

After the assessment, Mary scored the two observations using the standardised criteria of the AMPS. The information that Mary analysed and later collated with regards to motor and process performance skills is listed here using the global skill categories of the AMPS. Definitions of motor and process skills can be found in Table 16.1.

*See http://www.innovativeotsolutions.com/content/amps.

Body position: David had some difficulty maintaining an upright posture while standing at the sink; he propped on the countertop while standing and walking *(stabilises)*. He also had some difficulty *positioning* his body effectively at the refrigerator and the lower cupboard units, which caused him some difficulty obtaining tools and materials from the lower shelves. Ellen hovered nearby and attempted to support David while standing at the sink and while walking, thus impeding his ability to demonstrate the quality of his standing and walking skills and his ability to maintain his balance *(stabilises)* while interacting in the task environment.

Obtaining and holding objects: David was able to *reach* for and *bend* his trunk to obtain objects with minimal effort. He had weak grasp *(grips)* in his left hand making it difficult to hold and *manipulate* small objects such as cutlery, especially when he coordinated two hands together as when opening the juice container and screwing the top back onto the milk container *(coordinates)*.

Moving self and objects: David was able to open doors and drawer without undue effort *(moves)* but used two hands to *lift* heavier objects such as the milk container and teapot (when washing the dishes). He walked safely using one walking stick *(walks)*, but this impeded his ability to *transport* items in the kitchen as he could not carry more than one object at once. Stiffness of movement of his left hand and wrist *(flows)* caused difficulty while washing dishes and his ability to grade the force of movement *(calibrates)* when placing objects on the countertops or dish drainer.

Sustaining performance (motor): David's performance slowed over time *(paces)* and, as a result of physical fatigue, he asked to sit down during the second task observation *(endures)*.

Sustaining performance (process): David maintained focused attention *(attends)* for the majority of the task. On a couple of occasions he did look away from what he was doing towards Ellen, who made a suggestion and made an attempt to help him. He completed both tasks as agreed *(heeds)*.

Applying knowledge: David chose all needed tools and materials *(chooses)* and *used* them appropriately. He had difficulty supporting and stabilising larger objects *(handles)* such as the juice container during bilateral actions. He did not need to seek out additional information *(inquires)*.

Temporal organisation: David was seen to hesitate before starting steps *(initiates)*; he interrupted action sequences on a number of occasions *(continues)*, ordered steps in a logical *sequence* and spent a long time washing some of the dishes *(terminates)*. This led to steps taking longer to complete and performance being moderately inefficient.

Continued on following page

David *(Continued)*

Organising space and objects: David was able to *search for and locate* all task objects and *gather* them into the workspace appropriately. However, his workspace at times was crowded *(organises)*, resulting in him bumping into objects *(navigates)*, and at other times he arranged tools and material between two workspaces *(organises)*, resulting in slowed and moderately inefficient performance. Ellen stepping in to pass things to him also impeded his ability to demonstrate the quality of his organising skill. He *restored* all items at the end of both tasks.

Adapting performance: David was delayed in responding to water running out of the washing up bowl *(notices/responds)* and he *adjusted* the taps constantly during the washing up task. He had limited ability to modify his actions (motor and process) in response to problems occurring *(accommodates)*

and some problems *(stabilising, positioning, manipulating, coordinating, transporting, handling, organising)* persisted through the task performances *(benefits)*.

After the task observations Mary sat down with David and Ellen and discussed with David the occupational performance analysis that she had carried out. The summary of the AMPS earlier describes the areas of difficulty that most affected David's occupational performance (with the motor and process skill items in italics or in parentheses). Next Mary discussed with David what he had found difficult and the reasons for this. A left-sided weakness after the stroke had resulted in a number of motor-sensory and perceptual body function impairments. Body function and body structure impairments that negatively affected performance can be found in Table 16.6.

TABLE 16.6

Person Factors for David, Including Body Functions as Described by the ICF – Motor, Process and Social Interaction Skills in Italics

1. Client Factors

Values	Values his role as a husband as it increases his sense of commitment and belonging but has difficulties in expressing his views in a polite and respectful way, which interferes with effective social exchanges *(questions, replies, disagrees, transitions, times response, takes turns)*
Beliefs	Has difficulty expressing his views regarding his expectation that he should contribute towards the household tasks and duties impedes his ability to say what his priorities are *(replies, disagrees, times response, takes turns, clarifies, accommodates)*
Spiritual	High levels of motivation and personal investment in maintaining prior roles give meaning and purpose

2. Neuromusculoskeletal and Movement-Related Functions

Mobility of joints	Range of motion and postural alignment *(aligns)* did not appear impaired
Muscle power	Weakness of left hand *(grips)* and arm affected ability to *lift* heavier items; tended to slide these items *(moves)* Reduced postural control (balance) of left side of trunk *(stabilises)* and left lower limb weakness *(walks)* noted
Muscle tone	Increased muscle tone and spasticity in left wrist and hand affects smoothness of movement *(flows)*. On the left side of the trunk it affects *reaching* and *bending* into cupboards and *positioning* body at the units
Movement functions	Poor bilateral integration and hand–eye coordination noted when manipulating small objects using two hands (or two body parts) together *(manipulates, coordinates, handles)*. Reduced ability to control force of movement when using left hand *(calibrates)* noted. Lurching gait and walking pattern *(walks)* cause some instability when transporting items *(transports)*
Involuntary movements	Occasional poor righting reactions were noted during standing and reaching, resulting in transient loss of balance *(stabilises)*. Slight tremor was noted in left hand when pouring *(flows)*

3. Cardiovascular Functions

Heart	Poor physical endurance and stamina led to a slowing down during both task *(paces)*. Fatigue led to a need to sit during the second task *(endures)*

4. Sensory Functions

Seeing function	*Noticing/responding* to the water running from the left tap and bowl may have been affected by hemianopia

David (Continued)

TABLE 16.6
Person Factors for David, Including Body Functions as Described by the ICF – Motor, Process and Social Interaction Skills in Italics (Continued)

Touch/sensation	Mild loss of sensitivity to touch resulted in some fumbling of small objects with left hand (*manipulates*)
Proprioceptive function	Poor joint position sense of left upper limb resulted in bumping into items (*navigates*)

5. Mental Functions of Perception and Cognition

Energy	Maintained motivation to complete task but slowed as tasks progressed (*paces*)
Attention	Generally sustained focus attention but looked away from the task towards comments made by spouse (*attends*). Completed both task as intended (*heeds*)
Memory	Able to search for and find needed tools and materials (*searches/locates*). No need to ask for information or any need for verbal prompts (*inquires*). Completed the tasks without prompts (*heeds*), including putting everything away (*restores*)
Emotional functions	Not always able to control the range and regulation of emotions and self-control (*regulates, expresses emotion, disagrees, acknowledges and encourages, empathises*)
Visuospatial functions	Reduced awareness of left side of space resulted in a tendency to bump into objects (*navigates*) and have items crowded on the right side of space (*organises*)
Time management	Gathering items to nonadjacent workspaces (*gathers*) delayed task progression. Able to *sequence* steps in an efficient and appropriate order and without interruptions (*continues*)
	Takes longer to *produce speech and speak fluently* and to express his views in a mature, respectful and polite manner, easily becoming frustrated when he is not able to do this effectively (*replies, disagrees, times response, takes turns*)
Decision making	Some hesitations noted or slow to begin (*initiates*) or end (*terminates*) actions – washing and washing dishes
	Slow to end social exchanges (*concludes/disengages*)
	A tendency to be dominated by others during a conversation (*takes turns*) and problems adapting performance when problems were encountered during social exchanges (*accommodates*)
Regulation of motor response to events	Turning off taps was delayed or sometimes random (*adjusts*). Delayed in responding to the water running out of the washing up bowl (*notices/responds*)
Problem solving	A tendency to persist in discussion the same topic or a delay moving on with the conversation (*transitions*)
	Difficulty in anticipating and changing actions in response to problems encountered and during social exchanges (*accommodates; benefits*)

The cluttered worktops (physical environment) and the input from Ellen (social environment) also negatively affected his performance. Ellen reported that she helped as she felt David needed assistance. David did not initially respond, but his nonverbal body language suggested he did not agree and when asked directly he indicated that this was the case. Activity and environmental demands can be found in Table 16.7.

OCCUPATIONAL PERFORMANCE ANALYSIS: SOCIAL INTERACTION SKILLS

Evaluation of Social Interaction (ESI)*

Mary had noted some friction between David and Ellen when they talked to each other about what David could (and could not) do. In particular, David found it difficult to express his needs to Ellen and Ellen did not always listen to what David was trying to say. After some discussion,

Mary used the ESI to observe David *sharing information* with Ellen about what kind of household tasks he would like to help her with now that he was back home; and for the second observation she observed David, Ellen and Kate (their daughter) engage in casual conversation while eating lunch together. Using the ESI she was able to observe the two social exchanges, SI-1 and CS-1 (Intended Purposes definitions can be found in Table 16.3) and analyse the quality of David's social interaction skill and the impact of the social partners during both social exchanges. She was keen during their discussion before the observations to ensure that these two intended purposes were what David perceived as difficult (and not what Ellen wanted him to do) and to ensure that he engaged in the two social interactions with typical social partners (his wife and daughter) in a naturalistic context (his home).

*See http://www.innovativeotsolutions.com/content/esi.

Continued on following page

David (Continued)

TABLE 16.7
Contextual and Activity Demands for David

Objects and their properties	Familiar objects supported performance overall but impairment of left side (and left hand in particular) required the provision of different or adapted equipment for more efficient performance (nonslip mat, stabilising devices, etc.)
Physical spaces	Small kitchen area and cluttered worktops impeded performance (organises)
Cultural	Familiar role as a husband had been disrupted and no longer supported effective social exchanges
Social	Presence of spouse did not support performance or provide supervision/assistance appropriately if required Presence of spouse impeded polite and respectful expression of views during social exchanges
Sequence/timing	Previous habits and routines (rigid adherence to previous methods) slowed performance (paces) and impeded polite and respectful social exchanges (questions, replies, disagrees, transitions, times response, takes turns)

After this assessment, Mary scored the two observations using the standardised criteria of the ESI. The information that Mary analysed and later collated with regards to social interaction skills is listed next using the global skill categories of the ESI. Definitions of social interaction skills can be found in Table 16.2.

Initiating and terminating social interactions: David had no difficulty *initiating* conversation and there was no problem with either social exchange. However, when David tried to *terminate* the conversation, in both social exchanges Ellen continued to talk and David unnecessarily extended the conversation, resulting in a delay in ending it.

Producing social interaction: David did not always articulate some words clearly and occasionally he mumbled so that it was difficult for Ellen and Kate to hear him *(produces speech)*. He spoke slowly with pauses during some messages *(speaks fluently)* and used some *gestures* (frowning and shaking his head) that were unclear in the social context and did not always support the message he was sending.

Physically supporting social interaction: David turned his body but not his face towards Kate and he turned away from

Ellen at times *(turns towards)*, impeding any further social interaction with her at that point. He *looked* down or out of the corner of his eye when Ellen was talking. He was also observed to speak in a loud voice and drum his fingers on the chair arm *(regulates)* on several occasions when Ellen was talking. He *placed himself* at an appropriate distance from Ellen and Kate and there was no need for *touch* during either social exchange.

Shaping content of social interaction: David asked no *questions* at all in the second social exchange (questions are required for this Intended Purpose; see Table 16.3 for CS-1). He did not *reply* to many of Ellen's questions or suggestions and when he did they were very brief *(times duration)*. He used an irritated tone of voice *(expresses emotion)* when Ellen interrupted him and frequently *disagreed* with her suggestions by responding in a defensive or argumentative way. He did not make any belittling comments about others *(discloses)* and there was no need to *thank* his social partners.

Maintaining flow of social interaction: David frequently persisted in discussing an earlier topic and repeatedly asking the same question *(transitions)* after the conversation had moved on. He constantly interrupted Ellen when she was talking *(times response)* and did not always *reply* to her comments. He did not always finish his sentences, leaving some 'hanging in the air' *(times duration)*, and did not always *take turns* in the conversation, allowing Ellen to dominate, which on several occasions results in the social exchange breaking down.

Verbally supporting social interaction: David sometimes used a whining tone of voice *(matches language)* when responding to Ellen and did not *acknowledge or encourage* her to participate in the ongoing discussion. He did not *empathise* or send any messages of support to Kate when she expressed discomfort or *clarify* which tasks he wanted to do when Kate was unsure.

Adapting performance: David stayed on topic *(heeds)* in both social exchanges but had many problems in modifying his social interactions in anticipation of many problems that arose *(accommodates)*. He had problems turning towards and looking at his social partners, not replying to their questions or suggestions, and expressing emotion and disagreeing in a respectful, polite and mature way; he did not always take his turn in the conversation and allowed himself to be dominated by one social partner (Ellen). He repeatedly interrupted one social partner (Ellen), resulting in disrespectful and impolite social interactions. His problems persisted *(benefits)* throughout both social exchanges.

After her observation of two social exchanges, Mary used the ESI results to discuss the outcome of her observations with David and Ellen and their daughter Kate, who had stayed for the afternoon's discussion. The ESI highlighted many instances where there was a breakdown in social interactions between David and Ellen and this negatively affected David's ability to

PRACTICE STORY 16.1

David *(Continued)*

express his needs and preferences. This was especially seen when Ellen wanted to make all the decisions for David and David was clearly frustrated but unable express himself in a polite and respectful way. Mary was able to identify specific skills to work

on as part of her occupation-based intervention plan. She concluded that the reason for David and Ellen's many difficulties related to their social interaction problems but did not see this with Kate.

 http://evolve.elsevier.com/Curtin/OT

REFERENCES

American Occupational Therapy Association (2014). Occupational therapy practice framework: Domains and processes, 3rd edition. *American Journal of Occupational Therapy, 68*(Suppl. 1), S1–S48.

Brown, T., & Chien, C. W. (2010). Top-down or bottom-up occupational therapy assessment: Which way do we go? *British Journal of Occupational Therapy, 73*(3), 95.

Canadian Association of Occupational Therapists (2012). *Definition of occupational therapy.* Retrieved from, http://www.caot.ca/default.asp?pageid + 1344.

Cantin, N., & Polatajko, H. (2013). Occupation-focused intervention approaches for children and youth. *Ergoterapeuten, 6,* 28–34.

Cavallin, U. (2011). *The impact of the environment on the quality of social interaction.* Unpublished master's thesis, Sweden: Umea University Cited in Fisher, A. G., & Griswold, L. A. (2015). *The evaluation of social interaction* (3rd ed. rev.). Fort Collins, CO: Three Star Press.

Christiansen, C. H., Baum, C. M., & Bass-Haugen, J. (Eds.). (2005). *Occupational Therapy: Performance, Participation and Well-being.* (3rd ed.). Thorofare, NJ: Slack.

Christiansen, C. H., & Townsend, E. A. (Eds.). (2004). *Introduction to occupation: The art and science of living.* Upper Saddle River, NJ: Prentice Hall.

College of Occupational Therapy (2012). *Assessments and outcome measures: Good practice briefing.* London: COT.

College of Occupational Therapy (2015). *Definitions of occupational therapy: Essential briefing.* London: COT.

Connelly, K., & Dalgleish, M. (1989). The emergence of a tool-using skill in infancy. *Developmental Psychology, 25,* 894–912.

Crepeau, A. B. (2013). Analysing occupation and activity: A way of thinking about occupational performance. In E. B. Crepeau, E. S. Cohn, & B. A. B. Schell (Eds.), *Willard & Spackman's occupational therapy.* Philadelphia: Lippincott Williams & Wilkins.

Diamantis, A. (2010). Defending occupation in paediatric practice. *British Journal of Occupational Therapy, 73*(8), 343.

Dunn, W. (2000). Habits: What's the brain got to do with it? *Occupational Therapy Journal of Research: Occupation, Participation & Health,* (Suppl. 1), 6S–20S.

Fisher, A. G. (1998). Uniting practice and theory in an occupation framework: Eleanor Clarke Slagle Lecture. *American Journal of Occupational Therapy, 52,* 509–520.

Fisher, A. G. (2009). *Occupational therapy intervention process model: A model for planning and implementing top-down, client-centred, and occupation-based interventions.* Fort Collins, CO: Three Star Press.

Fisher, A. G. (2013). Occupation-centred, occupation-based, occupation-focused: Same, same or different? *Scandinavian Journal of Occupational Therapy, 20,* 162–173.

Fisher, A. G., & Griswold, L. A. (2015). *Evaluation of social interaction* (3rd ed. rev.). Fort Collins, CO: Three Star Press.

Fisher, A. G., & Jones, K. B. (2012). *Assessment of motor and process skills: Volume 1* (7th ed., rev.). Fort Collins, CO: Three Star Press.

Fisher, A. G., & Jones, K. B. (2014). *Assessment of motor and process skills: Volume 2* (8th ed.). Fort Collins, CO: Three Star Press.

Hocking, C. (2001). Implementing occupation-based assessment. *American Journal of Occupational Therapy, 55*(4), 463–469.

Ideishi, R. I. (2003). Influences of occupation on assessment and treatment. In P. Kramer, J. Hinojosa, & C. B. Royeen (Eds.), *Perspectives in human occupation: Participation in life.* Baltimore, MD: Lippincott Williams & Wilkins.

Kielhofner, G. (2008). *Model of human occupation: Theory and application* (4th ed.). Baltimore, MD: Lippincott Williams & Wilkins.

Law, M., Cooper, B., Strong, S., Stewart, D., Rigby, P., & Letts, L. (1996). The person-environment-occupation model: A trans-active approach to occupational performance. *Canadian Journal of Occupational Therapy, 63,* 9–23.

Nelson, D., & Thomas, J. J. (2003). Occupational form, occupational performance, and a conceptual framework for therapeutic occupation. In P. Kramer, J. Hinojosa, & C. B. Royeen (Eds.), *Perspectives in human occupation: Participation in life.* Baltimore, MD: Lippincott Williams & Wilkins.

O'Toole, G. (2011). What is occupation analysis? In L. Mackenzie, & G. O'Toole (Eds.), *Occupation analysis in practice.* Chichester, UK: Blackwell Publishing.

Pierce, D. (2001). Untangling occupation and activity. *American Journal of Occupational Therapy, 55,* 138–146.

Polatajko, H., Davis, J. A., Hobson, S. J. G., et al. (2004). Meeting the responsibility that comes with the privilege: Introducing a taxonomic code for understanding occupation. *Canadian Journal of Occupational Therapy, 71*(5), 261–264.

Polatajko, H. J., Mandich, A., & Martini, R. (2000). Dynamic performance analysis: A framework for understanding occupational performance. *American Journal of Occupational Therapy, 54*, 65–72.

Reed, K. I. (2005). An annotated history of the concepts used in occupational therapy. In C. H. Christiansen, M. C. Baum, & J. Bass-Haugen (Eds.), *Occupational therapy: Performance, participation, and well-being*. Thorofare, NJ: Slack.

Rodger, S. (2010). Introduction to occupation-centered practice with children. In S. Rodger (Ed.), *Occupation-centered practice with children*. Wiley Blackwell: Oxford, UK.

Segal, R. (2004). Family routines and rituals: A context for occupational therapy interventions. *American Journal of Occupational Therapy, 59*(5), 499–506.

Simmons, C. D., Griswold, L. A., & Berg, B. (2010). Evaluation of social interaction during occupational engagement. *American Journal of Occupational Therapy, 64*(1), 10–17.

Townsend, E. A., & Polatajko, H. J. (2007). *Enabling occupation II: Advancing an occupational therapy vision for health, well-being, & justice through occupation*. Ottawa: Canadian of Association Occupational Therapists.

Trombly, C. (1993). Anticipating the future: Assessment of occupational function. *American Journal of Occupational Therapy, 47*(3), 253–257.

Weinstock-Zlotnick, G., & Hinojosa, J. (2004). Bottom-up or top-down evaluation: Is one better than the other? *American Journal of Occupational Therapy, 58*(5), 594–599.

World Federation of Occupational Therapists (2012). *Definition of occupation. Retrieved from,* http://www.wfot.org/AboutUs/AboutOccupationalTherapy/DefinitionofOccupationalTherapy.aspx.

World Health Organization (2001). *International classification of functioning, disability & health (ICF)*. Geneva, Switzerland: WHO.

17

PERCEIVE, RECALL, PLAN AND PERFORM (PRPP) SYSTEM OF TASK ANALYSIS AND INTERVENTION

CHRIS CHAPPARO ■ JUDY L. RANKA ■ MELISSA THERESE NOTT

Abstract

This chapter focuses on the place of cognitive strategies in occupational therapy assessment and management of reduced physical capacity and the way cognition may hinder or enhance physical aspects of performance. This chapter describes an ecological standardised measure of cognitive strategy use, the Perceive, Recall, Plan and Perform (PRPP) System of Task Analysis and Intervention. An example of how the PRPP Assessment could be employed as an observational assessment format is provided. Information processing theory is coupled with notions of occupational performance to demonstrate how difficulty with learning new skills affects occupational performance.

KEY POINTS

■ The Perceive, Recall, Plan and Perform (PRPP) System of Task Analysis and Intervention represents a contemporary shift in occupational therapy towards a more ecological and dynamic style of practice where assessment and intervention are mutually informative and where the focus is on the particular occupational needs of particular people in particular contexts.

■ The PRPP System of Task Analysis and Intervention focuses on cognitive strategy use in the context of tasks and activities that are meaningful and relevant to the person.

■ The PRPP Assessment is an ecologically valid, process-oriented, criterion-referenced assessment that employs task analysis methods to determine problems with occupational performance.

■ The PRPP Intervention is a task-oriented information processing approach that simultaneously focuses on task training and strategy training within the context of everyday performance.

■ The interaction between reduced cognitive ability and physical impairment can compound the impact of each of these disorders on occupational performance.

INTRODUCTION

Assessment and intervention is a dynamic process, based on observation of the interaction between people and their environments, with effective performance supported by a number of sensorimotor, biomechanical and cognitive capacities (Chapparo & Ranka, 1997a). Physical participation in occupational performance requires that people are able to engage in everyday occupational roles by learning what they have to do (work, leisure, social and self-maintenance occupations), knowing when and where they have to do things (situating their roles in the space and time of the day), and attributing meaning to why they do things (Chapparo & Lowe, 2011). Learning or relearning to accomplish the purposeful motor skills that enable participation in daily life activities is a primary goal of occupational therapy for people with physical disorders that affect occupational performance (Shumway-Cook & Woollacott, 2001).

Of particular relevance to this chapter are the cognitive or 'thinking' strategies used to process salient information for coordinated and effective physical performance during everyday activities. Cognition has been defined in many ways. In this chapter, it is defined as an interaction of processes that involve all forms of awareness and knowing such as perceiving, conceiving, insight, remembering, questioning, reasoning, judging, problem solving and decision making (VandenBos, 2015). Simply put, *cognition* refers to the functions of the mind that result in thought and goal-directed action. Cognition not only influences what a person chooses to do, it also determines how physical experience is remembered and interpreted, and as such, it contributes to sense of self (Radomski & Morrison, 2014). Compared with able-bodied peers, people who sustain physical impairments may have to think harder about how, when and where to move their bodies for optimum occupational performance. Moreover, an accompanying neurocognitive deficit might compound difficulties experienced. This chapter focuses on the place of cognitive strategies in occupational therapy management of reduced physical capacity and the way cognition may hinder, or be used purposefully to enhance, physical aspects of performance.

Reduced physical ability can originate from many sources. First, some central nervous system disorders such as traumatic brain injury, stroke, multiple sclerosis, and Parkinson's disease directly affect central nervous system (CNS) structures that organise motor performance, including the primary motor cortex, cerebellum and brainstem, resulting in changes to a person's capacity to move (Shumway-Cook & Woollacott, 2007). This type of physical disorder is often associated with concomitant neurocognitive deficit that may include difficulty thinking about and planning movements, relearning movement or learning new movements, maintaining goal-directed movements, or using sensorimotor feedback systems to adjust the quality of physical actions (Wolpert, Diedrichsen, & Flanagan, 2011). The interaction between reduced cognitive ability and physical impairment can compound the impact of each of these disorders on occupational performance.

Second, people who have a physical impairment caused by musculoskeletal disorders such as upper-limb amputation, injury caused by falls, back injury and hand injury have to 'reset' their thinking about how to move. Indeed, many such physical impairments arise when people move without thinking, misjudge their physical abilities, or fail to consider their limitations (Bootes & Chapparo, 2010). Even in the absence of a neurocognitive deficit, motor relearning for occupational performance requires that people with a musculoskeletal disorder use thinking strategies to learn how to move again, move in a different way or compensate for lost movement.

Third, people who experience fluctuating systemic disorders that reduce physical performance, such as chronic fatigue syndrome and rheumatoid arthritis, depend on use of their cognitive strategies to monitor performance and compensate for day-to-day changes in physical capacity (Abeare et al., 2010). Finally, physical capacity alters with increasing age, mirroring structural changes to the CNS, peripheral nervous system and musculoskeletal system function (Alcock, O'Brien, & Vanicek, 2015), and results in reduction in strength, speed and dexterity during everyday performance. Compounding physical changes are age-related changes in problem solving, reasoning, memory and attention, usually after 70 years of age but sometimes appearing before then (Banich & Compton, 2011; Riddle, 2007). These scenarios suggest that occupational therapy for people with compromised physical capacity should include assessment of how cognitive strategies might impact physical performance and how they may be utilised to optimise outcomes of physical skills intervention. Moreover, although people bring their own neuromotor, experiential, and sociocultural predispositions to how they process cognitive information for physical activity, their performance at any given time is mediated by the task they have to do and the context in which it is done (Hardwick, Rottschy, Miall, & Eickhoff, 2013). This means that the most meaningful assessment of cognition is one that is carried out with reference to ecological variables, namely, the particular functional performance that is of concern to the person's situation, and in the context performance is required (Burgess et al., 2006).

The purposes of this chapter are to: (1) describe elements of information processing theory and cognitive strategy application for occupational performance; (2) describe one example of an ecological standardised measure of cognitive strategy use – the Perceive, Recall, Plan and Perform (PRPP) Assessment (Chapparo & Ranka, 1997b); and (3) illustrate the use of the PRPP System of Task Analysis and Intervention with practice examples of people who have occupational performance restrictions as a result of physical impairment in the presence or absence of neurocognitive deficit.

The following three assumptions underlie the use of the PRPP System of Task Analysis and Intervention. First, information processing during occupational performance is determined by the processing demands of the task, the performance context and the processing capacity of the person doing the task. Second, the application of cognitive strategies can be behaviourally observed during everyday occupational performance. Third, a generic set of cognitive strategies is adapted by people for use across a range of daily occupations.

INFORMATION PROCESSING AND COGNITIVE STRATEGIES FOR OCCUPATIONAL PERFORMANCE

Information processing theory is an ecological, inclusive model of cognition that can be used to explain disorders in motor learning evident during occupational performance (Schmidt & Wrisberg, 2008). Using principles from information processing theory, occupational therapists can structure their observations of how people do everyday tasks and plan intervention to enhance the thinking that supports performance. People participate in tasks that occur in specific contexts such as their home or workplace. As described earlier in this chapter, the physical ecology of task performance is a critical element of successful participation, reinforcing the notion that context-based performance (what a person actually does in his or her own environment) may be quite different to clinic-based capacity (a person's ability to perform a task at the highest probable level of functioning). For this reason an ecological approach to assessment is needed that describes the discordance between a person's capacity to engage in performance and the expectations of the performance context.

Models of information processing such as the one illustrated in the central boxes of Fig. 17.1 trace the staged flow of information from initial reception, through several processing points, to the final response and monitoring of that response (Bohannon & Bonvillian, 2005; Friedenberg & Silverman, 2012). The human brain, or information processor, takes in information (sensing), stores and relocates it (memory or recall), organises the information by means of various strategies for problem solving and decision making (planning), and generates responses to the information (planning and output monitoring).

Despite the remarkable power and flexibility of the human brain, its capacity to process information is surprisingly limited. Decisions are made at all stages of processing about the importance of information relative to salient conditions (what is happening here and now) and its *worth* (the goal or purpose for processing) (Buschman, Siegel, Jefferson, & Miller, 2011). Information that is not regarded as 'important' is discarded. What is processed and the quality of processing throughout the whole system is therefore controlled by an executive system that monitors and regulates these processes in order to engage in corrective strategies when processing is not going smoothly and to evaluate outcomes and decisions (Huitt, 2003). This has been referred to as 'metastrategic control' in people's ability to apply the thinking strategies that process new information (Couchman, Coutinho, Beran, & Smith, 2010; Demetriou & Kazi, 2006; Kieran & Christoff, 2014).

Metastrategic control assists people to cope with the many problems of performance that arise during their everyday round

of activity and allows people to not just 'do what they know' but to figure out the most effective way to perform under conditions of change such as that experience with reduced physical capacity. Cognitive strategies are goal directed behaviours that people use to do the following (Siegler, 2007):

1. Identify important or difficult information
2. Understand and retain information
3. Retrieve information from memory
4. Apply relevant information
5. Plan responses
6. Simultaneously cope with internal and external distractions during performance of a task

Cognitive strategies have been defined as either external, when people use external sources such as memory diaries, mind maps and mnemonics to support cognitive aspects of task performance (Katz, Baum, & Maeir, 2011), or internally generated thinking processes that are part of the process of thinking through task performance (Toglia, Rodger, & Polatajko, 2012). Within a physical rehabilitation setting, the strategies referred to are often external and are learned as compensatory behaviours for residual cognitive impairments. They are often viewed as the end product of intervention (Giles, 2011; Katz et al., 2011; Koh, Hoffmann, Bennett, & McKenna, 2009). For example, a person may learn a unilateral dressing strategy to compensate for one-sided weakness or use an electronic device to assist memory for timing of daily activities.

Internal cognitive strategies are the focus of this chapter and are depicted in the outer boxes in Fig. 17.1. When applied to motor learning, these strategies enable people with physical impairments to acquire new skills or adapt to a challenging activity or problem (Toglia, 2005). Internally generated cognitive strategies can be general (applied to any task) or more specific (used to process a unique task such as making a soufflé or water skiing). The PRPP System of Task Analysis and Intervention focuses on how people can use general internal thinking strategies in specific situations of occupational performance.

It has been suggested within the field of neural science that in the presence of limited capacity to process information people 'share' cognitive strategies across tasks. For everyday tasks, this means people use a general set of cognitive strategies across all tasks. Research during the early development of the PRPP System of Task Analysis and Intervention confirms that people use the same set of cognitive strategies to solve problems of everyday life but apply them differently depending on salient conditions (e.g. perceived importance, timing, expected quality, safety, disability) (Chapparo, 2011). Cognitive strategy use implies salience or use of known strategies in the 'here and now'; it is the ability to choose and apply the 'best' strategy to fit a particular situation. Effective cognitive strategy use is defined as the simplest and most efficient means of processing information relative to a situation (Siegler, 2007) and enables a person to participate in everyday activities without having to 'think too hard'.

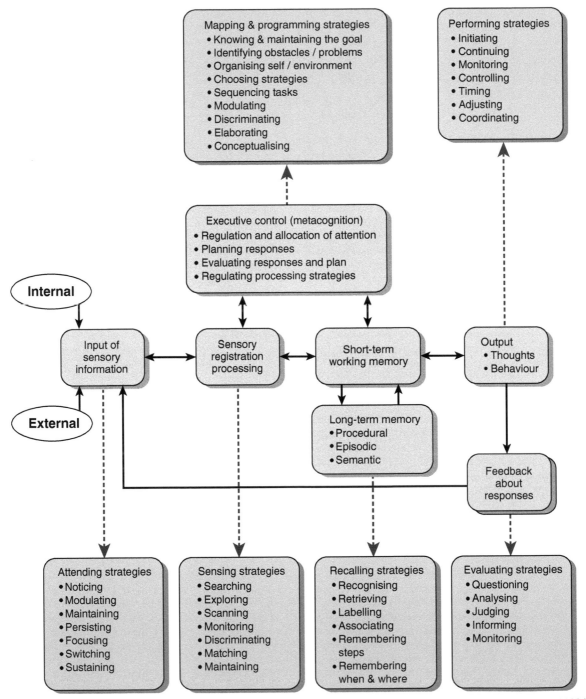

FIG. 17.1 ■ Information processing model with associated processing strategies. *(Reprinted with permission from Nott, 2008.)*

COGNITIVE STRATEGY USE AND THE PRPP SYSTEM OF TASK ANALYSIS AND INTERVENTION

Relative to occupational performance, cognitive strategies are defined by the four information processing quadrants of the PRPP System of Task Analysis and Intervention. Strategies are aligned with attention and perception (Perceive); learning, memory and recall (Recall); planning, decision making and judgement (Plan); and the ability to act on a decision and follow through with plans (Perform). When using the PRPP Assessment, occupational therapists can assess the extent to which people with physical impairments are able to use cognitive strategies in a variety of home, work and community occupations. Cognitive strategies used during occupational performance are determined largely by the processing demands of the occupation, the performance context and the processing capacity of the person doing the occupation. At times of stress or illness, people experience difficulty processing the information needed for occupations. Although for most people this is temporary, people who have sustained significant physical or neurological impairments are likely to experience a persistent processing disorder resulting in a long-term impact on occupational performance. The nature of the disorder is not viewed as a deficit in cognition per se, but an inability to apply cognitive processing strategies to occupations in context.

People have individual ways of performing occupations, and occupational therapists increasingly are coming to understand the limitations of traditional deficit-specific approaches to assessment that measure impairment in isolation from daily occupation (Burgess et al., 2006; Chapparo, 2010; Chapparo & Ranka, 1997b; Fisher, 1993). Performance of each task throughout the day poses unique demands on information to be processed and used for a specific purpose. This is particularly true when learning new or adaptive processes for task performance or relearning occupational tasks in the presence of physical impairments. A new set of motor tactics has to be chosen, constructed, processed, stored, recalled and organised with reference to the context in which occupation will occur (Morris & Ward, 2004).

For example, Bryce is a 32-year-old male who sustained a traumatic transhumeral amputation in a motor vehicle crash. Bryce is married and has a young child. His wife works night shift. Bryce currently uses a hybrid prosthesis with a switch locking elbow, a friction wrist and a myoelectric hand. Bryce wears his prosthesis most days and, although he can operate the prosthesis, he has limited use of the prosthesis in functional tasks. Bryce identified the occupational goal of picking his daughter up from her cot at night when his wife was at work. Bryce demonstrated difficulty monitoring his body and arm position during this task, did not organise himself or the task environment before beginning the task and did not choose the best approach to take. He was unable to analyse the errors he was making and

so did not adjust how he performed the task. Bryce needed to learn a new set of motor tactics to position himself relative to his daughter's cot and store and retrieve this information on each occasion of task performance. The context in which this task occurred was specific and placed limitations on the range of movement available, the need for sensitive calibration and smooth motor performance. Dynamic cognitive strategies were required to monitor and make musculoskeletal adjustments in response to the task demands and in response to movements of his daughter during the task.

This ecological approach to evaluation and intervention is a fundamental and core aspect of the PRPP System of Task Analysis and Intervention. Further, the PRPP Assessment recognises and incorporates the individuality of occupational task performance by enabling the occupational therapist to observe a sample of occupations that are pertinent to the person's situation and judge whether performance is effective compared with the person's expectations of performance and expectations of others in the person's contexts, rather than constraining the evaluation of performance to a set of standard occupations that all people do. The assumption underlying this assessment structure is that people, with or without disorders of cognition, use the same general set of cognitive strategies when they carry out everyday occupations (Aubin, Chapparo, Gélinas, Stip, & Rainville, 2009; Chapparo & Ranka, 1997b; Nott, Chapparo, & Heard, 2008).

PRPP ASSESSMENT

The PRPP Assessment is conducted in two stages. In Stage One, a *behavioural* task analysis is used to break down everyday occupation into steps for the purpose of identifying errors. An overall measure of mastery for specific and relevant occupations is computed (Kirwan & Ainsworth, 1992). Stage Two focuses on information processing strategies required for performance by using a *cognitive* task analysis. Cognitive task analysis is a family of assessment methods that describe the cognitive processes that underlie performance of occupations within real-world situations (Militello & Hutton, 1998; Schraagen, Chipman, & Shalin, 2000). This chapter focuses on the use of Stage Two of the PRPP Assessment as an observational instrument when evaluating adults with physical impairments.

The PRPP [Stage Two] conceptual model (Fig. 17.2) is centred on four processing quadrants with multidirectional arrows that mirror the multistaged flow of information in theoretical models of information processing. These quadrants include attention, sensory perception (Perceive), memory (Recall), response planning and evaluation (Plan) and performance monitoring (Perform).

The four central quadrants are further divided into 12 subcategories that can be seen in the middle ring of Fig. 17.2. Key descriptive words used to name and frame information processing strategies that are observable during task performance are

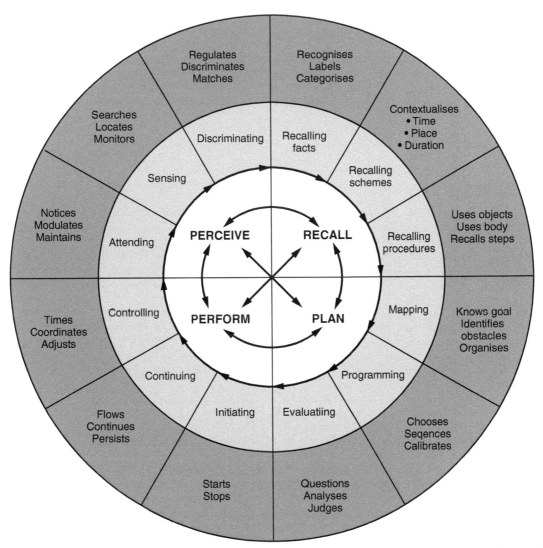

FIG. 17.2 ■ The PRPP System of Task Analysis [Stage Two] Conceptual Model. *(From Chapparo & Ranka, 2011.)*

termed *descriptors*. These form the outer layer of the system. Each descriptor is rated on a 3-point rating scale relative to the task criterion for that descriptor: (1) descriptor performance does not meet criterion expectations and inhibits performance; (2) descriptor performance meets criterion expectations but concerns indicated because of safety, timing or prompts needed; and (3) descriptor performance meets criterion expectations, reasonable time, without assistance or prompts.

An underlying assumption of the assessment system is that a person's capacity to process the demands inherent in everyday tasks can be observed, identified and used to determine the need for occupational therapy intervention (Chapparo & Ranka, 1997b; Chrenka, Hutton, Klinger, & Aptima, 2001). The purpose

of the assessment is to identify difficulties in application of specific information processing strategies during task performance and to provide a focus for intervention (Fry & O'Brien, 2002; Nott & Chapparo, 2008, 2012; Nott et al., 2008).

PRPP INTERVENTION

The PRPP Intervention is a task-oriented information processing approach that simultaneously focuses on task training and cognitive strategy training within the context of everyday performance (Chapparo, 2010; Chapparo & Ranka, 2007; Nott et al., 2008). It is an extension of the 'Stop Think Do' programme developed for use with children and adolescents

(Beck & Horne, 1992; Murphy & Cooke, 1999). The core intervention principles in PRPP Intervention are defined in Table 17.1.

Occupational therapy using PRPP Intervention focuses on teaching people to apply a sequence of processing strategies to 'Stop/Attend, Sense, Think, Do' – that is, gain the required level of arousal/attention for the task (Stop/Attend), perceive sensory information relevant to the task (Sense), engage in recall (Think to remember) or planning strategies to develop a plan of action (Think to problem solve), then implement the plan (Do/monitor). People learn to apply these strategies to their task performance by initially observing and modelling the therapist. The therapist's role as a cognitive mediator fades as the person begins to internalise the strategies and apply them across a range of tasks and settings.

The prompts of 'Stop, Attend, Sense, Think, Do' (given via verbal, visual, gestural and/or physical modes) are used as content-free 'metaprompts' to focus on the information processing task requirements rather than procedural or skill-based task requirements. Content-free prompts have been shown to enhance monitoring of current and future goals in performance, as well as the strategies necessary to achieve these goals (Fish et al., 2007). This approach extends traditional skills training to improve performance. In other words, gaining the capacity to do a task does not necessarily result in mastery. Instruction

is also needed that will support a person's capacity to think about doing in many different occupational contexts so that the skill learned may be generalised throughout their occupational life. These global prompts are followed up with more specific content-based behavioural prompts, selected by the therapist based on findings from the assessment component of the system. One or two descriptor strategies from each processing quadrant for 'Stop, Attend, Sense, Think, Do' are selected by the therapist to prompt a sequence of information processing.

USING THE PRPP SYSTEM OF TASK ANALYSIS AND INTERVENTION: JONAS

Before observing a person's occupational performance, therapists should have a clear understanding of the type and level of information processing required to perform the target occupations. The goal of observation is to determine whether people are able to process information required by a particular occupation in a particular context. In other words, successful observation is referenced to particular criteria that are determined by the nature and complexity of the occupation, the expectations

TABLE 17.1	
Core Principles of PRPP Intervention	
Principle	**Definition**
Intervention goal is task mastery	■ Expected outcome is improved functional performance in everyday tasks required by the person's occupational roles and context.
	■ Intervention success is therefore measured by increased functional performance.
Application of evidence-based principles of systematic instruction	■ Goal of intervention is clear to person.
	■ Least to most prompt hierarchy is used.
	■ Multiple opportunities for practice of the task and target cognitive strategies are offered and performance errors are prevented.
	■ Learning occurs across natural contexts and tasks to promote generalisation.
	■ Feedback is specific to task mastery and the cognitive strategy that is the target of intervention.
Target descriptors (cognitive strategies) are behaviourally defined and measurable	■ Descriptors required for task performance are identified using the PRPP Assessment (outer ring, Fig. 17.2) and their effectiveness measured before and throughout intervention.
'Chunking' of descriptors across multiple PRPP quadrants is planned	■ Starting with 'Stops' to correct errors, one or two descriptors only are targeted from each processing quadrant for 'Attend/Sense' (Perceive quadrant), 'Think to remember' (Recall quadrants), 'Think to evaluate' (Plan quadrant) and 'Do' (Perform quadrant).
	■ Training in single descriptors is not used.
	■ A line of processing required for the task mirrors the direction of arrows in the centre of the PRPP Model (see Fig. 17.2).
Focus of intervention is on application of cognitive strategies (descriptors) to real-world performance	■ The descriptor behaviours form the central verbal, physical or visual prompts given during performance and are modelled by the therapist if required.
	■ The person is taught to self-instruct in the strategies if possible.

PRPP, Perceive, Recall, Plan and Perform.

of the person and other people in the performance context and the sensorimotor characteristics of the task context. This approach differs from a norm-referenced model of assessment that specifies one general standard of performance against which everyone's performance capacities are measured.

Three questions guide therapists' observations of ability in information processing:

- What type of processing does this occupation demand?
- What type of processing does the performance context demand?
- Is there evidence (through observation or inquiry) that the person is processing to the level needed to perform this particular occupation?

Jonas' story (Practice Story 17.1) is used to illustrate how observations of everyday function can be interpreted using the PRPP System of Task Analysis and Intervention.

PRACTICE STORY 17.1

Jonas

Jonas was 60-year-old man who sustained a right hemisphere cerebrovascular accident (CVA). Jonas was found in bed by his son with a dense left hemiparesis, slurred speech and facial droop. Computed tomography scanning revealed a right frontoparietal intraparenchymal haemorrhage that was surgically evacuated. Jonas was initially admitted to inpatient rehabilitation with a dense left hemiparesis, left-sided sensory impairment and left visuospatial deficits and inattention. He spent 4 weeks on an inpatient rehabilitation ward before being transferred to a transitional living unit (TLU).

On admission to the TLU Jonas's Functional Independence Measure (FIM) total score was 76 (motor = 54; cognitive = 22). Higher FIM scores indicate greater level of independence with motor tasks such as showering/bathing, upper- and lower-body dressing and transfers, and cognitive abilities, including memory and attention. Scores range from 18 to 126. Jonas required assistance of one person for showering and dressing; he was able to eat his food using his right upper limb, without assistance, once all food had been prepared (e.g. cut to size and packages opened). He was able to ambulate with a four-point stick and near supervision. He did not have any residual expressive or receptive language deficits. During the day and when he went on weekend leave he experienced significant fatigue.

His programme goal was to be discharged home where he lived with his wife and adult son. He was employed full time as a bus driver before his stroke. At this stage of his rehabilitation, Jonas had not decided if he would resume employment in the future or if he would retire.

Perceive: Observing Sensory Processing Strategies During Occupation

Once sensory input captures a person's attention and that person focuses on it, details of the information are registered and the person creates sensory pictures of occupation. Sensory registration serves to interpret and maintain the information from the input receptors long enough for it to be perceived and analysed. It becomes sensory perception, registered sensory input that is meaningful. Information processing research has demonstrated how copies of sensory images are stored very briefly, for seconds only (Huitt, 2003). Unless there is an effort to pay attention to sensory images, the information is lost from the sensory register.

In the top left hand quadrant of Fig. 17.3 specific behaviours from the PRPP Assessment associated with this Perceive stage of information processing are outlined. These behaviours are observable signs that people are attending to and purposefully dealing with specific sensory input that is needed for the particular occupations being performed (Chapparo & Ranka, 1997b).

The Perceive assessment findings for Jonas are presented in Box 17.1 along with related intervention implications.

Recall: Observing Information Storage and Retrieval Strategies During Occupation

In the second stage of information processing, incoming sensory images are transferred to short-term working memory, the temporary information processing storage facility. Working memory is what a person is thinking about at any given time. It is created when a person pays deeper attention to sensory input, or a thought that 'comes to mind' (Ranka, 2005). Working memory has a limited capacity, so incoming information continually replaces information that is already in this short-term storage. It will initially last somewhere around 15 to 20 seconds unless it is repeated, at which point it may be available for use for up to 20 minutes, the length of a typical therapy session early in rehabilitation. If information is not placed into long-term storage for use at a later time, it fades.

Long-term memory storage is where people store their wealth of occupational experience, bringing pertinent information back into working memory for use when they need it (Levy, 2011; Nee et al., 2013; Smith & Jonides, 1999; Sodorow & Rickabaugh, 2002). Each person has a unique occupational memory, a platform of knowledge from which information is retrieved for quick and automatic performance, allowing a person to 'think' and 'do' simultaneously. This automatic process breaks down when a person needs to engage in new learning (e.g. learning a compensation strategy in the presence of physical impairment) or relearning occupations that have been done successfully for years when the task procedures have been forgotten (e.g. in neurocognitive disorders).

Memory for occupational performance involves two important information processing operations: *recognition*, or the capacity to perceive something previously known, and *retrieval*, or the

As the person is doing an occupation, does he/she ... ?

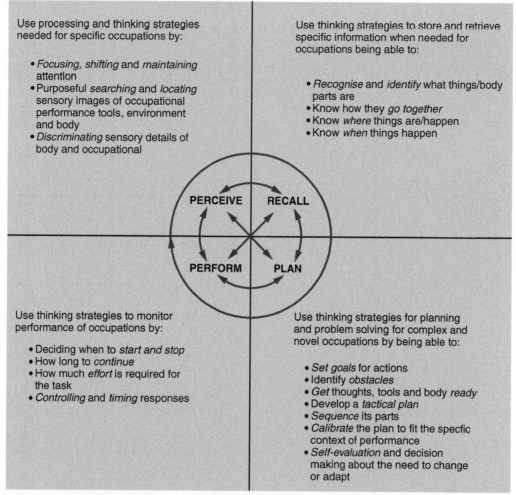

Use processing and thinking strategies needed for specific occupations by:

- *Focusing, shifting* and *maintaining* attention
- Purposeful *searching* and *locating* sensory images of occupational performance tools, environment and body
- *Discriminating* sensory details of body and occupational

Use thinking strategies to store and retrieve specific information when needed for occupations being able to:

- *Recognise* and *identify* what things/body parts are
- Know how they *go together*
- Know *where* things are/happen
- Know *when* things happen

PERCEIVE   **RECALL**

PERFORM   **PLAN**

Use thinking strategies to monitor performance of occupations by:

- Deciding when to *start and stop*
- How long to *continue*
- How much *effort* is required for the task
- *Controlling* and *timing* responses

Use thinking strategies for planning and problem solving for complex and novel occupations by being able to:

- *Set goals* for actions
- Identify *obstacles*
- *Get* thoughts, tools and body *ready*
- Develop a *tactical plan*
- *Sequence* its parts
- *Calibrate* the plan to fit the specfic context of performance
- *Self-evaluation* and decision making about the need to change or adapt

FIG. 17.3 ■ Information processing strategies observed during occupations performance. *(From Chapparo & Ranka, 2005.)*

BOX 17.1
PERCEIVE: JONAS'S ASSESSMENT FINDINGS AND INTERVENTION IMPLICATIONS

PERCEIVE: ASSESSMENT FINDINGS

When Jonas was observed making a sandwich in the transitional living unit kitchen, he had difficulty:

- noticing incoming sensory information on his left-hand side towards the end of the task;
- changing the focus or modulating his attention from small details in front of him (one object in the pantry) to the 'big picture' of the task context (kitchen, his four-point stick and the general layout of the environment);
- searching for and locating the objects he needed (systematically searching for the knife and chopping board); and

- monitoring use of his body (mainly lower limbs) and his four-point stick (bumping into fridge door, pantry door when opening).

The occupational therapist could hypothesise that part of the reason Jonas was not performing to expectations in a well-known task was because he was not processing some of the necessary sensory information in the first stage of information processing. He did not have some of the critical attention and sensory processing strategies in place to give him updated information about what he had to do, how to do it in an unfamiliar kitchen and when to use some unfamiliar tactics to accommodate his reduce physical ability.

Continued on following page

BOX 17.1
PERCEIVE: JONAS'S ASSESSMENT FINDINGS AND INTERVENTION IMPLICATIONS *(Continued)*

Based on this finding the therapist might decide to assess how Jonas did the same task in his own kitchen where the need to search and find sensory information would be reduced.

Jonas's noticing and attending met task requirements at the commencement of the task; however, this reduced towards later stages of task performance as fatigue began to affect Jonas's ability to use these cognitive strategies in occupational performance.

PERCEIVE: INTERVENTION IMPLICATIONS

Jonas had to learn to process the information needed to think about where and how to look for things required for

performance, and how to shift the focus of his attention from the small details to the broader environment and back as he proceeded through the task. Jonas's relatives could be given concrete ideas about how to encourage him to think about how he needs to look for things during home and community tasks (e.g. shopping) for safe and effective performance. Most importantly Jonas could be taught more effective 'search and find' strategies to direct his own performance when he 'got lost' in a task (Nott et al., 2008).

---

capacity to regain stored memories. Both recognition and retrieval are dependent on adequate prior processing of sensory information, successful storing of information and purposeful use of strategies that allow a person to access stored information and answer the question, 'Do I know …?' (Chapparo, 2010; Ranka, 2005). The purpose of occupational therapy assessment is, in part, to determine what people have learned (know), how their knowledge is constructed and how functional it is for everyday living.

Three broad categories of memories are stored and retrieved for use during every task (Nee et al., 2013). These are factual memories, schematic memories and procedural memories. These are reflected by the subquadrants of the top right hand quadrant (Recall). Specific behaviours from the PRPP Assessment associated with this stage of information processing are outlined in Fig. 17.3.

- *Recalling facts:* Memory for factual information enables people to determine 'Do I know WHAT…' Knowing what things are, what they are called, what they go with and what they are used for is the basis for recognition and retrieval during occupational performance. When factual information is not stored or coded correctly, people may make mistakes of recognition during occupation. They will call things by the wrong name, put things together the wrong way or use things the wrong way.
- *Recalling schemes:* Schematic memory represents what people have learned about where, when and how long something happens. It answers the questions 'Do I know WHERE…', 'Do I know WHEN…', 'Do I know HOW LONG…'. Schematic information provides people with a personally constructed 'map' or a model for how, when, and where to act. When people are unable to develop stable schematic memory, their behaviour will not match the context. People may act impulsively, erratically or engage in tasks not suitable for their level

of current ability and skills. Although people may be able to do what is required, they are unable to either retrieve the contextual rules for behaviour (now/not now, here/not here) or use metacognitive strategies to assess the appropriateness of behaviours across different contexts.

- *Recalling procedures:* Procedural memory enables us to automatically determine 'Do I know HOW…?' based on past experience. Procedural memory has been shown to be the most resistant to forgetting in people with CNS disorders (Sodorow & Rickabaugh, 2002). Examples of tasks that people do every day that rely on procedural memory are dressing, brushing teeth, and driving a vehicle. People can usually do these things without thinking because they have learned them so well. After a physical injury people may have difficulty storing and retrieving procedural knowledge; their movements may seem clumsy even when doing familiar tasks, because they are unable to remember how to use their bodies in the most efficient manner. They may consistently forget steps of previously well-learned tasks or steps of newly learned methods of task performance that compensate for physical impairments. These recall errors are more evident in the presence of pain or fatigue (Sanchez, 2011).

The Recall assessment findings for Jonas are presented in Box 17.2 along with related intervention implications.

Plan: Observing Strategies for Organising Information and Problem Solving During Occupation

Inability to plan significantly influences social participation, daily activity and functional outcome (Goverover, 2004; Reeder, Newton, Frangou, & Wykes, 2004). There is often

BOX 17.2
RECALL: JONAS'S ASSESSMENT FINDINGS AND INTERVENTION IMPLICATIONS

RECALL: ASSESSMENT FINDINGS

When Jonas was observed engaging with his wife in a community leisure task (going out for lunch), he had difficulty:

- categorising food items into similar groups (when ordering from the menu);
- contextualising to place: not knowing the correct place (here/not here) to set himself up to complete the task (positioned himself in wheelchair in central thoroughfare of café);
- contextualising to duration: unaware of time passing and the duration of task performance (nil comparison between own pace of performance and task partners); and
- recalling the procedures for using his body and task objects: not knowing how to position himself to avoid bumping into the edges and legs of the café table.

Jonas experienced memory related difficulties across the three subquadrants of recalling facts, recalling schemes, and recalling procedures. Performance errors that underpinned recognition, retrieval and categorisation led to Jonas ordering items from the incorrect section of the menu. Although Jonas was able to perform most aspects of this task competently, he was unable to either retrieve the contextual rules for behaviour in this context or use metacognitive strategies to assess the appropriateness of his own behaviour. He positioned his wheelchair in the central thoroughfare of the café, blocking access for other patrons, but

was unaware of the implications of his choice. The interaction between Perceive and Recall was evident when Jonas attempted to recall the strategy for positioning himself in his wheelchair at the café table. His visual perceptual difficulties and reduced recall of procedures led to performance errors bumping his foot plates into the café table legs on several occasions.

RECALL: INTERVENTION IMPLICATIONS

A significant focus of intervention for adults who have sustained significant physical impairments involves enabling them to establish functional memory stores of how to 'do' occupations when needed. This has been referred to as 'skills training' or 'task specific instruction' (Hubbard, Parsons, Neilson, & Carey, 2009; Larkin & Parker, 2002). Efficient motor performance requires selection of information most relevant for the immediate performance situation — for example, remembering 'how to' use task specific objects including new objects such as adaptive aids and equipment, and also 'how to' use body parts in different movement patterns that may be necessitated after physical impairment (Schmidt & Wrisberg, 2008). Processing of information in long-term storage requires specific strategies for controlled and often effortful processing, involving rehearsal and making specific connections between new and previously learned information. People need to 'know the facts' before they can recall 'the facts' required for occupational performance.

---

dissociation between what a person wants to do and actually does (Eriksson, Tham, & Borg, 2006, Eriksson, Aasnes, Tistad, Guidetti, & Von Koch, 2012). Planning functions may be masked during familiar occupations but are most apparent when a person is required to function in situations that are difficult, less structured, require multitasking or require dealing with novelty and unexpected situations (Bootes & Chapparo, 2010; Burgess et al., 2006; Ranka & Chapparo, 2010). Examples of these latter types of occupations might include catching public transport, operating workplace plant and equipment, selecting and purchasing grocery items at the supermarket or organising a daily routine of occupations at home or work.

Planning requires thinking strategies such as organisation problem solving, decision making, insight, and purposeful allocation of attention, all referred to as executive functions within the information processing system. This third stage of information can be thought of as the 'rules of operation' that people apply to problem solving and analysing information in any occupation. They are not linked to any particular type of sensory information or ability but are applied to all information that has to be organised for use. Every day, people rely on their executive skills by applying thinking strategies to what they do. This

strategy application capacity allows people to orchestrate multiple occupations and parts of occupations into a seamless whole. Research suggests that people with neurocognitive disorders almost universally have difficulty with some aspect of planning and problem solving, giving rise to difficulties coping when occupation becomes complex (Burgess et al., 2006).

During the occupations that people do in every minute of every day, information flows into the processing system and presents it with a problem to solve. What is that object? What was I told to do? How can I do it differently? How much do I need to do? How can I do it without making a mistake? How does my work compare with others? Is that safe? Will it work? These are just a few of the typical problems that require the use of higher order information processing such as critical thinking, decision making and planning.

To engage in problem solving, planning and self-evaluation, people must construct and evaluate their own goal-oriented strategies for action. This means that they process information with reference to a particular goal, an idea, an understanding of what has to happen. People who have sustained significant injuries or acquired significant physical disabilities may have difficulty constructing an idea or a goal; they may have an incomplete idea of the expected outcome; or the idea may fade when they begin to act, as performance becomes increasingly influenced by other motivations. When people engage in goal-oriented occupation, they initiate executive thinking operations that prepare them to put a plan into action. These strategies are different to mere memory retrieval and involve 'figuring out' extensions or elaborations to habitual responses that may be demanded by the occupation. People have to solve the following problems before, during and on review as they do complex tasks:

- What obstacles might/did get in the way?
- How can I get ready for action?
- What is the best choice of action, place and tool to use for this specific task?
- How do I have to sequence the task?
- What do I have to do to make my responses fit the expectation/context/my abilities?

In general, everyone wants to be responsible for their own engagement in occupation. This happens when they are able to reflect, evaluate their own plans and performance and make considered decisions about satisfaction, effectiveness and the need for correction or change. This evaluative thinking involves metacognition, where people think about their thinking. It is a type of cognitive monitoring that involves questioning, analysing their ideas and performance of occupation and making final judgements about their worth. Three thinking strategies appear to be critical for each person being able to evaluate their own performance:

- Being able to question whether their performance matched the expected outcome
- Being able to further analyse the reasons why they did or did not meet their goals
- Being able to make decisions about the need to carry on or change the goal and the plan
- Observations of a person's planning, problem solving and decision making can be guided by asking how well the person seems to know the answers to questions in the bottom right hand quadrant of Fig. 17.3 (Plan).

The Plan assessment finding for Jonas are presented in Box 17.3 along with related intervention implications.

BOX 17.3
PLAN: JONAS'S ASSESSMENT FINDINGS AND INTERVENTION IMPLICATIONS

PLAN: ASSESSMENT FINDINGS

Completing meal preparation activities in the unfamiliar transitional living unit (TLU) kitchen, in combination with recently acquired sensorimotor impairments, required Jonas to engage a number of executive processing strategies. Jonas was able to remember most processes (Recall); however, he could not rely on memory alone. He had to make an overall mental plan for what had to be done that would draw many sensing and thinking strands together into a coherent whole.

Jonas had difficulty with the basic executive functions required for this task:

- He was very slow to identify obstacles to task completion or generate an alternative plan around these.
- He was unable to organise his thoughts or actions and 'get ready' to complete the task in the required task environment.
- He was slow to sequence the steps without help and step transitions required prompting and additional time.
- He did not choose the best strategy or tactics for place, procedures or use of objects.
- His safety was questionable, highlighting difficulty with analyses and judgements.

Jonas had significant difficulty getting organised in his head before commencing this task. He had difficulty making a mental plan that integrated prior knowledge of how he had made lunch in the past, while adapting for his current sensorimotor deficits. This is an essential cognitive strategy for initiating and maintaining goal-directed occupational performance. He had difficulty figuring out or choosing where to do the task (e.g. on the kitchen bench or on a plate) and how to position himself (including a four-point stick) relative to the bench. His reduced decision making led to slowed performance and long pauses between task steps while Jonas tried to figure out what to do next or how to do the next task step. He had to purposefully shift his attention between each one of these operations in an ordered sequence and not get distracted by people moving around him in the TLU. As his performance continued, his ability to filter peripheral stimuli reduced, leading to increased distractibility and safety concerns during task performance.

PLAN: INTERVENTION IMPLICATIONS

Assessment of Jonas's performance indicated that simply practicing a variety of occupations would not help him. He needed to practice *thinking* about what he had to do, what he was doing and what he had done so that he could learn from his own occupational experience. Jonas needed to learn more effective ways of thinking that could assist him in solving the problems that arise for him during everyday occupations. Rather than simply direct his action, modelling of thinking from the therapist, together with scaffolding of thinking skills required to solve problems, was viewed as a 'best practice' instruction technique (Greber, Ziviani, & Rodger, 2007). In this approach, the therapist acts as a model who overtly and explicitly verbalises the strategic metacognitive strategies needed for successful performance. This would be done through teaching Jonas how to process information strategically and figure out solutions to problems and complexities that arise while he is doing daily occupations.

Perform: Processing Output and Performance Feedback

The last stage of information processing focuses on using thinking strategies to perform, or create output responses. Numerous researchers have linked reduced thinking strategies and reduced speed of processing to inefficient response control and timing (e.g. Schmidt & Wrisberg, 2008). Actively responding to information that is processed requires being able to plan and initiate both starting and stopping of action. Responses generate further input into the information processing system and result in the ability to self-monitor. Motor programmes operate within the motor system with feedback from sensory systems to produce skilled actions. It has been demonstrated that people adjust and slow their movements when interacting with task objects that require greater control (e.g. a full water glass) or when performing tasks with their nondominant limb (Schmidt & Wrisberg, 2008). This has implications for cognitive strategy use with adults who have physical impairments that may require a change in upper-limb dominance as a result of injury, amputation or paresis.

Observations of a person's performance monitoring strategies can be guided by the information processing behaviours listed in the bottom left hand quadrant (Perform) in

Fig. 17.3. These information processing behaviours are dependent on the formation of an adequate plan, knowing the purpose of responses, and rapid and accurate processing of the changing body and contextual sensory details that are critical to task performance.

The Perform assessment findings for Jonas are presented in Box 17.4 along with related intervention implications.

CONCLUSION

This chapter described how an occupational therapist can employ elements of the PRPP System of Task Analysis and Intervention. Through the story of Jonas, this chapter explored a range of information processing problems that people with physical impairments may experience at home or in the community, and brief examples of intervention were given. The approach presented in this chapter is consistent with contemporary shifts in occupational therapy towards a more ecological and dynamic style of intervention where assessment and intervention are mutually informative and where the focus is on the particular occupational needs of particular people in particular contexts.

BOX 17.4
PERFORM: JONAS'S ASSESSMENT FINDINGS AND INTERVENTION IMPLICATIONS

PERFORM: ASSESSMENT FINDINGS

Jonas was very slow in his task performance and had difficulty with his initiation of a task. Based on observations listed in Fig. 17.3, Jonas had difficulty with the following information processing strategies:

- He had difficulty starting and restarting after distractions from other transitional living unit (TLU) residents.
- He had significantly reduced flow – starting, stopping and pausing between most task steps, often seeking reassurance from staff.
- He required verbal prompting to continue and keep his thinking 'on task'.
- He did not make the necessary motor adjustments to place his body in the correct position relative to task objects or environmental features such as the fridge door or café table.

Jonas's initiation difficulties may be closely linked to the observed difficulties in the Plan quadrant that highlighted poor thought or action organisation relative to the task goal. This links to poor initiation as Jonas did not have a clear mental picture of how to perform the task with his current sensorimotor deficits. Consistent with the research reported earlier, Jonas used motor control techniques that led to slowed performance when interacting

with task objects that require greater control, such as a four-point stick for indoor mobility and a manual wheelchair for outdoor mobility. As reported in earlier areas of this assessment (Perceive and Plan), Jonas relied on external prompting to maintain task attention and modulate attention to reduce the impact of distractors. This linked with observed task difficulties in the Perform quadrant, requiring external supports to continue task performance and keep his thinking on track.

PERFORM: INTERVENTION IMPLICATIONS

Jonas's performance indicated that strategy training should not target relearning of specific tasks but should focus on teaching Jonas new ways to cognitively manage the problems resulting from his impairments. The cognitive strategies that he needed to practice thinking about were general cognitive strategies such as: 'When should I start/stop/resume task performance?' 'Am I on-track?' 'Do I finish now or keep going?' 'Do I move like this or like this?' 'What adjustments can I make?' These cognitive strategies would enable Jonas to apply relevant information to task performance, select and monitor his responses and simultaneously cope with internal and external distractions during task performance (Siegler, 2007).

http://evolve.elsevier.com/Curtin/OT

REFERENCES

Abeare, C. A., Cohen, J. L., Axelrod, B. N., Leisen, J. C. C., Mosley-Williams, A., & Lumley, M. A. (2010). Pain, executive functioning, and affect in patients with rheumatoid arthritis. *The Clinical Journal of Pain, 26*(8), 683.

Alcock, L., O'Brien, T. D., & Vanicek, N. (2015). Age-related changes in physical functioning: Correlates between objective and self-reported outcomes. *Physiotherapy, 101*(2), 204–213.

Aubin, G., Chapparo, C., Gélinas, I., Stip, E., & Rainville, C. (2009). Use of the perceive, recall, plan and perfom system of task analysis for persons with schizophrenia: A preliminary study. *Australian Occupational Therapy Journal, 56*(3), 189–199.

Banich, M. T., & Compton, R. J. (2011). *Cognitive neuroscience* (3rd ed.). Belmont, CA: Wadsworth Publishing.

Beck, J., & Horne, D. (1992). A whole school implementation of the stop, think, do! Social skills training program. In B. Willis, & J. Izard (Eds.), *Student behavior problems: Directions, perspectives and expectations.* Hawthorn, Victoria: Australian Council for Educational Research.

Bohannon, J. N., & Bonvillian, J. D. (2005). Theoretical approaches to language acquisition. In J. B. Gleason (Ed.), *The development of language* (6th ed., pp. 230–291). Boston: Pearson/Allyn and Bacon.

Bootes, K., & Chapparo, C. (2010). Difficulties with multitasking on return to work after TBI: A critical case study. *Work, 36*(2), 207–216.

Burgess, P. W., Alderman, N., Forbes, C., et al. (2006). The case for the development and use of measures of executive function in experimental and clinical neuropsychology. *Journal of the International Neuropsychological Society, 12*(02), 194–209.

Buschman, T. J., Siegel, M., Jefferson, E. R., & Miller, E. K. (2011). Neural substrates of cognitive capacity limitations. *Proceedings of the National Academy of Sciences of the United States, 27,* 11252–11255.

Chapparo, C. (2010). *Perceive, recall, plan and perform (PRPP): Occupation centred task analysis and intervention system. In S. Rodger (Ed.), Occupation centred practice with children: A practical guide for occupational therapists* (pp. 183–202). Hoboken, NJ: Wiley-Blackwell. Retrieved from, *http://CSUAU.eblib.com/patron/FullRecord.aspx?p=485688.*

Chapparo, C. (2011). Section ten: Instrument development. In C. Chapparo, & J. Ranka (Eds.), *The PRPP system of task analysis: User's training manual – Research edition.* Lidcombe, Australia: Occupational Performance Network, School of Occupation & Leisure Sciences, The University of Sydney.

Chapparo, C., & Lowe, S. (2011). School: Participating in more than just the classroom. In S. J. Lane, & A. C. Bundy (Eds.), *Kids can be kids: A childhood occupations approach* (pp. 83–101). Philadelphia: FA Davis.

Chapparo, C., & Ranka, J. (1997a). *Occupational performance model (Australia), monograph 1.* Sydney: Total Print Control.

Chapparo, C., & Ranka, J. (1997b). The perceive, recall, plan and perform system of task analysis. In C. Chapparo, & J. Ranka (Eds.), *Occupational performance model (Australia), monograph 1* (pp. 189–198). Sydney: Total Print Control.

Chapparo, C., & Ranka, J. (2007). *The PRPP system: Intervention.* Lidcombe, Australia: Discipline of Occupational Therapy, Faculty of Health Sciences, The University of Sydney.

Chapparo, C., & Ranka, J. (Eds.). (2011). *The PRPP system of task analysis: User's training manual – Research edition.* Lidcombe, Australia: Occupational Performance Network, School of Occupation & Leisure Sciences, The University of Sydney.

Chrenka, J., Hutton, R. J., Klinger, D. W., & Aptima, D. A. (2001). Focusing cognitive task analysis in the cognitive function model. *Proceedings of the Human Factors and Ergonomics Society 45th Annual Meeting, 5,* 1738–1742.

Couchman, J. J., Coutinho, M. V. C., Beran, M. J., & Smith, J. D. (2010). Beyond stimulus cues and reinforcement signals: A New approach to animal metacognition. *Journal of Comparative Psychology, 124*(4), 356–368.

Demetriou, A., & Kazi, S. (2006). Self-awareness in G (with processing efficiency and reasoning). *Intelligence, 34*(3), 297–317.

Eriksson, G., Aasnes, M., Tistad, M., Guidetti, S., & Von Koch, L. (2012). Occupational gaps in everyday life one year after stroke and the association with life satisfaction and impact of stroke. *Topics in Stroke Rehabilitation, 19*(3), 244–255.

Eriksson, G., Tham, K., & Borg, J. (2006). Occupational gaps in everyday life 1-4 years after acquired brain injury. *Journal of Rehabilitation Medicine, 38*(3), 159–165.

Fish, J., Evans, J. J., Nimmo, M., et al. (2007). Rehabilitation of executive dysfunction following brain injury: 'Content-free' cueing improves everyday prospective memory performance. *Neuropsychologia, 45*(6), 1318–1330.

Fisher, A. G. (1993). The assessment of IADL motor skills: An application of many-faceted Rasch analysis. *American Journal of Occupational Therapy, 47*(4), 319–329.

Friedenberg, J., & Silverman, G. (2012). *Cognitive science: An introduction to the study of mind* (2nd ed.). Thousand Oaks, CA: Sage Publications.

Fry, K., & O'Brien, L. (2002). Using the perceive, recall, plan and perform system to assess cognitive deficits in adults with traumatic brain injury: A case study. *Australian Occupational Therapy Journal, 49*(4), 182–187.

Giles, G. M. (2011). A neurofunctional approach to rehabilitation after brain injury. In N. Katz (Ed.), *Cognition, occupation and participation across the life span: Neuroscience, neurorehabilitation and models of intervention in occupational therapy* (3rd ed., pp. 351–381). Bethesda, MD: AOTA Press.

Goverover, Y. (2004). Categorization, deductive reasoning, and self-awareness: Association with everyday competence in persons with acute brain injury. *Journal of Clinical and Experimental Neuropsychology, 26*(6), 737–749.

Greber, C., Ziviani, J., & Rodger, S. (2007). The four-quadrant model of facilitated learning (part 2): Strategies and applications. *Australian Occupational Therapy Journal, 54*(Suppl. 1), S40–S48.

Hardwick, R. M., Rottschy, C., Miall, R. C., & Eickhoff, S. B. (2013). A quantitative meta-analysis and review of motor learning in the human brain. *NeuroImage, 67,* 283–297.

Hubbard, I. J., Parsons, M. W., Neilson, C., & Carey, L. M. (2009). Task-specific training: Evidence for and translation to clinical practice. *Occupational Therapy International, 16*(3–4), 175–189.

Huitt, W. (2003). *The information processing approach to cognition. Educational psychology interactive.* Retrieved from, http://chiron.valdosta.edu/whuitt/col/cogsys/infoproc.html.

Katz, N., Baum, C., & Maeir, A. (2011). Introduction to cognitive intervention and cognitive functional evaluation. In N. Katz (Ed.), *Cognition, occupation and participation across the lifespan: Neuroscience, neurorehabilitation and models of intervention in occupational therapy* (3rd ed., pp. 3–12). Bethesda, MD: AOTA Press.

Kieran, C. R. F., & Christoff, K. (2014). Metacognitive facilitation of Spontaneous thought processes: When metacognition helps the wandering mind find its way. *The Cognitive Neuroscience of Metacognition*, 293–319.

Kirwan, B., & Ainsworth, L. K. (1992). *A guide to task analysis.* London: Taylor & Francis.

Koh, C., Hoffmann, T., Bennett, S., & McKenna, K. (2009). Management of patients with cognitive impairment after stroke: A survey of Australian occupational therapists. *Australian Occupational Therapy Journal*, 56(5), 324–331.

Larkin, D., & Parker, H. (2002). Task-specific intervention for children with developmental coordination disorder: A systemic review. In S. Cermak, & D. Larkin (Eds.), *Developmental coordination disorder* (pp. 234–247). Albany, NY: Delmar Thomson Learning.

Levy, L. L. (2011). Cognitive aging. In N. Katz (Ed.), *Cognition, occupation, and participation across the life span: Neuroscience, neurorehabilitation, and models of intervention in occupational therapy.* Bethesda, MD: AOTA Press.

Militello, L. G., & Hutton, R. J. B. (1998). Applied cognitive task analysis (ACTA): A practitioner's toolkit for understanding cognitive task demands. *Ergonomics*, 41(11), 1618–1641.

Morris, R., & Ward, G. (2004). *The cognitive psychology of planning.* Abingdon, UK: Taylor & Francis.

Murphy, D. P., & Cooke, J. (1999). Traffic light lessons: Problem solving skills with adolescents. *Community Practitioner*, 72(10), 322–324.

Nee, D. E., Brown, J. W., Askren, M. K., et al. (2013). A meta-analysis of executive components of working memory. *Cerebral Cortex*, 23(2), 264–282.

Nott, M. T. (2008). *Occupational performance and information processing in adults with agitation following traumatic brain injury.* PhD dissertation, Australia: The University of Sydney.

Nott, M. T., & Chapparo, C. (2008). Measuring information processing in a client with extreme agitation following traumatic brain injury using the perceive, recall, plan and perform system of task analysis. *Australian Occupational Therapy Journal*, 55(3), 188–198.

Nott, M. T., & Chapparo, C. (2012). Exploring the validity of the perceive, recall, plan and perform system of task analysis: Cognitive strategy use in adults with brain injury. *The British Journal of Occupational Therapy*, 75(6), 256–263.

Nott, M. T., Chapparo, C., & Heard, R. (2008). Effective occupational therapy intervention with adults demonstrating agitation during post-traumatic amnesia. *Brain Injury*, 22(9), 669–683.

Radomski, M. V., & Morrison, M. T. (2014). Assessing abilities and capacities: Cognition. In M. V. Radomski, & C. A. Trombly (Eds.), *Occupational therapy for physical dysfunction* (7th ed., pp. 121–143). Philadelphia: Wolters Kluwer Health.

Ranka, J. (2016). Section Six: Stage Two analysis: The Recall Quadrant. In C. Chapparo, & J. Ranka (Eds.), *The Perceive, Recall, Plan & Perform System Assessment course manual.* Sydney, Australia: Occupational Performance Network.

Ranka, J., & Chapparo, C. (2010). Assessment of productivity performance in men with HIV associated neurocognitive disorder (HAND). *Work: A Journal of Prevention, Assessment, & Rehabilitation*, 36(2), 193–206.

Reeder, C., Newton, E., Frangou, S., & Wykes, T. (2004). Which executive skills should we target to affect social functioning and symptom change? A study of a cognitive remediation therapy program. *Schizophrenia Bulletin*, 30(1), 87–100.

Riddle, D. R. (2007). *Brain aging: Models, methods, mechanisms.* Boca Raton, FL: CRC Press/Taylor Francis.

Sanchez, C. (2011). Working through the pain: Working memory capacity and differences in processing and storage under pain. *Memory*, 19(2), 226–232.

Schmidt, R., & Wrisberg, C. (2008). *Motor learning and performance* (4th ed.). Champaign, IL: Human Kinetics.

Schraagen, J. M., Chipman, S. F., & Shalin, V. (2000). *Cognitive task analysis.* Mahwah, NJ: Lawrence Erlbaum Associates.

Shumway-Cook, A., & Woollacott, M. H. (2001). *Motor control: Theory and practical applications* (2nd ed.). Baltimore, MD: Lippincott Williams & Wilkins.

Shumway-Cook, A., & Woollacott, M. H. (2007). *Motor control: Translating research into clinical practice* (3rd ed.). Philadelphia: Lippincott Williams & Wilkins.

Siegler, R. S. (2007). Cognitive variability. *Developmental Science*, 10(1), 104–109.

Smith, E. E., & Jonides, J. (1999). Storage and executive processes in the frontal lobes. *Science (New York)*, 283(5408), 1657.

Sodorow, L. M., & Rickabaugh, C. A. (2002). *Psychology* (5th ed.). Boston: McGraw Hill.

Toglia, J. P. (2005). A dynamic interactional approach to cognitive rehabilitation. In N. Katz (Ed.), *Cognition and occupation across the life span: Models for intervention in occupational therapy* (2nd ed., pp. 29–72). Bethesda, MD: American Occupational Therapy Association.

Toglia, J. P., Rodger, S. A., & Polatajko, H. J. (2012). Anatomy of cognitive strategies: A therapist's primer for enabling occupational performance. *Canadian Journal of Occupational Therapy*, 79(4), 225–236.

VandenBos, G. R. (2015). *APA dictionary of psychology* (2nd ed.). Washington, DC: American Psychological Association.

Wolpert, D. M., Diedrichsen, J., & Flanagan, J. R. (2011). Principles of sensorimotor learning. *Nature Review Neuroscience*, 12(12), 739–751.

18 ASSESSING THE ENVIRONMENT

GUNILLA CARLSSON ▪ AGNETA MALMGREN FÄNGE

CHAPTER OUTLINE

Abstract
The environment provides the context in which people engage in their occupations. This engagement takes place in many different environments, such as a person's home or the homes of family and friends, workplaces, public places, and a variety of locations where social and cultural events occur. Sometimes environments can prevent people from engaging in their necessary or desired occupations. Therefore from an occupational therapy perspective, each assessment related to the environment should aim to identify issues within the environment that affect the occupational engagement of individuals, groups or societies. Accordingly, the assessments selected will depend on whether the individual, group or societal level is in focus, and whether objective or subjective assessments, or a combination of both, should be used.

KEY POINTS

- Physical, social, cultural and institutional aspects of the environment influence occupational engagement.
- The effect of a person's illness, injury or impairment can vary considerably between individuals and therefore it is important to consider functional capacity as well as individual preferences when assessing the environment.

- When choosing how to assess the environment, the occupational therapist has to consider if the focus of the assessment is at the level of the individual, group, community and/or society.
- To deal with environmental assessments and interventions, occupational therapists need to obtain and apply knowledge from different scientific areas.
- When considering subjective and objective aspects of assessing the environment, it is important to distinguish between the assessment and the outcome.

ENVIRONMENTAL ASPECTS OF OCCUPATIONAL ENGAGEMENT

Engagement in occupations is known to have a positive effect on people's health and sense of well-being. Occupational engagement encompasses all that people do to become occupied and can occur in a huge range of different environments. Different environmental aspects, such as the physical, social, cultural and institutional aspects, influence engagement (Canadian Association of Occupational Therapists (CAOT), 2007). For example, what and how a person eats may vary in experience and performance depending on whether the person is in a restaurant with his colleagues or on a hike in the forest with friends and will vary across different cultures. The environmental effect on occupational engagement also changes over the life course as a result of age-related changes in the activity repertoire, the use of new physical and social arenas and because people may relocate to another home. New technologies that are continually being developed can support occupational engagement but can also be a major challenge and increase the environmental demands for many people. Thus in order to understand occupational engagement, in individuals or groups of people the role and characteristics of the environment in which the occupation is being performed need to be considered in addition to the physical, cognitive and affective performance components.

The environment can be considered on an individual level – for example, a person's own home or the home of a person's family and close friends. The individual level has long been the prevailing interest within occupational therapy; for instance, interventions have focused on adaptations based on an individual's needs and risks by means of the provision of assistive devices and home modifications (Ekstam, Carlsson, Chiatti, Nilsson, & Malmgren Fänge, 2014). The therapeutic, restorative use of the environment for individuals has also been a fundamental consideration from the very early stages of occupational therapy practice, in mental health hospitals and veteran clinics (Meyer, 1922), and still forms a central tenant for today's occupational therapy practice (Fisher, 2009). An example of this is the use of therapeutic gardens for people who have a mental health or cognitive impairment (Adevi & Lieberg, 2012; York & Wiseman, 2012).

Today, because of international recognition for supportive environments for health, the occupational therapy profession is increasingly taking on the challenge of working with a public health agenda. In 1991 the World Health Organization (WHO) introduced a greater focus on public health matters, stressing the need for supportive environments and encouraging health promotion in different environmental arenas (World Health Organisation, 1991). This statement has been followed by several other documents (e.g. United Nations (UN), 1993, 2006, 2015; World Health Organization & World Bank, 2011), each of them acknowledging the importance of the environment for health. In practice, this means that occupational therapists need to contribute to the development of sustainable environments designed to meet the needs of whole populations (e.g. Risser, Månsson Lexell, Bell, Iwarsson, & Ståhl, 2015; Thompson & Kent, 2014) and can play a role in response to environmental disasters (Sinclair, 2014).

The environment is thus targeted in many different ways from an individual to societal level as an important means to increase and improve health and well-being. Given the crucial role of the environment for occupational engagement, thorough assessment of the environment is necessary for the planning of occupational therapy interventions. Depending on the purpose of the assessment, different qualitative and quantitative methods have to be used, targeting objective and subjective outcomes.

The Environment: Theoretical Background and Models

As the effect of the environment on occupational engagement is complex, it is essential to be systematic in gaining an understanding of this effect. One way to classify the environment is in terms of social, cultural, physical and institutional elements, as in the Canadian Model of Occupational Performance and Engagement (CAOT, 2007). Another way is to focus on levels, in terms of individual and societal level as in the International Classification of Functioning, Disability and Health (ICF) (WHO, 2001). In some models, assistive devices are classified as an environmental factor, as in the ICF (WHO, 2001), whereas in other models, such as the Human Activity Assistive Technology Model (Cook & Oolgar, 2008), such devices are considered as a separate unit. The value of classifying the environment is not that the complexity is reduced; instead the different perspectives that should be assessed are articulated in the dynamic relationships among person, environment and occupation.

In the ecological model (Lawton & Nahemow, 1973), further developed in the Ecological Model of Aging (Scheidt & Norris-Baker, 2003), the dynamic relationships between person and environment are described and used to highlight the balance between competence of the person and environmental demands. Medium and high demands might be inspiring and challenging for people with higher levels of functioning, whereas too high or too low environmental demands might have a negative effect on the behaviour or occupational engagement. People with lower levels of functioning may be more sensitive to the demands of the environment than people with higher levels of functioning. The concept of accessibility is based on this theoretical model (Iwarsson & Ståhl, 2003), whereas the concept of usability explicitly targets effectiveness, efficiency and satisfaction with using physical features (International Organization for Standardization (ISO, 2015) – that is, the person–environment–occupation relationships. Overall, what needs to be considered is the complex interaction among the person, environment and occupation and how this affects occupational engagement. This means that occupational therapists need to draw on knowledge from a range of sciences, including occupational, medical, technical, psychological and social sciences, to increase their understanding of the environmental effect. This will then influence how occupational therapists assess the effect of the environment on occupational engagement.

The Complexity of Environmental Arenas

People organise their lives through their daily occupations and move around in different physical, social, cultural and institutional environments. As a result, there are a multitude of environmental arenas for occupational engagement, and if the environment is supportive, it increases the possibility for occupational engagement. The concept of supportive environments for health refers to the physical and social aspects of the surroundings, embracing the home, local community and work and play environments for all age groups (WHO, 1991). Within public transport planning, the expression 'travel chain perspective' has been introduced to emphasise the complexity of an individual's travel and used as an approach for exploration of travel. A travel chain is defined as the actual chain of events that occurs while moving from origin to destination

(Risser et al., 2015). Irrespective of whether the occupation includes travelling or not, several environmental arenas are linked to each other when a person is engaged in occupations; this perspective can be applied when exploring occupational engagement as well. To illustrate the complexity of environmental arenas for everyday occupations and the nature of a supportive environment, an example of John grocery shopping is provided:

> John walks through the entrance to his home, maybe via some stairs. He then walks along the pedestrian path to the bus stop near his house. He catches the bus and disembarks at the bus stop closest to the grocery shop, where he meets a friend and has a short conversation. After entering the shop, he walks around the numerous aisles pushing a shopping trolley and collecting his groceries from the shelves. He purchases his groceries with a credit card, packs them in his backpack and walks to the bus stop to catch a bus back towards his home. He steps off the bus at the stop closest to his home and then walks on the pedestrian path towards his home. When he reaches his home he walks along his garden path to his front door and then enters the house. John may do this trip by himself or with his partner. He feels comfortable enough to make this trip as he is very familiar with the environments and with the occupation of grocery shopping. Thus it can be seen that the current physical, social and cultural environments affect John's occupation of going grocery shopping, as does his familiarity with the occupation and his physical and cognitive capacities. Changes within the environments or the occupation or with John's physical and cognitive capability (Brorsson, Öhman, Cutchin, & Nygård, 2013; Risser et al., 2015) could affect his ability to do the grocery shopping.

In a person's home, the decision on how to use and furnish the environment is very much up to the people who own or who live in the house. That is, the power to govern daily life within the home is framed within the ownership of the environment. The home has a symbolic meaning for individuals, and therefore, in spite of the fact that individually tailored housing adaptations can be made in order to increase occupational engagement, changes to the physical design of the building can affect the perception of the home negatively (Aplin, de Jonge, & Gustafsson, 2013; Ekstam, Malmgren Fänge, & Carlsson, Submitted for publication). When illness, injury or impairment increasingly challenge a person's occupational engagement, relocation to another living arrangement might be suggested. In such situations, the fear a person has over losing control of his or her life situation is commonly negotiated against increased care needs and the possibilities of being able to remain in his or her home (Löfqvist et al., 2013).

Moving to a nursing or care home is intended to increase the opportunities to be active and to participate even when facing major care needs; however, to a large extent this move may constrain the possibilities for occupational engagement. Given the fact that nursing homes and sometimes a person's own home are not only the homes of the people living there but also the workplace for care staff, conflict can arise as to who owns the final decision on how to furnish and equip the environment. When the needs of the staff are prioritised above the needs and preferences of the people living there, the environmental demands on the people living there increase and vice versa.

A change in environmental effect can be slow, but the change can also be very dramatic and specific in some situations, as, for example, among asylum seekers (Morville et al., 2015). The context for refugees is totally different from the situation in their home countries, often negatively influencing the well-being and structure of their daily life. That is, their physical, social, cultural and institutional environments have changed dramatically and new strategies to live their lives need to be developed.

Further increasing the complexity of the environment as a prerequisite for occupational engagement, the use of the public environment is often problematic for people with reduced capacity (e.g. Brorsson et al., 2013). An individual's needs, such as tailored adaptations, often cannot be accommodated. Instead, the environmental challenges that hinder people's occupational engagement have to be taken to the group or societal level to be solved. Therefore, when designing public environments the diversity of the population needs to be considered and the environments have to be designed so that it can be used by as many people as possible.

Including and Excluding Environments

All environments, whether physical or social, should enable equal participation for all people, and therefore features and conditions that include and exclude people from occupational engagement have to be considered. In the built environment, for example, it is obvious that the environment is not inclusive when steps to the entrance of a building prevent a person using a wheelchair from entering. To be inclusive, all people should be able to enter a building comfortably through the same entrance. Physical exclusion might lead to social exclusion, but social exclusion can also occur as a result of negative attitudes in society. Even some specific environmental solutions implemented with the intention of including people with impairments can be stigmatising, such as when a person who uses a wheelchair cannot sit together with his or her friends in the cinema and instead is directed to the space allocated for wheelchair users. Further, poorly designed environments might also become stigmatising, such as the design of some cash and ticket machines that are confusing and difficult to use by people who have a mild cognitive impairment.

Universal design has become a worldwide movement that aims to create physical environments, products, services and technology that are usable, accessible, safe and convenient for the vast majority of people (Mace, 1985). Although the principles of universal design elucidate important aspects in the design process, the wide range of people who use and experience a specific environment at a specific time makes it difficult to define valid and reliable asessments. As a result, currently there are no reliable and valid criteria for evaluating 'universally designed' buildings and devices (O'Shea, Paviaa, Dyer, Craddock, & Murphy, 2016). Instead, when assessing the design of the environment, the aim is to determine how best to design or adapt it to make it more *accessible, usable* and *safe/secure* for a single individual or a group of people with similar capacity and functional restrictions.

Accessibility and *usability* are anchored in the planning and building legislation in many countries, and accordingly buildings are meant to fulfil such requirements. *Accessibility* is a relative concept denoting the relationship between a person's functional capacity and the prevalence of environmental barriers (Iwarsson & Slaug, 2010). *Usability* targets the possibility that the environment offers for performing specific occupations (Oswald et al., 2006). According to the ISO, *usability* is defined as 'the extent to which a product can be used by specified users to achieve specified goals with effectiveness, efficiency and satisfaction in a specified context of use' (ISO, 2015). The qualitative aspect of usability is how easy and comfortable a person finds it to perform different tasks and activities in a certain environment and with different human-made objects, whereas the quantitative aspect is demonstrated by the frequency and consistency with which the person participates in different kinds of activities (Arthanat, Bauer, Lenker, Nochajskia, & Wub, 2007).

Inclusive environments also acknowledge the need for ensuring the *safety* and *security* of the people using it. It is essential to avoid danger or unnecessary risk for people. An example of this would be the need for homes and sheltered housing to be friendly and accommodating for people with dementia (Struckmeyer & Pickens, in press) and public environments that are built to reduce the risk of people falling (Gillespie et al., 2012).

ASSESSMENT

According to the Oxford Learners Dictionary the definition of *assessment* is the act of judging or forming an opinion about somebody or something (Oxford Learners Dictionary, 2016). That is, assessments can be both subjective and objective, and the outcome can be both subjective and objective as well.

Objective assessment of, for example, accessibility and usability is about the strength of the validity, reliability and other psychometric aspects of the assessment (Wahl, Fänge, Oswald, Gitlin, & Iwarsson, 2009). When considering the psychometric properties of objective assessments, there is also a need to consider sources of inconsistency (e.g. the raters, the examination and the context) (Jette, 1989; Slaug et al., 2011). Objective outcomes have an existence independent of the perception of the individual, such as the actual height of the working surface, whereas subjective outcomes depend on an individual's perception, such as the experience of using a high or low working surface.

Subjective assessment, such as an nonstandardised self-report during an interview or a diary, can focus on the same outcomes, but the psychometric properties are not established. A subjective outcome is 'the subjective state of a person, where the entity results from the feelings of the subject or person, or where an entity is perceptible only to the person being assessed' (Jette, 1989, p. 580).

To understand occupational engagement and the effect of the complexity of the environments involved, different assessments are needed, from subjective and objective assessments of personal experiences to systematic inquiries. Assessment instruments explicitly focusing on different aspects of the environment are used within occupational therapy, and such instruments are predominantly based on concepts relating to accessibility, usability and safety. In other assessments the environment is more or less explicitly considered. In assessments of activities of daily living, for example, the environment is usually measured indirectly, in spite of the central role it plays in the theory and models guiding the profession (CAOT, 2007). On the other hand, in assessments of physical activity the environment is increasingly considered (Gray, Zimmerman, & Rimmer, 2012). When deciding which instrument to use, it is important to make sure that the instrument is valid for the purpose and target group for the assessment, and that, when it comes to assessment of objective outcomes, the instrument sound pyschometric properties. Social and cultural environments are rarely assessed in themselves; instead informal consideration of these environments are integrated in assessments of occupational engagement.

Assessing Environmental Effect on Occupational Engagement

Occupational therapists use different methods to assess the effects of the environment on occupational engagement. In spite of the fact that models and theory guiding the profession put equal importance on all environmental aspects, methods assessing the physical environment dominate.

Some instruments assessing the physical environment are in fact checklists of physical features or barriers with unknown psychometric properties, whereas others have sound pyschometric properties. Physical environmental barriers have to be assessed according to national standards for housing design, and thus the definition of what actually constitutes an environmental barrier can differ depending on the national context. However, these instruments just focus on the environment and do not assess the effect on occupational engagement. Environmental features are also essential in the design of restorative environments and are mainly used in architecture and landscape architecture. Then the environmental qualities for different groups of individuals are focused on in terms of proximity, closeness, safety, and social opportunities (see e.g. Bengtsson & Grahn, 2014; Nejati, Shepley, Rodiek, Lee, & Varni, 2016).

Accessibility is more complex to assess than environmental barriers, because a person's or group's functional capacity has to be considered in relation to the environmental barriers. Together, the personal component and the environmental component lead to accessibility problems. Thus the magnitude of accessibility in a given environment differs depending on the capacity of a person or a group of people (Iwarsson & Slaug, 2010). Checklists and instruments in which the outcomes are targeting environmental barriers and accessibility problems are necessary in physical planning of housing and public environments to ensure the validity of the planning process and to acquire systematic knowledge about how the environment is designed. For occupational therapy intervention purposes, such instruments are only useful for walk-through assessments. Most importantly, occupational therapists have to consider many more aspects relating to occupational engagement, such as the effect of housing adaptations.

To enhance occupational engagement, environmental assessments that encompass activity and participation are necessary. These types of assessments target the complex transaction of person–environment–occupation and are useful for the planning of effective interventions to enhance occupational engagement. For example, before and after a housing adaptation that is explicitly aimed at enabling a person to engage in occupations within the home, the design and planning of the house and the extent to which it supports or enhances occupational performance and engagement (i.e. the usability of the home) needs to be assessed (Fänge & Iwarsson, 2005). Whereas accessibility is measured from a professional, objective, perspective, usability is generally assessed from an individual, subjective perspective.

Assessment of assistive device needs and use poses a particular challenge for occupational therapists. Assessments need to target the outcomes of the assistive device for participation in the home as well as in other areas (Brandt et al., 2008) as the device is prescribed to compensate for lack of functioning, while at the same time interacting with environmental features. That is, assistives devices are integral both to the person and the environment to enhance occupational engagement.

In assessments of risks of falling and fear of falling, the environment is often implicit and not geographically defined. Although data about the person's fear of falling when, for example, buying some groceries or climbing stairs (Yardley et al., 2005) are obtained during an assessment, often little specific information about the different environment the person moves in is obtained. Hence, depending on the purpose of the assessment, additional assessments may be needed to collect this information.

The social environment refers to the people that an individual connects with, such as family and friends, as well the help received from caregivers. Social aspects of the environment are predominantly subjective in character. For assessment purposes, qualitative methods such as semistructured interviews are most commonly used to gather this type of information.

The use of information and communications technology (ICT)–based media for assessments is increasing rapidly with technical developments. Photographs, video clips and real-time surveillance systems can be used to assess implicit aspects of the environment, such as activity and participation, as well as falls in certain environments (Robinovitch et al., 2013).

Assessment at Individual Level

The choice of assessment method and instruments focusing on environmental aspects of occupational engagement must be made consciously. In many cases – for example, in relation to adaptations of the home or workplace – detailed assessment of the environment is necessary. Even though such assessments focus on environmental barriers, accessibility, usability or safety/security, it is important to note that within occupational therapy each assessment should originate from a defined difficulty that a person has with occupational engagement. It is also important to note that not all aspects of the environment can be assessed simultaneously or be assessed by the use of one single assessment instrument. Instead, several assessments must be used to capture the complexity of the environment in relation to occupational engagement.

Assessment at Group and Societal Levels

Although occupational therapists mostly target the individual level in their assessments, a similar reasoning can be applied to the group and societal levels. However, the complexity of the environment is increased when considering group and societal level assessments as the effect of individual differences have to be taken into account as well as differences in culture, design, and the variety of ways in which activities are performed.

It is possible to identify groups of people with similar conditions and needs in relation to the physical environment. One such group is older people using rollators, who require ramps and threshold-free entrances to buildings; another group is people with severe loss of sight, who require good contrasts to be able to see and orientate themselves in the surroundings. The consequences of an illness, injury or impairment can vary considerably between different individuals and therefore the diagnosis is of less importance. Thus regarding environmental assessment related to occupational engagement, the impairments and the capacity of the individual need to be considered instead of the diagnosis. For example, an individual who had a cerebrovascular accident might have paresis or cognitive dysfunction; the two impairments pose completely different demands on environmental design to support occupational engagement. As a result of the paresis, he or she might use a wheelchair, which has to be considered when designing the environment to ensure that it is accessible for a wheelchair. If the individual instead has a cognitive deficit, the requirements for designing the environment are different, ensuring that the environment is easy to understand, interpret and negotiate and that key aspects of the environment are clearly signposted.

Insights and knowledge generated on an individual level provide a sound basis for developing knowledge at the group and societal levels. This knowledge can be generated, for example, from databases comprising high-quality data on large groups of people.

CONCLUSION

Assessments in which the outcomes target the environment are only part of what occupational therapists need to consider for intervention planning. Within occupational therapy, each assessment should originate from an identified difficulty of occupational engagement at individual, group or societal level. Whether more traditional or ICT-based assessments are used, it is most important to consider what perspective is taken in the assessment, if objective or subjective assessments should be used, and if the outcomes are objective or subjective.

 http://evolve.elsevier.com/Curtin/OT

REFERENCES

Adevi, A. A., & Lieberg, M. (2012). Stress rehabilitation through garden therapy. A caregiver perspective on fators considered most essential to the recovery process. *Urban Forestry & Urban Greening, 11*, 51–58.

Aplin, T., de Jonge, D., & Gustafsson, L. (2013). Understanding the dimensions of home that impact on home modification decision making. *Australian Occupational Therapy Journal, 60*(2), 101–109.

Arthanat, S., Bauer, S. M., Lenker, J. A., Nochajskia, S. M., & Wub, Y. W. B. (2007). Conceptualization and measurement of assistive technology usability. *Disability and Rehabilitation. Assistive Technology, 2*(4), 235–248.

Bengtsson, A., & Grahn, P. (2014). Outdoor environments in healthcare settings: A quality evaluation tool for use in designing healthcare gardens. *Urban Forestry & Urban Greening, 13*(4), 878–891.

Brandt, Å., Löfqvist, C., Jóndottir, I., Sund, T., Salminen, A.-L., Werngren-Elgström, M., et al. (2008). Towards an instrument targeting mobility-related participation: Nordic cross-national reliability. *Journal of Rehabilitation Medicine. 40*(9), 706–772.

Brorsson, A., Öhman, A., Cutchin, M., & Nygård, L. (2013). Managing critical incidents in grocery shopping by community-living people with Alzheimer's disease. *Scandinavian Journal of Occupational Therapy, 20*, 292–301.

Canadian Association of Occupational Therapists (CAOT). (2007). In E. Townsend, & H. Polatajko (Eds.), *Enabling occupation II: Advancing an occupational therapy vision for health, well-being & justice through occupation*. Ontario: Canadian Association of Occupational Therapists.

Cook, A. M., & Oolgar, J. M. (2008). *Cook & Hussey's assistive technologies principles and practice*. St Louis: Mosby Elsevier.

Ekstam, L., Carlsson, G., Chiatti, C., Nilsson, M. H., & Malmgren Fänge, A. (2014). A research-based strategy for managing housing adaptations: Study protocol for a quasi-experimental trial. *BMC Health Services Research, 14*, 602.

Ekstam, L., Malmgren Fänge, A., & Carlsson, G. (2016). Negotiating control i everyday life when deciding to apply for a housing adaptation. *Housing for the Elderly, 30*(4), in press.

Fänge, A., & Iwarsson, S. (2005). Changes in accessibility and usability in housing: An exploration of the housing adaptation process. *Occupational Therapy Internationl, 12*(1), 44–59.

Fisher, A. (2009). *Occupational therapy intervention process model*. Fort Collins, CO: Three Star Press.

Gillespie, L. D., Robertson, M. C., Gillespie, W. J., et al. (2012). Interventions for preventing falls in older people living in the community. *Cochrane Database of Systematic Reviews, 9*. CD007146.

Gray, J. A., Zimmerman, J. L., & Rimmer, J. H. (2012). Built environment instruments for walkability, bikeability and recreation: Disability and universal design relevant? *Disability and Health Journal, 5*, 87–101.

International Organisation for Standardization. (2015). *Human-centred design for interactive systems*. ISO 9241–210.

Iwarsson, S., & Slaug, B. (2010). *The housing enabler: An instrument for assessing and analysing accessibility problems in housing*. Nävlinge & Staffanstorp, Sweden: Veten & Skapen HB & Slaug Enabling Development.

Iwarsson, S., & Ståhl, A. (2003). Accessibility, usability and universal design – Positioning and definition of concepts describing person-environment relationships. *Disability and Rehabilitation, 25*, 57–66.

Jette, A. (1989). Measuring subjective outcomes. *Physical Therapy, 69*, 580–584.

Lawton, M. P., & Nahemow, L. (1973). Ecology and the aging process. In C. Eisdorfer & M. P. Lawton (Eds.), *The psychology of adult development and aging*. Washington, D. C: America Psychological Association.

Löfqvist, C., Granbom, M., Himmelsbach, I., Iwarsson, S., Oswald, O., & Haak, M. (2013). Voices on relocation and aging in place in very old age—A complex and ambivalent matter. *The Gerontologist, 53*(6), 919–927.

Mace, R. (1985). *Universal design: Barrier free environments for everyone*. Los Angeles: Designers West.

Meyer, A. (1922). The philosophy of occupational therapy. *Archives of Occupational Therapy, 1*, 1–10.

Morville, A.-L., Amris, K., Eklund, M., Danneskiold-Samsøe, B., & Erlandsson, L.-K. (2015). A longitudinal study of changes in asylum seekers ability regarding activities of daily living during their stay in the asylum center. *Journal of Immigrant and Minority Health, 17*(3), 852–859.

Nejati, A., Shepley, M., Rodiek, S., Lee, C., & Varni, J. (2016). Restorative design features for hospital staff break areas: A multi-method study. *Health Environments Research & Design Journal, 9*(2), 16–35.

O'Shea, E. C., Paviaa, S., Dyer, M., Craddock, G., & Murphy, N. (2016). Measuring the design of empathetic buildings: A review of universal design evaluation methods. *Disability and Rehabilitation. Assistive Technology, 11*, 13–21.

Oswald, F., Schilling, O., Wahl, H.-W., Fänge, A., Sixsmith, J., & Iwarsson, S. (2006). Homeward bound: Introducing a four domain model of perceived housing in very old age. *Journal of Environmental Psychology, 26*, 187–201.

Oxford Learners Dictionary. (2016). *Assessment*. Retrieved from http://www.oxfordlearnersdictionaries.com/definition/english/assessment?q=assessment.

Risser, R., Månsson Lexell, E., Bell, D., Iwarsson, S., & Ståhl, A. (2015). Use of local public transport among people with cognitive impairments – A literature review. *Transportation Research Part F: Traffic Psychology and Behaviour, 29,* 83–97.

Robinovitch, S. N., Feldman, F., Yang, Y. , et al. (2013). Video capture of the circumstances of falls in elderly people residing in long-term care: An observational study. *Lancet, 381,* 47–54.

Scheidt, R. J., & Norris-Baker, C. (2003). The general ecological model revisited: Evolution, current status and continuing challenges. K. Warner Shaie (Ed.), *Annual review of gerontology and geriatrics: Vol. 23* (pp. 34–57).

Sinclair, K. (2014). Global policy and local actions for vulnerable populations affected by disaster and displacement. Editorial. *Australian Occupational Therapy Journal, 61,* 1–5.

Slaug, B., Schilling, O., Helle, T., Iwarsson, S., Carlsson, G., & Brandt, Å. (2011). Unfolding the phenomenon of interrater agreement: A multicomponent approach for in-depth examination was proposed. *Journal of Clinical Epidemiology, 65*(9), 1016–1025.

Struckmeyer, L. R., & Pickens, N. D. (2015). Home modifications for people with Alzheimer's disease: A scoping review. *American Journal of Occupational Therapy, 70,* 7001270020p1-7001270020p9. doi: 10.5014/ajot.2015.016089.

Thompson, S., & Kent, J. (2014). Healthy built environments supporting everyday occupations: Current thinking in urban planning. *Journal of Occupational Science, 21*(1), 25–41.

United Nations. (1993). *Standard rules on the equalisation of opportunities for persons with disabilities.* New York: UN.

United Nations. (2006). *The Convention on the Rights of Persons with Disabilities.* New York: UN.

United Nations. (2015). *Transforming our world: The 2030 Agenda for Sustainable Development.* New York: UN.

Wahl, H. W., Fänge, A., Oswald, F., Gitlin, L. N., & Iwarsson, S. (2009). The home environment and disability-related outcomes in aging individuals: What is the empirical evidence? *Gerontologist, 49*(3), 355–367.

World Health Organisation (WHO). (1991). *Sundsvall Statement on Supportive Environments.* June 9–15, 1991 Sundsvall, Sweden. Geneva: WHO.

World Health Organization. (2001). *International classification of functioning, disability and health (ICF).* Retrieved from. http://www.who.int/classifications/icf/en/.

World Health Organization & World Bank. (2011). *World report on disability.* Retrieved from. http://www.who.int/disabilities/world_report/2011/en/index.html.

Yardley, L., Beyer, N., Hauer, K., Kempen, G., Piot-Ziegler, C., & Todd, C. (2005). Development and initial validation of the Falls Efficacy Scale-International (FES-I). *Age and Ageing, 34,* 614–619.

York, M., & Wiseman, T. (2012). Gardening as an occupation: A critical review. *British Journal of Occupational Therapy, 72*(2), 76–84.

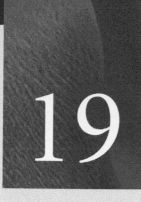

19

REASONING UNDERPINNING ASSESSMENTS FOR PEOPLE EXPERIENCING NEUROLOGICAL CONDITIONS

MARY EGAN ■ LISE ZAKUTNEY

CHAPTER OUTLINE

Abstract

Occupational therapists carry out formal and informal assessments as they seek to learn more about the person who has a neurological condition and determine how best to support function and valued occupation. Keeping in mind the 'who', 'what', 'why' and 'where' of information gathering helps the occupational therapist select appropriate assessment procedures. In addition, the selection of assessment tools will be dependent on whether the person is in acute care, rehabilitation or a community-based setting, as the focus of assessment will be different in each setting.

KEY POINTS

- Assessment in neurology begins with considering the person who is being assessed. The occupational therapist should have a good understanding of the person's history, goals and concerns.

- An assessment tool should be selected for its ability to measure the construct, its appropriateness for describing, evaluating or predicting, and its feasibility for the setting.

- Assessment procedures require consent. The occupational therapist must explain the assessment and any potential negative repercussions in an understandable and straightforward manner.

- Occupational therapists are increasingly involved in completing assessments mandated by the facility or the funder. Information from these assessments may need to be supplemented by other assessment information to ensure occupational therapy is person-centred.

INTRODUCTION

The goal of this chapter is to provide general guidelines for the complex process of selecting assessment tools and interpreting and sharing assessment results when working with people

265

who have neurological problems. Occupational therapists are increasingly moving from a mechanistic, biomedical approach in their assessments to one that is more holistic and occupation-focused. In addition, assessment is increasingly understood as a joint endeavour between the occupational therapist and the person. Confirmation that issues are being addressed that are important to the person, seeking informed consent, and communicating assessments results in an accurate and understandable manner are all critical. Additionally, assessment procedures must be appropriate for the person's age, culture, and communication and cognitive abilities.

Before carrying out an assessment, the notes of other health care providers, contained in paper or electronic medical records, should be reviewed for the information already collected. Although the occupational therapist will confirm any critical information with the person, it is important to make every effort to ensure that similar questions or tests are not duplicated by multiple assessors. This not only helps coordinate the work of the health care team, it also decreases burden on the people being assessed, while demonstrating that they can trust that their health care team is working together and attending to and sharing pertinent information about them. Where it is desirable and feasible, portions of assessments could be carried out in conjunction with another member of the team. For example, the occupational therapist and physiotherapist who are just beginning to work with a person experiencing neurologically related mobility problems may coordinate with each other to assess the person's current ability to get out of bed. Finally, it must be kept in mind that assessment of the person is only one aspect of enabling occupation; a similar level of attention must be given to examining the occupation and the environment.

With these principles in mind, broad strategies for thinking about assessment in the context of acute care, inpatient rehabilitation and community settings are provided. It is suggested that each setting has a primary issue that may influence the focus of assessment. In acute care, the focus is often on prevention of further problems, facilitating early mobilisation and providing information that is essential to discharge planning. In inpatient rehabilitation, the focus is often on improving a person's ability to perform activities of daily living and instrumental activities of daily living in preparation for returning to the community. In community care, the focus is often on engagement and reengagement in personally valued occupations. Regardless of the setting, assessments are carried out to guide and support transitions to the next setting or, in the case of assessments in the community, to promote reengagement in valued occupations within valued environments.

Within this chapter a number of assessments are mentioned. These assessments are only referred to as examples. The assessments mentioned may not meet the exact assessment needs of a given person. Also, further research may demonstrate important limitations of these assessments or indicate that other assessments are better suited to particular assessment situations.

It is worth noting that there are a number of excellent websites that describe assessment tools relevant for work with people who have neurological issues. For example, StrokeEngine (http://www.strokengine.ca/) can be found on the Canadian Partnership for Stroke Recovery website and contains descriptions and reviews of assessment tools relevant for work with people who have experienced stroke. The Centre for Outcome Management in Brain Injury (COMBI) website (http://www.tbims.org/combi/) contains descriptions and reviews of tools relevant for work with people who have experienced head injury.

Sites such as StrokeEngine and the COMBI websites contain both tools developed within the profession and tools developed outside of the profession. When using tools developed outside of occupational therapy, it is particularly important that the therapist has an excellent understanding of what it is they are attempting to measure and for what ultimate purpose, so that it is clear that the tool can respond to the particular needs of the occupational therapy assessment.

GENERAL ASSESSMENT CONSIDERATIONS

The 'Who' of the Assessment Process

Although it sounds almost too simple to mention, any assessment procedure must begin with an excellent sense of what the therapist is trying to discover. To select the best assessment tool, justify the use of less structured methods of assessment, or interpret the results of any assessment procedure, the occupational therapist must have a clear understanding of the question he or she is trying to answer. What needs to be kept in mind, though, is that assessment begins and ends with a person who is unique and affected by assessment procedures. Therefore the first step to any assessment is to start to learn about the person.

Any element of person-centred occupational therapy proceeds from a keen interest in the person with whom the therapist is working. What has brought this person to this encounter? What are his or her previous experiences with occupational therapy? Many people will have had no prior experience with occupational therapy. To be able to consent to and fully engage in assessment, they must first understand what occupational therapy is and what it might be able to offer to them in the particular health care setting they are in. A simple and clear explanation of the occupational therapy lens and the general goals of intervention will help people understand the reasons for assessment.

Furthermore, to ensure that intervention goals and assessment procedures are relevant to the person, the therapist must explore the person's aspirations and apprehensions. What are his or her hopes for what will be accomplished in occupational therapy and what are his or her primary concerns about therapy? These and other questions make up the 'who' of the assessment process that must be considered before turning to the 'what', 'why' and 'where' of assessment.

The 'What' of the Assessment Process

In quantitative assessment the 'what' is generally referred to as the measurement 'construct'. The most critical step in selecting an assessment is having a well-reasoned understanding of what should be measured. That is, what is the construct of interest? Constructs related to performance components that are commonly assessed by occupational therapists include things such as movement, sensation, affect, perception and cognition. Constructs related to occupation include such things as priority occupational performance issues and occupational balance. In addition, there are a number of constructs often used in rehabilitation that relate to issues typically associated with activities of daily living.

The 'Why' of the Assessment Process

The 'why' relates to the purpose of the assessment tool. Assessment tools are generally developed to respond to one of three purposes: description, evaluation or prediction. Because tools are generally built to respond to one of these tasks, they do not usually work that well for others. Hence, it is important to select a tool designed for the purpose for which you will use it.

Descriptive Assessment Tools

Descriptive assessment tools include screening and diagnostic tools. Screening tools indicate the need for further assessment to definitively determine whether the problem is present. Diagnostic tools indicate the presence or absence of a problem. For example, an occupational therapist may use a screening tool such as the star cancellation test (Halligan, Wilson, & Cockburn, 1990) to screen for the presence of spatial neglect – that is, to determine whether there is enough evidence to suspect this problem to warrant further testing. If this assessment indicates neglect may be present, the occupational therapist can then carry out the Catherine Bergego Scale (Azouvi et al., 2003) to confirm that the person is experiencing spatial neglect.

When considering whether an assessment is a good tool for screening, the therapist would look for evidence that the tool rapidly identifies people who might have the problem. When considering whether an assessment is a good tool for 'diagnosis', the therapist would look for evidence that the tool accurately identifies whether the person really has that problem. Occupational therapists do not diagnose medical conditions but may be called upon to provide an expert opinion about the presence of certain types of problems. Both types of descriptive tools should be accurate in indicating whether a characteristic or condition is present or absent; however, screening tools provide a quick first step to determine who may or may not need further testing and for this reason favour speed over accuracy.

Evaluative Assessment Tools

Evaluation tools indicate whether a construct has changed after intervention. Use of these tools are extremely helpful in providing encouragement to people regarding their progress, indicating to the occupational therapist that a change in the intervention may be necessary when progress has plateaued, or illustrating the effectiveness of occupational therapy to administrators and funders. In addition to truly reflecting change of a specific construct as opposed to measuring change of another construct (i.e. the tool should be valid), evaluation tools should be able to identify change that is meaningful to the person (i.e. the tool should be responsive to change that would be considered important to the person). In addition evaluation tools work better to reflect change when changes in scores are indicative of real change in the construct, rather than random differences from one measurement period to another (i.e. the tool should be reliable).

The Canadian Occupational Performance Measure (COPM) (Law et al., 2014) is an example of a tool that was developed to have two functions. That is, it allows for the identification of occupational performance issues of importance to the person and therefore provides a description of these to support person-centred occupational therapy goal setting. A person's perception of performance in and satisfaction with performance of these occupations before and after intervention provides an evaluation of these areas.

Predictive Assessment Tools

Predictive tools indicate the likelihood of a future event. This is perhaps the greatest area of caution for occupational therapists – indeed for all health professionals. Although there is often a temptation to try to predict future events from standardised assessments, few tools have been examined for their ability to accurately predict future outcomes. Where studies have been carried out to examine predictive ability, the results are often disappointing (Barry, Galvin, Keogh, Horgan, & Fahey, 2014).

The 'Where' of the Assessment Process

The 'where' of assessment is also essential to consider. Assessments that provide the information that the therapist is looking for but that require more time, training or specialised equipment than is available in the therapist's particular setting will not be feasible. Therefore it is important to consider these and other aspects of clinical utility (Smart, 2006) when selecting assessment procedures.

Of course, occupational performance is the product of interaction between the person, the environment and the occupation. Because of this, assessment of occupational performance in an artificial environment will not always reflect the person's performance in his or her home (Provencher, Demers, Gagnon, & Gélinas, 2012).

As previously noted, before beginning assessment and intervention it is critical to learn about each person's understanding of their situation, their most pressing concerns and what they currently see as the best approach to addressing these concerns.

There is no standard tool that provides this type of information. A relaxed, open-ended interview, perhaps from an ethnographic perspective (Gitlin, Corcoran, & Leinmiller-Eckhardt, 1995), is likely the most effective way to gather this information.

ASSESSMENT REASONING RELATED TO THREE PRACTICE SETTINGS: ACUTE CARE, INPATIENT REHABILITATION, AND COMMUNITY

Acute Care Settings

In occupational therapy, assessment is not generally an isolated step that is fully completed before intervention begins. In any setting, assessment typically proceeds as an iterative process of observing function, forming hypotheses about underlying performance components and experimenting with adjustments to tasks to improve occupational performance and carrying out more targeted assessments where necessary. During any assessment, but particularly when people are acutely ill, the therapist should be alert for signs that the person is experiencing a dangerous amount of cardiovascular stress. Such signs include chest pain, shortness of breath, wheezing, changes in colour or substantial fatigue. If any of these things occur, the therapist should discontinue the assessment and alert nursing staff. The therapist should also monitor for less severe fatigue and ensure that the person has adequate opportunity to rest. Scheduling assessments for times of the day that the person is less tired and assessing in shorter sessions is also important.

Joint Movement, Muscle Tone, Skin Breakdown, and Consciousness

As noted earlier, assessment and intervention in acute care are often targeted towards prevention of further problems, facilitating early mobilisation and providing information that is essential to discharge planning. People who are experiencing a severe neurological problem and have been hospitalised on an acute care unit may be relatively immobile. Prevention of further problems may require assessing joint mobility and muscle tone to determine whether joints need to be protected through positioning interventions. The constructs of interest here include range of motion, muscle tone (low tone or spasticity), and skin breakdown. Regarding range of motion, the purpose is to describe the degree of potential joint movement (e.g. Is it less than typical?) and evaluate this movement (e.g. Is it decreasing or increasing over time?). Describing range of motion as typical or limited is often carried out through visual inspection while moving each joint through its range. Regarding muscle tone, the purpose is to describe (e.g. determine the presence of low tone or spasticity) and evaluate (e.g. determine severity of abnormal tone). The Modified Ashworth Scale (Gregson et al., 1999) can be used for both purposes.

Regarding skin breakdown, the purpose is to predict future problems (e.g. If no action is taken to prevent it, is this person likely to have skin breakdown?) and to evaluate (e.g. What is the current condition of the skin?). The Braden Scale (Bergstrom, Braden, Laguzza, & Holman, 1987) is used to identify people who may be at greater risk for skin breakdown and should therefore have preventative measures put in place. This scale is often carried out by or in conjunction with nurses. The European Pressure Ulcer Advisory Panel classification system for pressure ulcers (Black et al., 2007) may be used to evaluate the severity of existing pressure ulcers, so that the effectiveness of measures to heal these lesions can be evaluated.

Sometimes people who are hospitalised for neurological problems are not fully conscious when seen by an occupational therapist. There are important principles to keep in mind while assessing someone who appears have a decreased level of consciousness. The occupational therapist first sees if simple communication can be established through asking the person to move a body part or to blink or nod his or her head to signal a yes or no answer. When people cannot follow these commands, they still may be able to hear what is going on around them and understand what is being said (Andrews, Murphy, Munday, & Littlewood, 1996). It is therefore always important for therapists to introduce themselves and explain all procedures as they are being carried out. Speaking and moving calmly helps ensure that verbal and nonverbal communication is reassuring (Geraghty, 2005). Also, it is critical that the occupational therapist remain aware of and understand the purpose and positioning of all medical equipment, such as intravenous lines, Foley catheters and feeding tubes, to ensure that these are not disturbed. If equipment is accidentally upset or disconnected, the therapist should immediately seek help from nursing staff.

As the person's level of consciousness improves, it is still critical to maintain a calm and respectful tone during assessment procedures. Many people hospitalised for acute neurological problems are experiencing a sudden and frightening change in their health, as a result of an illness or injury. In addition, acute neurological problems are often accompanied by a degree of slowing of thought processes and fatigability as well as possible problems with attention and memory. Calmness on the part of the therapist, and allowing additional time for responses, is important. Simplification of questions and instructions without infantilising communication is also critical. The therapist should position himself or herself at a person's eye level; maintaining good eye contact is essential, unless there are specific reasons against doing so (such as knowledge that for this particular person this might be threatening or culturally insensitive).

Communication

Before engaging the person in assessment, it is critical to have an excellent understanding of any potential communication issues. After confirming the languages the person uses and obtaining help for translation if the therapist and the person do not share a common language, the therapist reviews notes from the physician, nurse or speech-language pathologist that relate to receptive communication. If no information is available, communication can be screened by asking the person to follow simple verbal or written instructions, depending on the type of receptive communication of interest.

When the person is experiencing communication problems related to neurological issues, the occupational therapist should use measures to enable the person's full participation in the assessment process. The Aphasia Institute provides an excellent web-based resource to help health professionals develop the skills necessary to have supportive conversations with people experiencing aphasia (http://www.aphasia.ca/home-page/health-care-professionals/). Important principles include entering conversations with the expectation that the person will be able to make personal ideas known; using respectful, age-appropriate language; allowing adequate time for responses; and facilitating responses through pictures and written cues (Kagan et al., 2008).

The therapist must seek the person's consent for all procedures, including assessment. If the person is unable to provide consent because of problems with communication or cognition, consent should be sought from the person's substitute health decision maker. In either case, it is the therapist's responsibility to describe procedures in ways that are easily understood and outline any important negative outcomes that could arise as a result of the assessment. Assessments related to cognitive status are particularly relevant here, as negative results may trigger withdrawal of driving permits, present barriers to referral for further rehabilitation services or lead to pressure on the person to consider a move to residential care.

Mobility

Through knowledge of pathology, the occupational therapist first assesses performance components important for basic mobility that might be affected by the illness, injury or impairment. Depending on the type of neurological problem the person is experiencing, this might include strength testing of affected limbs and screening for visual and sensory deficits. Again, it is important that these assessments not be redone if they have already been carried out by another team member such as the physiotherapist. Early assessment of mobility (e.g. getting out of bed and into a wheelchair or walking to the bathroom) should be carried out with another person if it is not yet clear how much assistance the person might need. Ideally early assessment of mobility is carried out jointly with the physiotherapist or rehabilitation assistant to make best use of the person's energy and attention and share expertise.

It is important to note that many people who are hospitalised because they are experiencing neurological problems do not demonstrate obvious difficulties with movement or basic functional activities. However, they may be experiencing subtle problems with perception and cognition that need to be identified in acute care so that adequate rehabilitation follow-up can be planned. All people who potentially may have such subtle problems should be adequately screened and assessed where indicated by screening results.

Discharged Location

The function of an acute hospital unit is generally to stabilise the person medically. The person is usually discharged as quickly as possible after medical stability is achieved. People are typically discharged to their homes (with or without home care services), a rehabilitation hospital or unit or a long-term care facility.

Home. When the discharge destination is the person's home, or a retirement home without extensive assistive services, the foremost question in the therapist's mind is what processes can be put in place to ensure that the person is able to manage at home. Standardised assessments have been designed to describe a person's basic functional abilities, with the goal of determining whether these abilities are adequate to allow the person to manage at home. For example, the Barthel Index (Mahoney & Barthel, 1965) provides a description of the person's ability to eat, bathe, groom, dress, go to the toilet, get in and out of bed, walk and climb stairs. Other scales, such as the Nottingham Extended Activities of Daily Living Scale (Nouri & Lincoln, 1987), include instrumental activities of daily living such as obtaining groceries, paying bills and doing laundry. Increasingly the Functional Independence Measure (FIM) (Keith, Granger, Hamilton, & Sherwin, 1987) is used to support decision making regarding services on discharge.

Although such assessments include many activities that the person may be required to carry out independently at home, their scores do not unequivocally demonstrate whether someone will be able to comfortably manage at home. Appreciating that occupational performance is a result of the interaction among the person, the environment and the occupation, the occupational therapist understands that good knowledge of the environment and the person's occupations within that environment are necessary to determine what further help or services may be important to the person once he or she is home.

For example, a person may have a fairly sedate lifestyle and quite a bit of assistance at home, or physically taxing responsibilities and very little help. Formal or informal supports may be easier or more difficult to obtain and welcomed or unwelcomed by the person. For these reasons, standardised assessments will not provide an adequate picture of how well a particular person will be able to manage at home. Thorough investigation of the person's occupations and physical, social, cultural and institutional environments are critical. These are generally best carried out through discussion with the person and, with the person's consent, his or her partner or other key care partners. Assessment of more complex environments may require a home visit or referral to a community-based occupational therapist. In many hospitals, there is a 'discharge planner', a member of the team, often a nurse or social worker, responsible for coordinating discharge plans.

Rehabilitation Hospital or Unit. When the person's discharge destination is a rehabilitation hospital or unit, the occupational therapist typically shares his or her acute care assessments with the occupational therapist on the rehabilitation unit. This is done so that previously attained function can be maintained. More complex assessment of performance components and function are generally carried out by the occupational therapist at the rehabilitation facility.

Long-term Care Facility. When the discharge destination is a residential care facility with extensive assistive living services, the occupational therapists shares assessment reports with health care providers in that facility. These reports focus on how best function and further recovery can be supported. If there is no occupational therapist within this facility, this assessment information should be sent to the person or people who will coordinate further care, such as the nurse, primary care physician, family member, or the person himself or herself. It is important to ensure that this information has been received by, and is clear to, the reader.

Inpatient Rehabilitation Settings

As noted earlier, the focus of inpatient rehabilitation tends to be on maximising basic function. Typically this work is carried out by a team that may include physicians, nurses, occupational therapists, physical therapists, speech-language pathologists, rehabilitation assistants, social workers, psychologists, therapeutic recreation specialists and others. There is often a highly structured assessment process designed to meet the administrative needs of the facility and funders, as well as the health care needs of the person. Additional assessments may be required to ensure that services enable occupation while promoting recovery of function. It is important for occupational therapists to understand the reasoning behind mandated assessment procedures, as well as their strengths and limitations. In this way, the occupational therapist ensures that additional assessment procedures complement rather than overlap with existing information.

For example, in many provinces in Canada, the FIM (Keith et al., 1987) is a government-mandated tool for documenting functional gains made by people over the course of rehabilitation. Facilities must ensure this assessment is carried out within the required time limits by professionals who have been properly trained to use the tool. The components of the assessment completed by occupational therapists vary from facility to facility, but all occupational therapists are involved in some aspects of FIM assessment.

Carrying out components of the initial FIM assessment (or similar mandated assessments) provides the occupational therapist with valuable information regarding the person's current level of function in terms of mobility, memory, communication and activities of daily living. In addition, observation of the person during the assessment will provide important insights into possible performance component issues underlying current

difficulties. For example, the person who attempts to sit on the toilet before pulling down pants and undergarments may be having difficulty sequencing.

However, it is critical to note that additional assessments may be required to ensure that care is occupation-focused and person-centred. In addition to ensuring that all of the issues around function outlined in the previous section are addressed, it is also important that the occupational therapy assessment includes identification of the person's significant roles, occupations and occupational performance concerns. Significant roles and occupations could be discovered through procedures such as the Elicitation module of Personal Projects Analysis (Egan, Scott-Lowery, De Serres Larose, Gallant, & Jaillet, 2016; Little, 1989) or more informally through discussion of occupations within a typical day or month. Occupational performance concerns can be identified using the COPM (Law et al., 2014).

Through such assessment procedures and related discussion with the person, therapy goals are developed. In facilities where goals are developed by the team, these goals can be included within the team goals. After goal setting, further assessments are carried out to collect information helpful to the process of achieving these goals. Again, there is often an iterative process of assessments and interventions. Evidence of performance component problems can be observed during performance of occupations, or therapists may carry out a Dynamic Performance Analysis to pinpoint barriers to performance that could be overcome through changes to the environment or occupation (Polatajko, Mandich, & Martini, 2000). As noted in the previous section, environmental assessment is also important to the problem solving necessary to achieve goals.

Assessment at the end of the person's stay is important to document progress made and determine outstanding issues that must be addressed to support the person's continued recovery and ability to engage in personally valued occupations. Interestingly, goal setting at the completion of inpatient rehabilitation may be an effective strategy of helping ensure that progress continues, even in the absence of follow-up services (Brock et al., 2009). Readministration of the COPM and review of personal projects may assist in this goal setting. The occupational therapist may also be involved in readministering mandated assessments such as the FIM to determine the overall functional progress made by the person during inpatient rehabilitation.

Community Settings

People experiencing neurological problems may be referred to outpatient or home-based occupational therapy services after discharge from hospital or an inpatient rehabilitation centre, or they may be referred to these services directly from the community. As noted earlier, community-based assessment generally focuses on reengagement in roles and valued activities. This might include global assessments of occupational engagement or participation or more specific assessment of particular occupations.

Global assessments of occupational engagement or participation measure the extent to which the person is taking part in a range of occupations. These assessments are all based on a structured interview. Some are assessments of independence in occupations relative to a particular criterion (such as whether something is done or not or the amount of help required to carry out the occupation). An example of such an assessment is the Assessment of Life Habits (LIFE-H) (Noreau, Fougeyrollas, & Vincent, 2002). Others consider the person's satisfaction with current function, so that scores can be achieved in the presence of different performance levels. That is, if a person is satisfied with his or her current ability in a certain type of occupation, a good score is given even if the person is not independent or involved in this occupation. An example of this kind of assessment is the Reintegration to Normal Living Index (Wood-Dauphinee, Opzoomer, Williams, Marchand, & Spitzer, 1988). A third type of participation assessment combines both types of scoring. An example of this type of assessment is the Craig Handicap Assessment and Reporting Technique (CHART) (Hall, Dijkers, Whiteneck, Brooks, & Krause, 1998). Global participation measures may be helpful in demonstrating changes in occupational engagement after intervention.

These global assessments may be helpful in identifying particular aspects of occupational engagement that are problematic for the person. Alternatively, the COPM or a semistructured interview may also be used to determine which areas of occupational performance are of greatest concern to the person. Ethnographic interviewing (Gitlin et al., 1995) can be very helpful to determine how individuals view their current occupational challenges, what successful reengagement looks like to them, how they view their current difficulties with these valued occupations and what has been attempted to date to address these difficulties.

Once the areas of concern are identified, performance in community-based activities are ideally assessed in a person's natural environment and include consideration of the physical, social, cultural and institutional aspects of the environment that may help to facilitate performance and engagement.

The opportunity to examine occupational performance in the person's natural environment is one of the greatest advantages of community-based occupational therapy. When another person plays a significant role in self-care activities, the occupational therapist, with the person's consent, should include this other person in the assessment. When the person's goal is increased independence, assessment may focus on determining maximum current abilities and the impact of adaptation of the occupation or environment to maximise independence. When the goal is for a person to increase comfort and minimise effort from a care partner or minimise effort to save energy for other activities, the focus of the assessment will be on opportunities to minimise pain and conserve energy, again through adaptation of the occupation or environment.

Assessment to support engagement in productivity and leisure occupations are also ideally carried out in the community environment where they are to take place. Similarly to self-care, these occupations are ideally assessed through discussion with the person and observation in the specific environment that the work or leisure activity takes place.

CONCLUSION

Occupational therapists working with people with neurological problems use a variety of formal and informal assessment methods. These methods are applied to a wide range of potential problems from issues with sensation and movement to higher level cognitive functioning and participation in valued occupations. Selection of assessment methods will need to consider what is to be assessed, why and where. However, all assessment procedures must begin with an appreciation of the person as a unique individual who has hopes and anxieties concerning an illness, injury or impairment and the assessments and interventions that may take place.

http://evolve.elsevier.com/Curtin/OT

REFERENCES

Andrews, K., Murphy, L., Munday, R., & Littlewood, C. (1996). Misdiagnosis of the vegetative state: Retrospective study in a rehabilitation unit. *BMJ (Clinical Research Edition)*, 313(7048), 13–16.

Azouvi, P., Olivier, S., De Montety, G., Samuel, C., Louis-Dreyfus, A., & Tesio, L. (2003). Behavioral assessment of unilateral neglect: Study of the psychometric properties of the Catherine Bergego Scale. *Archives of Physical Medicine and Rehabilitation*, 84(1), 51–57.

Barry, E., Galvin, R., Keogh, C., Horgan, F., & Fahey, T. (2014). Is the timed up and go test a useful predictor of risk of falls in community dwelling older adults: A systematic review and meta-analysis. *BMC Geriatrics*, 14. 14-2318-14-14.

Bergstrom, N., Braden, B. J., Laguzza, A., & Holman, V. (1987). The Braden Scale for predicting pressure sore risk. *Nursing Research*, 36(4), 205–210.

Black, J., Baharestani, M. M., Cuddigan, J. , et al. (2007). National pressure ulcer advisory panel's updated pressure ulcer staging system. *Advances in Skin & Wound Care*, 20(5), 269–274.

Brock, K., Black, S., Cotton, S., Kennedy, G., Wilson, S., & Sutton, E. (2009). Goal achievement in the six months after inpatient rehabilitation for stroke. *Disability & Rehabilitation*, 31(11), 880–886.

Egan, M., Scott-Lowery, L., De Serres Larose, C., Gallant, L., & Jaillet, C. (2016). The use of personal projects analysis to enhance occupational therapy goal identification. *The Open Journal of Occupational Therapy*, 4(1), 4.

Geraghty, M. (2005). Nursing the unconscious patient. *Nursing Standard*, 20(1), 54.

Gitlin, L. N., Corcoran, M., & Leinmiller-Eckhardt, S. (1995). Understanding the family perspective: An ethnographic framework for providing occupational therapy in the home. *American Journal of Occupational Therapy*, 49(8), 802–809.

Gregson, J. M., Leathley, M., Moore, A. P., Sharma, A. K., Smith, T. L., & Watkins, C. L. (1999). Reliability of the Tone Assessment Scale and the Modified Ashworth Scale as Clinical Tools for Assessing poststroke spasticity. *Archives of Physical Medicine and Rehabilitation, 80*(9), 1013–1016.

Hall, K., Dijkers, M., Whiteneck, G., Brooks, C., & Krause, J. S. (1998). The Craig Handicap Assessment and Reporting Technique (CHART): Metric properties and scoring. *Topics in Spinal Cord Injury Rehabilitation, 4*(1), 16–30.

Halligan, P. W., Wilson, B., & Cockburn, J. (1990). A short screening test for visual neglect in stroke patients. *International Disability Studies, 12*, 95–99.

Kagan, A., Simmons-Mackie, N., Rowland, A. , et al. (2008). Counting what counts: A framework for capturing real-life outcomes of aphasia intervention. *Aphasiology, 22*(3), 258–280.

Keith, R. A., Granger, C. V., Hamilton, B. B., & Sherwin, F. S. (1987). The functional independence measure: A new tool for rehabilitation. In M. G. Eisenberg & R. C. Grzesiak (Eds.), *Advances in clinical rehabilitation* (pp. 6–18). New York: Springer.

Law, M., Baptiste, S., Carswell, A., McColl, M. A., Polatajko, H., & Pollock, N. (2014). *Canadian occupational performance measure (COPM).* Canadian Association of Occupational Therapists (CAOT).

Little, B. R. (1989). Personal project analysis: Trivial pursuits, magnificent obsessions, and the search for coherence. In D. M. Buss & N. Cantor (Eds.), *Personality psychology: Recent trends and emerging issues* (pp. 15–33). New York: Springer-Verlag.

Mahoney, F. I., & Barthel, D. W. (1965). Functional evaluation: The Barthel Index. *Maryland State Medical Journal, 14*, 61–65.

Noreau, L., Fougeyrollas, P., & Vincent, C. (2002). The LIFE-H: Assessment of the quality of social participation. *Technology and Disability, 14*(3), 113–118.

Nouri, F., & Lincoln, N. (1987). An Extended Activities of Daily Living Scale for Stroke Patients. *Clinical Rehabilitation, 1*(4), 301–305.

Polatajko, H. J., Mandich, A., & Martini, R. (2000). Dynamic performance analysis: A framework for understanding occupational performance. *American Journal of Occupational Therapy, 54*(1), 65–72.

Provencher, V., Demers, L., Gagnon, L., & Gélinas, I. (2012). Impact of familiar and unfamiliar settings on cooking task assessments in frail older adults with poor and preserved executive functions. *International Psychogeriatrics, 24*(05), 775–783.

Smart, A. (2006). A multi-dimensional model of clinical utility. *International Journal for Quality in Health Care, 18*(5), 377–382.

Wood-Dauphinee, S. L., Opzoomer, M. A., Williams, J. L., Marchand, B., & Spitzer, W. O. (1988). The Reintegration to Normal Linving Index. *Archives of Physical Medicine and Rehabilitation, 69*, 583–590.

20

REASONING UNDERPINNING ASSESSMENTS FOR PEOPLE EXPERIENCING MUSCULOSKELETAL CONDITIONS

TANJA A. STAMM ■ STEFANIE HAIDER ■ SIMONE LUSCHIN ■ AGNES STURMA

Abstract

People with musculoskeletal disorders are often referred to occupational therapists. Before any therapeutic intervention is started, an assessment is done. Most commonly, occupational therapists address occupational or functional performance as outcomes. Assessments can be classified into certain types, such as generic versus disease-specific, standardised versus nonstandardised and performance-based versus self-reported assessments. Despite the usefulness of nonstandardised assessments, it is often recommended to use standardised assessments to achieve comparable results and a solid basis for evaluation. Standardised assessments fulfil certain psychometric properties, such as reliability, validity and responsiveness. The most commonly used assessments in occupational therapy in musculoskeletal dysfunction are interviews, observations, functional range of motion and goniometry, assessments that assess occupational and/or functioning performance in the activities of daily living, assessments of hand, motor or sensory functions, muscle function tests and assessments that assess quality of life and pain.

KEY POINTS

- In musculoskeletal dysfunction, occupational therapists most often address occupational and/or functional performance as outcomes.

- Different types of assessments exist to measure these outcomes, such as generic versus disease-specific, standardised versus nonstandardised and performance-based versus self-reported assessments.

- Assessments need to fulfil certain psychometric properties, such as reliability, validity and responsiveness.

- A standardised assessments is administered and scored in a consistent, well-defined way.

- Despite the usefulness of nonstandardised assessments, it is often recommended to use standardised assessments to achieve comparable results and a solid basis for evaluation.

- Generic assessments are used independently of a specific disease, whereas disease-specific assessments are developed for specific health conditions only. Occupational performance assessments are commonly considered generic.

- Performance-based assessments are used to assess a person's ability to perform a task or an activity. Self-reported assessments involve people assessing themselves on the extent of a certain problem, rating their level of pain, functioning, ability to work or quality of life.

- The most commonly used assessments in occupational therapy in musculoskeletal dysfunction are interviews, observations, functional range of motion and goniometry, assessments that assess occupational and/or functioning performance in the activities of daily living, assessments of hand, motor or sensory functions, muscle function tests and assessments that assess quality of life and pain.

INTRODUCTION

People with musculoskeletal disorders are commonly referred to occupational therapists. Before any therapeutic intervention is started, an assessment is done (Townsend & Polatajko, 2007). To select an appropriate assessment, outcomes must be identified. Outcomes in health relate to clinical signs and symptoms and results that are important to people referred for health services, such as level of pain, functioning in daily life, occupational and functional performance, quality of life and so on.

Assessments are structured forms of gathering information or measurements of signs, symptoms and other results of interest. In occupational therapy, a person's level of occupational performance is considered an important outcome (Wilcock, 2006).

To classify outcomes in rehabilitation, the World Health Organization's (WHO) International Classification of Functioning, Disability and Health (ICF) (WHO, 2001) is commonly used as a frame of reference. The ICF is a classification that includes categories and codes of problems that people may have related to their activities of daily living including categories for body functions and structures and environmental factors. The ICF is not an assessment as such, but allows therapists and other health professionals to link the results of their assessments to a common frame of reference. The ICF is often used for team meetings as a common terminology because different professional terminologies can be translated into the categories of the ICF. To measure the extent of problems in certain ICF categories, assessments are needed. For example, when a person is referred because of fine motor hand function difficulties, this is related to the ICF category d440 – fine hand use. The occupational therapist consequently selects an appropriate assessment to measure fine motor hand function.

For the assessment of people with musculoskeletal disorders, several standardised assessments exist and numerous articles have been published that compare these assessments (Stamm, Cieza, Machold, Smolen, & Stucki, 2004). Out of the large number of assessments (an) appropriate assessment has to be selected. In this chapter, the process of how to select an appropriate assessment is described. However, a wide range of assessments are used in musculoskeletal occupational therapy (Prior & Duncan, 2009).

There are two main factors that can structure and shape the process of selecting an assessment and collecting information in occupational therapy:

1. The selection of a model to guide practice can lead to specific assessments being used. Conversely, some standardised assessments originate in conceptual models of occupational therapy. An example is the Canadian Occupational Performance Measure (COPM) (Law et al., 1994), which originated from the Canadian Model of Occupational Performance (Law, Polatajko, Baptiste, & Townsend, 1997). Hence, many assessments that focus on occupational performance originate somehow in a model of occupational performance because the measurement of occupational performance depends on how this concept is defined and which components are considered to make up occupational performance. Therefore isolated measurements of grip strength, muscle power, range of motion, and so on are not commonly done by occupational therapists who have occupational performance as a target outcome in their mind.

2. The area of practice an occupational therapist is working in influences the selection of assessments. When

working with people who have musculoskeletal conditions, an occupational therapist's knowledge of anatomical structures, biomechanics and the impact of conditions and injuries will guide assessment selection. However, even if functioning is the main target outcome of therapy, occupational therapists commonly consider a more holistic picture of a person's occupational performance. Assessments thus do not focus solely on biomedical variables.

The focus of this chapter is on musculoskeletal occupational therapy and applies mainly an orthopaedic and rheumatological perspective with a particular focus on upper limb assessments.

TYPES OF ASSESSMENTS

Different types of assessments can be used to determine the occupational performance of a person with a musculoskeletal disorder: generic and disease specific; nonstandardised and standardised; and performance-based and self-reported.

Generic and Disease-specific Assessments

Generic assessments are used independently of a specific disease, whereas disease-specific assessments are developed for specific health conditions only. Occupational performance assessments such as the COPM or the Assessment of Motor and Process Skills (AMPS) (Fisher, 2003) are commonly considered generic. Disease-specific assessments such as the Health Assessment Questionnaire (HAQ) (Fries, Spitz, Kraines, & Holman, 1980) are only used with people who have a specific health condition; the HAQ is used with people who have a rheumatic condition. It is a self-reported questionnaire that focuses on eight domains of functioning in daily life. In general, occupational therapists focus on a person's occupations and occupational performance rather than on the specific symptoms of a disease. Therefore a large number of occupational therapy assessments would be considered generic (Stamm et al., 2004).

Nonstandardised and Standardised Assessments

A standardised assessment is administered and scored in a consistent, well-defined way. Administering, scoring procedures and, if applicable, questions and interpretations are determined and defined, and definitions and instructions are accessible to users of these assessments. Some standardised assessments require training for correct administration, scoring and interpretation. An example of an assessment that requires therapists to be trained to be able to administer the assessment is the AMPS (Fisher, 2003).

A nonstandardised assessment may produce different results when administered another time or by another health professional. An example is an initial open or semistructured interview. This interview is used to gather disease-specific information from a person (in German/Latin, *anamnesis*); however, it does not follow a fully standardised structure. Another example of a nonstandardised assessment is informal or semi-structured observation of a person. This is part of every therapeutic interaction but can be more formalised and used as a part of an assessment. Informally, these observations can support the therapist in planning, applying, monitoring and evaluating assessments and interventions. Especially in therapy planning, nonstandardised instruments can be a suitable tool to gather relevant information.

Despite the usefulness of nonstandardised assessments, it is often recommended to use standardised assessments to achieve comparable results and a solid basis for evaluation. Nonstandardised assessments lack intrarater and interrater reliabilty as the motivations of the person being assessed and the assessor, and the ways in which it is administered often vary. However, it is not only important to select standardised assessments, it is equally important to apply them in a standardised way. The advantages of using standardised assessments in the appropriate ways are described in Table 20.1.

In professional practice, standardised assessments are required to be used in a standardised way in order to produce comparable results. Even nonstandardised ways of generating and acquiring data should be done in a systematic manner. For example, when gathering information about people's occupational biographies, each person can be asked to tell his or her life story with a single narrative-inducing question (Breckner, 1998; Stamm et al., 2008a, 2008b; Wengraf, 2001): 'Please tell me your life story – all the events and experiences which were important to you. Start wherever you like. Please take the time that you need. I'll listen first. I won't interrupt. I'll just take some notes for getting back to what you said after you have finished telling me about your experiences'. In this method, the initial question and the probing questions need to be worded in a similar way so that results are comparable. Furthermore, there are assessments that include certain qualitative elements, such as structured interviews in combination with self-reported scale such as the COPM (Law et al., 1990).

Likewise, obtaining medical, contextual and biographical data, such as in the context of an open interview/anamnesis, also requires structured procedures: it is not sufficient if medical and biographical data, which are essential for future treatment and intervention, are left out. An approach to structure these kinds of assessments is to use a checklist. Checklists should ensure that all relevant information is obtained and can be self-developed.

Performance-based and Self-reported Assessments

Another way to classify assessments is performance-based versus self-reported. Performance-based assessments are used to assess a person's ability to perform a task or an activity. People with a musculoskeletal disorder are asked to complete a certain task,

TABLE 20.1
Comparison Between Standardised and Nonstandardised Assessments

Statement	Explanation
Standardised assessments that fulfil psychometric properties ensure accurate measurement.	The assessment fulfils validity (truth) and reliability (the assessments can be repeated by the same or another assessor with the same or similar result).
Applying assessments in a standardised way makes data comparable.	Assessments should be applied always in the way outlined in the manual in which how it should be administered is described. This is also important in terms of determining scores in a certain scale. Standardised assessments usually include specific details on how to score a person's performance.
Using the same assessment at different time point establishes long-term data.	Using the same assessment at different times during the intervention process enables the impact of an intervention to be monitored and progress measured and recorded.
Even more unstructured assessments require certain elements of structure.	Often informal assessments, such as anamneses, follow a certain structure so that they are applied in the same way (e.g. the same topics are addressed, questions are worded in a similar way). This ensures that we are able to compare between time points and between people receiving occupational therapy services.
A team of trained persons conducts the assessments.	Ideally some assessments may even perform better if the same person or, more realistically, a team of trained persons administers the assessment. There are different approaches to increase assessment quality: ■ Definition of terms and scores so that assessors know when to allocate a certain score. ■ Training of assessors to achieve similar results. ■ Calibration of assessors regarding scores: an example is the AMPS, where assessors are given their individual scoring key to ensure consistency between assessors. ■ Quality checks: team members assess the same person and discuss discrepancies.
The context is also important – the situation and the conditions under which an assessment is administered.	Occupational therapists need to comply with standardised situations and conditions to administer the assessments as this contributes to the results of the assessment being based on a person's actual performance rather than because of the context.
Environmental factors regarding living conditions should be considered.	Environmental factors specific to the living conditions of people can go into assessments and may be important additional information; however, these information should also be obtained in a standardised way.

and their performance is then subjected to a clinimetric measurement. Clinimetric measurements are any forms of body measurements in professional practice. Examples of performance-based assessments include the Jebsen Taylor Hand Function Test (Jebsen, Taylor, Trieschmann, Trotter, & Howard, 1969) and the AMPS (Fisher, 2003), as well as grip strength or range of motion measurements (Stamm et al., 2002). These assessments can be performed in standard settings (in a clinic) or in a real-life setting (at the person's home or workplace).

Self-reported assessments involve people assessing themselves on the extent of a certain problem, rating their level of pain, functioning, ability to work or quality of life. These assessments include questionnaires, numerical rating scales or visual analogue scales.

Numerical rating scales ask people to select the number on a scale that best fits their perspectives, level of functioning, satisfaction, quality of life, level of pain and so on. Visual analogue scales do not use numbers, but a 100-mm horizontal line on which people are asked to mark the appropriate levels of pain, fatigue, disease activity and so on. Numerical rating scales

and visual analogue scales produce comparable results; however, numerical rating scales are easier to administer.

QUALITY CRITERIA OF ASSESSMENTS

Assessments need to fulfil certain measurement properties. To have a common terminology, the consensus-based standards for the selection of health measurement instruments (COSMIN) standard for *self-reported health-related* assessments was developed (www.cosmin.nl). In a checklist, measurement properties and criteria were defined. The COSMIN checklist was developed as a result of an international multidisciplinary Delphi study and can be used to evaluate the measurement properties of self-reported assessments. Commonly, three quality domains are addressed: reliability, validity and responsiveness. Each domain contains one or more measurement properties. These three domains equally apply to performance-based assessment. *Reliability* means that the assessment leads to a similar result if the same assessor (intrarater reliability) or a different assessor (interrater reliability) applies the assessment at another time. *Validity* determines whether an assessment measures what it is intended to measure; for example, an occupational performance assessment should measure occupational performance 'in a holistic sense' rather than hand movement and function. *Responsiveness* refers to whether an assessment measures a potential change, even if only small changes occur within therapy.

Before selecting a standardised assessment, occupational therapists should determine whether the assessment is acceptable in terms of its reliability, validity and responsiveness. In addition, literature should be consulted on whether an assessment is appropriate for the cultural context and available in the necessary language. Although COSMIN was developed for self-reported assessments, reliability, validity and responsiveness are common quality criteria that all standardised assessments should fulfil. Before using an assessment, it is recommended that therapists do a literature search on a database such as PubMed, search for the name of the assessment together with one quality criterion (e.g. reliability) and see whether there are studies showing good or acceptable quality.

COMMONLY USED OCCUPATIONAL THERAPY RELATED ASSESSMENTS IN MUSCULOSKELETAL DISORDERS

A large number of assessments exist that are commonly used by occupational therapists when working with people who have a musculoskeletal disorder. A selection of these assessments is presented in Table 20.2. The table can be used to assist with the selection of an assessment for a specific situation/question/person. In addition, therapists are encouraged to search for further literature for more information about the assessment. For example, when using Table 20.2, it can be seen that the Nine-hole Peg Test (Oxford Grice et al., 2003) can be excluded if a therapist wants to measure the ability to complete activities of daily living (ADL). In this case an assessment that covers ADL performance could be recommended, such as the AMPS.

Please note that the selection of assessments presented in Table 20.2 has been derived from the practice experience and research work of the authors. This list is not to be considered to be complete or exhaustive.

KEY ASSESSMENTS USED FOR PEOPLE WITH MUSCULOSKELETAL DISORDERS: DETAILED DESCRIPTION OF SELECTED ASSESSMENTS

In the following section selected assessments are described in more detail to provide an impression about what is assessed and what requirements there are to ensure appropriate use. After each description a short summary of possible strengths and weaknesses is given. Administration duration; materials, training and preparation required; necessary expenses; psychometric properties; and focus of the assessment have been taken into account. Those short summaries should provide an idea on practical implications when choosing an appropriate assessment.

Interview

An interview is always dependent on a person's ability to express him- or herself verbally (or at least in writing). In addition the interviewer needs to have certain skills regarding conversation techniques to obtain useful and meaningful information from the interviewee. Those are the fundamentals to be considered when using interviews for assessment purposes. Even though there are strictly structured or even preformulated interview assessments, the interview process requires competent conversational skills, the ability to create a basis of trust and an understanding atmosphere to gain honest insight in a person's point of view of his or her own occupations and abilities. Often semistructured interviews are used to guide an interview. Semistructured interviews are applied in health services to gather relevant biographical and medical history of people. A semistructured interview can ensure that all important aspects are covered.

Observation

In musculoskeletal conditions, the therapist observes a person's quality of movement, range of motion, posture, use of hands and/or performance capabilities. Facial expressions, appearance and demeanour can help to generate hypotheses concerning how the illness, injury or impairment affects daily occupation performance (Creek & Bullock, 2008). Observing the person during the first appointment in an informal way provides useful indications for choosing appropriate and diagnostically conclusive assessments that prevent quick 'preconclusions' based on unreliable data. In Practice Story 20.1A the therapist's observation of unexpected behaviour (e.g. avoidance of shaking hands, taking off her jacket primarily using the left hand, etc.) led to further nonstandardised assessments (interview) and standardised assessments (Visual Analogue Scale, Kapandji Index).

Functional Range of Motion and Goniometry

In the following section, the two most common ways of measuring range of motion are described.

Functional Active Range of Motion Scan (Without Exact Measurements)

A functional active range of motion (AROM) scan is a preliminary evaluation that provides the therapist with a quick overview of the mobility of a person's extremities and trunk as well as the use of range of motion during activities rather than measuring single joints. This provides a quick impression of the person's movement range, allows a right–left comparison

TABLE 20.2
Commonly Used Musculoskeletal Assessments by Occupational Therapists

Name of Assessments	POPULATION				FOCUS		TYPE				This Assessment Measures:
	Children	Adolescents	Adults	Older Adults	Disease Specific	Generic	Self-Reported	Interview	Observation-/Performance-Based	Technology-Assisted	
Assessment of Motor and Process Skills (AMPS) (Fisher, 2003)	•	•	•	•		•			•	•	Occupational performance/ADL
Biometrics E-LINK Evaluation & Exercise Systems (www.biometricsltd.com)	•	•	•	•		•			•	•	Hand function
Canadian Occupational Performance Measure (COPM) (Law et al., 1994)	•	•	•	•		•		•			Occupational performance/ADL
Disability of Arm, Shoulder and Hand (DASH) (Drummond, Sampaio, Mancini, Kirkwood, & Stamm, 2008; Gummesson, Atroshi & Ekdahl, 2003)		(•)	•		•		•				Person's perception of arm and hand function
Figure-of-eight method (Leard et al., 2004) (https://www.youtube.com/watch?v=M-iOb8v8MXw)	(•)	•	•	•		•			•		Measurement of oedema with a measurement tape applied on the hand in a figure of eight
Goniometry (Armstrong et al., 1998; Lewis et al., 2010)	•	•	•	•		•			•	(•)	Range of motion
Health Assessment Questionnaire (Bruce & Fries, 2003, 2005) (http://aramis.stanford.edu/HAQ.html)		•	•	•		•	•				Functional performance
Jamar Adjustable Hand Dynamometer (Hogrel, 2015; Mathiowetz, 2002)		•	•	•		•			•	(•)	Hand function – grip strength
Jebsen Taylor Hand Function Test (Jebsen et al., 1969)	•	•	•	•		•			•		Hand function
Kapandji Index (Kapandji, 1986)	•	•	•	•		•			•		Hand function
Box and Block Test (Hebert & Lewicke, 2012; Mathiowetz, Volland, Kashman, & Weber, 1985)		•	•	•		•			•		Hand function
(Modified) Moberg Picking Up Test (Stamm et al., 2003)		•	•	•		•			•		Hand function
Nine-hole Peg Test (Oxford Grice et al., 2003)			•	•		•			•		Hand function
Semmes-Weinstein Monofilaments / Aesthesiometer (Weinstein, 1993) (http://www.sorribauru.com.br/Arquivos/English223.pdf)	•	•	•	•		•			•		Sensory function of hand innervation

PRACTICE STORY 20.1A

Assessment of a person with hand osteoarthritis after surgery

Mrs Samson was a 64-year-old former administration secretary who lived in a terraced house with her husband. She loved gardening and was often busy keeping her garden and house orderly.

For 2 years – before seeing an orthopaedic specialist – Mrs Samson found it had become more and more difficult for her to keep up her routines because the symptoms of thumb osteoarthritis had been steadily worsening in her right hand; the pain and weakness in her right thumb had increased. The orthopaedic specialist referred her to surgery for a trapeziectomy and ligamentoplasty. Slips of the flexor carpi radialis tendon were sutured with the abductor pollicis longus tendon, which allowed her to maintain a distance between the scaphoid and the base of the first metacarpal bone and stabilised the metacarpal at the base of the thumb.

After surgery a thumb cast was made, which Mrs Samson was asked to wear for 3 weeks. The occupational therapist provided her with specific finger exercises to do while she wore the thumb cast, as well as information on oedema prevention and treatment. After 3 weeks she was issued with an occupational therapy custom-fabricated splint to wear for a further 3 weeks, which she could remove for skin care and specific exercises. From the seventh week after surgery she was instructed to wear the occupational therapy custom-fabricated splint only during heavy activities and at night.

Eight weeks after the surgery, when Mrs Samson attended her occupational therapy appointment, the occupational therapist observed the following:

- Mrs Samson avoided shaking hands.

- She removed her jacket primarily using her left hand.
- She opened her bag using her right forearm for holding the bag, and closed the zipper with her left hand.

Based on these observations the therapist generated a hypothesis about an underlying comorbidity being the cause for this unusual behaviour of Mrs Samson. The therapist conducted a pain assessment using the Visual Analogue Scale, examined the appearance and sensitivity of the skin and conducted an anamnesis on functional impairments in daily life. In addition, the therapist observed Mrs Samson's functional range of motion of the joints in her right hand in a nonstandardised way and measured her active range of motion of the thumb by goniometry and the Kapandji Index. The therapist concluded that Mrs Samson had developed a complex regional pain syndrome in the right upper extremity and adjusted her intervention accordingly.

In this practice story, the *observation of unexpected behaviour* (Mrs Samson avoided shaking hands, removed her jacket primarily using her left hand, etc.) led to the following:

A. *Further semistandardised assessments* (anamnesis on functional impairments in daily life)
B. *Further standardised assessments* (pain assessment using the Visual Analogue Scale, range-of-motion assessment using goniometry assessment and the Kapandji Index)

These assessments confirmed the therapist's hypothesis about an additional comorbidity and the impact this was having on Mrs Samson's ability to perform daily life activities. The outcomes of these assessments were used to make changes to her interventions.

---

and identifies certain limitations. The results of the preliminary evaluation may suggest other specific assessments to be conducted.

In conducting a functional AROM scan, it is helpful to select a starting point in order to be systematic, to ensure that important movements associated with certain tasks are observed and to keep the scan efficient. A guideline may be to evaluate motions from proximal to distal and from cranial to caudal. In the following section, examples of a functional AROM scan of the upper extremity are provided, including suggestions for phrasing instructions for the person.

When conducting a functional AROM scan, the following points should be considered:

- The person should be seated on a bench/plinth or stool, if possible, to ensure that movement is not impeded by the

seating support (e.g. a chair with arms will impede active movement of the upper limbs).
- The person should perform the requested movements bilaterally. If this is not possible, a baseline can be set by first observing the AROM of the unimpaired or less impaired side of the body.
- The therapist observes the active range of the movement and whether the movements are symmetrical and performed in a timely manner.
- If the person does not understand what is being requested because of a language barrier or cognitive deficits, the therapist can demonstrate the required movements.

Examples of the verbal instructions that can be used when conducting a functional AROM scan can be found in Table 20.3.

TABLE 20.3

Examples of Verbal Instruction To Use When Conducting a Functional Active Range of Motion (AROM) Scan

Shoulder	Motion
'Lift your arms straight up in front of you and reach for the ceiling.'	Flexion
'Touch the back of your head with both hands.'	External rotation
'Put your hands behind your back, like you are tucking in your shirt.'	Internal rotation
'Stretch out your arms to your sides (up to shoulder level).'	Abduction
'Put your stretched arms down again.'	Adduction

Elbow	Motion
'Put your arms straight down by your sides.'	Extension
'Bend your elbows so you can touch your shoulders.'	Flexion

Forearm and Hand	Motion
'With your arms at your side and the elbow flexed to 90 degrees, show me your palms and now turn them down to face the floor.'	Supination/pronation
'Move your wrists up and down.'	Wrist extension/flexion
'Make a fist and then open your fingers again.'	Finger flexion/extension
'Touch every fingertip with your thumb.'	Thumb opposition

If the therapist observes any deviations between right and left in quality or amount of movement within this scanning process, further assessments are needed (Practice Story 20.1B). Some illness, injury or impairment may only affect one side of the body. This should be kept in mind. Detailed measurements of the joints affected can be taken. This is commonly done by goniometry.

Goniometry

A goniometer is an instrument used to measure range of motion by measuring joint angles. Goniometers can capture objective information on decreased range of motion and monitor a person's progress during rehabilitation. The therapist uses a goniometer to measure the range of motion of all affected joints before starting an intervention. The therapist will repeat measurements at regular intervals to evaluate the progress being made.

The advantages of using goniometry include the following:

- Quick measurement of range of motion (ROM) for selected joints
- Good/acceptable intrarater reliability (between time points of measurement for one therapist)

The limitations of using goniometry include the following:

- Moderate to poor interrater reliability (between therapists) because of difficulties with different therapists placing the goniometer in the same position
- A lack of high-quality reference data

Before beginning to take ROM measurements using a goniometer, the therapist should be familiar with the anatomical structures, such as the bony landmarks related to each joint, joint axis, joint and muscle function, end-feel and recommended positioning of self and the person, as well as the procedure of ROM measurement. The therapist should be skilled in correct positioning, alignment and stabilisation and should be familiar with palpation of bony landmarks related to each joint and with handling of the goniometer. Measurements should be recorded accurately (Killingsworth, Pedretti, & Pendleton, 2013).

A standard goniometer is the most common tool used for measuring joint range of motion of the upper extremity. Various types of goniometers exist that are different in size and material (plastic or metal), but they all have two arms with a centre line and an axis. The axis is the centre of the protractor. The use of a goniometer to measure range of motion of the upper limb and its parts are illustrated in Figure 20.1.

Another device for measuring ROM is a gravity goniometer/inclinimeter, which uses gravity to determine the ROM from the starting position to the end of movement range. The gravity goniometer consists of a handle, a 360 degree protractor (divided into two 180-degree sections). The gravity line coincides with the neutral-zero position. This device is useful for reliably measuring pronation and supination of the forearm (Laupattarakasem, Sirichativapee, Kowsuwon, Sribunditkul, & Suibnugarn, 1990; Urban, Kalberer, Roos, & Dumont, 2002). The use of a gravity goniometer is illustrated in Figure 20.2. An essential condition for using the gravity goniometer is that

PRACTICE STORY 20.1B

Mrs Samson showed signs of nonuse of her right hand and protective posturing after the postsurgical phase of immobilisation. This behaviour also led to a loss of motion and other symptoms in shoulder and elbow. It was therefore appropriate to screen shoulder and elbow range of motion by bilateral comparison to ensure motion ranges were within normal limits and to determine whether other symptoms were triggered when conducting these movements. If any abnormalities were observed by the therapist, a thorough measurement of the affected joints and assessment of surrounding areas would be recommended.

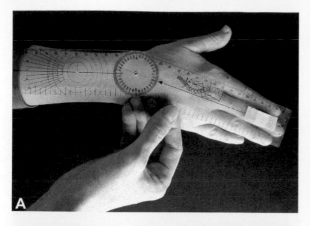
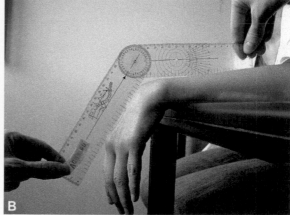
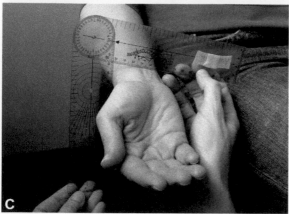
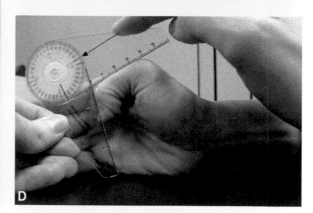

FIG. 20.1 ■ Range-of-motion measurements using goniometry.

A, Wrist ulnar deviation.

Position of the person: Seated at a table with forearms placed comfortably on the surface of the table without raising shoulders; forearm and hand are placed in pronation on the table, wrist in neutral position, fingers in extension.

Position of the goniometer:

Axis   On the dorsum of the wrist in extension of the third metacarpal, over the capitate bone
Stationary arm   Over the distal midline of the forearm
Moveable arm   Placed over the third metacarpal

B, Wrist flexion.

Position of the person: Seated at a table with forearms placed comfortably on the surface of the table without raising shoulders; forearm is placed on the table surface in pronation, wrist flexed over the edge of the table.

Position of the goniometer:

Axis   At the dorsum of the wrist in extension of the third metacarpal, over the capitate bone
Stationary arm   On edge over the midline of the forearm
Moveable arm   On edge over the third metacarpal

C, Supination and pronation of the forearm.

Position of the person: Seated on a straight chair without armrests, shoulder adducted, elbow flexed to 90 degrees, and the forearm in mid position.

Position of the goniometer:

Axis   The goniometer is aligned with the medial aspect of the distal forearm.
Stationary arm   Perpendicular to the floor
Moveable arm   Placed on the edge along the proximal wrist crease so that the goniometer arm is in contact with the middle half of the wrist

D, Thumb interphalangeal flexion.

Position of the person: Seated at a table with forearms placed comfortably on the surface of the table without raising shoulders; forearm and hand are placed on the table surface in supination, fingers in extension.

Axis   Perpendicular over the dorsal surface of the interphalangeal joint
Stationary arm   On edge over the midline of the proximal phalanx
Moveable arm   Over the distal phalanx

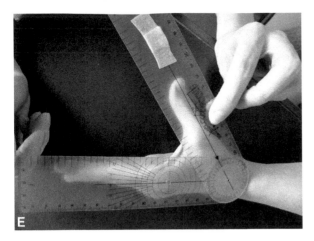

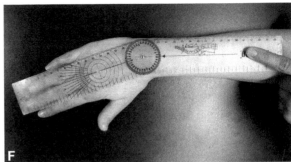

FIG. 20.1—CONT'D

E, Palmar abduction.

Position of the person: Seated at a table with forearms placed comfortably on the surface of the table without raising shoulders; forearm and hand are on the table resting on the ulnar side, wrist at 0 degree, fingers in extension.

Axis	Over the trapezium (on the dorsal side)
Stationary arm	Along the radial surface of the second metacarpal
Moveable arm	Over the first metacarpal

F, Radial abduction.

Position of the person: Seated at a table with forearms placed comfortably on the surface of the table without raising shoulders; forearm and hand are placed on the table surface in pronation, fingers in extension.

Axis	Over the carpometacarpal joint at the base of the first metacarpal
Stationary arm	On the dorsal surface of the second metacarpal
Moveable arm	On the ulnar surface of the first metacarpal

the person undertaking the assessment is able to grasp the handle appropriately. Please note that movement substitution can bias the result of measurement. In Figure 20.3 the person increases supination and pronation with additional movements of fingers and wrist (see Fig. 20.3A and B) and elbow abduction (see Fig. 20.3C).

Range-of-motion measurement is a commonly used musculoskeletal assessment. The protocol for range-of-motion measurements vary with each protocol, providing guidance on where to position the arms of the goniometer in attempt to provide consistency of placement. Although studies have indicated moderate interrater reliability when therapists follow measurement protocol when using a goniometer (Armstrong, MacDermid, Chinchalkar, Stevens, & King, 1998; Lewis, Fors, & Tharion, 2010), differences in measurement between therapists of 10 degrees and more are not uncommon. In general, intrarater reliability for range-of-motion measurements is better than interrater reliability in all the studies addressing this matter (Armstrong et al., 1998; Burr, Pratt, A. L., & Stott (2002); Ellis & Bruton, 2002; Lewis et al., 2010; Macionis, 2013; Pratt, Burr, & Stott, 2004). Measurement error of range-of-motion measurements was found to be 5 degrees (Killingsworth et al., 2013). The implications of measurement error are that in order to record a real difference in outcome, the difference in range of motion needs to be greater than the stated measurement error (i.e. 5 degrees) to represent real change. This means, if a person shows, for example, 45-degree flexion in the proximal interphalangeal (PIP) joint of the left ring finger at the initial assessment and a 50-degree flexion in the same joint after five occupational therapy units, it is unclear whether this is a real improvement of ROM or if the improvement is just derived out of a measurement error produced by the therapist. Actual improvement of ROM in the PIP joint can only be assumed when the improvement is more than 5 degrees compared with the initial assessment.

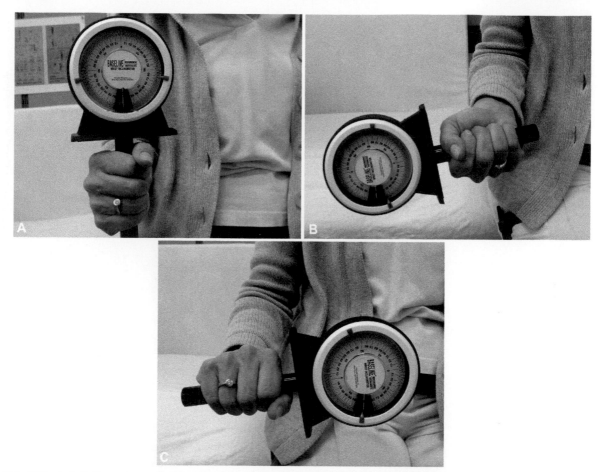

FIG. 20.2 ▪ A–C, Pronation and supination of the forearm measured with a gravity goniometer.
Position of the person: Seated on a straight chair without armrests, feet flat on the ground, shoulder adducted, elbow flexed to 90 degrees, and the forearm in mid position.

To improve psychometric properties, technological products have been developed which can assist with range-of-motion measurements; for example, people are positioned in a more standardised way and data from electronic or digital goniometers are automatically stored so that the therapist does not have to read scores from the goniometer. Motion capture systems, such as the Vicon system, are commonly and mainly used for the lower extremity and for gait analysis. However, range of motion of small hand joints using validated protocols has been carried out by occupational therapists (Adams, Metcalf, & Macleod, 2008). The systems commonly require that markers are placed on the body. Marker-free systems, such as the Kincet sensor or leap motion, cannot be used for measurements because of the lack of accuracy.

Research on technology-assisted range-of-motion measurement has been increasing over the years along with the progress of technological capabilities (Hoffmann, Russell, & Cooke, 2007; Rettig, Fradet, Kasten, Raiss, & Wolf, 2009).

Technical devices, apps and other innovations have been and are currently being developed to provide accurate and reliable range-of-motion measurement (Cools et al., 2014; Kim et al., 2014; Shin, Ro du, Lee, Oh, & Kim, 2012; Watanabe & Saito, 2011; Werner et al., 2014). Those include devices such as the Biometrics E-LINK Evaluation & Exercise System and electronic inclinometers. However, currently no technical solution exists that fulfils all quality criteria for a reliable standardised range-of-motion measurement.

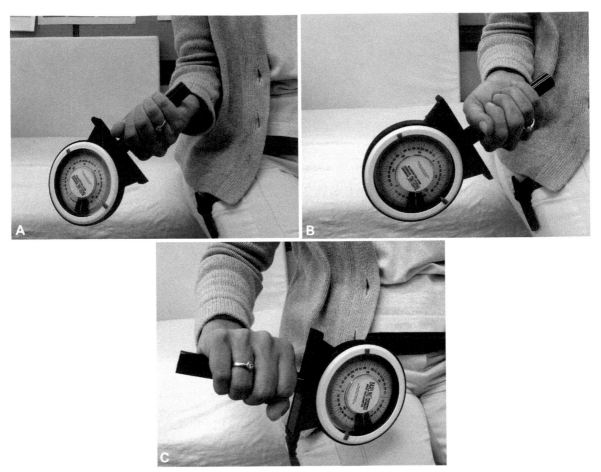

FIG. 20.3 ■ A–C, Pronation and supination of the forearm measured with a gravity goniometer: common movement substitutions. The three figures show possible substitutions the therapist should be aware of and ask the person to correct position if any of these types of movements are observed.

Technology-assisted Assessments Such As the Biometrics E-LINK Evaluation & Exercise System

Assessments are considered technology assisted when certain (electric) measuring instruments are used, either to assist in the measurement itself or in calculating scores. If the therapist wants to use such an assessment, the instruments have to be available and fully operative, which in some cases requires regular maintenance. Furthermore, the person administering the assessment has to be trained and experienced in order to obtain reproducible and reliable results.

The Biometrics System (www.biometricsltd.com) was one of the earliest technology-assisted systems developed for rehabilitation. Its primary application is in the fields of hand therapy and

stroke/neurological rehabilitation. The evaluation components of the Biometrics System include a dynamometer, pinch meter, electronic goniometer and force plates. All measurements are automatically entered into the provided software by the click of a button and can therefore easily be compared over time and used as starting values for the comprised exercises (Fig. 20.4).

An electro-goniometer consists of two arms like every analogue goniometer. Electro-goniometers do not usually display a degree scale because measurements are taken by sensors, which directly send the information to software where the values are automatically captured. It is also usual for all the other electronic evaluation devices to have no scales on them because data are captured electronically and need not to be read by the therapist.

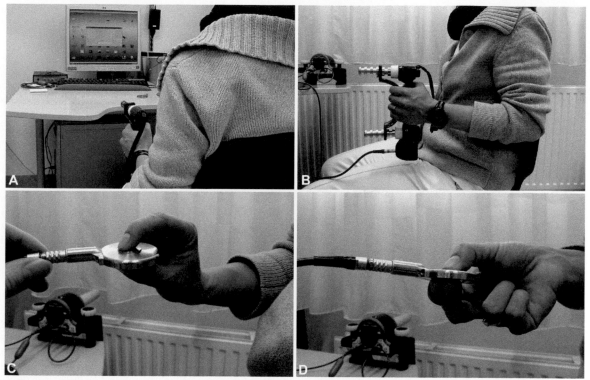

FIG. 20.4 ▪ A, Biometrics E-LINK Evaluation & Exercise Systems. B, Electronic dynamometer. C and D, Electronic pinch meter.

The advantages of these electronic assessment instruments include the following:

- Assessments and intervention tools are combined in one system.
- The software allows additional collection of manually entered data in standardised formats for health and medicolegal reports and outcomes purposes.

The weaknesses and limitations of this assessment include the following:

- It requires expensive equipment.
- Psychometric properties have not yet been sufficiently examined.
- Only a few studies have been conducted so far using the electro-goniometers.

Grip Strength: Jamar Adjustable Hand Dynamometer

The Jamar dynamometer is a standardised measurement of grip strength (Fig. 20.4B shows a digital version of this dynamometer; the analogue version of a Jamar dynamometer is similar in appearance). Grip strength has also been measured often using a vigorimeter, where people are asked to grip and squeeze a rubber bulb that has been selected to fit their hand size (Jones et al., 1991; Kleven, Russwurm, & Finsen, 1996). In an earlier study on hand osteoarthritis, the middle-sized rubber bulb (Ø 43 mm) was used for all people (Stamm et al., 2002). In rheumatic diseases, further instruments for grip strength include the Gripit (Nordenskiold & Grimby, 1993). When using the Jamar dynamometer or the virgorimeter, the following protocol is commonly applied: person in a sitting position, shoulders in a neutral position, elbow at 90 degree flexion, forearm in a neutral position, thumb upwards and outside of the fist. Resting the arm on a table is not permitted. People are encouraged to squeeze as firmly as possible.

The advantages of both the Jamar dynamometer and the vigorimeter include the following:

- They are quick to apply and there are reference values for gender and age.

The limitations include the following:

- Some people are not able to hold the Jamar dynamometer in the correct position because of its weight.
- The Jamar dynamometer needs calibration at regular intervals.
- There is no calibration for the virgorimeter.

Kapandji Index

The Kapandji Index is a quick and simple assessment to measure opposition of the thumb. No measurement tool is required as the system of reference is the hand itself on which opposition is tested. With the tip of the thumb the person is asked to touch the volar surface of each of the long fingers on the same hand. Scoring ranges from 0 to 10; scores are allocated as follows and are shown in Figure 20.5 (0 = impossible to do):

1. The lateral side of the middle phalanx of the index finger is touched with the tip of the thumb.
2. The lateral side of the distal phalanx of the index finger is touched with the tip of the thumb.
3. The tip of the index finger is touched with the tip of the thumb.
4. The tip of the middle finger is touched with the tip of the thumb.
5. The tip of the ring finger is touched with the tip of the thumb.
6. The tip of the little finger is touched with the tip of the thumb.
7. The distal interphalangeal crease of the little finger is touched with the tip of the thumb.
8. The proximal interphalangeal crease of the little finger is touched with the tip of the thumb.
9. The metacarpophalangeal crease of the little finger is touched with the tip of the thumb.
10. The distal volar crease of the hand below the little finger is touched with the tip of the thumb.

Every stage of the test has to be performed to obtain a valid result, as there is the possibility the thumb is moved across the palm by adduction rather than opposition (Kapandji, 1986). No disadvantages in using the Kapandji Index have been found, as it is simple and quick to perform and a reliable way to evaluate an important part of hand function, as the opposition of the thumb is necessary for functional grip.

Assessment of Motor and Process Skills

The Assessment of Motor and Process Skills (AMPS) (http://www.innovativeotsolutions.com/content/amps/) was designed to evaluate if a person can independently live at home and to determine the quality of performance in basic and instrumental activities of daily living. The therapist and the person to be assessed choose together two challenging tasks for the person to be completed based on the ability of the person. There are 120 internationally standardised, culturally adapted and well described tasks to choose from. After an initial interview in which the person has expressed concerns about his or her occupational performance in ADL tasks, the occupational therapist proceeds to determine which ADL tasks are presenting a challenge to the person. The chosen tasks can be carried out in a familiar environment to the person.

After the observation of each AMPS task, the therapist scores the person's quality of performance on each of 16 motor and 20 process items (i.e. occupational performance skills) according to the standardised criteria in the AMPS manual. Each task performance observed is scored separately and each ADL skill is rated using a 4-point ordinal scale. For valid and reliable use, the developers recommend that it is performed by a trained occupational therapist, whose ratings have been calibrated (Fisher, 1995). The AMPS can furthermore assist in planning intervention and is used to compare reevaluation results to determine the success of intervention.

The characteristics of this assessment are as follows: extensive training is required for using the assessment properly. The software needed for score calculation is based on Rasch analysis, which is an advanced statistical analysis. No special equipment is needed for conducting the tasks because the ADL tasks are usually carried out in 'natural' environments. The psychometric properties are well established and it is validated as a cross-cultural measure for use with people older than 2 years of age.

Canadian Occupational Performance Measure

The Canadian Occupational Performance Measure (Law et al., 1994) evaluates the performance, satisfaction and importance in up to five 'problems' that the individual has to identify in the areas of everyday life. Self-care, productivity and leisure are addressed in a semistructured interview. Individuals rate their performance and satisfaction on the self-selected activities on a 10-point Likert scale. The COPM is a semistandardised, person-centred assessment that is based on the underlying Canadian Model of Occupational Performance (Law et al., 1997). The test–retest reliability was 0.63 for performance and 0.84 for satisfaction. Validation studies have been done in a

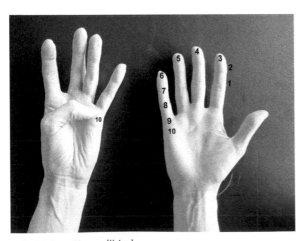

FIG. 20.5 ■ Kapandji Index.

variety of practice settings. Average time to administer is 40 minutes. The COPM has been linked to the ICF (Stamm et al., 2004).

The COPM can be used in people with various illnesses, injuries or impairments; has good psychometric properties; and is person-centred. However, the therapist requires training and good communication skills to be able to use the COPM effectively.

Disabilities of Arm, Shoulder and Hand Questionnaire

A widely used questionnaire, designed to measure physical function and symptoms in people with musculoskeletal disorders of the upper limb, is the Disability of the Arm, Shoulder and Hand (DASH) outcome measure (Davidson, 2004; Gummesson, Atroshi & Ekdahl, 2003). It consists of 30 items and takes about 10 minutes to complete. The items include questions about difficulties in performing physical activities and symptoms such as pain, weakness and stiffness, but also the impact on social activities, work, sleep and self-image (Kennedy, Beaton, Solway, McConnell, & Bombardier, 2011). Disability is reflected by a score from 0 (no disability) to 100. According to Gummesson, Atroshi, and Ekdahl (2003), a difference of 10 points may be considered as minimal important change. Because the DASH is suitable to measure disability in different upper extremity disorders, it also allows comparisons among different conditions (Hudak, Amadio, & Bombardier, 1996). The questionnaire is available in many languages, including English, German, Spanish, French, Italian, Dutch and Swedish. Also studies on the reliability and validity have been published for those versions (http://dash.iwh.on.ca/).

Health Assessment Questionnaire – Disability Index

The HAQ (Fries et al., 1980) (http://aramis.stanford.edu/HAQ.html) is a standardised questionnaire which is most commonly used for people who have rheumatic diseases. The disability assessment component of the HAQ, the HAQ-DI, assesses a person's level of functional ability and includes questions of fine movements of the upper extremity, locomotor activities of the lower extremity and activities that involve both upper and lower extremities. Twenty questions are grouped within the following eight categories: dressing, rising, eating, walking, hygiene, reach, grip and usual activities. Each item refers to the past week and people are asked to score their performance level on a particular task. The person's responses are made on a scale from 0 (no disability) to 3 (completely disabled). In addition, people can indicate whether they use equipment and assistive devices and help from another person to do activities.

The advantages of this assessment include the following:

- It is person-reported.
- It has been validated in a wide variety of rheumatological and nonrheumatological conditions and in studies of normal aging.

- It has good psychometric properties.
- It can be administered in 5 to 10 minutes (paper, online or interview).

A limitation, however, is that it has a commonly occurring ceiling effect in people with low levels of functional limitation.

Assessments of Hand, Motor or Sensory Functions

Several assessments exist that assess certain hand, motor or sensory functions. Commonly they focus exclusively on these functions, which is a limitation but also a strength if they are applied together with other assessments (Stamm et al., 2004). Some of them are more comprehensive than others. An example of a comprehensive generic hand function test is the Jebsen-Taylor Hand Function Test (JTHFT) (Jebsen et al., 1969), which includes various components of hand function and can be used to determine the impact injury or impairment has on a person's hand function. The JTHFT takes about 40 minutes to administer. It consists of seven subtests that are all timed with a stopwatch and summarised to obtain the total score: writing, turning cards (simulated page turning), picking up small objects, simulated feeding with beans and a spoon, stacking checkers upon each other, placing large light objects on a board and placing large heavy objects on a board. The JTHFT is a unilateral test in which each hand is measured separately. The total scores are calculated by summing up the scores of the seven subtests from both hands (Jebsen et al., 1969).

In addition to the JTHFT, other assessments that can be used to assess specific hand functions are the Box and Block Test, the (Modified) Moberg Pick-Up Test (Fig. 20.6) (Stamm, Ploner, Machold, & Smolen, 2003), the Nine-Hole Peg Test (Fig. 20.7) and the Semmes-Weinstein Monofilaments Aesthesiometer (Fig. 20.8); this last assessment is used to assess sensory functions of hand innervation after nerve damage.

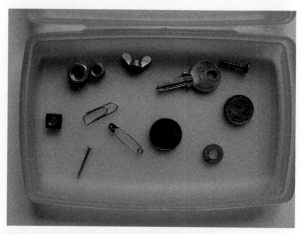

FIG. 20.6 ■ (Modified) Moberg Pick-up Test.

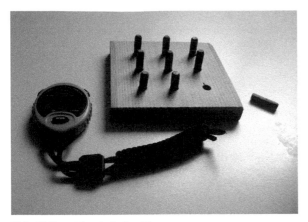

FIG. 20.7 ■ Nine-hole Peg Test.

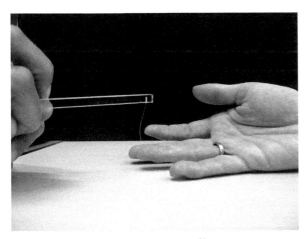

FIG. 20.8 ■ Semmes-Weinstein Monofilaments Aesthesiometer.

Manual Muscle Testing

The assessment of muscle strength is a key component in a physiotherapy assessment and less often used by occupational therapists. Muscle testing assesses muscle strength. A number of different methods can be used. A commonly used method of evaluating the muscle strength of muscle groups or individual muscles is the manual muscle test (MMT) (Palmer & Epler, 1990; Wintz, 1959). Muscle weakness is by far the most common negative symptom reported by a person with muscle disease and MMT is a relatively simple method of diagnosing the muscle strength.

MMT is used to determine five grades of strength in people with pathological problems ranging from low back pain to neck

pain and is also used for foot, knee and shoulder pain after fractures, postsurgical impairments or neurological injuries like amyotrophic lateral sclerosis and muscular dystrophy to name just a few. MMT measures effective performance of a movement in relation to the forces of gravity and manual resistance (Palmer & Epler, 1990).

For MMT a number of grading systems exist. The chart in Table 20.4 is based upon data from the Medical Research Council (MRC) Scale and can be used to grade manual muscle testing results. When using the MRC procedure for MMT, antigravity positions are those positions in which a body part is lifted against the force of gravity; gravity-minimised positions are those when movement of a body part is assisted or helped by gravity.

Although a MMT can provide information on the muscle strength, it is important for occupational therapists to also

| | **TABLE 20.4** | |
| | **Manual Muscle Testing** | |
MRC	Explanation	Position
5	Holds test position against maximal resistance	Antigravity position
4+	Holds test position against moderate to strong pressure	
4	Holds test position against moderate resistance	Antigravity position
4−	Holds test position against slight to moderate pressure	
3+	Holds test position against slight resistance	
3	Holds test position against gravity	Antigravity position
3−	Gradual release from test position	
2+	Moves through partial range of motion (ROM) against gravity or moves through complete ROM gravity eliminated and holds against pressure	
2	Able to move through full ROM gravity eliminated	Gravity-minimised position
2−	Moves through partial ROM gravity eliminated	
1	No visible movement, palpable or observable tendon prominence/flicker contraction	Gravity-minimised position
0	No palpable or observable muscle contraction	Gravity-minimised position

Modified from Palmer & Epler, 1990, and Rider et al., 2010.
MRC, Medical Research Council Scale.

consider using performance-based assessments such as hand function tests and ADL assessments when determining the impact of an illness, injury or impairment on a person.

Assessments in Upper Limb Function for People Wearing a Prostheses

The following section provides an overview of special assessments for people who use upper limb prosthetics. Prosthetic hand function can either be evaluated by objective hand function tests or by self-reported questionnaires that measure perceived impairment.

The DASH outcome measure described earlier can also be used in this field. Although its use is not restricted to prosthetics, it can easily provide information about functional limitations and disability in daily life for people with upper limb loss.

In contrast to the DASH, the Upper Extremity Functional Scale (UEFS) is specifically designed to be used for people with an upper limb prosthetics. It is a module of the Orthotic and Prosthetics Users Survey (OPUS), which is used with people who use lower limb prostheses. UEFS has 23 items (Heinemann, Bode, & O'Reilly, 2003) and focuses on self-care, productive work and leisure (Burger, Franchignoni, Heinemann, Kotnik, & Giordano, 2008; Heinemann, Connelly, Ehrlich-Jones, & Fatone, 2014).

The Trinity Amputation and Prosthetics Experience Scale – Revised (TAPES-R) is a multidimensional assessment to evaluate psychosocial processes of a person after amputation and subsequent prosthetic fitting and use. It also evaluates device satisfaction, impairment in daily life, phantom limb and stump pain, as well as other medical conditions. The questionnaire can be completed within 15 minutes (Desmond & McLachlan, 2005).

Another questionnaire that can be used for people with upper limb prostheses is the Nottingham Health Profile (NHP). The first part of this questionnaire consists of 38 items, including pain, mobility, sleep, social interaction, emotional health and energy. The second part focuses on the influence of health issues on daily life. It is possible to use both parts of the assessment or to only use the first part. However, as the NHP mainly focuses on functions of the lower extremity, it might not be the optimal assessment for upper extremity amputation (Demet, Martinet, Guillemin, Paysant, & Andre, 2003).

Widely used observational tests for prosthetic function include the Action Research Arm Test (ARAT), Southampton Hand Assessment Procedure (SHAP), Assessment of Capacity for Myoelectric Control (ACMC), Activities Measure for Upper Limb Amputees (AM-ULA) and Box and Blocks Test. The ARAT is an observational test used to determine upper limb function. The test consists of 19 items grouped in several subtests (grasp, grip, pinch and gross arm movement). Performance of each item is rated on a 4-point scale ranging from 0 (no movement possible) to 3 (movement performed normally) (Platz, Pinkowski, van Wijck, Kim, di Bella & Johnson, 2005).

The SHAP is a clinically validated hand function test that was originally developed to assess the effectiveness of upper limb prostheses but has now been applied to assessment of musculoskeletal and neurological conditions as well. It is made up of eight abstract objects (each one as heavy and light object) and 14 tasks that mimic daily living, with each task timed by the people doing the assessment themselves. Normal hand function is regarded as equal to 100 points (Bouwsema, Kyberd, Hill, Corry & Bongers, 2012; Kyberd et al., 2009).

The ACMC provides an assessment that reflects real-life tasks. While the person is doing one of several standardised tasks (e.g. repotting a plant or packing a bag), the tester evaluates the use of the prosthesis in bimanual tasks. Therefore a scale from 0 (not capable) to 3 (can do task very well) is used. Six factors are assessed: use of appropriate force, external support provided by the unaffected arm, prosthetic function in different arm positions, readjustment of grip, coordination of both sides and need for visual feedback (Hermansson, Bodin & Eliasson, 2006; Hermansson, Fischer, Bernspang, & Eliasson, 2005; Lindner, Linacre & Hermansson, 2009).

Similarly, the AM-ULA evaluates performance in activities of daily living. It consists of many items of self-care such as eating with a spoon and fork, dressing and undressing, tying shoes or doing hair. In some tasks the person is asked to only use the prosthetic hand, whereas in other tasks bimanual hand use is expected. The quality of prosthesis use within the task is rated using a scale from 0 to 4 (0 = unable, 1 = poor, 2 = fair, 3 = good, 4 = excellent) (Resnik et al., 2013).

A simple way to test prosthetic function is the Box and Blocks Test. It is a timed test in which the person is asked to move as many little wooden blocks as possible from one box to another with a divider between them. The test time is usually 1 minute (Kuiken, Miller, Lipschutz, Stubblefield, & Dumanian, 2005). Another option to perform this test is by having a defined number of blocks and measuring the time it takes to put them to the other side (Hebert & Lewicke, 2012).

Assessments of Pain and Quality of Life

When determining the level of pain a person is experiencing and the impact their illness, injury or impairment has on their quality of life, a number of assessments can be used. Quality of life and pain influence occupational and functional performance. The same is true for fatigue in chronic rheumatic diseases or other symptoms of health conditions that influence functioning and occupation. In occupational therapy, these assessments can be used in addition to occupational performance measurements to clarify levels of such things as pain and quality of life. Four of these assessments are briefly presented in the next paragraphs.

The Short Form 36 Health Survey (SF-36) is the gold standard for measuring a person's health status. It includes eight sections: vitality, physical functioning, body pain, general health perceptions, physical role functioning, emotional role functioning, social role functioning and mental health (Ware & Sherbourne, 1992). The SF-36 is a self-reported questionnaire.

WHO Quality of Life (WHOQOL-BREF) is an international cross-culturally comparable quality-of-life assessment that assesses individuals' perceptions of their quality of life in the context of their culture and value systems and their personal goals, standards and concerns (http://www.who.int/substance_abuse/research_tools/whoqolbref/en/). The WHOQOL-BREF is a self-reported questionnaire.

The Visual Analogue Scale (VAS) is often used for the fast evaluation of pain status. People are asked to define their pain between 0 (no pain) and 10 (worst pain possible). Likewise, VAS can be used for assessment of disease activity in rheumatic diseases (Studenic, Stamm, Smolen, & Aletaha, 2015).

The Multidimensional Pain Inventory (MPI), as published by the Central Institute of Mental Health in Mannheim, Germany, assesses phantom limb pain and neuroma pain, including the impact of these types of pain on daily life (Flor, Rudy, Birbaumer, Streit, & Schugens, 1990).

CONCLUSION

Occupational therapy commonly starts with an assessment. Occupational therapists focus on and assess occupational performance as an outcome of their therapy. However, especially for people who have musculoskeletal conditions, functional performance is also an important outcome. Standardised assessments are needed to obtain reliable and valid data, as well as long-term data that allow comparison between time points. Nonstandardised assessments like open interviews and informal observation produce also relevant information and should be used together with standardised assessments. Although generic assessments can be used in various health conditions, some assessments have been developed to assess signs, symptoms and levels of occupational performance as well as quality of life related to specific illnesses, injuries or impairments.

 http://evolve.elsevier.com/Curtin/OT

REFERENCES

Adams, J., Metcalf, C., Macleod, C., et al. (2008). Three dimensional functional motion analysis of silver ring splints in rheumatoid arthritis. Paper presented at the British Society of Rheumatology Annual Meeting. Retrieved from http://eprints.soton.ac.uk/265631/.

Armstrong, A. D., MacDermid, J. C., Chinchalkar, S., Stevens, R. S., & King, G. J. (1998). Reliability of range-of-motion measurement in the elbow and forearm. *Journal of Shoulder & Elbow Surgery, 7*(6), 573–580.

Bouwsema, H., Kyberd, P. J., Hill, W., Corry, K. S., & Bongers, R. M. (2012). Determining skill level in myoelectric prosthesis use with multiple outcome measures. *Journal of Rehabilitation Research & Development, 49*(9), 1331–1347.

Breckner, R. (1998). The biographical-interpretative method – Principles and procedures. *Sostris Working Paper, 2*, 91–104.

Bruce, B., & Fries, J. F. (2003). The Stanford Health Assessment Questionnaire: A review of its history, issues, progress, and documentation. *Journal of Rheumatology, 30*(1), 167–178.

Bruce, B., & Fries, J. F. (2005). The Health Assessment Questionnaire (HAQ). *Clinical and Experimental Rheumatology, 23*(5 Suppl. 39), S14–S18.

Burger, H., Franchignoni, F., Heinemann, A. W., Kotnik, S., & Giordano, A. (2008). Validation of the orthotics and prosthetics user survey upper extremity functional status module in people with unilateral upper limb amputation. *Journal of Rehabilitation Medicine, 40*(5), 393–399.

Burr, N., Pratt, A. L., & Stott, D. (2002). Inter-rater and intra-rater reliability when measuring interphalangeal joints. *Physiotherapy, 89*(11), 641–652.

Cools, A. M., De Wilde, L., Van Tongel, A., Ceyssens, C., Ryckewaert, R., & Cambier, D. C. (2014). Measuring shoulder external and internal rotation strength and range of motion: comprehensive intra-rater and inter-rater reliability study of several testing protocols. *Journal of Shoulder & Elbow Surgery, 23*(10), 1454–1461.

Creek, J., & Bullock, A. (2008). Assessment and outcome measurement. In J. Creek, & L. Lougher (Eds.), *Occupational therapy and mental health* (pp. 81–108). Edinburgh: Churchill Livingstone.

Davidson, J. (2004). A comparison of upper limb amputees and patients with upper limb injuries using the disability of the arm, shoulder and hand (DASH). *Disability and Rehabilitation, 26*(14–15), 917–923.

Demet, K., Martinet, N., Guillemin, F., Paysant, J., & Andre, J. M. (2003). Health related quality of life and related factors in 539 persons with amputation of upper and lower limb. *Disability and Rehabilitation, 25*(9), 480–486.

Desmond, D. M., & MacLachlan, M. (2005). Factor structure of the trinity amputation and prosthesis experience scales (TAPES) with individuals with acquired upper limb amputations. *American Journal of Physical Medicine & Rehabilitation/Association of Academic Physiatrists, 84*(7), 506–513.

Drummond, A. S., Sampaio, R. F., Mancini, M. C., Kirkwood, R. N., & Stamm, T. A. (2008). Linking the disabilities of arm, shoulder, and hand to the international classification of functioning, disability, and health. *Journal of Hand Therapy, 20*(4), 336–344.

Ellis, B., & Bruton, A. (2002). A study to compare the reliability of composite finger flexion with goniometry for measurement of range of motion in the hand. *Clinical Rehabilitation, 16*(5), 562–570.

Fisher, A. (1995). *Assessment of motor and process skills.* Fort Collins, CO: Three Star Press.

Fisher, A. (2003). *AMPS assessment of motor and process skills.* Fort Collins, CO: Three Star Press.

Flor, H., Rudy, T. E., Birbaumer, N., Streit, B., & Schugens, M. M. (1990). The applicability of the West Haven-Yale multidimensional pain inventory in German-speaking countries. Data on the reliability and validity of the MPI-D. *Der Schmerz, 4*(2), 82–87.

Fries, J. F., Spitz, P., Kraines, R. G., & Holman, H. R. (1980). Measurement of patient outcome in arthritis. *Arthritis and Rheumatism, 23*(2), 137–145.

Gummesson, C., Atroshi, I., & Ekdahl, C. (2003). The Disabilities of the Arm, Shoulder and Hand (DASH) outcome questionnaire:

Longitudinal construct validity and measuring self-rated health change after surgery. *BMC Musculoskeletal Disorders, 4*(1), 11.

Hebert, J. S., & Lewicke, J. (2012). Case report of modified Box and Blocks test with motion capture to measure prosthetic function. *Journal of Rehabilitation Research and Development, 49*(8), 1163–1174.

Heinemann, A. W., Bode, R. K., & O'Reilly, C. (2003). Development and measurement properties of the Orthotics and Prosthetics users' Survey (OPUS): A comprehensive set of clinical outcome instruments. *Prosthetics and Orthotics International, 27*(3), 191–206.

Heinemann, A. W., Connelly, L., Ehrlich-Jones, L., & Fatone, S. (2014). Outcome instruments for prosthetics: Clinical applications. *Physical Medicine and Rehabilitation Clinics of North America, 25*(1), 179–198.

Hermansson, L. M., Bodin, L., & Eliasson, A. C. (2006). Intra- and inter-rater reliability of the assessment of capacity for myoelectric control. *Journal of Rehabilitation Medicine, 38*(2), 118–123.

Hermansson, L. M., Fischer, A., Bernspang, B., & Eliasson, A. C. (2005). Assessment of capacity for myoelectric control: A new Rasch-built measure of prosthetic hand control. *Journal of Rehabilitation Medicine, 37*(3), 166–171.

Hoffmann, T., Russell, T., & Cooke, H. (2007). Remote measurement via the Internet of upper limb range of motion in people who have had a stroke. *Journal of Telemedicine and Telecare, 13*(8), 401–405.

Hogrel, J. Y. (2015). Grip strength measured by high precision dynamometry in healthy subjects from 5 to 80 years. *BMC Musculoskeletal Disorders, 16*, 139.

Hudak, P. L., Amadio, P. C., & Bombardier, C. (1996). Development of an upper extremity outcome measure: The DASH (Disabilities of the Arm, Shoulder and Hand) [corrected]. The Upper Extremity Collaborative Group (UECG). *American Journal of Industrial Medicine, 29*(6), 602–608.

Jebsen, R. H., Taylor, N., Trieschmann, R. B., Trotter, M. J., & Howard, L. A. (1969). An objective and standardized test of hand function. *Archives of Physical Medicine and Rehabilitation, 50*(6), 311–319.

Jones, E., Hanly, J. G., Mooney, R. , et al. (1991). Strength and function in the normal and rheumatoid hand. *Journal of Rheumatology, 18*(9), 1313–1318.

Kapandji, A. (1986). Clinical test of apposition and counter-apposition of the thumb. *Annales de Chirurgie de la Main, 5*(1), 67–73.

Kennedy, C. A., Beaton, D. E., Solway, S., McConnell, S., & Bombardier, C. (2011). *Disabilities of the arm, shoulder and hand (DASH). The DASH and QuickDASH outcome measure user's manual* (3rd ed.). Toronto: Institute for Work & Health.

Killingsworth, A. P., Pedretti, L. W., & Pendleton, H. M. (2013). Joint range of motion. In L. W. Pedretti, H. M. Pendleton, & W. Schultz-Krohn (Eds.), *Pedretti's occupational therapy: Practice skills for physical dysfunction* (7th ed., pp. 497–528). St. Louis: Elsevier.

Kim, T. S., Park, D. D., Lee, Y. B. , et al. (2014). A study on the measurement of wrist motion range using the iPhone 4 gyroscope application. *Annals of Plastic Surgery, 73*(2), 215–218.

Kleven, T., Russwurm, H., & Finsen, V. (1996). Tendon interposition arthroplasty for basal joint arthrosis. 38 thumbs followed for 4 years. *Acta Orthopaedica Scandinavica, 67*(6), 575–577.

Kuiken, T., Miller, L., Lipschutz, R., Stubblefield, K., & Dumanian, G. (2005). Prosthetic command signals following targeted hyper-reinnervation nerve transfer surgery. *Conference Proceedings: … Annual International Conference of the IEEE Engineering in Medicine & Biology Society, 7*, 7652–7655. http://dx.doi.org/10.1109/IEMBS.2005.1616284.

Kyberd, P. J., Murgia, A., Gasson, M., et al. (2009). Case studies to demonstrate the range of applications of the Southampton Hand Assessment Procedure. *British Journal of Occupational Therapy, 72*(5), 212–218.

Laupattarakasem, W., Sirichativapee, W., Kowsuwon, W., Sribunditkul, S., & Suibnugarn, C. (1990). Axial rotation gravity goniometer. A simple design of instrument and a controlled reliability study. *Clinical Orthopaedics & Related Research,* (251), 271–274.

Law, M., Baptiste, S., Carswell, A., McColl, M., Polatajko, H., & Pollock, N. (1994). *Canadian occupational performance measure – Manual.* Toronto: Canadian Association of Occupational Therapists.

Law, M., Baptiste, S., McColl, M., Opzoomer, A., Polatajko, H., & Pollock, N. (1990). The Canadian occupational performance measure: An outcome measurement protocol for occupational therapy. *Canadian Journal of Occupational Therapy, 52*, 82–87.

Law, M., Polatajko, H., Baptiste, S., & Townsend, E. (1997). Core concepts of occupational therapy. In E. Townsend (Ed.), *Enabling occupation: An occupational therapy perspective* (pp. 29–56). Ottawa: Canadian Association of Occupational Therapists.

Leard, J. S., Breglio, L., Fraga, L. , et al. (2004). Reliability and concurrent validity of the figure-of-eight method of measuring hand size in patients with hand pathology. *Journal of Orthopedic and Sports Physical Therapy, 34*(6), 335–340.

Lewis, E., Fors, L., & Tharion, W. J. (2010). Interrater and intrarater reliability of finger goniometric measurements. *American Journal of Occupational Therapy, 64*(4), 555–561.

Lindner, H. Y., Linacre, J. M., & Hermansson, L. M. (2009). Assessment of capacity for myoelectric control: Evaluation of construct and rating scale. *Journal of Rehabilitation Medicine, 41*(6), 467–474.

Macionis, V. (2013). Reliability of the standard goniometry and diagrammatic recording of finger joint angles: A comparative study with healthy subjects and non-professional raters. *BMC Musculoskeletal Disorders, 14*(1), 1–11.

Mathiowetz, V. (2002). Comparison of Rolyan and Jamar dynamometers for measuring grip strength. *Occupational Therapy International, 9*(3), 201–209.

Mathiowetz, V., Volland, G., Kashman, N., & Weber, K. (1985). Adult norms for the Box and Block test of manual dexterity. *American Journal of Occupational Therapy, 39*(6), 386–391.

Nordenskiold, U. M., & Grimby, G. (1993). Grip force in patients with rheumatoid arthritis and fibromyalgia and in healthy subjects. A study with the Grippit instrument. *Scandinavian Journal of Rheumatology, 22*(1), 14–19.

Oxford Grice, K., Vogel, K. A., Le, V., Mitchell, A., Muniz, S., & Vollmer, M. A. (2003). Adult norms for a commercially available nine hole peg test for finger dexterity. *American Journal of Occupational Therapy, 57*(5), 570–573.

Palmer, M. L., & Epler, M. (1990). Principles of examination techniques. In M. L. Palmer, & M. Epler (Eds.), *Clinical assessment procedures in physical therapy* (pp. 8–36). Philadelphia: Lippincott.

Platz, T., Pinkowski, C., van Wijck, F., Kim, I., di Bella, P., & Johnson, G. (2005). Reliability and validity of arm function assessment with standardized guidelines for the Fugl-Meyer test, action research arm test and Box and Block test: A multicentre study. *Clinical Rehabilitation, 19*(4), 404–411.

Pratt, A. L., Burr, N., & Stott, D. (2004). An investigation into the degree of precision achieved by a team of hand therapists and surgeons using hand goniometry with a standardized protocol. *British Journal of Hand Therapy, 9*(4), 116–121.

Prior, S., & Duncan, E. A. S. (2009). Assessment skills for practice. In E. A. S. Duncan (Ed.), *Skills for practice in occupational therapy* (pp. 75–90). London: Churchill Livingstone Elsevier.

Resnik, L., Adams, L., Borgia, M. , et al. (2013). Development and evaluation of the activities measure for upper limb amputees. *Archives of Physical Medicine and Rehabilitation, 94*(3), 488–494.

Rettig, O., Fradet, L., Kasten, P., Raiss, P., & Wolf, S. I. (2009). A new kinematic model of the upper extremity based on functional joint parameter determination for shoulder and elbow. *Gait & Posture, 30*(4), 469–476.

Rider, L. G., Koziol, D., Giannini, E. H. , et al. (2010). Validation of manual muscle testing and a subset of eight muscles for adult and juvenile idiopathic inflammatory myopathies. *Arthritis Care Research (Hoboken), 62*(4), 465–472.

Shin, S. H., Ro du, H., Lee, O. S., Oh, J. H., & Kim, S. H. (2012). Within-day reliability of shoulder range of motion measurement with a smartphone. *Manual Therapy, 17*(4), 298–304.

Stamm, T. A., Cieza, A., Machold, K. P., Smolen, J. S., & Stucki, G. (2004). Content comparison of occupation-based instruments in adult rheumatology and musculoskeletal rehabilitation based on the International Classification of Functioning, Disability and Health (ICF). *Arthritis and Rheumatology, 51*(6), 917–924.

Stamm, T. A., Lovelock, L., Stew, G. , et al. (2008a). I have a disease, but I am not ill: A narrative study of occupational balance in people with rheumatoid arthritis. *OTJR: Occupation, Participation and Health, 29*(1), 32–39.

Stamm, T. A., Lovelock, L., Stew, G. , et al. (2008b). I have mastered the challenge of living with a chronic disease: The life stories of people with rheumatoid arthritis. *Qualitative Health Research, 18*(5), 658–669.

Stamm, T. A., Machold, K. P., Smolen, J. S. , et al. (2002). Joint protection and home hand exercises improve hand function in patients with hand osteoarthritis: A randomized controlled trial. *Arthritis & Rheumatism, 47*(1), 44–49.

Stamm, T. A., Ploner, A., Machold, K. P., & Smolen, J. S. (2003). Moberg picking-up test in patients with inflammatory joint diseases: A survey of suitability in comparison to button test and measures of disease activity. *Arthritis & Rheumatism, 49*(5), 626–632.

Studenic, P., Stamm, T., Smolen, J. S., & Aletaha, D. (2015). Reliability of patient-reported outcomes in rheumatoid arthritis patients: An observational prospective study. *Rheumatology (Oxford)*.

Townsend, E., & Polatajko, H. (2007). *Enabling occupation II: Advancing an occupational therapy vision for health, well-being & justice through occupation.* Ottawa: CAOT Publications ACE.

Urban, V., Kalberer, F., Roos, M., & Dumont, C. E. (2002). Reproduzierbarkeit der Messung der aktiven Unterarmdrehung: Vergleich von 3 Methoden. [Reliability of active range-of-motion measurement of the rotation in the forearm: comparison of three measurement devices]. *Zeitschrift für Orthopädie und Ihre Grenzgebiete, 140*(01), 72–76.

Ware, J. E., & Sherbourne, C. D. (1992). The MOS 36-item short-form health survey (SF-36). A conceptual framework and item selection. *Medical Care, 30*, 473 483.

Watanabe, T., & Saito, H. (2011). Tests of wireless wearable sensor system in joint angle measurement of lower limbs. *Conference Proceedings: ... Annual International Conference of the IEEE Engineering in Medicine & Biology Society*, 5469–5472.

Weinstein, S. (1993). Fifty years of somatosensory research: From the Semmes-Weinstein monofilaments to the Weinstein enhanced sensory test. *Journal of Hand Therapy, 6*(1), 11–22 discussion 50.

Wengraf, T. (2001). *Qualitative research interviewing: Biographic narratives and semi-structured methods.* London: Sage Publications.

Werner, B. C., Holzgrefe, R. E., Griffin, J. W. , et al. (2014). Validation of an innovative method of shoulder range-of-motion measurement using a smartphone clinometer application. *Journal of Shoulder & Elbow Surgery, 23*(11), e275–e282.

Wilcock, A. A. (2006). *An occupational perspective of health.* Thorofare, NJ: Slack.

Wintz, M. N. (1959). Variations in current manual muscle testing. *Physical Therapy Reviews, 39*, 466–475.

World Health Organization (2001). *ICF – International classification of functioning, disability and health.* Geneva: World Health Organization.

21

REASONING UNDERPINNING ASSESSMENTS FOR PEOPLE EXPERIENCING MEDICAL CONDITIONS AND CONDITIONS REQUIRING SURGERY

DEIDRE MORGAN ▪ CELIA MARSTON ▪ JENNI BOURKE

Abstract
Professional reasoning in acute general medical and surgical settings is influenced by a number of factors. Assessment needs to take into consideration the complexity of people's multiple comorbidities, the fast-paced nature of admission and a focus on occupational performance factors that influence decisions about discharge destination. Although the occupational therapist seeks to adopt an occupational and person-centred focus to assessment, this can be challenging to achieve in a biomedical setting. Decision making that requires consideration of ethical and other complex issues in a person's care is best done within the context of interdisciplinary and senior occupational therapy support. Assessments in these settings need to be conducted in a timely manner to ensure best possible outcomes.

Observational assessment of occupational performance and predicting the impact of the discharge environment on a person's performance is the primary focus of assessment. Observational assessments are often augmented by assessment using standardised screening tools. Although occupational therapists should aim to support a person's autonomy and choice, they should also seek to minimise risk to a person's well-being and occupational performance where this is possible.

KEY POINTS

▪ Assessment in acute general medical and surgical settings is fast paced but should strive to maintain a person-centred focus.

293

- Assessment focuses on those areas that will enable occupational participation, minimise deconditioning and promote discharge home.

- Early assessments are particularly crucial to managing risk and autonomy and determining best possible outcomes.

- Timing of home assessments is crucial as a person may not be performing at his or her optimal physical and cognitive level if conducted too early.

- Although standardised screening tools may provide the occupational therapist with valuable information about factors influencing occupational performance, they augment but *do not* replace observational assessments of occupational performance.

- Observing a person's occupational performance and relevant performance components increases the accuracy of a therapist's overall assessment and ability to predict safety and care needs for discharge from hospital.

- Although occupational therapists seek to support a person's autonomy and choice, they have a duty of care to mitigate risks wherever possible. Decisions about complex scenarios should be made in conjunction with team members and senior occupational therapists wherever possible.

INTRODUCTION

Assessments used by occupational therapists when working with people admitted to acute general medical and surgical units, with a particular focus on performance decline and the elderly, is the focus of this chapter. The majority of people admitted to acute general medical and surgical units are living with complex and chronic disease. Subsequently, an admission to hospital can result in a significant decline in occupational performance, which is often referred to as deconditioning (Kortebein, 2009). Understanding the underlying causes for, and the person's experience of this decline in occupational performance is the key factor that informs an occupational therapist's assessment choice in this acute setting. An overview of the societal and practice contexts occupational therapists are required to work within and the impact this has on the professional reasoning of occupational therapists is also presented in this chapter. The biomedical and discharge-focused context of a medical and surgical inpatient setting influences not just the final choice of assessment but how assessment of this population is approached and delivered (Britton, Rosenwax, & McNamara, 2015).

Key principles that underpin the professional reasoning used to determine and undertake assessment in medical and surgical wards are identified. These principles include a person-centred approach that minimises burden and maintains a focus on the person's occupational priorities; timeliness and coordination of assessment; and discharge-focused assessments that promote autonomy and safety.

Finally, an overview of current and evidence-based types of assessment commonly used by occupational therapists working in medical and surgical wards is provided, including a description of the information these assessments provide and how this information contributes to professional reasoning. A practice story that appears through the chapter overviews the experiences of Bert, an older man living with cancer and admitted to hospital for surgery, providing an example of how the principles and processes presented in this chapter can be applied by occupational therapists working in these inpatient settings.

Understanding the Societal and Practice Contexts

Although occupational therapists are trained to consider each person as an occupational being, practice contexts do not always support this approach. This next section explores the biomedical context of medical and surgical wards and how this influences occupational therapy assessment in this setting.

Working in a Biomedical Context

People are typically admitted to general medical or surgical wards for medical treatment or procedures for conditions that require immediate attention. The majority of people admitted to these wards are elderly and have multiple comorbidities, chronic diseases such as diabetes, chronic obstructive airways disease and life-limiting illnesses like cancer and dementia. These health conditions commonly contribute to the illness that has led to the hospital admission for medical or surgical treatments (Australian Institute of Health and Welfare, 2014). An example of comorbidities is provided in story of Bert, a man requiring surgery after a diagnosis of cancer (Practice Story 21.1).

PRACTICE STORY 21.1

Bert: Medical Condition and Surgery

Bert is a 78-year-old gentleman who presented to his general practitioner with increasingly loose bowel motions, faecal incontinence and melaena. He had experienced rectal bleeding and weight loss of 22 kg over the last year. He was subsequently diagnosed with a large rectal adenocarcinoma. He had a history of diabetes, chronic obstructive pulmonary disease and peripheral neuropathy. Bert was initially treated with radiotherapy and chemotherapy as an outpatient before being admitted to hospital for surgery for the formation of a stoma and colostomy. The surgery was considered a curative measure for Bert's cancer. Although Bert had experienced substantial weight loss, diarrhoea and rectal bleeding, he was still physically active, completing the weekly shopping with his wife Joan and attending to his vegetable garden. Bert managed his diarrhoea with continence pads, but it was now starting to limit his time away from the house. His overall health and activity levels made him a suitable candidate for surgery.

Working from an occupation-based framework within a biomedical model can be challenging for occupational therapists and raises ethical issues (Bushby, Chan, Druif, Ho, & Kinsella, 2015) but is possible (Robertson & Finlay, 2007; Wilding & Whiteford, 2007). Occupational therapists working in biomedical settings are expected to understand what is happening to the individual from a disease perspective and from the perspective of the person experiencing the illness (Roberts & Robinson, 2014). Understanding implications of the underlying physiological symptoms a person is experiencing, how these change over time and what type of recovery is predicted will help occupational therapists start to identify potential occupational performance issues that warrant further assessment (Eyres & Unsworth, 2005).

In the case of Bert, an understanding of the cancer disease trajectory, the side effects of cancer treatments, and the expected recovery from surgery, as well as Bert's individual response to his illness, will enable the occupational therapist to generate some initial hypotheses regarding potential occupational issues. Undergoing surgery with a curative focus indicates that there are likely to be positive changes to Bert's occupational performance such as overcoming his previous symptoms of faecal incontinence and subsequent loss of weight. However, these symptoms as well as his other medical conditions have contributed to decreased occupational performance before surgery. As a result the impact of this decreased occupational performance on his recovery time needs to be considered.

Occupational therapists should consider what problems the people receiving occupational therapy services may be experiencing in relation to their comorbidities during their admission and after their discharge. Bert's history of chronic obstructive pulmonary disease and peripheral neuropathy is likely to result in a slower recovery time compared with a person without these chronic illnesses.

Working within an acute medical hospital setting means that once the symptoms of disease or illness have been properly managed and no longer require acute medical attention and care, there is an expectation that people will be discharged in a timely and effective manner (Roberts & Robinson, 2014). Occupational therapy assessment predominantly focuses on capturing people's occupational performances once their acute illness has been treated and their conditions are considered stable in order to identify potential occupational issues that could affect discharge planning.

Unexpected acute illnesses can occur during admission, such as delirium in Bert's case (Practice Story 21.2). This can alter the occupational therapist's expectations of the recovery trajectory and the timing and focus of assessment. Conducting an in-depth cognitive assessment and making predictions about a person's capacity to manage at home should wait until this acute medical condition has resolved. Bert's experience of delirium may also lead to a greater loss in his performance status compared with a healthier person undergoing the same surgery. This raises the issues of deconditioning and functional decline, which, as previously indicated, the occupational therapist must take into

---

PRACTICE STORY 21.2

Bert: Postoperative

Bert successfully underwent surgery for formation of a stoma and a colostomy. He was slow to recover from his surgery and was observed by nursing staff to be confused and agitated, particularly at night. He was diagnosed with a resolving delirium.

---

consideration when assessing a person in an acute hospital setting.

Deconditioning and Functional Decline

Deconditioning is a term used often to describe functional decline or reduced ability to perform tasks of everyday living as a result of decrement in physical or cognitive functioning. Deconditioning is commonly associated with an acute hospital stay. It may be a result of the illness or injury or because of extended periods in bed and prolonged periods of inactivity (Eyres & Unsworth, 2005; Kortebein, 2009).

For some the functional decline associated with deconditioning may be reversible (e.g. postoperative recovery for a person who was previously well before surgery). However, for the older person or someone who is contending with breakdown across a range of body systems (e.g. musculoskeletal, circulatory, nervous and autoimmune systems), prolonged bed rest can have significant negative ramifications on occupational performance. It can influence the person's potential to return home and may lead to adverse outcomes such as falls, pressure injuries, delirium and incontinence (Department of Health, 2012; Kortebein, 2009; Victorian Quality Council, 2003). Understanding the nature and impact of this decline and its interaction with a person's acute or chronic condition contributes to the therapist's ability to generate hypotheses around the reasons for the decline in occupational performance and what focus assessment should take place (Robertson & Blaga, 2013).

PRINCIPLES OF ASSESSMENT

Although an occupation focus is integral to all occupational therapy assessments, there are some principles underlying acute assessments that are specific to a medical and surgical environment. These factors will be considered as they relate to a person-centred approach, joint interdisciplinary assessments, the taking of an occupational profile and assessment of occupational performance. The occupational therapist plays a key role in enabling people to make autonomous decisions about their place of care. How this is achieved and the impact it has on occupational therapists warrants exploration.

A Person-centred Approach to Assessment

A person-centred approach to assessment influences interactions with people admitted for assessment and also the interdisciplinary team. This approach drives the timing and choice of assessment employed by the occupational therapist. It is imperative the occupational therapist develops an understanding of each individual's response to illness, their expectations of themselves and their recovery or prognosis (Townsend & Polatajko, 2013). People undergoing medical or surgical treatments typically have a response to the acute and immediate nature of their illness or condition. They have to contend with loss of function in a busy and intrusive hospital environment and are subjected to multiple assessments from multiple health professionals. Occupational therapists need to consider whether their choice of assessment and assessment process minimises burden and is respectful of the autonomy of persons they are assessing (Moats & Doble, 2006; Robertson & Blaga, 2013). Although the person must remain central in the assessment process, the occupational therapist has to do this within the constraints of an environment that often promotes organisational needs over individual ones (Mortenson & Dyck, 2006).

Conducting Joint Interdisciplinary Assessments

An interdisciplinary approach to assessment is recommended within medical and surgical inpatient settings (Dainty & Elizabeth, 2009). These types of assessments have been shown to improve a person's function, or occupational performance outcomes, and satisfaction with care (Wells, Seabrook, Stolee, Borrie, & Knoefel, 2003). The team gathers initial information regarding a person's premorbid and social history, anticipated goals and preferred discharge destination. This informs more detailed assessment of a person's occupational performance and evaluation of the person's response to illness. For example, an interdisciplinary initial assessment can involve the individual and/or family being interviewed about the individual's premorbid and social and occupational history by one of the allied health team members. This information can then be used by team members to inform their approach to assessment. When done well, this successfully avoids duplication of information documented in the history as well as reducing the likelihood of the person and the person's family having to participate in multiple assessments that divulge similar information.

Occupational therapists and physiotherapists commonly carry out assessments of a person's physical performance collaboratively. This has the benefit of minimising fatigue and taps into the shared and unique expertise of each discipline. For example, a person on a general medical or surgical unit may be moving out of bed for the first time. The occupational therapist and physiotherapist can work together to assess the person's abilities in transferring from the bed to chair and consider the subsequent implications for discharge and the need for additional assistance and aides.

Two important factors are essential to enable an interdisciplinary approach to assessment. First, each therapist must be competent in his or her own professional role. Team members need to be confident in their reasoning for including, excluding and sharing aspects of the assessment skill set (Craig, Robertson, & Milligan, 2004). This confidence evolves and develops over time but is enhanced by the support of skilled supervisors and engagement in reflective practice (Robertson & Finlay, 2007). It is common for new graduate therapists to lean towards a more discipline-specific approach to ensure they are providing a thorough assessment and to assist them in their intervention planning. However, experienced health professionals have been found to conduct more person-centred and occupationally focused assessments (Crennan & MacRae, 2010). Second, it is important for health professionals to have a clear understanding of other health professionals' roles in order to decide where blurring of roles may occur (Robertson & Finlay, 2007). This is a dynamic process that requires ongoing review as other health professionals' comfort with the type and scope of role blurring may change as team members rotate.

Conducting an Occupational Assessment

Occupational therapists working in acute hospital settings typically use brief, nonstandardised assessments over standardised assessments (Craig et al., 2004; Crennan & MacRae, 2010; Robertson & Blaga, 2013) to predict the implications a person's occupational performance issues may have on the discharge plan. Informal initial interviews and observational assessment of functional tasks like self-care are the preferred methods to meet the time pressure demands on decision-making in medical and surgical settings (Craig et al., 2004; Robertson & Blaga, 2013). Assessment of a person's performance in self-care tasks is commonly used by occupational therapists in these settings to determine a person's level of occupational performance (Crennan & MacRae, 2010; Eyres & Unsworth, 2005; Roberts & Robinson, 2014). Although people may have difficulty participating in a range of valued occupations because of illness, capacity to manage self-care is the primary occupation that determines a person's ability to return home from an acute hospital setting. Consequently, occupational performance around self-care is considered a strong indicator of what a person's anticipated discharge plan may be (Dainty & Elizabeth, 2009; Wells et al., 2003).

Professional experience in a specialist area like general medicine or surgery can equip therapists to predict potential discharge plans early in the initial interview process. However, actually observing a person's occupational performance and relevant performance components increases the accuracy of a therapist's overall assessment and ability to predict safety and care needs for discharge from hospital (Robertson & Blaga, 2013).

Standardised assessments are used less often in the acute general medical and surgical settings by occupational therapists. When they are used, they are used to measure specific performance components like cognition and upper limb function to complement the observational functional assessments and inform more complex discharge decision making (Douglas, Liu, Warren, & Hopper, 2007; Robertson & Blaga, 2013). For example, a person may be observed having difficulty planning and sequencing basic self-care tasks on the unit, which raises concerns about how the person will manage at home after discharge. A standardised cognitive assessment can confirm these problem areas and potentially identify other cognitive components that require addressing, such as orientation and recall. Standardised assessment tools are also considered useful in communicating outcomes to other professionals; however, it is acknowledged that standardised assessments may be less person-centred than an informal interview or observational assessment (Robertson & Blaga, 2013). For example, a person's score on the Functional Independence Measure (FIM) may inform other health professionals of the levels of assistance required for someone to transfer out of bed. However, it does not consider the person's response to this assistance and how it interacts with other performance components like cognition.

Understanding the limitations of standardised assessment tools is an important part of the professional reasoning process for occupational therapists, particularly across the diverse populations seen in general medicine and surgical settings. For example, the Mini-Mental State Examination (MMSE) (Folstein, Folstein, & McHugh, 1975) is a universally adopted tool for screening for cognitive impairment. However, it is not sensitive in detecting executive dysfunction and mild cognitive impairment (Ismail, Raji, & Shulman, 2010). Other assessment tools such as the Montreal Cognitive Assessment (MoCA) (Freitas, Simões, Alves, & Santana, 2013) and the Rowland Universal Dementia Assessment Scale (RUDAS) (Limpawattana, Tiamkao, & Sawanyawisuth, 2012) are more sensitive to these variables (Atwal, Wiggett, & McIntyre, 2011; Ismail et al., 2010).These assessment tools are discussed in more detail in Scope and Types of Assessments Used in Acute Settings.

Enabling Autonomy and Facilitating Safety

Ethical Issues

Occupational therapists play a major role in assessing a person's potential safety to return home. This can be particularly challenging in medical and surgical settings. The occupational therapist may experience pressure from the team to expedite a discharge because a person is 'medically stable' or prevent a discharge because the team considers a person's choice to return home unsafe. Occupational therapists often make professional decisions based on their assessments about a person's safety when attempting to meet both the team and the individual's needs. These needs are often competing and at times mutually exclusive (Moats, 2006; Moats & Doble, 2006).

The challenge for occupational therapists is to consider whether their decision making around return to home supports the person's values when these values are in contrast to the team's perspective (Bushby et al., 2015; Douglas et al., 2007; Durocher & Gibson; Moats, 2006; Robertson & Blaga, 2013). Therapists need to clearly articulate the professional reasoning underpinning their decisions and be prepared to discuss their rationale with other team members.

Supporting a person's autonomy and safety can be experienced as an ethical dilemma for occupational therapists (Durocher & Gibson, 2010). Atwal and Caldwell (2003) note that upholding a person's autonomy may be in conflict with the ethical principle of doing no harm if discharge home is perceived to be placing a person at risk. Active support by senior occupational therapists and shared decision making with other team members can assist less experienced therapists with these sorts of ethical dilemmas (Atwal & Caldwell, 2003; Atwal et al., 2011; Bushby et al., 2015).

Older people who have a chronic disease often live in environments that represent individual choice and well-being even though they are not always environments that are supportive of their care needs. This means that the occupational therapist needs to carefully consider discharge options that, although safe, may remove individual choice and autonomy. If a person is deemed to be cognitively intact or competent by a team and wants to return home to a physically unsafe environment, he or she has the right to do so (State Government of Victoria, 2013). Although occupational therapists seek to support personal autonomy and choice, they have a duty of care to mitigate risks wherever possible (Atwal & Caldwell, 2003).

Unplanned Readmissions

Irrespective of whether discharge home is driven by the organisation or the individual, premature discharge home may lead to unplanned readmissions to hospital and other adverse events such as falls (Roberts & Robinson, 2014). Older people with chronic disease have a high readmission rate to hospital. The reasons for these readmissions are complex and varied but may include premature discharge home, acute exacerbations of disease, further functional decline and inadequate support systems (Australian Institute of Health and Welfare, 2014; DePalma et al., 2013; Roberts & Robinson, 2014). One way to manage this uncertainty is to commence comprehensive assessment for discharge planning soon after admission. Early discharge planning has been found to be associated with lower readmission rates (Fox et al., 2013).

Many people admitted to medical and surgical wards have dementia and other cognitive impairments. These people are often excluded from discharge decision-making processes (Moats & Doble, 2006). When working from a person-centred model of care, it is imperative the individual is included as much as possible in the negotiation process so that decisions on goals and preferences are collaboratively made. This is described as negotiated decision making (Moats, 2007). A power of attorney may need to be appointed to advocate for the person with cognitive impairment when making the final decision around discharge. For people who have no-one to represent their best interests, the team may need to consider arranging for a legally recognised guardian to make these decisions on their behalf (e.g. a public advocate).

Occupational therapists working on medical and surgical wards should seek to conduct person-centred assessments that support a person's occupational autonomy and choice wherever possible. Effective communication, joint assessments and shared decision making with other health professionals and early discharge planning are particularly crucial to managing risk and autonomy and determining best possible outcomes in these acute settings (Atwal et al., 2011; 2012; Bushby et al., 2015). This next section addresses the specific types of assessments occupational therapists may use in an acute setting.

SCOPE AND TYPES OF ASSESSMENTS USED IN ACUTE SETTINGS

The process an occupational therapist undertakes to act upon referrals received for people admitted to medical and surgical wards is presented in this section. After a referral, therapists engage with individuals to identify initial goals and potential occupational issues, and then, guided by their experience, frames of reference, knowledge of best practices and practice contexts (Townsend & Polatajko, 2013), the therapist determines the most appropriate assessments to use.

Enter/Initiate or Responding to Referrals

When a person is initially admitted to a general medical or surgical ward there is often a period where the person is acutely unwell, such as when recovering from recent surgery or undergoing numerous investigations. Occupational therapy referrals are typically initiated once the person is considered medically stable enough for discharge planning or sometimes immediately before discharge.

Referrals for occupational therapy can be requested early in the acute stages of admission. The interdisciplinary team may request baseline information to inform the team assessment process and develop an early discharge plan or to address issues related to a person's acute stay and performance on the unit. These referrals are often linked to factors contributing to a person's performance decline such as pressure care, cognition and functional transfers.

Once a referral is received, occupational therapists gather preliminary information to determine the appropriate timing of their assessment (Townsend & Polatajko, 2013). This relies on the occupational therapist's knowledge of the acute illness trajectory and presenting issues, effective liaison with the interdisciplinary team regarding a person's anticipated discharge plan (i.e. estimated date and expected destination), and contact with the person and the person's caregivers regarding expectations of the occupational therapist's role.

There is evidence of this process in Bert's story where the occupational therapist made initial contact with Bert and his wife to ascertain their preference for discharge (Practice Story 21.3). Details from Bert's medical history indicated that he was still experiencing acute delirium and was not well enough to warrant assessment that focused on matching his current performance status with what was required to return home.

PRACTICE STORY 21.3

Bert: Referral to Occupational Therapy

Bert was referred to occupational therapy five days after his operation by the nurse unit manager to review his suitability for discharge home. The occupational therapist reviewed Bert's medical history and noted he had diabetes, peripheral neuropathy and chronic obstructive pulmonary disease and was a heavy smoker in the past. He had also been diagnosed with acute delirium and was being treated with intravenous antibiotics. Before seeing Bert, the occupational therapist talked with his treating nurse, who described him as disoriented overnight. Although able to ambulate, he was unable to find the toilet and had been incontinent of urine. She reported he required full assistance to manage his colostomy. The occupational therapist also talked with the physiotherapist who provided Bert with a walking frame; she stated that Bert kept forgetting to use the frame.

When the occupational therapist met Bert, his wife, Joan, was sitting beside his bed. The occupational therapist commenced her initial interview with Bert and Joan and they talked about how the two of them were managing at home before Bert came to hospital. This included information about Bert's occupational performance (i.e. he was independent with his self-care, mobility and transfers). Bert helped his wife hang out the washing at home and did the vacuuming. Their son helped with the lawns. Bert drove an old, automatic utility and accompanied Joan each week to do the weekly shopping in town, along with the banking and paying bills.

Bert said he was very keen to return home as soon as possible. The occupational therapist acknowledged this and explained that completing this interview would help with working towards his discharge. After the interview the occupational therapist wrote her notes at the nurse's desk. Joan appeared and asked if she could talk with her. She expressed her concerns and stated that she did not know how she was going to cope. Joan said Bert was really forgetful and she was worried he would forget his walker and fall.

Teams plan to discharge people admitted to medical and surgical wards as soon as practicable. Occupational therapists will typically prioritise people who are identified by the team as being imminent discharge candidates. People deemed at risk of functional decline related to their acute presentation or underlying comorbidities are also prioritise for assessment. Early assessment is crucial to identify strategies that will prevent complications that may increase their length of stay and delay discharge (Department of Health, 2012; Shearer & Guthrie, 2013). As Bert was being treated for his delirium and it was expected that the delirium would be resolved, the occupational therapist and the team initially decided to work towards Bert being discharged to his home. As a result, an early assessment of his premorbid history and he and his wife's expectations regarding discharge was commenced. It was identified during this early assessment that Joan was concerned about Bert returning home if he remained confused and alerted the occupational therapist to this being a potential barrier to discharge.

The occupational therapist may also receive referrals or uncover issues for assessment not directly related to discharge planning or the acute admission such as driving or major home modifications. These issues should be addressed after the acute hospital stay. The acute occupational therapist will refer on to community or subacute occupational therapists to address these ongoing issues.

Setting the Stage/Initial Interview
Obtaining a Premorbid History

Assessment within a medical and surgical setting relies on the occupational therapist obtaining information from multiple sources at the initial contact stage and throughout engagement with the person. Identification of priority occupational issues and possible goals, particularly preferred discharge plans, involves collaboration with a range of sources. These include but are not restricted to medical histories, interdisciplinary team members, external service providers, the person and the person's family. The occupational therapist's decision to use specific sources will depend on the nature of information required, the medical and cognitive status of the person, the stage or purpose of assessment and the consent of the person. The needs of the caregiver are also central to the choice of assessment and intervention and are an important source of information in these settings (Moats & Doble, 2006). For example, assessment of Bert's wife's needs became more apparent when she had the opportunity to talk to the occupational therapist alone.

Gathering information before conducting formal assessments is important as it determines the reason for and appropriateness of referral to occupational therapy. It also determines the timing of the first assessment. Understanding of the occupational therapist's role and triggers for referral for assessment in medicine and surgery settings can vary greatly among members of the multidisciplinary team. It is important for occupational therapists to effectively communicate the scope and remit of their role to other team members in order to elicit timely referrals (Robertson & FInlay, 2007). In the case of Bert, the occupational therapist could inform the nurse unit manager that assessment of Bert's suitability for discharge home is limited until his delirium has resolved.

To understand the impact acute illness has had on a person's occupational performance, it is vital to establish the person's previous level of occupational performance along with any environmental considerations. A person's previous level of occupational performance is dependent on the progression of preexisting chronic or advanced illness, the rate of associated functional decline and the level of support from families or caregivers. This means that the person is likely to have preexisting

issues with his or her occupational performance. Bert was independent in his self-care and mobility and shared domestic and community-based occupations with his wife. It would be important for the occupational therapist to ascertain how his wife was coping with providing any assistance required and what performance level Joan and Bert anticipated he would return to. In addition, consideration would have to be given as to whether Bert's past care needs were the result of his loss of weight and general decline because of the impact of his cancer or because of other factors and whether his care needs change after his medical and surgical treatments.

Discharge Planning

Occupational therapists in medical and surgical settings work in an interdisciplinary discharge-driven context. Professional reasoning and assessments that inform discharge planning must be completed quickly, and this time pressure can be experienced as stressful by therapists (Britton et al., 2015; Durocher & Gibson, 2010; Robertson & Blaga, 2013). However, evidence supports an individualised approach to discharge planning and implementation (Dainty & Elizabeth, 2009; Fox et al., 2013; Shepperd et al., 2010). Estimation of discharge date and destination on admission is common, and evidence suggests this early discharge planning leads to a shorter length of stay and a reduction in readmission rates (Roberts & Robinson, 2014). This plan is informed by multidisciplinary team assessment and the person's response to the medical and surgical treatment over the course of admission.

Occupational therapists identify potential barriers to discharge related to a person's occupational performance and environment. Professional reasoning must constantly link current occupational performance to what would be required for a safe or effective discharge, adapting plans to anticipated progress and potential recovery or decline. It is the task of the occupational therapist to consider all aspects of a person's performance and how this may affect a return to the premorbid environment. Assessment of discharge needs determines a person's capacity to return home independently, the need for additional supports (and what they may be) and indicators for rehabilitation or palliative care (inpatient- or outpatient-based), where the person lives, and what is available in his or her local area.

Assessment Commonly Used by Occupational Therapists in Medical and Surgical Settings
Occupational Performance and Performance Components

In medical and surgical settings occupational therapists primarily analyse a person's occupational performance by observing a person completing self-care tasks (Robertson & Blaga, 2013) (i.e. a hands-on assessment of showering, dressing or toileting capacity). The professional reasoning used to justify this focus is that self-care tasks are easily observable and assessed in a ward environment and are key indicators of a person's suitability to return to his or her predischarge environment. In Bert's case, a comprehensive self-care assessment may contribute to the overall picture of how his recent episode of delirium and surgical procedure may have affected his performance and how this translates into other occupations and his potential discharge destination (Practice Story 21.4). However, to ensure a person-centred approach, therapists need to carry out this assessment in different ways. This can include observation, self-report, and by-proxy report from family, nursing staff and other health professionals (Robertson & Blaga, 2013).

The different areas of self-care, such as showering, grooming, feeding and toileting, usually do not all need to be formally assessed for each person and will be determined by that person's immediate and anticipated discharge needs and the therapist's available time. For example, a person who receives help with showering and dressing from a formal service at home, and reports minimal change to his or her overall performance in self-care, may not require a formal observational assessment. In another case, a comprehensive self-care assessment may contribute to the overall picture of how a person's recent cognitive decline affects performance and how this translates into other occupations and potential discharge destination.

Occupational therapists working in acute hospital settings will also assess the physical, cognitive, affective components of the person that contribute to occupational engagement (Townsend & Polatajko, 2013). Mobility and transfers, cognition and upper limb function are the most common areas addressed in these settings (Robertson & Blaga, 2013).

Cognitive Assessments

The occupational therapist may be asked to conduct a cognitive assessment to determine a person's capacity to return home. Cognitive deficits are associated with poorer rehabilitation outcomes and ability to return home (Lenze et al., 2004). However, before the occupational therapist makes a judgement about whether a person is safe or unsafe to return home, each individual must be considered within the context of his or her illness and the environment the person may be returning to. Importantly, the presence of family and carers may enable a person with impaired cognition to still return home.

PRACTICE STORY 21.4

Bert: Ready for Discharge

The medical team said that Bert was medically ready for discharge and his delirium had essentially resolved. The physiotherapist recommended that Bert return home with the four-wheeled frame, and the social worker suggested that formal services be put in place to assist Joan with his care. Joan wanted to try having Bert at home but she was nervous about how they would both manage.

It is imperative to rule out an acute delirium as the underlying cause of cognitive changes as this will compromise a person's occupational performance. Understanding the differences between a delirium and a preexisting cognitive deficit will inform the choice of occupational therapy assessment and team approach. A comprehensive assessment of a person's cognition to establish intact and impaired domains is vital to inform intervention strategies to optimise occupational participation. This may entail an observational assessment of a person's cognition during occupational performance and/or the use of standardised assessments. The differences between delirium and other types of cognitive dysfunction and possible assessment approaches are outlined in the following sections.

Delirium is an acute condition that has a rapid onset and a time-limited, although variable, course. It is characterised by disturbances of consciousness and cognition (Siddiqi, Holt, Britton, & Holmes, 2007). In most cases the cause of delirium is an underlying physical illness such as an infection that is often treatable and, once resolved, a person's occupational performance can improve (AHMAC Health Care of Older Australians Standing committee, 2011). Risk factors for delirium in surgical units include preexisting cognitive impairment, including dementia, severe medical illness, age older 70 years, adding three or more medications during admission, visual impairment and use of indwelling catheters (AHMAC Health Care of Older Australians Standing committee, 2011; Siddiqi et al., 2007).

Regular ongoing assessment is essential to monitor effects of delirium on occupational performance and subsequent discharge plans. Evidence-based guidelines recommend that a formal, diagnostic assessment is undertaken by medical staff to identify delirium and its causes (AHMAC Health Care of Older Australians Standing committee, 2011). However, the interdisciplinary team members' informal observations also help develop a picture of how delirium may be influencing a person's behaviour. The MMSE has been found to have some utility in detecting delirium but is not reliable (Brown, 2015; Mitchell, 2013).

It is important for the occupational therapist to note that older people with dementia who present with an acute episode of delirium may experience decline in cognitive and physical function that does not resolve to a premorbid level. Further, although the medical causes of delirium are often treatable, those without dementia may experience detrimental effects on cognition and function that can last for up to 12 months after the episode. Experiencing an episode of delirium may also predispose the person to future episodes (Irwin, Pirrello, Hirst, Buckholz, & Ferris, 2013).

Assessment of Cognition

If delirium has been ruled out, then cognition should be assessed, initially within the context of occupational performance. In a general medical or surgical environment, this may be done by assessing a person's ability to manage components of self-care (Crennan & MacRae, 2010) or a simple occupational task like making a sandwich or cup of tea. Formal cognitive assessments used by occupational therapists in acute general medical and surgical settings include the MMSE, MoCA and RUDAS (Crennan & MacRae, 2010).

The Mini-Mental State Examination is used in many hospitals to assess for dementia and delirium (Folstein et al., 1975; Mitchell, 2013). Although the MMSE is accepted as a gold standard for assessment of dementia and is effective at detecting this, it should be used with caution and not as the sole diagnostic tool for detecting cognitive deficit. Correlations have been found between the MMSE, FIM and functional performance of people with dementia (Brown, Joliffe, & Fielding, 2014). However, a person may perform poorly on the MMSE, which may not be reflected in their occupational performance. An occupational therapist may choose to complete an MMSE because it is the preferred assessment used by the team or because they are assessing a person with suspected dementia. However, when reporting back MMSE results, it is important to do so in conjunction with reports about what is observed when the person engages in occupational tasks. Assessments of occupational performance should always supplement a standardised assessment (such as the MMSE) and inform professional reasoning and decision making about capacity and discharge (Robertson & Blaga, 2013).

The Montreal Cognitive Assessment (Atwal & Caldwell, 2003; Freitas et al., 2013; Larner, 2012; Nasreddine et al., 2005) and the Rowland Universal Dementia Assessment Scale (Limpawattana et al., 2012; Pang, Yu, Pearson, Lynch, & Fong, 2009) have been found to be effective in detecting mild cognitive impairment and impairments in executive dysfunction; these impairments are not always detected by the MMSE (Mitchell, 2013). Of the three assessments, RUDAS has been developed and validated for assessment of mild cognitive impairment with culturally and linguistically diverse populations (Basic et al., 2009; Naqvi, Haider, Tomlinson, & Alibhai, 2015). As there is limited evidence to support the correlation of numerical test scores with functional capacity, the occupational therapist must weigh these scores up against assessment of occupational performance. In Bert's case, his delirium has reportedly resolved and thus a standardised cognitive assessment could be conducted to identify any residual cognitive impairment in conjunction with an observational assessment of him carrying out his self-care tasks on the ward. This latter assessment would enable the occupational therapist to identify the potential impact his cognitive impairment may have on his occupational performance and his care requirements after discharge. A summary of key tasks included in the MMSE, MoCA and RUDAS is included in Table 21.1.

Occupational theory encourages consideration of the environmental impact on a person's occupational performance (Kielhofner, 2008). Functional assessments in familiar (e.g. home) environments should be conducted with people with dementia if there is uncertainty about whether they are safe to return home. Their performance in a familiar environment can be markedly better than in an unfamiliar hospital setting. A person who presents with significant deficits in this familiar space will be unlikely to return home to live alone.

Pressure Care

Occupational therapists, along with other members of the interdisciplinary team, have a role in the early identification of pressure ulcer risk (Jaul, 2010). Standardised risk screening tools are commonly used to evaluate the risk of adverse outcomes related to hospitalised deconditioning (Macens, Rose, & Mackenzie, 2011). For example, pressure risk assessments such as the Braden or Waterlow screens may be used on admission to a general medical or surgical unit to identify risk of pressure injury development (Giesbrecht, 2006; Macens et al., 2011). Results of this screening tool may trigger a referral to an occupational therapist for comprehensive assessments factors that may contribute to compromised pressure care. These may include physical factors such as how a person is transferring (i.e. assessing for shear on fragile skin as a person moves across a surface like a bed) or assessment for excess moisture, such as from incontinence, that may lead to skin breakdown. Environmental factors that also warrant assessment include seating surfaces of a chair, toilet or wheelchair and the assessment for pressure-relieving devices such as cushions and air mattresses. Cognitive factors that may affect skin care also need to be taken into consideration during assessment, such as poor recall of transfer techniques to minimise skin shear.

Home Environment

The occupational therapist needs to determine whether a home assessment is indicated to effect a discharge home. In the acute settings, a home assessment is conducted to assess potential risk, including falls risk. It aims to determine how well a person's occupational performance (physical and cognitive) matches with the environment the person is being discharged to (Welch & Lowes, 2005). Traditionally home assessments involve occupational therapists observing the person performing relevant occupations and skills within his or her physical home environment. In an acute medical or surgical setting this is often achieved through interview-based assessments with the person and his or her caregivers. If an observational home assessment is indicated, the next critical thing to determine is the timing of this assessment.

Home assessments related to medical and surgical needs may occur predischarge or postdischarge (Welch & Lowes, 2005). Home assessment related to longer-term occupational performance needs will be referred to the local community services where they exist. Rate of falls in the community and falls risk has been found to be lower in people who have received a home assessment and appropriate home modifications. Effectiveness of these interventions has also found to be higher when conducted by an occupational therapist (Gillespie et al., 2012).

TABLE 21.1
Key Areas Assessed by the Mini–Mental State Examination, Montreal Cognitive Assessment and Rowland Universal Dementia Assessment Scale

Mini–Mental State Examination (MMSE)	Montreal Cognitive Assessment (MoCA)	Rowland Universal Dementia Assessment Scale (RUDAS)
Orientation ■ Year, season, date, day, month ■ State, country, town, hospital, floor	*Visuospatial/Executive* ■ Track route ■ Copy cube ■ Draw clock	*Memory* ■ List of four grocery items given; person asked to repeat list three times; five practice reminders allowed
Registration ■ Name three objects, repeat until all objects remembered, count trials	*Naming* ■ Three animals	*Visuospatial Orientation* ■ Identify different body parts (maximum required is five)
Attention and Calculation ■ Serial 7s, starting at 100, stop after five answers *or* ■ Spell *WORLD* backwards	*Memory:* ■ Immediate recall (two trials, no score)	*Praxis* ■ Copy action with hands and repeat until asked to stop
Recall ■ Recall of three objects, no cueing allowed	*Attention: Three Tasks* ■ Five digits forwards; three digits backwards ■ Listen to list of letters and tap at each letter A ■ Serial 7s starting at 100, stop after five answers	*Visuoconstructional Drawing* ■ Copy cube
Language ■ Name pencil and watch ■ Repeat short sentence: 'No ifs ands or buts'	*Language* ■ Sentence repetition ■ Fluency: as many words starting with F as possible in 1 minute	*Judgement* ■ Describe how to cross road safely in absence of pedestrian crossing and traffic lights
Language ■ Follow three-step command ■ Read command and complete it	*Abstraction* ■ Similarity between train and bicycle, watch and ruler	*Memory/Recall* ■ Asked to recall shopping list, one prompt only
Language ■ Write a short sentence ■ Copy two intersecting pentagons	*Delayed Recall (five words)* ■ Uncued ■ Category cue ■ Multiple choice cue Scored for uncued only *Orientation* Date, month, year, day, place, city	*Language* Name as many animals as possible in 1 minute
Score Out of 30 24–30: normal 18–23: mild impairment 10–17: moderate impairment ≤9: severe impairment Assess for level of consciousness	*Score Out of 30* 27/30: normal 18–26: mild impairment 10–17: moderate impairment <10: severe impairment Three paper versions in English, available in multiple languages Not available as electronic assessment yet but development underway (http://www.mocatest.org/)	*Score Out of 30* ≤23 indicates possible cognitive impairment and requires further investigation Less language focus, developed for use with multicultural populations (https://www.health.qld.gov.au/tpch/html/**rudas**.asp)

The timing of a home assessment is related to the level of risk identified during the discharge planning process. It may be appropriate to conduct a predischarge home assessment in instances when there are concerns about the person's physical and cognitive capacity or concerns about the home environment. If a home assessment is conducted too late in the admission, it may slow down discharge. Equally, if it is conducted too early, a person's occupational performance may not be at the anticipated level required for discharge (Atwal, McIntyre, Craik, & Hunt, 2008).

However, observing a person within his or her home environment provides optimal insight into the potential physical, social, cognitive and occupational barriers to discharge. There is also evidence to support its impact in reducing the risk of falls on discharge and assisting carers in preparing for discharge (Atwal et al., 2008; Crennan & MacRae, 2010). A home assessment may also assist the occupational therapist to identify additional factors that will support a discharge home. When assessing suitability and safety of a home environment, the occupational therapist must also evaluate carer expectation and capacity to provide care and whether the home environment can support a person to maintain his or her physical, mental and emotional health.

ASSESSMENT FOR CARE REQUIREMENTS POST DISCHARGE

The majority of people who are not discharged to residential care have needs that continue in the community. It is important for the occupational therapist to assess for a person's ongoing care needs in the mid- to long-term after discharge. For example, a postdischarge referral may be made to the local community occupational therapist to address strategies to manage activities of daily living that extend beyond self-care required for discharge. Knowledge of discharge options such as support services, rehabilitation streams and residential care alternatives inform therapists' development of discharge plans. This knowledge can also assist people and their families in setting their own goals for discharge. For example, some people may not be aware of options available to them for rehabilitation. Explaining this earlier in the admission will enable a person and the person's caregivers to participate in informed decisions about future care to meet their preferred goals and discharge options (Roberts & Robinson, 2014).

CONCLUSION

This chapter has described the factors that characterise occupational therapy assessment and professional reasoning in acute general medical and surgical settings. Occupational therapists play an important role in the assessment of persons to optimise occupational participation, minimise deconditioning and promote discharge home. A person-centred approach underpins these assessments, although this can be challenging to maintain

consistently in fast-paced, biomedical-focused medical and surgical settings. The support of senior occupational therapists and other interdisciplinary team members can aid junior therapists as they develop professional expertise to work in medical and surgical settings.

 http://evolve.elsevier.com/Curtin/OT

REFERENCES

AHMAC Health Care of Older Australians Standing committee. (2011). *Delirium pathways.* Canberra: Commonwealth of Australia.

Atwal, A., & Caldwell, K. (2003). Ethics, occupational therapy and discharge planning. *Four broken Australian Occupational Therapy Journal, 50*(4), 244–251.

Atwal, A., McIntyre, A., Craik, C., & Hunt, J. (2008). Older adults and carers' perceptions of pre-discharge occupational therapy home visits in acute care. *Age and Ageing, 37,* 72–76.

Atwal, A., McIntyre, A., & Wiggett, C. (2012). Risks with older adults in acute care settings: UK occupational therapists' and physiotherapists' perceptions of risks associated with discharge and professional practice. *Scandinavian Journal of Caring Sciences, 26*(2), 381–393.

Atwal, A., Wiggett, C., & McIntyre, A. (2011). Risks with older adults in acute care settings: Occupational therapists' and physiotherapists' perceptions. *British Journal of Occupational Therapy, 74*(9), 412–418.

Australian Institute of Health and Welfare. (2014). *Australia's health 2014.* Canberra: AIHW.

Basic, D., Khoo, A., Conforti, D., et al. (2009). Rowland Universal Dementia Assessment Scale, Mini-Mental State Examination and general practitioner assessment of cognition in a multicultural cohort of community-dwelling older persons with early dementia. *Australian Psychologist, 44*(1), 40–53.

Britton, L., Rosenwax, L., & McNamara, B. (2015). Occupational therapy practice in acute physical hospital settings: Evidence from a scoping review. *Australian Occupational Therapy Journal, 62*(6), 370–377.

Brown, J. (2015). The use and misuse of short cognitive tests in the diagnosis of dementia. *Journal of Neurology, Neurosurgery, and Psychiatry, 86*(6), 680–685.

Brown, T., Joliffe, L., & Fielding, L. (2014). Is the Mini Mental Status Examination (MMSE) associated with inpatients' functional performance? *Physical and Occupational Therapy in Geriatrics, 32*(3), 228–240.

Bushby, K., Chan, J., Druif, S., Ho, K., & Kinsella, E. A. (2015). Ethical tensions in occupational therapy practice: A scoping review. *British Journal of Occupational Therapy, 78*(4), 212–221.

Craig, G., Robertson, L., & Milligan, S. (2004). Occupational therapy practice in acute physical health care settings: A pilot study. *New Zealand Journal of Occupational Therapy, 51*(1), 5–13.

Crennan, M., & MacRae, A. (2010). Occupational therapy discharge assessment of elderly patients from acute care hospitals. *Physical and Occupational Therapy in Geriatrics, 28*(1), 33–43.

Dainty, P., & Elizabeth, J. (2009). Timely discharge of older patients from hospital: Improving the process. *Clinical Medicine, 9*(4), 311–314.

DePalma, G., Xu, H. P., Covinsky, K. E., et al. (2013). Hospital read-mission among older adults who return home with unmet need for ADL disability. *Gerontologist, 53*(3), 454–461.

Department of Health. (2012). *Best care for older people everywhere. The toolkit 2012.* Victoria, Australia: Department of Health & Human Sevices. Retrieved from, *www.health.vic.gov.au/older.*

Douglas, A., Liu, L., Warren, S., & Hopper, T. (2007). Cognitive assessments for older adults: Which ones are used by Canadian therapists and why. *Canadian Journal of Occupational Therapy, 74*(5), 370–381.

Durocher, E., & Gibson, B. E. (2010). Navigating ethical discharge planning: A case study in older adult rehabilitation. *Australian Occupational Therapy Journal, 57*(1), 2–7.

Eyres, L., & Unsworth, C. (2005). Occupational therapy in acute hospitals: The effectiveness of a pilot program to maintain occu-pational performance in older clients. *Australian Occupational Therapy Journal, 52*(3), 218–224.

Folstein, M. F., Folstein, S. E., & McHugh, P. R. (1975). Mini-Mental State: A practical method for grading the cognitive state of pati-ents for the clinician. *Journal of Psychiatry Research, 12,* 189–198.

Fox, M. T., Persaud, M., Maimets, I., Brooks, D., O'Brien, K., & Tregunno, D. (2013). Effectiveness of early discharge planning in acutely ill or injured hospitalized older adults: A systematic review and meta-analysis. *BMC Geriatrics, 13,* 70.

Freitas, S., Simões, M. R., Alves, L., & Santana, I. (2013). Montreal Cognitive Assessment (MoCA): Validation study for mild cogni-tive impairment and Alzheimer's disease. *Alzheimer's Disease and Associated Disorders, 27*(1), 37–43.

Giesbrecht, E. (2006). Pressure ulcers and occupational therapy practice: A Canadian perspective. *Canadian Journal of Occupa-tional Therapy, 73*(1), 56–63.

Gillespie, L. D., Robertson, M. C., Gillespie, W. J., et al. (2012). Interventions for preventing falls in older people living in the community (review). *Cochrane Collaboration, 9,* 1–416.

Irwin, S. A., Pirrello, R. D., Hirst, J. M., Buckholz, G. T., & Ferris, F. D. (2013). Clarifying delirium management: Practical, evidenced-based, expert recommendations for clinical practice. *Journal of Palliative Medicine, 16*(4), 423–435.

Ismail, Z., Raji, T. K., & Shulman, K. I. (2010). Brief cognitive screen-ing instruments: An update. *International Journal of Geriatric Psy-chiatry, 25,* 111–120.

Jaul, E. (2010). Assessment and management of pressure ulcers in the elderly – Current strategies. *Drugs and Aging, 27*(4), 311–325.

Kielhofner, G. (2008). *Model of human occupation: Theory and appli-cation* (4th ed.). Baltimore, MD: Lippincott Williams & Wilkins.

Kortebein, P. (2009). Rehabilitation for hospital-associated decondi-tioning. *American Journal of Physical Medicine and Rehabilitation, 88*(1), 66–77.

Larner, A. J. (2012). Screening utility of the Montreal Cognitive Assessment (MoCA): In place of – or as well as – The MMSE? *International Psychogeriatrics, 3,* 391–396.

Lenze, E. J., Munin, M. C., Dew, M. A., et al. (2004). Adverse effects of depression and cognitive impairment on rehabilitation partic-ipation and recovery from hip fracture. *International Journal of Geriatric Psychiatry, 19*(5), 472–478.

Limpawattana, P., Tiamkao, S., & Sawanyawisuth, K. (2012). The performance of the Rowland Universal Dementia Assessment

Scale (RUDAS) for cognitive screening in a geriatric outpatient setting. *Aging Clinical and Experimental Research, 24*(5), 495–500.

Macens, K., Rose, A., & Mackenzie, L. (2011). Pressure care practice and occupational therapy: Findings of an exploratory study. *Aus-tralian Occupational Therapy Journal, 58*(5), 346–354.

Mitchell, A. J. (2013). The Mini-Mental State Examination (MMSE). An update on its diagnostic validity for cognitive disorders. In A. J. Lamer (Ed.), *Cognitive screening disorders. A practical approach* (pp. 15–46). London: Springer.

Moats, G. (2006). Discharge decision-making with older people: The influence of the institutional environment. *Australian Occupa-tional Therapy Journal, 53,* 107–115.

Moats, G. (2007). Discharge decision-making, enabling occupa-tions, and client-centred practice. *Canadian Journal of Occupa-tional Therapy, 74*(2), 91–101.

Moats, G., & Doble, S. (2006). Discharge planning with older adults: Toward a negotiated model of decision making. *Canadian Journal of Occupational Therapy, 73*(5), 303–311.

Mortenson, W. B., & Dyck, I. (2006). Power and client-centred practice: An insider exploration of occupational therapists' expe-riences. *Canadian Journal of Occupational Therapy, 73*(5), 261–271.

Naqvi, R. M., Haider, S., Tomlinson, G., & Alibhai, S. (2015). Cog-nitive assessments in multicultural populations using the Row-land Universal Dementia Assessment scale: A systematic review and meta-analysis. *Canadian Medical Association Journal, 187*(5), E169–E176.

Nasreddine, Z. S., Phillips, N. A., Bédirian, V., et al. (2005). The Montreal Cognitive Assessment, MoCA: A brief screening tool for mild cognitive impairment. *The American Geriatrics Society, 53*(4), 695–699.

Pang, J., Yu, H., Pearson, K., Lynch, P., & Fong, C. (2009). Compar-ison of the MMSE and RUDAS cognitive screening tools in an elderly inpatient population in everyday clinical use. *Internal Medicine Journal,* 411–414.

Roberts, P. S., & Robinson, M. R. (2014). Occupational therapy's role in preventing acute readmissions. *American Journal of Occupa-tional Therapy, 68*(3), 254–259.

Robertson, L., & Blaga, L. (2013). Occupational therapy assessments used in acute physical care settings. *Scandinavian Journal of Occu-pational Therapy, 20,* 127–135.

Robertson, C., & Finlay, L. (2007). Making a difference, teamwork and coping: The meaning of practice in acute physical settings. *British Journal of Occupational Therapy, 70*(2), 73–80.

Shearer, T., & Guthrie, S. (2013). Facilitating early activities of daily living retraining to prevent functional decline in older adults. *Australian Occupational Therapy Journal, 60,* 319–325.

Shepperd, S., McClaran, J., Phillips, C. O., et al. (2010). Discharge planning from hospital to home (review). *Cochrane Collaboration, 1,* 1–75.

Siddiqi, N., Holt, R., Britton, A. M., & Holmes, J. (2007). Interven-tions for preventing delirium in hospitalised patients (review). *Cochrane Collaboration,* 1–41.

State Government of Victoria.(2013). *Responding to hoarding and squalor. Retrieved from, www.health.vic.gov.au/agedcare/publications/hoarding.htm.*

Townsend, E., & Polatajko, H. (2013). *Enabling occupation II: Advancing an occupational therapy vision for health, well-being, and justice through occupation.* Ottawa: CAOT Publications ACE.

Victorian Quality Council. (2003). *VQC state-wide PUPPS report.* Melbourne: Victorian Quality Council.

Welch, A., & Lowes, S. (2005). Home assessment visits within the acute setting: A discussion and literature review. *British Journal of Occupational Therapy, 68*(4), 158–164.

Wells, J. L., Seabrook, J. A., Stolee, P., Borrie, M. J., & Knoefel, F. (2003). State of the art in geriatric rehabilitation. Part I: Review of frailty and comprehensive geriatric assessment. *Archives of Physical Medicine and Rehabilitation, 84*(6), 890–897.

Wilding, C., & Whiteford, G. (2007). Occupation and occupational therapy: Knowledge paradigms and everyday practice. *Australian Occupational Therapy Journal, 54*(3), 185–193.

ASSESSMENT - EXCERPTS FROM BONUS PRACTICE STORIES

 [Read the full practice stories on Evolve at http://evolve.elsevier.com/Curtin/OT]

 ### MRS TREMBLAY: A PRACTICE STORY OF A PERSON EXPERIENCING REHABILITATION FOLLOWING A STROKE - ASSESSMENT

DOROTHY KESSLER, KATRINE SAUVÉ-SHENK, & VALERIE METCALFE

Part 1: Acute Care

Assess and Evaluate. Following the interview, I evaluated Mrs Tremblay using direct observations and Dynamic Performance Analysis (DPA). I focused on functional tasks that could be completed within her current hospital environment ...

 To read the full Practice Story and complete a reflective exercise please visit Evolve at http://evolve.elsevier.com/Curtin/OT

KARIN: A PRACTICE STORY OF A PERSON EXPERIENCING RHEUMATOID ARTHRITIS - ASSESSMENT

MATHILDA BJÖRK & INGRID THYBERG

Part 1: Initial Diagnosis

Assess and Evaluate. During the interview Karin made it clear that even though she felt worried she did not want to have a lot of contact with health care services. The only thing she wanted my help with was her aching wrist ...

 To read the full Practice Story and complete a reflective exercise please visit Evolve at http://evolve.elsevier.com/Curtin/OT

ANGELA: A PRACTICE STORY OF A PERSON EXPERIENCING PALLIATIVE CARE - ASSESSMENT

DEIDRE MORGAN & CELIA MARSTON

Assess and Evaluate. My initial discussion with Angela occurred in her room. The interview was deliberately unstructured to assist with developing rapport with her. Rapport was established by engaging in conversation with Angela about her recent contact with the music therapist. During this time she reflected on her love of music and her past life roles and valued occupations ...

 To read the full Practice Story and complete a reflective exercise please visit Evolve at http://evolve.elsevier.com/Curtin/OT

Section 5 GOALS

22

WRITING OCCUPATION-FOCUSED GOALS

JULIA BOWMAN ■ LISE MOGENSEN ■ NATASHA A. LANNIN

CHAPTER OUTLINE

Abstract

Planning the implementation of enabling strategies is an essential process in the practice of occupational therapy. It is much more than a sequence of steps therapists employ to provide a service for individuals. It is an organisational structure that facilitates the occupational reasoning process for conducting assessments, identifying goals, selecting strategies and evaluating outcomes. This chapter provides a linear structure for developing occupation-focused enabling strategies. This approach has been specifically developed to assist therapists to identify and write occupation-focused goals and link strategies and evaluation methods directly to the occupational engagement or performance outcome. If occupational therapy strategies are not carefully planned, they may lack focus on occupation, fail to directly address goals and be ineffective in achieving desired occupational engagement or performance outcomes. Therefore planning is a skill all therapists must master to ensure appropriate and effective service provision to individuals.

KEY POINTS

When setting occupation-focused goals, do the following:

- Collaborate with individuals and consider the Person–Environment–Occupation fit.

- Focus on occupation and tailor goals to a person's unique occupational needs.

- Apply the principles of the International Classification of Functioning, Disability and Health (ICF).

- Clearly identify and define the desired outcome of enabling strategies.

- Use SMART goals to direct occupation-focused strategies.

- Incorporate outcome measures to quantify change over time in a person's body structure and functions, activity or participation.

- Clearly document each step of the process and progress towards goal attainment.

BACKGROUND

Occupational therapists have claimed that occupation as a therapeutic medium is core to their practice (Emerson, 1998; Rebeiro & Cook, 1999). Today, the World Federation of Occupational Therapists describes occupational therapy as a profession 'concerned with promoting health and well-being through occupation' (World Federation of Occupational Therapists, 2012). As such, it is important that occupational therapy strategies have occupation as the central focus.

Occupational therapists believe people, their environment and the occupations in which they engage are closely interrelated. Consequently therapists need to be aware of factors that may influence this finely balanced relationship. The Person–Environment–Occupation (PEO) model (Law et al., 1996) acknowledges the complexity of people performing occupations within broad environments. As such the model provides a sound theoretical framework to assist therapists to account for these interrelated constructs when planning strategies. The PEO model assumes that a person and the person's environment and occupations interact continuously across time and space. Therefore the greater the congruence between these elements, the closer the individual is to a desired level of occupational engagement and performance. The PEO model directs therapists to think about strategies that target the person, occupation and environment in different ways. Therapists are also challenged to identify multiple options to elicit change in occupational engagement and performance. As the relationship between the person, environment and occupation is dynamic and constantly changing, the PEO model advocates the ongoing monitoring of strategies to ensure progress towards goal attainment is being made.

Another model designed to assist the intervention planning process is the International Classification of Functioning, Disability and Health (ICF) developed by the World Health Organization (WHO, 2002). The ICF framework was designed to facilitate the conceptualisation, classification and measurement of disability. Within this framework, disability is recognised as a multidimensional experience with participation viewed as a component of health rather than a consequence of disease. Use of the ICF by therapists promotes an integrated approach to gathering and sharing information, professional decision making and evaluating the efficacy and effectiveness of interventions (Australian Institute of Health and Welfare (AIHW), 2003). As such, the ICF has specific application to the intervention planning process in occupational therapy. According to the ICF framework, a person's level of participation is conceived as a dynamic interaction between health conditions and personal and environmental factors (Fig. 22.1).

Once therapists have a clear understanding of the ICF framework they can use it to guide intervention planning. Through the assessment and goal-setting process therapists identify the desired outcome of intervention. Consideration is then given to which aspect of health (body structure and function, activity or participation) will be targeted by the enabling strategy.

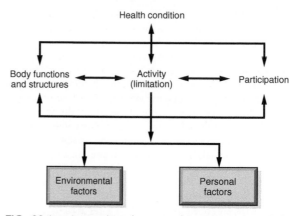

FIG. 22.1 ■ Interactions between the components of the International Classification of Functioning, Disability, and Health. *(From Australian Institute of Health and Welfare (AIHW), 2003.)*

Appropriate enabling strategies are selected to facilitate goal attainment, and finally outcome measures are used that evaluate performance at the target level of health (Australian Institute of Health and Welfare (AIHW), 2003).

Intervention plans consist of a series of enabling strategies to facilitate achievement of desired occupation-focused goals. To construct enabling strategies that are tailored to meet a person's unique occupational needs, therapists require sound occupational reasoning skills. Occupational reasoning is essentially the way therapists think about, develop and modify their actions and plans during all phases of intervention planning and delivery (Schultz-Krohn & McHugh Pendleton, 2011). Therapists use a combination of deductive and inductive reasoning to aid the strategy planning process. Deductive reasoning (e.g. scientific, procedural, hypothetical or diagnostic reasoning) is used to apply general knowledge, theories and scientific evidence to specific practice situations. Inductive reasoning (e.g. interactive, conditional or narrative reasoning) is used by therapists to assist in understanding each person and help each therapist to learn from specific practice situations (American Occupational Therapy Association, 2010). It has been well established that therapists integrate information from a variety of sources when planning strategies for individuals (e.g. Duncan, 2011; Fawcett, 2002; Hocking, 2009; Neistadt, 1995; Schultz-Krohn & McHugh Pendleton, 2011; Radomski, 2002). Therefore therapists must effectively synthesise the information gathered in order to formulate sound aims and set goals that are person-centred, propose strategies to achieve desired occupation-focused goals, make decisions about each person's progress and evaluate the overall effectiveness of their strategies.

Detailed documentation of each step of the process is essential to maintain a record of progress, change and development.

Documentation may occur in different formats such as file notes, assessment forms, progress reports, outcome measure score sheets and evaluation forms. Not only is documentation and record keeping a legal requirement, it is an effective means of communicating progress and status to the individual and members of the interprofessional team. Record keeping promotes continuity and supports effective evaluation of occupational therapy services. Without adequate documentation from the occupational therapist, other members of the interprofessional team may assume that assessments, strategies and evaluations have not taken place and there may be uncertainty about the person's current circumstances.

OCCUPATION-FOCUSED PLANS: AN OVERVIEW

In occupational therapy literature the occupational therapy process has been described both in a linear fashion (e.g. Radomski, 2002; Schultz-Krohn & McHugh Pendleton, 2011) and in a cyclical fashion (e.g. Duncan, 2011; Schultz-Krohn & Pendleton, 2006). In reality, the process does not take place in a linear or cyclical fashion but is influenced by many changing and intervening factors. However, a linear approach is the most suitable method to facilitate knowledge and skill acquisition in student and novice therapists. Therefore this chapter will describe each step of the process in a tangible and linear way.

Developing enabling strategies is pertinent in all occupational therapy settings. The process is collaborative and involves the person, the person's family and other team members (American Occupational Therapy Association, 1998). However, enabling strategies are also multifaceted with several steps that require careful consideration. As such, the occupational therapist is typically the initiator and facilitator of each step in the process. These steps include accepting and prioritising referrals, conducting assessments and identifying the occupational aims and goals, followed by the selection of occupation-focused strategies and evaluating the effectiveness of the plan as a whole (Radomski, 2002; Schultz-Krohn & McHugh Pendleton, 2011). Clear links between these steps should be evident in the plan. An overview of the process is illustrated in Fig. 22.2. Each step of the occupational therapy process is described here in more detail. Two practice stories have also been included to illustrate the occupational therapy process in practice.

REFERRAL TO OCCUPATIONAL THERAPY

Referrals are verbal or written requests for service. To effectively manage their caseloads, therapists should develop a method to screen and prioritise referrals. Once a referral has been accepted

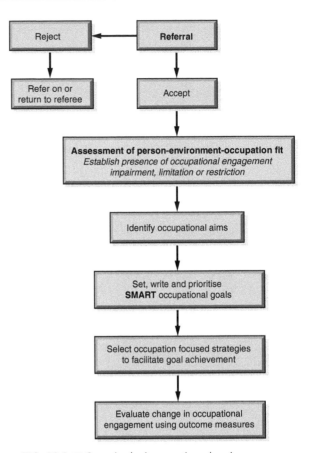

FIG. 22.2 ■ Steps in the intervention planning process.

the therapist will proceed with relevant assessments to establish the balance between the person, environment and occupation and impairment, limitation or restriction in occupational engagement.

Assessing the Person–Environment–Occupation fit

Thorough occupational therapy assessment facilitates the development of effective occupation-focused enabling strategies that will result in improved engagement in daily occupations and an enhanced quality of life (Fawcett, 2002; Hocking, 2009). The purpose of assessment in occupational therapy is to establish a clear picture of an individual's person–environment–occupation fit and identify the presence of any impairment, restriction or limitations in occupational engagement. Therapists analyse the specific skills and abilities the person requires to meet intrinsic needs and achieve his or her goals. Additionally, therapists identify enabling or constraining environmental

---

BOX 22.1
ASSESSMENT OF THE PERSON–ENVIRONMENT–OCCUPATION FIT

KEY STEPS

- Gather information before meeting the person.
- Gather information from the person, family and caregivers.
- Establish an occupational engagement history.
- Establish person–environment–occupation fit.
- Identify occupational impairment, restrictions, limitations or deprivation.

- Use occupational analysis to identify component skills required to perform desired daily self-care, productivity or leisure occupations.
- Evaluate enabling or constraining effects of the environment.
- Measure baseline occupational engagement before participation in intervention.

---

factors within the occupational engagement context. Occupational therapists are encouraged to use standardised instruments to ensure their assessments are valid and reliable and to enable the evaluation of outcomes (Fawcett, 2002; Hocking, 2009). However, it is important to remember that the assessment process should be viewed as the starting point for identifying aims and setting goals, and not as an end in itself (Duncan, 2011). The key steps in the assessment of an individual's person–environment–occupation fit are summarised in Box 22.1.

WRITING OCCUPATION-FOCUSED AIMS

Identifying occupation-focused aims is a shared effort among the occupational therapist, the individual and often the individual's family. Aims are established as a result of the synthesis of information collected from both objective and subjective assessments. The purpose of aims is to provide a broad and overarching statement about the person's desired occupational engagement outcome. Therefore articulation of clear aims sets the course or provides direction for the implementation of enabling strategies. As aims are broad, overarching statements, they contain few specific details, and as such they are difficult to address with one particular strategy. For example, an individual's aim may be to return home and live independently after having a stroke. The aim statement articulates the individual's desired outcome; however, detailed occupational goals are required to specify how these outcomes will be achieved. The key steps that should be followed when establishing occupational aims are summarised in Box 22.2.

SETTING OCCUPATION-FOCUSED GOALS

Goal setting is the cornerstone of the occupational therapy process as goals are a prerequisite to selecting appropriate enabling strategies and evaluating outcomes (Duncan, 2011). Occupational

---

BOX 22.2
ESTABLISHING OCCUPATION-FOCUSED AIMS

KEY STEPS

- Synthesise information collected through subjective and objective assessments.
- Determine what the person would like to achieve as a result of the implementation of enabling strategies.
- Construct a statement that broadly describes the person's desired occupational engagement outcomes and provides direction for the intervention.

---

therapy goals must directly address the identified aims. Therefore the purpose of goal setting is to operationally define the specific desired outcomes and describe the factors involved in achieving the outcomes. Clearly articulated goals can provide an effective snapshot of the overall intervention plan.

Goals can be either long term or short term. Long-term goals have been described as the destination of therapy, whereas short-term goals are the pathways to get there (Foto, 1996). Short-term goals, where practical, should employ strategies that facilitate the person's engagement in occupation at an activity or participation level. However, short-term goals may address issues at the level of body function and structure. If this is the case, it is important that therapists clearly articulate how short-term goals contribute to the achievement of long-term occupation-focused goals.

Occupational therapists should work collaboratively with individuals to set goals. Research has shown that increased motivation in individuals is related to active participation in identifying goals (Latham, 2004; Locke & Latham, 2002). Individuals are also more committed if they have been involved in goal setting and as a result make significant gains in self-care and living skills occupations (Neistadt, 1995). Issues identified during the assessment phase should be considered carefully when setting goals.

To assist individuals to prioritise their goals, the occupational therapist should explore issues related to the general health, safety, independence, social support networks and cultural and social values. The therapist should also seek to understand each individual's view on his or her current situation and the person's expectations for the future. Synthesis of this information into appropriate occupation-focused goals can be a complex process. Thus it is important that occupational therapists follow a systematic method to assist them to write goals that are clear and measurable and reflect the wishes of the people for whom the goals are directed. Selection of a valid and reliable method will also help therapists to avoid setting goals that are vague and ambiguous.

Tools such as the Canadian Occupational Performance Measure (Law et al., 1990) and the Goal Attainment Scale (Kiresuk & Sherman, 1968) were developed to assist therapists to collaboratively set and prioritise goals with the people with whom they are working.

Writing SMART Goals

Goals should be documented in the individual's intervention plan. Currently there is no universally agreed method to guide therapists in writing goals (Levack et al., 2006; Siegert, McPherson, & Taylor, 2004). Several studies have shown that there is a need for occupational therapists to become skilled at writing clear, occupation-focused goals (Bowman, 2006; Bowman & Llewellyn, 2002; Bowman, Mogensen, Marsland, & Lannin, 2015, Neistadt, 1995; Northern et al., 1995). To assist occupational therapists to write appropriate occupation-focused goals, a structured method was developed by the authors of this chapter based on the SMART goal concept commonly described in psychology, education and rehabilitation literature (Bowman et al., 2015). The SMART goal method addresses five domains: Specific, Measurable, Activity-based, Review and Time frame, and clearly illustrates the steps required for writing clinically useful goals. The requirements of each domain are described in detail next. Each criterion will be demonstrated using examples of short-term goals in two practice stories (Practice Story 22.1 and 22.2).

Specific (S)

Writing specific goals reduces ambiguity, discrepancy and individual interpretation of achievement expectations. To be *specific*, a goal must address three criteria. The goal must do the following:

1. Include a verb that describes the person's desired occupational engagement or performance outcome in terms of *observable behaviour;* for example, the person will *walk* (desired performance behaviour)
2. Include the *conditions* that are required for performing or maintaining the goal behaviour (e.g. with use of equipment, assistance, independently, with verbal cues, or requires supervision)

3. State the performance *context,* meaning the environment within which the desired behaviour be performed (e.g. the hospital ward or rehabilitation gym, the person's home or workplace, or local shops)

Measurable (M)

A goal must be measurable to objectively determine whether the strategy has had an effect. The goal should indicate how achievement will be measured. Outcome measures can be standardised instruments or self-determined scales. It is particularly important that the method selected to measure the person's behaviour targets the appropriate level (body function and structure versus activity versus participation) of that behaviour. For example, if the person wants to be able to walk from his or her house to the local shops and back, the measure should determine an increase in distance walked within an acceptable time frame. To be *measurable,* a goal must address two criteria. The goal must do the following:

1. State *how* performance will be *measured* (e.g. using standardised outcome measurement instrument or by measuring distance, time and frequency, the reduction in the level of pain experienced or the number of cues or level of assistance needed)
2. Specify the *criteria for an acceptable standard of the behaviour performed*; the goal should specify how much, how fast, how long, how often or how accurate the behaviour needs to be (e.g. within 10 seconds, in half an hour, no more than two prompts, within 10 seconds after verbal prompt, for at least 20 minutes, to complete within 10 minutes on five consecutive occasions, 8 out of 10 correct responses or with 80% accuracy, on each occasion, on five consecutive occasions, daily).

Evaluation and outcome measurement are discussed in greater detail in a later section of this chapter.

Activity-based Strategies (A)

Activity-based strategies are interventions that will effect behaviour change and lead to goal achievement. A strategy must be selected to address the specific occupational impairment, limitation or restriction at the appropriate level of body function and structure, activity or participation. To be *activity-based* the goal must address one criterion. The goal must do the following:

1. State *how* the person will achieve the goal by describing a strategy (e.g. by wearing a compression bandage, participate in weekly relaxation groups, use self-calming techniques, practice or part practice of an activity/task such as sit to stand).

Review (R)

The review domain focuses on the regular monitoring of the person's progress towards achievement of the desired goal outcome. When planning the intervention programme, a schedule for review and administration of outcome measures should be specified. It is essential that baseline measures are taken before commencement of strategies to enable review of occupational performance progress. Scheduled reviews also assist the therapist to determine whether the goal is realistic and if the strategies are suitable or whether modification is required (e.g. increase the time frame for goal achievement) (see Box 22.2). To ensure review of progress occurs, the goal must address one criterion. The goal must do the following:

1. Include planned *progress review(s)* (e.g. within 1 week, weekly, after 4 sessions or 3 months).

Time Frame (T)

Time frame refers to the overall expected time limit for goal achievement. If no time frame is set for achieving the desired goal outcome, there is no direction for intervention intensity. This may cause costs to inflate unnecessarily. Additionally, a person's motivation may decline if there is no view to goal completion. The *time frame* domain includes one criterion. The goal must do the following:

1. Include the *time frame* within which the *desired outcome should be achieved* (e.g. by a specified date, in 1 week or by the end of the year).

Following a structured method such as writing SMART goals assists therapists in the planning of strategies and evaluation. Without specific goals, the occupational therapy process is likely to become directionless and may continue indefinitely. The key steps required for writing SMART goals are summarised in Box 22.3.

BOX 22.3
WRITING SMART GOALS

KEY STEPS

Specific
- Describe the person's desired occupational performance outcome in terms of *observable behaviour using a verb*.
- State the *conditions* that are required for performing or maintaining the goal behaviour.
- State the *environmental context* – that is, the environment within which the desired behaviour will be performed.

Measurable
- State *how* the behaviour will be *measured*.
- Specify the *criteria for an acceptable standard of the behaviour performed*.

Activity-based
- State *how* the person will achieve the goal by describing an intervention activity that addresses the desired occupational engagement or performance outcome.

Review
- State when progress reviews are planned.

Time Frame
- State the time frame within which the desired outcome should be achieved.

PRACTICE STORY 22.1

Michelle

Michelle (Fig. 22.3) is a senior occupational therapist with more than 14 years of experience in neurological rehabilitation. Michelle is currently employed within a community rehabilitation service, where she works with young adults who have a brain injury either as a result of trauma (such as a motor vehicle accident) or a nontraumatic cause (such as stroke). The people Michelle works with are both varied and unique, making setting individualised goals of critical importance.

The focus of occupational therapy services within this context is to extend rehabilitation into the home and community setting. The aim of therapy is to enhance occupational engagement and independence through both remedial and compensatory methods. Therapy may include prescription of complex equipment and assistive devices, environmental modification, community-based self-care retraining, carer

training (within the home or residential setting), community access skills training and return to work programmes. Michelle typically sees people for 6 to 12 weeks, although therapy is not time limited; rather, it is dictated by the person's need and progress made.

Michelle is a keen advocate of goal-directed therapy, a vision shared by the service, in which person-driven goals are the focus of all interventions. Michelle has been an integral part of establishing processes across the community team to incorporate the use of the Goal Attainment Scale (Kiresuk & Sherman, 1968) as routine practice for initial contact with people who received services from the team. Once a person's goals are obtained, each treating therapist in the team builds a structured intervention plan around the person. For Michelle, the Person–Environment–Occupation (PEO) model provides

Continued on following page

Michelle *(Continued)*

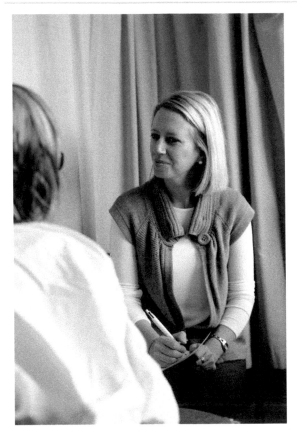

FIG. 22.3 ■ Michelle (occupational therapist) setting goals with Lucy.

structure to her occupational therapy intervention planning. Michelle always encourages people to set their own goals for community rehabilitation and encourages the contribution of family and carers in setting these goals. It is important to Michelle that everyone feels included in the team.

Each person typically receives 60 to 90 minutes of occupational therapy weekly. Michelle attends a community team meeting where the progress of people having therapy is discussed. The meeting's agenda centres on review of the individual's goals that acts as a guide to structure team discussion. Michelle monitors progress in occupational engagement towards goal achievement, plans for therapy sessions, and modifies goals or strategies based on the team meeting review. Workplace leadership and practices of occupational therapists like Michelle illustrate how the use of simple yet effective strategies can assist to ensure a collaborative, systematic and occupation-focused approach with intrinsic meaning to each person.

Goal examples 1 and 2 are the types of goals that Michelle may develop when working with people in the neurological rehabilitation setting.

EXAMPLE GOAL 1

By October 2015 **(T)**, Mr Lewis will be able to independently **(S2)** use public transport (train) **(S1)** to travel six train stops to his favourite coffee shop **(S3)**. Mr Lewis will receive training in public transport use by employing pause, prompt, praise retraining strategies and a graded approach **(A)**. Mr Lewis's progress will be monitored once per week **(R)** by his occupational therapist by comparing the number of errors and prompts required each week within the task **(M1)**. Mr Lewis expects to be able to independently catch the train to his favourite coffee shop 100% of the time after 8 weeks of therapy **(M2)**.

EXAMPLE GOAL 2

By the end of the year **(T)**, Lucy will return to her place of employment **(S3)** in a full-time capacity **(S1)**, with the support of her workplace team leader and occupational therapist **(S2)**. Lucy will gradually increase her daily work hours **(M1)** from 2 hours to 7 hours **(M2)** and decrease rest break duration **(M1)** from 15 minutes for every 2 hours of work, to 5 minutes **(M2)**. Her daily attendance will increase from 2 hours to 3 hours after 4 weeks, 4 hours after 8 weeks, 5 hours after 12 weeks, 6 hours after 16 weeks and 7 hours after 20 weeks. Duration of rest breaks will decrease to 10 minutes after 8 weeks and 5 minutes after 20 weeks, without increasing levels of fatigue **(M2)** on the Visual Analogue Scale (VAS) and the Fatigue Severity Scale (FSS) **(M1)** (Krupp, LaRocca, Muir-Nash, & Steinberg, 1989). Lucy's graded return-to-work programme and fatigue/energy levels will be reviewed weekly by the community rehabilitation occupational therapist **(R)** using the FSS. Ongoing progress will be monitored collaboratively (among Lucy, the occupational therapist and the workplace team leader) on a weekly basis using the VAS for fatigue management.

PRACTICE STORY 22.2

Kate

Kate is an occupational therapist who works in the area of aged care within a busy metropolitan hospital. Her caseload typically includes older adults who have been acutely ill (such as with pneumonia) and require an extended hospital stay to determine whether they will return to their own home or transition to living in supported aged care accommodation. Her occupational therapy role is therefore one of assessment, life planning and rehabilitation. Goal setting is a critical component of her occupational therapy role, as she sets both long-term and short-term goals to assist people to return to living life as independently as possible while aging.

Kate uses both remedial and compensatory methods to achieve an individual's goals, and therapy may include self-care retraining, prescription of equipment and assistive devices, home modification, and delivery of health promotion programmes, such as falls prevention and caregiver support. As an inpatient occupational therapist, Kate is often the first person who meets with the older person to discuss the person's goals for the future as he or she ages. She is thus an important member of the multidisciplinary team for the older person's admission because her focus is on both the short-term team goals (often centred around discharge planning from hospital) as well as long-term goals (often centred around the individual's preferences for remaining as active as possible and resuming important occupational tasks). Kate's role in the inpatient team demonstrates the importance of being person-centred in the health care system. Although Kate sets short-term goals that are often dictated by the health care system, she sets long-term goals with the older person to assist the person to return to a life that is as active as possible post discharge.

Goal examples 3 and 4 outline the type of goals that Kate may develop when working with older people. Mr Timmer identified his goal as being 'To live as a normal person and not to fall again'. To achieve this goal, Kate talked to Mr Timmer about his current abilities, his social situation and his planned length of stay in hospital (Fig. 22.4). Kate developed example goals 3 and 4 collaboratively with Mr Timmer. Setting small goals assists Mr Timmer to continue with his therapy both in hospital and after discharge. Having goals also help Mr Timmer to track his small but meaningful gains in resuming everyday tasks.

EXAMPLE GOAL 3

By discharge from hospital in 10 days' time **(T)**, Mr Timmer will be able to shower **(S1)** independently with equipment

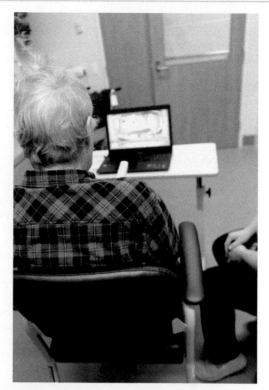

FIG. 22.4 ■ Kate (occupational therapist) setting goals with Mr Timmer.

(a shower chair) **(S2)** in the hospital bathroom **(S3)**. Mr Timmer will decrease the amount of setup assistance required **(M1)** from complete setup to partial setup by day 5 and from partial setup to no setup by day 10 **(M2)**. Mr Timmer will decrease the amount of supervision required **(M1)** from standby supervision to no supervision by day 10 **(M2)**. Mr Timmer will decrease the time taken to complete his shower **(M1)** from 30 to 20 minutes by day 5 and from 20 to 15 minutes by day 10 **(M2)**. Mr Timmer will shower daily, using a bag to carry his toiletries and clothes to the bathroom, and practice safe transfer techniques on and off the shower chair and apply falls prevention strategies taught by the occupational therapist **(A)**. The occupational therapist will monitor Mr Timmer's progress every second day **(R)**.

Continued on following page

EXAMPLE GOAL 4

Within 1 week after discharge **(T)**, Mr Timmer will walk **(S1)** independently using a walking stick **(S2)** from his front door to his mailbox to collect the mail **(S3)**. Mr Timmer will practice walking the route daily. He will gradually reduce the time taken **(M1)** from 10 minutes to 7 minutes after 3 days and 4 minutes after 1 week **(M2)** and reduce the number of rests required **(M1)** from 1 to 0 within 1 week **(M2)**. Mr Timmer will practice his leg strengthening exercises for 15 minutes daily and walk from his lounge chair to the front door and back twice daily to build his functional capacity and exercise tolerance **(A)**. Mr Timmer's progress will be reviewed twice weekly by the community occupational therapist **(R)**.

SELECTING OCCUPATION-FOCUSED STRATEGIES

Strategies in occupational therapy focus on the acquisition, remediation, improvement or maintenance of occupational performance, so that participation in life tasks, activities and occupational roles may be achieved (Schultz-Krohn & McHugh Pendleton, 2011). The process of selecting appropriate occupation-focused strategies is informed by the therapist's occupational reasoning skills, knowledge of occupation and conceptual models of practice (Duncan, 2011; Turner, 2002). When guided by the concepts of the PEO model and the ICF, occupational therapists should consider the transactional dynamics of the interdependent person–environment–occupation fit and the concepts of activity, participation and occupational roles when selecting strategies.

Occupational engagement and performance means different things to different people. Each person has a unique set of attributes such as life experiences, cultural traditions, values and beliefs that influence his or her life roles and occupations; other issues to consider when selecting strategies include age, gender, interests, skills and abilities (Foster, 2003; Law et al., 1996; Molineux, 2009). Strategies should be appropriate to these attributes to ensure that activities are meaningful to the individual. Meaningful activities have face validity and are more likely to be intrinsically motivating. Ultimately, strategies should be selected specifically to address the aims and goals of therapy. Further to this, the therapist needs to carefully match the strategy so that it targets the appropriate level of body function and structure, activities or participation. The format of strategies must also be carefully considered in order to facilitate the best occupational performance outcome (e.g. one-on-one therapy versus a group approach).

Occupational engagement and performance takes place within the context of an environment. Considerations should be given not only to an individual's physical and social environment but also to his or her socioeconomic, institutional and cultural environments (Law et al., 1996). Time and environment have a strong influence on enabling strategies. The management, availability and allocation of time present a constant challenge for occupational therapists. When planning a programme for an individual, the time of sessions must be carefully considered. For example, (a) What time of the day is the most suitable for the individual and their particular condition? (b) How much time can the person realistically spend on strategies? (c) Is it important to establish a routine for the individual? (d) Does timing of the session influence availability of the most suitable location for therapy, such as the home, workplace or the local community?

Environments can have enabling or restricting effects on a person. For example, a person may be able to transfer from a wheelchair into a hospital bed, where adjustable equipment and ample space is available, but have difficulty with the same task in his or her own home. At times, the environment may be more adaptable to change than the person. For example, an individual with a chronic or progressive illness or disability may not expect improvement at the body function level. In this case it would be appropriate to consider environmental modifications to achieve an occupational engagement or performance outcome at the activity or participation level. When selecting environmental strategies, it is important to consider the individual's current personal situation and the likelihood of any changes both in the short and long term.

Therapists need to prioritise strategies that are occupation-focused and facilitate change in occupational engagement. However, there are times where body function and structure must be addressed first to enable or improve occupational engagement at an activity or participation level. For example, increasing a person's muscle strength and joint range of motion may be necessary before the person can dress himself of herself, or improving sitting balance may be required before the person can sit at a table to eat a meal with his or her family. Where body function and structure is targeted by strategies, the link to activity and participation level goals should be explicit.

An important component of planning is to ensure, where possible, that occupation-focused strategies are evidence based. For therapists this means keeping up to date with the research being conducted within one's field of interest and implementing strategies that are supported by scientific evidence. The key steps in selecting occupation-focused strategies are summarised in Box 22.4.

EVALUATING THE PERSON–ENVIRONMENT–OCCUPATION FIT

There is increasing pressure for occupational therapists to demonstrate that the strategies they have selected achieve desired changes in occupational engagement and are cost efficient (Bowman, 2006; Bowman & Llewellyn, 2002; Gutman & Mortera, 1997; Kay, Myers, & Huijbregts, 2001; Landry & Mathews, 1998). Previously the allocation of occupational therapy services was largely based on therapists' personal and professional judgements and values. However, it is important to be responsive to all stakeholders in the health care system – that is, the individuals and their families, those who pay for the service and those who employ the therapists to provide the service (Foto, 1996). As such, evaluation of the outcome of strategies is a contemporary practice issue for all therapists. It is important then that therapists are competent in the skill of outcome measurement. An outcome can be defined as 'a characteristic or construct that is expected to change owing to a strategy, intervention or program' (Finch et al., 2002, p. 271). For example, range of motion may increase at a person's wrist joint as a result of wearing a splint, or a person may be able to independently catch the bus as a result of community travel training. Outcome measurement is the process of quantifying change in a characteristic or construct, using valid and reliable instruments (Austin & Clark, 1993; De Clive-Lowe, 1996). For example, an increase in range of motion can be measured using a goniometer, and a person's ability to independently catch the bus can be measured using the Goal Attainment Scale (Kiresuk & Sherman, 1968). Knowledge of the key steps in the evaluation process is essential if therapists are to choose and effectively use appropriate outcome measures with their clients. A number of authors have described in detail the outcome measurement process and issues to consider when selecting outcome measures appropriate to specific needs (e.g. Dittmar & Gresham, 1997; Finch et al., 2002; Law, 2001; Law, Baum, & Dunn, 2005). The key steps described in the literature are summarised in Box 22.5.

When evaluating a person's progress towards goal attainment, it is important to ensure that the outcome measure selected specifically quantifies change brought about by the enabling strategies used with that person. Where possible, outcome measures should be used that reflect a person's participation in daily occupations. Therapists should also develop the habit of reporting outcomes to others in occupational terms. This will reinforce the central role that occupation plays in occupational therapy practice.

CONCLUSION

Collaborative, occupation-focused planning is the foundation of occupational therapy practice. A strong emphasis has been placed on the need to consider the person, the person's occupational roles and his or her physical and social environment when planning an intervention programme. Collaboration was highlighted as essential to ensure therapy has intrinsic meaning to each individual to enhance the person's motivation to achieve his or her goals. Intervention planning was described in this chapter as a linear process to enhance the clarity of the requirements at each step of the process. The importance of linking each step of the process has also been stressed. Conducting subjective and objective assessments was illustrated to form the basis for identifying the broad overarching aims of intervention. SMART goals were clearly articulated and prioritised, leading to the selection of occupation-focused strategies to address impairment, limitation or restriction in occupational engagement. The importance of selecting appropriate outcome measures to measure change in occupational engagement was also described. Two practice stories have been used to demonstrate application of planning principles in two areas of practice. In summary, occupational therapists need to be skilled in all areas of planning to make certain that the services provided are effective, person-centred and occupation-focused.

 http://evolve.elsevier.com/Curtin/OT

REFERENCES

American Occupational Therapy Association (1998). Standards of practice. *American Journal of Occupational Therapy, 52,* 866–869.

American Occupational Therapy Association (2010). *Standards for practice for occupational therapy. Retrieved from,* http://www.aota.org/general/otsp.asp.

Austin, C., & Clark, C. R. (1993). Measures of outcome: For whom? *British Journal of Occupational Therapy, 56*(1), 21–24.

Australian Institute of Health and Welfare (AIHW) (2003). *ICF Australian user guide.* Version 1.0. Disability Series. AIHW Cat. No. DIS 33, Canberra: AIHW.

Bowman, J. (2006). Challenges to measuring outcomes in occupational therapy: A qualitative focus group study. *British Journal of Occupational Therapy, 69*(10), 464–472.

Bowman, J., & Llewellyn, G. (2002). Clinical outcomes research from the occupational therapist's perspective. *Occupational Therapy International, 9*(2), 145–166.

Bowman, J., Mogensen, L., Marsland, E., & Lannin, N. (2015). The development, content validity and inter-rater reliability of the SMART Goal Evaluation Method for evaluating clinical goals. *Australian Occupational Therapy Journal,* Retrieved from, http://onlinelibrary.wiley.com/doi/10.1111/1440-1630.12218/abstract.

De Clive-Lowe, S. (1996). Outcome measurement, cost-effectiveness and clinical audit: The importance of standardised assessment to occupational therapists in meeting these new demands. *British Journal of Occupational Therapy, 59*(8), 357–362.

Dittmar, S. S., & Gresham, G. E. (1997). *Functional assessment and outcome measures for the rehabilitation professional.* Gaithersburg: Aspen Press.

Duncan, E. A. S. (2011). *Foundations for practice in occupational therapy* (5th ed.). Edinburgh: Churchill Livingstone.

Emerson, H. (1998). Flow and occupation: A review of the literature. *Canadian Journal of Occupational Therapy, 65,* 37–44.

Fawcett, A. L. (2002). Assessment. In A. Turner, M. Foster, & S. E. Johnson (Eds.), *Occupational therapy and physical dysfunction: Principles, skills and practice* (5th ed., pp. 107–144). Edinburgh: Churchill Livingstone.

Finch, E., Brooks, D., Stratford, P. W., et al. (2002). *Physical rehabilitation outcome measures: A guide to enhanced clinical decision making* (2nd ed.). Hamilton: B C Decker.

Foster, M. (2003). Skills for practice. In A. Turner, M. Foster, & S. E. Johnson (Eds.), *Occupational therapy for physical dysfunction.* Edinburgh: Churchill Livingstone A. Turner, M. Foster, & S. E. Johnson (Eds.), *Occupational therapy for physical dysfunction* (5th ed.). Edinburgh: Churchill Livingstone.

Foto, M. (1996). Outcome studies: The what, why, how, and when. *American Journal of Occupational Therapy, 50*(2), 87–88.

Gutman, S. A., & Mortera, M. (1997). Applied scientific inquiry: An answer to managed care's challenge? *American Journal of Occupational Therapy, 51*(8), 704–709.

Hocking, C. (2009). Process of assessment and evaluation. In M. Curtin, J. Supyk, & M. Molineux (Eds.), *Occupational therapy and physical dysfunction: Enabling occupation* (6th ed.). London: Elsevier.

Kay, T. M., Myers, A. M., & Huijbregts, M. P. J. (2001). How far have we come since 1992? A comparative survey of physiotherapists' use of outcome measures. *Physiotherapy Canada, 53,* 268–275, 281.

Kiresuk, T. J., & Sherman, R. E. (1968). Goal attainment scaling: A general method for evaluating comprehensive community mental health programs. *Community Mental Health Journal, 4*(6), 443–453.

Krupp, L., LaRocca, N., Muir-Nash, J., & Steinberg, A. D. (1989). The fatigue severity scale: Application to patients with multiple sclerosis and system lupus erythematosus. *Archives of Neurology, 46,* 1121–1123.

Landry, D. W., & Mathews, M. (1998). Economic evaluation of occupational therapy: Where are we at? *Canadian Journal of Occupational Therapy, 65*(3), 160–167.

Latham, G. P. (2004). The motivational benefits of goal-setting. *Academy of Management Executive, 18*(4), 126–129.

Law, M. (2001). *All about outcomes: An educational program to help you understand, evaluate, and choose adult outcome measures (CD-ROM).* Thorofare, NJ: Slack.

Law, M., Baptiste, S., McColl, M. A., et al. (1990). The Canadian occupational performance measure: An outcome measure for occupational therapy. *Canadian Journal of Occupational Therapy, 57*, 82–87.

Law, M. C., Baum, C. M., & Dunn, W. (2005). *Measuring occupational performance: Supporting best practice in occupational therapy* (2nd ed.). Thorofare, NJ: Slack.

Law, M., Cooper, B., Strong, S., et al. (1996). The person-environment-occupation model: A transactive approach to occupational performance. *Canadian Journal of Occupational Therapy, 63*(1), 9–23.

Levack, W., Taylor, K., Siegert, R. J., et al. (2006). Is goal planning in rehabilitation effective? A systematic review. *Clinical Rehabilitation, 20*, 739–755.

Locke, E. A., & Latham, G. P. (2002). Building a practically useful theory of goal-setting and task motivation. *American Psychologist, 57*(9), 705–717.

Molineux, M. (2009). The nature of occupation. In M. Curtin, J. Supyk, & M. Molineux (Eds.), *Occupational therapy and physical dysfunction: Enabling occupation* (6th ed.). London: Elsevier.

Neistadt, M. E. (1995). Methods of assessing client's priorities: A survey of adult physical dysfunction settings. *American Journal of Occupational Therapy, 49*(5), 428–436.

Northern, J., Rust, D., Nelson, C., et al. (1995). Involvement of adult rehabilitation patients in setting occupational therapy goals. *American Journal of Occupational Therapy, 49*(3), 214–220.

Radomski, M. V. (2002). Planning, guiding and documenting therapy. In M. V. Radomski, & C. A. Trombly (Eds.), *Occupational therapy for physical dysfunction* (5th ed.). Philadelphia: Lippincott Williams & Wilkins. pp. xvii, 1155.

Rebeiro, K. L., & Cook, J. V. (1999). Opportunity not prescription: An exploratory study of the experience of occupational engagement. *Canadian Journal of Occupational Therapy, 66*, 176–187.

Schultz-Krohn, W., & McHugh Pendleton, H. (2011). Application of the occupational therapy practice framework to physical dysfunction. In H. M. Pendleton, & W. Schultz-Krohn (Eds.), *Pedretti's occupational therapy: Practice skills for physical dysfunction* (7th ed.). St Louis: Mosby.

Schultz-Krohn, W., & Pendleton, H. M. (2006). Application of the occupational therapy practice framework to physical dysfunction. In L. W. Pedretti, H. M. Pendleton, & W. Schultz-Krohn (Eds.), *Occupational therapy: Practice skills for physical dysfunction* (6th ed., pp. 28–52). St Louis: Mosby.

Siegert, R. J., McPherson, K. M., & Taylor, W. J. (2004). Toward a cognitive-affective model of goal-setting in rehabilitation: Is self-regulation theory a key step? *Disability and Rehabilitation, 26*(20), 1175–1183.

Turner, A. (2002). Occupation for therapy. In A. Turner, M. Foster, & S. E. Johnson (Eds.), *Occupational therapy for physical dysfunction*. Edinburgh: Churchill Livingstone.

World Federation of Occupational Therapists (2012). *What is occupational therapy? Retrieved from,* http://www.wfot.org/AboutUs/AboutOccupationalTherapy/DefinitionofOccupationalTherapy.aspx.

World Health Organization (2002). Towards a Common Language for Functioning Disability and Health ICF. Geneva, Switzerland: World Health Organization.

GOALS - EXCERPTS FROM BONUS PRACTICE STORIES

e [Read the full practice stories on Evolve at http://evolve.elsevier.com/Curtin/OT]

---

e **MRS TREMBLAY: A PRACTICE STORY OF A PERSON EXPERIENCING REHABILITATION FOLLOWING A STROKE - GOALS**

DOROTHY KESSLER, KATRINE SAUVÉ-SHENK, & VALERIE METCALFE

Part 1: Acute Care

Agree on objectives and plan. Mrs Tremblay and I reviewed my assessment findings, and we discussed what types of goals could be addressed in the acute care setting. Together, we established the following occupational therapy goals …

e **To read the full Practice Story and complete a reflective exercise please visit Evolve at http://evolve.elsevier.com/Curtin/OT**

---

e **KARIN: A PRACTICE STORY OF A PERSON EXPERIENCING RHEUMATOID ARTHRITIS - GOALS**

MATHILDA BJÖRK & INGRID THYBERG

Part 1: Initial Diagnosis

Agree on objectives and plan. Karin stated that her immediate focus was to be able to continue work and not be bothered by her painful wrist. She also wanted to be able to be able to sleep more restfully at nights; her sleep during the night had become regularly interrupted due to her wrist pain …

e **To read the full Practice Story and complete a reflective exercise please visit Evolve at http://evolve.elsevier.com/Curtin/OT**

---

e **ANGELA: A PRACTICE STORY OF A PERSON EXPERIENCING PALLIATIVE CARE - GOALS**

DEIDRE MORGAN & CELIA MARSTON

Agree on objectives and plan. Understanding a person's roles and motivations is crucial when developing intervention objectives and in an acute setting, to inform a discharge plan. Angela was determined to be as independent as possible but equally, she was determined not to go home as she was protective about her son and daughter and concerned about how they were coping …

e **To read the full Practice Story and complete a reflective exercise please visit Evolve at http://evolve.elsevier.com/Curtin/OT**

Section 6

ENABLING SKILLS AND STRATEGIES

23

OVERVIEW OF ENABLING SKILLS AND STRATEGIES

MICHAEL CURTIN

CHAPTER OUTLINE

Abstract

The concept of enablement is core to the practice of occupational therapy and underpins the overall goal of enabling people to achieve their occupational potential and be engaged in occupations that promote health and well-being. To achieve this goal, occupational therapists work in a complex and unique way and have to become critical thinkers when applying their enabling skills and planning, designing, implementing and evaluating their enabling strategies. The manner in which therapists work with people involves the use of at least 10 enabling skills: adapt, advocate, coach, collaborate, consult, coordinate, design/build, educate, engage, and specialise. The skills are used in a multitude of different ways when implementing six different strategies commonly employed by occupational therapists: remediation, compensation, education, community development, transformation and redistributive justice. These strategies embrace the traditional therapy focus of the profession, when working with individuals, groups and communities, as well as the more recent political focus, in which occupationally just societies are created for all community members.

KEY POINTS

- Occupation and its relationship with health and well-being underpin the practice and focus of occupational therapy.

- The overall goal of occupational therapy is to enable people to engage in occupations that promote health and well-being.

- The concept of enablement is the core foundation of occupational therapy.

- Occupational therapists must become *critical* practitioners to effectively apply their enabling skills and to plan, design, implement and evaluate their enabling strategies.

- Occupational therapists draw on at least 10 enabling skills, as proposed by Townsend et al. (2007), and six enabling strategies when working with individuals, groups and communities.

INTRODUCTION

The focus of this chapter is to provide an overview of the enabling skills and strategies that underpin occupational therapy interventions. Initially, a justification will be given as to why occupational therapists need to focus on occupation when working with people, followed by a discussion of the complexity of occupational therapy practice and the multitude of factors that should be considered when developing occupation-focused interventions. This section will include a discussion of the concept of being a critical occupational therapy practitioner. The concept of enablement is then presented, as this is considered the essence that underpins all skills and strategies of occupational therapists. Finally, the essential enabling skills of occupational therapists and suggested enabling strategies are briefly covered, providing an introduction to the more detailed discussion of these throughout the other chapters of this book.

FOCUS ON OCCUPATION

In the third edition of *An Occupational Perspective of Health*, Wilcock and Hocking (2015) provide a detailed analysis of the importance of occupation to the health and well-being of individuals, groups and communities, contesting that a lack of engagement in occupation contributes to ill health. Christiansen and Townsend (2010a,b) and Wilcock and Hocking (2015) suggest that competence in engaging in occupations contributes to the identity of a person, group or community and that the development of a satisfactory identity is essential to feelings of well-being. This is because occupations in which people engage are fundamentally driven by their aspirations, needs and environments and relate to their purposeful and meaningful use of time (Doble & Santha, 2008). Hence, when using an occupational lens, people are considered to be healthy when they have the choice and ability to actively participate in all aspects of daily living (Christiansen & Townsend, 2010a; Doble & Santha, 2008; Wilcock & Hocking, 2015).

This belief in occupation is shared by many leaders within the occupational therapy profession, who promote the move away from biomedical practice to an occupation-focused practice, a move that encourages occupational therapists to take an active and political role in building healthy communities by promoting engagement in meaningful and purposeful occupations for all citizens. This is exemplified by the embedding of an occupational perspective into the World Federation of Occupational Therapists' (WFOT's) 2002 Minimum Standards of Education of Occupational Therapists (Hocking, 2013). The move towards an occupational perspective is also clearly illustrated in the thought-provoking books edited by Kronenberg, Algado, Pollard and Sakellariou* that encourage occupational therapists to think differently about the work they do and the work they could do. This change in the focus of occupational therapy has resulted in the publication of the following political position statements by WFOT: community-based rehabilitation (2004), human rights (2006), diversity and culture (2010), human

---

*Kronenberg, F., Algodo, S., & Pollard, N. (2005). *Occupational therapy without borders: Learning from the Spirit of Survivors*. Edinburgh: Churchill Livingstone. Pollard, N., Sakellariou, D., & Kronenberg, F. (2009). *A political practice of occupational therapy*. Edinburgh: Churchill Livingstone. Kronenberg, F., Pollard, N. & Sakellariou, D. (2011). *Occupational therapy without Borders (Vol. 2): Towards an ecology of occupation-based practices*. Edinburgh: Churchill Livingstone.

displacement (2014a) and disaster preparedness and response (2014b).

Engagement in occupations is dependent on the dynamic and complex interaction among the type of occupation, the abilities, habits, skills and experience of the person, and the physical, geographical, cultural, attitudinal and social aspects of the environment (Christiansen, Baum, & Bass, 2015; Doble & Santha, 2008). Hence, the occupations people engage in are not static; they are dynamic, influenced by positive and negative experiences and factors throughout the lifespan, and contribute to the sense of 'doing', 'being', 'belonging' and 'becoming' (Doble & Santha, 2008; Wilcock & Hocking, 2015).

To account for the complexity of occupation Wilcock and Hocking (2015) use the terms 'doing, being, belonging and becoming [...] as a way to discuss the meaning given to occupation in relation to health' (p. 134). *Doing* refers to 'action, getting something done, carrying out, achieving, making, executing, performing, acting, completing, fixing, preparing, organising, and undertaking [...] exploits, deeds and accomplishments, and seeing to, sorting out, or looking after' (pp. 134-135). Doble and Santha (2008) suggest that the term 'doing is captured within the traditional practice models, that is, occupational performance' (p. 185).

Being refers to the personal, rather than social, aspect of occupation in which a person finds time for stillness and reflection. Wilcock and Hocking (2015) state that individually 'it is often a period of quiet contemplation about the self and about personal past, present and future pleasures, difficulties, and achievements' and for groups it refers to 'support and reflection, such as in prayer or grief or in times of great joy or celebration that affect a community at large' (p. 135). Doble and Santha (2008) summarise this by stating that 'occupation does not simply refer to what is done but to the process of doing or the here and now of individuals' occupational experiences' (p. 185).

Belonging accounts for the social nature of people and their need to affiliate with other people, places and things that have meaning to them (Wilcock & Hocking, 2015). Having a sense of belonging can contribute to a person feeling accepted, valued, secure, and happy and can facilitate engagement in occupations. Doble and Santha (2008) state that engagement in occupations provide 'opportunities to "belong" by developing and maintaining connections with others' (p. 185).

Becoming refers to the potential of people, the 'possibility, growth, and the ongoing evolution of individuals' occupational identities' (Doble & Santha, 2008, p. 185). Wilcock and Hocking (2015) state that 'the word "becoming" is linked with the idea of undergoing change, transformation, or development [...] coming to be, changing to, emerging as, or to metamorphose (turning or growing into something or becoming somehow different, more knowledgeable, or mature)' (p. 137).

The importance of occupation and its relationship with health and well-being underpins the practice and focus of occupational therapy. As stated in the WFOT (2012) definition of occupational therapy, 'The primary goal of occupational therapy is to enable people to participate in activities of everyday life. Occupational therapists achieve this outcome by working with people and communities to enhance their ability to engage in the occupations they want to, need to, or are expected to do, or by modifying the occupation or the environment to better support their occupational engagement'.

COMPLEXITY OF OCCUPATIONAL THERAPY PRACTICE

Occupational therapists assist individuals, groups and communities to identify practical options to adapt and overcome any occupational dysfunction, so that participation in all aspects of daily life is possible (WFOT, 2012). It is important to understand that occupational therapy is not about treating a disease, illness or an impairment; rather it is about assisting people to find fulfilment through engagement in meaningful occupation (Watson, 2006). This suggests that the meaning an individual, group or community finds during engagement in occupation can be more important than the outcome (Reed, Hocking, & Smythe, 2011).

As a result of the focus on the *doing, being, belonging* and *becoming* aspects of occupation (Christiansen & Townsend, 2010a; Doble & Santha, 2008), the finding that engagement in occupation is health giving (Wilcock & Hocking, 2015), and the dynamic interaction that occurs among the person, occupation and environment (Christiansen et al., 2015), the enabling skills and strategies that occupational therapists use are complex. These skills and strategies are complex because planning, designing, implementing and evaluating are nonlinear and unpredictable; they involve a continual shift of perspective that requires occupational therapists to engage in critical thinking (Robertson, Warrender, & Barnard, 2015). Robertson et al. (2015, p. 68) referred to the 'critical occupational therapy practitioner' as 'an individual equipped, through the adoption of a critical stance, to succeed in supercomplex environments such as those that exist in contemporary health and social care'.

Occupational therapists use a range of complex and dynamic enabling skills and strategies when working with people, and as a result there are myriad ways to plan, design, implement and evaluate interventions. This means that occupational therapists have to consider more than just their scientific thinking, the evidence base for practice (Layton, 2014; Robertson et al., 2015). This is to suggest that in addition to seeking out and, where appropriate, contributing to evidence for the strategies used, occupational therapists should also consider other forms of evidence, such as reflective experience, intuition, professional judgement, and consulting experts (Bannigan & Moores, 2009), leading to them becoming critical occupational therapy practitioners (Robertson et al., 2015) – therapists who are professionally engaged, critically self-reflective and informed by evidence. Being a critical occupational therapy practitioner encapsulates the process that occupational therapists undergo

when they are considering a multitude of information, including published research data and their reflections on practice, to develop effective and relevant enabling strategies for people and communities. Hence, the concept of an evidence base for practice is broadened. Through the process of self-reflection, consideration of research evidence and the outcome of consultations with others, occupational therapists become critical practitioners and are able to provide a clear, considered rationale for the strategies they use.

In spite of there being myriad ways to plan, design, implement and evaluate interventions, the occupational therapy focus or goal is clear and unequivocal. The overarching goal of occupational therapy is to enable people to engage in health-promoting and sustaining occupation; this is the core, the essence of occupational therapy and what makes the practice of occupational therapy different from the practice of other professions. Occupational therapists improve occupational performance and engagement, promote and maintain health and prevent disease and impairment through enabling engagement in occupations that are fulfilling, have personal meaning and provide opportunity to develop and express one's identity (Moyers, 2005). Occupational therapists address occupational dysfunction, and assist people to regain competence and a positive occupational identity, by using a range of enabling skills and strategies that often include adapting the demands of the occupation, altering the physical or social environment and teaching a person new skills or reestablishing lost skills (Duncan, 2012). Occupational therapists view people as occupational beings and, as a result, use enabling skills and strategies to address occupational performance and engagement difficulties that, if not addressed, may lead to greater dependence or a decline in health and well-being and an associated reduced quality of life (McColl & Law, 2015).

When enabling skills and strategies are based on occupation, people should be able to see how engagement in therapy is connected to performance in an occupation that they find meaningful and purposeful, an occupation that is centred on their needs, interests and priorities. Moyers (2005, p. 229) states that

> *Occupations are chosen because of their potential to remediate impaired capabilities; to facilitate transfer of capabilities to multiple contexts; to enhance motivation to change and adapt; to promote self-exploration and development of identity; to match current capabilities; to provide opportunities to practise skills and develop habits; to provide feedback; to experience success, pleasure and other emotions; to interact with others.*

THE CONCEPT OF ENABLING

When working with individuals, groups and communities, occupational therapists need to embrace the concept of 'enabling' (Townsend et al., 2007). Occupational therapists are considered to be enablers, as they empower people to engage in meaningful health-promoting and sustaining occupations. Townsend et al. (2007) state that enabling describes what occupational therapists actually do and consider it to be the core competency of occupational therapy. These authors go on to state that 'enablement is the professional identity and trademark of occupational therapists who engage others through meaningful occupation to pursue goals for health, well-being and justice through occupation' (p. 91).

Townsend and Polatajko (2007, p. 367) suggest that the skills required to be enabling 'are value-based, collaborative, attentive to power equities and diversity, and charged with visions of possibility for individual and/or social change'. In being enablers, occupational therapists become critically reflective and attentive to inequities, differing perspectives, conflicts, diversity and issues of choice, risk and responsibilities.

In their exploration of 'enabling' Townsend et al. (2007) propose some foundations to practising in this way. They suggest that working in an enabling way involves the following:

- Facilitating individual, group or community choice and involvement in just-right risk taking.
- Acknowledging the diversity, rights and responsibilities of the people with whom occupational therapists work.
- Implementing a person-centred approach in which effective collaboration between therapists and the people with whom they are working is established.

- Envisaging affirmative and optimistic futures that inspire confidence and resilience, fostering within people the notion that positive change and transformation are possible.

ENABLING SKILLS

Townsend et al. (2007) proposed 10 skills that occupational therapists require to enable occupation. Although these skills are not exclusive to occupational therapists, the focus on using these skills to promote occupational engagement is unique to the profession. These 10 skills are not exhaustive, but an attempt to encapsulate the essence of occupational therapy practice and to identify what Duncan (2012) refers to as the core skills required for enablement.

These enabling skills would usually be used in combination with each other, rather than separately, as the complexity of working with people means that several skills may be required at any one time. In addition, the skills used will vary throughout the time that the therapist and individual, group or community work together, corresponding to the changing emphasis of the strategies used to enable occupation. A brief overview of the skills is provided in Table 23.1, but reference should be made to Townsend et al. (2007) for further details. An example of how each skill may be used is also provided in the table, based on Practice Story 23.1.

PRACTICE STORY 23.1

Tilly

Tilly lived in a council house with her father, Bob, and younger brother, Matt. Her mother, Liz, left the family when Tilly started primary school, because she claimed that she could no longer cope, 'living with her two ungrateful children and a depressed husband who had turned to drink'. The family have had no contact with Liz since she left.

After Liz left, Bob gave up drinking and began attending a drug and alcohol addiction support group each week. He did some casual labouring work, helping out a friend who had a small building and maintenance company. However, he struggled to hold down a permanent job because of his depression, for which he was on medication. He found it difficult to be motivated to do things, and as a result Tilly used to do most of the cooking and house cleaning. Tilly and her brother struggled academically at school. They both tried to do well but, partly as a result of their home life, they had little time to study and do homework.

When Tilly was 11 she was diagnosed with acute lymphoblastic leukaemia. Her medical treatment included intrathecal therapy, a therapeutic strategy for maintaining remission in people with this condition. Complications arose after her last dose of intrathecal therapy, leaving Tilly with a permanent complete C3 tetraplegia. This occurred when Tilly was 15 years old. As a result of the tetraplegia, Tilly was unable to move and required 24-hour care for all her physical needs. She had limited neck, head and face movements, had difficulty swallowing and was only able to communicate in a weak whisper when she was not feeling tired. She used a respirator to assist her with breathing. This unexpected paralysis also left her emotionally vulnerable.

The hospital accepted fault for causing Tilly's tetraplegia and as a result Tilly was awarded significant financial compensation.

TABLE 23.1		
Enablement Skills Proposed by Townsend et al. (2007)		
Enablement Skill	**Description of Skill**	**Example of Skill When Working with Tilly**
Adapting	Refers to the ability of the therapist to change existing aspects of an occupation to meet a person's occupational performance needs. This skill involves breaking down tasks into 'just-right challenges' (Townsend et al., 2007, p. 117), problem-solving, reconfiguring an occupation or tailoring an occupation to the requirements of the person and/or environment in which the occupation is conducted.	*This skill will be required* when implementing strategies for Tilly to do and have control over her everyday occupations, as she will be dependent on her father, brother, and paid carers for her self-care, leisure and productive occupations. Tilly will need to change the way she relates to people around her and learn how to inform people how she would like things done so that she can have and maintain control over the things that people do for her (e.g. choice of clothes to wear, what and when to eat, deciding what to do during the day).
Advocating	Refers to the ability of the therapist to act in a political manner, on behalf of people requiring therapy services, lobbying to ensure a person's needs are met. This skill is political and can involve lobbying for policy change, when policies perpetuate inequities. This skill is key to addressing the concern occupational therapists have with 'health, well-being, inclusion, and justice for all in everyday occupations' (Townsend et al., 2007, p. 117).	*This skill will be required* when implementing strategies to empower Tilly to ensure that her choices and decisions are voiced and listened to by all those involved with her. This is especially the case as she is a teenager and most probably has not developed the skills required to be in control. This will include ensuring that she understands and has her say regarding issues such as housing (e.g. as she has a significant financial compensation she will be able to afford to have a house built to suit her needs, but as she has not ever been involved in designing a house, especially a house designed for a person with high-level tetraplegia, she will need an advocate to assist her to understand and make sound decisions); choice of carers (e.g. as she is going to work closely and intimately with the carers, it is important that she is involved in their employment and training); and equipment preference (e.g. she may prefer to be pushed around in a manual wheelchair rather than use a powered wheelchair with an adapted controller).
Coaching	Refers to the ability of the therapist to establish a partnership with a person, so as to, in a nonjudgemental manner, encourage, guide, mentor, reflect and facilitate that person in making his or her own decisions on how to achieve his or her occupational goals.	*This skill will be required* when implementing strategies to guide and encourage Tilly in many areas as she learns to live with her impairment. This will mean working with her when she wants to learn or do something new to enable her to develop the strategies and plans to engage in this new activity – to assist her to develop the problem-solving and planning abilities that she can apply to new situations. For example, if Tilly decides that she would go out with her friends or to have a sleep over, an occupational therapist using coaching skills will be able to assist Tilly to take control of the situation by encouraging her to ask and answer appropriate questions, to consider the factors involved and to take control of the planning of the activity, so that she decides the best way to achieve what she wants to do.
Collaborating	Refers to the ability of the therapist to develop a power-sharing, person-centred approach to practice. The therapist and the person work together to plan and implement strategies to achieve the person's goals. In a collaborative relationship there is a mutual sharing of expertise and of respect for the skills the	*This skill will be required* when implementing strategies that involve interaction with Tilly and her family. Tilly will probably feel little control over her situation initially, and the therapist will need to work with her to achieve a mutual power-sharing relationship. This will also be the case for Tilly's father and brother. In addition, many other health, social welfare, education and legal professionals, in addition to builders and

	TABLE 23.1	
	Enablement Skills Proposed by *(Continued)*	
Enablement Skill	**Description of Skill**	**Example of Skill When Working with Tilly**
	different partners have in the relationship. The skill of collaboration also refers to working together with other health and social welfare professionals for the benefit of the person.	other tradespeople and equipment suppliers, will be involved with Tilly. The therapist will need to collaborate with all of them to achieve Tilly's occupational goals.
Consulting	Refers to the ability of the occupational therapist to liaise with others involved in the care of the individual. Consultation may occur with team members, government personnel, business representatives, special interest groups, etc. In the role of a consultant the occupational therapist must integrate, synthesise and summarise multiple forms of data and put forward recommendations that may reframe the problems, issues, challenges and opportunities, as a way of stimulating a course of action.	*This skill will be required* when implementing strategies that involve liaison with a variety of people, mutually sharing expertise, to ensure Tilly's needs are being met. For example, when Tilly decides to return to school the occupational therapist will need to liaise with the teaching and support staff and students at the school to ensure that Tilly's needs will be accommodated and that her return to school will be successful. Another situation in which consulting skills will be used is when deciding on a wheelchair for mobility. The occupational therapist will need to ascertain from Tilly what her needs and expectations are and then consult with the wheelchair supplier, the respiratory specialist about the ventilator, the physiotherapist regarding seating posture, the builder regarding use of the chair within the house and the vehicle supplier to ensure the chair and Tilly can easily and safely be transported.
Coordinating	Refers to the ability of the therapist to manage and pull together the multiple factors required to achieve a person's goals (including the involvement of other professionals), to ensure that everyone is working towards the same purpose. Coordination can also refer to the management of services for the effective running of departments and faculties.	*This skill will be required* when implementing strategies that ensure the multiple professionals and people involved in working with Tilly work together. For example, arranging for all the people involved in building an appropriate house for Tilly and her father and brother, ensuring they are linked in and talking with each other, and that the house is ready when Tilly is discharged. Another example would involve bringing together all the people involved in assisting Tilly and her father and brother to organise a care package and the employment of carers when Tilly is discharged home.
Designing/building	Refers to the capacity of the therapist to accommodate the abilities of the person by changing/altering the physical environment (such as home modifications), providing assistive technology or splints, and/or designing and implementing programmes and services. The term *design* is also used to refer to the development of a plan or a strategy.	*This skill will be required* when implementing strategies for the planning and design of a house to accommodate Tilly and her father's and brother's needs. Also Tilly will require assistive technology such as a powered wheelchair and seating system for mobility, an environmental control system for controlling devices within the house (such as television, music system, lights), a vehicle to transport her while sitting in her wheelchair, and a computer system. This skill will also be evident in the plans developed for a safe discharge and reintegration into Tilly's community.
Educating	Refers to the ability of the therapist to transfer specific knowledge in a meaningful and appropriate manner to the person, the person's family, other professionals and the general public. Therapists need to draw on relevant educational theories and apply these to their work in enabling occupations. There are many ways in which education can be done, such as demonstration, practice, simulation, tutoring, etc. This skill is also evident in health promotion strategies to prevent occupational dysfunction.	*This skill will be required* when implementing strategies that inform Tilly and her family about her impairment. It is also required when exploring various equipment options (e.g. wheelchairs, beds, computer, environmental control system, etc.) to ensure Tilly and her father and brother understand the options, learn to use the equipment appropriately and can instruct others how to use the equipment. Many interactions with Tilly and her family will involve some degree of education. Health promotion will also be relevant for Tilly so that she is aware of the risk of pressure sores, respiratory, bowel and bladder complications, dietary considerations, vehicle travel safety requirements, etc.

Continued on following page

| | **TABLE 23.1** | |
| | **Enablement Skills Proposed by** *(Continued)* | |
Enablement Skill	Description of Skill	Example of Skill When Working with Tilly
Engaging	Refers to the ability of the therapist to create opportunities and to motivate a person to actively participate in occupations, to promote optimal performance and engagement related to the environment in which a person performs. The skill of engaging people in occupation is essential for health and well-being.	*This skill will be required* when implementing strategies to motivate Tilly to engage in occupations that are meaningful to her and to envisage a future full of potential and possibilities. The therapist will encourage Tilly to be actively involved in decisions that affect her and where possible to be in control of these decision, and to develop strategies to enable her to do the things she wants to do.
Specialising	This skill encompasses the many specific techniques that occupational therapists may use to achieve occupational goals. These techniques are usually developed through further training, related to an occupational therapist's area of practice. These techniques may be borrowed from other professionals and may not be occupational in nature, although they should be used to achieve occupational goals.	*This skill will be required* when implementing specific strategies to remediate and compensate for the effect the spinal cord lesion has on Tilly's body. This will include how to effectively reduce spasticity and prevent contractures, determining the most effective pressure relieving cushion and seating support system when sitting in a wheelchair, moving and handling techniques to ensure safe transfers between wheelchair and bed, etc. This could also involve having specialised knowledge regarding the assistive technology that may be appropriate for Tilly.

NB: As proposed by Townsend et al., the skills are listed alphabetically to demonstrate that there is no prioritisation of the skills; all are considered to be equally important. As these skills refer to what therapists do, the original skills proposed by Townsend et al. have 'ing' added to the words to emphasise the doing aspect of each skill.

ENABLING STRATEGIES

There are a number of ways in which to categorise the strategies used by occupational therapists. A simple way is to place the strategies into two major categories: top-down and bottom-up (Holm, Rogers, & Stone, 2003; Weinstock-Zlotnick & Hinojosa, 2004). Top-down strategies are generally considered to be more holistic, person-centred and suited to the occupation focus of occupational therapy. The focus of these strategies is on the social roles and responsibilities that define people's participation both at home and in the community. These approaches usually start by focusing on occupational roles and the meaning people assign to the occupations that are part of their roles; hence, occupational dysfunction or participation restriction is established first, and performance components, or a person's capabilities, are considered later. The rationale for this approach is that participation can be improved through adapted performance of occupations, even though impairments may not be remediated.

Bottom-up strategies generally focus on performance components and other foundational factors first, to obtain an understanding of a person's abilities and limitations. The rationale behind this approach is that body structures and functions support occupational performance and engagement, so by improving a person's abilities, there should be a corresponding improvement in the performance and engagement of occupations; hence, if impaired physical, psychological or cognitive skills are remedied or compensated for, then it is possible for the person to reengage in occupations.

Holm et al. (2003) state that top-down strategies are the most appropriate for occupational therapy practice. However, Weinstock-Zlotnick and Hinojosa (2004) suggest that each type of strategy used in isolation is insufficient and ineffective. They propose that a combination of both types of strategies is essential to be effective. It could be argued that whether a strategy is top-down or bottom-up is irrelevant as long as the ultimate focus is to enable occupation; as long as the focus is on the use of occupations meaningful to the person in order to promote and maintain health and well-being and to improve occupational performance and engagement (Moyers, 2005; Youngstrom & Brown, 2005).

Perhaps a more practical way of categorising strategies used by occupational therapists is to use the categories of remediation, compensation, and education (Moyers, 2005). Watson (2006) states that these three strategies can be referred to as 'therapy' and are the traditional strategies of therapists who focus on working occupationally with individuals and small groups. In addition to the 'therapy' strategies, she proposes three further strategies that occupational therapists use when working with communities and population: community development, transformation and redistributive justice. These three strategies point towards a political direction for occupational therapists, one in which they become social and political agents (Barros, Ghirardi, Lopes, & Galheigo, 2005; Kronenberg & Pollard, 2005). The reason for a move to a more political agenda is strongly put forward by Pollard, Alsop, and Kronenberg (2005, pp. 524-526):

Some [...] argue for an occupational therapy that reconnects with the culturally and spiritually significant aspects of occupation in areas of poverty and conflict, where health and social care services often do not reach. These voices can inform practice where social and economic deprivation limit access to occupation, where population is ageing and where physical disabilities combined with low income are apparent. Here the effectiveness of health and social care technologies is limited by the conditions in which people live. [...]

Occupational therapy has the potential to benefit the wider society as well as helping the individual and can engage with marginalised people to make connections with excluded communities.

Clearly these are important strategies for occupational therapists to use in their quest to create occupationally just societies for all community members. In Table 23.2 the three categories proposed by Moyers (2005) and the three by Watson (2006) are briefly explained and are related to the practice story.

It would be remiss not to mention that there are other ways of labelling/categorising the strategies that occupational therapists use, and of these other ways three are briefly defined in Tables 23.3 to 23.5. These are included in this chapter not to confuse the readers, but to offer alternative ways of thinking about enabling strategies, to assist readers to find a way of referring to the strategies that fits with their practice approach and reasoning.

TABLE 23.2		
Enabling Strategies		
Enabling Strategy	**Description of Strategy**	**Example of Strategy When Working with Tilly**
The following strategies are *usually* used when occupational therapists are working with an individual or small group (Moyers, 2005).		
Remediation	These strategies: focus on making changes in the person or population using approaches that remediate, restore or establish skills; refer to directly addressing the impairment, using activities so that a person can recover lost skills or attain new skills; and focus on identifying a person's skills and barriers to performance and then designing strategies that restore, maintain, develop and/or improve the person's abilities required for occupational performance and engagement. McColl and Law (2015) and AOTA (2014) refer to these types of strategies as training and skill development and establish/restore, and suggest that they can be used to prepare people for occupational performance and engagement. These activities may be considered preliminary to the use of meaningful occupation and may include exercises, facilitation and inhibition techniques, positioning, social and coping skills training, transfers, etc.	*This type of strategy may include (NB: many remedial strategies will be carried out by other health professional):* ■ Using hand splints and passive range of motion to prevent joint contractures. ■ Oral, facial and neck muscle exercises to maintain and improve muscle bulk and strength. ■ Sensory retraining to facilitate return of sensation where possible. ■ Awareness training to compensate for loss of sensation to body – increased use of auditory and visual senses. ■ Using visual imagery or breathing exercises as a relaxation technique. ■ Cognitive exercises to develop problem-solving skills. ■ Assertiveness training. ■ Study exercises and techniques to assist with education. ■ Business techniques to assist with the employment of carers.
Compensation	These strategies are directed at adapting the environment or the task to match a person's abilities and are referred to as compensatory or adaptive strategies. These strategies also include those not focusing on changing the person or adapting the environment, but on making the best person–environment fit. In this case the focus is on matching the abilities of the person/population with the environment or task that is most enabling. McColl and Law (2015) refer	*This type of strategy may include:* *Adapt/alter/modify task* ■ Employing carers to perform everyday activities and to assist with self-care needs. ■ Informing family/carers what she wants to do and how she wants things done – this can include giving instructions for self-care activities, cooking food, outings, etc. ■ Showering using a shower trolley. ■ Transferring between bed, wheelchair and/or shower-trolley, etc., using ceiling track hoist.

Continued on following page

	TABLE 23.2	
	Enabling Strategies *(Continued)*	
Enabling Strategy	**Description of Strategy**	**Example of Strategy When Working with Tilly**
	to these strategies as *task and environmental adaptation,* and AOTA (2014) refer to them as *modify.* The main focus of these strategies is to prevent or reduce occupational performance issues that may result from an impairment, to enable participation. When using compensation strategies changes may be made to the way the task is done, the tools required to do the task and/or the environment.	*Adapt/alter/modify tool/equipment* ■ Using a head control switch to manoeuvre a powered wheelchair, operate an environmental control system and access a computer. ■ Using a computer using switch access and appropriate software for writing and communication. ■ Using an environmental control system for controlling electrical appliances in the house, as well as for opening doors, windows, and using the telephone. ■ Using a powered wheelchair and seating system for independent mobility. ■ Using an adapted vehicle for safely transporting Tilly while sitting in her wheelchair. *Adapt/alter/modify environment* ■ Building a fully accessible house to accommodate her mobility needs – level floors, no steps, wide doorways, automatic opening doors, turning spaces, integrated environmental control system, ceiling hoists, etc.; the house needs to meet the needs of Tilly, as well as her father and brother, if they are to continue to live together. ■ Working with students and teachers at Tilly's school to ensure they understand how to accommodate her needs. ■ Working with local council to encourage local community services and shopping centres to be more accessible, where appropriate.
Education	These strategies are used as part of everyday practice to empower individuals by imparting knowledge, to enable them to change their behaviour, attitude, beliefs, confidence, skills and decision making ability. When designing education strategies, therapists need to understand education principles and consider various factors such as content, delivery mode and timing to ensure that it is relevant to an individual's circumstances. Education can include health promotion approaches that focus on the individual.	*This type of strategy may include:* ■ Informing Tilly, her father/brother, and carers about her impairment and the implications. ■ Demonstrating and training Tilly in how to use the assistive technology devices, such as the powered wheelchair, computer, environmental control unit, adapted vehicle, and ventilator. ■ Informing her teacher and students at Tilly's school about her needs. ■ Providing information, demonstrating and explaining to Tilly and her family how to reduce the risk of pressure sores. ■ Producing a DVD to use with new carers to demonstrate how to move and handle Tilly correctly and how to assist her with her self-care. ■ Explaining requirements for the house design to architects and builders.

The following strategies are *usually* used when occupational therapists are working with a community or population (Watson, 2006).

Community development	These strategies are indicative of a move away from one-to-one therapy, towards a community-based approached. Community development is a participatory approach that focuses on capacity building in which members of a community develop their own strategies to respond to the various local factors	*This type of strategy may include:* ■ Working with Tilly, her father and her brother, as a small community, to increase their capacity to accommodate her needs – where they become the experts. ■ Establishing support networks for the family – with friends, local service, charities, church groups, and drug and alcohol addiction support group – to provide assistance if required and accommodate needs.

TABLE 23.2
Enabling Strategies *(Continued)*

Enabling Strategy	Description of Strategy	Example of Strategy When Working with Tilly
	that affect their occupational engagement. This may include working in community-based rehabilitation and health promotion.	■ Working with Tilly's school community to increase their capacity to ensure that her social and educational needs are accommodated.
Transformation	These strategies involve the development of partnerships with groups who are marginalised, deprived and/or restricted, to develop services to meet their occupational needs. The aim of developing partnerships is ensure equity of service provision and opportunity. By developing these partnerships occupational therapists change the way they work, being led by the groups they are partnering with rather than by their own expertise/employers. The partnerships have the ultimate goal of facilitating participation.	*This type of strategy may include:* ■ Working with local disability groups to ensure the implementation of policy that promotes the rights of people who have an impairment – e.g. access to the school of choice, employment opportunities, accessible footpaths, availability of recreation and leisure facilities. ■ Developing the advocacy and lobbying skills of people who have an impairment to enable them to push for their rights. ■ Listening to and collaborating with Tilly to ensure her needs are voiced and met; it may also be appropriate to introduce Tilly to a support group of people who have an impairment so that her voice and needs can be considered as part of a collective.
Redistributive justice	These strategies refer to taking on direct and indirect action and advocacy through political intervention and policy implementation to develop the occupational rights of all citizens. These strategies are for the wider society rather than just for a specific community.	*This type of strategy may include:* ■ Writing letters to and personally lobbying members of parliament, local councillors and other relevant community leaders to develop policies promoting equity of services for people who have an impairment. ■ When working with Tilly ensure the fair implementation of policies, such as promoting a fair equipment provision scheme, so that she is not penalised from receiving essential government assessment for and provision of equipment because she has significant financial compensation.

TABLE 23.3
Law and McColl's (2010) Eight Types Of Occupational Therapy Strategies Based on Their Extensive Review of the International Literature

Type of Strategy	Brief Description of Strategy
Training	Strategies that focus on the remediation of deficits, such as restricted range of motion, using exercises that do not have an occupation focus or outcome.
Skill development	Strategies to improve performance of a specific task that has an occupation focus or outcome.
Education	Strategies that involve passing on relevant knowledge and information.
Task adaptation	Changing the way a task or activity is done to account for a person's abilities.
Occupation development	Strategies that promote participation in meaningful occupations.
Environmental modification	Adapting or modifying the physical environment to enable participation.
Support provision	Strategies that involve the therapist directly providing physical and/or emotional support to enable occupational performance.
Support enhancement	Strategies that involve the therapist facilitating a person's network to provide support to enable occupational performance.

TABLE 23.4

American Occupational Therapy Practice Framework's Five Enabling Strategies

Type of Strategy	Brief Description of Strategy
Create and promote (health promotion)	Strategies to encourage health promoting behaviours and attitudes.
Establish and restore (remediation, restoration)	Strategies to improve or reestablish or develop a person's ability and skill that may have been affected by an impairment.
Maintain	Strategies to ensure that a person is able to preserve his or her performance capabilities and/or that enable the person to continue to engage in occupations.
Modify (compensation, adaptation)	Strategies that change and alter a task/activity/occupation to suit the abilities and skills of a person.
Prevent (disability prevention)	Strategies that focus on eliminating or reducing the risk of occupational performance issues by addressing the personal and contextual factors that may contribute to the risk.

Modified from American Occupational Therapy Association, 2014.

TABLE 23.5

Bass, Baum, and Christiansen's (2015) Eight Types of Occupational Therapy Strategies (Approaches)

Type of Strategy	Brief Description of Strategy
Create/promote	Strategies that focus on enhancing well-being and quality of life.
Establish/restore	Strategies to recover or attain impaired physiological, neurobehavioural, cognitive and/or psychological performance capabilities.
Maintain/habilitate	Strategies that focus on maintaining a person's current abilities and capabilities.
Modify/compensate	Strategies that involve the use of assistive technologies or alterations of the environment to reduce the effects of a person's impaired performance capabilities when engaged in occupations.
Prevent	Strategies that focus on eliminating or restricting the effect of predicted difficulties and complications.
Educate	Strategies that involve passing on relevant knowledge and information.
Consult	Strategies that involve the therapist collaborating with the person to enable the person to develop effective problem-solving approaches.
Advocate	Strategies that involve the therapist working politically on behalf of, as well as with, the person 'to promote changes in policies, procedures and practices' (Bass et al., 2015, p. 64).

CONCLUSION

Occupational therapy enabling skills and strategies are complex. When applying their skills and planning, designing, implementing and evaluating strategies, occupational therapists have to be critical thinkers to address the occupational goals of the person, as there is no formula to follow when working with people. Practising in this way ensures that occupational therapists use their skills and strategies in an infinite variety of ways to promote and maintain the health and well-being of people, ultimately improving the occupational performance and engagement of individual, groups and communities.

 http://evolve.elsevier.com/Curtin/OT

REFERENCES

American Occupational Therapy Association (2014). Occupational therapy practice framework: Domains and process (3rd ed.). *American Journal of Occupational Therapy, 68*(1), S1–S48.

Bannigan, K., & Moores, A. (2009). A model of professional thinking: Integrating reflective practice and evidence based practice. *Canadian Journal of Occupational Therapy, 76*, 342–350.

Barros, D., Ghirardi, M., Lopes, R., & Galheigo, S. (2005). Social occupational therapy: A socio-historical perspective. In F. Kronenberg, S. Algado, & N. Pollard (Eds.), *Occupational therapy without borders: Learning from the spirit of survivors* (pp. 140–151). Edinburgh: Elsevier Churchill Livingstone.

Bass, J., Baum, C., & Christiansen, C. (2015). Interventions and outcomes: The Person-Environment-Occupation-Performance (PEOP) occupational therapy process. In C. Christiansen, C. Baum, & J. Bass (Eds.), *Occupational therapy: Performance, participation and well-being* (4th ed., pp. 57–79). Thorofare, NJ: Slack.

Christiansen, C., Baum, C., & Bass, J. (2015). The Person-Environment-Occupation-Performance (PEOP) model. In C. Christiansen, C. Baum, & J. Bass (Eds.), *Occupational therapy: Performance, participation and well-being* (4th ed., pp. 23–47). Thorofare, NJ: Slack.

Christiansen, C., & Townsend, E. (2010a). An introduction to occupation. In C. Christiansen, & E. Townsend (Eds.), *Introduction to occupation: The art of science and living* (pp. 2–34). Upper Saddle River, NJ: Prentice Hall.

Christiansen, C., & Townsend, E. (2010b). The occupational nature of social groups. In C. Christiansen, & E. Townsend (Eds.), *Introduction to occupation: The art of science and living* (pp. 175–210). Upper Saddle River, NJ: Prentice Hall.

Doble, S., & Santha, J. (2008). Occupational well-being: Rethinking occupational therapy outcomes. *Canadian Journal of Occupational Therapy, 75*(3), 184–190.

Duncan, E. (2012). Introduction. In E. Duncan (Ed.), *Foundations for practice in occupational therapy* (5th ed., pp. 3–7). Edinburgh: Elsevier Churchill Livingstone.

Hocking, C. (2013). Occupation for public health. *New Zealand Journal of Occupational Therapy, 60*(1), 33–37.

Holm, M., Rogers, J., & Stone, R. (2003). Person-task-environment interventions: A decision-making guide. In E. Crepeau, E. Cohn, & B. Schell (Eds.), *Willard and Spackman's occupational therapy* (10th ed., pp. 460–490). Philadelphia: Lippincott, Williams and Wilkins.

Kronenberg, F., & Pollard, N. (2005). Introduction: A beginning. In F. Kronenberg, S. Algodo, & N. Pollard (Eds.), *Occupational therapy without borders: Learning from the spirit of survivors* (pp. 1–13). Edinburgh: Churchill Livingstone.

Kronenberg, F., Algodo, S., & Pollard, N. (Eds.). (2005). *Occupational therapy without borders: Learning from the spirit of survivors.* Edinburgh: Churchill Livingstone.

Kronenberg, F., Pollard, N., & Sakellariou, D. (2011). *Occupational therapy without borders (Vol. 2): Towards an ecology of occupation-based practices.* Edinburgh: Churchill Livingstone.

Law, M., & McColl, M. (2010). *Interventions, effects, and outcomes in occupational therapy: Adults and older adults.* Thorofare, NJ: Slack.

Layton, N. (2014). Sylvia Docker lecture: The practice, research, policy nexus in contemporary occupational therapy. *Australian Occupational Therapy Journal, 61*, 49–57.

McColl, M., & Law, M. (2015). Occupational models of practice interventions. In M. McColl, & M. Law (Eds.), *Theoretical basis of occupational therapy* (3rd ed., pp. 125–130). Thorofare, NJ: Slack.

Moyers, P. (2005). Introduction to occupation-based practice. In C. Christiansen, C. Baum, & J. Bass-Haugen (Eds.), *Occupational therapy: Performance, participation and well-being* (3rd ed., pp. 221–234). Thorofare, NJ: Slack.

Pollard, N., Alsop, A., & Kronenberg, F. (2005). Reconceptualising occupational therapy. *British Journal of Occupational Therapy, 68*(11), 524–526.

Pollard, N., Sakellariou, D., & Kronenberg, F. (Eds.). (2009). *A political practice of occupational therapy.* Edinburgh: Churchill Livingstone.

Reed, K., Hocking, C., & Smythe, L. (2011). Exploring the meaning of occupation: The case for phenomenology. *Canadian Journal of Occupational Therapy, 78*(5), 303–310.

Robertson, D., Warrender, F., & Barnard, S. (2015). The critical occupational therapy practitioner: How to define expertise? *Australian Occupational Therapy Journal, 62*, 68–71.

Townsend, E., Beagan, B., Kumas-Tan, Z., et al. (2007). Enabling: Occupational therapy's core competency. In E. Townsend, & H. Polatajko (Eds.), *Enabling occupation II: Advancing an occupational therapy vision for health, well-being and justice through occupation* (pp. 87–135). Ottawa: CAOT Publications ACE.

Townsend, E., & Polatajko, H. (Eds.). (2007). *Enabling occupation II: Advancing an occupational therapy vision for health, well-being, and justice through occupation.* Ottawa: CAOT Publications ACE.

Watson, R. (2006). Being before doing: The cultural identity (essence) of occupational therapy. *Australian Occupational Therapy Journal, 53*, 151–158.

Weinstock-Zlotnick, G., & Hinojosa, J. (2004). Bottom-up or top-down evaluation: Is one better than the other? *American Journal of Occupational Therapy, 58*(5), 594–599.

Wilcock, A., & Hocking, C. (2015). *An occupational perspective of health* (3rd ed.). Thorofare, NJ: Slack.

World Federation of Occupational Therapists (2004). *Position statement: Community based rehabilitation. Retrieved from, www.wfot.org/ResourceCentre.aspx.*

World Federation of Occupational Therapists (2006). *Position statement: Human rights. Retrieved from, www.wfot.org/ResourceCentre.aspx.*

World Federation of Occupational Therapists (2010). *Position statement: Diversity and culture. Retrieved from, www.wfot.org/ResourceCentre.aspx.*

World Federation of Occupational Therapists (2012). *Statement on occupational therapy. Retrieved from, www.wfot.org/Portals/0/PDF/STATEMENT_ON_OCCUPATIONAL_THERAPY_300811.pdf.*

World Federation of Occupational Therapists (2014a). *Position statement: Human displacement. Retrieved from, www.wfot.org/ResourceCentre.aspx.*

World Federation of Occupational Therapists (2014b). *Position statement: Disaster preparedness and response. Retrieved from, www.wfot.org/ResourceCentre.aspx.*

Youngstrom, M., & Brown, C. (2005). Categories and principles of interventions. In C. Christiansen, C. Baum, & J. Bass-Haugen (Eds.), *Occupational therapy: Performance, participation and well-being* (3rd ed., pp. 397–411). Thorofare, NJ: Slack.

24

ADVOCACY AND LOBBYING

VALMAE ROSE ■ KEVIN COCKS ■ LESLEY CHENOWETH

CHAPTER OUTLINE

Abstract
This chapter is designed to introduce the concepts of advocacy
and lobbying as they pertain to the role of an occupational therapist. As professionals with a broad theoretical background and
a comprehensive understanding of the individuals with whom
they work, occupational therapists are in a key position to initiate, support and implement change for people experiencing
illness, injury or impairment. Advocacy and lobbying are
defined and contextualised through both real-world examples
and underpinning theoretical frameworks, and the skills,
knowledge and values critical to developing occupational therapists as agents of change are outlined. Finally, the dilemmas
and tensions that emerge when venturing into advocacy and
lobbying for change are explored.

KEY POINTS

- Occupational therapists, by virtue of their skills, knowledge
  and value base, are well positioned to advocate and
  lobby for individuals striving for an ordinary
  (or extraordinary) life.

- Defining disability as either a personal tragedy (moral
  model) or in terms of deficit (medical model) locates

disability within the individual and fails to address the
issue of disabling environments.

- The social model proposes that society creates physical
  and attitudinal barriers that prevent or limit a person's
  full participation in the society.

- For professionals working with vulnerable people, advocacy can be understood as the act of directly representing or defending those people.

- Lobbying involves taking direct action to influence a
  political decision, policy or law.

- There are three strategies for influencing policy and
  effecting change: the rational-empirical, the normative
  reeducation and the power-coercive strategies.

- Putting aside one's identity as a 'professional' or 'expert'
  to work *with* rather than *for* people experiencing illness,
  injury or impairment presents challenges for occupational therapists.

- Occupational therapists are in a position to extend the
  parameters of their practice moving beyond mere therapeutic strategies to consider the social and economic barriers to people's enjoyment of a full and rich life.

It is individuals who change societies, who give birth to ideas, who, by standing out against the tide of opinion, change them.
Doris Lessing

INTRODUCTION

Occupational therapists are professionals who go about their work equipped with knowledge, skills and, ideally, a value base that is consistent with the goal of being of service directly to individuals and indirectly to their families, friends and, ultimately, to the community. Occupational therapists apply creative solutions to somewhat defined needs with the aim of supporting people to independently engage in the community with the life roles they choose for themselves. They understand the value of meaningful relationships, support people to be connected to their community and inspire them in the direction of their own personal vision for the future.

Occupational therapists have an understanding of the following:

- The complex factors involved in living and working in the community without barriers
- The importance of having valued roles and of experiencing the ordinary rhythms and routines of life
- The ethical and moral right of all people to make and to experience the consequences of decisions about their own life; not just the everyday decisions but the big decisions – who to live with, where to live and how to define oneself
- The importance of being defined by one's own choices, desires and experiences, and not by a person's impairment or how a person responds to services offered

Occupational therapists, by virtue of their skills, knowledge and value base, are well positioned to support individuals striving for an ordinary (or extraordinary) life, advocating on their behalf against injustice or lobbying for change at a range of levels. Occupational therapists know the boundaries and limitations of their learning and values and, above all, their understanding of the lived experience of the people with whom they work. They do not pretend to understand the experience of the people they support and do not pass judgement. They trust the intuitive, self-determined actions and requests of people and comfortably work alongside those they support.

The purpose of this chapter is to introduce the concepts of advocacy and lobbying as they apply to the work of occupational therapists. Although often part of the system or service that needs changing, the occupational therapist is in a unique position to initiate, support and implement change at a range of levels. This chapter will define and contextualise advocacy and lobbying for the occupational therapist, propose a range of skills, knowledge and values considered critical to effective advocacy and lobbying, and begin to explore the dilemmas and tensions that arise when venturing into advocacy and lobbying.

UNDERSTANDING AND CONTEXTUALISING MODELS OF DISABILITY

Occupational therapists encounter a range of models that underpin their understandings of disability. These profoundly influence practice. Sometimes these models are implicit and therefore, if left unexamined, can give rise to tensions and incoherence in practice. In this section, three models that relate to disability and that can influence practice are explored.

Models of Disability

Throughout history disability has primarily been conceptualised as deviance from normalcy (Shakespeare, 2014). It is well recognised that the decision-making frameworks of people are significantly influenced by their personal values, belief systems and commonly held assumptions about class, culture, race, gender, sexuality and, in particular, disability (Brehm, Kassin, & Fein, 2002). Disability activists and academics have identified two dominant paradigms or models in the history of oppression and the disempowerment of people experiencing illness, injury or impairment: the *moral model* and the *medical model*. These two models can still be found in policy and practice; however, the third way', the *social model*, has gained prominence internationally and underpins many aspects of policy, legislation and programmes espousing a human rights approach.

The *moral model* is the oldest paradigm for understanding disability. Based in religious mythology, it regards disability as resulting from sin and shame and has led to the concealment and exclusion of individuals with impairments. People experiencing illness, injury or impairment are primarily seen as objects of suspicion and intolerance (Hughes, 2015). A positive outcome that has emerged as a reaction to the moral model includes the formation of principles that have led to human rights and social justice for socially excluded and marginalised people.

The *medical model* emerged as science took over from religion in the explanation of natural phenomena. The premise of the medical model is essentially that disability is the result of individual pathology, disease or injury; it is the problem of an impaired body or body function that requires attention (see e.g. Crinson, Duncan, & Yuill, 2010). When the cure is not forthcoming, issues relating to the disability are deemed to reside within the individual and to place no obligation on society in general. Support services tend to be limited and inadequate, and the lives of individuals with impairments are largely shaped by 'professionals' (Shakespeare, 2013).

Occupational therapy has been strongly aligned with the medical model in the past, before the 'renaissance of occupation,' a term coined by Whiteford, Townsend, and Hocking (2000). The interventions that stem from the medical model therefore are usually based on processes of assessment, therapeutic interventions and treatment of the individual (Kielhofner, 2004).

It is also important to recognise that every level of legislation, policy and practice brings its own definitions of disability and a list of criteria by which people can be included (or excluded) as relevant. Defining disability as either a personal tragedy (individual/moral model) or in terms of deficit (medical model) both locate disability within the individual and fail to address the real issues – that of disabling environments (Chenoweth, 2006).

Conversely, the *social model* comes from the perspective that disability is the result of social barriers and disabling environments. Here the problem lies in a society that creates physical and attitudinal barriers that prevent or limit a person's full participation in the society (see e.g. Crinson et al., 2010). The United Nations Convention on the Rights of Persons with Disabilities (CRPD; United Nations, 2006) heralded an official paradigm shift in attitudes towards people experiencing illness, injury or impairment and to respond to their concerns. The convention is based firmly on universal human rights. People experiencing illness, injury or impairment have the same rights and opportunities as all citizens and should not be regarded merely as charity or welfare recipients (Officer & Groce, 2009).

Occupational therapists may incorporate both the medical and social models into their practice. Both have legitimacy and play an important role, but it is important to understand and apply both perspectives appropriately. In acute settings, the *medical model* predominates and interventions need to address acute issues for an individual. However, beyond the acute stage, social forces and factors largely dictate what life will be like for a person with impairment. The occupational perspective on humans and health make occupational therapists well placed to respond to these social forces and factors.

Vulnerable Identities

It is widely acknowledged that throughout history and across cultures, people experiencing illness, injury or impairment have not been visible, their lives largely assigned to the margins of society (Norwich, 2007). The following ode symbolises, the reality of the lives often led by vulnerable and marginalised people experiencing illness, injury or impairment.

Ode to Vulnerable People's Lives

PINBALL LIVING
Balls in a pinball machine have no life of their own,
They are set into motion by someone else and
Then bounce from one place to another without any clear direction.
Sometimes even making big scores,
But then sinking into oblivion until someone sets them off again.

Anon

In general, society's beliefs and attitudes about disability are not mistaken in any simple way, as each assumption contains a kernel of experiential truth about encounters between those with authority and those with impairments. However, when tacit

theories and untested assumptions like these underlie public policy and social relations, they limit the life opportunities of people experiencing illness, injury or impairment, their families and allies (see e.g. Barnes, Oliver, & Barton, 2002). Several common negative assumptions about people experiencing illness, injury or impairment and the possible impact of these assumptions are listed in Box 24.1 (NB: In this box the term 'people with disability' is used to collectively refer to people experiencing illness, injury or impairment).

Historical and attitudinal factors have contributed to a failure of public policy dealing with disability in many jurisdictions. Services for people with disability have been primarily driven by

---

BOX 24.1
COMMON NEGATIVE ASSUMPTIONS ABOUT PEOPLE WITH DISABILITY AND THE IMPACT OF THESE ASSUMPTIONS

Common negative assumptions that restrict and restrain people with disability:

- Thinking of people with disability as partial, limited or lesser.
- Putting people with disability on a pedestal.
- Regarding people with disability as perfect objects of charity.
- Seeing disability as a sickness to be fixed.
- Stereotyping people with disability as a menace to themselves and society.
- Attributing 'special' talents to people with disability.
- Restricting the social circle of people with disability to other people with disability.
- Locating the problem within the individual rather than in societal attitudes or in the built environment.

Impact of negative assumptions on people with disability:

- Rejection by family, neighbours, and even paid carers and services.
- Isolation from nondisabled peers.
- Restricted options for development, growth and enrichment.
- Concentration of people with disability into social groupings of rejected people.
- A very circumscribed set of role options.
- Loss of control and autonomy.
- Material poverty, affecting health, housing and life expectancy.
- Diminished sense of individuality and uniqueness.
- Restricted social relationships, resulting in a lack of allies in times of need.
- Neglect, damage and abuse.

Adapted from Wolfensberger, W. (1983). Social role valorization: A proposed new term for the principle of normalization. *Mental Retardation, 21*(6), 234–239.

economic and fiscal policy, rather than social policy, and human rights frameworks have largely taken a back seat. Demand for greater accountability of public funds, increasing requirements for legislative and regulatory compliance, and a long history of underinvestment in disability services have resulted in crisis-driven rather than needs driven allocation of resources (Wills & Chenoweth, 2005).

The historic failures of public policy for people with disability, particularly with regard to housing, personal care and support services, transport and law, are well illustrated both in human rights reports and in anecdotal accounts of peoples' lived experience (see e.g. Kothari, 2007). People experiencing illness, injury or impairment have a much higher unemployment rate and a much lower workforce participation rate than their nondisabled peers. People with disability are much more likely to be homeless, be victims of crime (e.g. rates of sexual assault up to 10 times those in the general population), to underreport crime and to experience inadequate police follow-up (prosecution and conviction). In addition, incarceration rates of people experiencing illness, injury or impairment are up to 10 times greater than for people without experiencing illness, injury or impairment (Queensland Advocacy Incorporated, 2007).

In recent years, disability programmes have heralded more individualised approaches to service supports and funding. Based on choice and control and clearly in line with the CRPD, these programmes provide direct funding and/or increased control into the hands of people experiencing illness, injury or impairment and their families.

ADVOCACY AND LOBBYING

Advocacy

The concept of advocacy has primarily existed throughout recorded history as a concept in law and is derived from the Latin *advocare*, which means 'to be called to stand beside'. The right to legal representation dates from the system of law created by the Romans, and this right has existed in British law since the thirteenth century. The concept of guardianship also evolved through Roman law to ensure the best interest of those with diminished decision-making capacity were upheld. Over the past 100 years or so, as notions of human rights have become more established, advocacy has become increasingly widespread and its conceptualisation further refined. Formal industrial advocacy has been provided by trade and labour unions for more than 100 years. The women's suffrage movement advocated strongly for the rights of women to vote. More recent social rights movements – the civil rights movement in America, the antiapartheid movement in South Africa, and the Aboriginal and Torres Strait Islander peoples' land rights movement in Australia – have all helped to popularise ideas of rights.

Contemporary rights movements and protection regimes, such as those affecting children, older people and people with disability, have all led to the concept of advocacy for these groups. Early definitions of advocacy drew upon Wolfensberger's

(1998) work, which has shaped the advocacy movement in many Western democracies. By the early 1990s, in the human service arena it was common practice to incorporate the word *advocacy* into everyday language. In human service language, advocacy began to replace concepts such as lobbying, activism, community development and good job performance. The word *advocacy* almost seemed to have greater prestige for the user. Perhaps its usage reassured the practitioner that they were working within a social justice framework that validated their actions as being fair and ethical. Occupational therapists should take care not to use or practice the concept of advocacy loosely. A quote by an occupational therapist advocating for a disabled student in a mainstream setting reminds us of this.

> *Remember that as an advocate you are there to help represent the views, wishes and best interests of the person you are advocating for. As an occupational therapist it can be tempting to slip into the role of mediator and take into account and give credence to both sides. This is not advocacy and will lessen the effectiveness of your advocacy. While it is desirable to resolve the tensions of the situation, as an advocate, you cannot compromise your position. It is important to make it clear to all parties before commencing, exactly what the role of an advocate is.*
>
> **Gretel, Occupational Therapist**

Advocate is a widely used term which has many meanings depending on the context. The online Oxford Dictionary (n.d.) defines an advocate as (1) a person who publicly supports or recommends a particular cause or policy; and (2) a person who puts a case on someone else's behalf.

This definition situates advocacy as a process of pleading or arguing about an idea or a cause. For professionals working with vulnerable people, advocacy can be understood as the act of directly representing or defending those people. Different professional groups define and interpret advocacy and the advocacy role according to their own principles, knowledge and skill base. For example, lawyers have a strict legal notion of advocacy, whereas a social worker may see advocacy as including a broader range of activities. For occupational therapists, advocacy may be a relatively new idea but one which has increasing legitimacy when working with and for people experiencing illness, injury or impairment. Different ways to define advocacy are defined in Table 24.1.

Lobbying

As well as different forms of advocacy, occupational therapists and other allied health professionals, such as social workers, are often engaged in other activities such as lobbying or activism. This might be as part of their paid role or it might be outside of work – something therapists engage with in a voluntary capacity as a concerned citizen.

Lobbying involves attempting to influence a political decision, policy or law. The exact origin of the word 'lobbying' is uncertain (Montpetit, 2004). Lobbying usually takes a direct form – that is,

TABLE 24.1	
Different Types of Advocacy	
Legal advocacy	Involves representation by legally qualified advocates, usually solicitors or lawyers.
Formal advocacy	Sometimes called 'professional advocacy'; usually refers to schemes run by voluntary groups employing salaried coordinators and paid staff.
Citizen advocacy	A long-term, one-to-one partnership between user and advocate, usually as part of a coordinated scheme, with paid coordinator and volunteer partners.
Self-advocacy	A term used to describe people speaking out for themselves. 'People first' organisations are an example.
Peer advocacy	Defined as support from advocates who have themselves been service users.
Social advocacy	Speaking, acting and writing with minimal conflict of interest on behalf of the sincerely perceived interests of a disadvantaged person or group to promote, protect and defend their welfare and justice by: ■ being on their side and no one else's side; ■ being primarily concerned with their fundamental needs; and ■ remaining loyal and accountable to them in a way that is emphatic and vigorous and which is, or is likely to be, costly to the advocate or advocacy group (Wolfensberger, 1998).
Systems advocacy	Primarily concerned with influencing and changing the system (legislation, policy and practice) in ways that will benefit disadvantaged groups, particularly people experiencing illness, injury or impairment as a group within society. Systems advocates will encourage changes to the law, government and service policies and community attitudes. Usually systems advocacy agencies do not engage with individual advocacy. To do so can cause conflicts around the use of resources, focus and purpose. However, individual advocacy will highlight systems failure, thus informing systems advocates of emerging or existing areas requiring systemic reform.
Individual advocacy	Refers to action taken to encourage and assist individuals with an impairment to achieve and maintain their rights as citizens and to achieve equity of access and participation in the community. Strategies may include speaking or standing up for the person with impairment, supporting people to represent their own interests and making sure people know about the different ways they can have a say.

directly to the government official, the politician or the leader with power to make decisions. Often we lobby such people to vote or make a favourable decision on a new law or policy – for example, on an antidiscrimination law or on a new funding programme for people experiencing illness, injury or impairment. We can also lobby more broadly – perhaps to the general public before a referendum on accessible transport or labour laws.

Lobbying needs to be differentiated from activism, which refers to planned behaviour designed to achieve social or political objectives through activities such as consciousness raising, developing a coalition, political campaigning and producing publicity to influence social change. Activism is often undertaken as part of a bigger movement. For example, the community living movement, an international social movement for supporting people with disability and their families to live in the community rather than in institutions, often employed activist tactics to get their message across and bring about social change. People in this movement have held street marches, gathered petitions, held media conferences and even made documentaries to get their message across. All these activities were well planned and coordinated and all involved significant publicity. Many occupational therapists were involved as activists alongside people experiencing illness, injury or impairment, families and other professionals.

Lobbying is usually tactical in nature and focuses on a particular solution or course of action, rather than drawing attention to a problem (as in activism). Lobbying is about systematically persuading targeted, influential individuals or

agencies to make a decision. Most often it requires the 'lobbyist' to present a compelling, evidence-based case for action. This evidence may include data, research or story of lived experience framed in a way that supports the argument or case being made or illustrates the consequences of not taking a particular action. Effective lobbying also requires relationship and network building. The level of impact of lobbying efforts is often proportional to the quality of the respectful working relationship between the lobbyist and the decision maker or agency.

In the case of the Australian disability sector, significant social change has often been the result of a combination of an active social movement (activism), direct representation of individuals and families affected (advocacy) and strategic influencing of policy makers (lobbying).

THE OCCUPATIONAL THERAPIST AS AN AGENT OF CHANGE

By definition, an occupational therapist working within the context of a human service organisation cannot be considered an independent advocate. They can, however, advocate or lobby internally or externally for change to an organisation or on behalf of an individual or group.

Community service organisations often state advocacy as part of their organisational mission, but this is not to be confused with advocacy in its pure form. Specifically, these organisations refer to their role in educating the public and those who influence public policy about issues of concern to those the organisation serves.

Public policy (within a framework of legislation) reflects our beliefs, through government, about how resources should be allocated, to whom and on what basis. In doing so, they determine the balance of power, choice and opportunity for people who are disadvantaged (Hallahan, 2015).

In considering the respective roles of organisations and individual practitioners, with regard to influencing public policy (and ultimately outcomes for people experiencing illness, injury or impairment), it is important to understand the relationship among legislation, policy and practice. In simplest terms, legislation provides the foundation in law for public policy, which in turn drives resource allocation for programmes and practice. The scenario is made more complex by the fact that the legislation, policy and practice that affects a person arises from a multitude of government departments, across multiple jurisdictions in an ever-changing political environment.

As well as recognising the implications of how disability is defined at a legislative and public policy level, occupational therapists must also be discerning about the messages conveyed by the internal policy of their own organisation. To be effective, it is critical that occupational therapists not view the organisation as the passive context in which they operate (Jones & May, 1992). Irrespective of role, there will be many opportunities for occupational therapists to constructively challenge and potentially reshape organisational policy. Suggestions for successful advocacy and lobbying are provided in Box 24.2.

STRATEGIES TO EFFECT CHANGE

Change is often difficult and requires a strategic approach. Three strategies for influencing policy and effecting change are the rational-empirical, the normative reeducation and the power-coercive strategies (Burke, Lake, & Paine, 2009). All three strategies involve the exercise of power, authority and influence in varying ways to effect change.

The *rational-empirical strategy,* which exerts influence to resist or promote change through the planning, research and evaluation of policy, will be relevant where occupational therapists have policy development roles or the opportunity to give feedback on policy through the agencies continuous improvement processes. The following example illustrates this point.

The occupational therapist can significantly influence policy development by offering grounded examples, using real people and experiences, as evidence for why a particular policy direction will or won't work. A regular part of my work now is to gather disability service providers together to consider new government initiatives at an early stage. By giving service providers the chance to consider new initiatives early, they are able to give constructive feedback, using their current clients as evidence. Because the new policy is still in early draft stage and

---

BOX 24.2
TIPS FOR ADVOCATING AND LOBBYING

- Have a plan. Plan for incremental change to systems and policies that will result in sustainable change in people's lives.
- Regularly check your own intentions. Sometimes the personal agenda to influence can become bigger and more important than the goal.
- Work to build credibility. Always be able to back up argument with research and examples. Ensure your own behaviour reflects your arguments. Ensure all strategies are aligned to your stated goal and stated value base.
- Work to demonstrate integrity in lobbying. Respect confidentiality of information provided and keep all agendas on the table – that is, be transparent and communicate intention clearly.
- Manage the balance between gains for an individual versus gains for a group/community.
- Manage the balance between short-term and long-term gains. Have a clear plan for work and understand that compromise and patience will be required.
- Avoid discouragement by celebrating small gains and staying focused on the goal.
- Be prepared to be creative and flexible. If one strategy fails to deliver, be prepared to let it go and come up with another.
- Avoid confrontation. Avoid setting people up to be outraged and unhappy when their energy could be guided towards creating a solution.
- Build a network of supporters and actively support connections with and between them.
- Ensure supporters are given all the information and are empowered to come to their own conclusions about the evidence (not just the evidence that supports your argument).
- Avoid exploiting people who are already vulnerable in the interests of a short-term win.

---

the feedback is given in the spirit of being helpful, government is usually happy to accommodate the recommended changes. The overall result is more grounded, useful policy, and a higher level of ownership by the agencies who will be implementing the policy.

Vanessa, Occupational Therapist

The *normative reeducation strategy* focuses on the attitudes, values, skills and relationships within an organisation, and attempts to bring about change through education and training, as well as other organisation development techniques. This approach is a powerful and meaningful way for practitioners to inspire and implement change at a ground level. An example of how language can be a powerful strategy is found in the following quote.

> When I started working for a nongovernment agency about 4 years ago, I noticed that many of my peers used language that promoted difference – an us and them attitude to government and to some of the other stakeholder groups we dealt with. I made a deliberate attempt to introduce new language such as working toward alignment rather than demanding change, and sharing/being open to a range of perspectives to refer to differences in opinion. This new language was used consistently, in a broad range of forums and publications, resulting in a significant reduction in adversarial interactions and better relationships over time.
>
> *Vanessa, Occupational Therapist*

The *power-coercive strategy* requires more direct use of power, influence and authority to effect change in policy and/ or practice and may be less relevant to occupational therapists who operate at a ground level within the organisation.

A number of authors suggest the real point of influence for practitioners is at a practice level – the point at which policy is implemented (Chenoweth & McAuliffe, 2014). This is the point at which people gain access to services (and are supported to gain access to services). Practitioners, irrespective of their role, can use their discretion in applying rules and supporting people to make choices about the service they receive. It is at this point that occupational therapists demonstrate congruity between their values and beliefs and their actions as illustrated in Fig. 24.1. Here Gretel reflects on this congruence:

> *Always remain assertive in the face of discrimination. I am always astounded by attempts to discriminate against people with disability, especially when this is masked by a smile and the assertion of care e.g. we are only concerned about his safety. This is a very insidious form of discrimination indeed. This position was put to me when advocating for a young man with an intellectual impairment wanting to join his local football club. The club was concerned he may have a seizure (in spite of having no history of seizures) or be more vulnerable to injury during tackling.*
>
> *Gretel, Occupational Therapist*

MANAGING THE DILEMMAS AND TENSIONS ASSOCIATED WITH ADVOCACY AND LOBBYING

Working to effect change as a practitioner within human service organisations will potentially give rise to a range of tensions and dilemmas. Not the least of these is the dilemma of trying to change a system of which occupational therapists are also participants. The incongruence associated with espousing social justice and equity as the basis of a therapist's work yet failing to effect change is a potential source of frustration and discouragement for practitioners. Closely associated with this is the potential conflict between a therapist's own values and aspirations and those of the organisation. Having to put aside one's identity as a 'professional' or 'expert' to work *with* rather than *for* people experiencing illness, injury or impairment may also present a challenge for the new therapist. Shakespeare (2014)

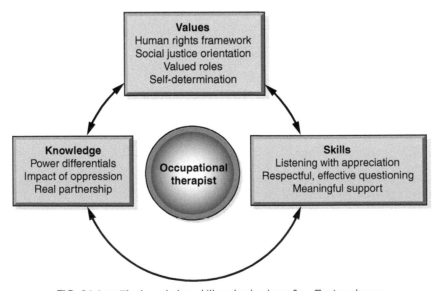

FIG. 24.1 ■ The knowledge, skill and value base for effecting change.

refers to the 'ethic of care', which relies on the person giving support finding out what people need to live with dignity and ensuring the interaction supports the interests of both parties. Approaches to ethical decision making can be useful here as a guide for beginning practitioners working through these dilemmas and tensions. One model for ethical decision making that takes into account the many factors professionals need to consider is the inclusive model. This model comprises four 'essential dimensions': accountability, critical reflection, cultural sensitivity and consultation. *Accountability* is about transparency and ability to justify decisions made. *Critical reflection* relates to the awareness of one's own patterning and the impact of one's values on practice. *Cultural sensitivity* focuses on respect for the worldview of others, whereas *consultation* refers to engaging with the wisdom of others in the interest of integrity in decision making. In combination, the four dimensions provide a strong foundation for ethical decision making (McAuliffe & Chenoweth, 2008).

CONCLUSION

The elements of advocacy and lobbying and their relevance to work in the disability field have been outlined in this chapter. The vulnerability of people experiencing illness, injury or impairment and the failure of many policies and services to address their needs create situations and contexts where a broader change is required. Occupational therapists are in a position to extend the parameters of their practice to make a real difference. This means moving beyond mere therapeutic strategies to consider the social barriers to people's enjoyment of a full and rich life. As Eric Dammann (1979) explains:

> *Belief in the values of the common people is our only hope. We cannot judge from how people behave under pressure of a society that forces them to compete for self interest or to be excluded. We must step out of our narrow social environment and learn to know the underprivileged who have never participated in our activities. When we have them with us that will be real change from below.*

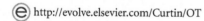 http://evolve.elsevier.com/Curtin/OT

REFERENCES

Barnes, C., Oliver, M., & Barton, L. (2002). *Disability studies today.* Cambridge: Polity Press.

Brehm, S. S., Kassin, S. M., & Fein, S. (2002). *Social psychology* (5th ed.). Boston: Houghton Mifflin.

Burke, W., Lake, D., & Paine, J. (2009). *Organisational change: A comprehensive reader.* San Francisco: Jossey-Bass.

Chenoweth, L. (2006). Disability. In W. Hong Chui, & J. Wilson (Eds.), *Social work and human services best practice.* Sydney: The Federation Press.

Chenoweth, L., & McAuliffe, D. (2014). *The road to social work and human service practice.* Brisbane: Cengage Learning Australia.

Crinson, I., Duncan, E., & Yuill, C. (2010). *Key concepts in health studies.* London: Sage Publications.

Dammann, E. (1979). *The future in our hands.* Oxford, UK: Pergamon Press.

Hallahan, L. (2015). *Australian Journal of Social Issues, 50*(2), 191–208.

Hughes, B. (2015). Disabled people as counterfeit citizens: The politics of resentment past and present. *Disability & Society, 30*(7), 991–1004.

Jones, A., & May, J. (1992). *Working in human service organisations: A critical introduction.* Melbourne: Longman Chesire.

Kielhofner, G. (2004). *Conceptual foundations of occupational therapy* (3rd ed.). Philadelphia: FA Davis.

Kothari, M. (2007). *Report of the special rapporteur on adequate housing as a component of the right to an adequate standard of living: Mission to Australia.* Geneva: United Nations.

McAuliffe, D., & Chenoweth, L. (2008). Leave no stone unturned: The inclusive model of ethical decision making. *Journal of Ethics and Social Welfare, 2*(1), 38–49.

Montpetit, E. (2004). Governance and interest group activities. In J. Bickerton, & A. G. Gagnon (Eds.), *Canadian politics.* Guelph, ON: Broadview Press.

Norwich, B. (2007). *Dilemmas of difference, inclusion & disability.* Philadelphia: Taylor & Francis.

Officer, A., & Groce, N. (2009). Key concepts in disability. *Lancet, 374*(9704), 1795–1996.

Oxford Dictionaries (n.d.). Oxford University Press. Web 11 September, 2016. http://www.oxforddictionaries.com/definition/.

Queensland Advocacy Incorporated (2007). *Disabled justice: The barriers to justice for persons with a disability in Queensland.* Brisbane, Queensland: Queensland Advocacy Incorporated.

Shakespeare, T. (2013). The social model of disability. In L. David (Ed.), *The disability studies reader* (4th ed.). London: Routledge.

Shakespeare, T. (2014). *Disability rights and wrongs revisited.* London: Routledge.

United Nations (2006). *Convention on human rights for persons with disability.* New York: UN.

Whiteford, G., Townsend, E., & Hocking, C. (2000). Reflections on a renaissance of occupation. *Canadian Journal of Occupational Therapy, 67*(1), 61–69.

Wills, R., & Chenoweth, L. (2005). Support or compliance. In P. O'Brien, & M. Sullivan (Eds.), *Allies in emancipation: Shifting from providing services to being of support* (pp. 49–64). South Melbourne: Thomson Dunmore Press.

Wolfensberger, W. (1998). *A brief introduction to social role valorization. A higher-order concept for addressing the plight of societally devalued people, and for structuring human services.* Syracuse, NY: Trinig Institute for Human Service Planning, Leadership and Change Agentry (Syracuse University).

25

EDUCATION

TAMMY HOFFMANN ■ SALLY EAMES

CHAPTER OUTLINE

Abstract

Occupational therapists provide education to individuals as part of everyday practice. If occupational therapists are to use education effectively in their daily practice, they need to be knowledgeable about relevant theories and models, which can provide therapists with useful guidelines for planning and implementing education strategies. The concept of therapists working in a collaborative partnership with individuals is also an underpinning principle that should guide education strategies. In addition to incorporating theoretical principles into the design and implementation of education strategies, therapists also need to make considered decisions about the content, format, timing, and evaluation of the strategies as well as acknowledging and accommodating individuals' health literacy and any impairments they have that may affect the understanding of information. The aim of this chapter is to provide guidelines and principles for occupational therapists to use to develop effective educational strategies.

KEY POINTS

■ Education is a core component of all areas of occupational therapy practice and should be treated like other strategies, with appropriate consideration given to its planning and evaluation.

■ As well as imparting knowledge, education can also aim to alter individuals' behaviour, attitude, beliefs, confidence, skills and decision-making ability.

■ Appropriate education empowers individuals and enables them to take responsibility for and participate in their health care.

■ Educational theories, models and principles can serve as useful guides for therapists when they are planning education strategies.

■ When planning an education strategies there are many decisions that therapists need to make, and deliberation should be given to issues related to the content, format, timing and evaluation of the intervention, as well as individuals' health literacy and any impairments that may affect understanding information.

INTRODUCTION

Education is an indelible component of occupational therapy practice. Occupational therapists continuously use education strategies in their day-to-day work with individuals. A survey of the intervention methods used by Australian occupational therapists who work with adults with physical impairment found that education and counselling were the most commonly used strategies, with three quarters of participants indicating that they use these often or most of the time (McEneany, McKenna, & Summerville, 2002). The widespread use of education was further confirmed by the finding that education and counselling were one of the top five strategies with participants from all caseloads except those working with older people, where they were rated sixth.

Despite the prevalence with which education is used by occupational therapists in their daily work with individuals, it is often not given the same thoughtful consideration as other strategies. Although the reasons for this are not clear, according to McKenna and Tooth (2006), there are a number of possible explanations for this, such as therapists:

■ Considering education to be a basic and straightforward skill that does not require specialised planning or consideration;

■ Not perceiving education to be a specific type of intervention and considering it secondary to 'real' interventions that directly relate to the care and treatment of individuals; and/or

■ Lacking an understanding of educational theories and principles and the crucial role that education can have in empowering individuals.

However, the success of many occupational therapy interventions depends on the use of sound education strategies; if occupational therapists are to use education strategies effectively in their daily practice, they need to understand the theories of education and be knowledgeable about the practical considerations associated with providing education. The aim of this chapter is to provide guidelines and principles for developing effective educational strategies for use in practice.

WHY DO OCCUPATIONAL THERAPISTS EDUCATE?

Education is far more than just imparting knowledge to individuals. In health fields, education has been defined as 'a planned learning experience using a combination of methods such as teaching, counselling, and behaviour modification techniques that influence [clients'] knowledge and health behaviour' (Bartlett, 1985, p. 323). The definition continues and highlights that education is '… an interactive process which assists [clients] to participate actively in their health care' (Bartlett, 1985, p. 323). From this definition it is clear that influencing the knowledge, attitudes and behaviour of individuals is at the centre of education. To engage an individual and allow them make informed decisions about their own health behaviour, education strategies may be used to build an individual's confidence and facilitate the acquisition of skills. Numerous systematic reviews have concluded that education that is specific to an individual's condition or disease can improve their knowledge, self-efficacy to manage chronic conditions and short-term behaviour change, improve quality of life and reduce morbidity and health care utilisation (Boyde, Turner, Thompson, & Stewart, 2011; Ronco, Iona, Fabbro, Bulfone, & Palese, 2012; Waller, Forshaw, Bryant, & Mair, 2014).

At various times, an occupational therapist will provide education for one or more of these reasons. Consider the following examples of education commonly provided by occupational therapists: teaching an individual who has had a stroke how to perform hand strengthening exercises; demonstrating to an individual how to use newly prescribed assistive equipment; educating people about their chronic health conditions and how to manage it; facilitating a person to incorporate movement precaution strategies into daily life after a total hip replacement; tutoring an individual with low back pain about strategies to use to cope with the pain and enable performance of everyday activities; and educating an individual with diabetes about behaviours to prevent health problems and complications from developing. Some of these education strategies focus on influencing knowledge in the hope that this will also influence a specific behaviour; others focus on facilitating skill development, whereas the intention of still others is to additionally influence attitudes or beliefs and consequently lifestyle behaviours.

Education can take many forms. It can be incidental or planned, formal or informal. It is often a one-to-one interaction between just the therapist and the individual, or it may take the form of a formal group education programme that the therapist is conducting for a number of individuals who have similar educational needs. There are also various formats that can be used to provide education, such as verbal, written, audio, video, computer-based or a combination of these. Considerations for the use of each of these formats are discussed later in the chapter. As well as providing education to individuals they are working with, occupational therapists often need to provide education to each individual's family and friends as they also have informational needs. And as with the individuals that the therapists work with, the educational needs of family members often extend beyond acquiring new knowledge and may, for example, require the learning of a new skill, such as how to assist with car transfers.

THEORIES, MODELS AND PRINCIPLES THAT CAN GUIDE THE IMPLEMENTATION OF EDUCATION INTERVENTIONS

For a long time it was believed that, as with other strategies, theories and models should always be drawn on when planning education strategies. However, the evidence is not consistent or clear that theory-based strategies are more effective than education strategies that do not have an explicit theoretical basis, nor it is clear which theories are superior in which circumstances. Nonetheless, therapists might find some of the principles espoused by key theories and models useful when designing education strategies and providing a rational basis for selecting various components. An overview of some theories and models will be covered in the following section along with suggestions of the ways in which these can be practically applied. In the adult education and health behaviour change literature, the distinction between the terms *theory* and *model* is often not clear. Often strategies are designed by using a combination of approaches from more than one theory or model.

Adult Learning Theory

Regardless of the goal of education, it is important that education aimed at adults is built on the principles of adult learning. The central premise of the adult learning theory is that the learning process of adults differs from that of children, and for successful adult learning, adherence to these principles is necessary. The key principles are described next, along with some of the implications for practice:

- Adults *need to know why they need to learn something before beginning to learn it* (Knowles, Holton, & Swanson, 1998). Planning an education strategy should commence with an assessment of the needs of the individuals who are to receive the education. Education should meet the expressed needs of individuals and their families. Ironically, though, individuals often are not aware of their need for information, and if they do not know that they

are lacking information, they may not perceive a need for it (Buckland, 1994). Consequently, to facilitate an individual's engagement in the learning process, therapists may need to initially educate an individual about the reasons for needing to learn and the benefits of it before conducting a needs assessment.

- Adults need to be *actively involved in learning,* rather than passive recipients of information (Knowles, 1980), with the goal of empowering learners and encouraging them to become self-directed and responsible for their learning. This can be assisted by encouraging individuals to provide input into the design and delivery of educational experiences as much as possible and making sessions interactive – rather than didactic – in nature.
- Adults have a *problem-centred orientation to learning* (Knowles, 1980). It is important that the practical application of the concepts being learned is emphasised. This can be achieved by providing how-to information and opportunities for the practice of newly learned skills.
- Adults enter the learning process with *prior experience,* and it is important that learners' life experiences are acknowledged and utilised throughout the learning process (Knowles et al., 1998). Therapists should identify individuals' prior health experiences and other life experiences and establish their existing knowledge, skills and attitudes and plan education strategies accordingly.
- Adults' *readiness to learn* will affect the outcomes of their learning (Knowles, 1980). Consequently, education strategies should meet learners' expressed needs, be sequenced according to their readiness to learn and appropriately target the learners' current confidence levels.
- Adults are most *motivated to learn when they see the content as relevant* (Knowles et al., 1998). Providing education that meets individuals' expressed needs, explaining how the education they receive will help to achieve their goals and what practical steps they can take to implement the information that they are receiving, and providing feedback on their progress can all assist in enhancing individuals' motivation to learn.

Health Belief Model

According to the Health Belief Model (Becker, 1974; Champion & Skinner, 2008), individuals are more likely to change their behaviour if they believe the following:

- They are susceptible to the condition *(perceived susceptibility)*
- The condition is serious and if untreated will impinge on their lives *(perceived severity)*
- There are benefits of taking health action *(perceived benefits)*
- Any negative aspects of the health action or barriers to undertaking it are outweighed by the benefits of the action *(perceived barriers)*

Additionally, this model includes the concept of cues to action, which trigger the decision-making process that can ultimately lead to a change in behaviour (Becker, Drachman, & Kirscht, 1974) and can be either internal or external. As an example of how this model could be used, consider a therapist who wanted to facilitate behaviour change in an individual who had experienced a stroke. The education provided might address the four components of the model, such as the seriousness and life-altering consequences of stroke *(perceived severity);* his or her vulnerability to experiencing another stroke *(perceived susceptibility);* the powerful role that changes in behaviour can have in reducing the risk of a secondary stroke *(perceived benefits);* and an individualised action plan that contains specific how-to information (to assist to overcome *perceived barriers).* The therapist may also discuss potential barriers to implementation of the action plan and, together with the individual, brainstorm solutions to overcome or cope with them.

Self-efficacy Theory

As the Health Belief Model became used with groups where the focus was long-term changes in lifestyle behaviours, it was recognised that the concept of self-efficacy needed to be added to the model (Champion & Skinner, 2008; Rosenstock, Strecher, & Becker, 1988). Self-efficacy was first described by Bandura (1977) as a concept in social cognitive theory that is fundamental to behaviour change. *Perceived self-efficacy* refers to an individual's judgement of his or her ability to perform an action to reach a desired goal (Bandura, 1986). According to self-efficacy theory, a person is more likely to perform a particular behaviour if engaging in that behaviour is expected to result in desired outcomes (Bandura, 1986). Even if individuals recognised the value in changing their behaviour, they also need to develop the confidence to carry out the behaviour before attempting the behaviour (Bandura, 1986).

As one of the goals of health education is behaviour change, self-efficacy has an important role to play in health education. Self-efficacy has been found to be a major determinant in the initiation and maintenance of behavioural change (Bandura, 1997; Strecher et al., 1986). Self-efficacy influences the amount of effort that an individual will put into a task and the length of time that he or she will persevere with the task in the face of obstacles (Bandura, 1977). According to self-efficacy theory, self-efficacy can influence the acquisition of new behaviours, inhibition of existing behaviours and disinhibition of behaviours (Bandura, 1977). It has been demonstrated that self-efficacy can be enhanced through education and that higher self-efficacy is related to successful attempts at behaviour change and improved health status (Clark et al., 1992; Lorig et al., 1989).

It is important to note that self-efficacy refers to specific behaviours in particular situations (Bandura, 1977). It is not a global trait or personality characteristic. Unlike personality characteristics, which are difficult to alter, self-efficacy is malleable and able to be altered (Lorig & Holman, 1993). Therefore when a therapist is attempting to alter self-efficacy (using the strategies listed next) it is important that the therapist is specific about the change sought. For example, a therapist in a cardiac rehabilitation programme providing education to an individual about the need to make healthy lifestyle changes would need to address each specific behaviour (such as regular exercise, quitting smoking, managing stress levels and healthy eating) separately. Each specific behaviour requires separate discussion and action plans. There are a number of strategies that therapists can use to enhance an individual's self-efficacy (Prohaska & Lorig, 2001; Strecher et al., 1986), such as the following:

■ *Performance accomplishment or skill mastery:* This strategy involves using incremental goal-setting, breaking the desired behaviour down into smaller steps, and ensuring the individual achieves success in performing the easier steps before attempting the more difficult ones. An example of when a therapist may use this strategy would be when helping an individual with a lower limb amputation learn to independently perform self-care tasks such as dressing and showering. This strategy requires therapists to use their skills in activity analysis and grading, which are core occupational therapy skills.

■ *Modelling:* This strategy involves an individual observing other people who appear similar, such as peers, performing the desired behaviour. If written information is used as part of education, it is important that the modelling strategy is also applied to the written material and that it contains illustrations of people similar to the individual in terms of characteristics such as age, body shape, and ethnicity.

■ *Verbal persuasion:* In this strategy, therapists talk with individuals and emphasise the importance of performing the behaviour.

■ *Reinterpreting signs and symptoms:* In this strategy, therapists clarify information with an individual, correct any myths or misconceptions that they may have, and aim to lessen any fear and anxiety about physiological signs and symptoms by explaining how to reinterpret them. For example, the therapist working with an individual who has an upper limb burn and who needs to perform frequent gentle stretching exercises to prevent contractures from developing may need to explain to the person that feeling some pain or discomfort while doing the stretching is normal and that it is not harming, but helping, the burned area.

Transtheoretical Model

As highlighted earlier in this chapter, a characteristic goal of education is behaviour change. The transtheoretical model considers the transition points in behaviour change and the underlying factors that facilitate change from one stage to another (Prohaska & Lorig, 2001). According to the transtheoretical model, change is a process that consists of six discrete stages and individuals move through these stages, although not necessarily in a linear fashion, as they adopt a behaviour (Prochaska, Di Clemente, & Norcross, 1992). Another element of this model is the process of change component, which states that there are specific activities that individuals use to progress through the stages (Prochaska et al., 1992). The six stages, along with some strategies (Neufeld, 2006; Prochaska et al., 1992) that can be used to assist individuals to move through them are described in Table 25.1.

Theories of Reasoned Action and Planned Behaviour

According to the theory of reasoned action, a person's *intention* to perform a particular behaviour is considered the most important predictor of behaviour, and this intention is a result of both their attitude towards that behaviour and their perception of the social norm (Montano & Kasprzyk, 2008; Sharma & Romas, 2008). A person's *attitude* is a result of both a belief that a particular outcome will be achieved from a certain behaviour *(behavioural belief)* and the value the person attaches to that outcome *(evaluation)*. One's perception of the social norm – or the *subjective norm* – is a combination of a person's belief of whether other people think of the behaviour as desirable or not *(normative belief)* and the *motivation to comply* with what other people think. (Montano & Kasprzyk, 2008; Sharma & Romas, 2008). Additionally, other variables, such as demographics and personality, are acknowledged as influencing these constructs (Montano & Kasprzyk, 2008).

The theory of planned behaviour builds on the theory of reasoned action in that a person's *perceived behavioural control* is considered a third influence on intention. Perceived behaviour control is similar to self-efficacy and is described in this theory as being the extent to which a person feels in control of completing the particular behaviour. It is a combination of both the perceived effect of any internal or external factors that might make it easier or harder to change behaviour *(control beliefs)* and the perceived ease or difficulty of performing that behaviour under those conditions *(perceived power)* (Montano & Kasprzyk, 2008; Sharma & Romas, 2008). As a result, the practical implications of these theories include the use of brainstorming, discussion and role play to change behaviour; use of incentives and role models; and reducing barriers and breaking healthy behaviour

TABLE 25.1		
Stages of the Transtheoretical Model and Strategies That Can Be Used to Assist Individuals to Move Through the Stages		
Name of Stage	**Description of Stage**	**Aim of Strategies Used in This Stage**
Precontemplation	The individual has no intention to change behaviour within the next 6 months.	To increase awareness through activities such as providing information about the risk and the need for change.
Contemplation	The individual has an awareness of a problem that needs action and intends to take action within the next 6 months.	To increase the individual's confidence and motivation to change by reemphasising the benefits of change, discussing possible action plans along with potential barriers and solutions to coping with them, and, where appropriate, incorporating the support of family and friends.
Preparation	The individual intends to change behaviour within the next month and in the past year has taken significant action towards the desired behaviour.	To initiate action, through strategies such as deciding on an action plan, breaking it down into small steps and using goal setting to incrementally achieve each step.
Action	The individual has made observable behaviour change, to a specified criterion that is sufficient to reduce risks to health, within the past 6 months.	To help the individual commit to the change, by using strategies such as providing encouragement and support, discussing and problem-solving any difficulties that have arisen, enlisting the support of family and friends, and planning to prevent relapse.
Maintenance	The individual has changed behaviour for more than 6 months and is striving to prevent relapse.	To help the individual convert the new behaviour into a lifestyle habit, through activities such as joining self-help groups (if applicable), discussing and trialling coping strategies, and implementing steps to prevent relapse.
Termination	The individual has total self-efficacy regarding the behaviour and regardless of the situation, does not revert to previous undesirable behaviour.	Self-efficacy in this model refers to an individual's confidence to cope in high-risk situations and not revert to engaging in undesirable behaviours (Prochaska, Redding, & Evers, 2008).

down into smaller steps. Although the predictive power of the theory of planned behaviour exceeds that of the theory of reasoned action, there is evidence that they both can be used to predict health-related behaviour with greater effect than the Health Belief Model (Taylor et al., 2007).

The Behaviour Change Wheel

For education strategies where the goal is behaviour change, the behaviour change wheel (Fig. 25.1) may provide some useful guidance. Michie, van Stralen, and West (2011) drew on 19 existing frameworks to develop a behaviour change wheel framework. At the centre of this framework lies the Capability, Opportunity and Motivation Behaviour system (or COM-B), in which capability and opportunity both influence an individual's motivation and all three in turn can influence – and be influenced by – behaviour (Michie et al., 2011). Around the COM-B (in a middle 'layer' of the wheel) sit nine intervention functions: environmental restructuring, restrictions, education, persuasion, incentivisation, coercion, training, enablement and modelling. These address deficits in one or more of these conditions. In the 'outer layer' are seven categories of policy: fiscal measures, guidelines, environmental/societal planning, communication/marketing, legislation, service provision and regulation) that could enable those interventions to occur.

Unlike the *theories and models* described earlier in this section, which are a set of ideas used to explain or predict behaviour change, a *framework* is merely a structure to support the planning of behaviour change strategies, without the predictive nature of a model or theory. Theories/models and frameworks can be useful in planning education strategies.

PARTNERSHIPS AND SHARED DECISION MAKING BETWEEN THERAPISTS AND THE PEOPLE WITH WHOM THEY WORK

The importance of adults actively participating in their learning has long been recognised by adult learning theorists. Recognising the relationship between the individual and the occupational therapist as a *partnership* is a key element of the model of 'person-centred care'. This model also emphasises communication, respect, choice and empowerment and a focus on individuals rather than their specific medical condition (Groves, 2010). This model of care sits between the 'paternalistic' and 'informed patient or independent choice' models of care (Entwistle & Watt, 2006; Quill & Brody, 1996). In the 'paternalistic' model of care, the practitioner is in control, discloses information as

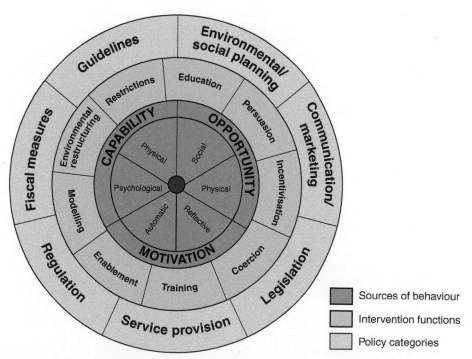

FIG. 25.1 ■ The behaviour change wheel. *(From Michie, S., van Stralen, M. M., & West, R. (2011). The behaviour change wheel: A new method for characterising and designing behaviour change interventions.* Implementation Science 6:42, *with acknowledgement of Biomed Central. Available at: http://www.implementationscience.com/content/6/1/42)*

and when he or she decides it is suitable to, and makes the decisions for the individual who is expected to be passive, unquestioning and compliant. In the 'informed patient or independent choice' model, the practitioner presents the facts and leaves the decision making solely up to the individual (Entwistle & Watt, 2006). Person-centred care has become the model that is advocated by health professionals and health professional associations.

Person-centred practice can increase the satisfaction and quality of life of the person receiving health services, reduce individuals' anxiety and improve symptom resolution, pain control, function and physiological measures and improve adherence to long-term medication use (Groves, 2010; Kahn et al., 2007). Central to person-centred care is treating people with dignity, responding quickly and effectively to individuals' needs and concerns (Coulter, 2002) and providing them with enough information to enable informed choices about their health care (McKenna & Tooth, 2006). Informed decision making can be facilitated by shared decision making, which involves the person and the health professional jointly participating in a health decision after discussing the options, the benefits and harms, and considering the person's values, preferences and circumstances (Hoffmann et al., 2014). It can be viewed as a continuum (Kon, 2010) along which the extent of responsibility for the decision making lies with either the person or the health professional varies. Shared decision making between health professionals and individuals has been linked with improved outcomes – for example, better compliance (Frosch & Kaplan, 1999; Wilson et al., 2010), greater family satisfaction with communication (White et al., 2007), improved emotional status (Stewart, 1995), improved use of medications (McWilliams et al., 2008), and reduced hospital admissions and health care costs (Wennberg et al., 2010).

Shared decision making is a process, which may be assisted by the use of decision support tools but does not require them. Decision support tools can help therapists and the people receiving therapy services to draw on available evidence when making decisions and include decision aids, evidence summaries, communication frameworks and/or question prompt lists (Kastner & Straus, 2012). Of these tools, decision aids have had the most research and have demonstrated effectiveness for increasing knowledge and risk-perception accuracy, improving communication, and reducing decisional conflict, feeling uninformed and passivity in decision making (Stacey et al., 2014).

Although active involvement of individuals in making decisions about their own care is ideal, shared decision making is not always possible. Many people and their families find it difficult to take an active part in health care decisions and not all individuals may desire this level of involvement, preferring a more passive role. This is a legitimate choice that should be respected (Coulter, 2002). However, the opportunity to be actively involved should be available for all who want to take it (Hoffmann et al., 2014). Therapists should be flexible and adapt their approach so that it meets individuals' preferences and needs. Further information on engaging people in collaborative goal setting is covered elsewhere in this book.

CONSIDERATIONS WHEN PLANNING AND IMPLEMENTING EDUCATION INTERVENTIONS

When planning an education strategy, there are many other decisions a therapist needs to make. An overview of some of the key steps and decisions that a therapist should take during the planning process is provided in the following section.

Determine Educational Needs and Establish Objectives

For education to be person-centred, it must meet the needs of the individual. Generally the most effective way to establish individuals' educational needs is by asking them (Lorig, 2001). As well as establishing the content of individuals' educational needs (i.e. the topics or areas to be covered), therapists also need to determine their preferences regarding the format and timing of the education. To determine content needs, therapists may also wish to use a checklist of topics as a prompt to ensure that topics are not overlooked. The topics listed on the checklist can be derived by the therapist's experience, previous groups or individuals involved and relevant scientific literature. For many conditions and situations, formal studies of individuals' informational needs have been undertaken and are readily available in the literature. Therapists may also wish to use a more formal means of establishing informational needs such as a knowledge test, attitude scale or behaviour checklist. One advantage of using a formal assessment is that it can be used as baseline measurement and the assessment readministered after the education strategy has been implemented, as a way of evaluating the strategy (see the section later on evaluating the outcomes of education strategies).

The process of assessing individuals' educational needs is a continual one as needs change over time and depend on many factors, such as the nature and stage of their medical condition and their readiness to change. For example, an individual who has had heart surgery may initially be concerned about when he or she can return to self-care activities, whereas some weeks later the person may want to know about returning to driving.

After an individual's educational needs have been ascertained (Tlach et al., 2014), therapists need to, in conjunction with the individual, set goals. The SMART goal method addresses five domains (Specific, Measurable, Activity-based, Review and Time frame) and is a useful way to develop goals. The following example of an objective illustrates these components: after reading the instruction sheet and also having it explained by the therapist (*activity* and *review/time frame)*, Mr Jones will be able to explain the wearing regime and care guidelines for his wrist splint without prompting from the therapist (*specific* and *measurable* behaviour). By setting guidelines such as this, at the conclusion of the implementation of the education strategy, therapists are able to impartially ascertain if the goal has been met. Further information on SMART goal setting can be found elsewhere in this book.

Decide on Format for Providing Education

There are many formats that therapists can use to provide education. When deciding which format to use, there are a number of factors that therapists should consider, such as the educational resources available to the therapist and the type of content being provided. A systematic review of teaching strategies and methods of delivery of education that was structured, culturally appropriate and tailored to the individual was found to be better than ad hoc teaching or generalised teaching (Friedman, Cosby, Boyko, Hatton-Bauer, & Turnbull, 2011). Therefore factors about the individual also need to be considered such as cognitive ability, educational level, vision, hearing, communication skills, preferred learning style (e.g. visual or auditory), cultural background and primary language, as strategies will only be as effective as the individual's ability to use or access that format (Friedman et al., 2011).

Formats for providing education include traditional lectures, discussions, simulated games, computer technology, written material, audiovisual sources, verbal recall, demonstration, and role playing. Therapists should be aware that, where possible, using a combination of formats can often be more effective than using a single format (Friedman et al., 2011). Education will be more effective when individuals have the opportunity to hear information, see it, have it repeated and interact with it, than when they just, for example, hear it. Although verbal and written education are the two forms of education most commonly used by occupational therapists, there are other forms that therapists may find valuable in certain situations. The provision of information about some topics is particularly suited to a combination of verbal education, demonstration and written information. For example, when educating individuals about exercises to perform, adaptations to activities or how to use assistive equipment, demonstration is invaluable. Written materials, lectures, audiotapes and videotapes have been found to be more effective teaching strategies than only verbal teaching and discussions, with a positive effect on individuals' knowledge, anxiety and satisfaction (Friedman et al., 2011). However, a systematic review found that demonstration was the most effective teaching strategy and hence its use is recommended when appropriate.

Verbal

Partly because of its convenience, verbal education is the most commonly used format, although verbal teaching and discussions have been found to be the least effective strategies in a systematic review of education strategies (Friedman et al., 2011). One of the major problems with verbal education is that individuals often forget the information provided to them (Kitching, 1990), with estimations that most individuals remember less than a quarter of what they have been told (Boundouki, Humphris, & Field, 2004).

Combined Verbal and Written

Written information is a particularly valuable format that should ideally be used to supplement or reinforce information that is presented verbally (Friedman et al., 2011), as this has the potential to maximise an individual's knowledge. For example, a Cochrane systematic review that evaluated the effect of providing written summaries or recordings of consultations for people with cancer found that the majority of participants in the trials who received recordings or summaries used and valued them as a reminder of what was said during the consultation (Pitkethly, MacGillivray, & Ryan, 2008).

Written

Written materials have the advantage of being available to refresh an individual's memory as needed. They can also be useful if the individual thinks of a question *after* seeing the health professional. To some extent, written materials may be able to assist individuals in answering the questions that occur when they are not interacting with a health professional. Written materials have a number of advantages such as message consistency, reusability, portability, flexibility of delivery and permanence of information, and they are economical to produce and update. A further benefit of written materials is that individuals can choose the level and amount of information that best suits them as their level of coping changes. Of course, before deciding to use written materials with an individual, the therapist needs to consider the factors listed earlier, such as the individual's cognitive abilities, primary language, communication skills, vision and reading ability. If a therapist chooses to proceed and use written materials with an individual, it is essential that appropriate attention is given to the design of the written materials. This issue is explained further in the Content and Design Principles for Effective Written Health Education Materials section later in this chapter.

Audio-visual

Formats that contain audio and/or video can be a useful when providing education to individuals who are unable to read, whether this is because of illiteracy, a visual or perceptual impairment or some other reason. The use of digital video discs (DVD) that contain educational material can be particularly useful when the education involves demonstrations, such as of movements, techniques, exercises or activities. For example, a DVD on how to carry out joint protection and energy conservation techniques while performing self-care and household activities may be useful for a therapist to provide to individuals with arthritis to reinforce information that has already been provided face-to-face by the therapist. By also providing a DVD, individuals can review the information when and as many times as needed. DVDs can also be useful when the topic being covered requires graphics to more effectively explain the content, such as explaining to individuals what happens in hip replacement surgery so they can understand why postoperative movement precautions are important. Video presentation of information caters to individuals with auditory learning styles, as well as those with visual learning styles, and can assist individuals who have low functional health literacy or English as a second language to understand the content being conveyed.

Videos depicting 'real people' doing an activity are more effective in supporting individuals' to modify their behaviour than videos that provide only spoken or graphically presented health information (Abu Abed, Himmel, Vormfelde, & Koschack, 2014). Audio, video and written materials all have the added advantage that individuals can share them with their family members, so that even if family were not present when the therapist was providing the information, they can still receive the information.

Computer- or Internet-based

Computer technology can also be an effective teaching strategy, positively affecting knowledge, anxiety and satisfaction (Beranova & Sykes, 2007; Friedman et al., 2011). There are a number of ways in which computer programs and the Internet can be used as education strategies, such as e-health, providing individuals with interactive information, helping individuals to make health-related decisions (see e.g. Hochlehnert et al., 2006), or providing individuals with tailored printed information that is customised according to their informational and visual needs (see e.g. Hoffmann, Russell, & McKenna, 2004).

There is an increasing use of e-health, which can be defined as an interactive website used for 'monitoring, treatment instructions, self-management training and general information and communication' (Eland-de Kok, van Os-Medendorp, Vergouwe-Meijer, Bruijnzeel-Koomen, & Ros, 2011, p. 2997) between individuals and their health professional. A systematic review of e-health interventions for individuals with chronic conditions concluded that when offered instead of or in addition to usual care, they resulted in small to moderate positive effects on health outcomes (Eland-de Kok et al., 2011). Interactive computer-based health information interventions can have a positive effect on health knowledge, social support and behavioural outcomes for individuals with chronic diseases (Murray et al., 2005). Compared with standard verbal or written methods of providing information, interactive computer-based information has been found to significantly increase patients' knowledge, understanding and satisfaction (Beranova & Sykes, 2007).

Tailored information is customised according to an individual's characteristics or preferences. There is evidence that tailored print information is better remembered, read and perceived as relevant or credible than nontailored information (Noar, Benac, & Harris, 2007). There is preliminary evidence that computer-tailored education materials can be effective in changing various health-related behaviours (Bailey et al., 2010; Kroeze, Werkman, & Brug, 2006; Neville, O'Hara, & Milat, 2009; Short et al., 2011). Tailored information is also more likely to result in greater satisfaction with the information that is provided and better met informational needs (Hoffmann et al., 2007; McPherson, Higginson, & Hearn, 2001). However, the effectiveness of tailored information is moderated by a number of variables such as the type of health behaviour, individual differences, and theoretical concepts that are being tailored (Noar et al., 2007).

Although it depends on the features of the software being used, the advantages of using computer programs to provide information can include the following:

- Enabling individuals to interact with the information, to view it at their own pace, and view only information that is relevant to them
- Often containing graphics that individuals can interact with, which can assist with understanding the information
- Incorporating learning tools such as knowledge quizzes
- Enabling printing out the information viewed on screen, providing a resource that can be referred back to at any time

Computer programs should be designed so that they are user-friendly and able to be operated by individuals who do not have computer experience. Although computer-based education should not be a substitute for interaction with therapists, it can be useful for supplementing or reinforcing information that is provided by therapists.

As well as computer-based programs, the Internet can also be a valuable source of information for individuals; health information is one of the most commonly searched topics on the Internet (McMullan, 2006). Individuals who wish to be active consumers of health information will have a need to seek out their own information either before or after they have seen their therapist (McMullan, 2006). Therapists may find that individuals will come to them with information that they have found on the Internet that they wish to discuss. Therapists need to be aware that 'Internet-informed' individuals will affect the traditional therapist–person relationship. Therapists should acknowledge individuals' search for information, answer questions they have about the information that they have found, assist individuals by directing them to reliable and accurate Internet sites (McMullan, 2006), and, as needed, evaluate the health information from the Internet that patients may bring with them (Grant, Rodger, & Hoffmann, 2015). (See the DISCERN website in the Further Reading section for a checklist that can be used to evaluate health information websites.)

Group-based

Although most education is provided on a one-to-one basis, providing education in a group format can be a time-effective method of providing information to individuals who have similar educational needs. For example, group-based diabetes self-management education can result in improvements in behaviour changes, health and psychosocial outcomes compared with routine interventions (Steinsbekk et al., 2012). The information that is provided in a group format is typically generic information and therefore group education should also be supplemented by a one-to-one consultation between each individual and the therapist to allow for provision of information that is specific to each individual's needs and situation. When deciding whether group education is appropriate for an individual, consideration of factors such as the individual's roles and responsibilities (such as full-time work), personality and level of anxiety is important. Some individuals will benefit from the group process and being able to share and discuss issues with other group participants; others may not feel comfortable doing this. Although group education has advantages, this format also has potential disadvantages as it can be resource intensive, involve significant preparation time for the therapists and requires group leadership skills. Refer to the Further Reading section at the end of this chapter for citation details of a chapter (Lorig & Harris, 2001) that provides details about the steps that health professionals should take when planning and conducting group education sessions.

Decide When to Provide the Information

Providing appropriate education to individuals at the appropriate time is critical and can greatly affect the effectiveness of education strategies. The extent of information that is provided at any point will vary according to many factors. When seriously ill, individuals may only want to receive brief information that is relevant to their immediate concerns. Later, individuals may want to receive more detailed information. Anxiety can prevent individuals from absorbing and processing information. Therapists should consider individuals' coping level and style each time that they provide information and be guided by individuals' readiness to digest information. There are no guidelines as to the optimum time to provide information as this varies according to the individual, the individual's circumstances and needs and the type of information being provided. Therapists need to be sensitive to and guided by individuals' needs. To assist with the comprehension and recall of information, therapists should provide the information in more than one format (such as verbal and written), repeat information over time and provide opportunities for reinforcement, clarification and questions. For example, in between therapy sessions or appointments, individuals may be given written information to read or videos to watch or be referred to recommended Internet sites.

Consider Impairments That May Affect Receiving and/or Understanding Information

Individuals may have one or more impairments, such as a hearing, visual, cognitive, or speech and language impairment, that will affect how they are able to process information. These impairments may be preexisting (such as hearing loss associated with aging) or a result of the health condition for which they are seeing the therapist (such as aphasia after a stroke). Therapists' choices of formats for providing information need to consider any impairments individuals have. For example, the use of written information is not appropriate for an individual who has a severe visual impairment that can not be corrected (such as with corrective lenses) and information that is provided verbally should be supplemented by some other means, such as audio-recorded information. There are a range of strategies that

therapists can use to facilitate communication with individuals who have one or more of these impairments, and further reading related to strategies specific to each impairment type is recommended. (Please refer to Further Reading section at the end of this chapter for details.)

Consider Health Literacy

If written health education materials are used to provide information or supplement information that is provided verbally, the literacy level of the individuals receiving the information needs to be considered. The written material will not benefit individuals if they are unable to understand it. There are various definitions of health literacy. The US Institute of Medicine has defined health literacy as the degree to which individuals have the capacity to obtain, process and understand the basic information needed to make appropriate decisions about their health (Institute of Medicine, 2004). Low health literacy is associated with poorer knowledge of health conditions (Al Sayah, Majumdar, Williams, Robertson, & Johnson, 2013), increased hospitalisations and emergency department care use, lower use of preventative health care and screenings, poorer ability to take medications or correctly read labels and health messages and – among older individuals – poorer overall health status and higher mortality (Berkman et al., 2011). People with poor literacy may try to hide their literacy problems and be reluctant to ask questions so that they do not appear ignorant (Wilson & McLemore, 1997). Health professionals should be aware of the literacy skills of individuals so that they can alter the education strategy accordingly.

A person's level of health literacy may not be reliably linked to the level of their general literacy skills or their years of education (Effective Health Care Program, 2010). Instead, a health literacy screening tool can be used and many have been developed. Two examples are the Rapid Estimate of Adult Literacy in Medicine (REALM) (Murphy et al., 1993) and the Test of Functional Health Literacy in Adults (TOFHLA) (Parker et al., 1995). These tests evaluate an individual's ability to understand medical terminology and language and are quick and easy to administer. Additionally, with the increasing use of computer- and Internet-based education, the development and validation of computer-based health literacy screening tools continues to evolve (Collins, Currie, Bakken, Vawdrey, & Stone, 2012). The principles for designing effective written health education materials, which are also generally applicable to online information, are described next.

Content and Design Principles for Effective Written Health Education Materials

When written health education materials are designed, there are a number of principles that should be followed to maximise their effectiveness. Put simply, for written information to be effective, it needs to be read, understood and remembered. Studies have reported a mismatch between the reading level of written materials and the reading ability of the individuals who received the materials (Griffin, McKenna, & Tooth, 2006;

Hoffmann & McKenna, 2006a; Morony et al., 2015). The reading level, or readability, of a material refers to how easy it is to read. Written materials should be written simply, at a fifth- to sixth-grade reading level (Doak, Doak, & Root, 1996). There are a number of readability formulas that can be used to quickly and easily determine the readability of written material, such as the SMOG (Simple Measure of Gobbldygook) (McLaughlin, 1969) or the Flesch Reading Ease formula (Flesch, 1948). The latter is available through some word processing programs such as Microsoft Word.

Although the readability of written materials is very important, there are many other features that contribute to the suitability of written materials, and they can be grouped into the following categories: content, language, organisation, layout and typography, illustrations, and learning and motivation. After reviewing literature concerning the design of written health education materials, Hoffmann and Worrall (2004) compiled a list of recommended content and design features that should be followed when designing written materials. The principles are shown in Box 25.1. Checklists are available for therapists to use

---

BOX 25.1

RECOMMENDATIONS FOR DESIGNING EFFECTIVE WRITTEN HEALTH EDUCATION MATERIALS

- Involve all key stakeholders, including the person receiving occupational therapy services, in the development and testing of the written material

CONTENT

- Clearly state the purpose of the material.
- Provide information that is behaviour-focused (e.g. 'It is important that you do the exercises every day').
- Ensure that the content is accurate, up-to-date, and evidence-based and that sources are appropriately referenced
- Include the authors' names on the material and the publication date.

LANGUAGE

- Avoid judgemental or patronising language.
- Aim for a fifth- to sixth-grade reading level.
- Use short sentences, expressing only one idea per sentence.
- Use short words, preferably one to two syllables, where possible.
- Use common words wherever possible. Avoid the use of jargon or abbreviations. Include a glossary if jargon or unfamiliar words are necessary.
- Write in the active voice and in a conversational style.
- Write in the second person (e.g. 'you' rather than 'the client').
- Structure sentences so that the context or old information is presented before new information. (e.g. 'To lower your risk of stroke [context], you will need to make changes to what you eat' [new information]).

ORGANISATION

- Sequence the information so that the information that individuals most want to know is at the beginning.
- Use subheadings.
- Present the information using bulleted lists where possible.
- Group related information into lists, with no more than five points in each list, and label each list descriptively.
- Keep paragraphs short and express only one idea per paragraph.
- Summarise the main points, either at the end of sections or end of the material.

LAYOUT AND TYPOGRAPHY

- Use a minimum 12-point font size.
- Avoid the use of italics and all capitals.
- Only use bold type to emphasise key words or phrases.
- Ensure good contrast between the font colour (e.g. black) and the background (e.g. white).

ILLUSTRATIONS

- Only use illustrations if they will enhance the reader's understanding.
- Use simple line drawings that are likely to be familiar to the reader.
- Use an explanatory caption with each illustration.
- Refer to the illustration in the text.

LEARNING AND MOTIVATION

- Incorporate features that actively engage the reader (e.g. blank space to write questions down, short quiz, 'list three things that you should do').

Modified from Hoffmann, T., & Worrall, L. (2004). Designing effective written health education materials: Considerations for health professionals. *Disability and Rehabilitation, 26,* 1166-1173, with permission from Taylor and Francis Journals. Available at: http://www.informaworld.com.

to evaluate the suitability of the written materials they are considering using, whether self-designed or from other sources. Two of these checklists are the Suitability of Assessment of Materials (SAM) (Doak et al., 1996) and a checklist of content and design characteristics that was developed by Pau, Redman, & Sanson-Fisher (1997).

Evaluating the Outcome of Education Interventions

Although therapists are accustomed to measuring outcomes and evaluating the effectiveness of the strategies that they implement, they often do not apply the same process to education strategies. Therapists should evaluate the outcome of any education strategy they implement, as they would after implementing any other strategy, to determine whether the education had the intended effect and whether the stated goals have been met. This information enables therapists to decide whether further education or reinforcement of the content is needed and whether the objectives, content or delivery methods of subsequent education strategies should be altered to improve effectiveness (Hoffmann & McKenna, 2006b).

Evaluating the outcome of education strategies can be done informally or formally, and this usually depends on factors such as the objectives of the strategy, the purpose of the evaluation, and the time and resources available. Methods of informal evaluation include seeking feedback from individuals and ascertaining if they have understood the information that the therapist has provided to them, if their informational needs have been met and if they have any unanswered questions. Individuals' satisfaction with the process of receiving education can also be assessed simply by asking them. Informal evaluation may be as simple as, for example, asking an individual who has had a stroke to correctly demonstrate to the therapist the adapted technique that he or she was taught to use when putting a shirt on. Even if formal methods of evaluation are used, informal questions relating to whether individuals have understood the information provided and if they have further informational needs should always be asked by the therapist.

Formal evaluation typically requires administration of formal outcome measures and therapists must decide which outcomes they will measure, which outcome measure they will choose, and when and how the outcome measure will be administered. Decisions about which outcomes to measure should be guided by the goals of the education strategy. For example, if the objective is to improve an individual's knowledge about the risk factors for coronary artery disease, then a knowledge test is an appropriate outcome measure. However, if the objective of the strategy is to assist an individual to change his or her behaviour – for example, incorporating regular exercise into his or her week – then an outcome measure that assesses behaviour change is needed.

Decisions about which outcome measures to use will depend on whether there is an existing outcome measure that is appropriate for a therapist's needs. There are many published health education measures (such as measures of knowledge for various conditions, satisfaction, self-efficacy, health behaviour, emotional health and quality of life) and many of these are freely available. The Redman (2003) resource that is listed in the Further Reading section at the end of this chapter overviews many of the published health education measurement tools. However, for many education strategies implemented by occupational therapists, an existing outcome measure will not be sufficient. In this case therapists will need to adapt an existing outcome measure or create their own. There are some general guidelines to follow when adapting or creating outcome measures, and these are described in the Hoffmann and McKenna (2006b) reference that is listed in the Further Reading section at the end of this chapter and summarised briefly here:

- Ensure that the outcome measure is kept as simple as possible and that there is no ambiguity or unnecessarily complex words or long sentences.
- Do not use biased or leading questions or items.
- Follow the guidelines in Box 25.1 to ensure that the measure is formatted in a 'user-friendly' manner.
- Obtain feedback on the measure from colleagues and alter as necessary.
- Pilot the measure with the type of individuals with whom it will be used and alter as necessary.

After deciding which outcome measure to use, therapists also need to decide when the measure will be administered. Decisions about timing will be guided by the original objectives that were set for the education strategy. For example, for education strategies to improve knowledge, it is appropriate to evaluate them shortly after, such as on the same day, the education has been provided, whereas it may be more appropriate to evaluate an education strategy to change behaviour at a later time, such as a number of weeks, after the strategy has been implemented, so that individuals have the chance to apply what they have learned. An advantage of formal evaluation is that therapists can readminister the same formal assessment that was used earlier when they were establishing individuals' educational needs, and then compare changes in individuals' performances on the assessment (a pretest–posttest approach) that likely occurred as a result of the education strategy. Because the same outcome measure may be used at both the beginning and the end, when initially planning an education strategy, therapists should also plan how they are going to evaluate the strategy.

However, not all evaluations need to be done before and after the implementation. Evaluating education strategies partway through its delivery can also be valuable as this allows therapists to respond to individuals' feedback and progress and adjust the strategy accordingly. This applies to both individual and group education strategies where, for example, a therapist may administer a brief questionnaire after two of the four scheduled classes have been held.

Before proceeding with the evaluation, therapists also need to decide how it will be administered. There are many available methods, and the choice will depend on factors such as the information sought, the individuals' needs and abilities, and the time and resources available (Hoffmann & McKenna, 2006b). Use of a combination of methods is often most appropriate. Some of the most common methods of measuring outcomes include observation, interview, individual self-report, open-ended questioning, questionnaires, scales, tests, and diaries (Hoffmann & McKenna, 2006b).

CONCLUSION

Education is an important component of all areas of occupational therapy practice and should be considered as a specific and valid strategy in its own right. As such, therapists should be knowledgeable about relevant educational theories, models and principles and be guided by them when planning education strategies. When planning and implementing these strategies, therapists also need to make many other decisions such as those related to the content, format, timing and evaluation of the strategy. Practice Story 25.1 illustrates the application of some of the principles that have been described in this chapter. With appropriate consideration of the principles and guidelines discussed in this chapter, therapists can aim to provide effective education strategies to the individuals they work with, thus enabling them to participate fully in their own health care.

PRACTICE STORY 25.1

Education About Performing Daily Living Skills After a Total Hip Replacement

Mr Williams is a 78-year-old man who was first seen by an occupational therapist 4 days after he had undergone total hip replacement surgery on his right hip. The occupational therapist conducted an initial interview with Mr Williams to gather background information regarding his previous and current performance abilities and occupational roles, home environment and understanding of hip movement precautions. The therapist also wished to identify and prioritise Mr Williams' current occupational issues and goals while in rehabilitation.

Before his surgery, Mr Williams lived alone and was independent in performing basic activities of daily living such as self-care tasks and most of his own domestic tasks such as cooking, doing the laundry and light cleaning, and he enjoyed taking part in the leisure occupations of gardening and lawn bowls. During the interview, the therapist also learned that Mr Williams was highly anxious about learning to do things 'exactly right' after surgery and was fearful of hip dislocation and any setbacks to his recovery. He reported that several friends had given him advice on what to do and what not to do and he was confused about how he should go about doing daily tasks without risking the dislocation of his hip. The therapist also established that he had forgotten a lot of what he had been told before surgery about hip precautions and was not confident in his ability to manage his self-care tasks at home upon discharge.

Together, the therapist and Mr Williams established that his goals before discharge were to be able to walk independently, get in and out of bed and chairs independently and complete his own personal self-care tasks and light meal preparation. To achieve these goals, one component of the agreed upon plan was the provision of education related to hip precautions and the impact that they will have on Mr Williams' occupational roles. In this instance the desired outcomes of education strategies were for Mr Williams to have (a) sufficient knowledge of the necessary hip precautions after surgery; and (b) the skills and confidence to independently and safely complete his personal self-care tasks while also adhering to the relevant hip precautions.

The therapist proposed to use a combination of education materials with Mr Williams. As the therapist wanted to use written information, she administered the REALM to Mr Williams and established that he had approximately an eight reading grade level (in the Australian education system, this is typically equivalent to 13 years of age). After this, the therapist provided him with a well-designed information booklet ('Things You Need to Know About Hip Replacement Surgery') that contained both written information and clear, useful illustrations. The booklet had previously been assessed using the SMOG readability formula and had a reading level of grade 6. The therapist used the information booklet as a teaching guide and explained the hip anatomy and the surgical procedure using the illustrations in the booklet to support the explanations. The therapist then explained the practical implications of hip precautions using examples relevant to Mr William's own personal circumstances and acknowledged the presence of his anxiety about dislocating his hip. At his bedside, the therapist demonstrated the use of long-handled dressing and showering assistive devices to Mr Williams and he then had the opportunity to practise using these devices, ask questions, and undertake practical problem solving in relation to these tasks. The therapist provided Mr Williams with feedback and encouragement as he practised using these assistive devices, and Mr William's confidence in his ability to undertake these tasks grew as he experienced success in performing them safely.

The following day, the therapist conducted an activities of daily living assessment with Mr Williams and observed him perform showering, dressing, and transfer tasks while using the appropriate assistive devices. The therapist provided Mr Williams with feedback about his adherence to movement precautions while performing the tasks. Over the following days, other

Continued on following page

PRACTICE STORY 25.1

Education About Performing Daily Living Skills After a Total Hip Replacement (Continued)

members of the multidisciplinary rehabilitation team such as nurses and physiotherapists also provided Mr Williams with consistent instruction and reinforcement of these same techniques. This contributed to Mr William's mastery of transfers and daily living skills and also built his confidence in his ability for independent with his self-care after discharge and reduced his anxiety.

A few days before discharge, the occupational therapist invited Mr Williams to participate in a small-group education session that was being held for people in hospital who had undergone hip surgery. Spouses and carers were also invited to attend the group. The group was led by the occupational therapist and used DVD-based movie images of scenarios to illustrate techniques for completing personal and domestic tasks at home after hip surgery. There was also some discussion about these issues and the group concluded with each participant completing a short quiz to gauge his or her level of understanding of and ability to apply the information to practical daily life scenarios. Before his discharge, the therapist completed another activities of daily living assessment (this time it also included the preparation of a small meal) with Mr Williams and observed that he was able to safely and independently perform self-care activities and light domestic tasks, adhered to movement precautions throughout all activities, and was confident in his ability to manage these tasks at home.

 http://evolve.elsevier.com/Curtin/OT

REFERENCES

Abu Abed, M., Himmel, W., Vormfelde, S., & Koschack, J. (2014). Video-assisted patient education to modify behaviour: A systematic review. *Patient Education and Counselling, 97*(1), 16–22.

Al Sayah, F., Majumdar, S. R., Williams, B., Robertson, S., & Johnson, J. A. (2013). Health literacy and health outcomes in diabetes: A systematic review. *Journal of General Internal Medicine, 28*(3), 444–452.

Bailey, J., Murray, E., Rait, G., et al. (2010). Interactive computer-based interventions for sexual health promotion. *Cochrane Database of Systematic Reviews*. CD006483.

Bandura, A. (1977). Self-efficacy: Toward a unifying theory of behavioural change. *Psychological Review, 84*, 191–215.

Bandura, A. (1986). *Social foundations of thought and action: A social cognitive theory*. Englewood Cliffs, NJ: Prentice Hall.

Bandura, A. (1997). *Self-efficacy: The exercise of control*. New York: W.H. Freeman.

Bartlett, E. (1985). At last, a definition. *Patient Education and Counselling, 7*, 323–324.

Becker, M. (1974). The health belief model and personal health behaviour. *Health Education Monographs, 2*, 324–508.

Becker, M., Drachman, R., & Kirscht, J. (1974). A new approach to explaining sick-role behaviour in low-income populations. *American Journal of Public Health, 64*, 205–216.

Beranova, E., & Sykes, C. (2007). A systematic review of computer-based softwares for educating patients with coronary heart disease. *Patient Education and Counselling, 66*, 21–28.

Berkman, N. D., Sheridan, S. L., Donahue, K. E., et al. (2011). Health literacy interventions and outcomes: An updated systematic review. *Evidence Report/Technology Assessment, 199*, 1–941.

Boundouki, G., Humphris, G., & Field, A. (2004). Knowledge of oral cancer, distress and screening intentions: Longer term effects of a patient information leaflet. *Patient Education and Counselling, 53*, 71–77.

Boyde, M., Turner, C., Thompson, D. R., & Stewart, S. (2011). Educational interventions for patients with heart failure: A systematic review of randomised controlled trials. *Journal of Cardiovascular Nursing, 26*(4), E27–E35.

Buckland, S. (1994). Unmet needs for health information: A literature review. *Health Libraries Review, 11*, 82–95.

Champion, V. L., & Skinner, C. S. (2008). The health belief model. In K. Glanz, B. K. Rimer, & K. Viswanath (Eds.), *Health behaviour and health education: Theory, research and practice* (4th ed.). San Francisco: Jossey-Bass.

Clark, N., Janz, N., Dodge, J., et al. (1992). Self-regulation of health behaviour: The 'take PRIDE' program. *Health Education Quarterly, 19*, 341–354.

Collins, S. A., Currie, L. M., Bakken, S., Vawdrey, D. K., & Stone, P. W. (2012). Health literacy screening instruments for eHealth applications: A systematic review. *Journal of Biomedical Informatics, 45*(3), 598–607.

Coulter, A. (2002). *The autonomous patient: Ending paternalism in medical care*. London: The Nuffield Trust.

Doak, C., Doak, L., & Root, J. (1996). *Teaching patients with low literacy skills* (2nd ed.). Philadelphia: J.B. Lippincott.

Effective Health Care Program (2010). *Health literacy interventions and outcomes: An update of the literacy and health outcomes systematic review of the literature*. Retrieved from. http://effectivehealthcare.ahrq.gov/ehc/products/151/392/Health%20Literacy%20Protocol%20%282-9-2010%29.pdf.

Eland-de Kok, P., van Os-Medendorp, H., Vergouwe-Meijer, A., Bruijnzeel-Koomen, C., & Ros, W. (2011). A systematic review of the effects of e-health on chronically ill patients. *Journal of Clinical Nursing, 20*(21–22), 2997–3010.

Entwistle, V., & Watt, I. (2006). Patient involvement in treatment decision-making: The case for a broader conceptual framework. *Patient Education Counseling, 63*, 268–278.

Flesch, R. (1948). A new readability yardstick. *Journal of Applied Psychology, 32*, 221–233.

Friedman, A. J., Cosby, R., Boyko, S., Hatton-Bauer, J., & Turnbull, G. (2011). Effective teaching strategies and methods of delivery for patient education: A systematic review and practice guideline recommendations. *Journal of Cancer Education, 26*(1), 12–21.

Frosch, D., & Kaplan, R. (1999). Shared decision making in clinical medicine: Past research and future directions. *American Journal of Preventive Medicine, 17*, 285–294.

Grant, N., Rodger, S., & Hoffmann, T. (2015). Evaluation of autism-related health information on the web. *Journal of Applied Research in Intellectual Disabilities, 28*(4), 276–282.

Griffin, J., McKenna, K., & Tooth, L. (2006). Discrepancy between older clients' ability to read and comprehend and the reading level of written educational materials used by occupational therapists. *American Journal of Occupational Therapy, 60*, 70–80.

Groves, J. (2010). International Alliance of Patients' Organisations perspectives on person-centred medicine. *International Journal of Integrated Care, 10*(Suppl.), 27–29.

Hochlehnert, A., Richter, A., Bludau, H., et al. (2006). A computer-based information tool for chronic pain patients: Computerised information to support the process of shared decision-making. *Patient Education and Counselling, 61*, 92–98.

Hoffmann, T., & McKenna, K. (2006a). Analysis of stroke patients' and carers' reading ability and the content and design of written materials: recommendations for improving written stroke information. *Patient Education and Counselling, 60*, 286–293.

Hoffmann, T., & McKenna, K. (2006b). Evaluation of client education. In K. McKenna, & L. Tooth (Eds.), *Client education: A partnership approach for health professionals* (pp. 159–182). Sydney: University of New South Wales Press.

Hoffmann, T., Russell, T., & McKenna, K. (2004). Producing computer-generated tailored written information for stroke patients and their carers: System development and preliminary evaluation. *International Journal of Medical Informatics, 73*, 751–758.

Hoffmann, T., & Worrall, L. (2004). Designing effective written health education materials: Considerations for health professionals. *Disability and Rehabilitation, 26*, 1166–1173.

Hoffmann, T., McKenna, K., Worrall, L., et al. (2007). Randomised controlled trial of a computer-generated tailored written education package for patients following stroke. *Age and Ageing, 36*, 280–286.

Hoffmann, T., Légaré, F., Simmon, M., et al. (2014). Shared decision making: What do clinicians need to know and why should they bother? *Medical Journal of Australia, 201*(1), 35–39.

Institute of Medicine. (2004). *Health literacy: A prescription to end confusion*. Washington, D.C.: Institute of Medicine.

Kahn, K., Schneider, E., Malin, J., et al. (2007). Patient centred experiences in breast cancer: predicting long-term adherence to Tamoxifen use. *Medical Care, 45*, 431–439.

Kastner, M., & Straus, S. E. (2012). Application of the Knowledge-to-Action and Medical Research Council frameworks in the development of an osteoporosis clinical decision support tool. *Journal of Clinical Epidemiology, 65*, 1163–1170.

Kitching, J. (1990). Patient information leaflets: The state of the art. *Journal of the Royal Society of Medicine, 83*, 298–300.

Knowles, M. (1980). *The modern practice of adult education*. New York: Cambridge.

Knowles, M., Holton, E., & Swanson, R. (1998). *The adult learner* (5th ed.). Houston: Gulf Publishing.

Kon, A. (2010). The shared decision-making continuum. *Journal of the American Medical Association, 304*, 903–904.

Kroeze, W., Werkman, A., & Brug, J. (2006). A systematic review of randomised trials on the effectiveness of computer-tailored education on physical activity and dietary behaviours. *Annals of Behavioral Medicine, 31*, 205–223.

Lorig, K. (2001). *Patient education: A practical approach* (3rd ed.). Thousand Oaks, CA: Sage Publications.

Lorig, K., Chastain, R., Ung, E., et al. (1989). Development and evaluation of a scale to measure perceived self-efficacy in people with arthritis. *Arthritis and Rheumatism, 32*, 37–44.

Lorig, K., & Holman, H. (1993). Arthritis self-management studies: A twelve-year review. *Health Education Quarterly, 20*, 17–28.

McEneany, J., McKenna, K., & Summerville, P. (2002). Australian occupational therapists working in adult physical dysfunction settings: What treatment media do they use? *Australian Occupational Therapy Journal, 49*, 115–127.

McLaughlin, H. (1969). SMOG grading: A new readability formula. *Journal of Reading, 12*, 639–646.

McKenna, K., & Tooth, L. (2006). Client education: An overview. In K. McKenna, & L. Tooth (Eds.), *Client education: A partnership approach for health professionals* (pp. 1–12). Sydney: University of New South Wales Press.

McMullan, M. (2006). Patients using the Internet to obtain health information: How this affects the patient–health professional relationship. *Patient Education and Counselling, 63*, 24–28.

McPherson, C. J., Higginson, I. J., & Hearn, J. (2001). Effective methods of giving information in cancer: A systematic literature review of randomized controlled trials. *Journal of Public Health Medicine, 23*, 227–234.

McWilliams, D., Jocobson, R., Van Houten, H., et al. (2008). A program of anticipatory guidance for the prevention of emergency department visits for ear pain. *Archives of Paediatric Adolescent Medicine, 162*, 151–156.

Michie, S., van Stralen, M. M., & West, R. (2011). The behaviour change wheel: A new method for characterising and designing behaviour change interventions. *Implementation Science, 6*, 42.

Montano, D. E., & Kasprzyk, D. (2008). Theory of reasoned action, theory of planned behavior, and the integrated behavioral model. In K. Glanz, B. K. Rimer, & K. Viswanath (Eds.), *Health behavior and health education: Theory, research and practice*. San Francisco: Jossey-Bass.

Morony, S., Flynn, M., McCaffery, K. J., et al. (2015). Readability of written materials for CKD patients: A systematic review. *American Journal of Kidney Disease, 65*(6), 842–850.

Murphy, P., Davis, T., Long, S., et al. (1993). REALM: A quick reading test for patients. *Journal of Reading, 37*, 124–130.

Murray, E., Burns, J., Tai, S., et al. (2005). Interactive health communication applications for people with chronic disease. *Cochrane Database of Systematic Reviews*. CD004274.

Neufeld, P. (2006). The adult learner in client-practitioner partnerships. In K. McKenna, & L. Tooth (Eds.), *Client education: A partnership approach for health professionals* (pp. 57–87). Sydney: University of New South Wales Press.

Neville, L., O'Hara, B., & Milat, A. (2009). Computer-tailored dietary behaviour change interventions: A systematic review. *Health Education Research, 24*, 699–720.

Noar, S., Benac, C., & Harris, M. (2007). Does tailoring matter? Meta-analytic review of tailored print health behaviour change interventions. *Psychological Bulletin, 133,* 673–693.

Parker, R., Baker, D., Williams, M., et al. (1995). The Test of Functional Health Literacy in Adults: A new instrument for measuring patients' literacy skills. *Journal of General Internal Medicine, 10,* 537–541.

Paul, C., Redman, S., & Sanson-Fisher, R. (1997). The development of a checklist of content and design characteristics for printed health education materials. *Health Promotion Journal of Australia, 7,* 153–159.

Pitkethly, M., MacGillivray, S., & Ryan, R. (2008). Recordings or summaries of consultations for people with cancer. *Cochrane Database of Systematic Reviews.* CD001539.

Prochaska, J., Di Clemente, C., & Norcross, J. (1992). In search of how people change: Applications to addictive behaviours. *American Psychologist, 47,* 1102–1114.

Prochaska, J., Redding, C., & Evers, K. (2008). The transtheoretical model and stages of change. In K. Glanz, B. K. Rimer, & K. Viswanath (Eds.), *Health behaviour and health education: Theory, research and practice* (4th ed., pp. 99–120). San Francisco: Jossey-Bass.

Prohaska, T., & Lorig, K. (2001). What do we know about what works? The role of theory in patient education. In K. Lorig (Ed.), *Patient education: A practical approach* (pp. 21–25). Thousand Oaks, CA: Sage Publications.

Quill, T., & Brody, H. (1996). Physician recommendations and patient autonomy: Fnding a balance between physician power and patient choice. *Annals of Internal Medicine, 125,* 763.

Ronco, M., Iona, L., Fabbro, C., Bulfone, G., & Palese, A. (2012). Patient education outcomes in surgery: A systematic review from 2004 to 2010. *International Journal of Evidence-Based Healthcare, 10*(4), 309–323.

Rosenstock, I., Strecher, V., & Becker, M. (1988). Social learning theory and the health belief model. *Health Education Quarterly, 15,* 175–183.

Sharma, M., & Romas, J. A. (Eds.). (2008). *Theoretical foundations of health education and health promotion.* Sudbury: Jones and Bartlett.

Stacey, D., Légaré, F., Col, N. F., et al. (2014). Decision aids for people facing health treatment or screening decisions. *Cochrane Database Systematic Reviews.* CD001431.

Stewart, M. A. (1995). Effective physician-patient communications and health outcomes: A review. *Canadian Medical Association Journal, 152,* 1423–1433.

Short, C., James, E., Plotnikoff, R., et al. (2011). Efficacy of tailored-print interventions to promote physical activity: A systematic review of randomised trials. *International Journal of Behavioral Nutrition and Physical Activity, 8,* 113.

Steinsbekk, A., Rygg, L. Ø., Lisulo, M., et al. (2012). Group-based diabetes self-management education (versus routine treatment) in people with type 2 diabetes results in improvements in clinical, lifestyle and psychosocial outcomes. *BMC Health Services Research, 12,* 213.

Strecher, V., McEvoy, B., Becker, M., et al. (1986). The role of self-efficacy in achieving health behaviour change. *Health Education Quarterly, 13,* 73–91.

Taylor, D., Bury, M., Campling, N., et al., for the School of Pharmacy, University of London. (2007). *A Review of the use of the Health Belief Model (HBM), the Theory of Reasoned Action (TRA), the Theory of Planned Behaviour (TPB) and the Trans-Theoretical Model (TTM) to study and predict health related behaviour change.* London: The National Institute for Health and Clinical Excellence.

Tlach, L., Wüsten, C., Daubmann, A., et al. (2014). Information and decision-making needs among people with mental disorders: A systematic review of the literature. *Health Expectations, 18,* 1856–1872.

Waller, A., Forshaw, K., Bryant, J., & Mair, S. (2014). Interventions for preparing patients for chemotherapy and radiotherapy: A systematic review. *Supportive Care in Cancer, 22*(8), 2297–2308.

Wennberg, D., Marr, A., Lang, L., et al. (2010). A randomised trial of a telephone care-management strategy. *New England Journal of Medicine, 363,* 1245–1255.

White, D., Braddock, C., Bereknyei, S., et al. (2007). Toward shared decision making at the end of life in intensive care units: Opportunities for improvement. *Archives of Internal Medicine, 167,* 461–467.

Wilson, F., & McLemore, R. (1997). Patient literacy levels: A consideration when designing patient education programs. *Rehabilitation Nursing, 22,* 311–317.

Wilson, S., Strub, P., Buist, S., et al. (2010). Shared treatment decision making improves adherence and outcomes in poorly controlled asthma. *American Journal of Respiratory Critical Care Medicine, 181,* 566–577.

FURTHER READING

DISCERN instrument – quality criteria for online health information. 1997. Retrieved from www.discern.org.uk.

Fleming, J., & Onsworth, T. (2006). Educational partnerships with clients who have cognitive impairment. In K. McKenna, & L. Tooth (Eds.), *Client education: A partnership approach for health professionals* (pp. 246–269). Sydney: University of New South Wales Press.

Hickson, L. (2006). Educational partnerships with clients who have hearing impairment. In K. McKenna, & L. Tooth (Eds.), *Client education: A partnership approach for health professionals* (pp. 226–245). Sydney: University of New South Wales Press.

Lorig, K., & Harris, M. (2001). How do I get from a needs assessment to a program? Program planning and implementation. In K. Lorig (Ed.), *Patient education: A practical approach* (3rd ed., pp. 85–142). Thousand Oaks, CA: Sage Publications.

McKenna, K., & Liddle, J. (2006). Educating older clients. In K. McKenna, & L. Tooth (Eds.), *Client education: A partnership approach for health professionals* (pp. 183–205). Sydney: University of New South Wales Press.

Redman, B. (2003). *Measurement tools in patient education.* New York: Springer.

Worrall, L., Howe, T., & Rose, T. (2006). Educating clients with speech and language impairments. In K. McKenna, & L. Tooth (Eds.), *Client education: A partnership approach for health professionals* (pp. 206–225). Sydney: University of New South Wales Press.

PUBLIC HEALTH

RACHAEL DIXEY

Abstract

This chapter introduces concepts of contemporary health promotion, suggests ways in which occupational therapists can engage with health promotion and explores ways in which occupational therapy and health promotion have common aspects of practice philosophy. The chapter will provide a sense of the philosophy that health promoters have in terms of their orientation to the problem of helping people to improve their health, but it cannot hope but to skim the surface of this complex discipline. Health promotion can be seen as a social movement aimed at increasing health justice, and it uses many strategies and techniques to do so, including those included in other chapters in this book, such as health education, working with communities, and advocacy. The chapter is not intended as a 'how to do' health promotion guide, but it will provide a foundation in the key principles and point readers to further reading. The chapter also demonstrates that health promotion is already part of the everyday work of occupational therapists.

KEY POINTS

- Health promotion is a social movement aimed at increasing health justice and tackling health inequalities.

- The aims, philosophy and principles of health promotion align well with those of occupational therapy.

- Three key concepts – a social model of health, salutogenesis and upstream thinking – underpin modern health promotion.

- Health promotion, based on the Ottawa Charter, has moved further away from health education and behaviour change and more towards a settings approach, building healthy public policy, and creating active and empowered citizens.

INTRODUCTION

The aim of this chapter is to provide an orientation to current thinking in health promotion and to suggest links with the field of occupational therapy. It is evident since the last edition of this volume that occupational therapy as a discipline has moved further towards embracing health promotion as a key element of its practice. Wilson, Andrew, & Wilson, (2012, p. 36) assert that, 'The compatibility between health promotion and occupational therapy is well documented'. It is perhaps not surprising that the convergence of the two disciplines has come mainly from those countries where health promotion is particularly strong, such as New Zealand and Australia (Frenchman, 2014; Wilcock, 2006; Wilson et al., 2012; Wood, Fortune, & McKinstry, 2013). Discussion of how occupational therapists can play an active role in primary health care, public health and health promotion has increased, and the key ideas of health promotion have become more obvious in the occupational therapy discourse.

Parallels can be seen between the development of health promotion and the recent concerns of occupational therapy. Both have struggled to move away from a medical model of health and the dominance of medical clinicians in setting health agendas. Both are concerned with justice – in the case of occupational therapy, with occupational justice, and in the case of health promotion, with health justice. Indeed, it can be argued that health promotion is a social movement aimed at tackling health inequalities to bring about increased occupational justice. Both *occupational therapy* and *health promotion* are contested terms – that is, there is disagreement within the respective professions about the precise meanings of the terms used, but also more fundamentally, there are ideological and philosophical differences about the purpose, methods and values of the two disciplines. Moreover, there is a confusion among the general public and other health professionals about exactly what health promotion is, just as occupational therapy is often misunderstood or seen simplistically. Finally, both disciplines are concerned with enabling people to develop their future 'possible selves' (Oyserman, Bybee, Terry, & Hart-Johnson, 2004) – that is, with helping people to become all that they are capable of.

Occupational therapy has, arguably, a much narrower focus than health promotion, in that occupational therapy focuses on occupation as the means to attain health, whereas health promotion considers all aspects of life, and the full range of strategies at national, community and individual levels, in order to promote health. Specialist health promoters are most likely to work at a strategic or policy level, and less so with individuals. Health promotion *is* concerned with those who have lost their health but is more centrally concerned with whole, healthy populations, in order for all people to become as healthy as humanly possible. Health promotion, then, could be used with individuals who have suffered a heart attack, in order for them to return to fitness, but aims primarily to work with healthy populations on *prevention* (e.g. healthy eating, exercise, etc.). Health promotion would also encourage the pursuit of ever increasing levels of positive health as a 'good' in its own right. Likewise, occupational therapy has, in recent times, striven to assert its potential role with healthy individuals and communities to help them engage in life-enhancing occupations, rather than only playing a

rehabilitation role with people who have become ill or unhealthy. The latter is clearly important and necessary, but there are also opportunities to work in more creative, proactive ways to prevent ill health occurring in the first place and also to enable healthy people to pursue the highest possible level of occupational well-being. Just as health promotion sees health as a human right, the focus of occupational therapy is 'on the right of all people to participate in meaningful occupations, and proposes allegiance to occupational rights: the right of all people to engage in meaningful occupations that contribute positively to their own well-being and the well-being of their communities' (Hammell, 2008, p. 61).

Occupational therapy, then, is inherently health promoting. To take this further, it is useful to consider recent developments in the field of health promotion and how they apply to occupational therapy. A range of allied health professions have entered discussions on what their distinctive contribution is to health promotion (French & Swain, 2005; Ontario Physiotherapy Leadership Consortium, 2011). Within occupational therapy, Wilcock's (2006) work stands out as fostering discussion about the ways in which occupational therapy promotes health and well-being. There are also many examples of how occupational therapy works to *prevent* ill health with healthy communities (Pereira & Stagnitti, 2008) or to promote healthy aging (Clark et al., 1997, 2001). The American Occupational Therapy Association (2007) produced a useful position paper on health promotion that argues that the occupational therapist's role in health promotion is threefold: to promote healthy lifestyles, to emphasise occupation as an essential element of health promotion strategies, and to provide interventions with individuals and populations.

KEY IDEAS WITHIN HEALTH PROMOTION

Health promotion is a social movement with the central aim of tackling the social determinants of health to bring about greater social and health justice. The *social determinants of health* are those factors that enable people to live healthy and productive lives, including the obvious ones of decent housing, access to education, employment opportunities, nourishing food, well-functioning and accessible health care, cohesive communities, good systems of government and peaceful, safe nation-states. *Social justice* is harder to define and is often used interchangeably with related concepts such as *fairness, equality* and *equity*. The central concern with health equity has been present since the Ottawa Charter (World Health Organization (WHO, 1986), the founding document of modern health promotion, but was present in the WHO from 1946. According to Whitehead and Dahlgren (2007, p. 5), health equity implies that ideally everyone could attain their full health potential and that no one should be disadvantaged from achieving this potential because of their social position or other socially determined circumstance. This refers to everyone and not just to a particularly disadvantaged segment of the population. Efforts to promote social equity in health are therefore aimed at creating opportunities and removing barriers to achieving the health potential of all people. Health equity involves the fair distribution of the resources needed for health, fair access to the opportunities available, and fairness in the support offered to people when ill. The outcome of these efforts would be a gradual reduction of all systematic differences in health between different socioeconomic groups. The ultimate vision is the elimination of such inequities by levelling up to the health of the most advantaged.

Health promotion is thus centrally concerned with health equity, and in addition, there are three key concepts that need to be understood in order to comprehend the distinctiveness of health promotion: the social model of health, upstream thinking and salutogenesis. These will be discussed next.

Social Model of Health

A *social model of health* is demonstrated in the concern with health inequities. Over the last decade, this culminated in the global health promotion community welcoming the work of the Commission on Social Determinants of Health (CSDH). The Commission, chaired by Sir Michael Marmot, was established by the World Health Organization in 2005. It was essentially an independent enquiry into the social and environmental issues affecting health and planned to investigate actions with potential to promote greater health equity (Commission on Social Determinants of Health, 2008). The CSDH reported in August 2008 and concluded that social injustice is killing people on a grand scale. Publication was followed by a conference in London in November 2008, which constituted the first major international event to attempt to develop a global agenda to address the issues. The conference had the ambitious catchphrase 'closing the gap in a generation' and the optimistic task of turning the CSDH framework into practical action. This central concern with the social determinants of health is what distinguishes health promotion from public health. Health promotion takes a different approach from 'mainstream' public health, and thus health promotion is more a form of politics than a part of the medical enterprise and it is more allied to social policy than it is a profession allied to medicine.

The fact that people do not live in an equal and just society is easy to demonstrate. Data on inequalities in health abound, whether this is within rich countries such as the United Kingdom, between richer countries, such as the United States of America and Japan, or in poorer majority world countries. The reasons for the existence of these inequalities are more contentious. Wilkinson and Pickett (2009) in their book, *The Spirit Level,* claim to have produced an undeniable argument that inequalities in health within countries are explained by inequalities in wealth, not by the absolute wealth of that country, and that the more unequal a society, the more inequalities in health there are in that society. As epidemiologists who have researched health inequalities, Wilkinson and Pickett show the socially

corrosive impacts of inequality, continuing a concern with health inequalities that stretches back to the Black Report of 1980, which was the first major report in the United Kingdom to highlight how health is systematically related to social class. Later work refined analysis of health inequalities, and most notably the Marmot review of the social determinants of health highlights the role of psychosocial factors in explaining the fine gradients in health between social groups.

This concern with health inequalities is thus at the heart of the modern health promotion movement. Dahlgren and Whitehead's (1992) diagram (Fig. 26.1) is often reproduced to indicate the range of social determinants that interplay to determine any one individual's state of health.

Inequalities in health status are a constant feature of surveys in all countries. It is now incontrovertible that these inequalities are to do with the social and economic situation in which people live. Tackling inequalities is the starting point and the cornerstone of the value base of health promotion and leads logically to the targeting of health promotion efforts towards the most disadvantaged and marginalised. There have been a number of Western government attempts to reduce disparities in health, as evidenced by the United States's *Healthy People 2010* (US Department of Health and Human Services, 2000) and earlier in a Report to the Australian Government, "Goals and targets for Australia's Health in the Year 200 and Beyond" (Nutbeam, Wise, Bauman, Harris, & Leeder, 1993). A series of reports in the United Kingdom (Acheson, 1998; Marmot & Wilkinson, 2006; Townsend, 1988; Townsend, Davidson, & Whitehead, 1992) show a rather gloomy picture in that inequalities in health are persistent and difficult to reduce, let alone eradicate.

Upstream Thinking

The next key concept, that efforts to promote health need to be focused upstream, follows logically from the concern with inequalities. The catchphrase *focused upstream* has become common in public health circles and refers to the fact that many attempts to improve health only occur after the damage has happened – that is, attempts to improve health are focused on curative attempts to restore people to a state of health. Zola (1970) likened this to a person who is sitting on a riverbank, being called to rescue an individual who is clearly struggling in the water. The person hauls the individual out, and just as they both reach the riverbank safely, another person is seen struggling in the river, and so on and so on. That rescuer never has time to walk up the riverbank and find out who (or what) is pushing everyone in. The parallel with a doctor, nurse or other health professional who focuses on rescuing (curing) rather than on preventing is obvious. Health promoters try to focus their interventions on causes or determinants of ill health (whatever it is that makes people susceptible to illness in the first place), rather than on what might be happening 'downstream'. Of course, there will always be those who become ill, have accidents or

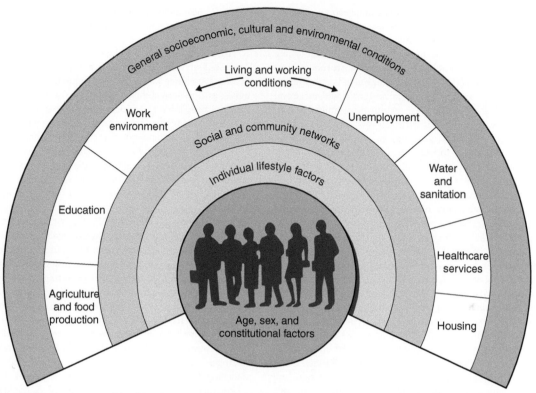

FIG. 26.1 ■ Determinants of health. (From Dahlgren & Whitehead, 1992. Reproduced with permission from the World Health Organization.)

develop illnesses about which the causes are little known (such as multiple sclerosis, Alzheimer's disease, etc.), and so it is not the case that health professionals with a curative focus are not needed. However, the adage that 'prevention is better than cure' means that a cadre of workers is needed to focus on how to prevent ill health before it occurs. This is what the health promotion profession can offer. Concern with determinants of health is central to that profession and to the focus on health inequalities.

Salutogenesis

Before going further, it would be useful to provide a model of health that suits the purposes of both health promotion and occupational therapy. To know what is being promoted, it helps to have an understanding of 'health'. Labonte's 1998 model of health (cited in Dixey, 2012) (Fig. 26.2) places well-being firmly at the centre, with key aspects, such as meaning and purpose, also prominent. This clearly goes beyond a medical model and is very much a social model of health, and illustrates how an occupational therapist could contribute to several of the dimensions, including 'ability to do things one enjoys', 'good social relations', creating 'meaning and purpose' and 'control over life'.

A key premise of health promotion is that the health of all individuals and groups *can* be improved and that health is

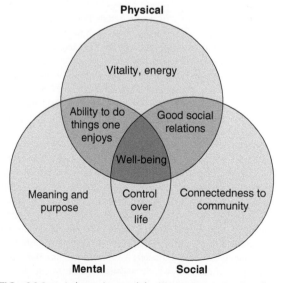

FIG. 26.2 ■ Labonte's model. (From Orme, J., Powell, J., Taylor, P., Harrison, T., & Grey, M. (2003). Public health for the 21st century. Buckingham: Open University Press. Reproduced with kind permission of Open University Press. All rights reserved.)

open-ended and positive. 'Health' is not simply about restoring a person to a 'normal' level of health or asserting that someone is well if he or she does not have an obvious disease or ailment. Health is about realising as much potential as possible and going on to become *more* physically fit, *more* emotionally robust, *more* socially happy. The WHO's (1986) definition of health – health is a state of complete physical, mental and social well-being and not merely the absence of disease or infirmity – might be utopian, but it also suggests that although this 'complete state' is difficult to achieve, as far as promoting health is concerned, the sky's the limit! The WHO (1986) has suggested that health is a resource for everyday life, not the objective of living, and Wilcock (2006, p. 315) follows by suggesting that an 'occupation-focused health promotion approach to wellbeing embraces a belief that the potential range of what people can do, be, and strive to become is the primary concern and [...] health is a byproduct'. Health, then, is not to be focused on for the sake of it, but so that it can enable a person to live a full, meaningful life. It goes without saying that the model of health adopted within a health promotion approach is a social model, not a medical one. The latter, with its disease focus, is narrow and does not enable illumination of the causes or determinants of health.

One of the key critiques of research investigating perspectives on health is that relatively few studies have actually examined concepts of *health* and instead have focused on aspects of illness (Becker & Rhynders, 2013; Hughner & Kleine, 2004). Clearly, health *can* be viewed in negative or positive ways, and the WHO definition of 1946 (cited in WHO, 1986) highlights how health should be seen as much more than the absence of illness, disease and disability. It is rather easier to frame health in negative rather than positive ways and easier to talk about those things that create ill health rather than those that create health – just as more has been written about what causes war rather than what causes peace. Biomedical accounts of health remain the most influential within Western contexts (Sidell, 2010), but salutogenic ways of thinking about health are more positive and focus on what creates health and well-being rather than on what causes ill health (Antonovsky, 1996). Logically, health promotion should align itself with more salutogenic ways of understanding and conceptualising health.

Salutogenesis is one attempt to capture a positive view of health and its causes and challenge negative ways of conceptualising health. It is the opposite of pathogenesis, which is the attempt to understand disease. Antonovsky (1996) coined the term *salutogenesis,* which asks the question 'What causes health?' and challenges the 'pathogenic' nature of the medical model of health by arguing that the focus should be on wellness, not illness. Rather than emphasising the biomedical dichotomy of health versus illness and disease, Antonovsky argues that people are all on a continuum, which he calls the 'health-ease-dis-ease' continuum, and that individuals move up and down this continuum all of the time, no one ever really achieving 'full' health. He argues that this is impossible given that people are all biological beings subject to the pathogenical forces of disease and

decay. He also called for a move away from the focus on the unwell and those deemed 'at risk', which is a key tenet of public health approaches.

Antonovsky further developed his ideas of what health is composed of with what he calls a Sense of Coherence. This encompasses three key elements: comprehensibility, meaningfulness and manageability. These relate, in turn, to the understanding people have of their world and making sense of their experiences, how they feel about these and to what extent they can cope with the demands that they face (Sidell, 2010). This idea becomes crucial in terms of understanding and accounting for their 'place' on the 'health-ease-dis-ease' continuum'; those with a stronger Sense of Coherence, Antonovsky argues, are more likely to be able to move towards the 'health' end of the continuum.

Kobasa, Hiker, & Maddi, (1979; Maddi, 2002) were the first to study hardiness as an aspect of personality, and they assert that *control* is one of three common factors in salutogenesis, the idea that an individual is able to influence the course of events. The other two factors are *commitment,* having a sense of curiosity for life and a sense of meaningfulness in life, and *challenge,* the expectation that life will change and that change is beneficial. Helping people to make appropriate changes is a key task of health promotion, with the aim of facilitating individual, community and societal change. Antonovsky's (1979) salutogenic concept of health, which was developed to try to understand what makes people healthy, as opposed to what makes them unhealthy, has been proposed as *the* key theory underlining health promotion.

THE IMPORTANCE OF THE OTTAWA CHARTER

Modern health promotion emerged in the 1980s from the Ottawa Charter. The fact that it was possible to promote and increase people's health has, of course, been known for much longer than this and can be seen in the attempts made by public health in most industrialised countries to promote health by providing better water and sanitation, enacting fair housing laws and workplace legislation, ensuring healthy diets, and so on. However, by the 1980s, these public health efforts to manage people's healthiness tended to take second place to the role of medicine, which had become spectacularly successful in many ways but was increasingly seen as unlikely to cope with the rise of preventable 'lifestyle disease' such as coronary heart disease, cancers and stroke. Medical costs could be infinite. A second strategy to deal with making the population healthier was health education. Health education, it was argued, would enable people to become informed about how to prevent lifestyle illnesses; once people understood, for example, the link between smoking and health, they would simply stop smoking, or if they knew the health benefits of eating fresh fruit and vegetables, then they would eat them. Clearly this is a gross underestimation of the complexities of human behaviour and also can be a form of victim blaming – if a family cannot afford fresh foods or does not know how to cook them, then there is no point educating about this in the absence of providing that family with the means and/or skills to carry out the required behaviour.

So the emphasis on the role of medicine and on health education was seen as insufficient in dealing with the population's health. The landmark report that highlighted this fact was Lalonde's (1974) report on the health of Canadians. The focus of this report was on the social and economic determinants of people's health, and it suggested that the key to improving health lay outside the health care sector (which is, on the whole, the illness or curing sector). Later, much of this thinking came together in the WHO conference held in Canada in 1986; this conference resulted in the Ottawa Charter on Health Promotion, which provides the foundation upon which the modern era of health promotion is built. The Charter shifted the main responsibility for improving health to policymakers, arguing that for people to be healthy, the right kind of public policy needs to be in place, together with the supportive environments that would address the environmental determinants of health. This newer emphasis became known as 'health promotion' as opposed to a health education approach that represented a narrower focus on behavioural determinants of health. It thus challenged the idea that health is determined by individual behaviours and actions that can be addressed by health education.

The Ottawa Charter argued for action in five areas:

1. Building healthy public policy
2. Creating supportive environments
3. Strengthening community action
4. Developing personal skills
5. Reorienting health services

The Ottawa Charter provided a much broader base for promoting health by moving beyond merely encouraging individuals to change their behaviour, to place the responsibility on governments to make healthier public policy and to locate the source of health *outside* the health care/illness sector. Canada continues to play a lead role in health promotion (Pederson, Rootman, & O'Neill, 2005), and the profession has developed substantially since 1986, in theoretical and academic ways and in its practice. The value base of health promotion as proposed by the Health Promotion Forum of New Zealand (2008) is stated on the Forum's website as follows:

Health promotion

- *works with people not on them;*
- *starts and ends with the local community;*
- *is directed to the underlying as well as immediate causes of health;*
- *balances concern with the individual and the environment;*
- *emphasises the positive dimensions of health;*
- *concerns and should involve all sectors of society and the environment.*

Health promotion is the process of supporting people to increase control over the factors that influence their health and quality of life. An important characteristic of health promotion is its focus on groups of people, either the whole population or specific subgroups. It places emphasis on changing the environment to enable behaviour to change. Health promotion draws upon principles of:

- *social change*
- *physical change*
- *policy development*
- *empowerment*
- *community participation*
- *equity and health*
- *accountability*
- *building partnerships and alliances between groups*

Health promotion draws on an explicit value base:

- *Individuals are treated with dignity and their innate self-worth, intelligence and capacity of choice are respected.*
- *Individual liberties are respected, but priority is given to the common good when conflict arises.*
- *Participation is supported on policy decision-making to identify what constitutes the common good.*
- *Priority is given to people whose living conditions, especially a lack of wealth and power, place them at greater risk.*
- *Social justice is pursued to prevent systemic discrimination and to reduce health inequities.*
- *Health of the present generation is not purchased at the expense of future generations.*

(Health Promotion Forum of New Zealand, 2008)

APPROACHES TO HEALTH PROMOTION

There are many writers (as evidenced in the Key References section at the end of this chapter) who have attempted to conceptualise health promotion, but most suggest that health promotion is complex and is *more* than only health education or attempts to change people's behaviour. However, health education and behaviour change do have a role to play; these two aspects are discussed next, before going on to argue that there are other essential features of health promotion.

Health Education

Health education has gained a reputation for 'victim blaming' and has been seen as a panacea when it could only ever be a partial solution to improving health. It was partly the deficiencies of health education as a sole approach that the Ottawa Charter was trying to remedy. If people are educated about an issue, they still might not be able to act on the knowledge for socioeconomic reasons, such as not being able to afford healthier foods, for example. A further weakness of health education is pointed out in the definition of health education by Keith Tones (1997, p. 37), one of the key academics writing about health promotion. He conceptualised health education as follows:

> *Health education is any intentional activity that is designed to achieve health- or illness-related learning, i.e. some relatively permanent change in an individual's capability or disposition. Effective health education may therefore produce changes in knowledge and understanding or ways of thinking. It may influence or clarify values; it may bring about some shift in belief or attitude; it may facilitate the acquisition of skills; it may even affect changes in behaviour or lifestyle.*

A key limitation is apparent – the stress is on 'may', but equally it 'may not' bring about required change, and the effect of increased knowledge on attitudes and behaviour is poorly understood and not especially straightforward. Clearly it is too simplistic to assume that if people are provided with correct information, they will act on it. Even if people are in the right environmental conditions to act upon advice and information, a complex series of psychological mechanisms can come into play that mean they do not act in the way the health educator would wish. Cognitive dissonance is one such psychological process, where new knowledge raises a sense of being uncomfortable with the status quo. An example might be where a person has his consciousness raised about his body mass index, perhaps through a healthy eating course, and begins to ponder whether he needs to lose weight. To reduce the dissonance, the individual either can dismiss the information or decide to lose some weight. Once having made the decision, of course, another series of complex processes come into play that will affect whether that person's intention is ever actually carried through.

The full complexity of the role of education in facilitating change will not be entered into here. The important point is that occupational therapists do not dismiss education, but rather think carefully about its use and limitations. Most importantly, consideration of how it can be used to good effect needs to be undertaken, because clearly there is a role for education in providing information and skills to individuals about their concerns. The adage 'knowledge is power' is still a powerful one.

When commenting on the role of occupational therapy for people with rheumatoid arthritis Adams and Pearce (2005, p. 145) note that 'participatory self-management education programmes will encourage the individual to change behaviour as well as improve their cognitive understanding of the disease'. They note that such programmes have been more effective in raising awareness than in creating long-term behaviour change, but a complete package of learning about psychological coping

skills, practising skills to reduce physical symptoms and improving anatomical knowledge can result in more effective self-management.

Behaviour Change

Behaviour change may be a key goal of health promotion, but as indicated earlier, the health promoter needs to be aware that people have differing socioeconomic circumstances, presenting different obstacles to change. For a woman living in difficult circumstances, perhaps on a low income, a single parent and with small children, trying to give up smoking or reduce weight, where smoking might be a coping strategy and the nearest shops offering fresh fruit and vegetables are out of easy reach, it would clearly be necessary to tackle some of those living difficulties first before attempting to address healthier behaviours. A critique of the social psychological models that attempt to explain the processes of behaviour change is that they often pay scant attention to these wider determinants of health. However, they also offer useful insights into health behaviours and provide a theoretical basis for planning interventions.

Health promotion has made great use of social cognition models such as the theory of reasoned action (Ajzen & Fishbein, 1980), later developed into the theory of planned behaviour (Ajzen, 1991). Social cognition models provide a theoretical account of how attitudes, motivations, subjective norms and behavioural intentions combine to predict behaviour. These are described as expectancy-value models, in that behaviour follows from what the individual expects will happen after a particular action; for example, 'If I work out at the gym I *expect* to get fitter'. According to the theory of planned action, intention to behave (a combination of motivation and effort) will be affected by subjective norms, or perceived pressure from significant others, and by attitudes, or salient beliefs about the health behaviour. Hobbis and Sutton (2005) point out the difficulties of using social cognition models to plan practical interventions or campaigns, but what these models perhaps help health promoters to do is to consider all the factors that might lead to an individual being able to overcome the obstacles to making changes – or not.

One model that has been extensively used in health promotion that attempts to understand the process of carrying out preventive health behaviours is Rosenstock's (1974) Health Belief Model. This model basically asserts that for individuals to carry out the proposed health behaviour, they need to perceive that they are susceptible to the health threat, that the health threat is serious, that there are perceived benefits to the action, and that there are minimal barriers or costs and there needs to be some kind of 'cue to action' (Rosenstock, 1974). The health promoter or occupational therapist can use these ideas to ascertain an individual's beliefs and then to work on the specific beliefs that hinder or help change. Rutter and Quine (2002) provide an in-depth discussion of the application of social cognition models to a range of health behaviours.

Another behaviour change model that has been applied a great deal in practice is the Stages of Change Model, also known as the Transtheoretical Model, developed by Prochaska, DiClemente, and Norcross, (1992). First used to help users of illegal drugs to stop their drug habit, this model has since been applied to helping people to stop behaviours (e.g. smoking cessation) and also to adopt behaviours (e.g. physical activity, condom use, etc.). The model can be used to assess readiness to change and to tailor an intervention to the appropriate stage; someone who is motivated to change, for example, will need a very different intervention from the person who is unaware or who is maintaining change and in need of support to do so. The idea is that people move through the stages, and the role of the therapist or health promoter is to facilitate successful movement through those stages. The model has been applied in a range of occupational therapy contexts, such as in mental health (Creek, 2011) or in helping older people to undertake home safety modifications (McNulty, Johnson, & Poole, 2004). The model has been subjected to a great deal of critique (see e.g. Povey, Conner, Sparks, James, & Shepherd, 1999) but it has been found to be useful in practice as a heuristic device. The use of these models in understanding health behaviours and in planning health promotion campaigns is provided by Green, Tones, Cross, & Woodall, (2015, Chapter 3) and Cross, O'Neil, and Dixey, (2012).

Painter et al. (2008), in a systematic review of the features of successful behaviour change interventions, suggest that when interventions are underpinned by a theoretical model of behaviour change, they are more likely to be effective. However, despite recommendations that theoretical models be used in the design of behaviour change interventions, the National Institute for Health and Care Excellence (NICE) guidelines (NICE, 2007) on behaviour change states that evidence to support the use of such models is inconsistent, and there is little to support the use of one over another; however, their guidance does provide a useful overview of behaviour change principles and practice.

More recently, there has been a move away from models that imply a somewhat mechanistic relationship among attitudes, knowledge and behaviours, and the focus shifted to more subtle approaches that capture the complexity of human motivations and actions with regards to behaviour change (Hart, 2015). 'Nudge theory' is a practical attempt to facilitate small steps towards behaviour change while avoiding the paternalism of many health campaigns (Marteau, Ogilvie, Roland, & Suhrcke, 2011). Behavioural economics is an emerging field that challenges the model of 'rational' people making decisions and enters into the complexity of human behaviour. A useful and concise outline of behavioural economics is provided by the New Economics Foundation (2007), and it fits with a more 'people-centred' approach to public health.

Health promotion might have had bad press in that it is seen as attempting to *stop* people doing things, such as to reduce fat and sugar in their diet, consume less alcohol, or give up smoking; but health promotion is far more than that. It is about creating the social conditions in which people can live life to the fullest, realise their potential, maximise their health and not be held back by the risk of poor health. What is clear is that action is required in an organised and concerted fashion to tackle any particular issue. To use the example of childhood obesity, there is little point encouraging families to change their eating and exercise habits without governments also taking action to curb advertising of 'unhealthy' foods, to produce school curricula where children can learn about food and learn how to cook, to work with the food industry and so on. There is evidence that obesity rates follow socioeconomic status, just as poorer people in general experience poorer health. Obesity strategies therefore need to tackle the social determinants of health.

Beattie (cited in Scriven, 2005) designed a model (Fig. 26.3) to conceptualise the full range of activities necessary to bring about healthy change. The model suggests that activity is required in each of the four sectors in order to bring about change. Again, using childhood obesity as an example, it might be that authoritative, top-down approaches that affect whole communities are needed to regulate the food industry, to ensure school meals meet certain standards or to make transport planners consider child safety to a greater extent, so as to encourage walking and cycling. Authority figures such as general practitioners might raise the issue with parents and caregivers on an individual basis, whereas using more negotiated approaches, a worker at a Children's Centre might work with groups of parents on aspects of healthy eating, starting a community garden to grow vegetables, or at an individual level the school nurse or youth worker might work with individual young people on how to be less sedentary.

This model can also be used to locate the positions of individual health workers, such as occupational therapists. Many may work primarily with individuals rather than with whole communities and primarily in a top-down rather than bottom-up way (i.e. in a more authoritative style rather than in a negotiated way). Nondirective counsellors might work in the bottom left quadrant, which is where occupational therapists might also be located.

Health promotion has an image that it is about producing leaflets and media campaigns to persuade a reluctant public to change their 'unhealthy' behaviours. This is as simplistic as thinking that occupational therapy is solely about assessing people's ability to negotiate steps. Modern health promotion, based on the Ottawa Charter, is characterised by complexity to such an extent that 'Complexity' has been proposed as a 'potential paradigm' for the health promotion discipline (Tremblay & Richard, 2011). An overview of the key elements of health promotion to create health and well-being is provided in Fig. 26.4. The figure illustrates that healthy settings, healthy public policy and active and empowered citizens are needed for effective health promotion. These elements will be outlined next.

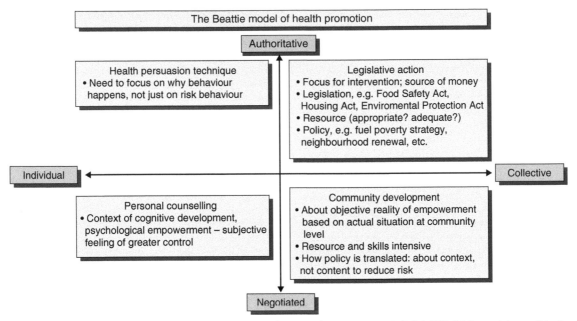

FIG. 26.3 ■ Beattie's Model of Health Promotion. *(From Gabe, M., Calnan, M., Bury, M. (Eds.) (1994). The sociology of the health service. London: Routledge, with permission.)*

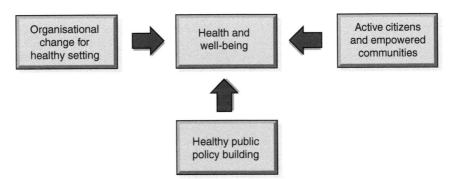

FIG. 26.4 ■ The key elements of health promotion.

Settings for Health Promotion

The Ottawa Charter and the subsequent conferences and declarations have argued that one way of giving health promotion a sharper focus is the development of the 'settings approach' (see Dooris, 2006; Green et al., 2015, Chapter 10; Whitelaw et al., 2001). The idea is that it would be useful to look at a 'setting', such as the workplace, a village, a school, clinic, and so on, and to consider *all* the people whose lives are affected within that setting and *all* the activities that take place within it, so as to consider how to make that setting healthier. The settings approach is now firmly in place within the health promotion field and has enabled the emergence of health-promoting schools and colleges, health-promoting hospitals, healthy workplaces, health-promoting prisons, healthier islands, and the Healthy Cities movement. It can lead to 'joined up thinking' as it places health on the agenda of all policymakers and all staff within an organisation. It enables people to think about contradictions; for example, in a school where children are taught about healthy eating in class, they are not then confronted with unhealthy choices for school lunch, as the purpose of the settings approach is to ensure that all aspects are thought about in an holistic manner.

A drawback of the settings approach is that individuals and groups outside various settings might be excluded, such as children who are not in school, people who are unemployed and so on. However, most public health programmes in most countries also have initiatives designed to include hard-to-reach groups or the socially excluded, in line with the concern with tackling health inequalities. This critique notwithstanding, the settings approach has added energy and systematic thinking to health promotion. Because of its focus on 'place', it provides tangible spaces within which health promotion can be highlighted and also enables professionals such as occupational therapists to physically locate themselves. Questions can be asked about how people are occupied within these places. For example, work has been done on creating health-promoting prisons (Woodall & Dixey, 2015); the setting of a prison certainly raises questions about how inmates can be purposefully occupied in order to be rehabilitated and to create healthier lives while imprisoned. For example, Baybutt's work shows how women in prison gain a sense of self-esteem and well-being through being occupied in gardening projects (Baybutt, 2013).

Building Healthy Public Policy

The role of healthy public policy was stressed in the Ottawa Charter, though it needs to be seen alongside the other four areas of action outlined in that Charter. Creating healthy public policies has been boosted by the Health in All Policies initiative, together with a 'whole of government' approach, which attempts to develop 'joined-up thinking' about health across government departments (WHO, 2014).

To use obesity once again as an example, not only has it been recognised that an 'obesogenic environment' has emerged, but also the solutions lie beyond individuals and lifestyle changes. It is necessary in countries with an 'obesity epidemic' to create supportive environments and therefore to develop, for example, transport policies that promote healthier ways of moving around and policies to control food advertising, regulate the food industry, and promote healthier eating and exercise in schools and workplaces. In addition, it is important to develop personal skills for healthier lifestyles and a role for health services to help those who struggle with weight gain. 'Healthy public policy' thus could do a great deal to tackle what the WHO calls the obesity crisis.

There are many examples of already enacted healthy public policies. The Framework Convention on Tobacco Control (Labonte & Laverack, 2010), which was the world's first *global* public health treaty, negotiated by the WHO in 2005, supported an internationally coordinated response to combating the use of tobacco. In the United Kingdom, the 2006 Health Act made it unlawful to smoke in almost all enclosed spaces and workplaces across the country. This healthy public policy aimed to reduce exposure to second-hand smoke for workers and the general public, with the secondary objective of reducing overall smoking rates. A similar ban was introduced in Spain in 2010, with much the same goals, and a large number of African countries have followed suit (Tumwine, 2011). There are global examples that can be regarded as healthy public policies, including the Kyoto Protocol on greenhouse gas emissions (Labonte & Laverack, 2010), which aims to reduce the levels of emissions at country level and as a result reduce climate change and potentially mitigate against the many health effects that are likely to ensue with changing temperatures across the globe.

A key strategy for building healthy public policy is that of advocacy, recognised and discussed within the Ottawa Charter as one of three major strategies for achieving health promotion goals (WHO, 1986). Advocacy can be defined in a number of ways, but essentially it is, according to Smithies and Webster's seminal work that reoriented passive recipients to active participants,

> *about people speaking up for or acting on behalf of themselves, possibly with the support of another person/group or 'advocate'. It is also about taking action to get something changed, in order to a take more control over our lives.*
>
> *(Smithies & Webster, 1998, p. 105)*

Advocacy may be undertaken by or on behalf of individuals or groups to create living conditions more conducive to health and healthier lifestyles. Advocacy for health therefore is about protecting those who are considered vulnerable, empowering people and tackling inequalities. Advocacy *can be* confrontational by challenging powerful commercial antihealth interests such as the tobacco lobby (Laverack, 2014b), or it can be about mediating and negotiating between opposing groups and positions to try to achieve positive health (Nutbeam et al., 1993). Advocacy may also have a capacity-building function, enabling individuals and groups to gain control over their lives and to improve their health by becoming effective policy advocates; health professionals such as occupational therapists can also become effective advocates (Lustig, 2012). Ultimately advocacy in relation to policy is about trying to influence the policy-making process so that healthier legislation and healthy public policies are introduced and implemented. Such advocacy can entail individuals and groups engaging in health activism, taking indirect or direct action, and perhaps leading to social health movements (Laverack, 2014a).

The centrality of healthy public policy to current health promotion can result in those working on the ground feeling disempowered, as they are often not in positions where they *can* influence policy. They may be working in what is really a health education role. Chapter 24 on advocacy and lobbying explains further how occupational therapists *can* carry out advocacy and lobbying.

Active and Empowered Citizens

Empowerment is seen as the key to promoting health. The Ottawa Charter states:

> *Health promotion works through effective community action in setting priorities, making decisions, planning strategies and implementing them to achieve better health. At the heart of this process is the empowerment of communities, and the ownership and control of their endeavours and destiny.*
>
> (WHO, 1986)

The implication is that participation must be a central principle of all health work. A focus on community health action is reflected in various global initiatives and statements from the WHO, such as in the Alma Ata declaration: 'people have a right and a duty to participate individually and collectively in the planning and implementation of their health care' (WHO, 1978). Similarly the WHO Regional Office for Europe argued that 'it is a basic tenet of the health for all philosophy that [...] health developments in communities are made not only for, but with and by, people' (WHO Regional Office for Europe, 1985).

In keeping with the social model of health, health promotion efforts should ensure that lay 'voices' and perspectives are 'heard'. In her important paper on shifting discourses within health promotion, Robertson (1998) commented that 'health promotion makes room for the stories which individuals and communities tell about their everyday experience of health, which legitimises them as being important to our understanding of health as statistics on morbidity and mortality rates'.

In moving towards greater room for lay involvement in creating health, and lay epidemiologies, it needs to be acknowledged first that people's understandings of health are what health promoters need to start with, rather than trying to change them or suggest that they are 'wrong'. Second, often lay opinion is not in tandem with public health and health promotion opinion, as, for example, professional priorities might differ from community priorities.

Putting people at the heart of health promotion and public health has gained momentum recently (South, White, & Gamsu, 2013). Initiatives such as Health Trainers, Community Health Champions and a range of other projects that enable people to become involved in public health roles (Woodall, White, & South, 2013) are changing the landscape of public health and facilitating increased civic engagement with health. These volunteering roles have been shown to improve the health of the volunteers, as well as that of the community members with whom they are engaged. This aspect of fruitful occupation has been examined by South, Branney, & Kinsella (2011), in two studies of volunteers in health projects 'bridging the gap', between what governments can provide and what is needed in communities. Other successful health promotion projects have used 'occupation' to improve health, including the Wye Wood project, which is an English initiative enabling people from disadvantaged backgrounds or experiencing mental health difficulties to work on forestry projects (Dixey, 2012).

THE ALIGNMENT BETWEEN HEALTH PROMOTION AND OCCUPATIONAL THERAPY

Considerable alignment between health promotion and occupational therapy is apparent from the discussion so far, and it can be inferred what health promotion can bring to the profession of occupational therapy and also what insights occupational therapy can offer to health promotion.

Scaffa and Brownson (2004, p. 485) note that 'community-level interventions are not as familiar to occupational therapy practitioners' but argue that they have an opportunity to 'respond to and help resolve the community health problems of the twenty-first century, including poverty, joblessness, inadequate day care and parenting skills, homelessness, substance abuse, mental illness, chronic disease and disability, unintentional injury, violence and abuse, and social discrimination' (p. 487). This opportunity to 'step outside of the box' of traditional occupational therapy (Withers & Shann, 2008) was discussed by Baum and Law (1998), and as far back as 1972 Finn offered a list of issues which occupational therapy needed to address for the profession to be able to contribute successfully to community health, arguing that it had a unique perspective to do so. This 'wish list' included learning about communicating with communities, having a secure professional identity and embracing health promotion (Scaffa, 2001). More recently, Fisher and Hotchkiss (2008) have discussed working with marginalised communities using a model of occupational empowerment in their work with women living in homeless shelters in the United States, illustrating that in some spheres at least, there is scope for occupational therapists to work at community level. The American Occupational Therapy Association (2007) suggests ways in which occupational therapists can contribute at community level. Health promoters more often than not work at community level, and there is scope for occupational therapists to join in existing teams.

The New Zealand Health Promotion Forum's outline of the value base of health promotion, provided earlier in this chapter, resonates with the client-centred practice base of occupational therapy, as described in *Enabling Occupation II* (Townsend & Polatjako, 2007). Client-centred practice features largely in the codes of ethics for occupational therapy (College of Occupational Therapists, 2005) and also within attempts to align the occupational health and health promotion agendas, such as in *For the Health of It: Occupational Therapy Within a Health Promotion Framework* (Letts, Fraser, Finlayson, & Walls, 1996). Sumsion (2005) suggests that client-centred occupational therapy practice hangs on the ideas of partnership, communication, choice, and power, and these resonate with key health promotion principles.

Within health promotion, the discourse around 'partnership' with communities and individuals is likely to be framed in terms of 'participation', 'collaboration' and 'involvement'. Peckham (2003, p. 70) argues that 'in adopting a more enlightened public health perspective, individuals and communities need to be seen as equal partners in promoting and producing health'. This equality of partnership implies a shift in the balance of power between lay people and professionals.

For health promotion to 'work', people need to be equal partners in all stages – top-down initiatives are likely to be resisted or ignored, and they are diametrically opposed to the key value of empowerment. A gradient of participation can be seen to increase empowerment (Fig. 26.5). A model which involves participation and empowerment clearly also involves the issue of choice and emphasises the importance of voluntarism – that is, of individuals not being coerced, but engaging willingly in activities that promote their health.

Empowerment within health promotion has been well explored by Laverack (2004), and it is becoming increasingly common to assert that empowerment is *the* central task of health promotion. Although the term *empowerment* has arguably been so overused that it has lost its initial radical intent (Woodall, Warwick-Booth, & Cross, 2012), if people are genuinely empowered, they acquire increased power and control, which is at the heart of the most well-known definition of health promotion, framed by the WHO (1986): 'the process of enabling people to increase control over, and to improve, their health'. This logically leads health workers, such as occupational therapists, into asking what constitutes empowerment and how they can facilitate the process of the people who receive their services becoming empowered. Scriven (2005) suggests that there are three important facets of personal development linked to empowerment:

1. Psychological perception involving enhancing self-esteem, self-efficacy and internal locus of control.
2. Cognitive development involving increasing awareness of health information and raising a 'critical consciousness'.
3. Life skills, including decision making, assertiveness and interpersonal skills.

Internal locus of control refers to the sense that individuals have of being in charge of their lives and is the opposite of being helpless or disempowered. It is the opposite of an external locus of control, which implies that individuals feel their lives are controlled by factors external to themselves, such as by fate or by other people. *Self-efficacy* refers to the belief people have in their ability to achieve or to carry out what they want to, such as giving up smoking, making more efforts to be sociable and less lonely or improving fitness. A model of empowerment increasingly used in England, adopted by the Altogether Better initiative (Fig. 26.6), also adds the all-important element of using personal skills and confidence to challenge systems (Woodall, Raine, South, & Warwick-Booth, 2010).

Harries (2005, p. 134) demonstrates how occupational therapy can help young people with eating disorders by 'building self-image, self-worth, communication skills, stress management skills and media awareness'. These ingredients are the standard fare of many health promotion interventions, but linking these aspects to a 'return to valued occupational engagement' (Harries, 2005, p. 131) is the occupational therapist's unique contribution.

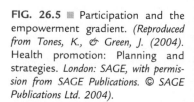

FIG. 26.5 ■ Participation and the empowerment gradient. *(Reproduced from Tones, K., & Green, J. (2004). Health promotion: Planning and strategies. London: SAGE, with permission from SAGE Publications. © SAGE Publications Ltd. 2004).*

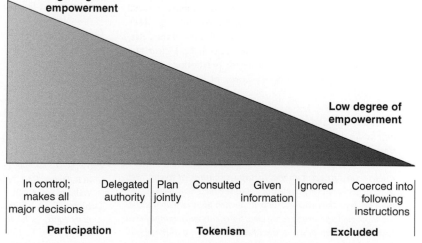

EMPOWERMENT MODEL

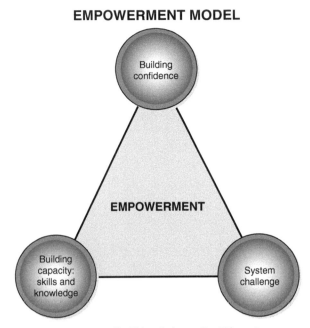

Empowerment = Healthier choices = Healthier outcomes

FIG. 26.6 ■ The Altogether Better empowerment model.

CONCLUSION

This chapter has shown that concerted action is needed at all levels – national, community and individual – to promote health. Health promotion 'is equally and essentially concerned with creating the conditions necessary for health at individual, structural, social, and environmental levels through an understanding of the determinants of health: peace, shelter, education, food, income, a stable ecosystem, sustainable resources, social justice, and equity' (Trentham & Cockburn, 2005, p. 441). 'Meaningful occupation' could be added to this list of the determinants of health. Occupational therapists have a clear and obvious contribution to make to health promotion, and it is appropriate to sum up with the words of Thelma Sumsion (2005, p. 107):

> There is a clear and positive link between client-centred practice and health promotion. The concepts of partnership, communication, choice and power are foundational to both client-centred practice and health promotion and must be implemented by occupational therapists committed to ensuring that clients have every chance of obtaining their health goals. The links between the two are strong, and when these two approaches are supported and clearly connected, the clients will be empowered to assume responsibility for their health, which is a unifying goal in both health promotion and client centred practice.

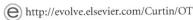

http://evolve.elsevier.com/Curtin/OT

REFERENCES

Acheson, D. (1998). *Independent Inquiry into Inequalities in Health Report.* London: The Stationery Office.

Adams, J., & Pearce, S. (2005). Occupational therapists and the promotion of psychological health in rheumatoid arthritis. In A. Scriven (Ed.), *Health promoting practice; the contribution of nurses and allied health professionals* (pp. 138–151). Basingstoke: Palgrave MacMillan.

Ajzen, I. (1991). The theory of planned behaviour. *Organisational Behaviour and Human Decision Making Processes, 50,* 179–211.

Ajzen, I., & Fishbein, M. (Eds.), (1980). *Understanding attitudes and predicting social behaviour.* Englewood Cliffs, NJ: Prentice Hall.

American Occupational Therapy Association. (2007). *Occupational therapy in the promotion of health and the prevention of disease and disability [electronic version].* Retrieved from, (2007). http://www.aota.org/Practitioners/Resources/Docs/Adopted/40983.aspx.

Antonovsky, A. (1979). *Health, stress, and coping: New perspectives on mental and physical well-being.* San Francisco: Jossey-Bass.

Antonovsky, A. (1996). The salutogenic model as a theory to guide health promotion. *Health Promotion International, 11,* 11–18.

Baum, C., & Law, M. (1998). Community health: A responsibility, an opportunity, and a fit for occupational therapy. *American Journal of Occupational Therapy, 52,* 7–10.

Baybutt, M. (2013). *Health, inclusion and citizenship: An ethnographic study of female prisoners' experiences of environmental work in the prison setting.* PhD thesis, University of Central Lancashire, UK.

Becker, C., & Rhynders, P. (2013). It's time to make the profession of health about health. *Scandinavian Journal of Public Health, 41*(1), 1–3.

Clark, F., Azen, S., Carlson, M., et al. (2001). Embedding health-promoting changes into the daily lives of independent-living older adults: Long-term follow-up of occupational therapy intervention. *Journal of Gerontology: Psychological Sciences, 56B*(1), 60–P63.

Clark, F., Azen, S., Zemke, R., et al. (1997). Occupational therapy for independent-living older adults. *Journal of the American Medical Association, 278*(16), 1321–1326.

College of Occupational Therapists (2005). *College of occupational therapists code of ethics and professional conduct.* London: College of Occupational Therapists.

Commission on Social Determinants of Health (2008). *Closing the gap in a generation: Health equity through action on the social determinants of health. final report of the Commission on Social Determinants of Health.* Geneva: World Health Organization.

Creek, J. (2011). *Occupational therapy and mental health: Principles, skills and practice* (3rd ed.). Edinburgh: Churchill Livingstone.

Cross, R., O'Neil, I., & Dixey, R. (2012). Communicating health. In R. Dixey (Ed.), *Health promotion: Global principles and practice.* Wallingford: CABI.

Dahlgren, G., & Whitehead, M. (1992). *Policies and strategies to promote equity in health.* Copenhagen: World Health Organization.

Dixey, R. (2012). *Health promotion: Global principles and practice.* Wallingford: CABI.

Dooris, M. (2006). Health promoting settings: Future directions. *Promotion and Education, 13*(1), 2–4.

Fisher, G., & Hotchkiss, A. (2008). A model of occupational empowerment for marginalised populations in community environments. *Occupational Therapy in Health Care, 22*(1), 55–71.

French, S., & Swain, J. (2005). The culture and context for promoting health through physiotherapy practice. In A. Scriven (Ed.), *Health promoting practice; the contribution of nurses and allied health professionals* (pp. 155–167). Basingstoke: Palgrave MacMillan.

Frenchman, K. (2014). The health promoting role of occupational therapy in primary health care: A reflection and emergent vision. *New Zealand Journal of Occupational Therapy, 61*(2), 64–69.

Green, J., Tones, K., Cross, R., & Woodall, J. (2015). *Health promotion: Planning and strategies.* London: Sage.

Hammell, K. (2008). Reflections on…well-being and occupational rights. *Canadian Journal of Occupational Therapy, 75*(1), 61–64.

Harries, P. (2005). Health promotion in eating disorders: The contribution of occupational therapists. In A. Scriven (Ed.), *Health promoting practice; the contribution of nurses and allied health professionals* (pp. 127–137). Basingstoke: Palgrave MacMillan.

Hart, D. (2015). Behavioural approaches to health and well-being. In F. Wilson, M. Mabhala, & A. Massey (Eds.), *Health improvement and well-being* (pp. 80–96). Maidenhead: Open University Press.

Health Promotion Forum of New Zealand (2008). What is health promotion? Retrieved June 19, 2008, from http://www.hpforum.org.nz/page.php?7.

Hobbis, I., & Sutton, S. (2005). Are techniques used in cognitive behaviour therapy applicable to behaviour change interventions based on the theory of planned behaviour? *Journal of Health Psychology, 10*(1), 7–18.

Hughner, R. S., & Kleine, S. S. (2004). Views of health in the lay sector: A compilation and review of how individuals think about health. *Health: An Interdisciplinary Journal for the Social Study of Health, Illness and Medicine, 8*(4), 395–422.

Kobasa, S., Hiker, R., & Maddi, S. (1979). Who stays healthy under stress? *Journal of Occupational Medicine, 21*(9), 595–598.

Labonte, T., & Laverack, G. (2010). Capacity building in health promotion, Part 1: For whom? And for what purpose? *Critical Public Health, 11*(2), 111–127.

Lalonde, M. (1974). *A new perspective on the health of Canadians: A working document.* Ottawa: Ministry of National Health and Welfare.

Laverack, G. (2004). *Health promotion practice: Power and empowerment.* London: Sage.

Laverack, G. (2014a). *A to Z of health promotion.* Basingstoke: Palgrave MacMillan.

Laverack, G. (2014b). *Health activism: Foundations and strategies.* London: Sage.

Letts, L., Fraser, B., Finlayson, M., & Walls, J. (1996). *For the health of it: Occupational therapy within a health promotion framework.* Toronto: Canadian Association of Occupational Therapists.

Lustig, S. (2012). *Advocacy strategies for health and mental health professionals. From patients to policies.* New York: Springer.

Maddi, S. R. (2002). The story of hardiness: Twenty years of theorizing, research, and practice. *Consulting Psychology Journal, 54*, 173–185.

Marmot, M., & Wilkinson, R. (2006). *Social determinants of health* (3rd ed.). Oxford, UK: Oxford University Press.

Marteau, T. M., Ogilvie, D., Roland, M., & Suhrcke, M. (2011). Judging nudging: Can nudging improve population health? *British Medical Journal, 342*, 263–265.

McNulty, M., Johnson, J., & Poole, J. (2004). Using the transtheoretical model of change to implement home safety modifications with community-dwelling older adults: An exploratory study. *Physical and Occupational Therapy in Geriatrics, 21*(4), 53–66.

National Institute for Health and Care Excellence. (2007). *Behaviour change: The principles for effective interventions.* London: NICE. Retrieved from http://www.nice.org.uk.

New Economics Foundation. (2007). *Economics as if people and the planet mattered.* London: New Economics Foundation.

Nutbeam, D., Wise, M., Bauman, A., Harris, E., & Leeder, S. (1993). *Goals and targets for Australia's health in the year 2000 and beyond.* Canberra: AGPS.

Ontario Physiotherapy Leadership Consortium. (2011). Physiotherapists in health promotion: Findings of a forum. *Physiotherapy Canada, 63*(4), 391–392.

Oyserman, D., Bybee, D., Terry, K., & Hart-Johnson, T. (2004). Possible selves as roadmaps. *Journal of Research in Personality, 38*, 130–149.

Painter, J. E., Borba, C. P. C., Hynes, M., et al. (2008). The use of theory in health behavior research from 2000 to 2005: A systematic review. *Annals of Behavioral Medicine, 35*, 358–362.

Peckham, S. (2003). Who are the partners in public health? In J. Orme, J. Powell, P. Taylor, T. Harrison, & M. Grey (Eds.), *Public health for the 21st century.* Buckingham: Open University Press.

Pederson, A., Rootman, I., & O'Neill, M. (2005). Health promotion in Canada: Back to the past or towards a promising future? In A. Scriven & S. Garman (Eds.), *Promoting health: Global perspectives* (pp. 255–262). Basingstoke: Palgrave MacMillan.

Pereira, R., & Stagnitti, K. (2008). The meaning of leisure for well-elderly Italians living in an Australian community: Implications for occupational therapy. *Australian Occupational Therapy Journal, 55*(1), 39–46.

Povey, R., Conner, M., Sparks, P., James, R., & Shepherd, R. (1999). A critical examination of the application of the Transtheoretical Model's stages of change to dietary behaviours. *Health Education Research, 14*(5), 641–651.

Prochaska, J. O., DiClemente, C. C., & Norcross, J. C. (1992). Measuring processes of how people change: Application to addictive behaviours. *American Psychologist, 47*, 1102–1114.

Robertson, A. (1998). Shifting discourses on health in Canada: From health promotion to population health. *Health Promotion International, 13*, 155–166.

Rosenstock, I. M. (1974). The Health Belief Model and preventive health behaviour. *Health Education Monographs, 2*, 354–386.

Rutter, D., & Quine, L. (2002). *Changing health behaviour: Intervention and research with social cognition models.* Milton Keynes: Open University Press.

Scaffa, M. (2001). Community-based practice: Occupation in context. In M. Scaffa (Ed.), *Occupational therapy in community-based practice settings* (pp. 3–18). Philadelphia: FA Davis.

Scaffa, M., & Brownson, C. (2004). Occupational therapy interventions: Community health approaches. In C. Christiansen, C. Baum, & J. Bass-Haugen (Eds.), *Occupational therapy: performance, participation, and well-being* (3rd ed., pp. 477–492). Thorofare, NJ: Slack.

Scriven, A. (2005). Promoting health: Perspectives, policies, principles, practice. In A. Scriven (Ed.), *Health promoting practice; The contribution of nurses and allied health professionals* (pp. 1–16). Basingstoke: Palgrave MacMillan.

Sidell, M. (2010). Older people's health: Applying Antonovsky's salutogenic paradigm. In J. Douglas, S. Earle, S. Handsley, L. Jones, C. Lloyd, & S. Spurr (Eds.), *A reader promoting public health, challenge and controversy* (2nd ed., pp. 27–32). London: Sage.

Smithies, J., & Webster, G. (1998). *Community involvement in health. From passive recipients to active participants.* Aldershot: Ashgate.

South, J., Branney, P., & Kinsella, K. (2011). Citizens bridging the gap? Interpretations of volunteering roles in two public health projects. *Voluntary Sector Review, 2*(3), 297–315.

South, J., White, J., & Gamsu, M. (2013). *People-centred public health.* Bristol: Polity Press.

Sumsion, T. (2005). Promoting health through client centred occupational therapy practice. In A. Scriven (Ed.), *Health promoting practice; the contribution of nurses and allied health professionals* (pp. 99–112). Basingstoke: Palgrave MacMillan.

Taylor Gregg, J., O'Hara, L., & Barnes. (2014). Health promotion: A critical salutogenic science. *International Journal of Social Work and Human Services Practice, 2*(6), 283–290.

Tones, K. (1997). Health education as empowerment. In M. Siddell, L. Jones, J. Katz, & A. Peberdy (Eds.), *Debates and dilemmas in promoting health: A reader* (pp. 33–42). Milton Keynes: Open University Press.

Townsend, P. (Ed.). (1988). *Inequalities in health.* London: Penguin.

Townsend, E. A., & Polatajko, H. J. (2007). *EnablingOccupation II: Advancing an Occupational Therapy Vision for Health, Well-being, & Justice through Occupation.* Ottawa, ON: CAOT Publications ACE.

Townsend, P., Davidson, N., & Whitehead, M. (Eds.), (1992). *Inequalities in health.* London: Penguin.

Tremblay, M.-C., & Richard, L. (2011). Complexity: A potential paradigm for a health promotion discipline. *Health Promotion International,* http://dx.doi.org/10.1093/heapro/dar054.

Trentham, B., & Cockburn, L. (2005). Participatory action research: Creating new knowledge and opportunities for occupational engagement. In F. Kronenberg, S. Algado, & N. Pollard (Eds.), *Occupational therapy without borders: Learning from the spirit of survivors.* Churchill Livingstone: Edinburgh.

Tumwine, J. (2011). Implementation of the framework convention on tobacco control in Africa: Current status of legislation. *International Journal of Environmental Research and Public Health, 8*(11), 4312–4331.

US Department of Health and Human Services. (2000). *Healthy people 2010: Improving health and objectives for improving health.* Washington, D.C.: US Government Printing Office.

Whitehead, M., & Dahlgren, G. (2007). Concepts and principles for tackling social nequities in health. Levelling Up Part 1. *Studies on Social and Economic Determinants of Health, No. 2.* Liverpool:

WHO Collaborating Centre for Social Determinants of Health, University of Liverpool.

Whitelaw, S., Baxendale, A., Bryce, C., MacHardy, L., Young, I., & Witney, E. (2001). 'Settings' based health promotion: A review. *Health Promotion International, 16*(4), 339–353.

Wilcock, A. (2006). *An occupational perspective of health* (2nd ed.). Thorofare, NJ: Slack.

Wilkinson, R., & Pickett, K. (2009). *The spirit level. Why more equal societies almost always do better.* London: Allen Lane.

Wilson, V., Andrew, A., & Wilson, L. (2012). Health promotion: Future occupational therapy in an ageing New Zealand. *New Zealand Journal of Occupational Therapy, 59*(2), 36–38.

Withers, C., & Shann, S. (2008). Embracing opportunities: Stepping outside of the box. *British Journal of Occupational Therapy, 71*(3), 122–124.

Wood, R., Fortune, T., & McKinstry, C. (2013). Perspectives of occupational therapists working in primary health promotion. *Australian Occupational Therapy Journal, 60,* 161–170.

Woodall, J., & Dixey, R. (2015). Advancing the health promoting prison: A call for global action. *Global Health Promotion,* (Epub 2015 Jul 8.).

Woodall, J., Raine, G., South, J., & Warwick-Booth, L. (2010). *Empowerment & health and well being: Evidence review.* Leeds: Centre for Health Promotion Research, Leeds Metropolitan University.

Woodall, J., Warwick-Booth, L., & Cross, R. (2012). Has empowerment lost its power? *Health Education Research, 27*(4), 742–745.

Woodall, J., White, J., & South, J. (2013). Improving health and well-being through community health champions: A thematic evaluation of a programme in Yorkshire and Humber. *Perspectives in Public Health, 133*(2), 96–103.

World Health Organization (1978). *Declaration of Alma Ata.* International conference on primary health care, Alma-Ata, USSR, 6–12 September 1978, Geneva, WHO. http://www.who.int/hpr/NPH/docs/declaration_almaata.pdf.

World Health Organization. (1986). *The Ottawa charter for health promotion.* Geneva: World Health Organization.

World Health Organization. (2014). *Health in all policies: Framework for country action.* Geneva: World Health Organization.

World Health Organization Regional Office for Europe (1985). *Targets for Health for All: Targets in Support of the European Regional Strategy for Health for All.* Copenhagen: World Health Organization Regional Office for Europe.

KEY REFERENCES ON PUBLIC HEALTH

Dixey, R. (2012). *Health promotion: Global principles and practice.* Wallingford: CABI.

Green, J., & South, J. (2012). *Evaluation.* Milton Keynes: Open University Press.

Green, J., Tones, K., Cross, R., & Woodall, J. (2015). *Health promotion: Planning and strategies.* London: Sage.

Gregg, J., & O'Hara, L. (2007a). Values and principles evident in current health promotion practice. *Health Promotion Journal of Australia, 18*(1), 7–11.

Gregg, J., & O'Hara, L. (2007b). The Red Lotus Health Promotion Model: A new model for holistic, ecological and salutogenic health promotion practice. *Health Promotion Journal of Australia, 18*(1), 12–19.

Laverack, G. (2014c). *The pocket guide to health promotion.* Maidenhead: Open University Press.

Laverack, G. (2013a). *A to Z of health promotion.* Basingstoke: Palgrave MacMillan.

Naidoo, J., & Wills, J. (2000). *Health promotion: Foundations for practice.* London: Elsevier Health Sciences.

Nutbeam, D., Wise, M., & Harris, E. (2004). *Theory in a nutshell: A practical guide to health promotion theories.* Sydney: McGraw Hill.

Scriven, A., & Garman, S. (Eds.). (2005). *Promoting health: Global perspectives.* Basingstoke: Palgrave MacMillan.

Taylor Gregg, J., O'Hara, L., & Barnes (2014). Health promotion: A critical salutogenic science. *International Journal of Social Work and Human Services Practice, 2*(6), 283–290.

Thompson, S. (2014). *The essential guide to public health and health promotion.* London: Routledge.

WHO (2009). *Milestones in Health Promotion: Statements from Global Conferences.* Geneva: World Health Organization.

World Health Organization (2014). *Health in all policies: Framework for country action.* Geneva: World Health Organization.

27 COMMUNITY DEVELOPMENT

MARIE GRANDISSON ■ ANICK SAUVAGEAU

Abstract
Occupational therapists are expanding their scope of practice by engaging in community development. Here their role is to build community capacity to promote the participation of all members. In a community-centred and community-driven process, therapists help communities define their occupational issues and foster the development of necessary knowledge and skills, the creation of more supportive environments and the modification of occupational demands and opportunities. In this chapter, a practical approach using the Person–Environment–Occupation Model (Law et al., 1996) and the Canadian Practice Process Framework (Davis, Craik, & Polatajko, 2013) is proposed to guide occupational therapists engaging in community development. Practice stories illustrate how occupational therapists can be involved in community development.

KEY POINTS

- Occupational therapists can use community development strategies to intervene with groups or communities.

- In a collaborative process, community development practitioners conduct a needs assessment and then assist communities to solve their most important issues.

- Occupational therapists involved in community development enable community members to identify occupational priorities and build community capacity to promote the participation of all members.

- They achieve this by helping groups to develop skills and knowledge, create supportive environments and modify occupational demands and opportunities.

■ A community development intervention follows a similar process to an intervention for an individual but gives more emphasis to strengthening the community's capacity, using local resources and developing self-sustainable initiatives.

■ Outcome evaluation should follow community development interventions.

INTRODUCTION

Recent occupational therapy guidelines call for a shift in the way therapists view the people to whom they provide services; occupational therapists are encouraged to see beyond their focus on individuals, and to focus more broadly on groups, communities, organisations and populations (American Association of Occupational Therapy (AOTA), 2010; Townsend et al., 2013a). In community development, occupational therapists collaborate with organisations and communities to build capacity and foster the development of a more healthy and inclusive society, in which all members have decent opportunities to engage in meaningful occupations. In this chapter key concepts associated with community development are defined, occupational therapists' roles in this area are explored and a practical approach for occupational therapists to engage in community development is proposed.

KEY CONCEPTS

What Defines a Community and an Organisation?

Occupational therapists working in community development may be working with a community or an organisation. There is no universal definition of *community*. It is generally accepted that a community is a group of people sharing an occupational engagement, interest, identity, issue, a circumstances or geographical location in which to work, play or carry out other roles (Doll, 2009; Labonte, 1997; Restall, Leclair, & Banks, 2005; Townsend et al., 2013a). The group may live within a neighbourhood and share common services or it may be a virtual community interacting electronically. An organisation is a structure that manages functions: it may be a business, an agency, a club, a professional body, or a nongovernmental organisation (AOTA, 2010; Townsend et al., 2013a). Some communities may be regrouped under organisations, such as an association for people with disabilities. As Labonte (1997, p. 90) stated, 'We all belong to multiple communities at any given time'.

What Is Community Development?

According to Labonte (1997), community development is 'the process of organising and/or supporting community groups in their identification of important concerns and issues and their ability to plan and implement strategies to mitigate their concerns and resolve their issues' (p. 97). It is a collaborative process aimed at building a community's capacity to help 'people to help themselves' (Rothman, Erlich, & Tropman, 1995, p. 29). The community development practitioner generally acts as a facilitator. Community representatives are considered experts regarding their own situations and are invited to reflect and make decisions on how to address their difficulties. Community development requires sound cultural competence and the development of genuine partnerships with organisations or stakeholders belonging to the targeted community; partnerships in which everyone's contributions and opinions are valued (Doll, 2009; Labonte, 1997). In other words, community development is a community-centred and community-driven process aimed at providing greater opportunities for all to participate actively in their communities, including disadvantaged groups.

Community practice generally refers to interventions based in and carried out for a community. It is not a synonym for community development. Rather, community development is one stream of community practice in which interventions are carried out with community members. The focus of community development is supporting members in defining and solving their problems and building the community's capacity (Leclair, 2010).

Rothman et al. (1995) propose three levels of community intervention: locality development, social planning/policy, and social action. These are briefly summarised in Table 27.1, along with key words representing their common features with occupational therapy. Although locality development is more often associated with community development, a mixture of the three levels may be most effective (Rothman et al., 1995). These levels can help occupational therapists see a continuum of community development initiatives (Lauckner, Krupa, & Paterson, 2011) and draw on the approach or approaches that best suit their situation. Thus a community development practitioner may help community groups define their priorities and explore potential action plans, locate empirical data to choose a target group or to facilitate group decisions, build local capacity, or foster change by transferring knowledge and skills, referring to other resources or advocating.

OCCUPATIONAL THERAPY AND COMMUNITY DEVELOPMENT

Why Should Occupational Therapists Engage in Community Development?

There are four key reasons why occupational therapists should engage in community development:

1. Occupational therapists are invited to shift the focus of their practice from individuals to groups, organisations and communities (AOTA, 2010; Townsend et al., 2013a).
2. Community development fits with the core values of the profession: occupational justice to address inequities in access to and ability to engage in meaningful occupations, health promotion through occupation, community-centredness,

dignity and autonomy of all, empowerment, and respect for cultural diversity and marginalised groups (Banks & Head, 2004; Thibeault & Hébert, 1997).

3. Community development represents an opportunity to contribute to the creation of 'a just and inclusive society so that all people may participate to their potential in the daily occupations of life' (Townsend et al., 2013a, p. 154).

4. Through their understanding of the personal, environmental, and occupational factors influencing participation in meaningful roles, occupational therapists possess an excellent skill set 'to promote community participation by people of diverse abilities, cultures and interests' (Restall et al., 2005, p. 9).

TABLE 27.1

Levels of Community Interventions and Common Features with Occupational Therapy Based on Rothman et al. (1995)

Levels of Community Interventions	Practitioner's Role	Common Features with Occupational Therapy
Locality development	Enabler who brings community members together and builds their capacity to define and solve their own problems	Community-centred practice and capacity building
Social planning / policy	Expert who uses data to define problems and to propose empirically supported action plans to provide goods and services to those in need	Evidence-based practice
Social action	Advocate who draws on local and political knowledge to change social structures through advocating and redistributing decision-making power and resources to marginalised groups	Quest for social or occupational justice

What Is Occupational the Therapist's Role in Community Development?

Lauckner, Pentland, & Paterson, (2007) emphasise the importance of engaging in a collaborative and empowering process: they define community development from an occupational therapy perspective as 'a multilayered, community-driven process in which relationships are developed and the community's capacity is strengthened, in order to affect social change in their community that will promote the community's access and ability to engage in occupations' (p. 317). Boudreau and Donnelly (2013) suggest that therapists should work 'with communities to enable occupation through the creation of inclusive communities that support the occupational growth and development of all citizens, no matter what their age, levels of abilities, and socioeconomic status' (p. 236). Thus, occupational therapists partner with community representatives to help them identify occupational priorities and promote the participation of all community members, including those who are marginalised or who have an illness, injury or impairment. They achieve this by strengthening the community's capacity to develop accessible and inclusive environments and to create opportunities for all to develop their full potential and engage in meaningful occupations. Such work may include assisting community representatives in developing the knowledge, skills and opportunities needed to reach their occupational goals and providing them with further resources upon which to draw (Lauckner et al., 2011). Through the process, therapists favour local resources and aim to develop self-sustainable initiatives.

PRACTICAL APPLICATION OF COMMUNITY DEVELOPMENT TO OCCUPATIONAL THERAPY

In the following section a practical approach to guide occupational therapists engaging in community development is provided. This approach aligns with key principles of community development as well as occupational therapy models and processes. It is intended to offer guidance to facilitate occupational therapists' involvement in community development initiatives. However, flexibility and sensitivity to local characteristics are essential: this approach should not be rigidly followed, particularly as other models may be relevant.

Conceptualising with the Person–Environment–Occupation Model

This chapter follows recommendations for using the Person–Environment–Occupation (PEO) model (Law et al., 1996) to frame occupational therapy practice in community development (Broome, McKenna, Fleming, & Worrall, 2009; Restall et al., 2005; Ripat & Becker, 2012; Strong et al., 1999). This strategy can help therapists define and communicate their role (Law et al., 1996), focus on occupation-centred goals (Fazio, 2006), remain community-centred (Strong et al., 1999) and promote community participation through occupation (Banks & Head, 2004). Using the PEO model, therapists support community groups in identifying occupational issues affecting part of or the entire group. They then support them in deciding on the actions required to address these issues. Actions can target personal factors, occupational demands and opportunities or environmental supports and barriers (physical, social, institutional, cultural or socioeconomic). This vision of the role of occupational therapists in community development is illustrated in Fig. 27.1. Although each component of the PEO model is treated separately, occupational therapists are also expected to analyse the person–environment, person–occupation, environment–occupation, and person–environment–occupation interactions.

Occupational therapists use their knowledge of personal factors affecting participation in meaningful occupations to assist community groups in identifying the knowledge and skills needed by targeted community members. Occupational therapists may then join them in advocating for the needed resources to develop knowledge and skills, or they may provide training (Restall et al., 2005). Through their understanding of environmental barriers and supports to occupational performance, occupational therapists foster the development of more accessible, usable, supportive and inclusive environments (Boudreau & Donnelly, 2013; Broome et al., 2009; Doll, 2009; Lauckner et al., 2007; Restall et al., 2005). Finally, using their thorough understanding of occupational demands and of the value of occupations, occupational therapists help

community groups to discover, modify or create opportunities for meaningful occupational engagement for all (Restall et al., 2005). In other words, occupational therapists in community development aim to enable all to participate in meaningful occupations by building the community's capacity to develop the knowledge and skills of targeted community members, to create supportive environments and to modify occupational demands and opportunities.

As change agents, occupational therapists build the capacity of targeted community members or of people and organisations closely involved with targeted members. They can also advocate for and with them. When applying the PEO model to community development, it is essential to clearly define whose occupational performance is affected and targeted by the interventions. This will determine whether knowledge and skills are classified under the personal factors or under the environmental barriers and supports. Examples of interventions that may be done to help communities develop knowledge and skills, create supportive environments and modify occupational demands and opportunities are presented in Table 27.2. They were extracted from the literature, with formulations adapted to reflect enablement skills (Townsend, Cockburn, Thibeault, & Trentham, 2013b). Some examples could fit into more than one of the PEO components.

Following the Canadian Practice Process Framework

The Canadian Practice Process Framework (CPPF) (Davis et al., 2013) can be a helpful guide in community development

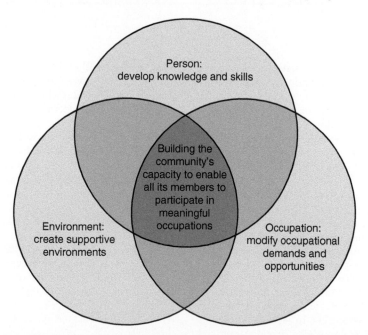

FIG. 27.1 ■ Occupational therapy contribution in community development.

TABLE 27.2
Examples of Community Development Interventions Associated with PEO Model Components (Law et al., 1996)

Person	■ Engage women in a residential area to help them identify the daily living skills they require and advocate for the needed resources to develop these skills (Restall et al., 2005).
	■ Educate tenants of a seniors' apartment building to enable them to respond to peers' health and quality of life needs (Cockburn & Trentham, 2002).
	■ Collaborate with people who have had a CVA, rehabilitation centre staff and a community partner to design a pilot peer-mentoring project for people who have had a CVA, and help them develop the skills needed to implement it (Lauckner et al., 2011).
Environment	■ Collaborate with individuals and municipal recreation facilities' staff to identify barriers to participation for all, then use universal design principles to remove barriers (Restall et al., 2005).
	■ Design a user-friendly tool for improving environmental accessibility in recreational programmes (Banks & Head, 2004).
	■ Educate summer recreation programme staff on the principles of inclusion (Banks & Head, 2004).
	■ Design age-friendly environments considering the entire bus transport chain, the consequences of aging on skills and on assistive devices use, and environmental factors. Act as a consultant and advocate for environmental changes (Broom et al., 2009).
	■ Advocate for playgrounds facilitating access and use by all children and caregivers, including those with illness, injury or impairment (Ripat & Becker, 2012).
Occupation	■ Collaborate with youth, community leaders and interested residents of a neighbourhood to create opportunities for youth to engage in healthier occupations by helping them identify a new occupation (i.e., creating art), and find the place and resources to carry it out (Restall et al., 2005).
	■ Coordinate services by linking seniors with volunteer opportunities in a community garden and a neighbourhood project (Lauckner et al., 2011).
	■ Collaborate with community members in identifying a shared occupation and engage them in developing opportunities for all to participate in it. Engage them in developing the community garden. Coordinate with organisations to obtain land, plants, benches or other resources (Leclair, 2010).
	■ Design an inclusive summer recreation programme (Banks & Head, 2004).
	■ Coach a group of outpatients to create meaningful work for themselves (Cockburn & Trentham, 2002).

CVA, Cerebrovascular accident.

work (Table 27.3). Following this framework can help occupational therapists remain community-centred, explicitly sharing decision making with community representatives. In a community development intervention, the therapists will also have a strong focus on building the community's capacity, using local resources and developing self-sustainable solutions. One or multiple cycles of evaluation and intervention may be completed with a community before concluding a partnership.

Occupational therapists involved in community development need to carry out needs assessments (Action Point 3). They can draw on a wide range of data collection methods to do so, including surveys, interviews, discussion groups and observations. To facilitate community engagement in the process, participatory tools can be used to assess needs (Action Point 3) or to establish the action plan (Action Point 4). Chevalier and Buckle's (2013) handbook of participatory tools and techniques may be useful to occupational therapists involved in community development. In Table 27.4, two tools inspired by their 'Tree of Problems', the 'Tree of Means and

Ends', and 'Hazards', are illustrated. These new tools were also inspired by Finlayson's (2007) asset-based needs assessment and Green and Kreuter's (2005) work on prioritising goals and objectives and tailored to occupational therapy in community development. Although these tools will not be relevant for all situations, they are provided as a practical option for occupational therapists to consider. When facilitating discussions using these tools, therapists may use flip charts, blackboards, or sticky notes on large sheets. Therapists are encouraged to adapt the tools to their needs and to the community they are working with and to look at Chevalier and Buckles' (2013) guide for other ideas for tools and ways to adapt them.

Two practice stories are included to illustrate community development initiatives in occupational therapy. Practice Story 27.1 describes the work of two occupational therapy students partnering with a regional association for people with traumatic brain injuries (TBIs). Practice Story 27.2 presents an occupational therapist collaborating with an agricultural college.

TABLE 27.3
How the Actions Points of the Canadian Practice Project Framework (Davis et al., 2013) Apply to Community Development

Action Points	How They Apply to Community Development Collaborating and sharing power with community representatives, the occupational therapist will:
1. Enter/initiate	■ Identify potential partners and create a first point of contact. ■ Communicate with community representatives to respond to a request.
2. Set the stage	■ Engage community members to clarify values and mutual expectations regarding occupational therapy's potential role. ■ Build rapport and collaborate to establish the partnership's boundaries.
3. Assess/evaluate	■ Coach the group in defining priority occupational issues affecting the community or a segment of the community. You may use the 'Tree of Occupational Goals' (see Table 27.4). ■ Assist the community in prioritising issues taking into account their importance and changeability and how the occupational therapist can help address the issues. You may use the 'Priority Scale' (see Table 27.4). ■ Collaborate to identify plausible causes of the occupational issues: personal factors, environmental barriers and supports, and occupational demands and opportunities. ■ Assess occupational performance in the priority issues. ■ Analyse findings to determine the most plausible explanation for occupational issues and share findings.
4. Agree on objectives and plan	■ Collaborate to formulate goals and objectives in occupational terms and clarify whether a subgroup should be targeted. You may use the 'Tree of Occupational Goals' or the 'Priority Scale' (see Table 27.4). ■ Discuss potential interventions and review the literature. Clarify whether the needed skills and resources are available and accessible. Identify stakeholders who have the power to change the situation. ■ Design and negotiate a sustainable action plan: occupational goals, action-based objectives to reach goals, modalities, stakeholders involvement, timeline, resources, reevaluation methods and plan for the future.
5. Implement the plan	■ Share responsibilities to implement the plan. ■ Use enablement skills. ■ Propose a tool to use or from which to build.
6. Monitor and modify	■ Informally monitor progress towards the objectives and goals. ■ Discuss with stakeholders whether adaptation is needed.
7. Evaluate outcome	■ Reevaluate to determine whether the goals and objectives have been met and whether further actions are required. ■ Present findings and help the group decide whether further evaluation or action is required or whether the partnership should end.
8. Conclude/exit	■ Communicate conclusions. You may provide documentation with recommendations for ongoing actions or tools built. ■ Clarify how the partnership could be reinitiated. ■ Reflect on the experience: What could be done differently next time? How does this project relate to occupational therapy skills and values?

TABLE 27.4
Suggested Tools

Tool 1: Tree of Occupational Goals[a] (Fig. 27.2)	■ Step 1: Draw a tree with a trunk and branches on a board, flip chart, or other material. ■ Step 2: Elicit major occupational issues and encourage group members to write them on large or small branches, depending on the importance of the issue. ■ Step 3: Discuss each occupational issue and define who is affected by it. Write key words on the branches to represent ideas. ■ Step 4: Prioritise one or two occupational issues with the group considering the importance of the issue and its modifiability, and circle them. Use the 'Priority Scale' if needed.

Continued on following page

TABLE 27.4

Suggested Tools (Continued)

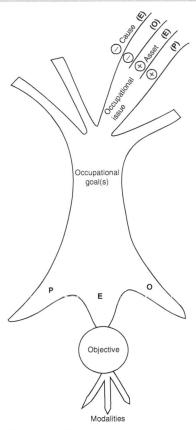

FIG. 27.2 ■ Tree of Occupational Goals.

- Step 5: Explore plausible causes and assets for each of the prioritised occupational issues on the corresponding branches. Invite group members to write causes on branches with a minus sign (−), and assets on branches with a plus sign (+). Ask the group: Why is this issue present? What are the assets available to tackle the issue? Who has the power to change the situation?
- Step 6: Collaborate with the group to identify how the causes and assets relate to the three components of the PEO (Law et al., 1996). Identify them with P, E or O.
- Step 7: Look at prioritised occupational issue(s) and assist the group in formulating measurable occupational goal(s). Invite group members to write them on the tree trunk.
- Step 8: Draw three main roots on the tree to facilitate discussions on the actions to be taken. Identify them with P, E, or O according to the PEO model (Law et al., 1996).
- Step 9: Review analysis of the main causes and assets, and discuss means to achieve the occupational goals. Invite and assist the group in writing action-based objectives on tree roots corresponding to personal (P), environmental (E), and occupational supports (O).
- Step 10: Prioritise one or two objectives considering how much they can contribute to the occupational goal(s) and how modifiable they seem.
- Step 11: Discuss potential modalities to achieve the objectives and write them on corresponding roots.

Tool 2: Priority Scale[b] (Fig. 27.3)

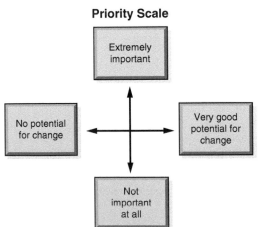

FIG. 27.3 ■ Priority Scale.

- Step 1: Draw a diagram in which a vertical line crosses a horizontal line of equal length. Indicate that the vertical line represents the importance of the issue or objective and that the horizontal line represents changeability.
- Step 2: Ask group members to rate how important the occupational issue or objective is. Invite them to consider how dissatisfied they are, the number of people affected and how much the problem contributes to the occupational issue. Invite them to place a dot on the vertical scale representing importance.
- Step 3: Ask group members to rate how changeable the issue or objective is. Invite them to consider which ones are most amenable to intervention, whether they were recently established or deeply rooted in cultural lifestyles, whether they include an addictive component and whether there are resources, legal levers or political desires to change the situation. Clarify how the occupational therapist has the skills required to facilitate change relating to the issue within the partnership's boundaries. Invite the group to place a dot on the horizontal scale representing changeability.
- Step 4: Draw a star at the junction between the importance and changeability dots for each issue or objective.
- Step 5: Invite the group to make a decision on what to prioritise, assisting them in realising that issues and objectives in the upper right quadrant are both important and amenable to change

CPPF, Canadian Practice Project Framework; PEO, person–environment–occupation.
[a]Steps 1–6 are related to the CPPF Action Point 3 (needs assessment), whereas steps 7–11 are related to the CPPF Action Point 4 (action plan).
[b]Steps 1–5 could be done for CPPF Action Point 3 (needs assessment) or CPPF Action Point 4 (action plan).

PRACTICE STORY 27.1

Partnering with a Regional Association for People with Traumatic Brain Injury

A regional association provides services to people with moderate to severe traumatic brain injury (TBI) who have severe cognitive and motor limitations. The goal of the services provided is to enable people with TBI to participate in meaningful occupations through adapted work, support meetings, board games, scrapbooking, cooking, painting, hockey and a monthly journal publication. Three staff members and 10 volunteers deliver most of the services.

Ann is an occupational therapist who often refers individuals to this association after rehabilitation. She contacted

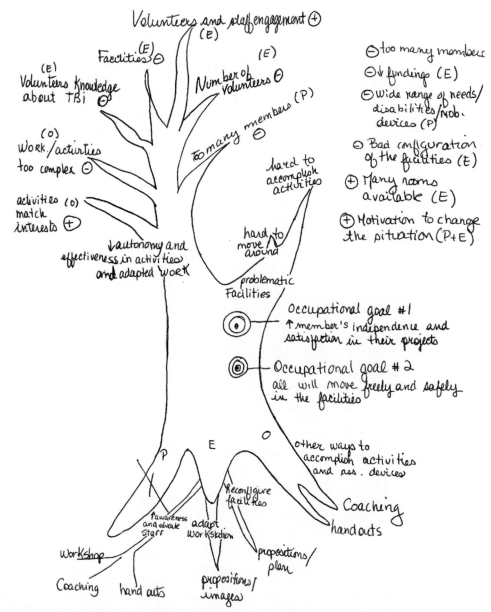

FIG. 27.4 ■ Example of completed Tree of Occupational Goals associated with Practice Story 27.1.

Continued on following page

Partnering with a Regional Association for People with Traumatic Brain Injury *(Continued)*

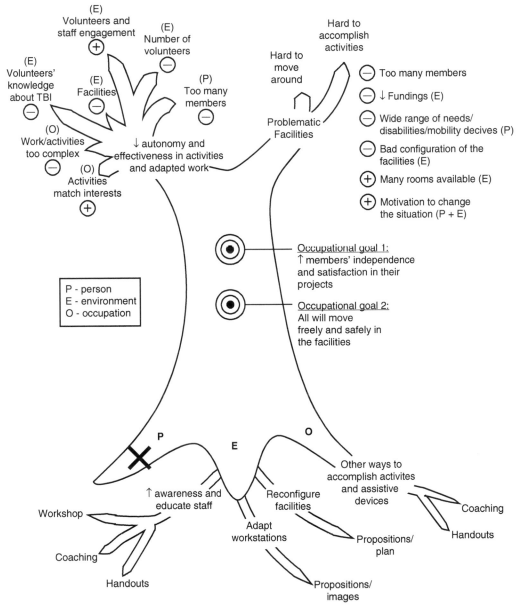

FIG. 27.4 —Cont'd

the manager of this association to determine whether two occupational therapy students could be involved in the association during an 8-week fieldwork placement focused on community development, which she would supervise. Upon agreement, the occupational therapy students, Sarah and Kathleen, started their placement by meeting the organisation's

staff members and volunteers and becoming familiar with the organisation's mission, services, target population and culture. The students then explained their vision of what they could contribute to the association. However, the students and the association's representatives struggled to understand occupational therapy's potential contribution to community

PRACTICE STORY 27.1

Partnering with a Regional Association for People with Traumatic Brain Injury (Continued)

development, as they were more familiar with occupational therapy's traditional roles in rehabilitation centres. Support from the students' supervisor was key at this point.

The students then spoke with association representatives, including members with TBI, staff members and volunteers, to clarify each other's expectations, conduct a needs assessment, and establish an action plan. Findings from the needs assessment and the action plan established are presented in the Tree of Occupational Goals in Fig. 27.4. The Priority Scale used to prioritise issues is included in Fig. 27.5. The action plan is further detailed next, including occupational goals, action-based objectives and chosen means.

- Occupational goal 1: Members with TBI will be more independent and satisfied in the different projects (courses, adapted work, etc.)
  - Objective 1.1 (Environment): Raise awareness and educate staff members and volunteers on strategies to encourage independence of individuals with TBI.
    □ Modalities: Workshop session, coaching, handouts
  - Objective 1.2 (Occupation): Identify alternative ways to accomplish the needed activities independently and with simple assistive devices.
    □ Modalities: Coaching, handouts specific to different activities
  - Objective 1.3 (Environment): Adapt workstations in the adapted work programme according to personal profiles and tasks accomplished.

    □ Modalities: Propositions made to staff and volunteers, including images showing workstation adaptations
- Occupational goal 2: Members with TBI, staff members and volunteers will move freely and safely within the association's facilities.
  - Objective 2.1 (Environment): Design a reconfiguration of the facilities taking into account how the rooms are used and the users' profiles (e.g. use of a wheelchair or a cane, visual impairment).
    □ Modalities: Propositions made to staff and members with TBI, including a detailed plan of the facilities

Sarah and Kathleen accomplished the different modalities planned and left tools with the association's representatives. Staff members and volunteers continued implementing the action plan in the months after the students' fieldwork (e.g. carrying out the reconfiguration, using the handouts when facilitating activities). As a result of the short length of the fieldwork placement, no evaluation of the outcomes was completed. However, it would have been relevant for Ann, the students' supervisor, to contact the association a few months later to evaluate whether the goals have been met and whether adjustments were needed.

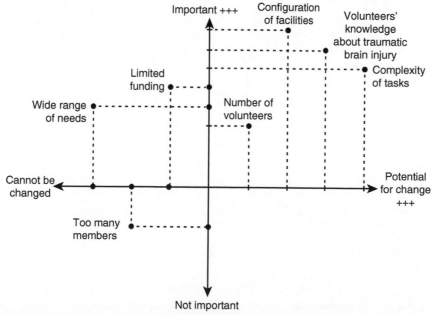

FIG. 27.5 ■ Example of completed Priority Scale associated with Practice Story 27.1.

PRACTICE STORY 27.2

Partnering with an Agricultural Vocational Training Centre

Samantha is an occupational therapist. She recently received a request from a youth safety advisor to develop a project with an agricultural vocational training centre in her community. This advisor regularly collaborates with various vocational schools to ensure that students received the necessary training in injury prevention. A meeting was convened between the occupational therapist, the safety advisor, and two teachers at the agricultural school to clarify needs and expectations. Estelle, a teacher in the horticulture programme of this school, was worried because many graduates injure themselves shortly after starting their work. Despite her efforts, she felt ill equipped to raise her students' awareness and help them gain healthy work habits. After the meeting, the group decided to establish a pilot project with Estelle's students to tackle the occupational issue identified: too many students sustained injuries shortly after starting work.

Samantha reviewed the literature to document the problem (prevalence of injuries in horticulture) and proven methods to enable students to apply injury prevention strategies. She then developed an action plan to discuss with the school's teachers. Samantha strongly believed that she needed to educate not only students but also teachers involved in the horticulture programme, in order for them to reactivate the strategies learned in all the practical courses. Teachers disapproved this idea and preferred that Samantha worked out what to do with the students. Samantha decided to follow their preference initially, hoping that she could propose her idea again when the partnership was stronger. The Tree of Occupational Goals completed with student participants is shown in Fig. 27.6, and the Priority Scale is presented in Fig. 27.7. Note that participants' perceptions of importance and changeability are illustrated.

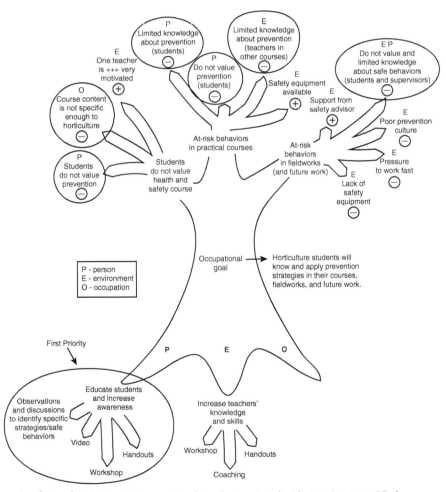

FIG. 27.6 ■ Example of completed Tree of Occupational Goals associated with Practice Story 27. 2.

PRACTICE STORY 27.2

Partnering with an Agricultural Vocational Training Centre (Continued)

The agreed-upon action plan follows:

■ Occupational goal 1: Horticulture students will know and apply injury prevention strategies in their courses, fieldwork, and future work.

    ■ Objective 1.2 (Person): Educate students on key injury prevention strategies specific to horticulture.

        □ Modalities: (1) Observations, literature review, and discussions to identify specific strategies; (2) theoretical and practical workshop for students; (3) video showing them applying the injury prevention strategies; (4) handouts

The students were very satisfied with the project. They took the initiative to form a health and safety committee and to nominate a student to be responsible for reminding his peers of the injury prevention strategies learned during their courses.

Teachers told the occupational therapist that they had noticed that their students applied prevention strategies in their courses after the initiative. To date, no study has been done to evaluate the outcomes of this project in fieldwork placements or the workforce. However, three other teachers from the agricultural school asked to replicate the experience with their cohort of students. The workshop and video will be offered in the weeks to come. This time, Samantha will make sure to further document the outcomes of the initiatives: she will ask students to sign an authorisation so that she can contact them after their first summer season in the workforce to evaluate the extent to which they have applied the injury prevention strategies and the percentage of them who got injured. She also hopes teachers will agree to be trained.

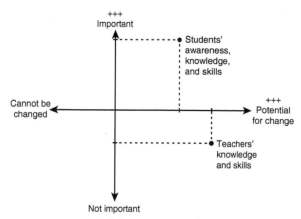

FIG. 27.7 ■ Example of completed Priority Scale associated with the Practice Story 27.2.

EVIDENCE FOR OCCUPATIONAL THERAPY IN COMMUNITY DEVELOPMENT

The evidence for occupational therapists' roles in community development comes from fieldwork placements (Banks & Head, 2004; Baril, Grandisson, & Cantin, 2013; Boudreau & Donnelly, 2013; Friedland, Polatajko, & Gage, 2001), educational experiences (Klinger & Bossers, 2009), case studies (Lauckner et al., 2007, 2011) and participatory action research (Cockburn & Trentham, 2002). The studies involve occupational therapists or occupational therapy students partnering with community groups or organisations to facilitate participation. Yet they represent different points on the continuum of community development approaches discussed earlier (Lauckner et al., 2007;

Rothman et al., 1995). They describe a range of community partners such as a municipal recreation programme, community college, housing support centre, association for children with disabilities, peer mentoring programme, and seniors volunteering programme. Although community-based rehabilitation is another strategy through which occupational therapists can foster inclusive community development for and by people experiencing illness, injury or impairment (WHO, UNESCO, ILO, & IDDC, 2010), it is not included here because it is the focus of Chapter 28 in this textbook.

What Are the Benefits?

Most of the benefits described in the literature refer to strengthening community groups' capacities in terms of knowledge, skills, tools, policies or funding requests. Knowledge and skills were mostly gained through needs assessments, programme evaluations and knowledge translation interventions (Baril et al., 2013; Cockburn & Trentham, 2002; Klinger & Bossers, 2009). Many emphasised the development of tools or resources for the organisation to use or from which to build (Banks & Head, 2004; Boudreau & Donnelly, 2013; Cockburn & Trentham, 2002; Friedland et al., 2001; Klinger & Bossers, 2009). These are congruent with developing self-sustainable solutions. Some examples include a user-friendly tool to assess environmental accessibility, an educational module on inclusion of people with disabilities and accessible information on home safety issues or transfer techniques. Other potential benefits include policies or procedures developed or funding requested (Cockburn & Trentham, 2002; Klinger & Bossers, 2009).

Klinger and Bossers (2009) evaluated community organisations' satisfaction with the involvement of occupational therapy students in community development initiatives and found very high satisfaction scores, with mean scores on their evaluation tool ranging from 28.9/32 to 30.8/32. In another study, community partners highly appreciated knowledge translation activities as they felt that the knowledge and skills gained were applicable to their realities (Baril et al., 2013). The literature also highlights the benefits for occupational therapists and students. Klinger and Bossers (2009) describe enhanced knowledge of community needs, resources and organisations. Others discuss the opportunity to take on evolving roles such as administrator, change agent, communicator, educator or facilitator (Baril et al., 2013; Lauckner et al., 2007).

What Are the Challenges?

The main challenges for occupational therapists in community development appear to be defining their role and coping with limited support. Friedland et al. (2001) explained that some students and community organisations found it difficult to specifically define the occupational therapy contribution. Lauckner et al. (2007) stress that many therapists felt unprepared and struggled to identify specific skills and theories from which to draw. Cockburn and Trentham (2002) explain that the tension therapists may feel between being a professional and a partner on equal ground might exacerbate this difficulty. Other challenges include the lack of support from other therapists and limited financial support (Lauckner et al., 2007).

In regards to student fieldwork in community development, authors suggest that some students were concerned with having insufficient opportunities to develop their traditional practice skills (Baril et al., 2013; Friedland et al., 2001). Friedland et al. (2001) also point to the difficulty of using traditional fieldwork evaluation instruments to assess students and to the challenge of developing sustainable formulas for these placements.

What Are the Facilitators?

A key feature of successful occupational therapy community development experiences is nurturing community partnerships (Lauckner et al., 2011). This includes sharing decision-making power, respecting and valuing everyone's contribution, addressing community concerns and clarifying roles and expectations (Cockburn & Trentham, 2002; Lauckner et al., 2011). Lauckner et al. (2011) emphasise that this may require therapists to let go some of their control and fully recognise community members as experts in their own experience. In addition, ongoing reflection can help therapists better understand their role: linking tasks with occupational therapy activities and values and focusing on occupations and assets (Banks & Head, 2004; Finlayson, 2007; Lauckner et al., 2011). Other facilitators include therapists immersing themselves in the organisation's culture by being part of the community team and having access to a workspace and resources (Banks & Head, 2004; Baril et al., 2013; Friedland et al., 2001), drawing on previous experiences and networks (Lauckner et al., 2007) and understanding historical and current relationships among health authorities, community members and community resources (Lauckner et al., 2011).

In respect to students' experiences, pairing to foster peer learning and support was seen as helpful in three studies (Banks & Head, 2004; Baril et al., 2013; Boudreau & Donnelly, 2013). In addition, 84% of students in Boudreau and Donnelly's (2013) study thought that the adapted fieldwork evaluation tool helped to identify the skills they were required to develop during their community development placement. Hence, such self-evaluation could be a relevant means to evaluate this type of fieldwork (Banks & Head, 2004; Boudreau & Donnelly, 2013). Lauckner et al. (2007) also suggested explicitly including community development in pre-professional training, and continuing education to prepare students and therapists for this emerging role.

CONCLUSION

Occupational therapists are being called to expand their scope of practice from individuals and groups to communities and organisations. With groups, communities or organisations, occupational therapists can play an important role in community development, enabling community partners to build their capacities to foster more supportive environments and to ensure all have opportunities to develop their potentials and engage in chosen occupations. Drawing upon recognised models and frameworks of occupational therapy practice (Davis et al., 2013; Law et al., 1996), a practical approach to achieve this work has been presented. It is anticipated that this will contribute to enhancing occupational therapists' desire and confidence to be engaged in community development. Further work evaluating occupational therapy community development experiences will help build the evidence base in this area and encourage others to take on this challenge.

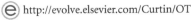 http://evolve.elsevier.com/Curtin/OT

REFERENCES

American Association of Occupational Therapy (AOTA). (2010). Standards of practice for occupational therapy. *American Journal of Occupational Therapy, 64*(Suppl), S106–S111.

Banks, S., & Head, B. (2004). Partnering occupational therapy and community development. *Canadian Journal of Occupational Therapy, 71*(1), 5–8.

Baril, N., Grandisson, M., & Cantin, N. (2013). Lessons learned from the establishment of a university occupational therapy clinic. *OT Now, 15*(1), 11–12. Retrieved from, http://www.caot.ca/default.asp?pageid=7.

Boudreau, M. L., & Donnelly, C. A. (2013). The community development progress and evaluation tool: Assessing community development fieldwork. *Canadian Journal of Occupational Therapy, 80*(4), 235–240.

Broome, K., McKenna, K., Fleming, J., & Worrall, L. (2009). Bus use and older people: A literature review applying the Person-Environment-Occupational model in macro practice. *Scandinavian Journal of Occupational Therapy, 16*, 3–12.

Chevalier, J. M., & Buckles, D. J. (2013). *Handbook for participatory action research, planning and evaluation.* Ottawa: SAS2 Dialogue. Retrieved from, *http://www.participatoryactionresearch.net/sites/default/files/sites/all/files/manager/Toolkit_En_March7_2013-S.pdf.*

Cockburn, L., & Trentham, B. (2002). Participatory action research: Integrating community occupational therapy practice and research. *Canadian Journal of Occupational Therapy, 69*, 20–30.

Davis, J., Craik, J., & Polatajko, H. J. (2013). Using the Canadian Practice Process Framework: Amplifying the process. In E. A. Townsend & H. J. Polatajko (Eds.), *Enabling occupation II: Advancing an occupational therapy vision for health, well-being, & justice through occupation* (2nd ed., pp. 247–272). Ottawa: CAOT Publications ACE.

Doll, J. (2009). *Program development and grant writing in occupational therapy: Making the connection.* Sudbury, MA: Jones & Bartlett Learning..

Fazio, L. S. (2006). *Developing occupation-centered programs for the community* (2nd ed.). Upper Saddle River, NJ: Pearson Prentice Hall.

Finlayson, M. (2007). Community-based practice: Assessing community needs and strengths. *OT Practice,* 29–31.

Friedland, J., Polatajko, H., & Gage, M. (2001). Expanding the boundaries of occupational therapy practice through student fieldwork experiences: Description of a provincially-funded community development program. *Canadian Journal of Occupational Therapy, 68*, 308–316.

Green, L. W., & Kreuter, M. W. (2005). *Health program planning: An educational and ecological approach* (4th ed.). New York: McGraw-Hill.

Klinger, L., & Bossers, A. (2009). Contributing to operations of community agencies through integrated fieldwork experiences. *Canadian Journal of Occupational Therapy, 76*, 171–179.

Labonte, R. (1997). Community, community development, and the forming of authentic partnerships: Some critical reflections. In M. Minkler (Ed.), *Community organizing and community building for health* (pp. 88–102). New Brunswick, NJ: Rutgers.

Lauckner, H. M., Krupa, T. M., & Paterson, M. L. (2011). Conceptualizing community development: Occupational therapy at the intersection of health services and community. *Canadian Journal of Occupational Therapy, 78*, 260–268.

Lauckner, H., Pentland, W., & Paterson, M. (2007). Exploring Canadian occupational therapists' understanding of and experiences in community development. *Canadian Journal of Occupational Therapy, 74*, 314–325.

Law, M., Cooper, B., Strong, S., Stewart, D., Rigby, P., & Letts, L. (1996). The Person-Environment-Occupation Model: A transactive approach to occupational performance. *Canadian Journal of Occupational Therapy, 63*(1), 9–23.

Leclair, L. (2010). Re-examining concepts of occupation and occupation-based models: Occupational therapy and community development. *Canadian Journal of Occupational Therapy, 77*, 15–21.

Restall, G., Leclair, L., & Banks, S. (2005). Inclusiveness through community development. *OT Now, 7*(5), 7–9. Retrieved from, http://www.caot.ca/default.asp?pageid=7.

Ripat, J., & Becker, P. (2012). Playground usability: What do playground users say? *Occupational Therapy International, 19*, 144–153.

Rothman, J., Erlich, J. L., & Tropman, J. E. (1995). *Strategies of community intervention: Macro practice* (5th ed.). Itasca, IL: F.E. Peacock.

Strong, S., Rigby, P., Stewart, D., Law, M., Letts, L., & Cooper, B. (1999). Application of the Person-Environment-Occupation Model: A practical tool. *Canadian Journal of Occupational Therapy, 66*(3), 122–133.

Thibeault, R., & Hébert, M. (1997). A congruent model for health promotion in occupational therapy. *Occupational Therapy International, 4*(4), 271–293.

Townsend, E. A., Beagan, B., Kumas-Tan, Z., et al. (2013a). Enabling: Occupational therapy's core competency. In E. A. Townsend & H. J. Polatajko (Eds.), *Enabling occupation II: Advancing an occupational therapy vision for health, well-being, & justice through occupation* (2nd ed, pp. 87–134). Ottawa: CAOT Publications ACE.

Townsend, E. A., Cockburn, L., Thibeault, R., & Trentham, B. (2013b). Enabling social change. In E. A. Townsend & H. J. Polatajko (Eds.), *Enabling occupation II: Advancing an occupational therapy vision for health, well-being, & justice through occupation* (2nd ed, pp. 153–171). Ottawa: CAOT Publications ACE.

World Health Organization, United Nations Educational, Scientific and Cultural Organization, International Labour Organization, and International Disability and Development Consortium (WHO, UNESCO, ILO, & IDDC). (2010). *Community-based rehabilitation: CBR guidelines.* Geneva, Switzerland: WHO Press. Retrieved from, *http://www.who.int/disabilities/publications/cbr/en/.*

28

COMMUNITY-BASED REHABILITATION

KIRSTY THOMPSON ■ CHRISTINA LARISSA PARASYN ■ BRIANA WILSON ■ BETH SPRUNT

• • • • • • • • • • • • • • • • • • •

CHAPTER OUTLINE

Abstract
Community-based rehabilitation (CBR) is a strategy that promotes collaboration among people with disabilities and their families, government and nongovernment stakeholders to promote an inclusive society that provides equal opportunities for all. Originally designed as a means of addressing the rehabilitation needs of people with disabilities in low- or middle-income countries, the strategy has evolved from a medically framed service delivery model to a community development approach grounded in human rights, empowerment, ownership and sustainability of a disability-inclusive community. Despite this conceptual evolution, in practice many CBR programmes continue with a traditional rehabilitation emphasis. The World Federation of Occupational Therapists recognises the coherence of CBR and occupational therapy approaches, promoting CBR as a means of facilitating access to occupation for all (World Federation of Occupational Therapists (WFOT), 2004b). There are shared beliefs in, for example, the importance of activity, participation, collaboration, and the environment. Occupational therapists are well positioned to contribute to the realisation of quality CBR initiatives in many ways. This may include, for example, working with people experiencing illness, injury or impairment and their families to identify and achieve their desired goals, provide direct therapy, and transfer of knowledge to other stakeholders. Importantly occupational therapists can act as facilitators by ensuring people experiencing illness, injury or impairment are key decision makers in their own lives and communities, as well as contributors to advocacy, policy, design and evaluation of CBR.

KEY POINTS

■ Community-based rehabilitation (CBR) is an evolving strategy, moving from more medically framed outreach services to a comprehensive community development strategy.

- CBR seeks to improve the lives of people experiencing illness, injury or impairment by promoting human rights, socioeconomic development and an inclusive society.

- CBR and occupational therapy are philosophically aligned, with a shared emphasis on, for example, occupation, the environment, collaborative relationships, rights and opportunities for meaningful participation.

- Occupational therapists' unique skills in enabling occupational engagement at an individual, community, and national level can play a crucial role in the realisation of CBR across multiple sectors, including, for example, health, education and employment.

- The CBR strategy challenges occupational therapists to strengthen skills in working with people experiencing illness, injury or impairment as active decision makers in all aspects of their lives. It challenges occupational therapists to work towards being resources who are 'on tap', supporting knowledge and skills development, disability rights awareness and collaboration in programme and policy development to ensure that rights are a reality.

- Occupational therapists need to further develop cultural awareness, research, policy, practice and education initiatives concerning the role of occupational therapy in CBR.

INTRODUCTION

Sheona comes from a small village in the Philippines. She has spina bifida. As a young girl, it was generally considered in her community that she would need to be 'looked after' all her life, and that education and expensive rehabilitation services and equipment would be wasted on her. She had gone to primary school but was withdrawn to 'provide what little help she could' in the family home, allowing her mother to earn much needed money by working in the fields. With limited mobility, she spent each day at home alone. This was her future – until a local community-based rehabilitation worker began working with Sheona and her family. Over time, Sheona accessed equipment to improve her mobility, small business training, and a US$100 loan to start a small general stall in her village. Today she is an esteemed member of her family and community. She returned to school and finished her education; the shop has expanded and she now employs both her parents. The extra family income has been used to ensure her siblings continue in school instead of leaving to work in the fields. Sheona is now working towards her goal of being a human rights lawyer. She wants to contribute to a better world for *all* people experiencing illness, injury or impairment.

Sheona's story is an example of what can be achieved through an investment and belief in the dignity and rights of all people to participate in everyday community life. Ideally, Sheona's story would be one of many among the estimated 15% of the world's population, or 1 billion people, who live with some form of impairment (World Health Organization (WHO) & World Bank, 2011). Approximately 80% of people impairment globally live in developing countries, where they constitute up to 20% of the poorest of the poor (WHO & World Bank, 2011). Many people experiencing illness, injury or impairment are commonly excluded from their right to access health, education and employment opportunities and services, resulting in higher rates of poverty, poorer health and education outcomes and less economic and political participation than people without disabilities (WHO & World Bank, 2011). For example, only 5% to 15% of people in low- and middle-income countries who require assistive devices or technologies receive the equipment they need to participate in and contribute to community life (WHO, 2015).

Community-based rehabilitation (CBR) commenced after the Declaration of Alma Ata in 1978 as an attempt to better meet the needs of the large population of people experiencing illness, injury or impairment in low- and middle-income countries (WHO, 2011). Since this time, the term *CBR* has been used to describe a wide range of services targeting people experiencing illness, injury or impairment in the community, including, for example, medical outreach services, self-help groups, vocational training and health promotion programmes. This led to confusion over what constitutes CBR. Recognising this, a joint position paper was issued by the International Labour Office, United Nations Educational Scientific and Cultural Organization (UNESCO) and World Health Organization in 1994 and revised in 2004, clarifying the CBR strategy (International Labour Organization et al., 2004). In that paper, CBR was defined as 'a strategy within general community development for the rehabilitation, equalisation of opportunities, poverty reduction and social inclusion of all people with disabilities. CBR is implemented through the combined efforts of people with disabilities themselves, their families, organisations and communities, and the relevant governmental and non-governmental health, education, vocational, social and other services' (p. 2). Framed within this paper, new guidelines have been developed for the implementation of CBR and are introduced later in this chapter (WHO, 2011).

As the context continues to evolve and change, so does CBR. With increased activity and discussion globally on inclusive development, there have been calls to revise CBR as community-based inclusive development (CBID), often using the CBR guidelines as a tool for this approach (International Disability and Development Consortium, 2012). This debate is not explored in this chapter. Rather, the implications of the principles underlying inclusive development and CBR for occupational therapy practice are explored.

CBR was founded in an attempt to meet the needs of people experiencing illness, injury or impairment, most of whom live in low- or middle-income or 'developing' countries. This is the focus on CBR taken in this chapter. However, it is acknowledged that people experiencing illness, injury or impairment living in more developed nations can also be subject to the conditions that CBR seeks to address, such as poverty, a lack of access to services, and compromises of basic human rights, including participating in the decisions that affect their lives, freely moving about their community or accessing employment.

UNDERSTANDING COMMUNITY-BASED REHABILITATION: AN EVOLVING STRATEGY

CBR is an evolving concept that seeks to promote the participation of people experiencing illness, injury or impairment in everyday community life. It continues to evolve from a medical, service-based orientation to a multisectoral, bottom-up strategy for meeting the basic rights and needs of people experiencing illness, injury or impairment through collaborative programmes focused on human rights, poverty reduction and inclusion and enabling access to health, education, social and livelihood opportunities (International Labour Office et al., 2004; WHO et al., 2011).

In this section the origins and motivations for the early development of CBR are explored. Despite the reconceptualisation of CBR, particularly in the context of the United Nations' Convention on the Rights of Persons with Disabilities (United Nations, 2006), in practice many CBR programmes continue to reflect traditional medically framed approaches (Iemmi et al., 2015). Accordingly, occupational therapists may still encounter programmes reflecting these early approaches and be involved in supporting the transition to CBR as a development approach. For occupational therapists to play a continued role in the evolution and realisation of CBR, they must understand and apply the principles of the Convention, be able to identify and understand the different expressions of CBR in practice and explore the potential roles that occupational therapists can play.

Early Community-based Rehabilitation

Early CBR was conceptualised and evolved primarily as an extension of the primary health care system to inexpensively deliver services, particularly in areas in low- and middle-income countries where there were inadequate resources for comprehensive institutional services (Helander, 2000; Thomas & Thomas, 2002, 2003; WHO, 1989). Hospitals and rehabilitation centres were considered costly to establish and maintain and were primarily located in large cities, providing often prohibitively expensive services. Services remained inaccessible for poorer families and those living in rural and remote areas. CBR covered a far wider geographical area and socioeconomic population at a reduced cost by shifting the responsibility of service delivery to minimally qualified 'nonprofessionals', including families and other volunteers from the community (Thomas & Thomas, 2002). Geographical distances and costs meant that, wherever

possible, local resources were used to make the required equipment. For example, buckets and sandbags may be used to make supportive seating and bamboo poles used to make parallel bars for practicing mobility exercises (Werner, 1998).

Despite this shift in responsibility to the community, the role and location of professionals like occupational therapists did not change drastically with the advent of CBR. 'Community' was mostly understood to be a geographical location for service delivery that specialists like occupational therapists visit. Occupational therapists mostly continued to work from centres or institutions, reaching out to communities to provide services such as basic training and support of CBR workers or home therapy programmes for parents and CBR workers to implement. Programmes were primarily initiated within communities by external agencies in what is known as a 'top-down approach' (Thomas & Thomas, 2002).

A medical understanding of disability framed the activities and goals of traditional CBR (Thomas & Thomas, 2003). Accordingly, professionals remained the experts and so determined the needs of people experiencing illness, injury or impairment. The programmes implemented by community workers were based on the assessments and recommendations of professionals. These programmes focused primarily on addressing impairments of the person's mind or body as a means of facilitating the person's participation in everyday community life. Therefore interventions were mainly positioned within the health sector. The role of occupational therapists largely focused on prescription of direct therapy programmes and adaptive equipment, for implementation in homes, schools and workplaces by local community workers.

In an international review of CBR that preceded the 2004 joint position paper, it was highlighted that most CBR programmes continued to primarily focus on health, and often exclusively on physical rehabilitation (WHO, 2003). Though some CBR programmes were found to also focus on education and income generation, these activities were run in isolation from health programmes. CBR focused only on a few aspects of occupation. This vertical, individual sector approach was considered counter to addressing the multidimensional need for achieving well-being in all aspects of life. People experiencing illness, injury or impairment themselves highlighted that the continued medical focus ignored their human rights and social and economic needs and those of their families (Disabled People's International, 2005). In the context of disabling policies, systems and physical and sociocultural environments, many people continued to experience occupational marginalisation, including limited engagement in social events, leadership, politics and, importantly, decisions that affected their lives (Wilcock & Townsend, 2000). Realising this, organisations like the Centre for Disability and Development Bangladesh (referred to in Practice Story 28.1) have focused on empowerment and leadership of people with disabilities, both male and female, to drive the change they want to see in their communities. This reflects the reconceptualisation of CBR outlined next.

PRACTICE STORY 28.1

The Active Involvement and Leadership of People with Disabilities in CBR

The Centre for Disability and Development (CDD) Bangladesh is a not-for-profit organisation established in 1996 to develop a more inclusive society for people experiencing illness, injury or impairment in Bangladesh. One of CDD's projects is Promoting the Human Rights of Persons with Disabilities, Bangladesh. This project works directly with people experiencing illness, injury or impairment to increase their empowerment and everyday functioning so that they can influence local and national government institutions, civil society organisations, employers, schools and the community at large to be more inclusive.

The project started with a focus on the development and empowerment of community self-help groups of people experiencing illness, injury or impairment and their families to bring about the change they wanted. This was significantly beneficial for women and girls experiencing illness, injury or impairment, who spent a large portion of their time inside the home, excluded from school and work. They were provided human rights and advocacy training, which increased their confidence and leadership to identify and advocate on key disability issues that they prioritised. Two members of each self-help group were elected to be part of an 'apex body' that represented people with disabilities at a district level. Actions taken at local and district levels also informed national level advocacy and resulted in the following, for example:

- People experiencing illness, injury or impairment accessing mainstream poverty reduction schemes by informing them about the schemes and influencing how they worked
- Local employment programmes including people experiencing illness, injury or impairment in training, such as cow rearing or mushroom cultivation, and allowing people experiencing illness, injury or impairment to access microcredit schemes
- Children experiencing illness, injury or impairment being identified in local school enrolment surveys and enrolled in school; teachers and schools were also provided inclusive education training
- Local government budgets including allocations for disability initiatives, expenditure guided by self-help groups
- Local authorities being informed and acting upon situations of abuse towards women and children experiencing illness, injury or impairment
- People experiencing illness, injury or impairment being included in disaster preparedness and response activities of the local government, so that people experiencing illness, injury or impairment would not be overlooked during evacuations from severe floods or storms

CDD also trained community disability resource people in basic rehabilitation and the provision of assistive devices to further enable participation by people with disabilities.

Bangladeshi and foreign occupational therapists played various roles, including the following:

- Contributing to curriculum design and training of community disability resource people
- A local occupational therapist from the assistive device centre resource team
- Working with CDD staff to facilitate reflection with staff, apex bodies and self-help groups on what was learned and to develop a strong strategy for a second phase, including discussions on how women and girls experiencing illness, injury or impairment, who experience disability- and gender-related discrimination, can benefit as much as men and boys experiencing illness, injury or impairment
- Working with CDD to design systems to monitor and evaluate project changes and ensure that the experiences of men, women, girls and boys experiencing illness, injury or impairment are captured and used to guide the project and inform other CBR initiatives

Community-based Rehabilitation Reconceptualised A Community-based Inclusive Development Strategy

The joint position paper on CBR identifies CBR as a *development strategy* that both improves the quality of life of people experiencing illness, injury or impairment and promotes the development of the community in which they live, thus also promoting an enabling environment for people with disabilities (International Labour Office et al., 2004). In particular, CBR initiatives or programmes were called upon to address the rights and broader needs of people experiencing illness, injury or impairment. This included ensuring that CBR contributed to reducing poverty, that people experiencing illness, injury or impairment and their representative organisations – or disabled people's organisations (DPOs) – were involved in decision-making processes, that community involvement and ownership were promoted, and that multisectoral collaboration and evidence-based practice were developed and strengthened (WHO et al., 2011). Some key conceptual changes underlying this evolution are outlined next and summarised in Table 28.1.

TABLE 28.1		
Evolution of CBR Concepts		
Concept	**Traditional CBR**	**'New' CBR**
Disability model	Medical	Social model; human rights
Rehabilitation concept	Primarily health sector; vertical sectors approach	Comprehensive, cross-sector
Primary implementer	Individual project/organisation	Multisectoral programme; networks between government and nongovernment stakeholders
Development approach	Needs based – identifying and meeting needs (service delivery)	Rights based – identifying rights and empowerment of community to exercise and realise these rights; poverty reduction
Drivers/ownership	Professionals	People experiencing illness, injury or impairment and wider community
Practice approach	Specialist and individual needs of people experiencing illness, injury or impairment	Inclusion through twin track – specialist and mainstream
Understanding of community	Geographical location for services	Wider community relationships are inclusive of people experiencing illness, injury or impairment (inclusive society)

CBR, Community-based rehabilitation.

A Social and Rights-based Approach to Disability

Reflecting the reorientation of disability as a social issue, CBR now frames disability within a social and rights-based model (International Labour Office et al., 2004; WHO et al., 2011). These models recognise that both medical impairment and social issues need to be considered in activities addressing disability (International Labour Office et al., 2004; Nagata, 2007; Shakespeare, 2009). The notion of disability is clearly explained in the CRPD, which describes disability as an evolving concept that results from the interaction between people experiencing illness, injury or impairment and attitudinal and environmental barriers that hinder full and meaningful participation in society on an equal basis with others (United Nations, 2006).

Human rights are a central tenant of CBR. The CRPD, a legally binding human rights and development instrument, provides CBR with the framework and standards to ensure that the rights of women, men, girls and boys with disabilities are promoted, protected and fulfilled on an equal basis with others in society. The Convention shifts the focus from people experiencing illness, injury or impairment being 'objects' of charity, medical treatment and social protection towards people experiencing illness, injury or impairment being seen as 'subjects' with rights in all aspects of life. As subjects with rights, people experiencing illness, injury or impairment are capable of claiming those rights and making decisions for their own lives (United Nations, 2013).

CBR principles are consistent with the principles of the Convention (Box 28.1), which emphasises that people experiencing illness, injury or impairment have equal rights to participate in,

BOX 28.1
GUIDING PRINCIPLES OF THE CONVENTION ON THE RIGHTS OF PERSONS WITH DISABILITY, ARTICLE 3

There are eight guiding principles that underlie the Convention and each one of its specific articles:
a. Respect for inherent dignity, individual autonomy including the freedom to make one's own choices, and independence of persons
b. Nondiscrimination
c. Full and effective participation and inclusion in society
d. Respect for difference and acceptance of persons with disabilities as part of human diversity and humanity
e. Equality of opportunity
f. Accessibility
g. Equality between men and women
h. Respect for the evolving capacities of children with disabilities and respect for the right of children with disabilities to preserve their identities

for example, school, work, social, economic, religious and political activities. CBR also seeks to advocate for and promote the application of these rights in government policies and budgets. A human rights approach is endorsed in the World Federation of Occupational Therapists (WFOT) position paper on CBR, which states that a core principle of occupational therapy is the right of all people to 'develop their capacity and power to construct their own destiny through occupation' (WFOT, 2004b, p. 1). The Convention is a useful tool to guide occupational therapists in ensuring person-focused and person-led practice.

Acknowledging the barriers that may inhibit full participation, the World Health Organization's International Classification of Functioning, Disability and Health (ICF), emphasises the relationship among function, activity and environment (WHO, 2001). This tool, often used by occupational therapists, notes that in addition to factors of body structure and function, there are five environmental factors that can limit activities or restrict participation: services, systems and policies; products and technology; natural environment and human-made changes to it; support and relationships; and attitudes (WHO, 2001). Although the term *occupation* is not used in ICF publications, the concept and the impact of the environment on occupational engagement are clearly present.

Empowerment of People Experiencing Illness, Injury or Impairment

Empowerment of people experiencing illness, injury or impairment is critical for the success of CBR. 'Nothing about us without us' is a slogan used by the international disability community. It means that nothing about people experiencing illness, injury or impairment can be decided without their involvement (International Disability Alliance, 2014) – the participation of the very people who know first-hand what enables and prevents their active participation in daily life. This mantra has been consecrated in the Convention:

> In the development and implementation of legislation and policies ... and in other decision-making processes concerning issues relating to persons with disabilities, States Parties shall closely consult with and actively involve persons with disabilities, including children with disabilities, through their representative organizations.
>
> *(United Nations, 2006)*

Therefore representative organisations of people experiencing illness, injury or impairment, also known as disabled people's organisations (DPOs) and self-help groups, must be present in all development and decision-making bodies at all levels (WHO et al., 2011). DPOs are organisations run by and for people experiencing illness, injury or impairment for the purpose of representing issues that affect their lives (Handicap International, 2011). They can be global, regional, national or local organisations. Despite statements about inclusion and participation, people experiencing illness, injury or impairment have largely remained invisible and outside of decision-making processes (Disability Rights Fund, 2013). As a result they continue to be excluded from the services and opportunities available to other citizens in the community. DPOs are also critical to occupational therapy practice to ensure people-led practice. The practice scenarios presented in this chapter are clear demonstrations of how leadership and participation of self-help groups and DPOs have been central to the success of CBR.

Disability and Poverty

CBR recognises the challenge of reducing the poverty experienced by so many people around the world unless people experiencing illness, injury or impairment are included in the socioeconomic development of their communities. There is an irrefutable link between poverty and disability, with poverty leading to higher rates of disability and disability increasing the risk of poverty (WHO & World Bank, 2011). There is a growing body of literature that explores this relationship (Banks & Polack, 2014; Groce et al., 2011; Hansen Chaki, & Mlay, 2013; Inclusion International, 2006; Mitra, Posarac, & Vick, 2013; Mizunoya & Mitra, 2013; Nagata, 2007). People living in poverty are more likely to be exposed to conditions that contribute to disability, such as poor nutrition and limited access to health service, poor housing and sanitation and unsafe working and living conditions (WHO et al., 2011). Conversely, people experiencing illness, injury or impairment and their families face significant barriers to accessing rehabilitation, education and employment, which can reduce poverty. Women and children experiencing illness, injury or impairment, people with intellectual and psychosocial impairments and elderly people often experience additional exclusion and marginalisation, pushing them further into the poverty cycle (WHO, 2011).

Community-based Rehabilitation in Practice

In 2011, CBR guidelines were launched to help stakeholders ensure that the benefits of the Convention reach people experiencing illness, injury or impairment at the local level and that these people are included in the development of their communities. The guidelines focus on some key components that need to become inclusive so that people experiencing illness, injury or impairment and their families become empowered and contributing members of their communities (WHO, 2011). These components are represented in the CBR matrix developed by the WHO (Fig. 28.1) and include health, education, livelihoods, social and empowerment. Each component comprises five elements that are fundamental to improving the quality of life of people experiencing illness, injury or impairment.

An effective CBR programme may contain these elements depending on local circumstances (WHO, 2005). It is not sequential, but rather a series of options from which communities and practitioners, in collaboration with people experiencing illness, injury or impairment and their families, can select. It is likely that only some of the components are addressed depending on local needs, priorities and resources. A CBR programme may start with a particular element, gradually expanding to encompass other elements through programme expansion and networking. In some instances, the programme may be led by one organisation but in many, a CBR programme frames the work of a range of connected organisations and initiatives.

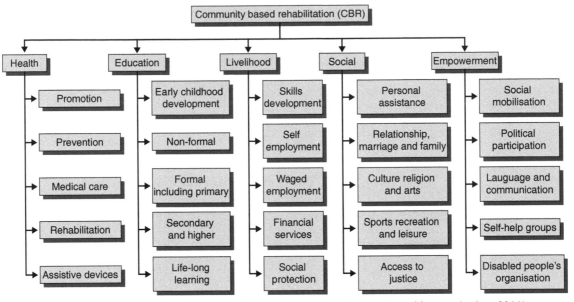

FIG. 28.1 ■ Community-based rehabilitation matrix (developed by World Health Organization, 2011).

Inclusion and empowerment requires CBR practitioners, including occupational therapists, to take a twin-track approach in their work, whereby they work to (1) integrate disability issues in mainstream development policies, systems and programmes, while at the same time (2) promote and support targeted activities that focus on enabling participation and inclusion of persons experiencing illness, injury or impairment (CBM Australia, 2012; WHO et al., 2011). For example, an occupational therapist may work with people experiencing illness, injury or impairment to ensure that education of children with disabilities is included in education sector strategies and teacher training programmes (mainstreaming). Simultaneously, he or she may work to ensure that children and adolescents experiencing illness, injury or impairment have access to the appropriate assistive technologies they require to attend and learn at their local school, such as an appropriately fitted wheelchair, sign language training or Braille education (disability targeted activities). Practice Story 28.2 shares the story of how the CBR unit in the Solomon Islands took a twin-track approach to improving wheelchair services, while increasing community participation and leadership by people who use wheelchairs.

CBR requires multisectoral partnerships and often involves collaboration from the national through to the community levels of each component to ensure consistent policy and practices and appropriate referral services. Collaboration at each level between the various stakeholders, such as ministries, non-government organisations, private sectors and DPOs helps ensure that an inclusive society is promoted in a comprehensive and coordinated way. This can include, for example,

involvement of health, education, employment and labour sectors; media, sports and recreations groups; and religious groups (Disabled People's International, 2005; International Labour Office et al., 2004; WHO, 2003, 2007, 2011). Practice Story 28.3 describes a cross-sector and multilevel CBR initiative in Pakistan in which occupational therapists have been involved at various levels. CBR also recognises that meaningful inclusion requires action in more than just the components outlined in the matrix. The practice stories have demonstrated the greater networks that need to be created for inclusion to happen. The guidelines remind practitioners about also building partnerships and alliances with other sectors not covered by CBR initiatives to raise awareness and ensure active participation by persons experiencing illness, injury or impairment and their families extends to all aspects of society.

OCCUPATIONAL THERAPY AND COMMUNITY-BASED REHABILITATION

Many authors have noted the synergy between features of occupational therapy and CBR (Barros, Ghirardi, & Lopes, 2005; Fransen, 2005; Sakellariou et al., 2006; Thomas & Thomas, 1996; Twible & Henley, 2000; WFOT, 2004b):

1. 'Occupation' is at the centre of occupational therapy practice (WFOT, 2004a) and so it aligns strongly with CBR, which is concerned with daily life and participation in activity.

PRACTICE STORY 28.2

A Twin-track Approach Empowering People Who Use Wheelchairs in Solomon Islands

The Community-based Rehabilitation (CBR) Unit within the Ministry of Health and Medical Services in the Solomon Islands is responsible for service delivery to the community, 80% of whom live in rural villages, spread across 10 provinces and many islands. A dispersed population creates a particular challenge for service delivery, as travel between islands is expensive. CBR staff are located across most provinces and provide rehabilitation services at the village level.

The CBR unit recognised that for children and adults with a mobility impairment, achieving a means of mobility was an essential step in rehabilitation, participation and inclusion and in exercising their rights. However, there was an unmet need for appropriate wheelchairs and wheelchair service provision, which led the CBR unit in 2008 to invite Motivation Australia to work with them to address it. Motivation Australia is a nongovernment organisation that works in developing countries to support and improve opportunities for children and adults with a mobility impairment.

Together with key stakeholders they embarked on a long-term vision to improve access by men and women who used wheelchairs living in the Solomon Islands to appropriate wheelchairs, training and support. They recognised that improving services and access to mobility devices was an ongoing process that took time and resources. By 2012, 400 wheelchair users across eight provinces were provided with a custom-fit wheelchair, 37% of whom were women and girls; 11% were custom wheelchairs for children. The actions to achieve such an outcome were supported by an occupational therapist at every stage and included the following:

TARGETED ACTIVITIES

- A feasibility assessment exploring the existing CBR system and resources, the needs of people who used wheelchairs, and how a system of wheelchair provision could be introduced sustainably, including contributions from the perspectives of the national DPO and individuals who used wheelchairs
- Basic level wheelchair service delivery training for CBR staff, including people who used wheelchairs
- Development of forms for assessment, prescription, fitting and follow up that focused only on information that was relevant to the Solomon Islands context
- Peer group training course for people who used wheelchairs to mentor and coach other people who used wheelchairs on personal health, all aspects of their wheelchair and its use

INTEGRATION INTO THE MAINSTREAM

- Awareness raising among decision makers about appropriate wheelchair service provision and appropriate wheelchairs for the Solomon Islands context
- Gaining government support through integrating wheelchairs into the existing government procurement system for medical devices, funding to cover training costs and creating a national wheelchair technician permanent post
- Integrating basic wheelchair service delivery training into the Solomon Islands Centre for Higher Education to increase the number and quality of local personnel trained
- Integrating access to mobility devices within the existing CBR system
- Awareness raising among health workers and individuals about the availability of the wheelchair service to enable referrals

2. Both occupational therapy and CBR emphasise the importance of the environment, while respecting the different cultural meaning placed on occupation (physical, social and political) as it interacts with individuals to inform occupation (Imms, 2006).

3. The right to occupation and opportunities, while respecting the different cultural meanings placed on occupation in each context, is fundamental to both occupational therapy and CBR (Pollard & Sakellariou, 2007). Indeed, the WFOT promotes CBR as the strategy through which to facilitate access to occupation for all (Sakellariou et al., 2006; WFOT, 2004b). Although occupational therapy has historically had a medical intervention focus, there has been a conceptual revival of socially and rights driven elements emerging in concepts like occupational justice (Al Heresh et al., 2013;

Lang, 2011; Pollard & Kronenberg, 2008; Thibeault, 2006; Watson, 2013).

4. Collaboration through enabling and empowering relationships is fundamental to successful CBR and occupational therapy practice. This includes sharing information and expertise and taking time to understand the story of the person or the wider community (Hansen et al., 2013). Both CBR and occupational therapy view the person or community as the central driver of this collaborative process, considering this essential to meaningful, purposeful and sustainable impact (Kuipers & Doig, 2010; WFOT, 2004a).

5. There is an emphasis on creatively adapting to the context in both occupational therapy and CBR (Fransen, 2005). This includes designing strategies and programmes that align with local priorities, needs and resources.

Multisector and Multilevel Engagement in CBR

In October 2005 an earthquake in the Himalayan ranges of Northern Pakistan left 79,000 people dead and thousands of people with physical injuries and impairments. Medical facilities were destroyed, and people were evacuated to cities for medical and rehabilitative services. Limited existing services saw hundreds of injured people in vulnerable situations, lying on concrete floors and contracting secondary complications, including pressure sores and infections. Occupational therapists worked to train local volunteers in basic mobility and daily living skills, but this was not enough.

Rehabilitation workers, including occupational therapists, began to advocate for the inclusion of people experiencing illness, injury or impairment at all levels of society. Key stakeholders, including DPOs, allied health professionals, government organisations, nongovernment organisations and community-based organisations, met for consultations to find ways to address the vulnerability and exclusion of people experiencing illness, injury or impairment. Stakeholders agreed that CBR was the most effective strategy to ensure the active participation of people experiencing illness, injury or impairment in community life. One such stakeholder, Handicap International, has developed CBR services in Northern Pakistan in partnership with the community, service providers and the government.

Handicap International, along with its partners, community-based organisations and DPOs, operate resource and information centres. The centres aim to do the following:

- Build capacity of community-level organisations to identify people experiencing illness, injury or impairment, provide basic therapy and coordinate referrals to rehabilitation centres
- Work with people experiencing illness, injury or impairment to have inclusive mainstream education and livelihood opportunities
- Provide technical advice for accessible construction of housing, public buildings and public transportation

- Raise awareness of communities regarding disability issues and the rights of people experiencing illness, injury or impairment
- Build capacity of local people experiencing illness, injury or impairment to form self-help groups for advocacy, including provision of small grants
- Offer a library of disability and development knowledge resources
- Build partnerships among people experiencing illness, injury or impairment, civil society organisations and government for enhanced information flow and comprehensive service delivery

Occupational therapists assisted in the development, coordination and continual improvement of information and resources. Facilitating community access to the centres and establishing linkages between community members and organisations was also a key role.

Partnerships with key rehabilitation services were formed and occupational therapists and other stakeholders facilitated curriculum development and training for community workers to assist in social change and provide adequate services. Consequently, the capacity of service providers to deliver quality, comprehensive rehabilitation services increased.

Handicap International and the government of Pakistan continue to strengthen the National Institute of Rehabilitation Medicine (a state-owned institute responsible for the provision of tertiary level services, human resource development and development and implementation of national policies and strategies on disability) by doing the following:

- Developing a strategy for the coordination, monitoring and evaluation of the CBR programme
- Developing effective communication pathways which ensure the rights of people experiencing illness, injury or impairment are addressed within policy development
- Promoting collaboration between all members of society

Therapists' skills in networking, advocacy, awareness raising and service delivery were critical in such ongoing processes.

Overall, CBR could be said to reflect what occupational therapists have described as 'community built' practice (Wittman & Velde, 2001). That is, practice using collaborative and interactive approaches, based on principles of community empowerment and engagement, and addressing the individual, social and environmental factors affecting health and participation, in a person- and community-focused way.

There are calls for occupational therapists to ensure that they understand CBR as a community development strategy, not a service delivery framework, and to ensure their practice is driven by the community and people experiencing illness, injury or impairment at all levels (Pollard & Sakellariou, 2008; Sakellariou et al., 2006). Occupational therapists may be involved in policy, advocacy, human rights awareness, and strengthening partnerships with mainstream development initiatives such as education, health, livelihood and leadership programmes, as well as participation in the development of national poverty reduction strategies and inclusive development policies and practices.

Though many programmes that align with the original concept of CBR still exist (i.e. focusing mainly on rehabilitation), others are moving to the more comprehensive social and rights-based CBR strategy. The compatibility of CBR and occupational therapy philosophies ideally positions occupational therapists to play an important role in the realisation of CBR.

Roles, Skills and Opportunities for Occupational Therapists in Community-based Rehabilitation

Fransen (2005) reviewed the literature and identified five roles for occupational therapists working in CBR:

1. Transfer of rehabilitation knowledge and skills
2. Provision of direct therapy
3. Referral services
4. Programme development and implementation
5. Facilitation of collaboration

Pollard and Sakellariou (2008) offer additional roles and skills critical for occupational therapy practice. These include actively facilitating and promoting participation of people experiencing illness, injury or impairment, being culturally aware, and contributing to inclusive policy and system development, implementation and evaluation. These and other roles are illustrated in the practice stories and explored in turn next.

Transfer of Rehabilitation Knowledge and Skills

At multiple levels, occupational therapists are involved in the transfer of basic rehabilitation skills and the creation of positive attitudes through training education and supervision (Fransen, 2005). Occupational therapists' unique skills in facilitating occupational engagement can play a crucial role in the realisation of CBR. Sharing and transferring skills in addressing impairments and adapting activities and environments to facilitate participation are vital. Transferring knowledge to others needs to be recognised by occupational therapists as a legitimate professional activity in its own right. It has been suggested that some occupational therapists have already identified this as a key role they play in CBR; however, the training these occupational therapists provided was primarily focused on addressing impairments (Sakellariou et al., 2006). With the reconceptualisation of CBR as a multisectoral community development strategy, it is important that traditional rehabilitation skills like these are still transferred and that community development skills in, for example, advocacy and community mobilisation are also developed and refined (WHO, 2010).

Occupational therapists need to develop or improve the skills required to be competent in transferring their knowledge and skills. Though 'teaching a skill' is not unfamiliar to occupational therapists, competent transfer of skills requires occupational therapists to understand and apply concepts of adult learning, including how to train trainers, how to work with groups and populations, and how to prepare and deliver culturally appropriate training materials. Ensuring the coordination and application of this knowledge in the community also

requires occupational therapists to have advanced skills in supervising, mentoring and coaching (Fransen, 2005; WFOT, 2004b).

The World Report on Disability (WHO & World Bank, 2011) recommended that the global health workforce be strengthened to ensure that people experiencing illness, injury or impairment are able to access health services, as one example. It has been noted that this strengthening provides a good opportunity to ensure that health staff working in CBR are equipped to implement CBR in the cross-sectoral manner described in the CBR guidelines. This could include training rehabilitation workers in all aspects of the CBR matrix to play a multipurpose and linking role. Training would draw from a range of disciplines, including occupational therapy (Mannan et al., 2013). Such a role calls for occupational therapists to strengthen skills in working collaboratively with other disciplines to design and implement training for multipurpose rehabilitation workers in a coordinated way (Mannan et al., 2013).

The Provision of Direct Therapy

Occupational therapists facilitate participation of people experiencing illness, injury or impairment through the provision of direct therapy when needed. This therapy can include the provision of rehabilitative equipment and teaching skills in advocacy and community awareness training (Fransen, 2005). The WFOT research project into CBR noted that direct therapy was a key service that occupational therapists were providing in CBR (Sakellariou et al., 2006). This encompasses activities that seek to prevent impairment as well as promoting occupational engagement through the programmes designed. Though more consistent with traditional CBR, occupational therapists may still be called on to provide services. However, this raises questions of sustainability if occupational therapists, local or expatriate, are the sole providers of services without ensuring their skills are transferred to the community.

Referral Services

Occupational therapists are also involved in the provision of referral services and guidance to help people negotiate their way through and articulate their rights and needs within service systems (Fransen, 2005). Within a multisector and multilevel CBR strategy, this requires occupational therapists to network with and have a good working knowledge of government and nongovernment providers across multiple sectors and at multiple levels.

Programme Development, Implementation and Evaluation

Fransen (2005) noted occupational therapists can facilitate the establishment, development and implementation of programmes at government and community levels. CBR emphasises the importance of evaluation as a means to improve the quality of CBR programmes and ensure evidence-based practice (WHO, 2011). Significantly, CBR now challenges occupational therapists to be directed by people experiencing illness, injury or impairment and their families in all stages of design, implementation and evaluation of CBR initiatives (Disabled People's International, 2005; WHO, 2006, 2007, 2011). This requires a shift in approach from 'professional as expert' to one where we act as resources when invited (Bury, 2005), working as partners and facilitators (Kuipers & Doig, 2010). Occupational therapists need to have effective listening skills and tools and practices for accessing and identifying community needs, priorities and resources. Such an approach by occupational therapists also necessitates good cross-cultural awareness. Cross-cultural understanding enhances occupational therapists' abilities to communicate effectively, to ensure there is good participation of all stakeholders and to support locally owned and designed CBR programmes (Pollard & Sakellariou, 2008; Sakellariou et al., 2006). Occupational therapists should be cautious about importing occupational therapy concepts that may not be culturally relevant to the communities they are working with (Hammell, 2009).

Occupational therapists can undertake roles in evaluating CBR and contributing to the evidence base about the outcomes of the CBR approach at individual, community and government levels (Bury, 2005). Practice Stories 28.1, 28.3 and 28.4 strongly illustrate this. Despite some progress, the continued need to develop an evidence base through evaluation and research of CBR at policy and practice levels has been well documented (Cleaver & Nixon, 2014; Disabled People's International, 2005; Iemmi et al., 2015; Kuipers & Harknett, 2008; WHO, 2011). Research is also needed to better understand the role of occupational therapists themselves in CBR (Sakellariou et al., 2006). Occupational therapists could be involved in research and evaluation, ideally employing participatory evaluation and research strategies that ensure people with disabilities, their families, and the wider community are involved (Kuipers & Harknett, 2009).

Facilitating Collaboration

Occupational therapists can also play a role in ensuring effective and efficient collaboration among the many stakeholders in CBR (Fransen, 2005; Hansen et al., 2013). This is a critical role

occupational therapists can play within the multisectoral, multi-level CBR strategy and is illustrated in Practice Story 28.3. The WFOT CBR data collection project, which surveyed many occupational therapists who have worked in CBR, raises some concerns about whether they are actually playing this collaborative role, given that few people surveyed mentioned involvement with other stakeholders (Sakellariou et al., 2006). This challenges occupational therapists to identify, listen and learn from others involved in CBR, particularly people with disabilities themselves (Pollard et al., 2008).

Other Roles

As demonstrated in all the practice stories, occupational therapists play a role in actively advocating and facilitating both with and for the equal participation of people experiencing illness, injury or impairment. Active participation of people experiencing illness, injury or impairment within CBR planning, implementation and evaluation is important in terms of empowerment, ensuring programmes are contextually and culturally relevant, and creating broader attitudinal change and stigma reduction (Sakellariou, Pollard & Kronenberg, 2008).

Occupational therapists are increasingly working at the policy level, influencing changes in policies and institutional systems that present barriers and continue to exclude or discriminate against people experiencing illness, injury or impairment. Occupational therapists are helping to broker relationships and facilitate consultations between, for example, governments, service providers and DPOs to identify ways policies, services and systems across a range of sectors can better include and benefit women, men, girls and boys with disabilities. Such a focus is not unfamiliar to occupational therapy practice and challenges occupational therapists to more strongly focus on the environmental areas that affect occupational performance. It also requires occupational therapists to strengthen their skills in policy development, implementation and evaluation. Practice Story 28.4 shares the story of an occupational therapist whose career in policy and practice has spanned the application of many of these roles from a local community level through to national and international levels.

PRACTICE STORY 28.4

A Career Reflecting and Shaping the Evolution of CBR

Kristen is an occupational therapist whose career to date, in many ways, has reflected and helped shape the evolution of CBR as a development approach. Her childhood experiences around the marginalisation, expectations and exclusion associated with both poverty and with disability have shaped her approach to inclusion in policy and practice.

Kristen's early career involved coordination and rehabilitation roles in disability and community health programmes with both government and nongovernment providers. She played similar roles in health and education for people experiencing illness, injury or impairment in her early experience in developing countries. With some additional study, she moved into a career

A Career Reflecting and Shaping the Evolution of CBR (Continued)

in international development, working largely for the Australian Government Aid programme – both at headquarters and in partner countries. Her role involved liaising with a range of stakeholders, including partner governments, politicians, nongovernment organisations, DPOs and other aid implementers. Although not always working in disability, she always tried to bring disability into the programmes she was engaged with as an advisor or manager. Kristen eventually led a team that developed and oversaw implementation of the Australian aid programme's first disability strategy (Government of Australia, 2008). Although this was not labelled as CBR, many of the objectives, principles and activities in this strategy reflect the principles and components of CBR.

More recently, Kristen has applied a broader inclusion lens to the health sector at an international level with the World Health Organization. In this role, she worked with a range of government and nongovernment stakeholders and national and international levels, including ensuring the input of people experiencing illness, injury or impairment in all policies and guidelines. She was integrally involved in the consultations and drafting of the WHO Disability Action Plan (WHO, 2014) and the development of rehabilitation guidelines. She now works with the Disability Rights Fund, once again supporting the central role of people experiencing illness, injury or impairment in development programmes.

Kirsten feels that combined with her personal experiences, the adaptable and well-rounded skill set acquired through occupational therapy has enabled her to practice aligned with the objectives and principles inherent in CBR. For example, functional assessment and task analysis skills have helped her to approach often complex tasks – from working with a child with severe autism to coordinating international development policy and action plans. The understanding of the clear steps involved, and how to assist different people, from individuals to organisations and government bodies, to achieve goals draws heavily on her skills as an occupational therapist. Similarly, the value of analytical skills and strong evidence-based approaches has strengthened her practice. She has also found the understanding of human behaviours (through psychology and sociology) helpful in communication and stronger collaborative work practices, which have been pivotal to her work to date.

CONCLUSION

CBR and occupational therapy are philosophically aligned. Clearly some knowledge and skills required within the CBR strategy are already part of occupational therapy. Other roles present challenges to occupational therapists to develop and foster new skills. Hartley, Kisanji, & Nganwa, (2002) highlighted that professionals involved in CBR need to change their attitudes – to be more humble about their achievements, more respectful, acknowledging that they can learn from others, and more willing to share their knowledge and skills with others. Pollard and Sakellariou (2007 & 2008) have highlighted the value of occupational therapists clearly understanding CBR and ensuring that people experiencing illness, injury or impairment and the community have a central role in the planning, design, implementation and evaluation of CBR.

We began this chapter with Sheona's story. Realisation of the CBR strategy in practice can help facilitate a more inclusive society for all people experiencing illness, injury or impairment, working towards Sheona's story becoming common rather than exceptional. The philosophy, concepts and skills underlying occupational therapy practice ensure occupational therapists are ideally positioned to continue to play a significant role in the development and implementation of community-based rehabilitation.

ⓔ http://evolve.elsevier.com/Curtin/OT

REFERENCES

Al Heresh, R., Bryant, W., & Holm, M. (2013). Community-based rehabilitation in Jordan: Challenges to achieving occupational justice. *Disability and Rehabilitation, 35*(21), 1848–1852.

Australia, C. B. M. (2012). *Inclusion made easy.* Retrieved from, http://www.cbm.org/Inclusion-Made-Easy-329091.php.

Banks, L. M., & Polack, S. (2014). *The economic costs of exclusion and gains of inclusion of people with disabilities: Evidence from low and middle income countries.* London: International Centre for Evidence in Disability, London School of Hygiene & Tropical Medicine. Retrieved from, http://disabilitycentre.lshtm.ac.uk.

Barros, D., Ghirardi, M., & Lopes, R. E. (2005). Social occupational therapy: A socio-historical perspective. In F. Kronenberg, S. Simó Algado, & N. Pollard (Eds.), *Occupational therapy without borders: Learning from the spirit of survivors* (pp. 140–151). Oxford, UK: Elsevier.

Bury, T. (2005). Primary health care and community based rehabilitation: Implications for physical therapy. *Asia Pacific Disability Rehabilitation Journal, 16*(2), 29–65.

Cleaver, S., & Nixon, S. (2014). A scoping review of 10 years of published literature on community-based rehabilitation. *Disability & Rehabilitation, 36*(17), 1385–1394.

Disability Rights Fund (2013). *One in seven: How one billion people are redefining the global movement for human rights.* Retrieved from, http://www.disabilityrightsfund.org/files/news/drf_report_oneinseven.pdf.

Disabled People's International (2005). *Disabled Peoples International position paper on community based rehabilitation (CBR)*. Retrieved from, http://www.aifo.it/english/resources/online/books/cbr/reviewofcbr/DPI%20on%20CBR.pdf.

Fransen, H. (2005). Challenges for occupational therapy in community based rehabilitation: Occupation in a community development approach to handicap in development. In F. Kronenberg, S. Simo Algado, & N. Pollard (Eds.), *Occupational therapy without borders: Learning from the spirit of survivors* (pp. 166–182). Sydney: Elsevier Churchill Livingstone.

Government of Australia (2008). *Development for All: Towards a disability-inclusive Australian aid program 2009–2014*. Retrieved from, http://dfat.gov.au/aid/topics/development-issues/disability-inclusive-development/Pages/disability-inclusive-development.aspx.

Groce, N., Kembhavi, G., Wirz, S., Lang, R., Trani, J., & Kett, M. (2011). *Poverty and disability – A critical review of the literature in low and middle-income countries*. Working Paper Series: No. 16, Leonard Cheshire Disability and Inclusive Development Centre. London: University College London & Leonard Cheshire Disability.

Hammell, K. W. (2009). Sacred texts: A sceptical exploration of the assumptions underpinning theories of occupation. *Canadian Journal of Occupational Therapy, 76*(1), 6–13.

Handicap International (2011). *Support to organizations representative of persons with disabilities*. Retrieved from, http://www.disabilityrightsfund.org/files/supporttodpo.pdf.

Hansen, A. M., Chaki, A., & Mlay, R. (2013). Occupational therapy synergy between comprehensive community based rehabilitation Tanzania and Heifer International to reduce poverty. *African Journal of Disability, 2*(1), 1–7.

Hartley, S., Kisanji, J., & Nganwa, A. (2002). Professionals participation in CBR programs. In S. Hartley (Ed.), *CBR: A participatory strategy in Africa* (pp. 72–85). London: The Centre for International Child Health.

Helander, E. (2000). Guest editorial: 25 years of community based rehabilitation. *Asia Pacific Disability Rehabilitation Journal, 11*(1), 12–14.

Iemmi, V., Gibson, L., Blanchet, K., et al. (2015). Community-based rehabilitation for people with disabilities in low- and middle-income countries: A systematic review. *Campbell Systematic Reviews, 2015*, 15.

Imms, C. (2006). The international classification of functioning, disability and health: They're talking our language. *Australian Occupational Therapy Journal, 53*, 65–66.

Inclusion International (2006). *Fact sheet on poverty and disability*. Retrieved from, http://www.inclusion-international.org/site_uploads/11223821811255806183.pdf.

International Disability Alliance (2014). *The post-2015 development agenda and the UN CRPD in Africa: Deepening dialogue between Africa stakeholders and global and regional DPOs to strengthen advocacy for inclusive development*. Retrieved from, http://www.internationaldisabilityalliance.org/en/article/ida-press-release-opening-conference-post-2015-development-agenda-and-un-crpd-africa-nairobi.

International Disability and Development Consortium (2012). *CBR guidelines as a tool for community based inclusive development*.

Retrieved from, http://iddcconsortium.net/sites/default/files/resources-tools/files/brochure_summary_bat.pdf.

International Labour Office, United Nations Educational Scientific and Cultural Organization, & World Health Organization (2004). *CBR: A strategy for rehabilitation, equalisation of opportunities, poverty reduction and social inclusion of disabled people*. Geneva, Switzerland: World Health Organization.

Kuipers, P., & Doig, E. (2010). Community-based rehabilitation. In J. Stone, & M. Blouin (Eds.), *International encyclopedia of rehabilitation* Retrieved from, http://cirrie.buffalo.edu/encyclopedia/en/article/362/.

Kuipers, P., & Harknett, S. (2008). Considerations in the quest for evidence in community based rehabilitation. *Asia Pacific Disability Rehabilitation Journal, 19*, 3–14.

Kuipers, P., & Harknett, S. (2009). Can we use the values and community orientation of community-based rehabilitation in its evidence base? *Development Bulletin, 73*, 90–93.

Lang, R. (2011). Community-based rehabilitation and health professional practice: Developmental opportunities and challenges in the global north and south. *Disability & Rehabilitation, 33*(2), 165–173.

Mannan, H., MacLachlan, M., & McAuliffe, E. (2013). The human resources challenge to community based rehabilitation: The need for a scientific, systematic and coordinated global response. *Disability, CBR & Inclusive Development, 23*(4), 6–16.

Mitra, S., Posarac, A., & Vick, B. (2013). Disability and poverty in developing countries: A multidimensional study. *World Development, 41*, 1–18.

Mizunoya, S., & Mitra, S. (2013). Is there a disability gap in employment rates in developing countries? *World Development, 42*, 28–43.

Nagata, K. K. (2007). Perspectives on disability, poverty and development in the Asian region. *Asia Pacific Disability Rehabilitation Journal, 18*(1), 3–19.

Pollard, N., & Kronenberg, F. (2008). Working with people on the margins. In J. Creek, & L. Lougher (Eds.), *Occupational therapy and mental health* (4th ed.). Philadelphia: Churchill Livingstone Elsevier.

Pollard, N., & Sakellariou, D. (2007). Occupation, education and community-based rehabilitation. *British Journal of Occupational Therapy, 70*(4), 171–174.

Pollard, N., & Sakellariou, D. (2008). Operationalizing community participation in community-based rehabilitation: Exploring the factors. *Disability & Rehabilitation, 30*(1), 62–70.

Sakellariou, D., Pollard, N., Fransen, H., et al. (2006). *Reporting on the WFOT-CBR Master Project Plan: The data collection subproject*. Retrieved from, https://www.researchgate.net/publication/257322846_Reporting_on_the_WFOT-CBR_Master_Project_Plan_the_Data-collection_subproject.

Sakellariou, D., Pollard, N., & Kronenberg, F. (2008). Time to get political. *British Journal of Occupational Therapy, 71*(9), 359–359.

Shakespeare, T. (2009). Disability: A complex interaction. In H. Daniels, H. Lauder, & J. Porter (Eds.), *Knowledge, values and education policy: A critical perspective*. London: Routledge.

Thibeault, R. (2006). Globalisation, universities and the future of occupational therapy: Dispatches for the majority world. *Australian Occupational Therapy Journal, 53*, 159–165.

Thomas, M., & Thomas, M. J. (1996). *The value of physiotherapy and occupational therapy in community based rehabilitation: Summary of discussion led by E. Henley & R. Twible.* Retrieved from, http://www.dinf.ne.jp/doc/english/asia/resource/apdrj/z13fm0100/zl13fm0105.htm.

Thomas, M., & Thomas, M. (2002). Some controversies in community based rehabilitation. In S. Hartley (Ed.), *CBR: A participatory strategy in Africa* (pp. 13–25). London: Centre for International Child Health.

Thomas, M., & Thomas, M. J. (Eds.). (2003). *Manual for CBR planners.* Bangalore: National Printing Press.

Twible, R., & Henley, E. (2000). Preparing occupational therapists and physiotherapists for community based rehabilitation. In M. Thomas, & M. J. Thomas (Eds.), *Selected readings in CBR* (pp. 243–273). Bangalore: National Printing Press.

United Nations (2006). *Convention on the rights of persons with disabilities.* New York: United Nations.

United Nations (2013). *Convention on the rights of persons with disabilities.* Retrieved from, https://www.un.org/disabilities/default.asp?navid=14&pid=150.

Watson, R. (2013). A population approach to occupational therapy. *South African Journal of Occupational Therapy, 43*(1), 34–38.

Werner, D. (1998). *Nothing about us without us: Developing innovative technologies for, by and with disabled persons.* Palo Alto, CA: Healthwrights.

Wilcock, A., & Townsend, E. (2000). Occupation terminology interactive dialogue: Occupational justice. *Journal of Occupational Science, 7*(2), 84–86.

Wittman, P. P., & Velde, B. P. (2001). Occupational therapy in the community: What, why and how? *Occupational Therapy in Health Care, 13*(3/4), 1–5.

World Federation of Occupational Therapists. (2004a). *Definition of occupational therapy.* Retrieved from, http://www.wfot.org.au/office_files/Definition%20of%20OT%20CM2004%20Final.pdf.

World Federation of Occupational Therapists. (2004b). *WFOT position paper on community based rehabilitation.* Retrieved from, http://www.wfot.org.au/officefiles/CBRposition%20Final.%20CM2004%281%29.pdf.

World Health Organization. (1989). *Training in the community for people with disabilities.* Geneva, Switzerland: World Health Organization.

World Health Organization. (2001). *International classification of functioning, disability and health.* Retrieved from, www.who.org.ch/icf.

World Health Organization. (2003). *International consultation to review community-based rehabilitation (CBR) (Report on International Consultation).* Geneva, Switzerland: World Health Organization.

World Health Organization. (2005). *Meeting report on the development of guidelines for community based rehabilitation (CBR) programmes (meeting report).* Geneva, Switzerland: World Health Organization.

World Health Organization. (2006). *Report on the 4th meeting on development of CBR guidelines.* Retrieved from, http://www.who.org.

World Health Organization. (2007). Community based rehabilitation: United National agencies work with civil society to draw up guidelines for implementing community based rehabilitation programmes. *WHO Newsletter on Disability and Rehabilitation, 3.*

World Health Organization. (2014). *WHO global disability action plan 2014-2021.* Retrieved from, http://www.who.int/disabilities/actionplan/en/.

World Health Organization. (2015). *Assistive devices/technologies.* Retrieved from, http://www.who.int/disabilities/technology/en/.

World Health Organization, International Labour Office, United Nations Educational Scientific and Cultural Organization & International Disability and Development Consortium. (2011). *Community based rehabilitation guidelines: Introductory booklet.* Geneva, Switzerland: World Health Organization.

World Health Organization, & World Bank. (2011). *World report on disability.* Retrieved from, http://whqlibdoc.who.int/publications/2011/9789240685215_eng. pdf.

29 COACHING

WENDY PENTLAND ■ AMY HEINZ ■ JEANETTE ISAACS-YOUNG ■ JEN GASH

CHAPTER OUTLINE

Abstract

Coaching is a specific type of relationship and conversation with people that fosters their ability to create a more fulfilling, meaningful and satisfying life. This chapter outlines what coaching is generally and in the context of occupational therapy. The chapter provides the theoretical background to coaching, explains how coaching aligns with occupational therapy practice, offers a model of coaching for occupational therapy and coaching competencies, describes the process of occupational therapy coaching for enabling positive change, offers example coaching questions occupational therapy practitioners can use in practice, and presents practice stories to illustrate the application of coaching.

KEY POINTS

- The coaching approach is entirely consistent with the aims and values of occupational therapy.

- Coaching focuses on three main areas: improving performance, learning, and life fulfilment.

- Coaching is a way for occupational therapy practitioners to communicate with people that shifts power and control to them and focuses directly on helping them to create and live a meaningful, fulfilled life through fostering personal awareness, choice making and self-trust.

- Coaching and occupational therapy operate using three mechanisms to enable occupational change: coaching mind set, relationship, and process.
- Coaching involves deep, active listening combined with intuitive, powerful questioning to enable people to generate their own solutions.

INTRODUCTION

Coaching is a specific type of relationship and way of communicating with people that enables them to create and sustain more of the life they want. This makes the coaching approach a valuable resource throughout the occupational therapy process, because much of what brings people to occupational therapy is about occupational transition, and desired occupational change. The coaching approach enables people to learn and grow, and provides an opportunity for reinvention and realignment of living with what really matters to them.

DEFINING COACHING

Coaching has been defined as 'partnering with clients in a specific conversation-based, thought-provoking and creative process that inspires them to move from their current state to a more desired future state' (International Coach Federation, 2011; Stober & Grant, 2006). The primary medium for coaching is the coach–person relationship and conversation process that incorporates powerful, provocative questions. Much of the power of effective coaching comes from the *coach–person relationship*, which is characterised by trust, openness and equality. The *coaching process* is person-centred, serves the person's agenda (not the practitioner's agenda), fosters self-directed learning and is grounded in self-awareness, personal values, strengths recognition, possibilities, choice, and self-responsibility. A primary focus is assisting people to discover and clarify what is important to them. They begin to bring more of their genuine self to the world, and this contribution from a place of personal authenticity gives them a greater sense of meaning and purpose. A summary of the distinguishing features of the coaching approach are included in Table 29.1.

According to Adler International Learning (2009), when working with a person, it is the coach's responsibility to

- Enable the person to discover, clarify and then to align with what he or she wants to achieve
- Invite and facilitate person self-discovery
- Elicit person-generated possibilities, solutions and strategies
- Hold the person as capable, responsible and accountable

Coaching goals and intentions typically fall into three areas: (a) performance, with goals that are oriented to behaviour change, achievement and results; (b) learning, with goals intended to gain new understandings, skills, attitudes and processes; and (c) fulfilment, with goals related to meaning, life

TABLE 29.1	
Distinguishing Features of the Coaching Approach	
Coaching Is Typified By:	**Coaching Is Not Typified By:**
Future focus	Past focus
Egalitarian, collaborative relationship	Expert approach
Powerful evocative questions	Advice
	Judging/evaluating/interpreting
Action–reflection–learning process	Problem-solving/weakness/fix or heal the past focus
Appreciative/strength/possibility focus	Prescribe/recommend
	Drive/achieve
Curiosity, create and invent	'You need my help'
	Assessments of compliance and cooperation
Championing/challenging	Professional evaluates success and outcomes
Accountability	
Person evaluates success and outcomes	

Adapted with permission from Adler Learning International (2009) and Pentland (2012).

balance and the desire for deeper satisfaction and sense of purpose in personal or professional occupations.

Coaching begins with the assumption that competency and success in designing and living a meaningful, fulfilling life are determined by awareness, choice making and self-trust (Adler Learning International, 2009). *Awareness* entails people being cognisant of:

- themselves and others;
- their effect on others and the effect of others on themselves;
- their habitual patterns of thinking and behaviour that get in the way;
- what's not working; and
- clarity about their values, what they really want and what is most important to them.

Choice refers to an individual's ability to see many possible attitudinal, behavioural and life choices, rather than seeing none or only one or two (notwithstanding that some of the choices may be difficult). Choice involves people recognising that they are always choosing and the need to take responsibility for the choices made.

Self-trust is the extent to which a person believes he or she deserves what he or she is wanting or working toward and that he or she is capable of creating it. Self-trust is similar to self-efficacy.

DIFFERENTIATING COACHING FROM THERAPY, MENTORING, CONSULTING AND TRAINING

Coaching is distinct from therapy, mentoring, consulting and training. Whereas therapy may deal with pain, dysfunction and healing from past experiences, coaching is forward-focused with the goal of assisting people to clarify what they really want and then moving towards that desired future. This is not to say that coaching and some therapeutic approaches do not have some common core elements. For example, acceptance and commitment therapy (ACT), like coaching, places importance on helping people clarify what is important to them, committing to that and then using mindfulness to recognise and accept inner resistance, such as anxiety and depression, that may get in the way, and not let it derail their desired behaviour and lifestyle changes (Eifert & Forsythe, 2005; Hayes, 2005). Furthermore, cognitive behavioural therapy (CBT) and coaching both help people to recognise the existence and impact of their thoughts, emotions and feelings on their behaviour (Segal, Williams, & Teasdale, 2002).

Where the coaching approach differs from other approaches is that it focuses on enabling people to generate their own solutions and thus increasing their capacity to deal independently with future problems. Although people definitely learn during coaching, they set their own learning goals and objectives for change; this learning does not follow any preset curriculum or linear learning path.

THE THEORETICAL UNDERPINNINGS OF COACHING

Like occupational therapy and most of the human service professions, coaching draws on an eclectic theory base. The key areas of theory underpinning the coaching approach can be grouped as follows: adult development theory; person-centred therapeutic theory; learning theory; postpositivism; appreciative, positive strengths-based approaches; and theories of human change.

Adult Development Theories

Adult development theories suggest that the issues and approaches to resolution of the paradoxical tension between the human need for self-expression versus integration change across the life course (Kegan, 1982, 1994; Vaillant, 2002). For example, tasks typically associated with young adulthood are reconciling social expectations of family and peers versus personal beliefs/desires, the need to work to earn income to live independently versus doing what you want to do, and establishing roles and relationships necessary to create and support stable social structures to raise children and sustain society. Tasks associated more with midlife and beyond (Corbett, 2013; Hollis, 2001) include individuation and authentic self-expression versus the pull of society's role and behavioural expectations. Tasks related to life integration, legacy and gerotranscendence become a focus in later life (Corbett, 2013; Ericksen & Ericksen, 1997; Tornstam, 2005). The coach and person partner to enable the person to design and live an optimal resolution to this differentiation versus integration tension given their particular lifestage.

Person-centred Therapeutic Theory

There is a particular therapist–coach mind set and cocreated relationship with a person in coaching that is totally person-centred and as such is entirely congruent with occupational therapy. The origins of person-centred practice lie in the person-centred approach first advanced by the psychologist Carl Rogers in the 1950s (Rogers, 1951). It forms the origins of the person-centred approach adhered to in occupational therapy as well as a number of other professions, including coaching. Rogers approached people from the perspective that humans have an innate tendency for growth and self-actualisation. He believed that all people have vast capacities for self-understanding and altering their self-concepts, attitudes and behaviours. These resources for personal change can be tapped if a climate of facilitative psychological attitudes can be provided.

Rogers (1951) stated that this growth-promoting climate requires three essential ingredients:

1. Therapist genuineness, realness, and congruence
2. Unconditional positive regard – acceptance, caring, prizing
3. Empathic understanding – accurately sensing a person's feelings and personal meanings and communicating this understanding to the person

As a result of the climate created that is characterised by these three ingredients, the therapist-client relationship becomes a growth promoting container that fosters person change. Through this type of relationship and being regarded positively by another, people tend to mirror the way they are being treated by the therapist. They become more aware of and able to listen to their own inner experiences, to be more self-accepting and self-compassionate, develop familiarity with and congruence in their inner self, and feel the freedom to be their true self. In this way, they become more and more of their own change-agent (Rogers, 1980).

Learning Theory

Theories based on the process of learning, reflection, change and, particularly, transformative learning also inform the coaching approach. Transformative learning theory focuses on those aspects of adult learning and knowledge construction that entail making meaning, particularly through becoming aware of the assumptions, habits of mind, values, expectations and purposes assimilated from others (Argyris & Schon, 1974; Mezirow, 2000). Transformative learning is often triggered by a sudden 'not knowing', or realisation of former 'knowing' no longer applying, or when faced with some form of personal crisis. The coach uses powerful, evocative questions that invite deeper insight and new awareness about personal values, assumptions, and expectations and how these currently define and frame issues and limit choices. This enhanced self-awareness alone is often sufficient to open the person to see and choose new options and possibilities.

Postpositivism

The coaching approach takes a postpositive worldview, as opposed to a positivist perspective. Positivism holds that the professional is independent and able to make truly objective observations that will reveal a single reality. Introspection and intuitive knowledge from the person receiving therapy are seen as having limited clinical value. Postpositivism holds that there is no single true reality; rather, people create their own reality with their thinking and the stories they tell themselves as they make meaning (Robson, 2002). It follows then that, once people 'wake up' by becoming aware of their personal constructions and stories, they realise they have power to reinvent their 'reality' by changing what thoughts they choose to focus on, or changing their thinking or their responses to it. This notion is not new and pervades various fields, including psychology (e.g. logotherapy; see Frankl, 1984; Glasser, 2000), Acceptance and Commitment Therapy (ACT) (see Eifert & Forsyth, 2005), Eastern religions such as Buddhism (see Kabat-Zinn, 2006; Thurman, 2005), and qualitative research methods such as the phenomenological and narrative approaches (see DePoy & Gitlin, 2005). Frankl refers to this ability to choose as the last of the human freedoms, 'that everything can be taken from a man but one thing: the last of the human freedoms—to choose one's attitude in any given set of circumstances, to choose one's own way' (Frankl, 1984, p. 86).

Coaches work with people to help them become more aware of how their thinking, language and personal stories are creating their outlook and experience. As people become more aware of how they limit themselves with their current thinking and realise they actually have far more choice in their attitude and responses than they were previously aware of, an increased feeling of personal agency and urge to make change often ensues.

Appreciative, Positive Strengths-based Approaches

Focus on a person's strengths and values rather than a primary orientation toward deficit and weakness is a notion fundamental to the coaching approach (Cooperrider & Whitney, 1999; Cooperrider, Whitney, & Stavros, 2003; Seligman, 2002). Coaching people who want to increase their sense of meaning and fulfillment begins first with assisting them to clarify their strengths and personal values and what is truly important to them and then helps them to evaluate the extent to which their current lifestyle is congruent with these. The coaching work then focuses on the person redesigning his or her occupational life to improve this congruence. Theoretical and empirical research on human flourishing informs this approach (Aspinall & Staudinger, 2003; Emmons, 2002; Keys & Haidt, 2003; Ryan & Deci, 2001; Seligman, 2002; Snyder & Lopez, 2002). This research provides more detailed accounts of human strengths, resilience, the importance of values, and the role of meaning for well-being. Positive psychologist Martin Seligman (2002) introduced a model of authentic happiness (subjective well-being) designed around the three constructs of (1) The "pleasant life", which is promoted by minimising negative emotions and maximising positive emotions; (2) "engagement", which occurs when persons find opportunities to use his or her strengths and (3) "meaning", which is experienced when the person believes he or she is using his or her strengths to make a contribution toward the greater good.

Theories of Human Change

The focus of coaching is human change, and this can include changes in self awareness, attitudes and behaviours. Consequently, a variety of theories of human change inform the coaching process. These include Argyris and Schon's Action-Reflection-Learning Model of Change (Argyris & Schon, 1974), Kolb's experiential learning theory (Kolb, 1984), Prochaska's Transtheoretical Model of Behaviour Change (Prochaska, DiClemente, & Norcross, 1992), Mezirow's transformative learning theory (Mezirow, 2000); Appreciative Inquiry (Cooperrider & Whitney, 1999) and Bridges' Life Transition Model (Bridges, 2004). Consistent with each of these theories, the coaching approach regards, and in fact expects and allows for, the human change process to be non-linear and iterative.

COACHING AND OCCUPATIONAL THERAPY

Coaching is a way of communicating and building relationships in occupational therapy that foster and enable positive occupational change. In the context of occupational therapy, coaching is defined here as 'a specific conversational partnership for enabling occupational change that assists clients to clarify what is important to them, access their strengths, resources and creativity, choose goals and design and follow a plan of action to get what they want' (Pentland, 2015). Although there is growing evidence, the conclusion of an integrative literature review conducted in 2013–2014 revealed a variety of coaching-based approaches but a general lack of explicit theoretical bases and models for coaching intervention in occupational therapy (Kessler & Graham, 2015). This lack of theoretical base and model for coaching intervention has led to the development of a Model of Coaching for Enablement in Occupational Therapy (Fig. 29.1).

The goal of occupational therapy coaching is to enable person-desired and person-driven occupational change that fosters optimal health and well-being. The distinguishing focus of occupational therapy coaching is its focus on occupational performance and occupational engagement. Occupational performance is the dynamic interaction of person, occupation and environment. The coaching process begins with deepening the person's self-awareness and understanding at the level of the person (affective, somatic, cognitive and spiritual). The coach then shifts the conversation focus to facilitating the person to expand his or her choices, and then to become accountable for taking actions. Through this repeated action–reflection–learning cycle (Schon, 1983) of the coaching process, the person begins to

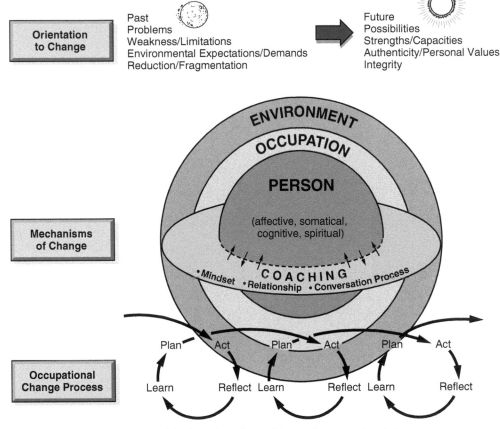

FIG. 29.1 ■ Model of coaching for enablement in occupational therapy.

create the occupational life they want and experiences changes at all three levels (person, environment, occupation).

Background to the Model of Coaching for Enablement in Occupational Therapy

The context for the model is informed by the Canadian Model of Occupational Performance – Enabling (Polatajko, Townsend, & Craik, 2007) and the Person–Environment–Occupation Model (Law et al., 1996). The Model of Coaching for Enablement in Occupational Therapy regards coaching as occurring across the interface of the person, the person's environment and the person's occupations. The occupational therapist coach is situated in the person's environment; the person is in the occupational therapist coach's (OT coach) environment; and engaging in coaching is an occupation for both the person and OT coach. As illustrated in the diagram, occupational therapy coaching is not done *to* the person but rather the person and the OT coach participate equally in the relationship and both are affected, influenced and changed by the process. Coaching can result in changes at all three levels of person, occupation and environment to some degree for both client and the OT coach.

Coaching has the capacity to addresses the affective, somatic, cognitive and spiritual realms of the person. As such, coaching operates and can effect change at the mind, body and spirit/soul places of the person. Indeed, coaching training prepares coaches to work at both the somatic and spiritual places in addition to the affective and cognitive realms, where occupational therapy traditionally has had more well-developed intervention approaches. In this sense, coach training expands the occupational therapists' abilities to work with people in a more holistic way.

The Model's Orientation to Occupational Change

The model is oriented towards occupational change and the occupational lifestyle that the person wants to create, rather than being past- and problem-focused. The goal is to enable people to experience a sense of living in integrity with their authentic self (Rogers, 1980). The focus is on what the person wants to be different as opposed to what is expected of them by their relationships and environment. The emphasis is on possibilities, strengths, opportunities and expanding choices versus the identification, assessment, analysis and solution of problems. This is not to say problems are ignored, but they are faced orthogonally rather than up front and head on. For example, the approach to a problem is more 'What do you want?' as opposed to 'What's wrong?' This is consistent with the Appreciative Inquiry approach to change (Cooperrider et al., 2003, 2008), where the focus is on people at their best, their strengths and capacities, what works well, creating best-case possibilities and then designing and organising actions to manifest them as opposed to trying to correct weaknesses and limitations.

The model's orientation to occupational change facilitates a person's authenticity and enables a person to become aware of and living in congruence with their personal values. Society does not typically encourage or offer opportunities for people to identify their values and strengths and what gives meaning for them. Instead, relationships and systems tend to reward conformity. So people live in a paradox between self-expression and embeddedness, and a continuous adult development life task involves each person differentiating from the need to receive external approval towards becoming aware of and taking a stand for who they are and their own values and beliefs (Laske, 1999; Lippmann, 1922; Mezirow, 2000). Occupational integrity and authenticity is the extent to which individuals can resolve that paradox in a way that honours their values and at the same time allows them to live in relationship with their environment (Pentland & McColl, 2009). Coaching focuses expressly on assisting people to be clear about who they are, what they value, what they stand for and what they want in life.

The Three Coaching Components in the Model that Enables Occupational Change

The model delineates three broad components through which change occurs in occupational therapy coaching: mind set, relationship and process.

Mind Set

Coaching is distinguished by a particular mind set. It is one of openness, curiosity, creativity, playfulness, genuineness and non-judgement and it is closely aligned with the hypotheses and definitions of person-centred therapy outlined by Carl Rogers beginning in the 1950s as essential for unleashing a person's innate yearning and capacities for self-understanding, growth and self-actualisation (Rogers, 1951, 1980). As people experience being regarded in this way, they in turn assimilate aspects of the mind set and begin to approach themselves and their world from this more accepting and open perspective. This enables them to be 'themselves' and expands their capacity to change.

Relationship

The coaching relationship is a unique and important container through which personal change is enabled. That container is a safe, honest and accepting space where each person feels accepted and championed and at the same time knows they will be challenged to

be their best. The coach–person relationship is cocreated to be in service of what the person wants. It is collaborative, time-limited and focused and occurs via meaningful conversations in which the coach manages the process that enables the person to lead in designing and implementing the actions necessary to achieve personal goals. When using the coaching approach it is important that occupational therapists adopt a collaborative stance and neutralise personal biases, so that they can work with people to identify and help them understand their issues from their own perspective. This may not always be easy for professionals who expect that as 'experts' they are obliged to identify the person's problems and the best approach to solve them.

Conversational Process

Coaching occurs over time via a process of numerous conversations that follow a particular format and include specific features. Individual coach–person conversations, and indeed the overall coaching engagement, can be regarded as following four guiding inquiries:

1. What do you want?
2. What works best?/What are your most powerful resources?
3. What gets in the way?/What smooths the way?
4. What do you need to do differently?

Unique to coaching is the importance of the coach and person establishing an 'agreement' or 'contract' at the beginning of their overall work together and at the beginning of each session. This agreement includes what the person wants to work on, what the person would like the outcome of the coaching to be, and how the person will know the outcome has been achieved. Without this agreement there is little creative tension and coaching may easily slip into noncoaching modes such as chatting, complaining, teaching and directing or advising.

The coaching conversation process has particular features that include powerful evocative questions and deep and generous listening. Fundamental to coaching are evocative, impactful questions that come from an attitude of curiosity rather than gathering data for the therapist to then interpret. There is deep listening where the coach's full awareness is on the person and not on how to interpret what the person has just said or on composing the next question. Listening in coaching includes deeper environmental listening for sight, sound, smell, feelings, intuition and what the person is *not* saying. The emphasis on impactful questions does not mean the coach never offers the person observations, feedback, other perspectives or suggestions. However, in all instances the coach remains *unattached* to whether the person accepts or agrees with these.

Powerful coaching questions are succinct, oriented to the person's goals and designed to take them into territory they have not yet explored. The answers are considered without judgement and the OT coach stays curious. The aim is not to gather information but to enable people to become astute self-observers and increase their self-awareness and understanding.

To help stay 'with' the person and go deeper, in each subsequent question the OT coach may use some of the words the person just used when responding to previous questions. For example:

> *Person:* 'I want more balance in my life'.
> *OT coach:* 'What would more balance give you?'

One method of developing and asking impactful questions is to use the I-C-A Map for coaching as illustrated in Table 29.2. In this instance, the "I" stands for Issue and Insight, the "C" for Choice and Commitment and the "A" for Action and Accountability. Examples of powerful coaching questions that could be used in practice are included in Table 29.3.

The coaching conversation includes many of the communication skills occupational therapists learn in their professional education, such as active listening and observing all dimensions of the person's communication (including tone, voice inflection, eyes, facial expression, body language and what saying not being said). *Coaching requires that therapists listen using both their "head" and their "gut" or intuition in order to hear what a person is really saying (in coaching this is referred to as level III listening)* (Kimsey-House, & Sandahl, 2011). The emphasis is on listening for what the person is *really* saying or wanting. In coaching conversations, paraphrasing and reflecting back are used less than they may be in therapy, and in their place the coach offers the

		TABLE 29.2	
		Overview of the I-C-A Map for Coaching	
Phase		**Focus**	**Example Questions**
I	**Issue**	Determine conversation focus: ■ Ask questions to identify the issue of focus for this coaching conversation. ■ Explore what the person's current situation is in relation to this issue/focus. ■ Explore specifically what the person wants to gain or walk away with from this conversation.	What's up? What do you want to work on?
	Insight	Enhance awareness and create new insight: ■ Explore the person's chosen focus in depth. ■ Ask questions to determine how the person is thinking and feeling about the situation/issue. ■ Generate insights, expand awareness and create learning through questioning, offering observation, exploring alternative perspectives, and reflecting back what you hear. ■ Help the person clarify his or her intention in light of the person's new awareness and insight.	What do you want? What's going on now?
C	**Choice**	Expand choices: ■ Generate a range of choices for achieving the intention through questioning and brainstorming. ■ What are ways to address this? What are some choices to consider? ■ Examine the pros and cons of the choices.	What choices do you see?
	Commitment	Commit to a choice for moving forward: ■ Help the person narrow down the choices to on which to move forward. ■ Explore what it would take to commit to this choice. ■ Support the person's commitment and trust in self to move forward by encouraging and acknowledging his or her choice.	What do you want to commit to?
A	**Action**	Design the next action: ■ Collaboratively design an action plan and choose the next steps for the person. ■ Ask: what, where, when, how? ■ Identify potential obstacles and how to handle them. ■ Explore what additional resources and support person needs.	What's next?
	Accountability	Determine accountability: ■ Ask how the person will hold himself or herself accountable for the commitment. ■ What structure can the person put in place to help do this? ■ Offer your support. ■ Agree on the next conversation.	How will you be held accountable?

© Adler International Learning. Adapted with permission from Adler Learning International (2009).

TABLE 29.3
Examples of Powerful Coaching Questions That Could Be Used in Practice

Focus of Conversation	Examples of Powerful Coaching Questions
Conversations for meaning and fulfilment	What do you really want? What makes your heart sing? What is the next chapter in your life? Going forward, what do you want the theme of your life to be? What is 'a good life' for you? How do you want the world to be different because you were in it? Where are you living in-line/not in-line with your values? What are you tolerating?
Conversations to expand self-awareness	What motivates you? What patterns in your life do you need to change? What repeated feedback are you receiving that you should attend to? What is your favourite way of sabotaging yourself? When are you unable to laugh at yourself? Is what you are doing right now life-affirming or life-numbing? Who are you at your best? How do you block yourself? What are your strengths/gifts? What are you grateful for? What is your gut telling you?
Conversations to expand choices	If you couldn't fail, what do you want your life to be like in 5 years? What might _____ (insert name) do? Where do we go from here? What are other possibilities?/What's just one more possibility? What happens if you choose to avoid change? If you had free choice in this, what would you do? What could happen if you make one small change? Want to brainstorm? [...] Let's come up with 20/30/40 possibilities.
Conversations for making choices and decisions	What are you assuming about all this which is not helpful? How do you usually make decisions? [...] What's another way to decide? What resources do you need to help you decide? What values are most important to you right now? How do you think it will all work out? What is your body telling you about this? How will you know you made the best choice?
Conversations for action	This time next week/month, what will you have done? What makes sense to do now? What's the next step for you? When we speak next, what will have happened? What needs to happen now? How can you make this be easy/fun? What are you committing to? What preparation do you need to do to move forward? How will you reward/acknowledge your steps forward? Who are your supports for taking action? How can you call on them to support you in your goal?
Conversations for the stuck client	What's not clear? What are the benefits for you of staying stuck? What does your intuition say about this? What are your assumptions? What seems to be the main obstacle? What do you already know that you will find out in a year's time? If you were at your best what would you do right now?

Continued on following page

TABLE 29.3	
Examples of Powerful Coaching Questions That Could Be Used in Practice *(Continued)*	
Focus of Conversation	**Examples of Powerful Coaching Questions**
	Where are you giving away your power?
	What price are you paying for not moving forward?
	Where are you holding back?
	What requests can be made to get you going?
	What will free you up?
	What if you do nothing?

person silence, slow pacing and deep listening to give the person a safe space to reflect and do his or her own thinking – to 'work'.

Proposed Competencies Related to Each Mechanism of Change for Coaching in Occupational Therapy

As a reminder, coaching in the context of occupational therapy can be defined as: 'A specific conversational partnership for enabling occupational change that assists clients to clarify what is important to them, access their strengths, resources and creativity, choose goals and design and follow a plan of action to get what they want' (Pentland, 2015).

As outlined in the Model of Coaching for Enablement in Occupational Therapy (see Fig. 29.1) coaching in occupational therapy is a conversational partnership having three unique mechanisms for change that can be translated into three competency areas for the OT coach: mind set, relationship and conversational process (Adler Learning International, 2009; Pentland, 2015). These three competencies for coaching in the context of occupational therapy are illustrated in Box 29.1.

The Process of Occupational Change Through Coaching

In coaching, much of the learning and work occurs between sessions in individuals' own lives in the real world, because they have the opportunity there to perform the actions they committed to in the coaching session and then begin to reflect and learn from their experience and then begin to plan what if anything they need or want to try differently next time. They then bring this feedback to their next coaching session where it is worked on in more depth with the coach following the same process. Over time the expectation is that as people experience and learn through the coaching process, deepen their self-awareness and insight and learn to access more of their own creativity and resourcefulness, they will graduate to more and more "self-coaching".

With any particular person, the occupational therapist might use coaching in conjunction with one or more of the other nine specified enablement skills (adapt, advocate, collaborate, consult, coordinate, design/build, educate, engage and specialise) (Townsend & Polatajko, 2013). To provide an idea of how this coaching conversation process might play out in

---

BOX 29.1
OCCUPATIONAL THERAPY COACHING COMPETENCIES

Mind set: Recognises that people's beliefs and assumptions about themselves, others and the world around them directly influence occupational behaviour and what they see as possible, and these beliefs and assumptions are amenable to change.

a. Demonstrates awareness of both their own and others' beliefs and assumptions about themselves, others and the world around them.

b. Recognises that people's experience of themselves and their environments are constructed by them based on these beliefs and assumptions.

c. Recognises the influence of these beliefs and assumptions on occupational choices and behaviour. Understands and recognises that humans are self-creating and construct their lives with the choices they make.

d. Recognises that people's beliefs and assumptions are not fixed but are amenable to change.

e. Recognises that people can choose to operate from a positive, appreciative, learner and strengths-based perspective.

f. Is able to model and facilitate people's access to and adoption of this mind set.

Relationship: Cocreates with the person and maintains an occupational therapist–person relationship that is designed to elicit and support what the person wants and is characterised by trust, openness, honesty, nonjudgement, curiosity, spaciousness and freedom to explore and live into possibilities.

a. Understands that the coaching process occurs in the relationship, which is a third system that is cocreated by the therapist and person and is greater than the sum of the two individuals.

b. Can identify and demonstrate interactions with the person that facilitate this type of relationship (curious, nonjudgemental, nondirective, deep listening, etc.).

BOX 29.1
OCCUPATIONAL THERAPY COACHING COMPETENCIES *(Continued)*

c. Recognises and manages the coaching process appropriately given the nature of both the intervention time frame and power balance that is unique to the occupational therapist–person relationship within that setting.

d. Approaches the occupational therapist coaching relationship as one that is time-limited and having as one of its goals the person's increased capacity to become his or her own agent of change.

e. Recognises their own limitations with respect to practicing only the coaching skills in which they are trained and competent and knowing when to seek further professional development to expand their coaching skill repertoire.

f. Understands the differences and relationships between coaching, counselling and psychotherapy and recognises when to refer a person for noncoaching services.

Conversational process: Within the cocreated occupational therapy coaching relationship, demonstrates competence in selected coaching skills designed to enable the person's forward movement toward desired occupational participation for greater health and well-being.

a. Contracts at the outset with the person.

b. Demonstrates powerful questioning and deep listening.

c. Minimises paraphrasing and reflecting back. Instead, offers the person silence, slow pacing and deep listening to provide a safe space to reflect and work.

d. Knows, follows and adapts the Issue/insight–Choice/commitment–Action/accountability (ICA) process as relevant in that situation. This ICA process refers to the content of the coaching conversations that typically begin with the people being coached obtaining clarity on their issues and what they are wanting, deepening their insight about what is going on and who they are being in the issues, expanding their choices and committing to an action(s), and then taking action and specifying how they will hold themselves accountable.

e. Demonstrates ability to use selected basic coaching techniques/concepts for each stage of the ICA process, such as working with the inner critic, brainstorming with person, 'yes but' listing, metaphor, goal-setting, committing, structures, accountability (see Kimsey-House et al., 2011, for more detailed instructions on these techniques).

f. Demonstrates ability to assist person in values identification, life purpose identification, and developing a personal vision.

g. Understands and can facilitate person change through the action–reflection–learning cycle.

Adapted with permission from Pentland (2015)

---

occupational therapy practice, the action–reflection–learning–revising cycle pictured in the Occupational Change Process section of the model in Fig. 29.1 has been expanded in Fig. 29.2. Depending on a person's needs, the OT coach may follow these steps in their entirety or just a few of them, and this might be done before or after steps in the problem-solving approach to intervention. Integrating coaching into occupational therapy may be as limited as beginning work with a person by asking what it is he or she wants to work on or take away from the session/occupational therapy, similar to the first step of the cycle illustrated in Fig. 29.2. This then becomes part of an 'agreement' as to what the therapist and person will focus on and what the person can expect to take away from working collaboratively with the occupational therapist. Or coaching may be integrated throughout with regular and repeated use of the steps in Fig. 29.2. At all steps in the cycle the therapist needs to allow space for the person to resist, relapse and 'fail', as this is where significant learning can occur. Assessments, tools and techniques are useful elements in the overall process, but ultimately they are only helpful in the context of a relationship of respect, partnership, trust and openness.

The model of coaching proposed here is intended to offer a template so that occupational therapists can include coaching skills into their practice with individuals. The same model can be adapted for occupational therapists to use when working with groups, organisations, and communities who want to improve their process, experience, performance and well-being.

It is hoped that as more occupational therapists incorporate and document their use of coaching approaches in practice, people will benefit and occupational therapy–specific coaching research will grow. This model offers a structure and language that may facilitate these outcomes.

APPLICATION OF COACHING IN OCCUPATIONAL THERAPY PRACTICE

Two brief practice stories to illustrate the application of coaching within occupational therapy practice areas are provided in Practice Stories 29.1 and 29.2. For each practice story coaching for enablement is presented to illustrate how it can be a powerful addition to the other strategies occupational therapists may use when working with people. A possible coaching contract/agreement between the therapist and the person receiving therapy is included, as well as some possible paths of inquiry.

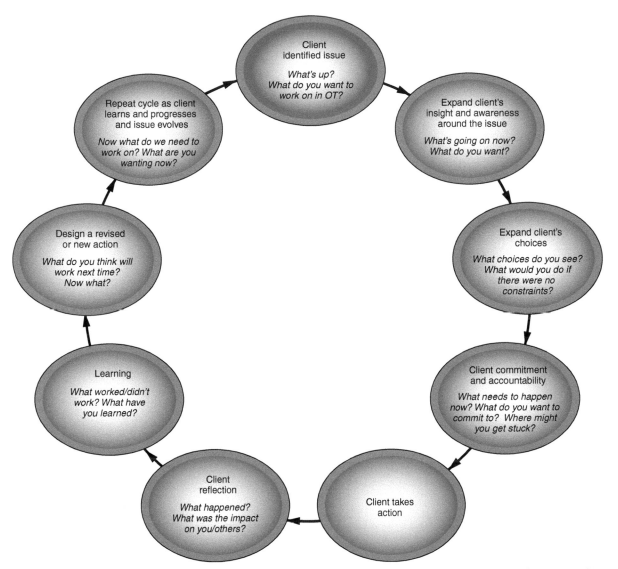

FIG. 29.2 ■ Action–reflection–learning–revising cycle of steps and example questions for each when applying a coaching approach in occupational therapy.

Olivia

Olivia is 38 years old and lives independently in an apartment in downtown Minneapolis. She was diagnosed with multiple sclerosis (MS) when she was 30. At that time she had only subtle symptoms of the condition such as occasional blurred vision and generalised weakness and fatigue. She has been managing well since her initial diagnosis, including working full time as an administrative assistant at a local law firm. More recently Olivia has noticed that her weakness and fatigue

PRACTICE STORY 29.1

Olivia (Continued)

are making her work challenging and leaving her little energy to complete household tasks and engage in leisure activities with friends and family. She has not shared these concerns with her friends and family. She does not like to ask for help or 'burden others with her problems'.

Olivia would also like a relationship. Although she has gone on a few dates, she has yet to be in a meaningful long-term relationship. This is something she longs for, and she is worried she will always be alone because of her MS.

Olivia is beginning to show signs of depression, including being less engaged in her daily routines. She recently had a visit with her primary care provider and was referred to an occupational therapist to address the progression of her MS, her feelings of depression, and the changes in her occupational participation.

EXAMPLES OF HOW COACHING WOULD BE APPLICABLE

- Assist Olivia in identifying what support she is willing to accept

- Explore ways for Olivia to ask for help that maintains her control and independence
- Analyse her daily routines and responsibilities to see how they may be adapted to accommodate for symptoms of MS

A POSSIBLE CONTRACT/AGREEMENT

Olivia might say the following:

- I want to feel in control of my circumstances.

POSSIBLE OCCUPATIONAL THERAPY COACHING QUESTIONS

- When do you feel most in control of your life? The least?
- What is your priority today?
- Where should we begin?
- What adaptations are you willing to make?
- What gets in the way of you asking for help?

PRACTICE STORY 29.2

Mr Bolton

Mr Bolton is a 67-year-old widower and retired chemical engineer with advanced amyotrophic lateral sclerosis (ALS). He has two grown married children and a 3-year old grandchild living in the same city. For 18 months he has been living in an acute care hospital, on a feeding tube and ventilator dependent via a tracheostomy. He is dependent for all activities of daily living and requires a two-person assist transfer. He has weak flexion and extension of his right index finger. With this movement he can activate a simple buzzer fixed to his wheelchair lap table. He communicates effectively in a soft voice. Mr Bolton wishes to move out of the hospital to a less institutional setting for his last days.

EXAMPLES OF HOW COACHING WOULD BE APPLICABLE

- Clarify what is important to him now and about how and where his death will be
- Identify what he is wanting from the move because some of that may in fact be able to be arranged immediately where he is now (i.e. more privacy)
- Engage him and his family in conversations that allow clarifying and sharing what is important to them right now

and going forward in order to assist with coping and remaining connected during the dying process

A POSSIBLE CONTRACT/AGREEMENT

Mr Bolton might say the following:

- I want to explore possible options for moving to a less institutional setting.

POSSIBLE PATHS FOR OCCUPATIONAL THERAPY COACHING QUESTIONS

- What's important to you about moving to a less institutional setting?
- What information do you need?
- Who else do you want to be part of this decision/choice/process?
- What is most important to you now? How might you get that here and now?
- How do you want this last time to be? If you could tell people what you want for your death, what would that be?
- What feels unfinished for you that you want to attend to?

Adapted from Canadian Occupational Therapy Foundation (1998). Case Review #42. Pentland & Heinz, (2016). Used with permission from the publisher CAOT-ACE.

CONCLUSION

Coaching offers occupational therapists a specific mind set, methods and process of enabling occupational change with people that starts directly with a person's self-awareness and helping the person to gain clarity on what is important and gives meaning. From here people are enabled to dream big and identify, design and implement options, choices and lifestyles for themselves they may never have thought possible. The coaching approach is entirely consistent with the aims and values of occupational therapy. Its use encourages people to shift from seeing the occupational therapist as a health professional involved with prescribing, recommending and guiding change and instead empowers people to regard and believe in themselves as the agents of change. There are increasing examples of coaching being applied in occupational therapy and occupational therapists adding coaching training to their toolkits. Next steps entail building a body of literature and research evidence to increase the understanding of the effects, outcomes and further potential use of coaching in occupational therapy.

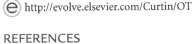 http://evolve.elsevier.com/Curtin/OT

REFERENCES

Adler Learning International (2009). *Positive change (course manual)*. Toronto: Adler International Learning.

Argyris, C., & Schon, D. (1974). *Theory in practice: Increasing professional effectiveness*. San Francisco: Jossey-Bass.

Aspinall, L. G., & Staudinger, U. M. (Eds.). (2003). *A psychology of human strengths: Fundamental questions and future directions for a positive psychology*. Washington, DC: American Psychological Association.

Bridges, W. (2004). *Transitions: Making sense of life's changes*. Cambridge, MA: DaCapo Press, Perseus Books Group.

Canadian Association of Occupational Therapists (2007). *Profile of occupational therapy practice in Canada (2007)*. Ottawa: CAOT Publications ACE.

Canadian Occupational Therapy Foundation (1998). *Case study review: Outcomes that matter*. Toronto, ON: Canadian Occupational Therapy Foundation.

Cooperrider, D. L., & Whitney, D. (1999). *Appreciative inquiry*. San Francisco: Berrett-Koehler Communications.

Cooperrider, D. L., Whitney, D., & Stavros, J. M. (2003). *Appreciative inquiry handbook*. San Francisco: Berrett-Koehler Publishers.

Cooperrider, D. L., Whitney, D., & Stavros, J. M. (2008). *Appreciative inquiry handbook* (2nd ed.). Brunswick, OH: Crown Custom Publishing.

Corbett, L. (2013). Successful aging: Jungian contributions to development in later life. *Psychological Perspectives: A Quarterly Journal of Jungian Thought, 56*(2), 149–167.

DePoy, E., & Gitlin, L. (2005). *Introduction to research: Understanding and applying multiple strategies* (3rd ed.). St. Louis: Elsevier Mosby.

Eifert, G., & Forsythe, J. (2005). *Acceptance and commitment therapy for anxiety disorders: A practitioner's treatment guide to using mindfulness, acceptance, and values-based behaviour change strategies*. Oakland, CA: New Harbinger Publications.

Emmons, R. A. (2002). Personal goals, life meaning and virtue: Wellsprings of a positive life. In C. L. M. Keyes, & J. Haidt (Eds.).

Ericksen, E., & Ericksen, J. (1997). *The life cycle completed: Extended version with new chapters in the ninth stage of development*. New York: W.W. Norton.

Frankl, V. (1984). *Man's search for meaning*. New York: Washington Square Press.

Glasser, W. (2000). *Choice theory: The new reality therapy*. New York: Harper Collins.

Hayes, S. (2005). *Get out of your mind and into your life: The new acceptance and commitment therapy*. Oakland, CA: New Harbringer Publications.

Hollis, J. (2001). *Creating a life: Finding your individual path*. Toronto: Inner City Books.

International Coach Federation (2011). *About*. Retrieved from http://www.coachfederation.org/about-icf/.

Keys, C. L. M., & Haidt, J. (Eds.). (2003). *Flourishing: Positive psychology and the life well-lived*. Washington, DC: America Psychological Association.

Kabat-Zinn, J. (2006). *Coming to our senses: Healing ourselves and the world through mindfulness*. New York: Hyperion.

Kegan, R. (1982). *The evolving self: Problem and process in human development*. Cambridge, MA: Harvard University Press.

Kegan, R. (1994). *In over our heads: The mental demands of modern life*. Cambridge, MA: Harvard University Press.

Kimsey-House, H., Kimsey-House, K., & Sandahl, P. (2011). *Co-active coaching: Changing business, transforming lives* (3rd ed.). Boston: Nicholas Brealey Publishing.

Kessler, D., & Graham, F. (2015). The use of coaching in occupational therapy: An integrative review. *Australian Occupational Therapy Journal, 62*, 160–176.

Kolb, D. A. (1984). *Experiential learning: Experience as the source of learning and development*. Englewood Cliffs, NJ: Prentice Hall.

Laske, O. (1999). An integrated model of developmental coaching. *Consulting Psychology Journal, 51*(3), 139–159.

Law, M., Cooper, B. A., Strong, S., Stewart, D., Rigby, P., & Letts, L. (1996). Person-environment-occupation model: Transactive approach to occupational performance. *Canadian Journal of Occupational Therapy, 63*(1), 9–23.

Lippmann, W. (1922). The mental age of Americans. *New Republic, 32*, 213–215.

Mezirow, J. (2000). *Learning as transformation: Critical perspectives on a theory in progress*. San Francisco: Jossey-Bass.

Pentland, W., & McColl, M. (2009). Another perspective on life balance: Living in integrity with values. In K. Matuska, & C. Christiansen (Eds.), *Life balance: Multidisciplinary theories and models* (pp. 165–180). Thorofare, NJ: Slack.

Pentland, W. (2012). Conversations for enablement: Using coaching skills in occupational therapy. *OT Now, 14*(2), 14–16.

Pentland, W. (2015). *Coaching and counselling for occupational change OT 853: Course manual*. Kingston, ON: Occupational Therapy Program, Queen's University.

Pentland, W., & Heinz (2016). What are some examples of coaching applied in occupational therapy? In W. Pentland, J. Isaacs-Young, J. Gash, & A. Heinz (Eds.), *Enabling positive change:*

coaching conversations in occupational therapy (pp. 71–88). Ottawa ON: CAOT-ACE.

Polatajko, H. J., Townsend, E. A., & Craik, J. (2007). Canadian Model of Occupational Performance and Engagement (CMOP-E). In E. A. Townsend, & H. J. Polatajko (Eds.), *Enabling occupation II: Advancing an occupational therapy vision for health, well-being, & justice through occupation (22–36).* Canadian Occupational Therapy Association: Ottawa.

Prochaska, J. O., DiClemente, C. C., & Norcross, J. C. (1992). In search of how people change: Applications to the addictive behaviours. *American Psychologist, 47,* 1102–1114.

Robson, C. (2002). *Real world research: A resource for social scientists and practitioner-researchers* (2nd ed.). Malden, MA: Blackwell.

Rogers, C. (1951). *Client-centred therapy, its current practice, implications and theory.* Boston: Houghton Mifflin.

Rogers, C. (1980). *A way of being.* Boston: Houghton Mifflin.

Ryan, R. M., & Deci, E. L. (2001). On happiness and human potential: A review of research on hedonic and eudaimonic well-being. *Annual Review of Psychology, 52,* 141–166.

Schon, D. A. (1983). *The reflective practitioner.* San Francisco: Jossey-Bass.

Segal, Z. V., Williams, J. M. G., & Teasdale, J. D. (2002). *Mindfulness-based cognitive therapy for depression: A new approach to preventing relapse.* New York: Guilford Press.

Seligman, M. E. P. (2002). *Authentic happiness: Using the new positive psychology to realize your potential for lasting fulfillment.* New York: The Free Press.

Snyder, C. R., & Lopez, S. J. (Eds.). (2002). *Handbook of positive psychology.* Oxford, UK: Oxford University Press.

Stober, D., & Grant, A. (2006). *Evidence based coaching handbook: Putting best practices to work for your clients.* Hoboken, NJ: John Wiley & Sons.

Thurman, R. (2005). *The jewel of Tibet: The enlightenment engine of Tibetan Buddhism.* New York: Free Press.

Tornstam, L. (2005). *Gerotranscendence: A developmental theory of positive aging.* New York: Springer.

Townsend, E. A., & Polatajko, H. J. (2013). *Enabling occupation II: Advancing an occupational therapy vision for health, well-being & justice through occupation* (2nd ed.). Ottawa: Canadian Occupational Therapy Association.

Vaillant, G. (2002). *Aging well.* Boston: Little, Brown & Company.

30 PSYCHOSOCIAL SUPPORT

JACQUELINE McKENNA

CHAPTER OUTLINE

Abstract
This chapter focuses on the provision of psychosocial support to individuals adjusting to illness, injury or impairment. The management of individuals with primary mental health needs is not discussed.

Adapting to capability, circumstance and environment after illness, injury or impairment is a complex and demanding task, not least in terms of emotional adjustment. To facilitate recovery using person-centred, occupation-based interventions, the occupational therapist must be mindful of psychosocial needs and the impact of these needs upon adjustment. The primacy of individual perspectives is assumed, and clearly linked to the identification of meaningful goals that accommodate changes in self, role and occupation.

A broad view of psychological functioning and adjustment is taken, acknowledging the psychosocial needs of the individual while focusing discussion on the essential nature of engagement and the development of an effective alliance that underpins the therapeutic process and specifically facilitates the provision of psychosocial support and participation in occupations. The use of communication skills and the development of collaborative relationships are specifically discussed alongside a consideration of the value of emotional intelligence in the management of emotional demand.

A brief consideration of the needs of those individuals with specific psychosocial issues is included and discussed within the context of well-being and adjustment to illness, injury or impairment. The support strategies that occupational therapists might provide are identified, and illustrative practice stories are presented.

KEY POINTS

■ The provision of psychosocial support requires a humanistic, holistic, person-centred, integrative and collaborative approach.

■ Adjustment to illness, injury or impairment requires consideration of emotional experiences and attendance to emotional well-being.

■ Acceptance of illness, injury or impairment is linked to adaptation, and adjustment is achieved by the use of a therapeutic alliance which enables coping strategies that facilitate engagement in meaningful occupations.

■ An understanding of the nature of occupation for individuals adjusting to illness, impairment or injury is essential in order to engage them in the process of occupational therapy.

■ Personal awareness and the therapeutic use of self are essential to the development of the efficacious, collaborative relationships that underpins engagement of individuals' in the process of occupational therapy.

■ An understanding and application of communication skills and related concepts underpin building of the therapeutic alliance, engagement and the achievement of the individual's goals.

■ Emotional intelligence abilities enhance self-awareness and the management of emotional demand. These skills can be developed and can positively affect both relationship development and the adjustment process.

INTRODUCTION

In considering the provision of holistic care, I recall my own experiences in a hospital-based mental health service. One referral made from the medical therapy team resulted in my sitting with a man with severe rheumatoid arthritis who had simply refused to engage, had stopped washing and cried frequently. The prospect of an adjunctive mental health issue pushed this individual outside the remit of the medical therapy team, who felt unable to commence rehabilitation until the mood disorder was addressed. Similarly an elderly woman with chronic obstructive pulmonary disease was referred because her shortness of breath was resulting in panic attacks. Again the psychological symptoms resulted in referral to a mental health service, based on a perception of more appropriate expertise. The individual was resistant to input from the mental health team, rejecting contact with 'psychiatrists', and consequently her anxiety was unmanaged. I introduce this anecdotal material not to imply criticism, but to provoke consideration of issues raised when reflecting on the application of person-centred principles within current occupational therapy roles, and asking if these management strategies focused on the whole person?

Occupational therapists are uniquely placed to facilitate a holistic approach to adjustment, having the specialist knowledge and skills required to provide both physical rehabilitation and management of psychosocial needs, supporting successful adaptation and recovery (Hannah, 2011). The essential elements of person-centred care for individuals experiencing illness, injury or impairment encompass respect and collaboration, coordinated care information and education, involvement of significant others, emotional support, and coping and working with the individual's beliefs and values to assist transition (Hammill, Bye, & Cook, 2014; Hewitt-Taylor, 2015; Pelzang, 2010). Satisfaction is clearly linked to levels of collaboration, communication and involvement of individuals in their own care (White et al., 2015).

Adjustment to the illness, injury or impairment is conceptualised as a process that is complex and continuous and is mediated by a wealth of individual and environmental factors. The therapist must acknowledge the potential effect of these factors upon each individual's psychological and emotional well-being and coping, engagement, relationship development and occupational participation (McKenna, 2007). The process of adjustment necessitates that the individual deals with emotional responses and their ramifications and requires that practitioners have greater flexibility within their physical field of practice to support application of psychosocial interventions (Jensen, Moore, Bockow, Ehdw, & Engel, 2011).

An occupational therapy service user consultation at the University of Salford (UK), identified that occupational therapists' abilities to develop effective, collaborative relationships with service users were vital (McKenna, Roberts, & Tickle, 2017). Findings suggested that communication, engagement, presence, commitment and emotion management were considered most important by service users in supporting participation in occupation-based interventions. Although service users recognised the value of applied knowledge and skills, connection and engagement outweighed any specific practice expertise (McKenna et al., 2017). Providing psychosocial support to facilitate adjustment necessitates truly holistic practice. It is imperative that this occurs within the context of an efficacious therapeutic alliance, as this is the foundation of the occupational therapy process.

Holistic Occupational Therapy Practice

The humanistic philosophy of occupational therapy necessitates the application of holistic, person-centred principles and practice. Each individual is viewed as unique and deserving of emotional connection, flexibility, personal control and actualisation (Taylor, 2008). The application of a holistic, biopsychosocial model that attends to physical, social and psychological ramifications is required in order to facilitate adaptation and adjustment (Hammill et al., 2014), and to meet the demands of the Code of Ethics and Professional Conduct (College of Occupational Therapists (COT), 2010). An empathic appreciation of the realities of living in an impaired or less able body (Coffee, Gallagher, & Desmond, 2014; Jensen et al., 2011; McKenna, 2007) will ensure that the focus of enabling strategies is determined by each individual's needs and their experience of the situation.

Psychosocial Adjustment

Adjusting to illness, injury or impairment will require time, space and support to adapt to the significant life changes occurring and their effect on occupational engagement and performance. The occupational therapist will work with individuals who are continually processing and responding to events and experiences and the effect of these upon their own lives and those of significant others. Although reactions are individualised, and are mediated by a range of biopsychosocial factors, the most common psychological sequelae include depression, anxiety, posttraumatic stress and self-image and identity issues (Hammill et al., 2014; World Health Organization, 2002). Specialist treatment may be required, and monitoring of psychosocial well-being and emerging psychosocial dysfunction is essential.

The management of psychosocial needs is imperative as ongoing adjustment issues are linked to less successful rehabilitation outcomes (Coffee et al., 2014; Sorensen et al., 2015) and increased costs in terms of long-term use of health and social care services (Cheng, Chair, & Pak-Chun Chao, 2014). The disruption of role poses a significant threat to identity, negatively affecting occupational engagement and well-being (Schier & Chan, 2007). The occupational therapist must remain cogent of the fact that an individual's emotional functioning, responses and coping skills, alongside the effectiveness of any support received, will mediate against or moderate development of psychosocial dysfunction and psychological ill health.

ENGAGEMENT AND THE THERAPEUTIC RELATIONSHIP

Engagement in this context refers to facilitation of an individual's involvement and participation in the occupational therapy process. Achieving engagement, for both the individual receiving therapy and the therapist, is essential and supports improved experience, outcomes and satisfaction (McKenna & Mellson, 2013; McKenna et al., 2017; Tickle-Degnen, 2014). Engagement is dependent on connection to an individual's priorities and needs (McKenna, 2007) and is concerned with the person's covert subjective experience (Wilcock, 2006). This is of particular relevance in the provision of psychosocial support that relies upon understanding each individual's subjective experience of any illness, injury or impairment, alongside their responses and adjustment to it.

The importance of a meaningful and collaborative relationship between the person and the therapist is fundamental to individualised, authentic and effective practice (Palmadottir, 2006; Tickle-Degnen, 2014). According to the College of Occupational Therapists (COT) (2014, p. 9) the occupational therapist must be able to 'build effective therapeutic relationships and collaborations as the foundation for occupational

therapy'. The therapeutic value of validation and acceptance is established (Tickle-Degnen, 2014), and the role of essential attitudes (caring), skills (communication) and values (professional, humanistic) in the development of a facilitative relationship that enables individuals to achieve health and well-being through occupational engagement is clear (Hewitt-Taylor, 2015; Tickle-Degnen, 2014).

To enhance and develop the collaborative relationship the therapist will apply humanistic, person-centred principles, using mutual trust, genuineness, warmth, collaboration, respect and a belief in the individual's potential for growth (Burnard, 2005; McKenna, 2007; Rogers, 2003). Schnur and Montgomery (2010) cite five elements of the therapeutic relationship: alliance, empathy, collaboration, consensus and cohesion. The value of partnership is supported by Sumsion (2006), who suggests that motivation for engagement is increased by involving the person in decision making and ensuring that the intervention is perceived as meaningful and purposeful.

The Intentional Relationship

A true collaborative alliance does not happen by chance, and simply caring is insufficient to facilitate this connection; a true collaborative alliance requires an intentional relationship. According to Taylor (2008) an intentional relationship recognises that every interaction is emotionally charged and has the potential to build or threaten the therapeutic relationship. An intentional relationship uses skills and interaction modes to develop an alliance capable of supporting efficacious occupational therapy practice. Taylor (2008) identified six interaction modes that underpin an intentional relationship: advocating (ensuring access to necessary resources), empathising (understanding the individual's experience), encouraging (positivity and encouragement), instructing (education), collaborating (application of person-centred practice) and problem solving (logical reasoning). Having awareness of these modes of interaction informs and encourages reflection and the development of the skills and knowledge that scaffold the development of a productive therapeutic alliance.

Meaningful Occupation and Mindful Practice

The concepts of meaning and purpose, passion, presence and mindfulness are inextricably linked when considering the occupational engagement of any individual. The essential nature of an understanding of meaning and purpose for the effective engagement of an individual in occupations is a key tenet of occupational therapy philosophy and practice (Polatajko, 2014; Wilcock, 2006). Meanings are subjective, unique and dynamic, mediated by individuals, their experiences and the context in which they exist (Molineux, 2010; Yerxa, 2011). An empathic understanding of the subjective reality of living with illness, injury or impairment is central to the engagement of the individual in meaningful and purposeful occupations within the process of authentic, individualised occupational therapy.

Wilcock (2006) postulated that the purpose of occupations can be aligned to a process of self-actualisation. This conceptualisation reflects the transformative potential of occupations for an individual transitioning through the adjustment process. Initially engagement in occupations would be used to exist and survive the trauma, moving on to engage in occupations that support skill development and coping, and finally using occupation to facilitate health and function by opening up possibilities and fulfilling personal potential. Adjustment requires commitment, persistence and resilience, and recognising the value of passion or a strong affinity with an activity (Mullen, Davis, & Polatajko, 2010) as a generator of meaning and purpose and a reenergiser or motivator for participation cannot be underestimated.

The value of mindful practice wherein the occupational therapist is present, active, aware and available to the individual in the present moment is well established (Reed, Hocking, & Smythe, 2011; Reid, 2009; Rogers, 2003). 'Being with' the individual facilitates connection and potentiates the value, purpose and meaning of the occupation. Relational mindfulness develops this concept, applying it specifically to interpersonal awareness within deliberate interactions, attending to warmth, acceptance, attunement and emotional intelligence (EI), which supports engagement and the development of the therapeutic relationship (Falb & Pargament, 2012; Reid, 2009). Presence is linked to mindfulness and supports true empathy and understanding, facilitating the respectful, sensitive, reflective, attuned and nonjudgemental practice that supports connection, engagement and the sharing of meaningful goals. The occupational therapist's connection with an individual will support subjective understanding of the challenges, resources and goals that emerge as the individual deals with adjustment to illness, injury or impairment. Becoming mindfully present (Reid, 2009) will help to forge a therapeutic bond, promoting relationship development, personal and affective growth and the engagement in meaningful activity that is necessary for psychosocial adjustment (McKenna et al., 2017; Weinstein, 2015).

THE THERAPEUTIC USE OF SELF AND SELF-AWARENESS

The therapeutic use of self is arguably one of the most important tools a therapist can employ (Duncan, 2006). The American Occupational Therapy Association (2008, p. 653) describes it as the 'planned use of personality, insights, perceptions and judgements'.

A solid therapeutic connection underpins the therapeutic process with mutuality and authenticity essential for both parties to be present, committed and able to coparticipate in a relationship that facilitates the application of occupational reasoning (Taylor, 2008; Tickle-Degnen, 2014). The use of unique abilities and characteristics as tools within the relationship can enable participation, enhancing outcomes and facilitating a focus on well-being and meaningful occupation (Rosa & Hasselkus, 2005; Sumsion, 2006; Weinstein, 2015). A positive,

genuine, flexible and resourceful therapist will engender the trust and motivation necessary for challenging interactions and creative problem solving.

A working alliance is more than simply a useful bond or connection and necessitates the use of self within therapy, fostering application of interactive reasoning and communication skills, facilitating connection and supporting development of shared, person-centred goals that are acted upon and linked to progress (Hammill et al., 2014; McKenna et al., 2017; Morrison & Smith, 2013). Occupational therapists may find it challenging to temper the pragmatic reasoning skills developed as problem solvers in order to listen effectively, rather than thinking about the most obvious or practical solution to the problem, and sound self-awareness is vital to the process of effective communication and consequently to the provision of psychosocial support.

The use of self is a conscious, guided and well-informed dynamic process wherein the therapist uses self-awareness, intuition, communication skills, EI, empathy and interpersonal skills to engage the individual, nurturing a meaningful, effective, person-centred affiliation (Hewitt-Taylor, 2015; McKenna & Mellson, 2013; McLeod & McLeod, 2011). Supervision should be used to deal with issues that arise, providing support, consultation, skill upgrading and opportunities for further development of personal awareness for the therapist (Burnard, 2005).

EMOTIONAL INTELLIGENCE

Evidence supports the belief that the single most important factor in superior performance and effectiveness for health care professionals is EI (Bailey, Murphey, & Porock, 2011). EI is a developed perspective in intelligence theory, drawn from Gardner's (1993) theory of multiple intelligences. The emotionally intelligent person is described as being better able to perceive, understand, integrate and use emotions, managing the emotions of self and others to promote emotional and intellectual growth (Brackett, Rivers, & Salovey, 2011; Mayer & Salovey, 1997).

The importance of an emotional connection between an individual and therapist in the process of engagement is acknowledged (Cherry, Fletcher, & O'Sullivan, 2014; McKenna et al., 2017,). EI skills mediate and manage emotional demand and support development of professional and therapeutic relationships, fostering the application of person-centred, holistic principles (McKenna, 2007). An emotionally intelligent occupational therapist understands and manages the emotions of self and others and enhances provision of psychosocial support by being warm, genuine, motivated, optimistic and persistent (Mayer & Cobb, 2000).

Development of EI abilities, including adaptability, responsiveness, creative problem solving and emotional resilience, supports psychosocial adjustment for the individual and enhances occupational therapy practice (Price, Kinghorn, Patrick, & Cardell, 2012; Reid, 2009). EI abilities facilitate creative and flexible problem framing and solving, which respects the emotional experience of self and others (Brackett et al., 2011), a key element of efficacious, individualised practice in the provision of psychosocial support. EI can be improved by using interventions that develop skills around the expression, perception, understanding, regulation and management of emotion-based material and the development of emotional resilience (Cherry, Fletcher, & O'Sullivan, 2014; Price et al., 2012).

Petrovici and Dobrescu (2014, p. 1409) describe effective communication as 'emotional intelligence in action', suggesting that the application of emotion management skills facilitates the adjustment of emotions to meet contextual demand and can significantly enhance the development of interpersonal relationships. Suhaimi, Marzuki, & Mustaffa (2014) suggest that an individual's psychological recovery from disaster-related injury experiences is supported by the use of effective communication skills and applied EI abilities. Further discussion of the application of EI within the process of psychosocial adjustment can be found later in this chapter.

APPLIED COMMUNICATION SKILLS

Communication is a dynamic, two-way process that involves the exchange of feelings, meanings and information via verbal and nonverbal methods (Burnard, 2005; McLeod & McLeod, 2011). It is affected by the experiences and perceptions, goals, reactions, responses and personal qualities of the communication participants, and the context and meaning in which the communication occurs (Hargie, 2011; McLeod & McLeod, 2011). Attending to these elements can positively affect both the interaction and the well-being of the person receiving occupational therapy services (McKenna, 2010).

Effective Communication within the Occupational Therapy Process

For the occupational therapist, effective communication is an essential tool that supports holistic practice (COT, 2010). Efficacious communication requires mastery of a range of skills and the application of essential attitudes and attributes, which when well applied will result in both the individual and the therapist experiencing responsiveness, positivity and a sense of motivation and progress toward goals. True rapport and collaboration is possible only when communication is open and honest and the therapist is charged with the responsibility of facilitating an effective interaction process. The therapist's ability to receive and interpret nonverbal and verbal information and their subsequent translation of observed behaviours to reflect a sense of an individual's thoughts and feelings is crucial for empathic understanding (Blanch-Hartigan, 2011).

Person-centred communication that is linked to emotional support and the involvement of the individual strengthens the therapeutic alliance and supports positive intervention outcomes (Pinto et al., 2012), with both parties experiencing high levels of positive connection. An individual's perception of the therapist's communication style relates directly to compliance and to health care satisfaction ratings (Pelzang, 2010; White et al., 2015). The therapist's presence and genuineness, listening and attendance skills, reading of nonverbal cues and ability to express and manage emotions within interactions are linked to the perceived efficacy of the relationship and to individual satisfaction and outcomes (McKenna et al., 2017; Tickle-Degnen, 2014).

Barriers to Communication

Illness, injury or impairment may affect a person's communication abilities. The therapist needs to be mindful of communication difficulties, ensuring time, space and skills are used for the development of the relationship and the application of functional communication strategies. For example, people who have neurological impairments may have difficulty with their concentration, nonverbal and verbal expression, fatigue and attentiveness (Lequerica, Donnell, & Tate, 2009); an elderly person recovering from surgery may have sensory deficits that can affect the recognition of nonverbal or verbal cues and their emotional connection; and an individual diagnosed with Parkinson's disease may have impeded motor-based facial expression capabilities (Tickle-Degnen, Zebrowitz, & Ma, 2011) that could result in communication misinterpretation and misjudgements, affecting connection and empathy. The individual may not be able to contribute equally to the development of rapport (Rosa & Hasselkus, 2005), and a coalition may be difficult to achieve. The therapist must be mindful of the potential for reduced collaboration, applying the skills necessary to support the alliance essential for relationship development and engagement (Palmadottir, 2006).

To be effective, an understanding of the impact of assumptions, beliefs, values and standards, skills, weaknesses and idiosyncrasies is necessary (Burnard, 2005; McLeod & McLeod, 2011). A person might challenge or contradict the therapist's world view or values, making relationship development more challenging. Developing self-awareness enhances insight and ensures management of any potential issues.

Sociocultural factors might affect communication and alliance development (culture, gender, race, religion, beliefs, values, experiences and environment), and the therapist must be aware of these factors and their context within the experience of the individual. For example, acceptable levels of emotional expression may be culturally driven and may influence what the person is willing or able to discuss with the therapist; likewise an individual's experience of pain may be linked to cultural expectations and norms.

Therapists need to be aware of their own assumptions and the needs of individuals, as these may affect the perception of the individual's narratives and the development of empathy and rapport (Tickle-Degnen et al., 2011). Although an individual's background should be acknowledged, therapists must not make assumptions. The relative importance of specific cultural knowledge versus adaptable communication expertise and personal awareness has been discussed by Burnard (2005), who suggests that misinterpretation occurs primarily because of assumptions of similarity, rather than problems communicating across different cultural orientations. The masterful use of a range of interpersonal skills will support trust development and ensure therapists' credibility in the eyes of the people receiving their services, facilitating communication across and through sociocultural differences.

Outcomes of Applied Communication Skills

The skills used by the occupational therapist working to support adjustment to illness, injury or impairment will have a communication focus and necessitate the ability to elicit personal experiences personal narratives. It is vital to facilitate the expression of feelings so that the transition to living with reduced or altered ability can occur. The provision of psychosocial support requires the use of open and honest communication to assist the individual with exploration of feelings, experiences, symptoms, expectations, goals and anxieties, supporting provision of the person-centred psychosocial support necessary. Providing a platform for communication and coalition empowers the individual to take an active role in therapy, facilitating negotiation of occupational goals and enabling both the individual and the process of therapy.

Factors that contribute to the application of effective communication skills in the context of the provision of psychosocial support are listed in Table 30.1.

Specific Skills for Effective Communication

The occupational therapist uses a range of communication skills to establish and maintain effective working relationships, establishing a platform that scaffolds provision of psychosocial support. The skills employed include environment-creating skills, relationship-building skills and advanced communication skills.

Environment-creating Skills

Occupational therapists communicate with individuals in all kinds of contexts. In an ideal world meeting an individual to discuss personal matters would take place in a private, neutral, safe, comfortable environment without distraction and interruption. In reality, interactions happen wherever they arise, planned and unplanned, triggered by questions, anxieties and responses both during and outside scheduled activities. The therapist is responsible for making the environment conducive to interaction and relationship-building skills, including management of the environment (COT, 2010).

Relationship-building Skills

To engage a person in a therapeutic alliance within which meaningful interventions can be negotiated and implemented, the occupational therapist needs to establish an understanding of

TABLE 30.1
Factors that Contribute to the Application of Effective Communication Skills in the Context of the Provision of Psychosocial Support

- Establishing a connection
- Building a relationship
- Demonstrating presence
- Exploring and understanding meaning, having meaningful interactions
- Engaging
- Exploring the individual's perspectives and experiences
- Facilitating engagement
- Validating
- Accepting
- Establishing available resources
- Motivating
- Sharing experiences
- Enabling individuals to share symptomatology and the impact of their illness, injury or impairment
- Discussing symptoms of illness, injury or impairment, including fatigue and pain
- Discussing reactions to illness, injury or impairment
- Facilitating clear expression of emotions

- Exploring social and relationship issues
- Expressing self-image perceptions
- Exploring cognitive appraisals
- Using interactive and narrative reasoning
- Conducting assessments
- Identifying and clarifying needs, wants, goals and motivators
- Collaborating on goal setting and decision making
- Prioritising actions, strategies and interventions
- Involving significant others
- Accessing, expressing, responding to, exploring and handling emotion
- Monitoring emotional functioning
- Providing support
- Providing information and education
- Reflecting and offering feedback on progress against goals

each individual and his or her personal experiences, meanings and perspectives (McKenna et al., 2017; McLeod & McLeod, 2011; Rogers, 2003). Rogers (2003) identified the core requirements necessary for the building of relationships: trust, respect, unconditional positive regard, empathic understanding and genuineness and warmth.

Trust is essential for an efficacious relationship and is contingent upon an individual being engaged enough to believe not only in the shared vision and its associated goals but also in the capabilities of the therapist. Building trust requires commitment, presence, respect, congruence, genuineness and honesty from both parties, as boundaries are explored and safety within the relationship is established (Hargie, 2011; McKenna et al., 2017). The relationship is authentic and productive for both the individual and the therapist and supports establishment of meaningful occupational goals (Burnard, 2005; McKenna et al., 2017; McLeod & McLeod, 2011).

Unconditional positive regard presumes a nonjudgemental attitude and is a powerful tenet of any therapeutic partnership. Respect is demonstrated alongside a belief that the individual is of value and has potential for growth and change (Burnard, 2005; McLeod & McLeod, 2011; Rogers, 1951). The individual can freely express his or her reactions to and experiences of illness, injury or impairment, without risk of judgement (McLeod & McLeod, 2011), fostering acceptance of and respect for the individual's unique subjective experience and supporting empathic understanding.

Unconditional positive regard and trust may be challenged if individuals behave in a way that therapists struggle to accept, if their values contradict those held by the therapists or if individuals lack expressive warmth (McLeod & McLeod, 2011; Thompson, 2015). The provision of committed and compassionate care for every individual makes significant emotional demands upon therapists, and the capacity of therapists for true empathy cannot be presumed (McKenna et al., 2017; Thompson, 2015; Tickle-Degnen, 2014). EI abilities can be useful in the management of emotional labour, protecting against stress, supporting flexible selection of coping strategies and thereby facilitating health and enhancing professional performance (Davis & Humphrey, 2012; Landa, Lopez-Zafra, Martos, & Aguilar-Luzon, 2008; McKenna & Mellson, 2013).

An empathic relationship fosters mutual trust and confidence and facilitates connection, fellowship and coalition (Burnard, 2005; Palmadottir, 2006). Empathy reflects an accurate perception of an individual's feelings and is developed by exploring, without judgement, the individual's world, using listening and attending skills to illuminate the subjective, lived experience of the individual and the effect of illness, injury or impairment. Responding to both explicit information and implicit cues facilitates development of relationships that deliver sensitive and caring management of emotional material and that empower, energise and engage the person (McKenna et al., 2017; Tickle-Degnen, 2014).

Genuineness requires honesty, approachability and openness (Burnard, 2005). Therapists cannot pretend to be interested; they must actually be interested, present and committed to involvement. This necessitates a willingness to be warm and nondefensive, using self-awareness, consistency, courage and a sharing of self to support connection and relationship development. Yerxa (2011) discussed the links between genuineness, warmth and mutuality and the value of an authentic relationship.

An authentic and genuine connection fosters partnership with the occupational therapist as the provider of rehabilitation and improves engagement with the health care system (Hewitt-Taylor, 2015; Palmadottir, 2006; Tickle-Degnen, 2014). Although a balance of power is difficult to achieve within the paternalistic, safety-focused and resource-constrained structure of most rehabilitation services (Burnard, 2005; McLeod & McLeod, 2011), achieving a true coalition will redress, to some extent, this power differential by working in partnership with the individual.

Advanced Communication Skills: Questioning, Listening and Working Through

Communication skills are divided into nonverbal (facial expression, eye contact, posture, gesture, touch) and verbal skills. Advanced communication skills are divided into listening, questioning and working through or exploring (Burnard, 2005; McKenna, 2010; McLeod & McLeod, 2011). A range of advanced communication skills drawn broadly from a Rogerian model of person-centred therapy are presented in Table 30.2 (Rogers, 1951, 2003), along with applied examples and their purpose within the context of illness, injury or impairment.

TABLE 30.2
Advanced Communication Skills

Skill	Definition (D), Applied Examples (AE) and Functional Purpose (FP) of Communication for Therapist and the Individual
Observation skills	**D:** Observation of people in terms of their presentation and verbal and nonverbal behaviour. Perceiving nonverbal cues and reactions can be indicators of mood, emotions and responses to therapist and content of discussion that may not be verbally articulated — posture, eye contact, gestures and facial expression. Be aware of incongruence, discomfort and patterns. Remember the individual might be in pain. **FP:** Information gathering, noting symptoms in evidence; congruence is checked.
Active listening skills	**D:** Using nonverbal skills, including body posture, facial expression, eye contact and gestures, to demonstrate that the therapist is listening. Drawing out skills will maintain the flow, offer encouragement to the individual to talk — nodding, smiling, and using eye contact and facial expression to convey interest. Problem identification necessitates attendance and responding to the individual's nonverbal communication during assessment. **AE:** *'Tell me more about the pain you are in; go on, uh hmm, ok'.* **FP:** Asking relevant questions, paraphrasing information, summarising information. Engagement commences, begin trust building, relationship building, accurate information pickup, sense making and understanding, empathy development and conveyance.

Continued on following page

	TABLE 30.2
	Advanced Communication Skills *(Continued)*

Skill	Definition (D), Applied Examples (AE) and Functional Purpose (FP) of Communication for Therapist and the Individual
Questioning skills	
Closed questions	**D:** Questions that will elicit a specific response used to check or clarify information, gain factual information are useful during interviews and assessments. Control of response is with the interviewer. **AE:** *'Did you come by bus today?'* *'Do you understand what the doctor told you?'* *'So who else knows about how bad the pain is?'* *'You say you don't like to be alone at night; is that why you live with your sister?'*
Open questions	**D:** Questions designed to help the individual explore, expand and explain – 'Who, Where, Why, What, How' questions, that encourage the expression of feelings. The control of the response is with the person receiving occupational therapy services. Can be broad or focused. **AE:** Broad: *'So what brings you to occupational therapy today?'* *'Tell me about your previous experiences with an occupational therapist?'* *'How does your fatigue affect you day to day?'* **AE:** Focused: *'So why did you refuse to let the occupational therapist into your house?'* *'How did you feel when the doctor gave you the diagnosis?'* *'What did you understand from the letter I sent you?'* *'Tell me what bothers you most about your restricted movement?'* *'When did you realise that you couldn't carry on with that job?'* **FP (for both closed and open questions):** Information is gathered and exchanged, clarifying symptoms, emotions, reactions and their impact; continue to build trust and relationship; encourage disclosure, sharing and intimacy, caring, commitment, connection and engagement. Explore occupational functioning and participation.
Working through/Exploring/Clarifying skills	
Reflection	**D:** Focusing on feelings, trying to identify feelings the person has and asking about this in a way that lets the person confirm or reject the therapist's suggestion, which is drawn from conversation so far (Rogers, 2003). **AE:** *'Would I be right in thinking you are very frustrated by this situation?'* *'It sounds to me like you felt humiliated by the lack of privacy?'* *'I'm wondering if you're feeling confused and overwhelmed by all the information about the Parkinson's disease.'* **FP:** Emotions explored and shared, experiences and emotions responded to, empathy demonstrated and information checked. Beliefs and values explored, experiences explored further, trust and relationship developed. Individual experiences sensitivity, caring and commitment, which deepens the connection. Individual makes sense of information.
Paraphrasing	**D:** Mini summary, question or comment that uses the person's own words to show active listening. **AE:** Person: *'Last night I had a lot of pain again, and I feel very angry because the medication didn't help me.'* Occupational therapist: *'So you are very angry because the medication didn't help your pain last night?'* *'You are very angry because the medication isn't working?'* **FP:** Listening is demonstrated, pushing the conversation forward, more information gathered, and empathy deepened. Detail and focus are checked. Individual experiences being listened to, being valued and contributing to connection and conversation.
Summarising	**D:** Useful to recap, gather and summarise information, pull material together so that both parties are clear. Used during conversations when there is a change of theme or large amounts of information have been presented, to capture what happened previously, at end of conversations and to close. Summary should be presented back to the individual so the individual can agree or amend information. **AE:** *'So we have discussed having to ask for help to use the toilet since you had the stroke, and how difficult you are finding this. You feel frustrated by your inability to do this for yourself but can't bring yourself to ask your husband to help as you feel scared he'll refuse, and you cannot see a way forward. Have I understood that right? Shall we start next time by focusing on talking to your husband about what is happening?'*

Continued on following page

	TABLE 30.2
	Advanced Communication Skills *(Continued)*
Skill	**Definition (D), Applied Examples (AE) and Functional Purpose (FP) of Communication for Therapist and the Individual**
	FP: Information is clarified and pulled together, preferences are clarified, understanding is clear for both parties. Trust and respect continue to build, partnership develops, starting points for problem solving and future directions emerge, and decisions take shape and are discussed and collaborated upon.
Concreteness	**D:** Asking for examples to make sure both the therapist and the individual are clear about what the individual is saying.
	AE: Person: *'I always feel like I do it wrong when I try to explain to my kids what is going to happen to me – they get really upset'* Occupational therapist: *'Give me an example of the last time you felt like you explained your illness and it went wrong'.* *'Explain to me what happened the last time you tried to explain to your kids about your cancer and it felt like you did it wrong'.* The therapist can also use concreteness to ensure dialogue is clear and unambiguous.
	FP: Information, experiences and reactions are made very clear, specific situations are explored, emotions are unpacked and understood, cognitive appraisals explored; uncertainties and new questions are raised, more information is provided. Relationship, engagement and collaborative partnership continue to develop.
Clarifying	**D:** Checking understanding of what the individual is saying (Burnard, 2005).
	AE: *'What do you mean when you say you are at the end of your tether with the pain in your hands?'* *'Can you help me understand what you mean when you say you just can't get over this injury to your back?'*
	FP: Meanings are individual and relative to each person. The therapist should not assume what the individual means. Use the person's words, stay within the person's frame of reference and meaning. The therapist can also ask if the person has felt like this before; this may help understanding of the feelings, clarify them and revisit how and why the feeling occurs. Meaning and understanding are the focus; clarity is essential to support goal development. The individual's role in goals and actions is made clear and used, supporting self-efficacy beliefs. Emotion management and emotional intelligence abilities are used. Trust and connection deepen further as deeper feelings are shared and explored and the individual experiences commitment and sensitivity.
Focusing	**D:** Helps the individual to focus on one issue or to identify which is the most pressing issue at present (Rogers, 1951, 2003).
	AE: *'So you say your husband's attitude, your level of pain and the medication you are on are all getting you down – which of those is getting you down the most?'* *'I understand that your nausea and the tiredness are really bothering you and your husband's fussing is not helpful, and it is important we talk about all of these issues. Here and now, though, today, which of these do you feel it is important to discuss first?'*
	FP: Individual has control of the agenda; trust and respect are enhanced and deepened. Values and beliefs are explored further, priorities are clarified, further information is gathered and given, exploration of emotional material and its management continue. Concordant goals and plans continue to take shape; self-management is enabled.
Confrontation	**D:** Can be used to suggest that something is being denied or an issue is being avoided, patterns of behaviour are occurring or there is incongruence (Rogers, 2003) – perhaps changing the subject, being evasive, avoiding answering questions. The pattern is pointed out or challenged.
	AE: *'You say you are OK, that you are relaxed, but I have noticed you are gripping the chair'.* *'When I ask you about using the wheelchair, you seem to change the subject'.* *'When we meet, you appear unwilling to talk about how angry you are about the way you were given this news'.* *'Every week you wait to discuss your feelings about your heart attack until we are almost out of time'.*
	FP: Avoidance is challenged, patterns are highlighted, therapist demonstrates commitment to problem solving and dealing with difficult emotional material. Connection and trust are strengthened and decision making and self-efficacy supported.
Handling silence	**D:** Allowing time to think can be useful for both parties (Burnard, 2005). Useful during interview when the individual has been asked a potentially difficult question, or if the therapist is delivering bad news. Silence can be very constructive; the individual could be making sense of thoughts and feelings, struggling to manage emotions, considering how much to tell the therapist or be unsure of how to answer the question. Be aware of the purpose of silences, the therapist must not let his or her own discomfort lead to filling the gaps or rushing in with another question. Genuineness is vital. If there is a long silence, the therapist can ask the individual what is going on.

Continued on following page

TABLE 30.2
Advanced Communication Skills (Continued)

Skill	Definition (D), Applied Examples (AE) and Functional Purpose (FP) of Communication for Therapist and the Individual
	AE: 'There has been a long silence, what are you thinking about?' 'Do you need time to think?' 'Do you feel able to pick up where we left off?' Silences can also provide time for the therapist to gather thoughts, check emotions, mentally recap and plan how to continue the interaction. **FP:** Respect and trust are enhanced, connection is deepened. Sharing of deep emotional material is encouraged and the individual's pace is accommodated, supporting disclosure of difficult experiences, reactions and emotions. Time and space are offered, validating and accepting the individual and empowering self-management.
Handling strong emotion	**D:** Self-awareness and reflection help the therapist handle his or her own emotions (Burnard, 2005). Use of emotional intelligence (EI) principles and abilities is required. All skills listed can be used here. Use appropriate nonverbal behaviour—therapist needs to be cautious with the use of touch, use touch for support if both parties are comfortable with it and it is culturally appropriate. Discomfort for either party will be obvious. Do not ignore the emotion; it is likely to be very important. Allow time, space and control. **AE:** 'Are you ok, do you want to carry on? 'You are obviously very angry/frightened about this information; are you able to talk to me about this diagnosis'. When breaking bad news, it can be useful to use a sandwich approach — prepare the individual, deliver the news, offer support. 'So as we discussed with the doctor this morning [...]; what has happened is serious [...]'. 'You have had a stroke. It is very unlikely that the damage this has caused to the sight in your left eye can be corrected [...].' 'This is very difficult [...]; it's a lot to take in [...]. It must be frightening/shocking [...]. I can try to help you get any information you need and will try to answer any questions you might have [...]. We can spend some time talking about how you feel and what you are most concerned about [...]'. **FP:** Time and space given to deal with emotionally charged material; this will be a constant feature of any adjustment process as the individual tries to make sense of the implications, experience or impact of his or her illness or injury. EI abilities are useful; connection and empathy are deepened and disclosure continues. The individual's pace is validated and expression is accepted using unconditional regard, confirming respect and trust.
Giving permission	**D:** Sometimes individuals struggle to express certain emotions or consider them to be unacceptable or embarrassing. Giving permission can be very powerful in assisting with emotional expression (Rogers, 1951, 2003). **AE:** 'It is ok to be upset and cry — this is a very difficult situation; coping with this news is very difficult, isn't it?' 'If you are angry about how your sister has responded to your illness, that is OK. Do you want to talk about it?' 'Tell me more about that feeling — maybe let it out'. 'It's normal to feel overwhelmed and frightened about the treatment choices you have been presented with; it's OK to feel like this'. Giving permission may elicit strong emotion. **FP:** Strong emotions are elicited and expressed. Genuineness is required and mutual respect and connection is enhanced as highly emotional material is expressed. Further information is gathered; insights into values and beliefs are generated. Trust, commitment, acceptance, presence and partnership are experienced, enhancing the relationship.
Immediacy	**D:** Focusing on the here and now (Burnard, 2005) is useful for any individual who finds it hard to express emotion or is stuck. Step out of the content of the conversation and ask: **AE:** 'How are you feeling right now, right this minute?' 'What are you thinking about right now?' **FP:** Creative problem solving, persistence and commitment are evident as the therapist looks for alternative ways to deal with information and issues. Motivation and reenergisation are sported by a change in tack or a switch of focus.

Definitions and skills have been informed by the evidence base and applied examples generated by the author.

PSYCHOSOCIAL SUPPORT AND ADJUSTMENT

The acceptance of the impact of illness, injury or impairment is recognised as an adaptive outcome for the adjustment process (Telford, Kralik, & Koch, 2006). Occupational therapists play a key role in facilitating adjustment by using enabling strategies and being mindful of the context of adjustment in terms of each individual's roles, values, meanings and beliefs, the realities of their limitations, and the social attitudes and reactions they experience (Hannah, 2011; Schier & Chan, 2007). Although the understanding and management of the emotions of self and others are essential for successful adaptation and adjustment to illness, injury or impairment, giving prominence to an emotional agenda challenges the outcome-driven, resource-focused reality of occupational therapy service provision (Ciechanowski & Katon, 2006; Jensen et al., 2011; Tickle-Degnen, 2014).

Strategies that manage both anticipatory and experienced distress and emotional responses draw broadly on cognitive behavioural, behavioural and psychodynamic techniques, including the following: exposure, cognitive restructuring and reframing, adaptive skills training, EI training, stress management, anger management, education, problem-solving and self-esteem and self-efficacy development (Cheng et al., 2014; Hannah, 2011; McKenna, 2007; Sorensen et al., 2015). These strategies are used in conjunction with occupation-based interventions and the use of meaningful activities focused on occupational functioning.

Interventions focused on development of cognitive and emotional strengthening and resilience, wellness, creative, expressive and healing arts, and transition management have been effective working with people who have a traumatic brain injury (Foote & Schwartz, 2012). The efficacy of group education and support that facilitate adjustment through the sharing of feelings, information and solutions is also well established (Cheng et al., 2014; Schreuer et al., 2006; Telford et al., 2006). The occupational therapist can also facilitate emotional resiliency by using personal narratives to explore individuals' journeys and their finding of meaning in their future identity, 'helping their clients to transcend the trauma' (Price et al., 2012, p. 111).

Emotional Intelligence, Coping and Adjustment

Negative affective experiences, including anger, fear, anxiety, frustration, uncertainty, confusion, despondency, despair and low mood, are noted as prevalent reactions to illness, injury or impairment, and individuals may oscillate between premorbid and postmorbid identities (Hannah, 2011; Sorensen et al., 2015; Telford et al., 2006). According to Schreuer et al. (2006, p. 201), 'severe physical disability is a long term stressor' which affects therapeutic engagement and adjustment. McKenna

(2007, p. 551) suggests that the experience of negative emotional responses is one of the most common responses to illness, injury or impairment and that this is 'linked to poor psychosocial adaptation and disability related stress'. Denial of illness, injury or impairment is linked to poor psychosocial adjustment, poor management and reported mental health problems (Sorensen et al., 2015), whereas acceptance and the identification of realistic goals aid adjustment and support engagement (Coffee et al., 2014; McKenna, 2007; Telford et al., 2006).

The individual's lived experience, cognitive appraisals and emotional responses are significant elements of the adjustment process, and the individual's resilience and self-management will mediate the challenges of living with the reality of a new identity, influencing rehabilitation outcomes (Price et al., 2012; Schreuer et al., 2006). Although coping styles vary, empirical evidence suggests that optimism and tempered emotional responses support resilience and adaptation, protecting against mental health problems and assisting the individual in adjusting to a new post illness, injury or impairment identity and related capabilities (Ciechanowski & Katon, 2006; McKenna, 2007; Price et al., 2012; Telford et al., 2006).

Within the occupational therapy process, emotion management and resilience support self-expression and expression of wants and needs, commitment to goals, self-efficacy, promotion of trust and engagement, reduction of frustration, promotion of health and resilience as well as protecting against psychological dysfunction, assisting with management of stress and anger, coping with the difficult situations likely to be encountered in the adjustment process, identity transition, and maintaining occupational functioning. Occupational therapists have the opportunity to identify and develop the EI abilities that support resilience and adjustment. Goleman (2006) claims that EI abilities can be developed and that competence enables resilience, survival, and self-protection alongside use of key emotional skills that include the following:

- Self-awareness and analysis
- Working in groups
- Identifying, expressing and managing feelings
- Impulse control
- Delaying gratification
- Handling stress and anxiety
- Negotiating solutions, goal setting and creative problem solving

The development of EI capabilities has significant potential to support individuals dealing with the psychosocial challenges of adjustment to illness, injury or impairment. Emotional resilience, self-management and adaptive coping can be supported by development of EI abilities (Price et al., 2012; Suhaimi, Marzuki, & Mustaffa, 2014). EI abilities can be facilitated both within a collaborative relationship and by engagement in specifically selected enabling strategies and activities (Cherry et al., 2014; McKenna, 2007; Price et al., 2012).

Examples of occupational therapy strategies used to develop EI abilities include the following:

- Communication skills, questioning skills, assertiveness
- Emotion identification, understanding and expression
- Empathy development, understanding and communicating feelings of self and others (discussing impact of diagnosis and reactions, understanding reactions of significant others)
- Role play and rehearsal of key conversations (e.g. giving family information about the diagnosis, explaining health needs to an employer)
- Self-esteem and self-efficacy building (problem solving, empowerment control and shared decision making
- Coping skills and techniques (emotion recognition, expression, priorities and meanings, activity for mood management, relaxation and stress management skills, emotional detachment and distraction techniques, energy redirection strategies, reframing)
- Self-monitoring and management – using narratives, diary keeping and review
- Group discussion, group working for education, sharing communication, problem solving and support
- Creative activity for expression, awareness, distraction and diversion

EI skills facilitate adaptive problem solving, helping to frame problems and use creativity and flexibility in solution finding (McKenna & Mellson, 2013), enhancing both the therapeutic outcomes and adjustment to illness, injury or impairment (McKenna, 2007; Telford et al., 2006).

Occupational Therapy for Psychosocial Support: An Overview

A broad overview of the occupational therapy strategies for psychosocial support can be found in Table 30.3. Some of these strategies clearly link or extend the communication activities outlined in Table 30.1, as these are inextricably linked within the process of relationship development, psychosocial support and the occupational therapy process.

Coping, functioning and emotional self-regulation are supported by personal choice and control, a sense of positivity, meaning and purpose and a clear focus on goal facilitation and problem resolution (Coffee et al., 2014; McKenna, 2007; Price et al., 2012). Person-centred interaction in the provision of emotional support facilitates involvement of the individual, fostering collaboration and enhancing the therapeutic alliance. Applying the principles of person-centred occupational therapy with a focus on the uniqueness of the individual experience will preserve the individual's autonomy, value, choice and commitment and will facilitate the self-efficacy, empowerment, resilience and perceived control necessary to support psychosocial adjustment (Hammill et al., 2014; Pelzang, 2010; Price et al., 2012).

TABLE 30.3

Occupational Therapy Strategies for Psychosocial Support and Well-being

- Engage the individual in an effective therapeutic alliance which maintains participation, motivation, involvement and autonomy
- Conduct assessments
- Collaborate to identify and clarify needs, wants, goals, priorities, motivators, actions, strategies and interventions
- Discuss emotional reactions to illness, injury or impairment
- Explore self-image
- Discuss symptoms of illness, injury or impairment including fatigue and pain
- Explore social and relationship issues
- Explore role and identity issues
- Access, express, respond to, explore and handle emotion
- Develop emotional intelligence abilities including self-/emotional expression and emotion management
- Explore and reframe cognitive appraisal
- Support acquisition of cognitive behavioural coping strategies and skills
- Support acquisition of stress and anger management skills
- Support acquisition of assertiveness skills
- Enable self-management strategies
- Support development of self-esteem through empowerment and involvement
- Provide information and psychoeducation
- Facilitate adaptive problem solving
- Enable participation in purposeful, meaningful occupations
- Support adjustment to physical dysfunction
- Monitor emotional health and mental health status

APPLICATION USING PRACTICE STORY

Practice Story 30.1 focuses on Claude, who had a neurological diagnosis and with a perceived significant change in personal identity, affecting role fulfilment and occupational participation, Claude's adjustment to his impairment using specific enabling strategies (EI training and cognitive behavioural intervention) to manage anxiety and emotional distress and promote occupational participation, is presented in this story.

CONCLUSION

Occupational therapists consider the physical, psychological and social elements of the individual and provide interventions that rely upon the use of a range of skills to enable the individual to overcome or adapt to injury or impairment. The provision of integrated, holistic, therapeutic interventions that meet psychosocial need enables adjustment, occupational functioning and

PRACTICE STORY 30.1

Claude

Claude was 32 years old, married, had two children (7 and 4 years old), and lived in a bungalow with his family. He was diagnosed with relapsing-remitting nonprogressive multiple sclerosis (MS) 4 years ago and had three exacerbations since then, the most severe of which necessitated that he use a wheelchair for 2 months.

Claude was admitted to a hospital ward after an exacerbation that had resulted in blurred vision in his right eye, bilateral dysesthesia, fatigue and reduced fine motor coordination. The referral read: '*OT assessment. Plus panic attacks, low mood – not coping'*.

Although Claude's presenting physical impairments were clear, his adjustment, emotional well-being, occupational roles, environment and social circumstances needed to be explored by the therapist. Jack, an occupational therapist, saw Claude on the ward.

ESTABLISHING TRUST

Claude initially refused to engage in any assessment, stating he was exhausted from lack of sleep. He was hostile and suspicious, accusing staff of keeping information from him. Jack used **clarification** and **immediacy** to explore what Claude meant when he talked about people keeping things from him and what thoughts he had 'right now'. Claude stated that he was concerned that he had been misdiagnosed and that he had a progressive form of MS and would not recover the neurological abilities currently compromised. Although medical evidence could have been used to challenge his perspective, Jack resisted the temptation to adopt an instructing mode of interaction (Taylor, 2008) to present information, instead demonstrating **respect** for the individual and his unique subjective experience, focusing on emotional expression and allowing fears and feelings vital time and space. A range of communication skills (**questioning, reflection, concreteness, clarification and confrontation**) were used to draw out the conversation, acknowledge Claude's fear, anger and frustration, and establish that he felt angry and resentful that he had this disease and that he was fearful of it becoming worse. EI abilities were used to recognise the emotionally charged material and manage the fear and hostility expressed with genuineness.

Focusing was used to identify that Claude was bothered most by the 'panics' he had been having; he reported feeling 'ashamed' that he could not control them. Claude's feelings were explored using **open questions, clarification, focusing,** and **reflection** and validated as real and important, establishing a connection, **empathy** and **nonjudgemental respect** (Rogers, 2003). **Concreteness** was used to explore situations when Claude had a panic attack and to clarify that he suspected that some panic symptoms related to his perception that his MS was worsening.

When asked about his family and his roles, Claude became tearful. Jack used **silence** to allow time and space for emotional expression, and Claude stated that he felt like a 'burden'. Occupations and roles were discussed, and the meaning and purpose of his roles as a freelance music teacher and carer to his two children were established. He described playing the guitar as a 'passion' and the thing he used to be good at, stating that it now felt 'pointless'. The therapist explored Claude's self-image, using **clarification, summarising, reflection, focusing** and **silence** to elicit feelings around his pre- and postimpairment self, the advancing and remitting nature of his condition and the importance of having a purpose to his well-being. The therapist recognised the effect this impairment was having upon his self-image and esteem, using **reflection, concreteness, confrontation** and **focusing** to explore feelings and identify priorities. EI was used to identify emotions, explore them and handle the high levels of emotion in a calm and measured way, expressing **empathy, genuineness** and **respect.**

Jack used some emotion identification and sharing exercises to begin building EI abilities and facilitate expression, exploration and understanding of feelings, supporting resilience. Claude identified feeling unable to discuss feelings with his wife, anticipating her distress. **Clarification** and **reflection** were used to explore anticipatory distress, and personal narratives explored his perspective, establishing that his real fear was facing his own and his wife's 'true' feelings.

The occupational therapist was aware of problems associated with MS in terms of fear of symptoms, reduced function, fatigue, relationship disruption and role strain, and their impact on adjustment. Professional reasoning skills were used to establish priorities and recognise the immediate need to address emotional resilience and anxiety, which was affecting all areas of occupational function. Claude had already identified the 'panics' as the most important problem, and the goal of addressing this issue was established collaboratively, motivating Claude and supporting the alliance and the meaning and purpose of interventions.

INTERVENTION TECHNIQUES

Problems were conceptualised and therapeutic goals were negotiated, following person-centred practice guidelines, to facilitate engagement and empowerment.

- Claude was offered a short, focused anxiety management programme using cognitive behavioural principles and strategies to assess and manage the behavioural and emotional components of his anxiety quickly and to begin cognitive appraisal and reframing to link thoughts, feelings and behaviours. Claude monitored his stress via diary keeping and managed physical symptoms using relaxation and breathing techniques. These interventions enabled acquisition of self-management

PRACTICE STORY 30.1

Claude (Continued)

skills, facilitated engagement in occupations and supported self-efficacy and esteem.

- EI training enabled Claude to develop skills in identifying, expressing and managing feelings; communication of emotion; goal setting; impulse control; assertiveness; handling stress; and development of self-protection, resilience and awareness.
- Selected activities, including music appreciation and music-related leisure activities with the family, were included in the occupational therapy programme to provide opportunity to reconnect with an occupation he had been passionate about and engage in occupations with meaning for leisure and enjoyment without the pressure of performance or product, supporting success and building confidence.
- A psychoeducation support group enabled Claude to gather information, develop confidence, planning and problem-solving skills, and share experiences with others outside his family, opportunities for honesty and self-expression, increasing flexibility and adaptation.
- Occupations related to purposeful role performance were encouraged while applying principles of self- and fatigue management; these included self-care and personal care of the children, planning and preparing simple meals and working with his children on their homework.

SUMMARY

- Applied advanced communication skills were used to build a trusting therapeutic relationship and enable a collaborative alliance that supported engagement.

- Psychosocial support was offered and specific issues addressed. Management of anxiety and emotions was prioritised to address acute emotional needs and facilitate assessment and engagement processes.
- Claude's engagement in the meaningful occupations that defined his key roles as husband, father, musician and worker were also being negatively affected by emotional issues, and so establishing a connection that would facilitate engagement and build resilience was prioritised.
- Claude was able to develop EI abilities, coping strategies and resilience to manage emotional issues.
- He engaged in support groups to facilitate education related to the condition, increasing his confidence, problem-solving skills and self-efficacious management of health.
- Enabling engagement in meaningful activities with the family (music, creative art), which had spiritual significance in terms of his sense of self, was crucial in maintaining self-esteem and meaning and occupational function.
- Meaningful occupation is viewed as a major mediator of adjustment to impairment and the restoration of health through the use of purposeful activity, and meaningful occupation remained central to the occupational therapy goals. The reestablishment of occupational function and roles within the family enhanced psychosocial well-being and facilitated adjustment and recovery.

---

well-being. The development of therapeutic relationships scaffold engagement in the occupational therapy process, and communication skills are used as a therapeutic tool that enables interaction within a therapeutic relationship, while supporting meaningful activity or occupation (Burnard, 2005; McLeod & McLeod, 2011; Whitcher & Tse, 2004).

Encouraging the participation of an anxious person in a group activity to better manage postsurgical pain, achieving a reliable kitchen assessment with a distressed and tearful person overwhelmed by a recent diagnosis of cancer, providing information relating to disease prognosis in a form that the person is able and willing to understand after a first exacerbation of multiple sclerosis, motivating a reluctant person to attend for splint refitting because of deteriorating rheumatoid arthritis, and securing access to the home of a person recently diagnosed with diabetes in order to complete a risk assessment are all more likely if appropriate skills are used effectively to connect with and engage the person in the occupational therapy process.

The skilled therapist will invest time in the application of these skills, aiming for masterful communication that facilitates authentic connections to support both the individual and the therapeutic process. The focus of therapy will be enabled and the individual will be engaged in meaningful and efficacious occupational therapy treatment.

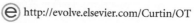 http://evolve.elsevier.com/Curtin/OT

REFERENCES

American Occupational Therapy Association (2008). Occupational therapy practice framework: Domain and process. *American Journal of Occupational Therapy, 62,* 625–683.

Bailey, C., Murphey, R., & Porock, D. (2011). Professional tears: Developing emotional intelligence around death and dying in emergency work. *Journal of Clinical Learning, 20,* 33–72.

Blanch-Hartigan, D. (2011). Measuring providers' verbal and non-verbal emotion recognition ability: Reliability and validity of the PECT. *Patient Education and Counselling, 82,* 370–376.

Brackett, M., Rivers, S., & Salovey, P. (2011). Emotional intelligence: Implications for personal, social and workplace success. *Social and Personal Psychology Compass, 5*(1), 88–103.

Burnard, P. (2005). *Counselling skills for health professionals* (4th ed.). Cheltenham, UK: Nelson Thornes Ltd.

Cheng, H. Y., Chair, S. Y., & Pak-Chun Chao, J. (2014). The effectiveness of psychosocial interventions for stroke family caregivers and stroke survivors: A systematic review and meta-analysis. *Patient Education and Counselling, 95,* 30–44.

Cherry, G. M., Fletcher, I., & O'Sullivan, H. (2014). Validating relationships among attachment, emotional intelligence and clinical communication. *Medical Education, 48,* 988–997.

Ciechanowski, P., & Katon, W. (2006). The interpersonal experience of healthcare through the eyes of patients with diabetes. *Social Science & Medicine, 63,* 3057–3078.

Coffee, L., Gallagher, P., & Desmond, D. (2014). A prospective study of the importance of life goal characteristics and goal adjustment capacities in longer term psychosocial adjustment to lower limb amputation. *Clinical Rehabilitation, 28*(2), 196–205.

College of Occupational Therapists (2010). *Code of ethics and professional conduct.* London: College of Occupational Therapists.

College of Occupational Therapists (2014). *Learning and development standards for pre-registration education.* London: College of Occupational Therapists.

Davis, S., & Humphrey, N. (2012). The influence of emotional intelligence on coping and mental health in adolescence: Divergent roles for trait and ability EI. *Journal of Adolescence, 35,* 1369–1379.

Duncan, E. (Ed.). (2006). *Foundations for practice in occupational therapy* (4th ed.). Edinburgh: Churchill Livingstone.

Falb, D., & Pargament, K. J. (2012). Relational mindfulness, spirituality and the therapeutic bond. *Asian Journal of Psychiatry, 5,* 351–354.

Foote, F. O., & Schwartz, L. (2012). Holism at the national intrepid centre of excellence. *Explore, 8*(5), 282–290.

Gardner, H. (1993). *Multiple intelligences.* New York: Basic Books.

Goleman, D. (2006). *Emotional intelligence – why it can matter more than IQ.* London: Bantam Press.

Hammill, K., Bye, R., & Cook, C. (2014). Occupational therapy for people living with a life-limiting illness: a thematic review. *The British Journal of Occupational Therapy, 77,* 582–589.

Hannah, S. (2011). Psychosocial issues after traumatic hand injury: Facilitating adjustment. *Journal of Hand Therapy, 1,* 95–103.

Hargie, O. (2011). *Skilled interpersonal communication: Research, theory and practice* (5th ed.). Hove, UK: Routledge.

Hewitt-Taylor, J. (2015). *Developing person centred practice: A practical approach to quality healthcare.* London: Palgrave.

Jensen, M., Moore, M., Bockow, T., Ehdw, D., & Engel, J. (2011). Psychosocial factors and adjustment to chronic pain in persons with physical disabilities: A systematic review. *Archives of Physical Medicine & Rehabilitation, 92,* 146–160.

Landa, J. M. A., Lopez-Zafra, E., Martos, M., & Aguilar-Luzon, M. (2008). The relationship between emotional intelligence and occupational stress and health in nurses: A questionnaire survey. *International Journal of Nursing Studies, 45,* 888–901.

Lequerica, A. H., Donnell, C. S., & Tate, D. G. (2009). Patient engagement in rehabilitation therapy: Physical and occupational therapy impressions. *Disability and Rehabilitation, 31,* 753–760.

Mayer, J. D., & Cobb, C. D. (2000). Educational policy on emotional intelligence – does it make sense. *Educational Psychology Review, 12*(2), 163–183.

Mayer, J. D., & Salovey, P. (1997). What is emotional intelligence? In P. Salovey, & D. Sluyter (Eds.), *Emotional development and emotional intelligence: Implications for educators.* New York: Basic Books.

McKenna, J. (2007). Emotional intelligence training in adjustment to physical disability and illness. *International Journal of Therapy and Rehabilitation, 14*(12), 551–556.

McKenna, J. (2010). Psychosocial support. In M. Curtin, M. Molineux, & J. Supyk Mellson (Eds.), *Occupational therapy and physical dysfunction enabling occupation.* London: Churchill Livingstone.

McKenna, J., & Mellson, J. (2013). Emotional intelligence and the occupational therapist. *British Journal of Occupational Therapy, 76*(9), 427–430.

McKenna, J., Roberts, S., & Tickle, E. (2017). *Engaging with Service Users.* In H. v. Bruggen, S. Kantartzis, & N. Pollard (Eds.) *'And a seed was planted...' Occupation based approaches for social inclusion.* London: Whiting and Birch.

McLeod, J., & McLeod, J. (2011). *Counselling skills: A practical guide for counsellors and helping professions* (2nd ed.). New York: Open University Press.

Molineux, M. (2010). The nature of occupation. In M. Curtin, M. Molineux, & J. Supyk Mellson (Eds.), *Occupational therapy and physical dysfunction: Enabling occupation.* London: Churchill Livingstone.

Morrison, T., & Smith, D. (2013). Working alliance development in occupational therapy: A cross-case analysis. *Australian Occupational Therapy Journal, 60,* 326–333.

Mullen, R., Davis, J. A., & Polatajko, H. (2010). Passion in the performing arts: Clarifying active occupational participation. *Work, 41*(1), 15–25.

Palmadottir, G. (2006). Client therapist relationships: Experiences of occupational therapy clients in rehabilitation. *British Journal of Occupational Therapy, 69*(9), 394–401.

Pelzang, R. (2010). Time to learn: Understanding patient centred care. *British Journal of Nursing, 19*(14), 912–917.

Petrovici, A., & Dobrescu, T. (2014). The role of emotional intelligence in building interpersonal skills. *Procedia, 116,* 1405–1410.

Pinto, R. Z., Ferreira, M. L., Franco, M. R. , et al. (2012). Patient-centred communication is associated with positive therapeutic alliance: A systematic review. *Journal of Physiotherapy, 58*(2), 77–87.

Polatajko, H. J. (2014). A call to occupationology. *Canadian Journal of Occupational Therapy, 8*(1), 4–7.

Price, P., Kinghorn, J., Patrick, R., & Cardell, B. (2012). 'Still there is beauty': One man's resilient adaptation to stroke. *Scandinavian Journal of Occupational Therapy, 19,* 111–117.

Reed, K. D., Hocking, C. S., & Smythe, L. A. (2011). Exploring the meaning of occupation: The case for phenomenology. *Canadian Journal of Occupational Therapy, 78*(5), 303–310.

Reid, D. (2009). Capturing presence moments: The art of mindful practice in occupational therapy. *Canadian Journal of Occupational Therapy, 76*(3), 180–188.

Rosa, S. A., & Hasselkus, B. R. (2005). Finding common ground with patients: The centrality of compatibility. *American Journal of Occupational Therapy, 59,* 98–208.

Rogers, C. R. (1951). *Service user-centred therapy.* London: Constable & Company Ltd.

Rogers, C. R. (2003). *Client centred therapy.* London: Constable and Robinson.

Schier, J. S., & Chan, J. (2007). Changes in life roles after hand injury. *Journal of Hand Therapy, 20,* 57–69.

Schreuer, N., Rimmerman, A., & Sachs, D. (2006). Adjustment to severe disability: Constructing and examining a cognitive and occupational performance model. *International Journal of Rehabilitation Research, 29,* 201–207.

Schnur, J. B., & Montgomery, G. H. (2010). A systematic review of the therapeutic alliance, group cohesion, empathy, and goal consensus/collaboration in psychotherapeutic interventions in cancer: Uncommon factors. *Clinical Psychology Review, 30,* 238–247.

Sorensen, S., White, K., Wingyun, M., et al. (2015). The macular degeneration and ageing study: Design and research protocol of a randomised controlled trial for a psychosocial intervention with macular degeneration patients. *Contemporary Clinical Trials, 3*(7), 2–30.

Suhaimi, A. W., Marzuki, N. A., & Mustaffa, C. S. (2014). The relationship between emotional intelligence and interpersonal communication in a disaster management context: A proposed framework. *Procedia, 155,* 110–114.

Sumsion, T. (Ed.). (2006). *Service user centred practice in occupational therapy: A guide to implementation.* London: Churchill Livingstone.

Taylor, R. R. (2008). *The intentional relationship: Occupational therapy and use of self.* Philadelphia: FA Davis.

Telford, K., Kralik, D., & Koch, T. (2006). Acceptance and denial: implications for people adapting to chronic illness: Literature review. *Journal of Advanced Nursing, 55*(4), 457–464.

Thompson, N. (2015). *People skills* (5th ed.). London: Palgrave.

Tickle-Degnen, L. (2014). Therapeutic rapport. In M. V. Radomski, & C. A. Trombly-Latham (Eds.), *Occupational therapy for physical dysfunction* (7th ed). London: Wolters Kluwer.

Tickle-Degnen, L., Zebrowitz, L. A., & Ma, H. (2011). Culture gender and healthcare stigma: Practioner response to facial masking experienced by people with Parkinson's disease. *Social Science and Medicine, 73,* 95–102.

Weinstein, E. C. (2015). Three views of artful practice in occupational therapy. *Occupational Therapy in Mental Health, 29*(4), 229–360.

Whitcher, K., & Tse, S. (2004). Counselling skills in occupational therapy: A grounded theory approach to explain their use within mental health in New Zealand. *British Journal of Occupational Therapy, 67*(8), 361–368.

White, R. O., Eden, S., Wallston, K. A., et al. (2015). Health communication, self-care and treatment satisfaction among low income diabetes patients in a public health setting. *Patient Education and Counselling, 98,* 144–149.

Wilcock, A. (2006). *An occupational perspective of health.* New York: Slack.

World Health Organization (2002). *ICD-10 Classification of behavioural and mental disorders: Clinical descriptions and diagnostic guidelines.* Geneva, Switzerland: WHO.

Yerxa, E. J. (2011). The 1966 Eleanor Clarke Slagle Lecture: Authentic occupational therapy. In R. Padilla, & Y. Griffiths (Eds.), *A professional legacy. The Eleanor Clarke Slagle Lectures in occupational therapy* (3rd ed., pp. 1955–2010). Bethesda, MD: AOT Press.

31

WORKING WITH GROUPS

CLAIRE CRAIG

CHAPTER OUTLINE

Abstract

Groups are a fundamental part of human existence with the potential to foster a sense of mutual sharing, support and collective problem solving. Therapeutically group work can offer a sense of community, promote engagement in meaningful occupations, provide an opportunity for the learning of new skills, build confidence, reduce isolation and create bridges to promote interaction. Group work can offer ways for participants to develop skills and techniques, promote health and well-being, and manage and adapt to physical and psychological impacts of their condition. However, for group work to be effective significant preparatory work needs to be completed, including identifying a need, envisioning the group, refining ideas, recruiting and reviewing. In addition, group sessions have to be sensitively and creatively facilitated to harness and manage the dynamic interactions between group members that evolve and change from the beginning phase until the ending phase of the group. The potential outcomes of group work are congruent with the philosophy of occupational therapy and skills in facilitating group work are core to occupational therapy practice.

KEY POINTS

- Group work has a role to play when working with people who have a physical illness, injury or impairment.

- Successful group work requires the creation of a supportive environment where individual members are able to give and take, express and listen, and offer and learn from each other and engage in the process of doing, being and becoming.

- Occupational groups are the domain of occupational therapists given their focus on encouraging the development or maintenance of healthy leisure, work and self-care occupations.

- Groups have the potential to foster a sense of community connectedness through enabling mutual sharing, support and collective problem solving.

- Occupationally focused groups provide opportunities for individuals to be creative and productive.

- Preparatory work needs to occur before a group can start, and this work can be divided into four pregroup stages: creating, recruiting, engaging and planning.

- Groups need to be actively managed throughout all stages of the group, with each stage raising different challenges and responsibilities for group leaders.

INTRODUCTION

Groups are a fundamental part of human existence (Lindsay & Orton, 2014) with the potential to foster a sense of mutual sharing, support and collective problem solving. When used therapeutically, groups can offer a sense of community, promote engagement in meaningful occupations, provide an opportunity for the learning of new skills, build confidence, reduce isolation and create bridges to promote interaction between generations. The aims of group work are therefore fully congruent with the core philosophy of occupational therapy, enabling individuals to recognise and build on their strengths and to act as a resource for themselves and others and in doing so to realise their occupational potential. It comes as no surprise that the World Federation of Occupational Therapists regards group work as a key skill of occupational therapists and includes it within its standards of proficiency (World Federation of Occupational Therapists, 2011).

However, group work for some years has been regarded very much as sitting almost exclusively within the domain of mental health. Although the contribution of group work here should not be underestimated, it is important not to limit it to this area. In physical rehabilitation group work can offer a way of enabling individuals to develop skills and techniques that can promote rehabilitation or manage and adapt to some of the physical and psychological challenges that living with a long-term condition can bring.

As health services are reconfigured to place more emphasis on self-management, disease prevention and recognising the importance of drawing on resources in the community, group work will play an increasing role across all occupational therapy practice and will assume a key role in the continued renaissance of our profession.

The primary aim of this chapter is to demonstrate the value of group work in physical rehabilitation and how it is practically applied in occupational therapy. This chapter begins by defining what is meant by group work, and more specifically therapeutic group work, before offering an overview of the broader evidence base to support its use in practice. The fundamental principles of group work are then described with a particular focus on ways of planning and facilitating groups. Finally the chapter concludes with a real-world example of an occupationally focused group with a focus on lifestyle management and health promotion aimed at community-living older people experiencing a range of long-term conditions.

SETTING THE SCENE, DEFINITIONS AND CLARIFICATION OF TERMINOLOGY

Groups come into existence when two or more individuals become linked in a relationship of some kind, where *relationship* implies interdependence and influence (Forsyth, 2006). Therapeutic groups harness the opportunities that are presented to engage multiple layers of relationships beyond one-to-one interactions with the therapist, and in doing so the group becomes the medium to support change (Ward, 2002). Group members are effectively instruments within their own therapy, contributing to and creating the group dynamic, which can potentially lead to transformation and sharing personal resources to facilitate learning in others.

Group work therefore reflects the holistic and person-centred philosophy of occupational therapy. Rather than the therapist holding the locus of control, group members themselves become the resource, modelling problem-solving techniques, sharing ideas of ways to overcome challenges, validating experiences and, through these elements, developing new roles, which can be transferred to other situations. At the heart of this process lies a strength- or asset-based approach where individuals are supported to draw on their existing skills.

Occupationally focused groups also provide opportunities for individuals to be creative and productive, which in turn can enhance individuals' sense of well-being and esteem while encouraging the development of skills and promoting change. All these values have been explored and solidly validated by research.

GROUP WORK IN PHYSICAL REHABILITATION

Given the potential that group work offers, it is puzzling as to why it is not a commonly employed intervention in physical rehabilitation. In part this is because much of the group work literature and practice mirrors the way that broader services have been configured, separating out the physical needs of individuals from their psychological and emotional needs. As a consequence, although an extensive history and literature around group work in the context of mental health exists, less is found in the literature relating to the evaluation of group work interventions within occupational therapy and physical rehabilitation.

A similar disconnect in relation to practice exists. Whereas in mental health it is established practice to see a range of groups using a number of models and frameworks (e.g. psychodynamic, cognitive behavioural, humanistic), the more typical picture of a group within physical rehabilitation is of people working on individual therapeutic exercises while seated together. An example of this is a 'rehab' or 'hand therapy' group with people sitting around a table and being treated by a therapist who goes round to each in turn. The parallel therapy being delivered in this way may be effective, but it is arguably not really *group* work – or at least it is not exploiting the rich potential of group work. It is also not exploiting the benefits of using meaningful occupation.

However, groups can offer people living with physical conditions the opportunity to share experiences and to develop techniques to help cope with the symptoms and challenges that living with the condition brings (Bertisch, Rath, Langenbahn, Sherr, & Diller, 2011). At a time when individuals may be experiencing a sense of occupational disconnect as a consequence of injury through trauma or through the symptoms of a long-term condition, the group experience can offer a context for the development and rehearsal of new roles. Here skills and ways of adapting and engaging with valued occupations can be acquired, and this mastery can then be generalised into other parts of their lives, including work environments as well as in relation to leisure and self-care.

There is good evidence to show the value of groups in helping individuals to make the significant psychological adjustments that living with a physical impairment or long-term condition can bring. These psychological aspects are important. Evidence shows, for example, that people living with a range of cardiovascular diseases are two to three times more likely than the general population to experience depression (Fenton & Stover, 2006; Welch, Czerwinski, Ghimire, & Bertsimas, 2009). There is an equally strong correlation between depression and diabetes (Simon et al., 2007; Vamos, Mucsi, Keszei, Kopp, & Novak, 2009) and up to 33% of women and 20% of men living with arthritis will also be diagnosed with comorbid depression (Sale, Gignac, & Hawker, 2008; Theis, Helmick, & Hootman, 2007). Sharpe (2014) has highlighted that 68% of people experiencing chronic mental health conditions also have a physical long-term condition. A raft of national and international policies which focus on a more integrated approach to physical and mental health services are consequently evolving.

In part this is in response to the growing voices of people who are showing that the separation of services into physical and mental health is no longer tenable. The narratives of individuals offer compelling support for the holistic philosophy and approach adopted by occupational therapists. This is illustrated by Inger Wallis, who described how she was 'discharged 3 weeks after major brain surgery with a booklet and a phone number' because she was deemed functionally able to undertake basic activities of daily living (National Health Service (NHS) England, 2014). However, before receiving the necessary psychological support, the physical changes she experienced after her cerebrovascular accident meant that she experienced loss of valued occupations and key roles including those of wage earner, mother and wife.

EVIDENCE FOR GROUP WORK

If this chapter has not already offered a compelling reason as to the importance of using group interventions to address both the emotional and physical needs of individuals, a closer look at the broader literature offers further evidence. Indeed, there is significant research supporting group-based interventions in the rehabilitation of individuals living with long-term neurological conditions and acquired brain injury (Flanagan, Cantor, & Ashman, 2008; Langenbahn, Sherr, Simon, & Hanig, 1999; Silver, McAllister, & Arciniegas, 2009).

Research undertaken by Gauthier, Dalziel, and Gauthier (1987), for instance, demonstrated the value of a group intervention aimed at supporting individuals living with idiopathic Parkinson's disease. Twenty hours of group occupational therapy was offered to each person with a focus on enabling participants to maintain their functional status. The results were positive. Participants who attended group rehabilitation experienced a reduction in bradykinesia and overall improvements in functional independence. Moreover, these improvements were sustained a year after participation in the group had ceased. Significantly, participants also reported increased psychological well-being.

Similar reports of improved psychological well-being have been identified by other studies relating to individuals engaged in physical rehabilitation groups in the context of acquired brain injury and long-term neurological conditions. A study undertaken by Bertisch, Rath, Langenbahn, Sherr, & Diller, (2011), for example, identified peer support and feedback as integral to the therapeutic benefits emerging through the study. Laing (2007) reported how participants who attended her group, which sought to improve communicative participation in people with dysarthria and multiple sclerosis, recognised the value of sharing experiences and learning with others. Both of these studies also identified a wide range of positive functional, physical, cognitive and social outcomes, including improvements in objective measures of attention, memory and reasoning; the acquisition of compensatory strategies; and increased social participation.

The authors of both studies separately conclude that the group approach intensifies and extends benefits obtained from individual interventions and achieves more behavioural changes than an individual, more dependent, person–therapist relationship would achieve. According to Bertisch et al. (2011) and Gauthier et al. (1987) part of the strength of the group lies in the creation of the dynamic within a supportive environment that facilitates interactions among peers, leading to the sharing of effective ideas and compensatory strategies. Both studies highlight the psychological and emotional benefits of being part of a group-based intervention, particularly in relation to improving motivation and reducing the social isolation that can so often occur when a person is living with a long-term neurological condition.

The potential of group work to facilitate transition is another theme that emerges from the literature. For instance, Nilsson and Nygard (2003) evaluated a predischarge occupational therapy group programme for older people. Older people in an inpatient rehabilitation setting attended group-based occupational therapy before discharge that sought to enable them to manage the discharge process from hospital to home. Findings from the study were again very positive. The group offered the opportunity for learning and reflection leading to the development of adaptive skills. Individuals shared how they found it easier to learn new things when doing something together rather than alone, and the sharing of experiences offered new insights into themselves. In some instances this led to new self-conceptions and confidence in relation to what individuals could achieve. Final interviews with participants identified the group dynamic as being key in creating this transformational understanding of the possibilities for adaptation. As a consequence techniques were not only learned but were internalised and attitudes changed because of the group experience as the group activities led them to reflect on who they were and on what was to come.

Other studies have identified the value of group work from the occupational therapists perspective. Cost-effectiveness and intensification of treatment effects are two broad benefits described by the literature. Research by Spilak (1999) has extended this discussion to suggest the use of the group as a predictive assessment of a person's function on return to the community. She proposes that group sessions provide opportunities to review each individual's motivation, frustration tolerance, 'problem-solving ability and interpersonal skills to determine how they will perform in their life roles outside of the treatment arena' (Spilak, 1999, p. 49). This is important if unnecessary readmission to hospital is to be prevented.

There is a growing interest in the potential of group work in enabling individuals to manage long-term conditions and in secondary and tertiary health promotion. For instance, a randomised controlled trial of six sessions of group intervention for people with low back pain in Sweden was found to lower the risk of long-term sick leave ninefold (Linton & Andersson, 2000).

The most significant evidence in favour of group work in relation to health promotion is the Well Elderly Study, an experimental, randomised controlled research conducted by Clark et al. (1997, 2001) in the United States. It took more than 3 years to complete the trial and involved 361 participants. The participants were randomly assigned to one of three cohorts: (1) a 9-month programme of group-based occupational therapy focused on lifestyle redesign; (2) a control condition where participants engaged in group-based activities, which were nonprofessionally led; and (3) no intervention. The results were powerfully consistent. Compared with the second and third cohort, the occupational therapy group produced clear benefits in numerous outcomes, including physical and social performance, mental health and vitality (Clark et al., 2001). Interestingly no difference was found between the group who received social activity and no intervention group, suggesting that activity alone is not necessarily therapeutic. Research by Clark et al. (1997) not only demonstrated that the health of the older people improved, they showed that the average savings in health care costs exceeded the cost of the occupational therapy itself.

Similar results are also reflected in other studies. For example, research by Okumiya et al. (2005) showed the value of group work using music therapy and handicrafts for older people living in the community who had age-associated cognitive decline or mild depressive moods. Improvements were observed in mood, quality of life and cognitive function.

Studies examining the potential of occupationally focused group work to enable individuals to manage their condition or in preventing health issues from developing are interesting for a number of reasons. Above all they highlight the shifting paradigm of health away from approaches that focus solely on addressing health problems as they arise to those that seek to promote health and well-being and to support the development of healthy coping skills.

Occupational therapists are in a position to work within such a paradigm. First and foremost the move towards preventing health issues from developing sits well with the profession's core philosophy and understanding of the importance of lifestyle and the relationship between what people do and their health and well-being. Occupational therapists recognise the importance of working holistically, the relationship between physical and psychological well-being and the importance of social participation. As occupational therapists continue to push the boundaries of practice forward and work in ever new and emerging areas of practice, the importance of and scope for occupationally focused group work will increase.

Group work therefore continues to occupy an important place in the occupational therapist's tool bag of therapeutic interventions. It is not surprising that group work is regarded as a core clinical skill. In the United Kingdom, the Standards of Proficiency published by the Health Care Professions Council, the professional regulatory body, identified the need for practitioners to understand group dynamics and roles and to be able to facilitate group work to maximise support, learning and change within groups and communities. It is to an exploration of these skills this chapter now turns.

CORE SKILLS AND REASONING IN GROUP WORK

Significant preparatory background work needs to occur before a group can begin. For the purposes of this chapter the preparatory work has been divided into five stages: identifying a need, envisioning the group, refining ideas, recruiting, and reviewing. Although these are described separately, in reality the stages blend into and inform each other.

Stage 1: Identifying the Need for the Group

The starting point is to first identify that there is a need for a group. Sometimes group interventions are preferred as there is an assumption that it is a more economical option because more people are treated at one time compared with individual interventions. However, groups are only cost effective if the intervention is effective as well. Groups must fulfil a particular need and there must be sufficient numbers of individuals with that need to warrant a group. Indeed, sometimes a group intervention might not be the most appropriate course of action and it may well be that a person's needs may be more simply and efficiently handled on an individual basis. The group should offer something that individuals would not gain from a one-to-one intervention.

To make a decision it will be necessary to undertake a needs analysis so that from the outset the overall purpose of the group and how it will enable the participants to meet their therapeutic goals is clear. The most successful forms of needs analyses are those that take into account the breadth of personal and community resources on which participants will be able to draw. At this point it is important to seek out precedents in the wider literature for a group of this nature and speak to colleagues regarding previous initiatives in order to understand more about the nuances of the local context in which the group will be running.

Stage 2: Envisioning the Group

Once a need for the group is established, then the process of envisioning or sketching out what a possible group may look like begins. This is necessary to identify whether the group will be feasible. Here decisions will be made about the broader group aims, the format, the proposed content and the context. At this point it will also be necessary to consider in more detail the resources that will be required to facilitate the group. Some of these will relate to physical resources, including the environment where the group will take place and the therapeutic media that may be needed. Other resources will relate to staffing of the group. It is important not to underestimate the resource. In addition to the time necessary to plan, physically facilitate and evaluate the group, it is also important to factor in time to see group members individually to prepare them for the group and to monitor progress.

Stage 3: Refining Ideas

It is important to engage in a process of refining ideas and grappling with the practicalities of what the group may look like. At this point the occupational therapist will begin to consider in more detail the practicalities of group membership. First, the size of the group needs to be planned, bearing in mind the number of facilitators needed or who are available. Decisions will be made based on the complexity of the participants' needs, the type of group and the experience of the therapists who are facilitating. Second, decisions need to be made regarding the mix of participants and parameters for inclusion. For example, individuals could be invited to participate in the group at a particular point in their rehabilitative journey to ensure that they have comparable goals and needs (Lindsay & Orton, 2014) or there may be merit in inviting people at different points of their journeys to participate, to act as role models for each other. This decision will be influenced by a third general consideration, which relates to the type of group that will be offered: will the group have an open membership or a closed and consistent membership? The latter of these, the 'closed group', can offer a more intensive group dynamic because members' progress through the group process

concurrently. As a result a more cohesive group can be formed. One advantage of a group with an open membership, the so-called open group, on the other hand, is that an ongoing group programme can be offered with participants joining at any time and attending sessions for as long as they require.

Stage 4: Recruiting

The next stage of the process involves gaining referrals and then choosing the people for the group. Before this can happen the group may need a campaign for advertising and marketing. Here the therapist may want to alert possible referral agents using letters and leaflets or perhaps use eye-catching posters to invite people to participate. The more professional and inviting the letters and posters look, the more likely it will be that appropriate referrals are made, which in turn will make the group more successful in the long run. So it is worth carefully planning this campaign in terms of timing and impact.

Having recruited the group members, each member needs to be assessed and, if he or she is thought to be suitable for the group, time needs to be spent engaging them. The prospective group members need to know what they are signing up to and how the group is going to be helpful to them. They need to be inspired to attend and participate actively. The therapist in turn uses this opportunity to assess the individual's needs for planning future interventions and to be aware of factors that might stop the individual from taking part. In effect, a contract to attend the group is established.

Stage 5: Reviewing

The final planning stage, which usually occurs as the group evolves over the weeks, is to review and specify aims, goals and objectives or outcomes for each group session. Linked to these aims, goals and objectives or outcomes, the therapist has to choose the group activity to fit the needs and abilities of the members – an activity that will be meaningful to the group members (Craig & Finlay, 2009). Then there are other practical planning decisions that need to be made to do with the required equipment and resources, how members are going to travel to the group and how the group environment will be set up. Care needs to be taken to consider any messages that are projected by the environment, which can set up certain expectations. Placing chairs in rows, for example, might signal that people are being invited to listen, whereas chairs in a circle suggest more active participation will be required. Creating a comfortable, welcoming area to greet members (e.g. offering coffee and biscuits) can help relax people at the start of the group.

FACILITATING A GROUP

Facilitating a group involves more than simply planning and running sessions. The complexity of what is involved should not be underestimated. Within the group context therapists need to be aware of the needs of individuals while also managing the dynamics and processes that occur when many personalities come together. It takes skill to learn to read a group and understand what might be happening below the surface of what people are doing.

Groups continuously evolve as relationships develop over time; at different points members can be seen to come together working cooperatively, whereas at other times they can seem to move apart through conflict and tensions. Group facilitators need to be able to understand what is happening and why as part of working towards enabling positive outcomes, and they need to adapt their role accordingly. These phases have been described in various ways (Bion, 1961; Tuckman, 1965; Yalom, 1985). Basically all groups have a beginning and ending phase and a middle phase occurs in between that may involve different degrees of both conflict and working effectively together. In each of these phases facilitators face certain tasks, challenges and responsibilities. How they handle these could make the difference between the success and relative failure of the group.

The Beginning Phase of the Group

During the beginning phase of a group, which usually includes the first few sessions, members tend to feel uncertain, possibly even anxious, about what the group is going to involve. Depending on their level of pregroup orientation, they may be approaching the group with anticipation or dread. They may feel shy about getting to know others in the group. The group facilitator's role during this phase is to assist members settle into the group, making them feel as comfortable and welcome as possible. Simple interventions such as providing housekeeping information and stating what is going to happen in the group and for how long can help settle members (Cole, 2011). Part of this job involves being clear about group roles, norms, expectations and ground rules so members know what they are supposed to be doing. Often the messages given early on can set the pattern for future sessions, so it is important to get the tone right. For example, a common trap facilitators can fall into is to do too much talking in the very first session. This can put the group members in a passive role, which may be counterproductive when the facilitator wants members to participate actively later. The other key part of the facilitator's role is to help facilitate group members to know and trust each other. Activities that encourage members to share their experiences are useful here, and it can help if the facilitator points out similarities in experiences between individual members.

The Middle Phase of the Group

The middle phase of the group will vary depending on the group, though it will probably include times when the group is working well together and times when there are some conflicts. When the group is working well together there is a feeling of cohesiveness as members cooperate and support each other. At other times the facilitator might be well advised to step back and allow group members to take on more responsibility. The key here is to keep the group members feeling safe (e.g. by having clear boundaries of confidentiality and keeping to agreed group rules such as accepting and respecting contributions from each member). The decisions about when to intervene are difficult. The facilitator does not want to take over completely as this may disempower group members, yet there is a balance to be found as members should not be left to flounder in discomfort for too long. Too much floundering is likely to encourage members to vote with their feet and not come back to the group. How much direction to give is a decision that can only be made in the context of the specific group.

Research, for instance, stemming from social identity theory (Tajfel & Turner, 1979) has shown that group members can be helped to identify with their group and that this has clear implications for the group's effectiveness and how cooperative/competitive or involved members are likely to be (Pratto, Sidanius, & Levin, 2006; Tyler & Blader, 2000). The facilitator can do two main things: mark the emerging boundaries of the group, and assist each individual member to feel positively included in the group community (Lizzio & Wilson, 2001; Stangor, 2004). Using language like 'us' and 'we' and 'our group' can help, as can noting emerging themes, such as saying, 'It seems that several of you are expressing the same point; who else feels the same?'

The Ending Phase of a Group

During the ending phase of a group, whether this is the last few minutes of the final session or the last few sessions, group members may well have mixed feelings, including feeling sad, worried and angry. Some tensions and conflicts may creep back into the group dynamics. At the same time some members may feel reluctant to acknowledge the group is finishing and try to find ways to prolong it. Depending on the type of group, the facilitator's responsibility is to find a gradual way to assist members to deal with the ending. The main aim should be to tie up loose ends to ensure members do not leave with a sense of unfinished business. Ideally there should be some consideration given to following up any gains made. For instance, how might members manage the transition between attending the group and accessing groups in the future once they find themselves in the community?

One positive approach the facilitator can make as a group is finishing is to ask group members to evaluate the effectiveness of the group. Precisely how this evaluation is carried out will depend on the requirements of the service concerned and the type of group work involved. In some places the main task may be simply to record each individual's progress. In other places a record of the evolution of the group as a whole may be useful. Often both forms of evaluation are used in combination. By combining these results it is possible to audit the effectiveness of the group overall and use this as the basis for further research.

Practice Story 31.1 contains a description of the development and facilitation of an occupationally focused group for community living older people. It illustrates the stages and offers an example of the practicalities of facilitating a group in practice.

PRACTICE STORY 31.1

Lifestyle Matters Group

Occupational therapists have an increasing role to play in the area of health promotion. The following narrative describes the journey taken to establish a community group with a focus on supporting community-living older people experiencing a number of long-term conditions to continue to engage in health-promoting meaningful occupation.

PREPARING FOR THE GROUP

Stage 1: Identifying a Need

A range of meetings were held with potential stakeholders (including older people, general practitioners and community nurses) and from these conversations and the evidence collected it was decided that a need for a group of this nature existed and that it should have a closed membership. Taking into account the resources available, a weekly group held over a period of 3 months seemed reasonable, although it was also decided to review the group with the participants after 1 month to see if the planned period was appropriate.

Stage 2: Envisioning the Group

It was always the intention that the group should be physically rooted in the community as it was envisioned that this would help members make links with community facilities and use the group as a springboard or a bridge to access these facilities. However, finding a community venue was more problematic. After trying a number of different places it was finally decided to use a small room at the back of a local church. The room had a loop system that was of great help to members with a hearing impairment. There were excellent toilet facilities, a seating area for coffee and light refreshments, and a small kitchen. It was private, inexpensive to hire and was on a main bus route and so could be easily accessed.

Stages 3 and 4: Refining and Recruiting

Resources were a challenge and it was therefore decided to enlist the support of a group of art students at a local college, who helped with the design and production of a range of posters, leaflets and fliers to advertise the group. They ensured that these had a professional look with clear, uncluttered text supported by pictures for participants with poor literacy. These were distributed across the town in the post office, local supermarket, college, fish shop, bookmakers and doctor's surgery — in fact, anywhere that the team involved with establishing the group thought older people regularly accessed.

When an older person expressed an interest, a meeting was arranged with the group facilitator at a mutually convenient time and place. This provided an opportunity to build a rapport, describe the aims of the group and provide a clear picture of what it was about. It also provided opportunity to find out more about the person and what he or she felt the group could offer. Practicalities such as transport and timing of the group were also discussed. In this way it was possible to undertake what was

effectively an initial assessment of the person's needs and each person could make an informed choice about attending.

As it was important that older people commit to attending a specified number of sessions, those interested in participating in the group were asked to sign a pregroup contract. Individuals were then left with written information about the group and contact details of the facilitator as a reminder for them and to show their families.

As there were only 10 places available it was important that places were offered to individuals on the basis of who could most benefit from the intervention. Where it was felt that the group was not appropriate for an individual, that person was guided to other relevant facilities or services. It was decided that, given the number of participants and the level of need identified, sessions would be facilitated by two occupational therapists. The final membership of the group is shown in Table 31.1.

TABLE 31.1
The Final Members of the Lifestyle Matters Group

Name[a]	Age	Reason for Attending
Phyllis	76	Difficulty in resuming roles after heart attack, struggling to cope with anxiety and loss of confidence
Kate	80	Reduced mobility and social isolation after fall; experiencing problems in managing pain caused by arthritis
Eileen	72	Poor coping skills after recent death of husband; struggling to manage her COPD
Grace	72	Reluctance to leave the house or engage in activity, leading to poor mobility and depression after CVA
Jacob	69	Increasing social isolation and withdrawal after diagnosis of Parkinson's disease, leading to reduced function
Ernest	74	Withdrawal, loss of motivation, decreased function after heart attack
Flo	82	Extreme social isolation after CVA
Jo	86	Depression as a consequence of arthritis; withdrawal from previous roles
Lucy	65	Loss of confidence after recent hip replacement
Alan	78	Poor coping skills, withdrawal and reduced function

COPD, Chronic obstructive pulmonary disease; CVA, cerebrovascular accident.
[a]To protect the identity of the individuals referred to in the practice story, pseudonyms have been used.

PRACTICE STORY 31.1

Lifestyle Matters Group *(Continued)*

Stage 5: Reviewing: Planning the Sessions

Although the overall aims of the group were clear, it was not possible to know the details of each sessions until all group members had been seen and their specific needs had been identified. This was tricky as often the first question participants asked was, 'What will you be doing in the sessions?' It was therefore necessary to have at least some idea about broad topic areas so that these questions could be answered effectively.

As the group was for community-living older people who had a long-term condition, it was apparent that membership would include people with a range of physical and emotional needs including those with histories of cerebrovascular accident, arthritis, anxiety, depression, heart disease and chronic obstructive pulmonary disease. Yet it was made clear from the outset that the focus was not on the health conditions of each member of the group but on assisting group members to understand the relationship among occupation, health and well-being, equipping them with necessary skills to make positive life changes.

Based on this, sessions in the following areas were offered:

■ Linking occupation, health and well-being
■ Transport
■ Leisure

■ Community connectedness: friends and social relationships
■ Maintaining mental well-being (including sleep as an occupation)
■ Managing pain
■ Home and community safety
■ Spirituality
■ Endings and new beginnings

Overall themes were identified through the pregroup interviews and the issues raised by individuals. This plan formed the starting point, but as time passed the group gradually took over the planning. The aim from the outset was that the locus of control would remain with the group members, so over time the facilitators gradually withdrew their level of direction and input. Instead of the spirituality sessions, for example, the group chose to look at memory and so a session was dedicated to exploring ways to improve memory. An example of a session plan can be seen in Table 31.2.

FACILITATION

One key message that was emphasised when establishing this group was that the older person was always the 'expert'. The focus was on enabling participants to recognise and utilise their skills and experience. Therefore each session

---

TABLE 31.2

Example of a Session on Physical Activity

Aims of the session	■ Explore the relationship between physical activity and health ■ Identify opportunities where physical activity could be incorporated into daily routine ■ Identify barriers to taking part in physical activity and explore ways to overcome these ■ Understand the factors that act as a source of motivation for being physically active ■ Participate in a range of leisure activities that are based on physical activity
Introductory exercises	■ Group members list the physical activities they have taken part in over the last week
Example of discussion questions	■ How can physical activity affect health and well-being? ■ Is exercise the only way to keep physically active or are there other ways to keep fit? ■ Apart from keeping fit, what other opportunities can taking part in physical exercise provide? ■ Are there any physical activities you would like to take part in but don't? What stops you from doing this? ■ Is it better to have an exercise regimen or to incorporate physical activity it into daily routines? ■ What qualities must a physical activity have for you to want to take part in it?
Group activity ideas	■ Explore how everyday activities can provide opportunities for physical activity. Discuss ways of incorporating activity into daily routines. After discussion, encourage each participant to identify one way that he or she could increase his or her level of physical activity on a daily basis. Work together over a series of sessions to create an 'active community' booklet that lists details of groups and facilities in the area. ■ Invite a local walking group to talk about the opportunities that exist in the community and ways to access these. This could form the focus of an outing. ■ Arrange for a t'ai chi or yoga teacher to take a session for the group. ■ Hold a tea dance where group members invite friends and family to join in, emphasising the social element of physical activity. ■ Organise a visit to a leisure centre where group members can try a range of activities, such as bowling, swimming or using the gym facilities.

Continued on following page

Lifestyle Matters Group (Continued)

involved some initial discussion and sharing of information (e.g. the principles of joint protection or the physiology of pain). At the same time the group included an element of 'doing', so each session included some time for active experimentation, allowing members to put theory into practice. Sessions then ended with more discussion to both evaluate what members enjoyed or gained and to make arrangements for the following week. Every third session there was the opportunity to try out these ideas more extensively through a visit to a local community facility or place of interest. This would often involve using public transport, reading timetables and asking for information.

Two hours were allocated for the weekly group meeting. However, the time allocated to the various activities within a weekly session varied. This meant that participants had enough time to explore quite significant issues in depth if they needed to, even though they were not expected to concentrate for longer than 15 to 20 minutes at any one time.

THE FIRST SESSION

There was an awareness that the first session was key. Cards were therefore sent to individual participants as a gentle reminder of the time and the date along with directions to the group.

It was recognised that for many of the participants, transport to the venue was a barrier. For the first few sessions group members were offered the option of travelling on local community transport. Transport was a theme that was addressed at a later point within the group, and so gradually over time responsibility was placed on group members to make their own arrangements.

The facilitators ensured that they arrived early to check that everything was in place and to arrange the space as they wanted. They understood the importance of the environment and the messages it can potentially communicate. As it was considered to be important to create an informal and relaxed atmosphere, the space was divided into two areas. In one area chairs were arranged in a circle to facilitate discussion. A flip chart was used to record ideas and to validate contributions from individual members. There was also an awareness of the importance of providing written cues for people with sensory impairments.

In the second area chairs were positioned around small circular tables with teacups and plates of biscuits and fruit. The aim was to make this seem inviting and welcoming. As people arrived informal conversation could occur over tea before moving to the other part of the room where the main business of the group took place.

CHALLENGES

The group did not have a promising start. The main challenge was balancing so many individual needs within the group and helping each member to trust the other members and the group process. There was friction at times. For example, during the session on pain the discussion spiralled out of control as Phyllis announced that women coped much better with pain than men and hinted that Ernest had not experienced what it was like to be in 'real pain'. In response Ernest stormed out. It was necessary to work quickly both to diffuse the situation and support Ernest and the group to move forward.

When the facilitators reflected on the session, they questioned how attentive they had been to the developing conflict as they had been rather too focused on following the session plan. This was a good reminder that the art of being a good facilitator required being able to read and interpret the group dynamics, to pick up on those nonverbal cues that denote whether someone is bored, tired, overwhelmed or angry, and to respond to these cues.

More challenging than this one incident were the evolving group dynamics where Lucy became overly dominant. With the rest of her life feeling out of control, she seemed to use the group as the one place to take control and exercise power. The initial response was to ignore this and to see how the group responded. However, very quickly there was a realisation that it was necessary to revisit the ground rules and to model to the group assertive behaviour. When this had little effect and she began to completely dominate discussion, the facilitators spoke to her individually to address some of the issues that she faced. A group session was then also dedicated to relationships and assertive behaviour.

In the early stages of the group, attendance was sporadic and difficult to manage. It was hard to tell whether the members had decided that the group just was not for them or whether there were genuine reasons why individuals did not attend. A closer investigation found the main reason for non-attendance related to problems accessing public transport as a consequence of recent changes by the bus company of familiar bus routes. This then became a focus of one of the group sessions and the group engaged in problem-solving skills, offering support to each other to overcome these challenges.

TRANSFORMATIONS

Over time the group assumed its own identity and group members began to draw strength from each other, sharing skills and resources and engaging in the process of group problem solving. The impact of this process on participants was transformative. For example:

- After an outing to the local leisure centre, Ernest began to bowl again and with encouragement from the group joined a local team. Between sessions Jo went along to offer him support, and the two developed a strong friendship.

PRACTICE STORY 31.1

Lifestyle Matters Group *(Continued)*

- Lucy started to attend adult literacy classes based at the local college and developed the confidence to offer her services as a volunteer. This provided the perfect outlet for her to channel her energy and to gain some control over certain areas of her life.

- Kate remained nervous when outdoors; however, the group outings improved her confidence and she began to walk to the local shops on her own.

- Flo still spent much of her day at home, but the strong social networks that were established meant that once a fortnight Kate, Eileen and Phyllis would visit her and they would share a meal together.

- The greatest changes observed were with June. She said that she had 'been asleep' for the last 2 years and now she was like a 'rosebud just waiting to bloom'.

Through understanding the relationship among occupation, health and well-being the group members were equipped to make informed choices and significant life changes. These changes were a testimony to the group and to the group work process, and to the incredible resources and resourcefulness of individuals, along with the involvement of the occupational therapy facilitators in unlocking this potential.

CONCLUSION

The value of group work associated with physical rehabilitation and how it is practically applied in occupational therapy has been presented in this chapter. Successful group work requires the therapist to create a space where individual members are able to give and take, to express and listen, and to offer and learn from each other in a mutually supportive environment, and in doing so to engage in the process of doing, being, becoming and belonging, which is at the heart of occupational therapy practice. Facilitating groups is challenging, exciting, sometimes frustrating and will draw on the sensitivity, creativity and ability to read and manage complex dynamics of the therapist. The ability to effectively facilitate a group is a skill to be mastered. However, when group work is used appropriately it can lead to changes of mammoth proportions and as such deserves a place in occupational therapists' tool bag of interventions when working with people attending physical rehabilitation.

 http://evolve.elsevier.com/Curtin/OT

REFERENCES

Bertisch, H., Rath, J. F., Langenbahn, D. M., Sherr, R. L., & Diller, L. (2011). Group treatment in acquired brain injury rehabilitation. *Journal for Specialists in Groupwork, 36*(4), 264–277.

Bion, W. R. (1961). *Experiences in groups.* London: Tavistock.

Clark, F., Azen, S. P., Zemke, R., Jackson, J., Carlson, M., Mandel, D., Hay, J., Josephson, K., Cherry, B., Hessel, C., Palmer, J., & Lipson, L. (1997). Occupational therapy for independent-living older adults. A randomized controlled trial. *JAMA, 278*(16), 1321–1326.

Clark, F., Azen, S. P., Carlson, M., Mandel, D., LaBree, L., Hay, J., Zemke, R., Jackson, J., & Lipson, L. (2001). Embedding health-promoting changes into the daily lives of independent-living older adults: long-term follow-up of occupational therapy intervention. *J Gerontol B Psychol Sci Soc Sci, 56*(1), 60–63.

Cole, M. (2011). *Group dynamics in occupational therapy: The theoretical basis and practice application of group intervention.* Thorofare, NJ: Slack.

Craig, C., & Finlay, L. (2009). Groupwork in physical rehabilitation. In M. Curtin, M. Molineux, & E. Supyk (Eds.), *Occupational Therapy and Physical Dysfunction.* Oxford: Elsevier.

Fenton, W. S., & Stover, E. S. (2006). Mood disorders: Cardiovascular and diabetes comorbidity. *Current Opinion in Psychiatry, 19* (4), 421–427.

Flanagan, S. R., Cantor, J. B., & Ashman, T. A. (2008). Traumatic brain injury: Future assessment tools and treatment prospects. *Neuropsychiatric Disease and Treatment, 4*, 877–892.

Forsyth, D. R. (2006). *Group dynamics.* London: Thomson Learning.

Gauthier, L., Dalziel, S., & Gauthier, S. (1987). The benefits of group occupational therapy for patients with Parkinson's disease. *American Journal of Occupational Therapy, 41*(6), 360–365.

Laing, C. (2007). Group therapy to improve communicative participation in people with multiple sclerosis and dysarthria. *Way Ahead, 11*(2), 8–10.

Langenbahn, D. M., Sherr, R. L., Simon, D., & Hanig, B. (1999). Group psychotherapy. In K. G. Langer, L. Laatsch, & L. Lewis (Eds.), *Psychotherapeutic interventions for adults with brain injury or stroke: A clinician's treatment resource* (pp. 167–189). Madison, CT: Psychosocial Press.

Lindsay, T., & Orton, S. (2014). *Groupwork practice in social work.* London: SAGE.

Linton, S. J., & Andersson, T. (2000). Can chronic disability be prevented? A randomized trial of a cognitive-behavior intervention and two forms of information for patients with spinal pain. *Spine, 25*, 2825–2831.

Lizzio, A., & Wilson, K. (2001). Facilitating group beginnings II: From basic to working engagement. *Group Work, 13*(1), 30–56.

National Health Service England (2014). *Better Outcomes, better value: integrating physical and mental health into clinical practice and commissioning.* London: National Health Service England.

Nilsson, I., & Nygard, L. (2003). Geriatric rehabilitation: Elderly clients' experiences of a pre-discharge occupational therapy group programme. *Scandinavian Journal of Occupational Therapy, 10*(3), 107–117.

Okumiya, K., Morita, Y., Nishinaga, M., et al.(2005). Effects of group work programs on community-dwelling elderly people with age-associated cognitive decline and/or mild depressive moods: A Kahoku Longitudinal Ageing Study. *Geriatrics and Gerontology International, 5*(4), 267–275.

Pratto, F., Sidanius, J., & Levin, S. (2006). Social dominance theory and the dynamics of intergroup relations: Taking stock and looking forward. *European Review of Social Psychology, 17,* 271–320.

Sale, J., Gignac, M., & Hawker, G. (2008). The relationship between disease symptoms, life events, coping and treatment, and depression among older adults with osteoarthritis. *Journal of Rheumatology, 35*(2), 335–342.

Sharpe, M., Walker, J., Holm Hansen, C., Martin, P., Symeonides, S., Gourley, C., Wall, L., Weller, D., & Murray, G. (2014). Integrated collaborative care for comorbid major depression in patients with cancer (SMaRT Oncology-2): a multicentre randomised controlled effectiveness trial. *The Lancet, 384*(9948), 1099–1108.

Silver, J. M., McAllister, T. W., & Arciniegas, D. B. (2009). Depression and cognitive complaints following mild traumatic brain injury. *American Journal of Psychiatry, 166,* 653–661.

Simon, G. E., Katon, W. J., Lin, E. H. B., et al. (2007). Cost-effectiveness of systematic depression treatment among people with diabetes mellitus. *Archives of General Psychiatry, 64*(1), 65–72.

Spilak, C. (1999). Incorporating occupational therapy group treatment in long-term care. *Topics in Geriatric Rehabilitation, 15*(2), 48–55.

Stangor, C. (2004). *Social groups in action and interaction.* Abingdon: Taylor and Francis Books.

Tajfel, H., & Turner, J. C. (1979). An integrative theory of intergroup conflict. In S. Worchel, & W. G. Austin (Eds.), *The social psychology of intergroup relations* (pp. 33–47). Monterey, CA: Brooks-Cole.

Theis, K. A., Helmick, C. G., & Hootman, J. M. (2007). Arthritis burden and impact are greater among U.S. women than men: Intervention opportunities. *Journal of Women's Health, 16*(4), 441–453.

Tuckman, B. W. (1965). Developmental sequences in small groups. *Psychological Bulletin, 63,* 384–389.

Tyler, T. R., & Blader, S. L. (2000). *Co-operation in groups: procedural justice, social identity and behavioural engagement.* Philadelphia, PA: Psychology Press.

Vamos, E. P., Mucsi, I., Keszei, A., Kopp, M. S., & Novak, M. (2009). Comorbid depression is associated with increased healthcare utilization and lost productivity in persons with diabetes: A large nationally representative Hungarian population survey. *Psychosomatic Medicine, 71*(5), 501–507.

Ward, D. (2002). Groupwork. In R. Adams, L. Dominelli, & M. Payne (Eds.), *Social work: Themes, issues and critical debates* (2nd ed.). Basingstoke: Macmillan.

Welch, C. A., Czerwinski, D., Ghimire, B., & Bertsimas, D. (2009). Depression and costs of health care. *Psychosomatics, 50*(4), 392–401.

World Federation of Occupational Therapists (2011). *Standards of Proficiency.* Forrestfield: World Federation of Occupational Therapists.

Yalom, I. D. (1975). *The theory and practice of group psychotherapy* (2nd ed.). New York: Basic Books.

32

ENABLING SEXUALITY

NARELLE HIGSON

Abstract
Sexuality is a central aspect of being human and closely related to quality of life and well-being. More than just sexual activity, *sexuality* refers to the way people perceive their sexual self and how they communicate this to others through roles and occupations that may be fluid and vary over time. The ability to express aspects of sexual identity, give or receive sexual pleasure or engage in roles and occupations of choice related to the expression of sexuality may be affected by illness, injury or impairment and environmental factors. Despite the fact that addressing challenges with sexuality is an integral part of a person-centred approach, this area of practice is often overlooked as a therapy concern in both health care and community settings. By taking steps to increase confidence and competence, occupational therapists are well placed to use their skills to address sexuality within a team approach.

KEY POINTS

- The experience and expression of sexuality is unique to the individual and the individual's life circumstances.

443

- Sexuality may influence all areas of life, including occupations related to personal expression, community connection and vocation, not just sexual activity.

- Individuals may not indicate the potential personal importance they place on sexuality unless given the opportunity to do so.

- Taking simple steps to ensure supports are in place can assist therapists to include sexuality in practice in a confident and comfortable manner.

- The Recognition Model provides a framework for addressing sexuality and promotes a team approach.

- Exploring the meaning and value the individual attributes to sexual occupations and roles allows for the identification of acceptable outcomes for intervention.

- Occupational therapists are well suited to addressing sexuality, which is an integral aspect of person-centred practice.

INTRODUCTION

Sexuality involves the body, mind and spirit. It encompasses how people identify as sexual beings and the way people communicate this to the world. The value and meaning people attribute to the various roles and occupations associated with sexuality are uniquely personal and shaped by many things, including the time and place in which they live, their life experiences, their relationship with and knowledge of their bodies, and the choices and opportunities available to them to explore this aspect of themselves and others.

In 2002, the World Health Organization (WHO) produced a working definition of sexuality. Although it does not represent an official WHO standpoint, it serves as a useful guide for this chapter:

> Sexuality is a central aspect of being human throughout life and encompasses sex, gender identities and roles, sexual orientation, eroticism, pleasure, intimacy and reproduction. Sexuality is experienced and expressed in thoughts, fantasies, desires, beliefs, attitudes, values, behaviours, practices, roles and relationships. While sexuality can include all of these dimensions, not all of them are always experienced or expressed. Sexuality is influenced by the interaction of biological, psychological, social, economic, political, cultural, ethical, legal, historical, religious and spiritual factors.
> (World Health Organization, 2006, p. 5)

With the profession's understanding of the complex interplay between the person, occupation, and environment, occupational therapists are well placed to support and affirm the sexual health and rights of individuals or groups who may be facing limited choice, control or challenges with sexuality because of illness, injury, impairment, or life circumstances.

Rather than covering the specifics of sexual function, for which there are many excellent sources of learning, this chapter seeks to describe an occupational therapy approach to addressing the area of sexuality within professional practice, an area closely connected with occupations that may hold immense value and meaning for those people occupational therapists aim to support, occupations that are often overlooked in the face of competing therapy priorities.

The word *sexuality* is used in this chapter to encompass sexual health and function, the experience of being a sexual being and the roles and occupations involved with sexual expression. There are many different terms related to sexuality that are commonly used; definitions of some of these terms can be found in Table 32.1.

The chapter begins with a discussion about the diversity of sexuality, exploring the factors that may affect the ability of people to engage in meaningful sexual roles and occupations. This is followed by a consideration of occupational therapists' roles and the potential barriers they may encounter when addressing sexuality in practice. Useful steps to develop a therapist's confidence and competence to address issues of sexuality are provided, with the Recognition Model presented as a potential framework for addressing sexuality within practice. Finally, a brief outline of strategies to address specific sexuality concerns will end this chapter. As it is not possible to cover every aspect of sexuality and an occupational therapist's role, it is anticipated that this chapter will encourage the reader to seek and embrace further learning related to this area of practice.

SEXUALITY: DIVERSITY OF EXPERIENCES, MEANINGS, PURPOSES AND VALUES

Sexuality as a human occupation includes an incredible diversity of experiences, meanings, purposes and values. If asked to describe their understanding and experience of sexuality, some people would speak of the importance of touch and connection, comfort, warmth and tenderness, pleasure or nurturing. Other people may mention vulnerability, excitement, freedom or power. Some people may speak with indifference, whereas other people may do so with passion, or with guilt, or with a sense of loss or longing. Some people consider this area deeply private and will choose not to answer at all. Many things affect the experience of sexuality, including the opportunities individuals have to learn about and take pleasure in their bodies, and their ability to exert choice and control in how they express their sexuality or engage with others in a sexual way. The experience of sexuality is fluid and can change with time and life circumstances. For some, the experience and expression of sexuality is a positive one. For others living with limited choice and control, sexuality may be associated with anxiety, shame, pain or fear.

The experience of sexuality may influence the occupational choices people make. The time and effort people take to present themselves to the world as sexual beings, the occupations and

TABLE 32.1	
Definition of Common Sexuality Terms	
Sexual activities:	Any activities, engaged in alone or consensually with another person (or other people), that are considered to be sexual by the people engaging in them (Silverberg, n.d.).
Intimacy:	The sharing of private thoughts, ideas or actions with another, which leads to developing a close emotional connection.
Sexual identity:	How people define themselves sexually, including the behaviours, roles and occupations they choose to engage in; their sexual orientation and desires.
Sexual esteem:	A person's sense of self as a sexual being, which contributes to feeling capable and loveable.
Sexual orientation:	The gender that a person is romantically, emotionally and sexually attracted to. Beyond sexual activity, it is often linked with social and emotional connection, personal and political identity, culture and community affiliation (Beagan et al., 2012). Different terms are used to identify a person's sexual orientation. These terms include the following: ▪ Homosexual/gay/lesbian: attracted to people of the same gender ▪ Heterosexual: attracted to people of the opposite gender ▪ Bisexual: attracted to people of the same gender *and* people of the opposite gender ▪ Pansexual: does not limit sexual choice to any gender or gender identity ▪ Asexual: a person with no sexual feelings or desires Note: These terms are a very simplistic attempt to categorise something that may be fluid or vary over time.
Gender identity:	A person's internal experience of gender; a person's sense of being a male, female or other. This does not necessarily match biological gender or gender expression. The term *transgender* refers to someone who identifies as a different gender from that assigned at birth.

activities they choose to do, with whom and when, and even their choice of vocation may be influenced by their sexuality, and the meaning and value their sexuality holds for them (Devine & Nolan, 2007). The types of sexual activities people find pleasurable and desirable differ between individuals and may vary with time and context. Sexual activities may be solo activities, be undertaken independently or with assistance, or occur with a partner or many partners; they may take place within formal or casual relationships, outside of relationships, or as a professional transaction. Although some people may need to feel an intimate connection with another before engaging in sexual activities, other people may seek intimacy through engagement in sexual acts. For other individuals, intimacy may play no part in sexual pleasure at all. A variety of roles, identities, occupations and activities related to sexuality are listed in Fig. 32.1.

ROLE OF OCCUPATIONAL THERAPISTS IN ADDRESSING OCCUPATION OF SEXUALITY

The expression of sexuality is regarded as a fundamental human right (World Association for Sexual Health, 2014). The opportunity to experience intimacy and give or receive desired sexual pleasure contributes to a person's quality of life (McCabe, Cummins, & Deeks, 2000; O'Dea, Shuttleworth, & Wedgwood, 2012) and has been reported to provide both physical and mental health benefits. Physical health benefits may include a strengthened immune system, lower blood pressure, pain reduction, improved sleep, improved pelvic muscle function and increased cardiovascular health and physical fitness (Jannini, Fisher, Bitzer, & McMahon, 2009). Mental health benefits may include reduced isolation, reduced anxiety and depression, improved self-esteem and body image and improved bonding within intimate relationships (Brody, 2010).

The expression of sexuality is considered by Pollard and Sakellariou (2007) to be both an important human occupation and an occupational health need. For some individuals, the ability to engage in roles and occupations related to sexuality may be of a higher priority than other activities of daily living commonly targeted in therapy, such as walking, transferring, eating or writing (Couldrick, 2005). As person-centred practice involves enabling individuals to engage in occupations of importance, meaning and value when illness or impairment affects participation, occupational therapists should ensure that issues related to sexuality are addressed.

Whenever illness, injury or impairment or environmental barrier affects a person's ability to engage in valued occupations related to sexuality, there is a potential role for occupational therapy to assist (Couldrick, 2005). Therapists working in a variety of practice areas, such as primary care, residential care, community rehabilitation, health promotion and hospital settings have the opportunity to offer a safe space for people of all sexual orientations, identities and genders to explore sexual concerns and challenges. Once personal, environmental and occupational barriers and enablers have been identified, therapists use the same skills and strategies employed when addressing other activities of daily living.

The strategies employed by occupational therapists aim to enable people to engage in sexual roles and occupations as they

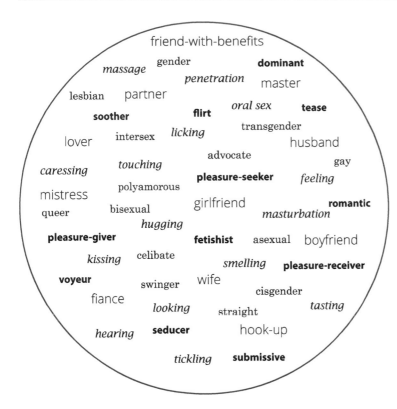

FIG. 32.1 ■ Roles, identities, occupations and activities related to sexuality.

would like in order to lead enjoyable and meaningful sexual lives. Despite the importance of this area, occupational therapists, and many other health professionals, often fail to address sexuality as a standard part of their practice (Dyer & das Nair, 2012; Hyland & McGrath, 2012; Kazukauskas & Lam, 2009). There are many reasons why professionals may not address sexuality as part of their practice; some of these reasons are listed in Box 32.1.

FACTORS THAT MAY AFFECT SEXUALITY

Personal Factors: Illness, Injury or Impairment

Living with illness, injury or impairment may have a profound impact on a person's self-esteem, body image, self-confidence and perception of attractiveness or worthiness as a sexual partner, which may lead to lower levels of well-being and sexual esteem (Brodwin & Frederick, 2010; Taleporos & McCabe, 2003). Changes in role dynamics, such as when an intimate partner transitions from a lover to carer role, may have a significant impact on personal relationships (Esmail, Esmail, & Munro, 2002; Hawkins et al., 2009). However, not all outcomes are negative. For some, the need for improved communication and the

exploration of different ways to experience sexual pleasure leads to gains in sexual self-acceptance, self-confidence and improved intimate relationships (Karlen, 2002).

Because of the diversity of human sexual experience, it is difficult to predict the potential impact illness, injury or impairment may have on an individual. A change in physical or cognitive function that creates barriers to participation for one person may have little impact on another person's ability to engage in roles and occupations of choice. Conversely, changes that may seem unimportant for one person may cause significant distress for another individual.

A useful method of exploring the potential impact of illness, injury or impairment on sexuality is to consider three levels of challenges: primary challenges, secondary challenges and tertiary challenges. Foley and Iverson (1992) originally presented these three levels as a conceptual model to describe the impact of multiple sclerosis on sexual activity. *Primary challenges* relate to changes in sexual response as a direct result of changes within the body's systems (e.g. nervous system, endocrine, cardiovascular), which directly affect the health and function of the genitals and sexual arousal system. *Secondary challenges* describe the impact of symptoms that are not directly related to sexual function or arousal but that may have significant impact on the ability to engage in sexual activities in an enjoyable and satisfying

BOX 32.1
BARRIERS THAT PROFESSIONALS MAY EXPERIENCE THAT WILL AFFECT ADDRESSING SEXUALITY ISSUES OF THE PEOPLE WITH WHOM THEY WORK

- Perceived lack of training and skills:
  - Not feeling equipped to confidently bring up the area without offending
  - Little knowledge regarding sexual expression and how illness, injury or impairment may affect sexual activities
  - Little exposure to relevant training; graduating from university without feeling equipped
- Cultural/religious values:
  - Fear of offending cultural/religious values of the individual
  - Therapist's own values and attitudes
- Assumed someone else will address the issues, or consider it to be someone else's role
- Fear of 'opening a can of worms':
  - Not able to assist/little knowledge of resources to assist
  - Causing harm to existing person–therapist relationship

- Not aware of potential importance:
  - Assumed it is not relevant/not a priority
  - Assumed if there were concerns they would be raised by the individual
- Not comfortable raising and talking about sexuality issues:
  - Allowing own values, attitudes and beliefs to affect intervention rather than honouring individual's concerns
  - Concerned about discussing intimate issues with a person who is a different age/gender than professional
- Unaware of policies (if they exist):
  - Unsure if intervention may be supported by the employer
- Lack of time/privacy

Sources: Dyer & das Nair, 2012; Gott, Galena, Hinchcliff, & Elford, 2004; Haboubi & Lincoln, 2003; Helland, Garratt, Kjeken, Kvien, & Dagfinrud, 2013.

way. *Tertiary challenges* describe the psychological, cultural and social impact of living with the condition and the toll this may take on sexual feelings and experiences.

It is important to note that the use of the words *primary, secondary* and *tertiary* does not imply that one area is more important than another. Examples related to each level of challenge are given in Table 32.2.

Environmental Factors

Environmental factors, whether cultural, institutional, physical or social, may act as an enabler or barrier to engaging in valued sexual occupations. Depending on a person's country of residence and the prevailing political, cultural or religious views, it may not be safe to openly engage in valued sexual roles and activities because of fear of discrimination or punishment. For people living in supported accommodation or reliant upon attendant care, the presence or absence of policies supporting sexual rights and the values and attitudes of staff may support or restrict the ability of residents to experience or express their sexuality. In addition, limited opportunities for socialisation, access to private space, time or practical assistance to engage in solo or partnered sexual activity may all affect a person's

TABLE 32.2
Examples Related to Foley and Iverson's (1992) Three Levels of Sexual Expression Challenges

Primary Challenges		Secondary Challenges	Tertiary Challenges
Male: - Difficulty attaining or maintaining an erection - Decrease in ejaculatory force or frequency Both genders: - Decrease or loss of sexual desire - Changes in genital sensation - Difficulties achieving orgasm	Female: - Reduced or absent lubrication - Decrease in clitoral engorgement	- Pain - Fatigue, reduced endurance - Tone changes, spasm - Movement limitations - Bladder and bowel issues - Sensory changes - Cognitive issues such as concentration, memory - Communication difficulties	- Changes in or loss of valued roles - Body image - Self-esteem - Mental health issues such as depression, anxiety - Sexual esteem - Sense of self

ability to exercise choice and control. Although people living with a visible physical impairment may face more social limitations and asexualising attitudes, those living with an invisible impairment (e.g. cognitive deficits after a brain injury) may be reluctant to put themselves in situations where they might encounter difficulties as a result of their impairment (Esmail, Darry, Walter, & Knupp, 2010). The introduction of assistive equipment into the physical environment, such as hospital-type beds, specialised seating, and mobility or communication aids, may affect the person's ability and desire to engage in sexual occupations and roles of choice (Taylor, 2011).

DEVELOPING READINESS TO ADDRESS SEXUALITY

To overcome some of the barriers therapists may face when addressing sexuality, it is useful to take some time to reflect, prepare and gather helpful resources. The Foundations for Addressing Sexuality Hierarchy (FAS Hierarchy), illustrated in Fig. 32.2, has been developed to assist therapists to become more equipped and ready to include sexuality as part of regular occupational therapy practice. Each of the levels of the hierarchy are explained in more detail next.

Values and Attitudes

Values and attitudes form the foundation of all levels of the hierarchy and influence practice. It is important to take time to become aware of and reflect on personal values and attitudes in relation to the expression of sexuality in all its diversity (Javaherian, Christy, & Boehringer, 2007; Kingsley & Molineux, 2000). This can be done through formal means, such as attending workshops or courses, or informal means such as reading and having discussions with

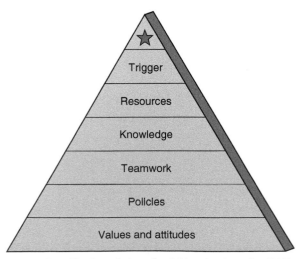

FIG. 32.2 ■ The Foundations for Addressing Sexuality (FAS) Hierarchy.

colleagues. The aim of this exploration is not to change a therapist's personal values or attitudes. Rather, the aim is for each therapist to recognise his or her own personal values and attitudes, to become aware of these and identify if and when these values and attitudes may affect working in a person-centred way.

Policies

Policies include not only the therapist's professional association and the work setting but also those governing the employment of support staff. If policies are not clearly stated and available, or are nonexistent, it will be left to individual therapists, teams or managers to determine what is appropriate in relation to supporting sexual expression (McConkey & Ryan, 2008); this may not always support the rights of the individual. To ensure health workers and support staff are supported in upholding sexual rights, it may be necessary to advocate for the development of policies where none exist.

Teamwork

As concerns related to sexuality may involve a complex interplay among biological, psychological and social factors, it is beneficial to draw upon the expertise of a multidisciplinary team to provide advice, support and an avenue for referral to address specific concerns when required (Couldrick, Sadlo, & Cross, 2010). Therapists working in isolated work settings may find it useful to develop connections through external or virtual networks to provide support and referral avenues.

Knowledge

To work in a holistic and inclusive way, it is useful to develop an awareness and understanding of the diverse range of occupations and roles related to sexuality and the way in which illness, injury or impairment might affect these. Is the illness, injury or impairment commonly seen in practice likely to affect sexual function, arousal or response, or will the challenges most likely be as a result of other personal issues, such as secondary or tertiary challenges? How might the different living environments play an enabling role or present barriers to engaging in desired sexual occupations? As with other activities of daily living closely linked with body functions (e.g. eating, toileting), it is useful to have a basic understanding of the body systems involved – in this case the physiological and psychological systems related to sexual function and arousal. Therapists are directed towards the many relevant written, online and course-based resources to develop their knowledge and understanding.

Resources

Resources that may be provided to individuals for learning and support include written, online and local services and peer support. It is important to check each resource for usefulness, as not all resources encourage recovery or address sexual concerns in a helpful manner (Hamam, McCluskey, & Cooper Robbins, 2013). Therapists should check if the information provided is useful, practical, relevant and written with the appropriate tone using accessible language. Many resources can be useful when introducing the topic or promoting discussion with a person's partner (Christopherson et al., 2006) but should not be relied upon as the sole source of information.

Therapists may develop a list of local services that can provide relevant information and support for people. Local services may include: sexual health services; relationship counselling; sex therapy services; physiotherapists specialising in pelvic issues or men's and women's health; lesbian, gay, bisexual, transgender, and intersex (LGBTI) support services; sex positive services, such as tantra coaches; and sex workers or sex work establishments with knowledge and experience in the disability sector.

Practical resources may relate to accessible equipment, such as toys and positioning aids. In addition to websites on these topics there are two downloadable publications developed by occupational therapists: *PleasurAble* and the *MA + Guide*. See the Further Reading section for information.

Trigger

Many health professionals find introducing the topic of sexual concerns more difficult than the discussion itself (Marsden & Botell, 2010). As a result, best intentions are often not enough to ensure the topic of sexuality is raised with every individual. There are a number of ways of formally building in opportunities to discuss sexual concerns in daily practice. Although formal prompts, such as including sexuality in assessments, may increase the likelihood that the topic will be raised (Marsden & Botell, 2010), informal methods of introducing the topic in conversation are also useful. Some examples of informal methods of introducing the topic in conversation can be found in Table 32.3.

A key message is 'never assume'. Never assume that it is not necessary to offer the opportunity to discuss sexual concerns because the individual may have other priorities or is too ill, old, tired, or impaired, or because of a person's relationship status. It is not possible to know if a person's sexuality and its expression is a significant and valued part of his or her life without consulting the person. It is also important not to make assumptions regarding sexual orientation, gender identity or preferences in sexual activities. The use of inclusive language, such as using the word *partner* until the gender of the partner is known, and ensuring that the pronouns individuals use to refer to themselves and their partners are used, is a way of developing respectful and inclusive practice habits.

Intervention

The star at the top of the hierarchy relates to implementation of the therapy process, which is described in the next section.

Once steps have been taken to become aware of personal values and attitudes, ensure that policies are in place, skills and resources of the team are identified, knowledge is developed, resources are gathered and a trigger is in place to assist with introducing the topic, the therapist will be in a sound position to use

TABLE 32.3
Examples of Triggers That Can Be Used to Initiate a Discussion Related to Sexuality Issues

Type of Trigger	Example of Using the Trigger
Part of role description	*'As an occupational therapist I am able to assist you in getting back to doing the occupations you would like to be able to do, such as returning to work, driving, sexual or intimate activities, meal preparation …'* Note: the choice of wording will vary according to context and the personalities involved. Including sexuality within the description of the occupational therapy role lets individuals know it is acceptable and appropriate to bring up concerns.
Normalising	*'Often people I see who have had a total hip replacement have questions about returning to intimate activities. If you would like to discuss this at any stage, please feel free to let me know.'*
Included as part of formal assessment	When using the Canadian Occupational Performance Measure, the person may need guidance or permission to include this under leisure/recreation or self-care or productivity.
Screening assessment/ checklists	Screening tools can be adapted to include items related to sexuality.
Posters/brochures	Advertising the possibility of discussing sexual concerns may be placed in prominent locations or provided to all service users.

enabling skills and strategies to address challenges related to sexuality with a greater degree of confidence and competence.

ADDRESSING SEXUALITY IN PRACTICE: THE RECOGNITION MODEL

The Recognition Model is a five-stage model developed by British occupational therapist Lorna Couldrick after her extensive study with community disability teams (Couldrick, Sadlo, & Cross, 2010). Couldrick et al. propose that if health professionals recognise that all people are sexual beings, they are more likely to introduce and address the area of sexuality in practice and be prepared for any unexpected questions related to sexual concerns (Couldrick et al., 2010). Couldrick et al. suggest that using the available skills of a multidisciplinary team enables most concerns to be dealt with without the need for referral to a specialist service. The stages of the Recognition Model are listed and applied to Jon and Cate in Practice Story 32.1 and Table 32.4.

PRACTICE STORY 32.1

Jon and Cate

Jon, 30 years old, lived with his fiancé, Cate. Jon was diagnosed with multiple sclerosis (MS) 2 months ago and had to stop working as a mechanic in the mining industry because of heat exacerbating his symptoms of leg weakness and vision loss. He was on the waiting list to see the MS counsellor to assist with depression. He watched TV all day and was unable to find motivation to leave the house.

During her initial home visit to Jon and Cate, Lisa, an occupational therapist, asked if the many challenges Jon was facing were having an impact on their intimate relationship. Cate answered, reporting that Jon had suggested she seek sex elsewhere, as he felt unable to satisfy her and things were not likely to improve. Cate was not interested in doing this and indicated that Jon's suggestion had dampened her desire.

When Lisa asked why Jon felt this way, he remarked that sexual activity had previously been a very important and regular part of their life together. He enjoyed taking an active role; however, he stated that he lost his erection and the sensation in his legs with no warning, often in 'mid-flight'. When this happened he said that he was unable to continue. Lisa asked if this happened every time, and Jon and Cate said that it happened often. They both recalled one time outside late at night when things had gone well (even though Cate 'was freezing!').

Lisa pointed out that MS symptoms often increased with heat or fatigue and asked if they thought this could be a factor; Jon and Cate agreed this was very likely.

Jon visibly relaxed and suggested that he might be able to take a less active role at times if that would help. The discussion became a brainstorming session around possible ways to keep cool. Lisa suggested trying positions where their bodies were farther apart when things heated up. Cate suggested using a pedestal fan, and Jon, smiling, remarked they could try outside again.

After this, Lisa outlined other options for managing Jon's erectile difficulties, which she explained might be directly related to his spinal lesions, which were also affecting his legs. Options included trying a penis ring, as they could be useful if a person was able to attain but not maintain an erection, and seeing his doctor if he wished to try oral medication. Lisa pointed out this medication only affected blood flow, not desire; hence mental or physical stimulation was required for the medication to work. She suggested that if Jon wanted to try these options he could try them alone first to see what it was like and to remove the need to 'perform'.

Cate remarked that for the first time in a long time Jon seemed enthusiastic about something.

TABLE 32.4

Applying the Recognition Model to Jon and Cate's Practice Story

Recognition Model Stage	Example of Stage When Working with Jon
Stage 1: Recognition of the service user as a sexual being	Recognising the fact that Jon is a sexual being helped Lisa become aware of and consider the potential impact of multiple sclerosis and resulting role changes on Jon's sexuality. Her acknowledgement of the fact that issues are to be expected normalised his concerns.
Stage 2: Permission to discuss sexual concerns	Lisa was able to use the informal nature of the setting and conversation to introduce the topic. If Jon had indicated that he did not wish to discuss his concerns, Lisa would have respected this and informed him that he could follow up in the future if desired (with another team member if preferred) and offered resources.
Stage 3: Exploration of sexual concern	Lisa was quickly able to determine that sexual activities were a central part of this couples' life, and being able to satisfy his partner sexually and take an active role in sexual activities was important to Jon. It became evident that some aspect of the environment or the activity (heat and fatigue) might be affecting Jon's ability to be active. It was also likely that personal factors, such as anxiety about his ability to satisfy Cate and depression as a result of his loss of roles, such as being an active worker and financial contributor to the house, added to his difficulties.
Stage 4: Addressing issues within the team's boundaries and expertise	Through collaboration with Jon and Cate, Lisa was able to discuss some potential strategies to enable Jon to address barriers and achieve his goal: to participate in sexual activities in the manner in which he would like. The usefulness and effectiveness of these strategies, to be followed up at their next meeting, would inform the direction of any future intervention.
Stage 5: Referral if necessary	As there were many possible contributing factors to Jon's erectile difficulties, including nerve damage, a trial of medication was suggested as an option, requiring referral to a medical practitioner. If Jon wished to investigate other options (e.g. injections), a referral to a urologist would be required.

Stage 1: Recognition of the Service User as a Sexual Being

The recognition of a person as a sexual being is the foundation for all areas of practice, enabling challenges related to sexuality to be acknowledged, normalised, validated and addressed in a proactive manner (Couldrick et al., 2010). Failure to recognise the sexuality of the person may result in an asexualising approach, even without intending to do so.

The following is an example of recognition:

▪ Acknowledging that replacing a double bed with a single adjustable bed may introduce a barrier to intimacy and discussing concerns and possible solutions to address this.

The following is an example of lack of recognition:

▪ A woman with incomplete tetraplegia being seen at home after discharge from rehabilitation reported to the community therapist that the only mention of sexuality in rehabilitation was in a group session, where they were advised that 'Women were fortunate, as nothing changes'. This view of sexuality, in which it is equated solely to reproduction or sexual function, fails to recognise the challenges presented by secondary and tertiary impacts of disability on the diverse experience and expression of sexuality.

Stage 2: Permission to Discuss Sexual Concerns

Individuals often expect health professionals to introduce the topic of sexuality (Gianotten, Bender, Post, & Höing, 2006). There are many ways of opening the discussion in a sensitive way that respects privacy if the person does not wish to discuss sexual issues. Some options are outlined in Table 32.3.

There is no clear guidance from research regarding the best time to address sexual concerns. Whereas some individuals would like information soon after the time of trauma, others prefer to access support just before discharge from hospital or shortly after (Leibowitz, 2005). Those living with chronic conditions may benefit from receiving support at any time (Kedde, Van de Wiel, Weijmar Schultz, Vanwesenbeek, & Bender, 2010). The most appropriate time is when it best suits the person.

It is important to inform each person that conversations will remain confidential and will not be disclosed to others without their expressed permission. Exceptions to this are where activities are outside the law or could endanger lives. In these cases it is important for therapists to refer to workplace policies for guidance.

It must be remembered that some people will not be interested in seeking assistance with concerns, or discussing matters related to sexuality. In this case it may be helpful to offer written resources and advise that assistance can be sought in the future.

Stage 3: Exploration of Sexual Concern/ Assessment

Whereas a sex therapy approach to initial assessment may be the taking of a detailed sexual history, occupational therapists typically reverse this and adopt a 'top-down' approach. Assessment is concerned with getting enough information to understand how the illness, injury or impairment may be affecting valued roles and occupations associated with sexuality. At this time there are no formal standardised assessments that specifically evaluate sexuality and intimacy from an occupational focus.

Evaluation may be an ongoing process if the practice setting permits. Thoughtful, respectful and sensitive enquiry may reveal more information with time, as some individuals require time and space to feel comfortable disclosing what is often seen as private information. Taking the time to listen in a nonjudgemental manner and resisting the urge to jump in with solutions is a skill that develops with practice and confidence and is an important part of the evaluation process. Examples of questions that may assist in determining the value and meaning of sexual expression and potential barriers and enablers to engaging in activities of choice are provided in Box 32.2.

Therapists will develop their own wording to guide enquiry that feels comfortable, which will vary according to the practice context. Even though taking time to practice asking questions

---

BOX 32.2
EXAMPLES OF GENERAL ASSESSMENT QUESTIONS THAT FOCUS ON POSSIBLE ISSUES OF SEXUALITY

▪ Are you able to participate in sexual activities of your choice in the way you would like? If not, is this a concern for you?
▪ Has this changed since your illness, injury or impairment? If so, is this a concern?
▪ What is it about this issue that causes the most concern?
▪ What are your goals?
▪ What is your understanding of the issue?
▪ Are you currently taking any medications?
▪ How long have you had this issue? Did anything happen around that time (life event/change in medication, etc.)?
▪ What have you tried to address the issue; what worked/what did not work?
▪ Who have you seen (e.g. urologist, counsellor) for assistance? Are they currently involved?
▪ Does your partner (if applicable) have any issues related to sexual activities?
▪ Is the issue always present, or only at certain times/in certain situations?
▪ Have you found anything that has made it better/worse (e.g. different timing, positions, etc.)?
▪ Do symptoms such as pain, fatigue, sensory changes or movement limitations ever interfere with satisfaction in sexual or intimate activities or participating in sexual activities of your choice as you would like?

like these of friends and family may seem awkward or artificial, it is a worthwhile exercise to develop comfort if these types of discussions are unfamiliar.

If it is determined at this stage that the team does not have the expertise to assist, referral to specialist services for further assessment or management may be appropriate.

Stage 4: Addressing of Issues Within the Team's Boundaries and Expertise

As with other areas of practice, the occupational concerns of the individual will inform therapy goals. Measurable occupation-focused goals developed in collaboration with the individual that related to sexuality may include the following:

- Developing knowledge of the impact of the illness, injury or impairment on sexual expression
- Developing strategies or procedures to overcome barriers and enable engagement in sexual occupations of choice
- Developing self-esteem, sexual esteem and body image
- Adapting to role changes
- Developing communication skills related to intimate matters
- Increasing repertoire of pleasurable behaviours and activities
- Reducing isolation by improving opportunities for socialisation

Examples of enabling skills and strategies that may be of use are outlined in the following section.

Stage 5: Referral as Necessary

Referral requires a knowledge of the wider services available that may be able to assist (see FAS Hierarchy: resources). This may involve advocating for accessible services where none currently exist or providing expertise related to the illness, injury or impairment to enable the person to gain the best outcome from using community sexuality services (Couldrick et al., 2010).

INTERVENTION: ENABLING SKILLS AND STRATEGIES FOR ADDRESSING SEXUALITY

Having introduced the subject of sexuality as a topic for discussion, identified barriers and enablers to engaging in related valued roles and occupations, and determined which outcomes are meaningful to the individual, intervention focuses on finding acceptable ways of achieving those outcomes.

Although occupational therapists may not be directly involved in the management of primary challenges related to sexual function, having an understanding of the various management options that may assist is useful for both discussion with the person and to determine when referral to other team members or specialist services is needed. An outline of primary sexual challenges management options are provided in Box 32.3.

BOX 32.3
INTERVENTION STRATEGIES TO ADDRESS PRIMARY CHALLENGES

ERECTILE DIFFICULTIES (ED)

- **Education/assessment:** Impact of the illness, injury or impairment and/or aging (may take longer to get an erection, may not be as firm, may not be maintained for penetration). Seek medical assessment to rule out cardiovascular disease or other health conditions, as erectile difficulties may be an early indicator.
- **Oral therapies:** Phosphodiesterase type 5 inhibitors prescribed by general practitioners are often the first treatment of choice. These drugs (e.g. sildenafil (Viagra), tadalafil (Cialis), vardenafil (Levitra)) work in similar ways, vary in half-life (6–24 hours) and require the individual to engage in sexual stimulation (mental or physical) to take effect. They do not increase libido.
- **Penis ring:** These may be of use if an erection can be attained but not maintained. A ring (stretchy or rigid) is placed around the base of the penis (some also surround the scrotum), which restricts blood flow out, maintaining the erection. Must not be left in place longer than 20–30 minutes; each person should ascertain their appropriate length of time.
- **Vacuum erection devices:** These produce an erection by using negative pressure to draw blood into the penis. A preloaded ring is then slipped onto the base of the penis.

- **Injection:** A smooth muscle–relaxing drug is injected into the side of the penis, resulting in increased blood flow and an erection. The discomfort caused by this has been likened to self-catheterising and is generally well tolerated. Usually highly effective and often trialled if oral medication is not useful.
- **Penile implant surgery:** This invasive, irreversible procedure is usually effective, producing reliable erections when desired. The corpora cavernosa within the penis are replaced with an inflatable or semi-rigid prosthesis.
- **Sex therapy/counselling:** This is particularly beneficial when the erectile dysfunction is thought to be due to psychological/relationship factors.
- **Pelvic floor exercises:** These may improve erectile and orgasmic response.
- **Vibrators:** These may induce erection/orgasm when used around the penis, perineum, anus or prostate area.
- **Strap-on dildos:** These may offer a suitable alternative for some wishing to engage in penetrative activities. They may be strapped over the flaccid or semi-erect penis or attached to another body part (e.g. thigh). See *PleasurAble* and the *MA + Guide* for examples.
- **Nonpenetrative activities**: These include sensual massage, exploring other areas of the body that may be receptive

> ## BOX 32.3
> ## INTERVENTION STRATEGIES TO ADDRESS PRIMARY CHALLENGES *(Continued)*
>
> to erotic touch, tantric sex practices, oral sex and mutual masturbation. The person may benefit from encouragement to look beyond the 'genital friction' view of sex and include a wider variety of sensual and sexual activities as part of sex play. Sex therapy may assist.
>
> ### DECREASED VAGINAL LUBRICATION
>
> - **Lubricants:** Commercially available water- or silicone-based lubricants have varying consistencies and drying times (5 minutes to >1 hour), which may suit different activities. Note: Silicone lubricant must not be used with silicone toys (as it will cause the silicone of the toy to break down).
> - **Hormone replacement therapy/oestrogen cream**: This is used if dryness is hormone or menopause related. Vaginal moisturisers may also be of use.
> - **Pelvic floor exercises:** May be of use to improve arousal and orgasmic response.
> - **Ensure adequate foreplay/arousal:** Many women require at least 20 mins of foreplay to ensure adequate arousal for comfortable penetration.
> - **Explore nonpenetrative activities:** See erectile difficulties.
>
> ### REDUCED LIBIDO
>
> - **Identify cause:** If possible. Sexual desire is a complex interplay of many factors, including medication, satisfaction with previous sexual encounters, physiological and psychological/relationship issues.
> - **Education:** Sexual desire is not a prerequisite for sexual pleasure; it is possible to experience sexual pleasure in the absence of desire, or for desire to develop in response to arousal. Referral to sex therapy/relationship counselling may be useful.
> - **Mindfulness techniques:** tuning in to arousal response of self and/or partner
> - **'Keep the battery charged':** Some find it useful to take time to regularly fantasise, read or view erotic material to boost or maintain desire.
> - **Environmental cues:** As identified by the individual, these may assist – for example, low light.
> - **Explore and prioritise:** If with a partner(s), explore activities enjoyed together that fostered an increase in desire early in the relationship. Plan opportunities to revisit these: date nights, scheduling time together, organising babysitters, etc.

Because of the shortness of this chapter, the following strategies primarily address practical concerns. However, it should be acknowledged that this is just one small part of sexuality. Issues such as self-esteem, body image, adapting to role changes and enabling opportunities to develop social and meaningful relationships are all appropriate areas for occupational therapists to make a significant and valuable contribution.

Education

Education is used to address gaps in knowledge and may include topics such as healthy sexual function, the potential impact of illness, injury or impairment on sexuality and its expression, safe sex practices and the impact of aging. It may be provided face-to-face, through virtual means (e.g. email, Skype), through resource provision or via contact with a peer mentor or peer group. Education may be targeted towards individuals, groups, partners or support staff.

The following are examples of education interventions:

- Group sessions addressing return to sexual activity after surgery
- The provision of resources related to how conditions such as diabetes, Parkinson's disease, arthritis or cancer and the treatment of these conditions may affect sexuality

- Training session for residential facility staff on sexual health and rights

Remediation

Remediation interventions that relate to sexuality issues may include improving a person's balance, strength, endurance or sensation and the development of motor and cognitive skills to enable participation in activities of choice.

The following are examples of remediation interventions:

- Practising transfers in and out of sexual positions after spinal cord injury
- Improving strength and balance to enable active participation in sexual activities after limb amputation
- Developing proficiency in using public transport after a stroke to enable participation in gay pride events and social groups

Compensation

Compensation strategies may aim at changing the task, introducing assistive equipment or changing the environment. This may include expanding the individual's view and repertoire of sexual activities, exploring alternative or adapted methods of experiencing and giving sensual and sexual pleasure, introducing positioning aids and negotiating practical support if required (Fig. 32.3).

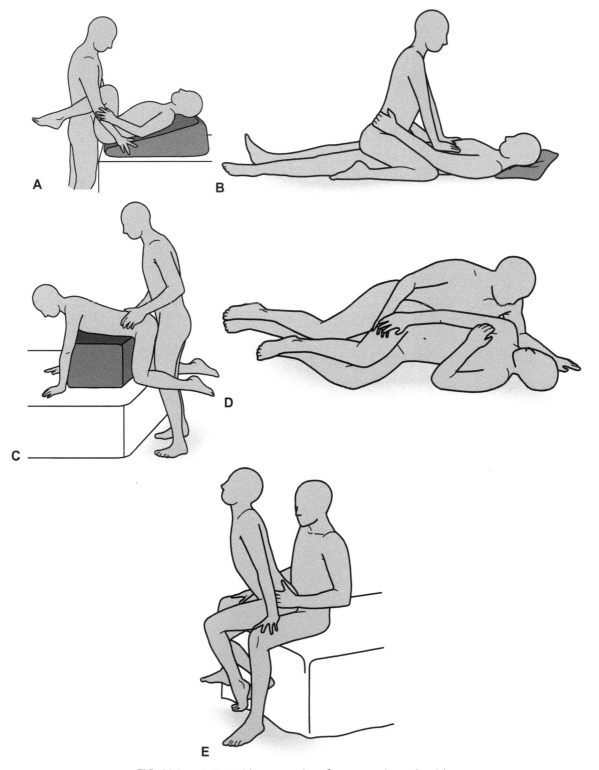

FIG. 32.3 ■ A–E, Position suggestions for partnered sexual activity.

The following are examples of compensation interventions:

- Body mapping to learn areas of pleasurable sensation after recovery from burns
- Exploring low-vision aids that may enable a transgender woman with vision impairment to apply makeup to her satisfaction
- The use of a vibrator to increase sensation for a woman with multiple sclerosis

A number of general compensation strategies that may be used to address challenges with sexual activity are listed in Table 32.5, with strategies to address specific areas of concern presented in Table 32.6.

Advocacy

The enabling skill of advocacy is useful when negotiating with services, health workers, or family regarding roles and responsibilities related to supporting sexual health and rights of individuals or groups.

The following are examples of using advocacy as an intervention:

- The right for residents to access erotica in supported accommodation
- Negotiating private time, space and practical support to allow a person to either self-pleasure or have time with a sexual partner
- Supporting an individual's right to make decisions and choices related to sexual expression

---

TABLE 32.5
General Compensation Strategies

Person Factors

Mindfulness training	Research suggests practicing mindfulness may enable tuning in to physiological arousal, body sensations, managing the sensation of pain, thoughts related to negative body image, anxiety, depression and overall well-being (Brotto et al., 2008; Silverstein, Brown, Roth, & Britton, 2011).
Body mapping	Body mapping refers to the systematic identifying of areas of the body that may be receptive to sensual/pleasurable touch and determining which type of touch is most pleasing (e.g. light, firm, soft or rough textures) in order to identify/reidentify pleasure zones. This information may then be shared with a partner if applicable.
Communication	The importance of clear communication related to sexual matters within a relationship to avoid misunderstanding, share concerns and seek or provide support cannot be underestimated. Individuals and partners may need support and assistance to develop communication skills.

Environment Factors

	Room temperature, ambient sounds and lighting may act as barriers or enablers to sexual expression.
	Sensory cues such as music, lighting, aromas, lingerie or visual / written / audio erotica may be useful. Privacy and the availability of practical assistance, if required, may need to be negotiated.

Occupation/Participation Factors

Toys	Toys are available in a variety of materials, shapes and sizes for use internally and externally and in solo or partnered play. Considerations about which toys to use include ease of use (e.g. managing controls, ease of holding on to/positioning, replacement of batteries/managing recharging), cleaning, privacy (noise, storage) and safety of construction materials. Toys may be useful to do the following: ■ Provide increased or varied sensation ■ Reduce dexterity or energy demands of the activity ■ Provide pleasure in solo or partnered play where motor control or reach may be limited ■ Introduce variety into sexual play Refer to Further Reading for more information.
Exploration of potential activities that may meet personal goals	Expanding the individual's view and repertoire of sexual activities and exploring alternative methods of experiencing and giving sensual and sexual pleasure (e.g. mutual masturbation, massage, 'cuddle date') can be helpful compensation strategies.

TABLE 32.6

Compensation Strategies for Specific Physical Issues

Issue	Compensation Strategy Suggestions
Bladder/bowel issues	■ Plan sexual activity around bladder/bowel routine; empty bladder and bowel before engaging in sexual activity, restrict fluids before planned activity. ■ Penetrative sexual activities are possible with an indwelling catheter. The catheter bag can be drained and secured to the thigh and tubing taped securely to avoid pulling. Refer to a continence specialist for further advice. ■ Using furniture protection such as bed pads, draw sheets and purpose-designed waterproof throws or towels may lessen washing and assist with continence concerns. ■ Experiment with positions to avoid placing pressure on bladder or catheter (see Fig. 32.3A–E).
Fatigue/reduced endurance	■ Investigate if sleep issues may be contributing to fatigue, such as poor sleep routines or insomnia. Many neurological conditions are associated with high prevalence of sleep disorders, so referral for sleep assessment may be appropriate. ■ If possible, plan sexual activity to coincide with the time of greatest energy (e.g. for some people, this may be the morning). Employ usual fatigue management strategies before planned activity (e.g. rest, use of assistive equipment to reduce effort throughout the day, pacing). ■ Use positioning supports such as firm cushions, adjustable bed if appropriate to support the body and lessen the energy demands (see Fig. 32.3A, B, and E). Alternate active positions/activities with less active positons/activities. ■ Assistive equipment such as the Intimate Rider or swings/slings may enable active participation while reducing energy demands. Similarly the use of toys, such as vibrators, may decrease energy or time requirements, which may be suitable for some individuals.
Pain/spasm	■ Medication for pain or spasm can be timed to ensure greatest effectiveness for planned sexual activity. Employ usual management strategies before activity that may be beneficial, such as stretches, massage, warm bath/shower. ■ Explore positions and/or positioning supports that may reduce spasm – for example, extensor spasm in the lower limbs may be reduced by choosing positions that involve hip and knee flexion (see Fig. 32.3A, C, and E). ■ Open communication with the partner is particularly valuable when pain is an issue.
Mobility/balance issues	■ Postural supports may assist when mobility limitations, balance, tone or reduced endurance cause challenges with attaining or maintaining positions. ■ Adjustable beds, cushions, pillows, rolled towels, rails and purpose-designed cushions may all be of assistance depending on the person's preferred activities. Other assistive technology such as off-the-shelf or customised slings, harnesses, swings, hoists, wheelchairs or specialised furniture may be useful. ■ Consider safety aspects such as load capacity. ■ Explore positions that offer stability, such as lying, leaning or all fours (see Fig. 32.3A–E). ■ Accessible toys may assist in overcoming dexterity or reach limitations affecting engaging in solo or partnered activities. Refer to Further Reading section for more information.
Sensory changes	■ Body mapping may be useful to identify areas of the body receptive to pleasurable touch (see Table 32.6). ■ If sensation is decreased, it is important to be aware of the possibility of skin or tissue damage. Experimenting with toys such as vibrators or textured fabrics may be of use. ■ Where increased sensation causes challenges, explore positions or alternative activities that reduce contact in those areas while still meeting personal goals.

CONCLUSION

The experience and expression of sexuality is unique to the individual.

Occupational therapists have a useful role to play in identifying valued occupations and roles related to sexuality that may be affected by a illness, injury or impairment and working with the person to achieve satisfactory outcomes. Although not all therapists feel comfortable addressing this area, sexual concerns may be a priority for the individual and acknowledging and addressing these in therapy is part of person-centred practice. As with other areas of occupational therapy, confidence and competence grows with practise and when therapists ensure work supports, knowledge and resources are in place. The Recognition Model provides a useful framework for addressing sexual concerns as part of a multidisciplinary team.

Although occupational therapy as a profession is well suited to play a significant role in addressing challenges related to sexuality from an occupational perspective, targeted research that may be used to inform evidence-based practice has not yet taken place, providing much potential for development of the role and value of occupational therapy and sexuality in the future.

 http://evolve.elsevier.com/Curtin/OT

REFERENCES

Beagan, B. L., Souza de, L., Godbout, C., et al. (2012). This is the biggest thing you'll ever do in your life': Exploring the occupations of transgendered people. *Journal of Occupational Science*, *19*(3), 226–240.

Brodwin, M. G., & Frederick, P. C. (2010). Sexuality and societal beliefs regarding persons living with disabilities. *Journal of Rehabilitation*, *76*(4), 37–41.

Brody, S. (2010). The relative health benefits of different sexual activities. *International Society for Sexual Medicine*, *7*, 1336–1361.

Brotto, L. A., Heiman, J. R., Goff, B., et al. (2008). A psychoeducational intervention for sexual dysfunction in women with gynecologic cancer. *Archives of Sexual Behavior*, *37*, 317–329.

Christopherson, J. M., Moore, K., Foley, F. W., & Warren, K. G. (2006). A comparison of written materials vs. materials and counselling for women with sexual dysfunction and multiple sclerosis. *Journal of Clinical Nursing*, *15*, 742–750. http://dx.doi.org/10.1111/j.1365-2702.2005.01437.x.

Couldrick, L. (2005). Sexual expression and occupational therapy. *British Journal of Occupational Therapy*, *68*(7), 315–318.

Couldrick, L., Sadlo, G., & Cross, V. (2010). Proposing a new sexual health model of practice for disability teams: The recognition model. *International Journal of Therapy and Rehabilitation*, *17*(6), 290–299.

Devine, R., & Nolan, C. (2007). Sexual identity and human occupation: A qualitative exploration. *Journal of Occupational Science*, *14*(3), 154–161.

Dyer, K., & das Nair, R. (2012). Why don't healthcare professionals talk about sex? A systematic review of recent qualitative studies conducted in the United Kingdom. *Journal of Sexual Medicine*, *10*(11), 2658–2670.

Esmail, S., Darry, K., Walter, A., & Knupp, H. (2010). Attitudes and perceptions towards disability and sexuality. *Disability and Rehabilitation*, *32*(14), 1148–1155.

Esmail, S., Esmail, Y., & Munro, B. (2002). Sexuality and disability: The role of health care professionals in providing options and alternatives of couples. *Sexuality and Disability*, *19*(4), 267–828.

Foley, F. W., & Iverson, J. (1992). Sexuality and multiple sclerosis. In R. C. Kalb, & L. C. Scheinberg (Eds.), *Multiple sclerosis and the family* (pp. 63–82). New York: Demos.

Gianotten, W. L., Bender, J. L., Post, M. W., & Höing, M. (2006). Training in sexology for medical and paramedical professionals: A model for the rehabilitation setting. *Sexual and Relationship Therapy*, *21*(3), 303–317.

Gott, M., Galena, E., Hinchcliff, S., & Elford, H. (2004). 'Opening a can of worms': GP and practice nurse barriers to talking about sexual health in primary care. *Family Practice*, *21*(5), 528–536.

Jannini, E. A., Fisher, W. A., Bitzer, J., & McMahon, C. G. (2009). Is sex just fun? How sexual activity improves health. *Journal of Sexual Medicine*, *6*(10), 2640–2648.

Haboubi, N. H. J., & Lincoln, N. (2003). Views of health professionals on discussing sexual issues with patients. *Disability and Rehabilitation*, *25*(6), 291–296.

Hamam, N., McCluskey, A., & Cooper Robbins, S. (2013). Sex after stroke: A content analysis of printable educational materials available online. *International Journal of Stroke*, *8*(7), 518–528.

Hawkins, Y., Ussher, J., Gilbert, E., Perz, J., Sandoval, M., & Sundquist, K. (2009). Changes in sexuality and intimacy after the diagnosis and treatment of cancer: The experience of partners in a sexual relationship with a person with cancer. *Cancer Nursing*, *32*(4), 271–280.

Helland, Y., Garratt, A., Kjeken, I., Kvien, T. K., & Dagfinrud, H. (2013). Current practice and barriers to the management of sexual issues in rheumatology: Results of a survey of health professionals. *Scandinavian Journal of Rheumatology*, *42*(1), 20–26.

Hyland, A., & McGrath, M. (2012). Sexuality and occupational therapy in Ireland: A case of ambivalence? *Disability and Rehabilitation*, *35*(1), 73–80.

Javaherian, H., Christy, A. B., & Boehringer, M. (2007). Occupational therapy practitioners' comfort level and preparedness in working with individuals who are gay, lesbian, or bisexual. *Journal of Allied Health*, *37*(3), 150–155.

Karlen, A. (2002). Positive sexual effects of chronic illness: case studies of women with lupus (SLE). *Sexuality and Disability*, *20*(3), 191–208.

Kazukauskas, K. A., & Lam, C. S. (2009). Importance of addressing sexuality in certified rehabilitation counselor practice. *Rehabilitation Education*, *23*(2), 127–140.

Kedde, H., Van de Wiel, H. B., Weijmar Schultz, W. C., Vanwesenbeek, W. M., & Bender, J. L. (2010). Efficacy of sexological healthcare for people with chronic diseases and physical disabilities. *Journal of Sex and Marital Therapy*, *36*(3), 282–294.

Kingsley, P., & Molineux, M. (2000). True to our philosophy? Sexual orientation and occupation. *British Journal of Occupational Therapy*, *63*(5), 205–210.

Leibowitz, R. Q. (2005). Sexual rehabilitation services after spinal cord injury: What do women want? *Sexuality and Disability*, *23*(2), 81–107.

Marsden, R., & Botell, R. (2010). Discussing sexuality with patients in a motor neurone disease clinic. *Nursing Standard*, *25*(15–17), 40–46.

McCabe, M. P., Cummins, R. A., & Deeks, A. A. (2000). Sexuality and quality of life among people with physical disability. *Sex and Disability*, *18*(2), 115–123.

McConkey, R., & Ryan, D. (2008). Experiences of staff in dealing with client sexuality in services for teenagers and adults with intellectual disability. *Journal of Intellectual Disability Research*, *45*(1), 83–87.

Pollard, N., & Sakellariou, D. (2007). Sex and occupational therapy: Contradictions or contraindications? *British Journal of Occupational Therapy*, *70*(8), 362–365.

O'Dea, S. M., Shuttleworth, R. P., & Wedgwood, N. (2012). Disability, doctors and sexuality: Do healthcare providers influence the sexual wellbeing of people living with a neuromuscular disorder? *Sexuality and Disability, 30*(2), 171–185.

Silverberg, C. (n.d.). *Sexual activities list.* Retrieved from http://sexuality. about.com/od/sexinformation/a/Sexual-Activities-List.htm.

Silverstein, R. G., Brown, A. H., Roth, H. D., & Britton, W. B. (2011). Effects of mindfulness training on body awareness to sexual stimuli: Implications for female sexual dysfunction. *Psychosomatic Medicine, 73*(9), 817–825.

Taleporos, G., & McCabe, M. P. (2003). Relationships, sexuality and adjustment among people with physical disability. *Sexual and Relationship Therapy, 18,* 25–43.

Taylor, B. (2011). The impact of assistive equipment on intimacy and sexual expression. *British Journal of Occupational Therapy, 74*(9), 435–442.

World Association for Sexual Health. (2014). *Declaration of sexual rights.* Retrieved from, http://www.worldsexology.org/wpcontent/uploads/2013/08/declaration_of_sexual_rights_sep03_2014.pdf.

World Health Organization. (2006). *Defining sexual health: Report of a technical consultation on sexual health 28-31 January 2002 (67).* Retrieved from, http://www.who.int/reproductivehealth/topics/gender_rights/defining_sexual_health.pdf?ua=1.

FURTHER READING

Joannides, P. J. (2013). *Guide to getting it on* (7th ed.). Waldport, OR: Goofy Foot Press.

Kaufman, M., Silverberg, C., & Odette, F. (2007). *The ultimate guide to sex and disability: For all of us who live with disabilities, chronic pain, and illness.* San Francisco: Cleis Press.

Kroll, K., & Levy Klein, E. (1995). *Enabling romance: A guide to love, sex, and relationships for the disabled (and the people who care about them).* Bethesda, MD: Woodbine House.

Tepper, M. (2015). *Regain that feeling. Secrets to sexual self-discovery: People living with spinal cord injuries share profound insights into sex, pleasure, relationships, orgasm, and the importance of connectedness.* North Charleston, SC: CreateSpace Independent Publishing Platform.

Accessible Assistive Technology

Higson, N. (2012). *The MA+guide: A guide to more accessible sexuality-related assistive technology. In The Multiple Sclerosis Society of Western Australia* Retrieved from, *http://ilc.com.au/resources/2/0000/0023/the_ma__guide.pdf.*

MacHattie, E., & Naphtali, K. (2009). *Pleasure able: Sexual device manual for people with disabilities.* Disabilities Health

Research Network. Retrieved from, *www.dhrn.ca/files/sexualhealthmanual_lowres_2010_0208.pdf.*

Resources: Useful Websites

About.com – Sexuality: Good general information related to disability, toys, seniors, etc. http://sexuality.about.com/.

Come As You Are: Inclusive Canadian sex toy store with good information regarding adapting toys, etc. http://www.comeasyouare.com/sex-information/sex-and-disability/.

SH&DA – *Sexual Health & Disability Alliance (UK): SH&DA was formed in 2005 by the Outsiders Trust to bring together professionals who work with disabled people. Useful section on developing policies. Minutes of meetings make interesting reading.* http://www.shada.org.uk/.

The Outsiders: Useful resource section. http://www.outsiders.org.uk/.

Webliographies

Bent: Another webliography, with a focus on the LGBTI community. http://www.bentvoices.org/bentlinks/linksblank.htm.

Disability and Sexuality Resources: A very comprehensive list of links! http://incurable-hippie.blogspot.com.au/2011/11/disability-and-sex-resources.html.

Guide to Getting It On: A useful webliography on all things disability/sexuality. http://www.goofyfootpress.com/links/disabled/.

The Center for Sexual Pleasure and Health. http://thecsph.org/sex-and-disability.

Podcasts

The Too Hard Basket. http://www.abc.net.au/radionational/programs/360/the-too-hard- basket/3093916.

Ouch BBC – Sex and Relationships Special. http://www.bbc.co.uk/news/blogs-ouch-24030101.

Online Videos

Dr. Mitchell Tepper's Videos: A range of videos related to sex and disability, including sexual positions for males and females with spinal cord injury. https://vimeo.com/drmitchelltepper/videos.

Research

(S)exploring Disability: Intimacies, Sexualities and Disabilities: A research summary by Kirsty Liddiard, MA. http://www.sciontario.org/news/sexploring-disability.

The Sexuality and Access Project. http://sexuality-and-access.com/the-survey/.

33 PERSONAL CARE

HELEN VAN HUET ■ TRACEY ELIZABETH PARNELL ■ VIRGINIA MITSCH

CHAPTER OUTLINE

Abstract

An overview of personal care occupations that people engage in every day, in particular bathing, toileting and dressing, is the focus of this chapter. Engagement in personal care involves a complex interaction between the occupation, the person, and the environment in which the occupation is performed. There are a range of enabling remediation, compensation and education strategies that can be chosen when working with people to enable them to perform their occupations of bathing, toileting and dressing. When working with people on their ability to do personal care occupations, occupational therapists must overcome any reservations they have and must maintain the dignity of the people with whom they are working. The goal of achieving full independence in performing personal care occupations as the desired outcome of occupational therapy interventions is often not realistic, achievable, desirable or culturally appropriate for many people who have an illness, injury or impairment. When achieving independence is not possible or culturally appropriate, the focus of enabling strategies should be on achieving interdependence. A practice story is provided detailing an intervention focused on the personal care occupations of a person with an orthopaedic condition to illustrate this area of occupational therapy practice.

KEY POINTS

- Engagement in personal care involves a complex interaction among the occupation, a person's sense of choice, motivation and meaning around the occupation, and the physical, social, cultural and institutional environment in which the occupation is performed.

- Independence in personal care may be the desired outcome of the therapist; however, interdependence may be the choice of the person engaged in the occupation.

- The importance of person-centred assessment and enabling strategies are critical to enablement.

- Clear and collaboratively determined goals are crucial to planning and selecting appropriate enabling strategies.

- There are a range of enabling remediation, compensation and education strategies to support people to perform their occupations of bathing, toileting and dressing.

INTRODUCTION

Historically the occupational therapy profession has predominantly been a Western, female-gendered, socially conservative profession. The profession has focused on the assessment and intervention of traditional occupational categories of self-care, leisure and work. These categories, or modifications of these categories, form the basis of many models and frameworks of occupational therapy practice, including the Person–Environment–Occupation–Participation Model (Christiansen & Baum, 1997), Canadian Model of Occupational Performance and Engagement (Polatajko, Townsend, & Craik, 2007a), Occupational Performance Model – Australia (Chapparo & Ranka, 1997) and Occupational Therapy Practice Framework: Domains and Process (2014) (American Occupational Therapy Association (AOTA), 2014).

The terminology used around the occupation of personal care has included personal activities of daily living (PADL) (James, 2009), which are the activities involved in a person taking care of his or her body, and the instrumental activities of daily living (IADL), which are 'activities to support daily life within the home and community' (AOTA, 2014, p. 19). These terms are used in health care settings and are often the cited acronyms found in occupational therapy assessment reports, in the health records of people receiving health services and in published journal articles (Sigurdardottir & Kåreholt, 2014). The use of PADL may have relevance for health care providers but often means little to recipients of health services, who may struggle with the acronyms encountered in health care. Also within the occupational therapy profession there is little evidence that supports the use of these categories and terms as being representative of what people do every day (Whalley-Hammell, 2009b). The term *personal care*, rather than *self-care*, is used in this chapter as it reflects the person-centred aspects of care of self and can be applied to a broad range of activities from showering and bathing to eating and managing medication.

The complexity of the actual doing of bathing, toileting and dressing involves a multiplicity of factors above and apart from a person's physical ability, sensorimotor skills, cognitive facilities and endurance, although these are, of course, important. In particular, the meaning, choice and motivation a person ascribes to engaging in an occupation underpins the values and beliefs, and the level of engagement, a person has in relation to that occupation (AOTA, 2014). In addition, consideration has to be given to the concepts of independence and interdependence, issues of routines and dignity, and the impact of the environment in relation to a person's ability to engage in personal care occupations. These factors and considerations are the focus of the following sections of this chapter.

MEANING

The meaning an individual assigns to a particular occupation influences the importance of this occupation in the individual's life. Meaning in relation to an occupation can be defined as the occupation having 'value, purpose and fulfilment' in a person's life (Aiken, Fourt, Cheng, & Polatajko, 2011, p. 299). Occupational theorists such as Kielhofner (2002) saw meaning as a primary factor that determined occupational engagement. Thus the meaning attached to an occupation acts as a motivator to actual performance of, or engagement in, that occupation. However, 'meaning and purpose are intimately linked and one cannot be known without the other' (Eakman, 2015, p. 315).

Although personal care occupations form an integral part of occupational therapy practice, they may not necessarily be satisfying and rewarding to an individual. Personal care activities have been described as 'routine', 'mundane or boring' (Whalley-Hammell, 2009b, p. 111) and 'everyday occupations [...] seen but unnoticed' (Hasselkus, 2006, p. 628). However, it is often not until an individual's engagement in these occupations is affected by illness, injury or impairment that the meaning of personal care becomes more apparent.

Therefore how occupational therapists communicate with a person in determining the meaning attached to, for example, the personal care occupations of bathing, toileting or dressing is worth considering. In terms of engaging with people collaboratively in establishing priorities for intervention, it would appear paramount to have an appreciation of not only the meaning of a particular occupation but also how this fits within the view a person has of his or her own identity and future life. Acknowledging a person's view of a situation and the meaning derived from engagement in an occupation can provide reaffirmation of a person's self-worth and provide opportunities to reestablish identities disrupted by injury, illness or impairment.

In addition to being a motivating force behind engagement in occupations, meaning has also been described as an 'outcome of occupational engagement' (Polatajko et al., 2007a, p. 60). Successful performance and achievement can act as a reinforcer of the importance of particular occupations for an individual and may have a positive influence on participation in other occupations (Rebeiro, 2000). The 'connection between actions [...] occupational performance and engagement' (Aiken et al., 2011, p. 300) may be a powerful motivator for people to participate in the therapy process, whereby a person contributing to his or her own personal care may still provide a positive experience. An example of this could be a person brushing his or her own hair with assistance or actively directing the doing of other personal care occupations such as putting on makeup.

Engaging in personal care needs to be balanced against the time cost involved in what may have been a previously simple, time-efficient task before the illness, injury or impairment. It may be expected that it would be difficult to maintain motivation towards independence in dressing if it took the person more than 1 hour each day to complete this occupation without assistance. This may particularly be the case if the person valued other occupations more highly (e.g. leisure occupations such as playing cards with friends or productive occupations such as paid employment or volunteer work) and if the completion of the personal care task left the person fatigued and unable to participate in other self-chosen preferred occupations.

CHOICE

The ability of a person to make and have choice in what that person will and will not do is seen as a fundamental human right. Townsend and Wilcock (2004) see choice as 'the means by which humans decide what occupations are priority and what occupations they consider the most useful and meaningful to them' (p. 260). Choice may be determined by survival needs (the need to find food) or be culturally defined (the choice of clothing worn to a particular event). Choice may also be mediated by the socioeconomic status of the individual (social position and financial resources) and political factors (influencing what people can and cannot do). Ultimately the concept of choice is one afforded to prosperous societies where the value of choosing what one will do is nurtured and supported. There is increasing evidence to suggest that making personal choices about daily occupations and engaging in those occupations is related to well-being (Krishnagiri, Fuller, Ruda, & Diwan, 2013; Whalley-Hammell, 2009b). Well-being relates to the meaning and satisfaction gained from engaging in everyday occupations that a person chooses to do and the contribution these choices make to a person's quality of life (Krishnagiri et al., 2013; Whalley-Hammell, 2009b).

Occupational therapists often work within health care institutions that prescribe assessments and interventions. Providing people with choice within institutional settings is often a low priority when precedence is given to adherence to care pathways in relation to completion of personal care assessments and interventions. To redress this, therapists could acknowledge the individuality of each person by asking simple questions such as if a shower or a bath is preferred, or what time would the person usually have a shower or bath at home. Being able to cater for the personal care requirements of individuals has the added benefit of providing a more realistic evaluation of their actual capabilities. By providing opportunity for choice the therapist can enhance a person's feelings of control over a situation. The provision of choice in addressing personal care activities is particularly important as personal care routines are often habitual and these activities help to ground each individual in the reality and usual structure to his or her day.

Providing choice does have the potential to bring both risk and responsibility to the therapist–person relationship. As emphasised by the Canadian Association of Occupational Therapists (2007), there is an ethical component to respecting people's views and allowing people to make choices that may carry inherent risks. The right to take risks and to experience the consequences of the outcomes of these risks might be considered to be central to person-centred practice (Whalley-Hammell, 2006). When collaborating with people so that they genuinely have choice and understand the possible implications of their decisions, occupational therapists aim to gauge acceptable risk to promote 'just right' risk taking (Townsend et al., 2007, p. 101). 'Just right' risk taking is the point where all risks have been taken into account and then balanced with the person's right of choice regarding a certain situation. For example, a person may

wish to return home early from hospital before the required home modifications have been completed. The therapist and the person may discuss temporary adaptive equipment that may not be ideal but would provide a degree of safety when doing personal care occupations; in looking into and being willing to discuss and consider alternative options the therapist respects the person's choice in making the decision to return home.

Developmentally people work towards gaining control and mastery over their environment as they engage in everyday occupations (Eakman, 2015). Control can be seen as a 'fundamental human need' (2015, p. 316) that is linked to the motivation to achieve desired goals. The impact of illness and impairment on a person's sense of control must be considered when occupational therapists are working to address any personal care issues. How people evaluate their performance of personal care may influence how they view themselves within the social world. Guidetti, Asaba, & Tham, (2007) examined the experience of 'recapturing self-care' after a having a stroke or spinal cord injury and reported that for some people the inability to undertake personal care occupations made them reflect on 'how closely this aspect of their daily life was linked with their former identities' (p. 308). Additionally, people who experienced occupational disruption as a result of illness, injury or impairment reported a reduced sense of being in control (Guidetti et al., 2007; Whalley-Hammell, 2006). For people with a life-limiting illness, maintaining normality and having choice and control over personal and other care with the support of others was identified as an important way of coping with the illness (Johnston, Milligan, Foster, & Kearney, 2012). Thus using a person-centred approach (where the individual is central in the decision-making process) to personal care intervention can assist in restoring a sense of control to the individual and the individual's ability to engage in and contribute to occupations that positively affect feelings of well-being (Eakman, 2015; Whalley-Hammell, 2009b).

MOTIVATION

Motivational factors play a critical role in personal care. Motivation can be both intrinsic (internal) or extrinsic (influenced by others). 'Intrinsically motivated behaviour or occupation refers to doing an activity for its own sake, for the satisfaction inherent in the doing' (Eakman, 2015, p. 317). External motivation may be the result of wanting to please others or be dictated by social obligations (Eakman, 2015).

If a person is not motivated towards a particular personal care occupation, the likelihood of engagement and successful completion is minimised. A person's degree of motivation to engage in personal care occupations requires the consideration of a range of factors that includes the person's interest in performing these occupations, how important these occupations are perceived to be and the person's sense of self-efficacy in completing these occupations (Kielhofner, 2008).

Personal values such as meaning and choice influence a person's motivation to engage in occupation by providing a sense of satisfaction and competence at being able to complete an occupation to an expected standard. These personal as well as social factors 'serve to motivate and sustain occupational performance' (Eakman, 2015). An example of this could be a person deciding what clothes to wear to a particular social event. Intrinsic motivators of pride in personal appearance and social motivators of being acceptable to other people attending the same social event influence the choice of clothing selected, the effort put into dressing and the outcome that meets the expected standard of the individual. Having the individual actively committed to the process provides the motivational drive required to direct a person's actions towards completing desired occupations (Creek, 2014).

INDEPENDENCE AND INTERDEPENDENCE

The concept of independence in occupation has contributed to the framework of occupational therapy practice since its inception as a profession. Within Western society, independence or self-reliance is valued and this stance has been reinforced by societal expectations (Reed, 2015).

As practitioners, occupational therapists base many of their interventions on facilitating independence in the performance of occupations. The health care institutions occupational therapists work in often demand independence as a requirement of completing care pathways and achieving discharge within set time frames.

A study by Hayase et al. (2004) showed that 'the sharpest growth in personal care abilities occurs between the ages of 3 to 6 years' (p. 192), and independence in personal care, once reached (around the age of 15), remains stable until about the age of 50, when deterioration begins to take place. As a person ages, being independent in everything one does may not be realistic or be seen as important as participating in other valued occupations. This is significant to consider given the increased longevity of the population. It has been predicted in Australia, for instance, that by 2055 the population of people living older than 65 will double and that those living to older than 100 years of age will number 40,000 people (Australian Government, 2015).

The cultural fit of the concept of independence requires attention as Western societies become increasingly multicultural, largely because of migration and the acceptance of refugees. The influx of different nationalities has meant a reconsideration of the concept of independence from a cultural perspective, as for people from many non-Western cultures interdependence is accepted as usual practice (Landi et al., 2006).

Interdependence can be defined as 'an interpersonal relationship [...] that is mutually beneficial or satisfying to both' (Reed, 2015, p. 581) that sees individuals seeking support through the development of reciprocal relationships with families and available services. Interdependence centres on relationships, goals and values, rather than on individual capabilities, and is based on respect and reciprocity where people may share the performance of different occupations (Beeber, 2008). A study of occupational engagement and health in older Southern Asian immigrants found that interdependence was related to relationship dynamics with extended family that reinforced cultural values and contributed to individuals' health (Krishnagiri et al., 2013).

Whalley-Hammell (2006) reflected that although independence is considered 'the norm', increasingly in contemporary society interdependence is 'the usual' (p. 128) and that 'occupations that promote interdependence contribute positively to well-being' (Whalley-Hammell, 2009a, p. 10) regardless of cultural background.

The importance of the caregiver within the concept of interdependence and as a standard consideration when discharge planning within health care has been highlighted as critical to adjustment to the home environment (Ockerby, Livingston, O'Connell, & Gaskin, 2013; Pereira & Rebelo Botelho, 2011). A study by Vellone et al. (2014) explored the relationship of people with heart failure and their carers to the level of personal care assistance required and quality of life for both. It found that better maintenance of personal care abilities was related to better mental quality of life for caregivers. Conversely it found that caregiver lack of confidence in supporting personal care was associated with 'poorer physical quality of life' (Vellone et al., 2014) for the people with heart failure. The authors noted the complex relationship between caregivers' quality of life and confidence and those they cared for in their ability to carry out personal care and their perceived quality of life.

To work effectively with people, occupational therapists need to explore what the concept of independence means to individuals and their caregivers including a thorough examination of the person's culture, role demands and personal values. Consideration of interdependence with others and how this is approached in the therapeutic relationship should also address individuals' ability to make decisions relevant to themselves in relation to others and to have control over their life.

ROUTINES

Routines are patterns of behaviour that are observable, regular and repetitive and include scheduled daily occupations (Segal, 2004) such as personal care occupations. Routines provide structure for daily life and a sense of stability and have also been linked to the maintenance of an individual's health and well-being (Kielhofner, 2002; Koome, Hocking, & Sutton, 2012). Routines are embedded in cultural and ecological contexts (Segal, 2004) and therefore can be influenced by and adapted in response to environmental factors (Walker, 2001).

The development, maintenance and, where necessary, adaptation of daily routines has been suggested to demonstrate a person's degree of control over daily life (Hasselkus, 2002; Koome et al., 2012; Walker, 2001). Koome et al. further proposed that the presence of routines in a person's daily life may contribute to his or her degree of well-being. Maintenance of personal routines during a period of ill health or after an injury can be challenging, particularly in an inpatient health care setting where the institutional routines often take precedence over those of the individual.

Occupational therapists are encouraged to consider how they can work with individuals to maintain or adapt daily routines to facilitate reengagement in personal care occupations.

DIGNITY

An important consideration when addressing the personal care issues of people is the issue of dignity. Performance of personal care occupations within a health care setting often provides opportunity for dignity to be compromised. Activities that have been identified as compromising dignity include 'support with hygiene and dressing', 'exposing procedures' (such as changing wound dressings), 'moving and handling' and even 'communication' (Baillie, Gallagher, & Wainwright, 2008, p. 17).

The health care environment does not always lend itself to privacy. Often people can be seen in cubicles from public corridors, and staff may inadvertently move the curtains around the bed when an individual is engaged in personal care occupations. As a safety measure, staff can access locked bathrooms and toilets in case of falls or medical emergencies; this access also has the potential to compromise dignity.

When facilitating personal care occupations there should be 'sufficient investment in health care settings to demonstrate that […] patients are valued and respected' (Baillie et al., 2008, p. 7). This includes ensuring that there is adequate space and equipment available for the personal care occupation to be carried out, that the person consents to being supervised or assisted during the activity and that there is a conscious effort to minimise situations where dignity could be compromised. Examples of respecting dignity include seeking the person's consent before the therapist observes the person dressing and making sure there are adequate towels or robes to cover the person once showering is completed.

Therapists can also find it confronting when working with people to achieve their goals in the area of personal care. In a qualitative study that explored the experience of new graduate occupational therapists undertaking their first shower assessment, Glenn and Gilbert-Hunt (2012) found that feelings of discomfort and awkwardness were common. They reported that 'occupational therapy programmes face practical and ethical dilemmas in replicating authentic practice experiences […] particularly in the more intimate areas of practice' (p. 188). As a consequence of their lack of exposure to these assessments, student and new graduate occupational therapists felt they lacked the necessary skills, knowledge and confidence to effectively address this common yet complex and challenging area of occupational therapy practice. Many participants also reported being unprepared for the emotional responses they experienced. To enhance the comfort and competence of occupational therapists when working with people to achieve their goals in the area of personal care, Glenn and Gilbert-Hunt recommended that 'early exposure to the practical methods of occupational therapy' (p. 195) through strategies such as simulation, experience on placement and direct supervision would be of benefit. They also suggested that improved understanding of the impact of social norms relevant to this area of practice would be of benefit.

Specific areas for consideration and strategies to assist with ensuring dignity and overcoming discomfort when working with people in the area of personal care are outline in more detail in Table 33.1 and Box 33.1, which are discussed and presented later in the chapter.

THE ENVIRONMENT AND PERSONAL CARE OCCUPATIONS

The environment is the context within which occupational performance takes place and can be considered to include physical, social, cultural and institutional factors (Polatajko et al., 2007b). Law et al. (1996) discuss the interactive, dynamic and complex relationship among the person, the environment, and the occupation and suggest that the environment can have either an enabling or constraining effect on an individual's performance of, and engagement in, occupations.

Occupational therapists have traditionally focused on the physical environment when working with people to enhance engagement in personal care occupations such as bathing, toileting and dressing (e.g. recommending and seeing the completion of home modifications). However, it is also important to consider social, cultural and institutional environmental factors that can affect each individual's level of independence, and their goals and future plans, and the meaning, choice and motivation they ascribe to engaging in their personal care occupations. These environmental factors have the potential to affect either directly or indirectly the person's level of engagement in personal care occupations.

The following example highlights the significance of giving due consideration to environmental factors in relation to personal care occupations. A middle-aged man was deemed by hospital outcome measures to be 'independent' in showering (as assessed within the hospital setting) but was unable to maintain the same level of independence when discharged. Review of the situation revealed that the person was, indeed, able to shower without assistance once he was in the bathroom setting. However, he was unable to negotiate the 50-metre walk on uneven terrain from his caravan (where he lived) to the amenities block.

The use of relevant assessment and enabling strategies is important. These strategies must be responsive to the needs of people and assist in achieving individual goals in personal care; this will require occupational therapists to consider each individual's environment in a comprehensive manner.

ADDRESSING PERSONAL CARE ISSUES

In the course of one chapter it is not possible to fully cover the range of issues related to personal care and the enabling strategies that may be facilitated by occupational therapists. Rather, the aim in this chapter is to provide a number of principles to guide intervention. The practical application of these concepts are further illustrated in Practice Story 33.1.

Please note, that it is important that therapists avoid applying any personal care assessment or intervention principles or

TABLE 33.1
Considerations in Undertaking Personal Care Interventions

Person		Environment	Occupation
Person Receiving Occupational Therapy Services ■ Age ■ Gender ■ Nature of diagnosis, prognosis, precautions, medications and contraindications ■ Current status and safety issues, including mobility, behaviour, cognition ■ Socioeconomic background, including supports available, living arrangements ■ Familial/cultural background ■ Care beliefs ■ Goals for the future ■ Discomfort or embarrassment undertaking bathing, toileting and dressing with another person present	*Therapist/Student* ■ Age ■ Gender ■ Familial/cultural background ■ Understanding of diagnosis and related factors ■ Previous experience in and reservations about working with people to address issues related to bathing, toileting and dressing ■ Ability to ensure dignity and modesty for person and establish trust and respect ■ Ability to overcome discomfort or embarrassment working with people undertaking bathing, toileting and dressing	*Practice Setting* ■ Familiarity of environment available for bathing, toileting and dressing ■ Lack of privacy in practice setting and impact on performance ■ Safety of practice setting ■ Comparison of practice setting with home setting ■ Home setting ■ Setup of home setting compared with practice setting (e.g. shower over the bath at home versus flat access shower with chair in hospital; see Figs. 33.1 and 33.2 for comparison) ■ Safety of home environment, including physical setup, supervision/assistance available ■ Environmental modifications/equipment required or available ■ Ability of person to translate strategies learned in practice setting to home environment	■ Nature of the occupation (bathing, toileting or dressing) ■ Complexity of occupation (may require task analysis) ■ Person's preexisting routine, including time of day he or she undertakes bathing, dressing and toileting, new routines that may need to be established ■ Comparison of performance in practice setting versus home setting ■ Frequency desired ■ Premorbid level of function ■ Consideration of other occupations person performs (i.e. What is the person's current and proposed occupational profile or repertoire?)

strategies prescriptively. Rather each person should be considered on an individual basis. An example of this is reflecting on what constitutes personal care for the individual. The importance that individuals place on their performance of different personal care occupations will vary. Take, for instance, the activity of grooming: a man might take pride in being cleanly shaven each day unless the man prefers to have a beard and as a result will not see shaving as an important activity.

Tips for Addressing Personal Care Occupations

It may be useful to have a checklist of items to consider and attend to before undertaking personal care interventions. This should include thinking about the person, the occupation and the environment factors that influence engagement and performance. Some guidelines to be considered are presented in Table 33.1.

To assist occupational therapists to prepare for the challenges of working with people to address areas of personal care, some specific resources may be useful. The occupational therapy team

at Princess Alexandra Hospital in Brisbane (Queensland, Australia) provides students with practice-based advice. One of these documents addresses personal care assessments in a mental health setting and is available on the Occupational Therapy Practice Education Collaborative – Queensland (OTPEC-Q) website. The content of the document is presented in Box 33.1. The document provides a list of suggestions collated from supervisors and students that may be useful for students and therapists to review in preparation for working with people to undertake personal care occupations. It is reproduced here with permission.

Enabling Strategies for Bathing, Toileting, and Dressing Occupations

The goal of any enabling strategy is to support people to perform their chosen occupations (Moyers, 2005). As discussed previously, people will choose the emphasis they place on the occupations of bathing, toileting and dressing, and this will influence their goals for engagement in personal care tasks.

There are a broad range of enabling strategies to support people to perform their personal care occupations. These

BOX 33.1
ADVICE TO STUDENTS: SHOWER ASSESSMENT

Aim:

To assess the ability of the patient[a] to manage personal care tasks. Components of performance such as cognition, sensation, perception and biomechanics are observed.

Time:

Scheduled in the mornings.

Where:

Assessments can be completed in the patient's en suite. If the patient's medical or mental health status is of concern, it is best to have your supervisor or a nurse present.

From your Supervisor:

- Always wear a duress alarm.
- Do not do personal care assessments on patients in the acute observation area (AOA). This would be inappropriate due to poor mental state and unstable nature of patients in this area.
- Notify patient of your intentions to assess them.
- Notify staff by writing in the communication book and speaking to contact nurse the morning of the assessment.
- Prepare everything you need before starting, and ensure that the bathroom/toilet is clean and ready for use.
- Ensure patient safety at all times. Do not allow the patient to do something if you are concerned they may fall, overexert themselves or put you at risk.
- Ask for help from the nursing staff to transfer the patient if needed.
- Check in the care plan and medical chart to ensure all is well with the patient, on the day.
- Double check how the patient should transfer and mobilise.

- Use universal precautions – gown, glove and booties. Always wash hands after removing gloves.
- Be prepared to provide assistance to the patient if required – this includes hygiene following toileting!
- Set the person up ready for the day following the shower – e.g. back in their room, nurse aware of location and outcome of assessment, etc., handy.
- Don't be embarrassed, or if you are don't let it show. If you are embarrassed then so will be the patient.

From Fellow Students:

- Be prepared! Nothing is worse than getting the patient showered and realising you forgot towels or their clean clothes.
- Plastic gown + booties – all patients lose control of the shower hose no matter how independent they are.
- Respect their dignity. To quote a nurse: 'Think about how you would like your mother/father, grandmother/grandfather to be treated'.
- Make the patient feel at ease.
- Try to have a sense of humour.
- Ask them to try to do as much as they can by themselves.
- Ask patients to participate in as much of the activity as they can. Let them know that you are there to observe and also help if they need it.
- Make sure you write that you will be doing a shower assessment on the patient on both the white board behind the nurse station and the therapy white board a day in advance.
- Discuss ADL ability of the patient with other team members.

ADL, Activities of daily living.
Format kindly provided by Simone Bartholomai, Ipswich Hospital. Edited for Princess Alexandra Hospital by Monique Kofler & Sue Holley. Available at http://www.qotfc.edu.au/mental-health/documents/advice/advice_to_students_personal_care_assessment.pdf.
[a]Although the *patient* is not the preferred term used in this book, it has been kept in this table as this is the term used by the authors of the checklist.

strategies may include adapting the demands of the occupation, altering the physical and social environment and teaching the person new skills or reestablishing lost skills (Duncan, 2006). Practice frameworks such as the Canadian Model of Occupational Performance and Engagement suggest a range of skills (including adapt, advocate, coach, educate and design/build) that occupational therapists can use to enable individual change and facilitate engagement in these occupations (Townsend et al., 2007). Therapists are encouraged to explore and develop the skills and strategies that best fit their practice settings.

The enabling strategies of remediation, compensation and education as they apply to bathing, toileting and dressing are

discussed using a practice story. *Remediation* refers to strategies that focus on the recovery of previous skills or the development of new skills. Compensatory strategies focus on environmental or occupational adaptation, whereas education has a teaching and learning focus specific to the individual's goals. Refer to Chapter 23, for more detailed information on these types of strategies. A therapist may commence intervention with a remedial approach and move to a compensatory approach if improvements have plateaued, time frames alter, or the person changes goals (Unsworth, 2010). A change in intervention strategy is illustrated in Bill's story (Practice Story 33.1).

Bill

INTRODUCTION

Bill was a 76-year-old man admitted to hospital with a fractured left neck of femur after a fall at home. Bill's medical history included multiple transient ischaemic attacks (TIA) over the past 5 years. Because of the nature of his injury, Bill underwent a left total hip replacement and was transferred from the surgical ward to the rehabilitation ward. Bill sat out of bed intermittently after his surgery; however, he required assistance with transfers and verbal prompting to adhere to his postoperative precautions. The focus of his rehabilitation was on increasing mobility, safety and independence in preparation for discharge to the home environment.

Before admission to hospital, Bill was living at home with his wife Margaret. Margaret was 63 years of age and was working part time as a counsellor. Margaret had been Bill's main carer. Margaret was responsible for most domestic and community activities for the couple and provided Bill with assistance with showering and dressing before his fall. Bill had been independent in his toileting needs and was able to prepare a light meal before his fall. He was also able to walk distances of up to 50 metres independently and negotiate steps with a handrail. Bill lacked confidence with community mobility and rarely went outside the home environment without his wife.

Bill outlined to the rehabilitation team that his goal was to return home to live with his wife. Margaret indicated to the team that Bill needed to be safe and independent with his toileting and light meal preparation, and be able to shower with minimal assistance, for her to feel comfortable for him to be discharged back to the home setting.

ASSESSMENT

Bill and Margaret agreed that to return home he needed to be able to shower with minimal assistance. The occupational therapist determined that it would be appropriate to assess Bill having a shower with the assistance of his wife. In preparing for this assessment, the occupational therapist considered the factors outlined in Table 33.1, in particular the differences between the hospital bathroom and Bill's bathroom at home (Figs. 33.1 and 33.2). The occupational therapist also considered issues related to Bill and Margaret being comfortable to complete the assessment by making them familiar with the shower space and ensuring that Bill's dignity and privacy was maintained. The occupational therapist also provided Bill and Margaret with a

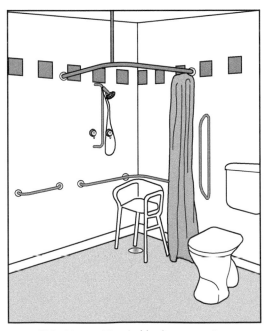

FIG. 33.1 ■ Hospital bathroom setting.

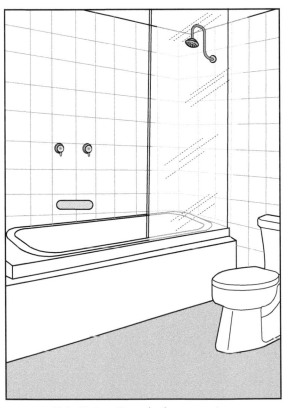

FIG. 33.2 ■ Home bathroom setting.

PRACTICE STORY 33.1

Bill (Continued)

choice about the timing of the assessment on the chosen day. Using a task analysis approach, the occupational therapist determined the steps involved in Bill showering.

During the assessment the occupational therapist observed Margaret's ability to provide Bill with assistance in a safe manner and determined both Bill and Margaret's awareness of postoperative precautions in a personal care context. Additionally, the assessment provided the occupational therapist with ideas regarding equipment that Bill may require in the home setting to be able to shower safely.

During the assessment the occupational therapist noted the following:

- Bill was able to reliably follow two-step instructions.
- Bill was able to walk from his bed on the ward to the bathroom (approximately 10 metres) with standby supervision.
- Bill was cooperative and willing to do as much as he was able to with regard to personal care.
- Bill was unsafe to stand while showering.

- Bill was unable to recall his postoperative precautions reliably and Margaret had limited knowledge of them.
- Bill required assistance with all lower limb washing, drying and dressing.
- Margaret was anxious about Bill falling.

During the assessment the therapist noted that Bill was experiencing difficulties with learning and independently following the postoperative hip precautions. Margaret reported that she did not have a clear understanding of the precautions and was happy to assist but would like Bill to be able to follow the precautions on his own if possible. Bill indicated that he was motivated to shower with minimal assistance. He was happy if Margaret checked on him and assisted with lower limb washing, drying and dressing but wanted to be able to initiate the activity himself.

The results of the assessment guided the occupational therapist's intervention strategies with Bill and Margaret. Some suggestions for remediation, compensation and education enabling strategies are listed in Table 33.2.

TABLE 33.2

Examples of Enabling Strategies That the Occupational Therapist May Use with Bill

INTERVENTION

Goals for Intervention	Enabling Strategy
To Be Able to Shower with Standby Assistance from Margaret	**Remediation** Using this approach, the therapist focused on the biomechanical components of the task, ensuring that Bill practised and repeated tasks/activities such as transfers with the aim of improving his physical capacity to perform specific tasks/activities. Intervention included the following: ■ Bill practising the correct way to place his feet when moving from sit to stand in order to maintain hip precautions ■ Improving Bill's standing balance to improve safety during showering ■ Increasing Bill's physical endurance to undertake the task in its entirety **Compensation** The therapist ensured the environment was set up to enable Bill to adhere to postoperative hip precautions and maximise his performance. Intervention included the following: ■ Safe setup of bathroom within both the hospital and the home environment ■ Use of rails and adaptive equipment within the hospital and home environment, including the use of a shower chair at the correct height to prevent hip flexion beyond 90 degrees (Fig. 33.3) ■ Close standby assistance from Margaret when Bill was standing and use of grab rails when standing ■ Long-handled aids to assist Bill to be able to wash and dry his lower limbs and feet (Fig. 33.4). ■ Practise and repetition of the techniques – consider if this can occur in home environment before discharge to ensure transfer of learning.

Continued on following page

TABLE 33.2
Examples of Enabling Strategies That the Occupational Therapist May Use with Bill *(Continued)*

INTERVENTION

Goals for Intervention	Enabling Strategy

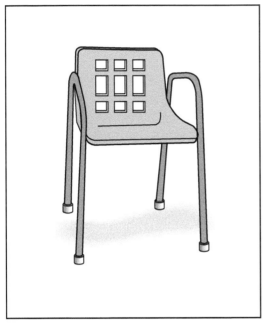

FIG. 33.3 ■ Example of shower chair.

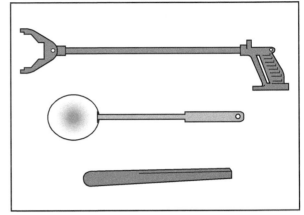

FIG. 33.4 ■ Example of long-handled equipment to assist with personal care.

Education

- Discussed falls prevention strategies with Margaret; provided written information.
- Discussed and demonstrated correct transfer techniques with Bill and Margaret.
- Discussed and demonstrated safe use of rails and equipment. Initially did this in the hospital and then did this in Bill's home to achieve greater compliance and carryover.

To Maintain the Stability of the Hip Prosthesis

Remediation

- It was decided that the use of remediation of memory and learning skills was not appropriate because of Bill's TIAs and subsequent memory deficits and the necessity for safety before discharge.

Compensation

- Considered what strategies Bill and Margaret previously used at home to assist him with recalling everyday matters of importance; for example, writing things down, reminders on the wall, alarms. Used Bill's established strategies to compensate for his preexisting memory loss to assist him to remember his hip precautions.
- Enabled Bill and Margaret to consider and choose strategies to recall precautions within their own environment.

Education

- Provided education to Margaret on the nature of Bill's surgery and the postoperative precautions. Provided information verbally and in writing. This information was reinforced when engaged in developing his performance capacity for his bathing, dressing and toileting occupations.
- Considered practice within the home environment and ensured any newly introduced strategies worked within the home environment.

TIA, Transient ischemic attack.

CONCLUSION

Facilitating a person's capacity to perform personal care occupations of bathing, dressing and toileting is an important focus of practice for many occupational therapists. When working with people who have difficulties with personal care occupations, an occupational therapist must take into consideration the meaning each individual attaches to, and their choice and motivation to engage in, particular occupations, as well as the environments in which the occupations are performed.

These factors and the professional reasoning skills the occupational therapists brings to the situation will influence the assessment and intervention strategies that are used. Whether the enabling strategies involve remediation, compensation or education, it is important that the occupational therapist collaborates with the person, and when appropriate with significant others. This ensures that person-centred goals are the focus of engagement in personal care occupations.

 http://evolve.elsevier.com/Curtin/OT

REFERENCES

Aiken, F. E., Fourt, A. M., Cheng, I. K. S., & Polatajko, H. J. (2011). The meaning gap in occupational therapy: Finding meaning in our own occupation. *Canadian Journal of Occupational Therapy*, *78*, 294–302. http://dx.doi.org/10.2182/cjot.2011.78.5.4.

American Occupational Therapy Association (2014). Occupational therapy practice framework: Domain and process (3rd ed.). *American Journal of Occupational Therapy*, *68*(Suppl 1), S1–S48.

Australian Government (2015). *2015 Intergenerational report: Australia in 2055*. Canberra: Australian Government.

Baillie, L., Gallagher, A., & Wainwright, P. (2008). *Defending dignity: Challenges and opportunities for nursing*. London: Royal College of Nursing.

Beeber, A. S. (2008). Interdependence: Building partnerships to continue older adults residence in the community. *Journal of Gerontological Nursing*, *4*(1), 19–25.

Canadian Association of Occupational Therapists (2007). *Canadian Association of Occupational Therapist Code of Ethics. Retrieved from(2007). www.caot.ca.*

Chapparo, C., & Ranka, J. A. (1997). *Occupational performance model australia, monograph 1*. Sydney: Sydney University Press.

Christiansen, C. H., & Baum, C. (1997). Person-environment occupational performance. In C. H. Christiansen, & C. Baum (Eds.), *Occupational therapy: Enabling functioning and well-being*. Slack: Thorofare, NJ.

Creek, J. (2014). The knowledge base of occupational therapy. In W. Bryant, J. Fieldhouse, & K. Bannigan (Eds.), *Creek's occupational therapy and mental health* (5th ed., pp. 27–48). London: Churchill Livingstone.

Duncan, E. A. (2006). Introduction. In E. A. Duncan (Ed.), *Foundations for practice in occupational therapy* (4th ed., pp. 24–57). Edinburgh, Elsevier Churchill Livingstone.

Eakman, A. M. (2015). Person factors: Meaning, sense-making, and spirituality. In C. H. Christiansen, C. M. Baum, & J. D. Bass (Eds.), *Occupational therapy: Performance, participation and well-being*. Slack: Thorofare, NJ.

Glenn, E. K., & Gilbert-Hunt, S. (2012). New graduate occupational therapists experience of showering assessments: A phenomenological study. *Australian Occupational Therapy Journal*, *59*, 188–196. http://dx.doi.org/10.1111/j.1440-1630.2012.01000.x.

Guidetti, S., Asaba, E., & Tham, K. (2007). The lived experience of recapturing self-care. *American Journal of Occupational Therapy*, *61*, 303–310.

Hasselkus, B. R. (2002). *The meaning of everyday occupation*. Thorofare, NJ: Slack.

Hasselkus, B. R. (2006). The world of everyday occupation: Real people, real lives. *American Journal of Occupational Therapy*, *60*(6), 627–640.

Hayase, D., Mosenteen, D., Thimmaiah, D., Zemke, S., Atler, K., & Fisher, A. G. (2004). Age-related changes in activities of daily living ability. *Australian Journal of Occupational Therapy*, *51*, 192–198.

James, A. B. (2009). Activities of daily living and instrumental activities of daily living. In E. B. Creqeau, E. S. Cohn, & B. A. B. Schell (Eds.), *Willard and Spackman's occupational therapy*. Philadelphia: Lippincott, Williams & Wilkins.

Johnston, B. M., Milligan, S., Foster, C., & Kearney, N. (2012). Self-care and end of life care – patients' and carers' experience. *Supportive Care in Cancer*, *20*(8), 1619–1627.

Kielhofner, G. (2002). Habituation: Patterns of daily occupation. In G. Kielhofner (Ed.), *A model of human occupation: Theory and application* (3rd ed.). Philadephia: Lippincott Williams & Wilkins.

Kielhofner, G. (2008). Volition. In G. Kielhofner (Ed.), *Model of human occupation: Theory and application* (4th ed.). Philadelphia: Lippincott, Williams & Wilkins.

Koome, F., Hocking, C., & Sutton, D. (2012). Why routines matter: The nature and meaning of family routines in the context of adolescent mental illness. *Journal of Occupational Science*, *19*(4), 312–325.

Krishnagiri, S., Fuller, E., Ruda, L., & Diwan, S. (2013). Occupational engagement and health in older South Asian immigrants. *Journal of Occupational Science*, *20*(1), 87–102.

Landi, F., Cesari, M., Onder, G., Tafani, A., Zamboni, V., & Cocchi, A. (2006). Effects of an occupational therapy program on functional outcomes in older stroke patients. *Gerontology*, *52*, 85–91.

Law, M., Cooper, B., Strong, S., Stewart, D., Rigby, P., & Letts, L. (1996). The person-environment-occupation model: A transactive approach to occupational performance. *Canadian Journal of Occupational Therapy*, *58*, 186–192.

Moyers, P. (2005). Introduction to occupation-based practice. In C. H. Christiansen, C. Baum, & J. Bass-Huagen (Eds.), *Occupational therapy: performance, participation and well being* (3rd ed., pp. 221–234). Thorofare, NJ, Slack.

Ockerby, C., Livingston, P., O'Connell, B., & Gaskin, C. J. (2013). The role of informal caregivers during cancer patients' recovery from chemotherapy. *Scandinavian Journal of Caring Sciences*, *27*(1), 147–155.

Pereira, H. R., & Rebelo Botelho, M. A. (2011). Sudden informal caregivers: The lived experience of informal caregivers after an unexpected event. *Journal of Clinical Nursing*, *20*(17-18), 2448–2457.

Polatajko, H., Townsend, E. A., & Craik, J. (2007a). Canadian model of occupational performance and engagement. In E. A. Townsend, & H. J. Polatajko (Eds.), *Enabling occupation: Advancing an occupational therapy vision of health, well-being & justice through occupation* (p. 23). Ottawa: CAOT Publications ACE.

Polatajko, H. J., Davis, J., Stewart, D., et al. (2007b). Specifying the domain of concern: Occupation as core. In E. A. Townsend, & H. J. Polatajko (Eds.), *Enabling occupation II: Advancing an occupational therapy vision of health, well-being and justice through occupation* (pp. 13–36). Ottawa: CAOT Publications ACE.

Rebeiro, K. L. (2000). Client perspectives on occupational therapy practice: Are we truly client-centred? *Candain Journal of Occupational Therapy*, *67*(1), 7–14.

Reed, K. L. (2015). Key occupational therapy concepts in the Person-Environment-Occupation-Performance Model. In C. H. Christiansen, C. M. Baum, & J. D. Bass (Eds.), *Occupational therapy: Performance, participation and well-being*. Slack: Thorofare, NJ.

Segal, R. (2004). Family routines and rituals: A context for occupational therapy interventions. *American Journal of Occupational Therapy*, *58*(5), 499–508.

Sigurdardottir, S. H., & Kåreholt, I. (2014). Informal and formal care of older people in Iceland. *Scandinavian Journal of Caring Sciences*, *28*(4), 802–811.

Townsend, E., Beagan, B., Kumas-Tan, Z., et al. (2007). Enabling: Occupational therapy's core competency. In E. A. Townsend, &

H. J. Polatajko (Eds.), *Enabling Occupation II: Advancing an occupational therapy vision for health, well-being & justice through occupation* (pp. 87–133). Ottowa: CAOT Publications ACE.

Townsend, E., & Wilcock, A. A. (2004). Occupational justice and client-centred practice: A dialogue in progress. *Canadian Journal of Occupational Therapy*, *71*(2), 75–87.

Unsworth, C. A. (2010). Cognitive and perceptual strategies. In M. Curtin, M. Molineux, & J. Supyk-Mellson (Eds.), *Occupational therapy and physical dysfunction: Enabling occupation* (6th ed., pp. 607–636). Edinburgh: Elsevier.

Vellone, E., Chung, M. L., Cocchieri, A., Rocco, G. R., Alvaro, R., & Riegel, B. (2014). Effects of self-care on quality of life in adults with heart failure and their spousal caregivers: Testing dyadic dynamics using the Actor–Partner Interdependence Model. *Journal of Family Nursing*, *20*(1), 120–141.

Walker, C. (2001). Occupational adaptation in action: Shift workers and their strategies. *Journal of Occupational Science*, *8*(1), 17–24.

Whalley-Hammell, K. (2006). *Perspectives on disability and rehabilitiation: Contesting assumptions, challenging practice*. Edinburgh: Elsevier.

Whalley-Hammell, K. (2009a). Sacred texts: A sceptical exploration of the assumptions underpinning theories of occupation. *Canadian Journal of Occupational Therapy*, *76*(1), 6–13.

Whalley-Hammell, K. (2009b). Self-care, productivity, and leisure, or dimensions of occupational experience? Rethinking occupational 'categories'. *Canadian Journal of Occupational Therapy*, *76*, 107–114.

34 LEISURE

RUTH SQUIRE ▪ LUCIA RAMSEY ▪ CAROLYN DUNFORD

Abstract

This chapter focuses on leisure occupations and the impact these occupations have on health and well-being. Leisure is defined as a nonobligatory activity that is intrinsically motivated and engaged in during discretionary time (American Occupational Therapy Association, 2014) with the purpose of enjoyment (e.g. socialising, creative expressions, outdoor activities, games and sport) (Townsend, 1997). The importance of leisure within contemporary occupational therapy practice is explored, highlighting the positive effects engaging in leisure can have on physical and mental well-being, with a particular focus on adults and older adults. An overview of the outcome measures used and factors to consider when assessing and working with individuals who have experienced some form of illness, injury or impairment that affects their leisure occupations is provided. Two practice stories provide examples of focusing on leisure when working with people.

KEY POINTS

- Leisure occupations are important for occupational therapists to consider when providing therapy services to people.

- Leisure is an occupational construct within the context of contemporary occupational therapy theory and practice.

- Recent legislation and policy calls for increased focus on recreational type occupations across all ages for increased health and well-being.

- Occupational therapists should aim to assess individuals' engagement in leisure in order to identify their leisure needs and include these within their intervention plans.

- Using leisure as an occupational therapy intervention can have positive impacts on physical and mental well-being and provide meaning to life.

INTRODUCTION

The primary goal of occupational therapy is to enable participation in occupations that a person wants to, needs to or is expected to do (World Federation of Occupational Therapists, 2012). Leisure occupations are an example of occupations that people want to do, and these must be balanced with the occupations they need to, and are expected to do.

In the early years of the profession the play spirit was considered essential for meaningful life (Primeau, 2009; Slagle, 1922). In the middle of the twentieth century scientific aspects dominated and play and leisure were seen as unscientific (Primeau, 2009). In the late twentieth century academics started to reclaim play and leisure as an essential part of occupational therapy (Crepeau, Cohn, & Schell, 2009). In the twenty-first century there has been a refocus on occupation-centred practice, which has raised awareness of the importance of play and leisure as occupational therapy domains (Johnson, 2009). However, some have seen leisure occupations as a luxury, with a preference for occupational therapists to focus on self-care and productivity occupations (Johnson, 2009). Nonetheless, leisure occupations can have significant, positive impacts on a person's physical and mental well-being as well as giving meaning to life.

Play and leisure occupations develop over the lifespan. Play dominates in early childhood and has been described as a primary occupation, and the work, of children (Bundy, 2012). It has also been recognised as a universal right for every child (United Nations, 1989). However, the concepts of play and leisure are intertwined, and it is unclear at what age people move from having play occupations to leisure occupations, particularly as adults are known to still engage in play occupations at times (Brooks & Dunford, 2014).

Missiuna and Pollock (1991, p. 883) define play occupations as 'spontaneous, intrinsically motivated, self-regulated, [that require] personal involvement of the child. [Play occupations] includes exploration, mastery, decision making, achievement, increased motivation and competency'. According to Bundy (2012) play is challenging to define, but she lists four primary characteristics: the transaction is framed as play, is relatively intrinsically motivated and internally controlled, and is free from some constraints of reality.

The World Health Organization's International Classification of Functioning, Disability and Health (ICF) (World Health Organization (WHO), 2001, 2007) includes leisure and recreation as part of community, social and civic life. Within the ICF leisure is defined as, 'Engaging in any form of play, recreational or leisure activity such as informal or organised play and sports, programmes of physical fitness, relaxation, amusement or diversion, going to art galleries, museums, cinemas or theatres; engaging in crafts or hobbies, reading for enjoyment, playing musical instruments; sightseeing, tourism and travelling for pleasure' (WHO, 2001, p. 186). Passmore (1998) proposes that there are three purposes of leisure: *achievement,* in which leisure occupations provide challenges and are demanding (e.g. sport and music), that

influence and are influenced by self-efficacy beliefs and self-esteem; *social,* in which leisure occupations provide opportunities for being with others, relationships and social acceptance; and *time-out,* in which leisure occupations provide opportunities for relaxation, which may have positive (e.g. rest) and negative (e.g. socially isolating, less demanding) effects.

Successful aging is a predominant concept in the literature and is positively linked with participation in leisure occupations (Adams, Leibbrandt, & Moon, 2011, Ricon, Weissman, & Demeter, 2013). In older age, leisure is often viewed as the antithesis of work and as a consequence plays a large role in the life of many older adults who are viewed as having more time for leisure. Many older adults also choose to stay in work, often in a reduced capacity, or participate in volunteering occupations, which have been found to have positive health benefits.

This chapter discusses some of the key theoretical ideas of engaging in leisure throughout the lifespan, focusing on adults and older adults. It looks at the research findings of participation within leisure and considers links between health and well-being, in addition to leisure after physical illness, injury or impairment. Factors to consider while assessing leisure, as well as leisure interventions, are outlined using the Person–Environment–Occupation (PEO) framework (Law et al., 1996). Two practice stories illustrate how leisure occupations can be woven into the intervention plans of the occupational therapist.

LEISURE THROUGHOUT THE LIFESPAN

Infancy, Early and Middle Childhood (Birth to Puberty)

In the early years of a person's life there is an emphasis on the physical development of the skills required for play and leisure occupations, with all the fundamental motor skills developed by 7 years of age. With increasing age the cognitive demands increase, with more complex and abstract rules for games and increasingly subtle nuances in social interaction; cognitive development continues into the mid-20s. As the focus of this chapter is on adulthood and older adults, those wishing to learn more about this early childhood period should refer to Brooks and Dunford (2014) and Case-Smith and Clifford O'Brien (2015) for an overview of the development of play occupations.

Adolescence

During early adolescence (from puberty to about 15 years) there is a focus on physical appearance and a shift to loose-knit, mixed-sex social groups with increased intimacy of individual friendships. There is a need for self-reliance and the beginnings of self-appraisal and consideration of the future. In late adolescence (from about 16 years onwards) independent living skills emerge alongside developing personal identity, morals and values, along with the emergence of the ability to express sexual needs. During this stage, adolescents can plan journeys and travel alone, further broadening their leisure horizons.

The cultural environment that people live in has an impact on how they spend their leisure time. Time use studies conducted with adolescents have shown differences between those who live in industrial and nonindustrial communities (Larson & Verma, 1999). Those who live in nonindustrial communities spend more time doing work occupations and therefore less time on leisure occupations, and when they are involved in leisure occupations, it is usually in an unstructured manner. Compared with those who live in industrial societies, those who live in nonindustrial communities spend less time doing work occupations and more in education occupations, with the time spent involved in leisure occupations varying among Europe, North America and East Asia (Larson & Verma, 1999). As an illustration of this, the comparative amounts of time adolescents spent involved in free time, watching television, sports, other active leisure and self-care occupations are illustrated in Table 34.1.

Adulthood

In early adulthood there is an emphasis on establishing occupational balance among leisure, productivity and self-care demands. Socialising and dating are important leisure activities. Some people partake in team sports and explore and pursue varying interests. Generally speaking it can be said that healthy adults participate in leisure pursuits that are wide ranging and diverse. However, the concept of leisure occupations and their impact on health and well-being are currently lacking in evidence within the occupational therapy profession (Hammell, 2009a; Law, Steinwender, & Leclair, 1998b; Suto, 1998). There are some studies emerging that have made links between health outcomes and leisure within specific communities of people with an illness, injury or impairment, like that of Buchholz et al. (2009), who found that adults with spinal cord injuries who participated in daily physical leisure occupations were less likely to develop cardiovascular disease and type 2 diabetes risk factors (Buchholz et al., 2009).

In relation to time spent on leisure occupations in adulthood, there is now an emerging pattern, arising from a number of epidemiological studies around the world, of a growing number of adults spending much of their leisure time sitting as opposed to engaging in physical forms of activity, which has been linked to increased morbidity, long-term illness and obesity (Patel et al., 2010). Patel et al.'s large-scale prospective study concluded that adults who spent 6 hours or more per day sitting for their leisure time, as opposed to 3 hours, had significantly higher death rates in both male (20%) and female (40%) populations (Patel et al., 2010). Similar epidemiological studies carried out in other developed countries, such as Australia, show comparable trends between the time adults spent sitting during leisure and increased detrimental health effects, as well as morbidity (Chau, van der Ploeg, Merom, Chey, Bauman, 2012). This phenomenon of a more sedentary leisure time is not unique to the Western world, as similar results can be seen in the study carried out in Brazil by Fernandes et al. (2010), who reported links to obesity and time spent watching television among adults.

Increasing obesity and its associated health concerns no doubt pose a challenge to contemporary occupational therapy practitioners who aim to underpin their practice with an ethos of promoting a healthy lifestyle and prevention of illness, injury or impairment (COT 2008). Coupled with this worrying trend in increasing obesity that is linked to a more sedentary lifestyle worldwide is the need for therapists to follow nationally recognised health and care guidance, which recently has specifically addressed the need to increase the general physical activity levels not only in adults but in children as well (National Institute of Clinical Excellence (NICE), 2015).

There have been other barriers identified for adults engaging in leisure time pursuits that may have an impact on how occupational therapists consider the leisure goals of the people receiving occupational therapy services. In their systematic review of the literature, Beenackers et al. (2012) observed that

TABLE 34.1
Estimates of Time Adolescents Spend in Activities (Larson & Verma, 1999)

Activity	TIME/DAY*			
	Europe	North America	East Asia	Nonindustrial Unschooled
Total free time	5.5–7.5 hours	6.5–8 hours	4–5.5 hours	4–7 hours
Television viewing	1½–2½ hours	1½–2½ hours	1½–2½ hours	Insufficient data
Sports	20–80 minutes	30–60 minutes	0–20 minutes	Insufficient data
Other active leisure	10–20 minutes	10–20 minutes	0–10	Insufficient data
Personal care	0.5–0.8 hours	No data	No data	No data
Eating	1.2 hours	No data	No data	No data
Sleep	8–9 hours	No data	No data	No data
Household labour	20–40 minutes	20–40 minutes	10–20 minutes	5–9 hours
Paid labour	10–20 minutes	40–60 minutes	10–20 minutes	0.5–8 hours
Schoolwork	4–5½ hours	3–4½ hours	5.5–7½ hours	NA

*Averaged across 7 days including weekdays and weekends.

socioeconomic factors play a significant role in the amount of time adults spend in leisure occupations, with those in higher economic positions spending more time on physical leisure activities. Therapists need to be aware of the cultural elements of this study when considering this evidence, as most of the studies meeting the inclusion criteria of this review came from Scandinavian countries (Beenackers et al., 2012).

Some researchers, including Gillen (2015), comment that specific condition-focused research, such as occupational therapy interventions after cerebrovascular accident (CVA), are narrowing the scope of the profession both from a research and a practice perspective by maintaining a focus on what are deemed essential areas of recovery, such as motor and cognitive function, and not extending intervention to social participation and leisure. Gillen challenges occupational therapy researchers across the globe to start using occupation-focused cognitive outcomes to demonstrate occupational therapists' unique contribution to health and social care delivery (Gillen, 2015). Others have found that people with multiple sclerosis engage in leisure occupations as often as their healthy counterparts, which led the researchers to conclude that occupational therapists should not assume the occupational engagement of people receiving occupational therapy services is necessarily shaped by impairment or that leisure be neglected within interventions (Brooke, Desmarais, & Forwell, 2007).

New theoretical frameworks are being introduced in occupational therapy that consider a more evidence-based approach to analysing occupations, such as the Canadian Association of Occupational Therapy Do-Live-Well framework (Moll et al., 2015). This framework encourages an exploration of the various dimensions of the experience of engaging in chosen occupations, and the activity patterns, as well as the health-related outcomes. Overarching this concept is the notion that there are a variety of complex intrapersonal and sociocultural elements that affect the quality of the occupational experience and outcome – some of which have already been alluded to earlier and will now be addressed further in the occupational science section.

Older Adults

When planning for older age, two predominant strategies have been identified in relation to the continuation of leisure occupations. These are continuity and innovation (Agahi, Ahacic, & Parker, 2006), with the preservation of individual and social identities being the motivation for participation. However, this is challenged by the prevalence of long-term and multimorbid conditions in older people, with 58% of people older than 60, compared with 14% younger than 40, having a range of these conditions (Department of Health, 2012).

Retirement from paid employment, deterioration in general physical and cognitive functioning and an often declining social network can severely restrict opportunities for engagement in leisure occupations for the older adult. Individual attributes such as gender and contextual variables such as meaning play a large part in influencing leisure choices. Further contextual factors influencing leisure choice include cultural norms, values, beliefs, spirituality, climate, cost, environment and correlational factors such as death of a spouse or friend who may have previously participated in a leisure pursuit with an individual. A recognition of the contextual factors that influence and shape the leisure choices of older adults who have a physical illness, injury or impairment must be acknowledged in the delivery of the occupational therapy process, in a similar way to that described earlier with adults.

The contribution of leisure to health and well-being in older adults is receiving growing attention within the literature (Chang,Wray, & Lin, 2014). Occupational therapists have traditionally been advocates of the link between engaging in meaningful occupations, including leisure, and health and well-being (Trombly Latham 2008). However, historically, more emphasis has been placed on maximising an individual's independence in self-care within occupational therapy practice after hospitalisation (Holm & Mu, 2012). Hartman-Maeir, Soroker, Ring, Avni, & Katz, (2007), in a study investigating the chronic consequences of CVA on activity limitations, found that there was a need for rehabilitation to focus on leisure in order to increase life satisfaction after CVA. They found that, on average, people who had a CVA gave up 57.2% of their leisure occupations. Within the ever-increasing elderly population there is a clear opportunity for occupational therapists to explore leisure as either a new domain of occupational performance or an expansion of previous meaningful leisure engagement.

AN OCCUPATIONAL SCIENCE PERSPECTIVE ON LEISURE

Contemporary theorists in occupational science find the traditional classifications of occupations of self-care, productivity and leisure (Creek, 2003; Townsend & Polatajko, 2007) problematic and reductionist (Hammell, 2009a) and advocate instead that an individual's diverse perspectives on defining occupations be taken into account both from a research and practice point of view (Hammell, 2009b). It is now more widely accepted among that it is the person's subjective experiences of doing or engaging in an occupation that reflects his or her state of health and well-being. In addition, there is acknowledgement of an interconnected nature to other individuals and a sense of belonging in society while engaging in valued occupations, as opposed to attempting to categorise occupations simplistically into areas of work, self-care or leisure (Borell, Asaba, Rosenberg, Schult, & Townsend, 2006; Hammell, 2009b). Defining occupations from an individual's perspective is deemed to be more helpful not only to align with the core philosophical beliefs of the profession but to avoid being economically or politically driven; indeed, there is now a change of thought within the literature in relation to frameworks of the profession that are being developed, such as the Do-Live-Well framework mentioned earlier, which should help shape the practice of occupational therapy for the future (Moll et al., 2015).

Engaging in Doing Occupations

As alluded to already, researchers are acknowledging the need to understand an individual's subjective experience of doing valued occupations, rather than necessarily categorising occupations into self-care, productivity or leisure. Central to this belief is the need to understand and unpack meanings that are attached to the occupation by the individual (Reed, Hocking, & Smythe, 2011). Care must be taken not to impose Western minority cultural views onto a person's experience of doing leisure occupations, as highlighted by Hammell (2009a) in her critique of underlying assumptions of many early occupational therapy advocates in relation to meanings attached to individuals and the occupations they are performing. For example, the meaning of doing a certain occupation for a person may not necessarily be positive and could result in boredom. Hammell is highly critical of the 'privileged triad' of self-care, productivity and leisure, concluding that attempting to define occupations in this manner is contestable (Hammell, 2009a, p. 10) and that leisure is an ableist concept, which is ultimately difficult to defend, advocating that the focus should be on consideration of factors like caring for others or spending time with relevant others who are valued.

Wallenbert and Jonsson (2005) carried out a small-scale qualitative study in Sweden looking at the recovery of seven people who had a CVA who ranged from 1.5 to 7 months post-discharge after rehabilitation, where they received occupational therapy interventions that focused on cognitive and motor recovery. The need for more planning from the participants' perspectives to engage in occupations was a recurring finding, and one participant in particular related this new level of planning with driving to the forest, which interfered with his ability to perform his leisure pursuit of hunting. This participant described the meaning of hunting to him as relaxing; however, after his CVA he had to arrange for lifts in advance, which affected his perception of doing the occupation. The message for occupational therapists here is that there is a role for empowering individuals to engage in their valued leisure occupations.

Restorative Occupations

Experiencing pleasure and joy while engaged in leisure pursuits has been linked with overall improved health outcomes, including emotional well-being (Pressman et al., 2009). In their review of the literature Pressman et al. (2009, p. 725) define leisure as:

> Pleasurable activities that individuals engage in voluntarily when they are free from the demands of work or other responsibilities. These might include hobbies, sports, socializing, or spending time in nature.

What is of note is how the authors broadened the scope of their review of literature beyond occupational therapy, taking on board studies from the field of psychology on coping and drawing on research in the field of leisure science. Results from this review should help occupational therapists underpin and justify their practice with evidence of the restorative and stress-relieving properties of activities deemed to require little mental effort or, in other words, during leisure occupations (Pressman et al., 2009).

The environment plays a major role in the enjoyment of leisure occupations, as does the meaning that the person attaches to that leisure pursuit. In a qualitative study of five individuals with rheumatoid arthritis, Squire (2012) concluded that the whole contextualised subjective experience of engaging in a person's leisure occupations, as well as embodying the richness of the specific environmental factors, need to be considered by the occupational therapist. Dave's story (Practice Story 34.1) illustrates his reasons for going freshwater swimming, highlighting the importance of the environment in his experience of engaging in his passion. For him it is not just about the health benefits of the physical exercise, which are part of his intrinsic motivation, but it is the psychological and sociological benefits of doing this hobby with friends that he finds most attractive.

PRACTICE STORY 34.1

Dave: Meanings of Occupations – Unique and Individual

Dave was a 40-year-old student who describes himself as an ex–civil servant who left his job to become a student again. When he was 37 years old he was diagnosed with rheumatoid arthritis (RA). His experience of the illness was very negative; he talked about how low he became after the initial diagnosis, especially as his mother had severe RA for many years and had many deformities as a result. Some of his key occupations included work (as a student), cycling (in relation to commuting), hill walking, gardening and cold-water swimming. Dave was not always a very physically active individual; however, since learning that he had a chronic health condition, his response was to become more physically active, including taking up cycling to and from his studies, as well as outdoor freshwater swimming. He stated that he loved swimming outside because

> It's not like a swimming pool or anything [....] I do it cause it's just really nice to be in the water, just surrounded by trees, with ducks and things [...] it's just lovely.

Nature has real meaning for him, and this is extended from the occupation of swimming into another of his leisure pursuits, gardening.

Modified from Squire (2012).

Temporal Aspects of Participating in Leisure Occupations

When living with a chronic or temporary illness, injury or impairment there may be a need to adapt the nature of engagement with the occupation over time. An individual may cease participation in chosen leisure pursuits for a number of months or even years at a time during periods of increasing symptoms or relapse of the chronic health condition but still feel connected to these leisure pursuits. Therefore the issue of time becomes less relevant in the narrative of how that person engages in leisure occupations. Occupational therapy practitioners should be mindful of this temporal aspect of engaging in leisure when working with people with fluctuating conditions, who may experience spells of reduced capacity, in order to encourage those who may have temporarily stopped doing a particular restorative occupation as a result of this reduced ability (Squire, 2012). To illustrate, Ann participates in watercolour classes as her main leisure hobby, but during periods of flare-up of her rheumatoid arthritis she is unable to either get to the classes or perform many of the tasks involved in painting and so she does not actively participate until her flare-up subsides. This often translates into returning to classes many months later. Her narrative about engaging in watercolour classes as a leisure occupation therefore covers a long period (Squire, 2012). While assessing people's level of participation in leisure, the therapist should consider the long-term narrative of the occupational engagement. This temporal aspect to leisure occupations is echoed in a phenomenological study of older adults after CVA recovery in Australia, where emerging themes included how participants reengaged in leisure activities over time and had internal hope for the future as a result of being able to take a longer term view of engaging in leisure pursuits (O'Sullivan & Chard, 2009).

Interconnectedness of Occupations

The interrelated nature of doing leisure occupations with significant others during all of the lifecycle stages is a core element in contemporary occupational therapy and has been well documented within the Do-Live-Well framework (Moll et al., 2015). In Dave's narrative (see Practice Story 34.1) his leisure activity revolved around his friends swimming with him (Squire, 2012). This interpersonal aspect is an important factor to explore with individuals experiencing interruptions and their motivations to engage in leisure.

CONTEXT OF LEISURE AND OCCUPATIONAL THERAPY IN PHYSICAL SETTINGS FOR ADULTS AND OLDER ADULTS

Majnemer (2010) argues that as part of everyday practice occupational therapists need to consider how the people they work with engage in leisure occupations. However, many occupational therapy practice contexts, such as acute care, are constrained by a variety of internal and external pressures placed on therapy services that narrow the agenda to simply focusing on self-care activities and safe discharge planning at the expense of working towards leisure occupations. Different practice settings will influence the choice of intervention. This can mean that enabling people to continue to participate in their valued leisure occupations can be neglected by occupational therapists. Yet if occupational therapists are to work in a holistic and person-centred manner, it is important to consider a person's leisure activities when conducting assessments and planning and implementing interventions. There has been a shift in the modern context of health care in the United Kingdom to health promotion, enablement or reablement and the ever-increasing move to working with people in their home environment where possible. Therapists working in rehabilitation and reablement (Social Care Institute for Excellence, 2011) will have more scope to include meaningful leisure occupations into their occupation-focused interventions.

Leisure is one of the core foci of occupational therapy; however, Stav, Hallenen, Lane, & Arbesman, (2012) point to a limited body of literature examining the effect of leisure on older adults' health. In the United Kingdom, inpatient and outpatient rehabilitation centres are traditionally the main location for older adults receiving occupational therapy interventions that related to leisure occupations. Occupations commonly offered are often limited to those readily available within the department, and as a consequence of reducing budgets occupational therapists must be ever more entrepreneurial in their approach to offering person-centred yet appropriate leisure occupations within their intervention.

The concept of well-being encompasses both physical and mental health domains (Chief Medical Officers of England, Scotland, Wales and Northern Ireland, 2011). It is therefore important for the occupational therapist to acknowledge the psychological impacts of illness, injury or impairment. The National Institute for Health and Clinical Excellence (NICE, 2008) highlight the importance of physical activity to maintain or improve mental well-being in the older population. This is particularly important if an individual is experiencing physical illness, injury or impairment, regardless of the life stage.

NICE (2008) have outlined the following recommendations for older adults in primary and residential care; however, the guidance could be considered relevant for all areas of occupational therapy practice with older adults (pp. 5–8):

- Offer regular sessions that encourage older people to construct daily routines to help maintain or improve their mental well-being. The sessions should also increase their knowledge of a range of issues, from nutrition and how to stay active to personal care.
- Offer tailored, community-based physical activity programmes. These should include moderate-intensity activities (such as swimming, walking, dancing), strength and resistance training, and toning and stretching exercises.

■ Advise older people and their carers how to exercise safely for 30 minutes a day on 5 or more days a week, using examples of everyday activities such as shopping, housework and gardening. (The 30 minutes can be broken down into 10-minute bursts.)

■ Promote regular participation in local walking schemes as a way of improving mental well-being. Help and support older people to participate fully in these schemes, taking into account their health, mobility and personal preferences.

■ Involve occupational therapists in the design of training offered to practitioners.

ASSESSMENT OF LEISURE OCCUPATIONS

During the assessment stage, the occupational therapist needs to obtain information from multiple sources in order to develop realistic, person-centred, collaborative goals. Self-report, observation and contact with relatives or carers can be triangulated in order to ensure a person-centred, occupation-based focus to intervention. A consideration of a prior level of functioning, the support system in the community and anticipated level of return to previous functioning will inform the assessment process (College of Occupational Therapists (COT), 2003). These basic concepts of assessment apply across all of the life stages.

As a result of the holistic nature of occupational therapy, the practitioners include consideration of the individual's leisure occupations when conducting assessments (McHugh Pendelton & Schultz-Krohn, 2013). Carrying out comprehensive assessment is supported by a range of evidence-based practice guidelines published by the COT in recent years. For example, in the COT (2012) guidelines for adults undergoing total hip replacement, recommendations 1 and 8 pertain specifically to the use of standardised assessment tools, and recommendation 24 highlights the need to encourage social reengagement after hospital discharge (COT, 2012). In the COT (2011) guideline for working with adults with lower limb amputation, there is specific reference made to the need for assessment of the individual's participation in recreational activities.

There are a diverse range of generic assessment tools available to the occupational therapist, including many that have a focus on leisure, such as the Canadian Occupational Performance Measure (Law et al., 1998a), a widely used tool that rates a person's performance and that person's satisfaction with performance in self-care, productivity and leisure occupations. Alternatively, there are those assessment tools that look more specifically at aspects of the person's performance skills, such as manual dexterity or cognition, the intention being that results are transferred to the different tasks required within the person's leisure pursuit to ascertain if engaging in that pursuit will be possible. An example would be the use of the Sequential Occupational Dexterity Assessment (Van Lankveld et al., 1996), a standardised tool developed in the 1990s for use with people with rheumatoid arthritis that requires the person to perform a range of hand function tasks to determine the quality of the person's hand dexterity. Many such commercially available assessments tools use timed tests as one method of the evaluation, which raises the question of how applicable they are to real-life engagement in leisure occupations.

Informal methods of assessment such as observation or interviews are utilised by many practitioners. The focus of these assessments tends to be on the person's ability to carry out activities of daily living, which translates into assessing the performance capacity of mobility and transfers, washing, dressing, toileting and eating activities as well as environmental assessment, often at the expense of exploring leisure. Turner, Chapman, McSherry, Krishnagiri, & Watts, (2000) revealed that there was less emphasis on leisure occupations within physical settings during assessment and the amount of assessment time spent on this area correlated to the value placed on leisure by the people receiving occupational therapy services. Moreover, they found that more value was attached to exploring leisure with people within psychosocial settings than in physical settings.

Wales, Clemson, Lannin, & Cameron, (2012) highlight the tendency for occupational therapists to choose nonstandardised over standardised assessments in this area of practice. Within acute care, Crennan and MacRae (2010) found that nonstandardised function-based assessments were the most commonly used assessment by occupational therapists. Similarly Carlill, Gash, & Hawkins, (2004) found that discharge from accident and emergency departments was predominantly based on nonstandardised function-based assessments not including leisure occupations. However, obtaining information on social engagement and participation in leisure can identify the need for increased community support (Crennan & MacRae, 2010). To demonstrate valid and reliable results, occupational therapists should, where possible, use available validated tools to assess and subsequently evaluate the effectiveness of interventions (COT, 2013a).

It is important to note that the assessment of sensory, movement-related and cognitive functions and awareness of deficits in relation to safety concerns will inform the occupational therapy process, and leisure will not usually receive a stand-alone assessment. Central to this is the exploration of older persons' feelings and awareness of their altered physical and psychological state after a health event. Only when this is accepted can a move to accepting adaptation, assistance or replacement in relation to leisure occupations occur.

The Interest Checklist (Matsutsuyu, 1969) is commonly used in practice and identifies the personal, occupational and environmental factors (Fazio et al., 2008) affecting older adults' participation in leisure. It has been further developed as the UK Modified Interest Checklist (Heasman & Salhotra, 2008).

Other checklists that can be considered for use are the Leisure Assessment Inventory (Hawkins et al., 2002), and the Leisure Interest Profile for Seniors (Henry, 1997). Occupational therapists must be mindful of the ability to comprehend the written word, possible visual difficulties and intact verbal memory when using questionnaires or checklists with the older adult.

The Activity Card Sort (Baum & Edwards, 2001) measures past and current leisure and sociocultural occupations. There are three versions for use with community-dwelling older adults, adults in hospital and older adults recovering from a health event. The original version has been modified and validated for use in several countries, including the United States of America, Puerto Rico and Australia (Eriksson et al., 2011). The Expanded Activity Card Sort (Ricon, Weissman, & Demeter, 2013) includes future planning, which allows the occupational therapist to establish client-centred treatment goals.

Some leisure assessments that are suitable to use with adults are listed in Table 34.2.

INTERVENTIONS THAT FOCUS ON LEISURE

An occupation-focused, person-centred approach to intervention is encouraged by COT (2015) and Crennan and MacRae (2010). Translating this into practice means that practitioners need to incorporate an individual's leisure pursuit within the intervention process, where possible, as a means to the end as well as the achievement of leisure goals being the product of intervention. Setting person-centred occupational goals follows on from the assessment phase of the occupational therapy process and should take into consideration many factors that can enable an individual to engage in leisure occupation.

TABLE 34.2
Selection of Occupational Therapy Leisure Assessments Suitable to Use with Adults

Assessment Tool	Outline of Use	Author(s)
Canadian Occupational Performance Measure (COMP)	An interview-style questionnaire where people with an occupational interruption identify and rate both their performance and their satisfaction with their performance.	Law et al. (1998; several updates since, including 2015 version)
Interest Checklist	Identifies personal, environmental and occupational factors affecting leisure occupations.	Matsutsuyu (1969)
Modified Interest Checklist	Records information on strength of interest and engagement in 68 past, current and possible future activities, focusing on leisure interests that affect activity choices.	Kielhofner and Neville (1983)
Modified Interest Checklist (United Kingdom)	Collects information on strength of interest and engagement in 74 activities in the past, current and future. Interests are listed in nine categories that focus on different types of activity choices.	Heasman and Salhotra (2008)
Leisure Assessment Inventory (LAI)	Measures leisure behaviours of adults.	Hawkins et al. (2002)
Leisure Interest Profile for Seniors	Used to select specific leisure activities with which to engage an older adult by assessing a person's interest and participation in leisure activities.	Henry (1997)
The Activity Card Sort (ACS)	Measure for evaluating past and current participation in instrumental, leisure and sociocultural activities.	Baum and Edwards (2001)
The Expanded Activity Card Sort	Includes a future planned activities sorting task in addition to the ACS.	Ricon et al. (2013)
The National Institutes of Health (NIH) Activity Record (ACTRE)	Users record participation in work, play or leisure activities by half-hour intervals throughout the day and record their pain, fatigue, level of difficulty, competence, value and enjoyment for each activity. Validated for use with people with rheumatoid arthritis.	Gerber and Furst (1992)
Leisure Competence Measure	Measures current level of functioning in relation to leisure using a rating scale and change over time. Validated for use with older adults.	Kloseck et al. (1996)
Possibilities for Activities Scale (PActS)	New assessment tool being developed for clinicians from research within occupational science. Looks at measuring the perceived occupational potential in older adults.	Pergolotti and Cutchin (2015)
Role Checklist & Role Checklist V2	Identifies an individual's roles and the value he or she attaches to them.	Scott et al. (2014)

The Person and Leisure Interventions

Leisure interventions are designed by the therapist based on information gained during the assessment of the performance capacities of the individual. Leisure interventions will usually form only part of an overall intervention plan. Older adults may struggle to return to participation in leisure occupations that may be key to recovery and maintenance of health after a health event (Hutchinson & Warner, 2014).

Therapists need to apply principles of underpinning theory to their practice, such as biomechanics or functional rehabilitation, to enable as full participation in leisure as possible. Biomechanical frameworks of reference make use of an individual's body movements, strength and endurance within the rehabilitation phase of intervention, and the creative therapist can apply these principles within an individual's meaningful leisure occupation so that these aspects are being improved while doing the occupation (Early, 2013). Central to occupational therapy interventions in this area is adaptation and pacing of leisure occupations, as increased fatigue levels are common after illness, injury or impairment disorders (Finsterer & Mahjoub, 2014).

Grading the activity to increase physical demands is one way in which to achieve biomechanical gain. For example, if someone's leisure pursuit involves baking, the therapist may start by engaging the person in short sessions of baking with very low level tasks, such as sifting the flour while seated, and then, as the person's movements, strength and endurance all improve, increasing the demands, such as with longer sessions and doing more physically challenging tasks like beating the butter and sugar by hand while standing. Core knowledge and skills of occupation/activity analysis will assist the therapist in devising such personalised interventions (Rybski, 2011).

Conversely, where there is limitation of movement, strength or endurance, or where the person is not expected to make any further improvement in any of these elements, it may be more appropriate for the therapist to take a compensatory approach to engaging the individual in his or her leisure occupations. This may result in adaptation of the environment or the occupation to enable participation. It is also worth noting at this juncture that when the person is experiencing psychological issues in addition to physical difficulties, a cognitive behavioural approach may also be required, as people must not be considered as purely machines without thoughts and feelings (Knudson, 2007).

Different practice settings will influence the choice of intervention. As noted earlier, within an acute care setting, goals are often prioritised to expectations for discharge, which commonly do not include leisure occupations. This may mean that therapists have to consider referring individuals to external agencies that can assist with reengagement in leisure occupations. Therapists working in rehabilitation and reablement (Social Care Institute for Excellence, 2011) will have more scope to include meaningful leisure occupations into their occupation-focused intervention plans.

Collaborative problem solving, with each individual having a realistic and safe expectation of his or her future level of functioning, is a key aspect of therapeutic intervention. However, the occupational therapist must be careful not to either overestimate or underestimate an individual's occupational performance abilities (Holm & Mu, 2012) and take into account cointerventions such as medication and resulting impairments such as pain and fatigue. A consideration of co- and multimorbidities resulting from the normal aging process will have an intensified effect on multiple performance areas after a health event.

The challenge for occupational therapists is to be leisure motivators or stimulators of return to leisure participation after a health event (Toepoel, 2013). Leisure motivation within the older adult population has been found to be influenced by social participation (Beggs, Kleparski, Elkins, & Hurd, 2014); loneliness and social isolation, experienced by an increasing number of older adults, have been independently associated with negative behaviour, which is more likely to put health further at risk (Shankar, McMunn, Banks, & Steptoe, 2011).

Leisure education has been highlighted as enhancing the ability of older adults to gain control over their leisure occupations (Chang et al., 2015). The importance of the use of education within occupational therapy practice to improve performance in occupations and facilitate successful lifestyle adjustments can be used for the older adults. This can take the form of a programme to improve attitudes to leisure, knowledge about leisure and capacity for leisure within the context of the older adult after a health event (Chang et al., 2015).

Group-based leisure interventions have been found to be beneficial to the health and well-being of individuals after spinal cord injury (Daniel & Manigandan, 2005). This study involved several groups of five people who had a spinal cord lesion resulting in paraplegia; they participated in group activities, including a trust-building warmup, games and homework that lasted up to 1 hour. The findings indicated significant improvement in quality-of-life outcomes after participation in leisure groups for these participants. However, caution is needed in designing leisure group interventions in order to avoid becoming therapist driven or moving away from the ethos of using meaningful occupations as intervention tools, as what one person considers enjoyable, like playing board games, for example, will not hold the same value to all group participants.

The Environment and Leisure Interventions

The environments in which people conduct leisure pursuits are very important to consider. Within the intervention phase, the occupational therapist needs to ensure interventions are implemented, where possible, within a real-life context. To illustrate, this may mean arranging for adaptions to the home environment to enable wheelchair access to the garden or ensuring there is adequate access to leisure centres to enable participation in yoga classes.

Physical, social and cultural environments will heavily influence an older person's ability and motivation to participate in leisure occupations after a health event. Whether someone is city or country dwelling influences participation in moderate to vigorous activity versus sedentary activity (Evenson, Morland, Wen, & Scanlin, 2014).

NICE (2008) recommend that occupational therapists be involved in designing and developing appropriate training schemes for care staff working with older adults. One reason for this is to enable staff to encourage independence in daily activities, including leisure (COT, 2013b). COT have developed the Living Well in Care Homes Toolkit (COT, 2014), which provides care homes with person-focused guidelines that can be tailored to their service and the activity choices of their residents.

Occupations as Intervention

Ideally the aim of therapy should be to use the person's meaningful leisure occupation as the intervention in order to reach the goals agreed with the individual. This may mean that the occupational therapist needs to be creative in how to engage the person who can no longer physically pursue previous pastimes because of illness, injury or impairment by looking at alternative ways to enable people to participate, such as using technology-based games. Education may play a key role in how the occupational therapists help individuals to engage in leisure occupations, encouraging them to embrace different roles within their former occupation or take up new occupations.

Studies have produced varying results in relation to which leisure occupations produce the highest level of well-being. Paillard-Borg, Wang, Winblad, & Fratiglioni, (2009), in a survey of older adults in an urban setting in Sweden, found that cognitive occupations such as reading and writing were the most popular and resulted in a higher level of well-being compared with social, physical, productive and recreational activities. Contrary to this, a review of the literature on social and leisure activity and well-being by Adams, Leibbrandt, & Moon, (2011) concluded that informal social activity promoted the best sense of well-being in later life. Overarching this is the person-centred nature of occupational therapy, which ensures that choices for leisure occupations will be central to an individual's personal goals and choices.

In a systematic review, Dorstyn et al. (2014) found that an improvement in physical, cognitive and psychological outcomes were attributable to the inclusion of leisure occupations within rehabilitation for people who had a CVA. Significant improvement in short-term mood and quality-of-life outcomes were evident. Regarding benefit gained, a further systematic review (Stav et al., 2012) identified that there was no gold standard in relation to specific occupations, their frequency and their intensity.

Ricon et al. (2013), in a study of 60 Israeli adults ages 55 to 74 years, found that older adults were more likely to continue with previous occupations than plan for new occupations, though there is some evidence to the contrary (Nimrod, 2008). Goal-setting discussions therefore should consider whether the person wants to continue with previous occupations or is interested in trying new occupations and experiences, such as use of the Internet (Nimrod, 2014), gaming technologies or Wii fit (Chan et al., 2012).

Leisure occupations explored in previous studies investigating health outcomes for older adults have included gardening, reading, visiting others, completing crosswords and playing games (Stav et al., 2012). These studies provide evidence for the use of leisure with this population but point towards the need for an expansion of the body of evidence for this area of practice. Gardening, woodwork and games are prominent within an occupational therapist's repertoire. Söderback (2009) presents an international perspective on the use of gardening or horticultural therapy for a range of individuals, including the older adult. It is low cost, has portability, uses the five senses, can be easily graded and is versatile and adaptable. The role of the occupational therapist in health promotion continues to grow. Clark et al. (2012), in the Well Elderly Lifestyle Redesign intervention, highlight the importance of assisting the older adult in overcoming 'mundane obstacles' such as body aches and transportation difficulties to be able to participate in occupations.

Practice Story 34.2, about Maria, illustrates how leisure occupations can be woven into the intervention plans of the occupational therapist.

PRACTICE STORY 34.2

Maria

Helen was an occupational therapist working in a community rehabilitation team. Maria was a 69-year-old retired media studies technician and was referred to Helen on discharge from an acute care hospital after a cerebrovascular accident (CVA). Maria progressed well in her rehabilitation; she had some residual speech and upper and lower limb movement difficulties on her dominant side, as well as mild attention and memory impairments. However, she was independent, if a little slow, in completing her self-care activities. She lived alone but had a close social circle centred on her photography club and a daughter with a young family who lived close by and helped with household management.

During completion of the COPM, Maria prioritised her desire to return to doing photography as this was what she was most passionate about. Maria was a keen photographer for many years and was a member of a very competitive

Maria (Continued)

photography club. She expressed worry about her ability to use her cameras effectively, being able to communicate clearly with her friends in the club, and being able to produce the same quality of photographs she had previously. Guided by the Canadian Practice Process Framework (Fazio et al., 2008) and the Person–Environment–Occupation Model (Law et al., 1996), Maria and Helen worked through the problems highlighted by Maria and explored options for returning to photography.

ASSESSMENT CONSIDERATIONS

Person

What were Maria's physical, psychological and psychosocial strengths and limitations?

Strengths. Maria was independent in her self-care activities and able to walk independently. She was motivated in her return to independence in all areas of occupation and had a very strong social network, including family who lived close by.

Limitations. Upper and lower limb movement difficulties and decreased strength and endurance provided challenges for carrying out photography at the pace Maria would have been used to before having a CVA. Expressive aphasia caused frustration when communicating with others. Attention and memory impairments affected daily routine, and Maria found she would often forget tasks that had to be completed or arrangements she had made with others.

COPM, Canadian Occupational Performance Measure.

Environment

What were the environmental factors within which the occupation of photography occurred that needed to be considered?

Factors to be considered included the following: the competitive culture within the photography club; multiple challenging environments to be negotiated depending on the subject being photographed; getting to and from the club and photography sites; manipulating the technology required to take and develop photographs.

Occupation

What were the physical steps, duration, complexity and demands of the tasks that made up the occupation of photography?

Therapist needs to conduct an activity and occupation analysis to determine the range of tasks Maria would need to complete when participating in photography.

Intervention Considerations

Helen attended a photography club session to assess the range of tasks Maria would be required to complete and identify where adapted equipment or techniques might assist her. She was able to talk with other members of the club to see where they might help Maria with tasks she found difficult or suggest specialist photography equipment to increase Maria's independence. She worked with Maria to create a routine for photography sessions, including the use of a diary as a memory aid. Energy conservation techniques, compensatory strategies and strength and endurance activities were used to improve function.

CONCLUSION

Leisure is a nonobligatory activity that is intrinsically motivated and engaged in during discretionary time with the purpose of enjoyment. A focus on the leisure occupations of people is important in contemporary occupational therapy practice because of the positive impact engaging in leisure can have on a person's physical and mental well-being. Where possible, occupational therapists should aim to assess people's engagement in leisure to identify their leisure needs and include these within their intervention plans. Exploring an individual's leisure occupations during assessment enables occupational therapists to more fully understand what is meaningful and of value to each individual with whom they are working and plan interventions in which leisure occupations can be used as a means to the end, as well as the achievement of leisure goals being the product of intervention.

Ⓔ http://evolve.elsevier.com/Curtin/OT

REFERENCES

Adams, K. B., Leibbrandt, S., & Moon, H. (2011). A critical review of the literature on social and leisure activity and wellbeing in later life. *Ageing & Society, 31*, 683–712.

Agahi, N., Ahacic, K., & Parker, M. G. (2006). Continuity of leisure participation from middle age to old age. *Journal of Gerontology: B Social Sciences, 61*, 340–346.

American Occupational Therapy Association (2014). Occupational therapy practice framework: Domain and process. *American Journal of Occupational Therapy, 6*(1), 1–48.

Baum, C. M., & Edwards, D. (2001). *Activity card sort (ACS). Test manual.* St. Louis: Washington University School of Medicine.

Beenackers, M. A., Kamphuis, C. B., Giskes, K., et al. (2012). Socioeconomic inequalities in occupational leisure-time, and transport related physical activity among European adults. *International Journal of Behavioural Nutrition and Physical Therapy, 9*(116), 1–23.

Beggs, B., Kleparski, T., Elkins, D., & Hurd, A. (2014). Leisure motivation of older adults in relation to other adult life stages. *Activities, Adaptation, & Aging, 38*(3), 175–187.

Borell, L., Asaba, E., Rosenberg, L., Schult, M.-L., & Townsend, E. (2006). Exploring experiences of 'participation' among individuals living with chronic pain. *Scandinavian Journal of Occupational Therapy, 13*, 76–85.

Brooke, K., Desmarais, C. D., & Forwell, S. J. (2007). Types and categories of personal projects: A revelatory means of understanding human occupation. *Occupational Therapy International, 14*(4), 281–296.

Brooks, R., & Dunford, C. (2014). Play. In W. Bryant, J. Fieldhouse, & K. Bannigan (Eds.), *Creek's occupational therapy & mental health* (5th ed). London: Churchill Livingstone.

Buchholz, A. C., Martin Ginis, K. A., Bray, S. R., et al. (2009). Greater daily leisure time physical activity is associated with lower chronic disease risk in adults with spinal cord injury. *Applied Physiology, Nutrition and Metabolism, 34*(4), 640–647.

Bundy, A. C. (2012). Children at play: Can I play too? In S. J. Lane, & A. C. Bundy (Eds.), *Kids can be kids: A childhood occupations approach*. Philadelphia: FA Davis.

Carlill, G., Gash, E., & Hawkins, G. (2004). Preventing unnecessary hospital admissions: An occupational therapy and social work service in an accident and emergency department. *British Journal of Occupational Therapy, 65*, 440–445.

Case-Smith, J., & Clifford O'Brien, J. (2015). *Occupational therapy for children and adolescents* (7th ed.). St. Louis: Elsevier.

Chan, T. C., Chan, F., Shea, Y. F., Lin, O. Y., Luk, J. K. H., & Chan, F. H. W. (2012). Interactive virtual reality Wii in geriatric day hospital: A study to assess its feasibility, acceptability and efficacy. *Geriatrics & Gerontology International, 12*(4), 714–721.

Chang, L., Yu, P., & Jeng, M. (2015). Effects of leisure education on self-rated health among older adults. *Psychology, Health & Medicine, 20*(1), 34–40.

Chang, P. J., Wray, L., & Lin, Y. (2014). Social relationships, leisure activity and health in older adults. *Health Psychology, 33*(6), 516–523.

Chau, J. Y., van der Ploeg, H. P., Merom, D., Chey, T., & Bauman, A. E. (2012). Cross-sectional associations between occupational and leisure-time sitting, physical activity and obesity in working adults. *Preventative Medicine, 54*(3–4), 195–200.

Chief Medical Officers of England, Scotland, Wales and Northern Ireland (2011). *Start active, stay active: A report on physical activity from the four home countries' Chief Medical Officers*. London: Department of Health, Physical Activity, Health Improvement and Protection.

Clark, F., Jackson, J., Carlson, M., et al. (2012). Effectiveness of a lifestyle intervention in promoting the well-being of independently living older people: Results of the Well Elderly 2 Randomised Controlled Trial. *Journal of Epidemiology & Community Health, 66*(9), 782–790.

College of Occupational Therapists (2003). *Occupational therapy defined as a complex intervention*. London: College of Occupational Therapists.

College of Occupational Therapists (2008). *Health promotion in occupational therapy*. London: College of Occupational Therapists.

College of Occupational Therapists (2011). *Occupational therapy with people who have had lower limb amputations*. College of Occupational Therapists: Evidence based guidelines. London.

College of Occupational Therapists (2012). *Occupational therapy for adults undergoing total hip replacement practice guideline*. London: College of Occupational Therapists.

College of Occupational Therapists (2013a). *Position statement. College of Occupational Therapists: Occupational therapists' use of standardized outcome measures*. London.

College of Occupational Therapists (2013b). *Occupational therapists work with people living in care homes*. London: College of Occupational Therapists (COT occupational therapy evidence – fact sheet).

College of Occupational Therapists (2014). *SNOMED subsets to support occupational therapy*. London: College of Occupational Therapists.

College of Occupational Therapists (2015). *Position statement. College of Occupational Therapists: Occupation-centred practice*. London.

Creek, J. (2003). *Occupational therapy defined as a complex intervention*. London: College of Occupational Therapists.

Crennan, M., & MacRae, A. (2010). Occupational therapy discharge assessment of elderly patients from acute care hospitals. *Physical and Occupational Therapy in Geriatrics, 28*(1), 33–43.

Crepeau, E. B., Cohn, E. S., & Schell, B. A. (Eds.). (2009). *Willard and Spackman's occupational therapy* (11th ed.). Philadelphia: Lippincott Williams & Wilkins.

Daniel, A., & Manigandan, C. (2005). Efficacy of leisure intervention groups and their impact on quality of life among people with spinal cord injury. *International Journal of Rehabilitation Research, 28*(1), 43–48.

Department of Health (2012). *Long-term conditions compendium of Information* (3rd ed.). London: Department of Health.

Dorstyn, D., Roberts, R., Kneebone, I. P., DPhil, K. P., Lieu, C., & Therapy, O. M. (2014). Systematic review of leisure therapy and its effectiveness in managing functional outcomes in stroke rehabilitation. *Topics in Stroke Rehabilitation, 21*(1), 40–51.

Early, M. (2013). *Physical dysfunction practice skills for the occupational therapy assistant* (3rd ed.). St Louis: Elsevier Mosby.

Eriksson, G. M., Chung, J. C. C., Beng, L. H., et al. (2011). Occupations of older adults: A cross cultural description. *Occupational Therapy Journal of Research, Occupation, Participation and Health, 31*, 182–192.

Evenson, K. R., Morland, K. B., Wen, F., & Scanlin, K. (2014). Physical activity and sedentary behavior among adults 60 years and older: New York City residents compared with a national sample. *Journal of Aging & Physical Activity, 22*(4), 499–507.

Fazio, K., Hicks, E., Kuzma, C., Leung, P., Schwartz, A., & Stergiou-Kita, M. (2008). The Canadian Practice Process Framework: Using a conscious approach to occupational therapy practice. *OT Now, 10*(4), 6–9.

Fernandes, R. A., Christofaro, D. G. D., Casonato, J., et al. (2010). Leisure time behaviors: Prevalence, correlates and associations with overweight in Brazilian adults. A cross-sectional analysis. *Revista médica de Chile, 138*, 29–93.

Finsterer, J., & Mahjoub, S. Z. (2014). Fatigue in healthy and diseased individuals. *American Journal of Hospice & Palliative Medicine, 31*(5), 562–575.

Gerber, L. H., & Furst, G. P. (1992). Validation of the NIH activity record: a quantitative measure of life activities. *Arthritis Care and Research, 5,* 81–86.

Gillen, G. (2015). What is the evidence for the effectiveness of interventions to improve occupational performance after stroke? *American Journal of Occupational Therapy, 69,* 6901170010.

Hammell, K. W. (2009a). Sacred texts: A sceptical exploration of the assumptions underpinning theories of occupation. *Canadian Journal of Occupational Therapy, 76,* 6–13.

Hammell, K. W. (2009b). Self-care, productivity, and leisure, or dimensions of occupational experience? Rethinking occupational 'categories'. *Canadian Journal of Occupational Therapy, 76*(2), 107–114.

Hartman-Maeir, A., Soroker, N., Ring, H., Avni, N., & Katz, N. (2007). Activities, participation and satisfaction one-year post stroke. *Disability and Rehabilitation, 29*(7), 559–566.

Hawkins, B. A., Ardovino, P., Rogers, N. B., Foose, A., & Olsen, N. (2002). *Leisure assessment inventory.* Ravensdale, WA: Idyll Arbor.

Heasman, D., & Salhotra, G. (2008). *Interest checklist guidance notes.* MOHO Clearinghouse: Moho Related Resources. University of Illinois.

Henry, A. (1997). *Leisure interest profile for seniors (research version 2.0).* Boston: University of Massachusetts.

Holm, S. E., & Mu, K. (2012). Discharge planning for the elderly in acute care: The perceptions of experienced occupational therapists. *Physical and Occupational Therapy in Geriatrics, 30*(3), 214–228.

Hutchinson, S. L., & Warner, G. (2014). Older adults' use of SOC strategies for leisure participation following an acute health event: Implications for recreation service delivery. *Journal of Park & Recreation Administration, 32*(1), 80–95.

Johnson, A. (2009). *Is leisure a luxury? Retrieved from, http://www.mstrust.org.uk/professionals/information/wayahead/articles/13032009_06.jsp.*

Kielhofner, G., & Neville, A. (1983). *The modified Interest Checklist.* Unpublished assessment. Chicago: University of Illinois at Chicago.

Kloseck, M., Crilly, R. G., Ellis, G. D., & Lammers, E. (1996). Leisure Competence Measure: Development and reliability testing of a scale to measure functional outcomes in therapeutic recreation. *Therapeutic Recreation Journal, 30*(1), 13–26.

Knudson, D. (2007). *Fundamentals of biomechanics.* New York: Springer.

Larson, R. W., & Verma, S. (1999). How children and adolescents spend time across the world: Work, play and developmental opportunities. *Psychological Bulletin, 125*(6), 701–736.

Law, M., Baptiste, S., McColl, M. A., Opzoomer, A., Polatajko, H., & Pollock, N. (1998a). The Canadian Occupational Performance Measure: An outcome measure for occupational therapy. *Canadian Journal of Occupational Therapy, 57*(2), 82–87.

Law, M., Cooper, B., Strong, S., Stewart, D., Rigby, P., & Letts, L. (1996). The Person-Environment-Occupation Model: A transactive approach to occupational performance. *Canadian Journal of Occupational Therapy, 63*(1), 9–23.

Law, M., Steinwender, S., & Leclair, L. (1998b). Occupation, health and wellbeing. *Canadian Journal of Occupational Therapy, 65*(2), 81–91.

Majnemer, A. (2010). Balancing the boat. Enabling an ocean of possibilities. *Canadian Journal of Occupational Therapy, 77*(4), 198–205.

Matsutsuyu, J. (1969). The Interest Checklist. *American Journal of Occupational Therapy, 23,* 323–328.

McHugh Pendleton, H., & Schultz-Krohn, W. (2013). The occupational therapy practice framework and the practice of occupational therapy for people with physical disabilities. In H. McHugh Pendleton, & W. Schultz-Krohn (Eds.), *Pedretti's occupational therapy. Practical skills for physical dysfunction* (7th ed., pp. 1–17). St. Louis. Mosby Elsevier.

Missiuna, C., & Pollock, N. (1991). Play deprivation in children with physical disabilities: The role of the occupational therapist in preventing secondary disability. *American Journal of Occupational Therapy, 45,* 882–888.

Moll, S. E., Gewurtz, R. E., Krupa, T. M., Law, M. C., Larivie, N., & Levasseur, M. (2015). 'Do-Live-Well': A Canadian framework for promoting occupation, health, and well-being. *Canadian Journal of Occupational Therapy, 82*(1), 9–23.

National Institute for Health and Clinical Excellence (NICE) (2008). *Occupational therapy interventions and physical activity interventions to promote the mental wellbeing of older people in primary care and residential care. NICE public health guidance 16.* London: NICE.

National Institute for Health and Care Excellence (NICE) (2015). *Maintaining a healthy weight and preventing excessive weight gain among adults and children. NICE public health guidance 7.* London: NICE.

Nimrod, G. (2008). In support of innovation theory: Innovation in activity patterns and life satisfaction among recently retired individuals. *Ageing and Society, 28,* 831–846.

Nimrod, G. (2014). The benefits of and constraints to participation in seniors' online communities. *Leisure Studies, 33*(3), 247–266. http://dx.doi.org/10.1080/02614367.2012.697697.

O'Sullivan, C., & Chard, J. (2009). An exploration of leisure activities post stroke. *Australian Occupational Therapy Journal, 57*(3), 159–166.

Paillard-Borg, S., Wang, H.-X., Winblad, B., & Fratiglioni, L. (2009). Pattern of participation in leisure activities among older people in relation to their health conditions and contextual factors: A survey in a Swedish urban area. *Ageing & Society, 29,* 803–821.

Passmore, A. (1998). Does leisure have an association with creating cultural patterns of work? *Journal of Occupational Science, 5*(3), 161–165.

Patel, A. V., Bernstein, L., Deka, A., et al. (2010). Leisure time spent sitting in relation to total mortality in a prospective cohort of US adults. *American Journal of Epidemology, 172*(4), 419–429.

Pergolotti, M., & Cutchin, M. P. (2015). The Possibilities for Activity Scale (PActS): Development, validity, and reliability. *Canadian Journal of Occupational Therapy, 82*(8), 85–92.

Pressman, S. D., Matthews, K. A., Cohen, S., et al. (2009). Association of enjoyable leisure activities with psychological and physical well-being. *Psychosomatic Medicine, 71*(7), 725–732.

Primeau, L. (2009). Play and leisure. In E. B. Crepeau, E. S. Cohn, & B. A. Boyt Schell (Eds.), *Willard and Spackman's occupational therapy* (11th ed.). Philadelphia: Lippincott Williams & Wilkins.

Rybski, M. (2011). *Kinesiology for occupational therapy*. Thorofare, NJ: Slack.

Reed, K. D., Hocking, C. S., & Smythe, L. A. (2011). Exploring the meaning of occupation: The case for phenomenology. *Canadian Journal of Occupational Therapy, 78*(5), 303–310.

Ricon, T., Weissman, P., & Demeter, N. (2013). A new category of 'future planning' in the activity card sort: Continuity versus novelty in old age. *Health, 5*, 179–187.

Scott, P. J., McFadden, R., Yates, K., Baker, S., & McSoley, S. (2014). The Role Checklist Version 2: Quality of Performance: Reliability and validation of electronic administration. *British Journal of Occupational Therapy, 77*(2), 96–106.

Shankar, A., McMunn, A., Banks, J., & Steptoe, A. (2011). Loneliness, social isolation and behavioural and biological health indicators in older adults. *Health Psychology, 30*(4), 377–385.

Slagle, E. C. (1922). Training aides for mental patients. *Archives of Occupational Therapy, 1*, 11–17.

Social Care Institute for Excellence (2011). *At a glance 46: Reablement: a key role for occupational therapists*. London: SCIE and College of Occupational Therapists.

Söderback, I. (Ed.). (2009). *International handbook of occupational therapy interventions*. New York: Springer Science + Business Media, LLC.

Squire, R. E. (2012). Living well with rheumatoid arthritis. *Musculoskeletal Care, 10*(3), 127–134.

Stav, W. B., Hallenen, T., Lane, J., & Arbesman, M. (2012). Systematic review of occupational engagement and health outcomes among community-dwelling older adults. *American Journal of Occupational Therapy, 66*, 301–310.

Suto, M. (1998). Leisure in occupational therapy. *Canadian Journal of Occupational Therapy, 65*(5), 271–278.

Toepoel, V. (2013). Ageing, leisure and social connectedness: How could leisure help reduce social isolation of older people? *Social Indicators Research, 113*, 355–372.

Townsend, E. (Ed.). (1997). *Enabling occupation: An occupational therapy perspective*. Ottawa: Canadian Association of Occupational Therapists.

Townsend, E. A., & Polatajko, H. J. (2007). *Enabling occupation II: Advancing an occupational therapy vision for health, well-being & justice through occupation*. Ottawa: CAOT Publications ACE.

Trombly Latham, C. A. (2008). Occupation: Philosophy and Concepts. In Vining Radomski, M. V., & Trombly Latham, M. V., 6th edition. *Occupational Therapy for Physical Dysfunction*. Baltimore: Lippincott Williams and Wilkins.

Turner, H., Chapman, S., McSherry, A., Krishnagiri, S., & Watts, J. (2000). Leisure assessment in occupational therapy: An exploratory study. *Occupational Therapy in Healthcare, 12*(2–3), 73–85.

United Nations Human Rights Office of the High Commissioner (1989). *Convention on the Rights of the Child*. New York: United Nations. Retrieved from, *http://www.ohchr.org/en/professionalinterest/pages/crc.aspx*.

Wales, K., Clemson, L., Lannin, N. A., & Cameron, I. D. (2012). Functional assessments used by occupational therapists with older adults at risk of activity and participation limitations: A systematic review and evaluation of measurement properties. *Systematic Reviews, 1*(45).

Wallenbert, I., & Jonsson, H. (2005). Waiting to get better: A dilemma regarding habits in daily occupations after stroke. *American Journal of Occupational Therapy, 59*, 218–224.

World Federation of Occupational Therapists (2012). *Definition of occupational therapy. Retrieved from, http://www.wfot.org/AboutUs/AboutOccupationalTherapy/DefinitionofOccupationalTherapy.aspx*.

World Health Organization (2001). *International classification of functioning, disability and health*. Geneva: World Health Organization.

World Health Organization (2007). *International classification of functioning, disability and health: Children and youth version*. Geneva: World Health Organization.

Van Lankveld, W., Van't Pad Bosch, P. J., Bakker, J., Terwindt, S., Franssen, M., & van Riel, P. (1996). Sequential occupational dexterity assessment (SODA): A new test to measure hand disability. *Journal of Hand Therapy, 9*, 27–32.

35 WORK

YELIZ PRIOR ■ ALISON HAMMOND

CHAPTER OUTLINE

Abstract
Work provides a path to social inclusion and is important for people's health and well-being. Work instability is a mismatch between a person's abilities and that person's job demands, which, if unresolved, can result in work disability, the ceasing of work before retirement age. Although common health conditions, injury and recovering from surgery can contribute to work absence and presenteeism, participation in work is complex and multifactorial. Work rehabilitation, a process to overcome the barriers people face when accessing, remaining or returning to work after illness, injury or impairment, can help people who have occupational performance problems that affect their ability to participate in work. Occupational therapists are well placed within health and social care settings to provide work rehabilitation as part of individualised complex intervention programmes in practice.

KEY POINTS

- Work is important for the health and well-being of individuals, regardless of whether it is a paid or unpaid occupation.

- A mismatch between a person's abilities and job demands results in work instability, which, if unresolved, can result in work disability.

- Work disability is multifactorial and not a direct result of an illness, injury or impairment.

- Work rehabilitation is an essential part of occupational therapy practice and is not necessarily an isolated intervention.

- Work rehabilitation can be provided for job retention and return to work after illness, injury or impairment that affects a person's ability to execute work-related tasks.

- Occupational therapists have the skills to conduct job analysis and devise complex interventions to facilitate work rehabilitation.

Everyone has been made for some particular work, and the desire for that work has been put in every heart.
Rumi, thirteenth-century poet, theologian, scholar and Sufi mystic

485

INTRODUCTION TO WORK AS OCCUPATION

Human occupations are often clasified into three broad domains: self-care, productivity and leisure (Christiansen, Baum, & Haugen, 2005). In this context, work, or productivity, is acknowledged as an important human occupation. Occupational therapists become involved when people experience difficulties at work as a result of physical, psychological or social dysfunction, which might result from illness, injury or impairment (Hammond, Jones, & Prior, 2016; Prior, Bodell, Amanna, & Hammond, 2014). Work as a human occupation is explored in this chapter, with a focus on work instability and disability in people with long-term physical conditions and work rehabilitation interventions provided by occupational therapists for people with musculoskeletal, neurological and general medical and surgical conditions.

Work, in its broadest sense, is defined as 'an activity involving mental or physical effort done in order to achieve a result' (Oxford Dictionaries, 2015). However, the concept of work can hold different meanings for individuals, ranging from paid employment to volunteering to being a person's purpose in life (Collins Dictionaries, 2013). Regardless of which meaning is used, work provides a structure to people's lives, helping them identify with a perceived role in society (Holmes, 2007) and a path to social inclusion (Waddell & Aylward, 2005).

The ability to participate in paid work is important for people of working age (working age is often considered to be between the ages of 18 and 65 years old in many Western countries), as they need to generate an income to sustain their lives (Holmes, 2007). Nevertheless, whether paid or unpaid, participation in work helps individuals to find their place in society, become involved in regular and structured social interaction, increase their potential for a better quality of life and develop their self-esteem and confidence. Being able to work is more often than not a necessity for adults. Therefore helping people to maintain and optimise their participation in productive activities through work rehabilitation is an important goal for occupational therapists. According to Black (2008), work rehabilitation is simply defined as any advice or intervention that could help people to remain or return to work after a period of illness or injury. According to the American Occupational Therapy Association (AOTA), work rehabilitation within an occupational therapy context aims to do the following (AOTA, 2011, p. 1):

- Maximise levels of function after [illness, injury or impairment] to maintain a desired quality of life for the worker
- Facilitate the safe and timely return of individuals to work after [illness, injury or impairment]
- Remediate and/or prevent future [illness, injury or impairment]
- Assist individuals in resuming their role as a worker

In spite of the occupational therapy profession's long history in providing work rehabilitation to individuals with work-related injuries (Cook & Lukersmith, 2010), the role of therapists in helping people with health-related work problems to stay at work or return to work after a period of ill health or unemployment is highly variable and not perceived as an intervention priority in many health and social care settings (Barnes, Holmes, & College of Occupational Therapists Specialist Section: Work., 2009; Hammond et al., 2016; Mcfeely, 2012; Prior et al., 2014). However, sociopolitical changes across the globe to tackle health inequalities in populations, coupled with the socioeconomic and health burden caused by work disability, have led to increased demand for health and social services to consider the consequences of health and injury on work participation. This provides an excellent opportunity for occupational therapists, whose profession has traditional values embedded in using occupation as a therapeutic medium, to drive and lead the delivery of work rehabilitation services across the globe.

A BIOPSYCHOSOCIAL APPROACH TO WORK DISABILITY

The World Health Organization (WHO) published the International Classification of Functioning, Disability and Health (ICF) (WHO, 2001), which defined disability as a complex interaction between a person (with a health condition) and that person's contextual factors (environmental and personal factors), thus proposing a biopsychosocial approach to disability, viewing this as a multifaceted process (Engel, 1980; Mosey, 1980). This is also in alignment with the occupational therapy approach, which proposes that participation in productive occupations (i.e. work) requires a person (i.e. worker) to interact with complex physical, psychosocial and environmental demands. Thus a mismatch between a person's abilities and the person's job demands results in *work instability* (Gilworth et al., 2003). If work instability is not resolved in a timely manner, it can result in *work disability,* which is broadly defined as ceasing to work before retirement age as a result of ill health (Allaire, Wolfe, Niu, & Lavalley, 2008).

The context of work disability is vast, with its impact transcending the individual and shaping the wider society as a result of its socioeconomic and cultural consequences. Therefore to measure the impact of work disability and suggest a range of potential health and social targets to implement interventions to reduce work disability in working age adults, researchers attempted to quantify this concept and introduced an array of new terminology specifically used to describe such phenomenon. Perhaps the most common and familiar notion in work disability is the quantification of the working hours or days lost as a result of illness, injury or impairment, when an employee is absent at work during a normally scheduled work period (i.e. off sick). This is referred as *absenteeism* in the literature. This is somewhat easier to measure than when people are at work but are unable to perform their tasks to the best of their ability because of illness, injury or impairment, resulting in *loss of productivity*. This is also referred as *presenteeism*. It is understood that frequent and unresolved presenteeism is a prelude to absenteeism, and prolonged absenteeism results in work disability. Definitions of common terminology used in the field of work rehabilitation are presented in Table 35.1.

Occupational therapy assessment of a person's work problems would typically consist of applying ergonomics (i.e. study of a person's efficiency in that person's work environment) with an emphasis on a biopsychosocial approach to examine the following:

■ The physical and psychological consequences of a person's health status on his or her activities at work (e.g. impact of the person's illness, injury or impairment on the person's physical functioning; impact of the person's mood, motivation and beliefs on undertaking certain tasks at work), and work participation (e.g. reduced productivity at work, increased absenteeism, work disability)

■ Contextual factors (personal and environmental factors) affecting an individual's work performance (e.g. personal factors such as being able to afford child care and environmental barriers such as difficulties in using public transport or driving to access work, mobility issues preventing the person from moving in and around the workplace)

After the work assessment, which can be conducted using standardised or nonstandardised assessments, an occupational therapist devises a work rehabilitation programme with the aim of enabling individuals to overcome barriers when accessing, remaining or returning to work after illness, injury or impairment. In this context work rehabilitation is conducted under two main umbrellas:

1. Job retention interventions: These interventions are aimed at people who are at work but experiencing problems affecting their productivity (e.g. work instability, presenteeism), which may have resulted in short-term sick leave (i.e. absenteeism).
2. Return-to-work intervention: These interventions are aimed at people who are either already on long-term sick leave (more than 3 months) or unable to work because of illness, injury or impairment (i.e. work disabled).

Once the type of intervention programme is identified, the occupational therapy work rehabilitation programme is devised as a complex and individualised intervention that can involve physical (e.g. hand exercises to improve range of movement and strength on hands; fatigue management through energy conservation and graded activity), psychological (e.g. self-management education, increasing self-efficacy using counselling skills to increase the person's belief in his or her own capabilities) and environmental interventions (e.g. advice on ergonomic equipment and advice on current work legislations, statutory and third sector employment, support and advisory services, and employee's rights).

Legislation, policies and services available greatly vary from one setting to another; thus it is not possible to cover all of these in the context of this chapter. However, it is important to understand that the aim of workplace legislation, policies and services is to facilitate work participation of people experiencing illness, injury or impairment that affects their ability to participate in work. It is therefore important that occupational therapists keep up-to-date with their local and national policies and services to ensure that they can support individuals they are working with to start, retain or return to work.

WORK DISABILITY IN PHYSICAL CONDITIONS

In the following section a brief overview of how musculoskeletal, neurological, and medical and surgical conditions can affect a person's ability to work is provided.

TABLE 35.1
Definition of Key Terms Related to Work

Key Terms	Definition Used in This Chapter
Work	Productive occupations performed within an employment setting.
Worker	A person who participates in paid or unpaid productive occupation.
Work instability	A mismatch between the duties and the abilities of an individual.
Work disability	Ceasing to participate in work before retirement age because of illness, injury or impairment.
Absenteeism	A state that occurs when an employee is absent from work during a normally scheduled work period.
Presenteeism	A loss of workplace productivity resulting from an employee's illness, injury or impairment, or personal issues.
Work rehabilitation	A process to overcome the barriers an individual faces when accessing, remaining or returning to work after injury, illness or impairment.
Job retention intervention	Interventions to help people with health problems overcome the barriers to stay at work.
Return-to-work intervention	Interventions to help people return to work after an injury, illness or impairment.
Ergonomics	The study of people's efficiency in their working environment.

Musculoskeletal Conditions

Musculoskeletal conditions are the most common cause of physical injury or impairment in the world, and the prevalence of these, along with associated impact on occupational performance, is estimated to increase in the next decade because of the aging population (Connelly, Woolf, & Brooks, 2006). Two musculoskeletal conditions that can significantly affect occupational performance are rheumatoid arthritis (RA) and osteoarthritis (OA) (Sullivan, Ghushchyan, Huang, & Globe, 2010). As a result the impact of RA and OA will be used as examples of musculoskeletal conditions that affect the ability of people to work.

RA can have a significant impact on a person's ability to work as it can cause pain, stiffness, joint tenderness and damage, deformities, fatigue and depression (Toussirot, 2010). Fatigue in RA characteristically differs from normal patterns of tiredness as it is described as unpredictable and overwhelming and is associated with negative feelings and declining self-esteem (Feldthusen, Bjork, Forsblad-d'Elia, & Mannerkorpi, 2013).

Paid work is positively linked to health-related quality of life for people with RA (Gronning, Rodevand, & Steinsbekk, 2010). However, many are unlikely to return to work once they stop working (Busch, Coshall, Heuschmann, McKevitt, & Wolfe, 2009; Langley, Mu, Wu, Dong, & Tang, 2011; Neovius, Simard, & Askling, 2011). Nearly three-quarters of people with RA are of working age at diagnosis (Neovius et al., 2011; Symmons et al., 2002) and most are likely to be in employment before disease onset (Laires & Gouveia, 2014). Up to 40% of people with RA stop working within 5 years of their diagnosis (Barrett, Scott, Wiles, & Symmons, 2000; Busch et al., 2009; Eberhardt, Larsson, Nived, & Lindqvist, 2007), with 60% of that work loss occurring in the first 3 years (Busch et al., 2009). Once unemployed, people with RA are unlikely to return to work (Verstappen et al., 2005).

Although improvements in the treatment of RA using biological agents (e.g. anti–tumour necrosis factor drugs) have decreased the impact of RA on physical functioning (Hallert, Husberg, & Bernfort, 2012; Rantalaiho et al., 2013), individuals still experience difficulties in performing many daily activities because of damage to their joints causing biomechanical difficulties with associated fluctuating levels of pain and stiffness (McArthur, Birt, & Goodacre, 2014). In addition, socioeconomic and environmental factors such as lack of access to medical treatments, a nonsupportive workplace and an inability to work flexible hours are important predictors of work disability (Gjesdal, Bratberg, & Maeland, 2009; Prior et al., 2014; Uhlig, 2010; Van der Meer et al., 2011). Occupational identity can be profoundly affected within the first year of RA diagnosis because of its impact on daily routines and participation caused by uncertainties associated with having good days and bad days, having to do things differently to protect joints and conserve energy (e.g. pacing), and changing views of self (McDonald et al., 2012). Work disability rates remain high for people

diagnosed with RA around the world (Sokka et al., 2010). Early recognition and rehabilitation of work instability is important in preventing work disabilities in people with RA.

The growing burden of noninflammatory arthropathies, chronic back pain and OA collectively result in a greater economic and human cost to society than inflammatory disease (Wilkie & Pransky, 2012). OA is the most common musculoskeletal condition and is strongly associated with increasing age and therefore accounts for greater disability in older people. With an aging workforce around the globe and the increasing pension age, it is more important than ever to consider the impact of musculoskeletal conditions on work (Palmer & Goodson, 2015). The prevalence of knee OA among working age people is expected to rise considerably in the next decade, with a significant proportion experiencing work disability as a result of OA (Gaudreault et al., 2014). The risk of hip OA is also increased for people in heavy manual occupations such as farming (Harris & Coggon, 2015). In the United Kingdom, people with OA are treated in primary care by general practitioners and do not necessarily receive specialist care from rheumatologists, specialist nurses, physiotherapists and occupational therapists unless they have severe pain or deformities that affect their daily life. This means it is even more difficult to identify those experiencing work instability. Severe OA can result in surgical procedures such as arthroplasty, which can have a negative impact on a person's work participation. Usually people have to take substantial time off to recuperate after surgery, which can be up to 6 weeks; therefore, if salaried extended sick leave or workplace support to facilitate return to work is not in place, working people will be at an increased risk of work disability.

To summarise musculoskeletal conditions are common in people of working age and have substantial impact both on presenteeism and absenteeism.

Neurological Conditions

Many neurological conditions have a significant impact on the ability of people to participate in work. For example, a brain injury is a common neurological condition that affects work ability. There are two main categories of brain injuries that can result in work disability: traumatic brain injury (i.e. an injury to the brain by an external force that may result from incidents such as traffic accidents, sport, head injuries and falls that involve striking the head) resulting in altered brain function; and acquired brain injury (i.e. brain injuries caused by cerebral vascular accidents (CVA) and hypoxic brain injury not the result of hereditary, congenital, degenerative or birth trauma causes). A significant number of people who sustain a brain injury have impaired self-awareness and work and social dysfunction and require long-term rehabilitation (Hommel et al., 2009). For the purposes of this chapter a brief focus on the impact of CVA is used to illustrate the impact of neurological conditions on work participation.

Twenty percent of people who have a CVA are of working age (Baldwin & Brusco, 2011). For most, return to work marks an important step in their emotional and functional recovery (Roth & Lovell, 2014). Those people who have had a stroke and who are older than 50 years of age have a higher risk of being unemployed compared with age-matched controls in the general population (Maaijwee et al., 2014). In addition, those people who had a CVA and who were from a lower socioeconomic background, with low levels of education (Brey & Wolf, 2015; Trygged, Ahacic, & Kareholt, 2011), and who were from an ethnic minority, who were female, or who were dependent in the acute phase reported having more difficulty returning to work (Busch et al., 2009). Return-to-work programmes appeared to have some impact on reducing the negative long-term effects unemployment has on life satisfaction and socioeconomic consequences (Brey & Wolf, 2015; Maaijwee et al., 2014). However, there is limited high-quality research evidence on which to make recommendations about what type of work rehabilitation programme increases the chances of returning to work for people after a CVA (Baldwin & Brusco, 2011).

Medical and Surgical Conditions

For the purposes of this chapter a brief focus on the impact of cancer will be used to illustrate the effect of medical and surgical conditions on work participation. Health conditions such as cancer can cause long-term disruptions to work participation. The proportion of working age people diagnosed with cancer is increasing, as is the number of people living with cancer as treatments have become more effective (de Boer, Taskila, Ojajarvi, van Dijk, & Verbeek, 2009; Schultz, Beck, Stava, & Sellin, 2002). Living with cancer involves undergoing treatments such as surgery, radiotherapy, and chemotherapy, which disrupt daily life and can negatively affect a person's ability to work (Gordon et al., 2011). Fatigue is a common and debilitating symptom of cancer and its treatment; fatigue levels provide a prediction of an individual's capacity to return to work (Spelten et al., 2003). Importantly, it is suggested that of those continuing to work who have cancer, 7.3% are faced with job discrimination, affecting their job satisfaction and motivation to work (Schultz et al., 2002). A better understanding of how cancer affects working adults and contributes to unwanted work cessation is required to identify individuals who may benefit from occupational rehabilitation programmes.

OCCUPATIONAL THERAPY AND WORK REHABILITATION

Occupational therapists are well placed to provide work rehabilitation because of their skills and expertise in analysing human occupation and biopsychosocial approach to their work (Prior et al., 2015). In the College of Occupational Therapists' (COT) Vocational Rehabilitation Strategy (2008) it is stated that therapists should routinely ask service users about work and offer work rehabilitation (COT, 2008). Work rehabilitation is defined as 'a process to overcome the barriers an individual faces when accessing, remaining or returning to work after injury, illness or impairment' (Department for Work and Pensions, 2004, p. 12). Work rehabilitation can influence many factors relating to work instability and work disability, including the following:

- Job-related factors, such as work limitations as a result of environmental barriers; lack of specialised equipment; physically demanding jobs; inflexible working hours; problems with transportation; long-term sick leave; and lack of employer/team support.
- Psychological factors, such as job strain, depression, lack of family/social support; poor work self-efficacy; lack of knowledge or advocacy skills to request and obtain help; and unwillingness to disclose condition and limited use of self-management strategies.
- Condition-specific factors, such as symptoms such as pain and fatigue relating to the specific health condition interfering with daily activities and work.

Occupational therapists should work collaboratively with individuals to address these factors when solving work-related problems. The process undertaken to assess, plan and deliver work rehabilitation interventions will differ from one setting to another, depending on the service provision, knowledge and experience of the team and cultural practices within that setting. Work rehabilitation is an essential part of occupational therapy practice and is not an isolated intervention (Waddell, Burton, & Kendall, 2008). A comprehensive discussion of all approaches to work rehabilitation, which include specialised services, standardised and nonstandardised assessments and interventions to meet individuals' different health and social care needs, is not possible in this chapter. The focus here is on work rehabilitation as part of the person-centred, holistic approach to occupational therapy.

Work Rehabilitation Delivery: Skills and Processes

For the occupational therapy process to be holistic and person-centred, therapists should ask individuals if they have problems at work, or access to work, to obtain a full picture of their daily lives. It is preferable to help people stay at work, as current evidence suggests that once out of work, people are much less likely to return to work (Busch et al., 2009; Verstappen, Jacobs, & Verkleij, 2004). Occupational therapists should aim to identify work problems even when these are not highlighted in the initial interview and goal-setting stage. This could be achieved through simply asking people the question, 'Does your health affect your work?' and screening for work instability using a standardised (e.g. RA Work Instability Scale [RA-WIS] (Gilworth et al.,

2003)) or nonstandardised outcome measure with a view to preventing work disability or maintaining or regaining work status. Therapists should explore the physical and psychosocial dimensions of jobs, the receptivity of the employer and the accommodations needed to promote a safe and timely return to work when creating a return-to-work transition for people with health conditions (Shrey & Mital, 2000).

Although work rehabilitation can be a stand-alone process in health and social care, for occupational therapists it can also be part of the individualised complex intervention provided to people with health problems and rehabilitation needs, tailored to suit the changing needs of the person as therapy progresses, with prevention of work loss as the primary outcome.

Aims and Objectives of Work Rehabilitation

The overall aim of work rehabilitation is to identify and overcome the health, personal/psychological and social/occupational obstacles to recovery and return to work (Waddell & Burton, 2004). In occupational therapy, work rehabilitation has two main objectives:

- To assist individuals to identify difficulties at work and employ a preventative approach to achieve job retention and avoid work loss
- To facilitate return to work after an illness, injury or impairment

The Work Rehabilitation Process

The work rehabilitation process in occupational therapy takes place when individuals identify problems at work or need help to enable them to return to work. The work rehabilitation process is illustrated in Practice Stories 36.1 to 36.3. Each of these practice stories is set around the use of a different initial assessment: the Canadian Occupational Performance Measure (COPM; Practice Story 35.1), the Model of Human Occupation Screening Tool (MOHOST) (Practice Story 35.2), and the ICF (Practice Story 35.3). These practice stories are intended to illustrate the potential scope and depth of the occupational therapists' roles within work rehabilitation.

Assessment of a person's work situation should start during the initial interview. This can be done by first establishing the person's work status and then by asking a question such as, 'Are you having any problems at work?' This question can be supported by further questions about the nature of the work (e.g. manual, professional or self-employed) and the identification of any areas for concern.

Effective work assessment requires a thorough job analysis to establish the impact of a person's health on the person's ability to perform their work role (Joss, 2007). Informally this could consist of a discussion about the person's physical work environment, role within the team or workplace, daily tasks and responsibilities, working hours, transportation, relationships with colleagues, culture at workplace, main stressors and knowledge of workplace policies to outline the support available for people when work performance is affected by illness, injury or impairment. If the person is currently not working, it is essential to understand whether this is by choice (i.e. he or she could take time out to study, care for dependents or for other personal reasons). Similarly, if the person is retired, it is imperative to establish whether retirement was a choice or caused by illness, injury or impairment to identify if return to work may be an appropriate goal at this time.

In this process, therapists can utilise standardised assessments to facilitate job retention and return to work and evaluate interventions. There are a number of standardised work assessments that could be used to identify a person's background, strengths, limitation, concerns and goals. An example of this is the COPM (Law et al., 2005), an individualised, person-centred outcome measure designed to detect change in a person's occupational performance. The COPM is administered using a semistructured interview format. It enables a person to identify occupational performance difficulties, prioritise these difficulties, and assist with determining goals for intervention. It is widely used in occupational therapy practice (Law, Baptiste, McColl, Polatajko, & Pollock, 1990). The COPM as an assessment for work rehabilitation is used in Melanie Turner's practice story (see Practice Story 35.1).

It is suggested that the Model of Human Occupation (Kielhofner & Burke, 1980) work assessments have good psychometric properties and are useful in evaluating work rehabilitation needs of individuals (Lee & Kielhofner, 2010). An example of these assessments are described in Table 35.2. The MOHOST is used in David Cook's practice story as an assessment for work rehabilitation (see Practice Story 35.2).

Another framework used in practice to facilitate work assessment is the WHO's International Classification of Functioning (WHO, 2001) (Fig. 35.1). The ICF offers the opportunity to develop an understanding of the individual's work problems through the biopsychosocial model proposed (see Fig. 35.1). This allows participation in work to be viewed as the outcome of the interaction between the individual and their environment. Therefore the ICF model may help to better identify potential targets to reduce work instability or facilitate a graded return to work when individuals are work disabled. The ICF as an assessment for work rehabilitation is used in Evrim Hepari's practice story (see Practice Story 35.3).

A number of other standardised assessments specifically aimed at measuring work outcomes that could be used by occupational therapists are listed in Table 35.3.

Although the provision of work rehabilitation is depicted as a standalone process in this chapter, it is important to understand that work rehabilitation could be undertaken by therapists as part of the complex interventions provided in day-to-day therapy settings. With this in mind, the assessments used in the work rehabilitation examples in the Practice Stories are based on common assessment tools used in occupational therapy worldwide.

TABLE 35.2
A List of MOHO Work Assessments

Name of MOHO Work Assessment	Description
Assessment of Work Performance (AWP) Version 1.0	This is an observation-based performance rating scale that assesses motor, process, communication and interaction skills within a work activity. This assessment could be used with anybody experiencing a work problem in any setting (Braveman & Page, 2012).
Work Environment Impact Scale (WEIS)	This is a semistructured interview and a rating scale to assess factors affecting performance at work. It is a particularly useful tool to identify the need for workplace accommodations. It is a suitable assessment to use for job retention programmes (Braveman & Page, 2012).
DOA: The Dialogue About Ability Related to Work	This is a self-assessment and professional observation tool to examine influence on volition, roles, physical ability and communication as well as interaction skills on work ability. This assessment is particularly useful for people with psychiatric or psychological problems which affect their work performance (Braveman & Page, 2012).
Worker Role Interview (WRI)	The WRI is a semistructured interview designed to be used as the psychosocial/environmental component of the initial rehabilitation assessment process for the injured worker or the worker with a long-term disability and poor/limited work history (Braveman & Page, 2012).
Occupational Performance History Interview (OPHI)	This scale is also administered as a semistructured interview, measuring three underlying constructs of occupational adaptation described by the authors as the occupational identity, occupational competence and occupational behaviour settings (Braveman & Page, 2012)
Occupational Self-Assessment (OSA)	The OSA is a self-assessment tool for people to capture their own performance and ability from a list of everyday occupations (Braveman & Page, 2012).
Model of Human Occupation Screening Tool (MOHOST)	This screening tool is another occupational therapy assessment used in practice and is based on the MOHO concepts of volition, habituation, skills and environment. It was developed in the United Kingdom and uses a variety of data collection methods. These determine individuals' motivations for and pattern of activities, as well as their communication, process and motor skills and environment. The assessment leads to goal setting, which is conducted using a predefined rating scale which includes four options: F=Facilitates occupational participation A=Allows occupational participation I=Inhibits occupational participation R=Restricts occupational participation

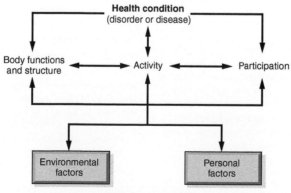

FIG. 35.1 ■ International Classification of Functioning, Disability and Health (ICF). *(From WHO, 2001.)*

TABLE 35.3		
Examples of Standardised Work Assessments		
Name of Work Assessment Scale	Author(s)	Description
Ergonomic Assessment Tool for Arthritis (EATA)	Backman, Village, & Lacaille, 2008	The EATA was developed to be used as an assessment for people with arthritis. It is individualised to each person through five screening questions: Does your work involve (a) Prolonged sitting? (b) Prolonged standing, kneeling, walking or stair climbing? (c) Gripping or grasping objects or hand tools? (d) Frequent lifting or carrying? (e) Pushing or pulling items?
Rheumatoid Arthritis Work Instability Scale (RA-WIS)	Gilworth et al., 2003	The disease-specific RA-WIS includes 23 yes/no scale questions that measure any mismatch between people's functional abilities and the demands of their jobs. Originally developed to measure work instability in people with RA, it has subsequently been validated for other musculoskeletal disorders.
Workplace Activities Limitations Scale (WALS)	Gignac et al., 2004	This 12-item questionnaire aims to measure the amount/level of difficulty in performing work tasks, with additional items for each question regarding whether the participant received help from others at work with the task or has any adaptation.
Work Environment Impact Scale	Braveman & Page, 2012	A semistructured interview and rating scale focusing on people with physical or psychosocial conditions and their work problems. There are 17 items to examine the social and physical environment, supports, changing demands, objects used, and daily job functions.
Work Experience Survey – Rheumatic Conditions (WES-RC)	Allaire & Keysor, 2009; Roessler, 1995	This is a structured interview for identifying barriers and formulate solutions for people with rheumatic conditions. The WES-RC can be administered through either face to face or telephone interview.
Work Limitations Questionnaire (WLQ)	Lerner et al., 2001	This 25-item questionnaire, with four subscales, measures physical work demands, time work demands, mental-interpersonal work demands and output work demands.

PRACTICE STORY 35.1

Melanie Turner: Therapeutic Work Rehabilitation Programme Using COPM

BACKGROUND

Referral

Diagnosis of rheumatoid arthritis (RA), hand pain and problems at work.

History of Present Condition

Melanie was a 37-year-old woman. Eighteen months before being seen by an occupational therapist she was diagnosed with RA. She reported pain, swelling and stiffness in her hands and knees, as well as severe fatigue. She also has developed severe back pain more recently, which was under investigation. She was under the care of a rheumatology consultant and had been stable on disease-modifying antirheumatic drugs (DMARDs) and nonsteroidal antiinflammatory drugs (NSAIDs), as well as tramadol (an opioid pain medication used to treat moderate to severe pain) for pain relief.

Domestic/Social Situation

She lived with her husband, a full-time accountant, and two children, ages 9 and 6 years, who both attended school. Before her condition worsened, she used to like socialising with friends, but at the time of the occupational therapy interview she reported that she stayed at home the majority of the time and rested her hands at every opportunity to allow her to continue to work.

Occupation (Work)

She worked at a secondary school for 10 years as a full-time art teacher. She was one of the two art teachers at the school and regularly worked long hours running after-school workshops, as well as holiday art clubs in school holidays. She was very passionate about her job and anxious to be able to continue to work. She had a 15-kilometre drive to and from work, which she said could take about 45 minutes in rush-hour traffic.

INITIAL ASSESSMENT

COPM Assessment: Problem Identification and Weighing

A summary of Melanie's ability to perform self-care, productivity and leisure occupations are presented in Table 35.4.

PRACTICE STORY 35.1

Melanie Turner: Therapeutic Work Rehabilitation Programme Using COPM (Continued)

TABLE 35.4
Melanie's Ability To Perform Self-Care, Productivity and Leisure Occupations

STEP 1A: Self-care

Personal Care (e.g., dressing, bathing, feeding, hygiene)	She was independent with all self-care activities.
Functional Mobility (e.g. transfers, indoor, outdoor)	She was independently mobile with all indoor and outdoor activities, but standing/sitting in the same position for long periods caused her pain and stiffness.
Community Management (e.g. transportation, shopping, finances)	Melanie struggled with long-haul driving (i.e. longer than 10–15 minutes) because of hand and knee pain and stiffness. When driving, her self-rated hand pain* is 8 and knee pain is 7. * The numerical rating scale (NRS) for self-rated pain: 0 = no pain, 10 = worst imaginable pain (1–3 = mild pain; 4–6 = moderate pain; 7–10 = severe pain)

STEP 1B: Productivity

Paid/Unpaid Work (e.g. finding/keeping a job, volunteering)	She was a secondary school full-time art teacher and loved her job. She found hand activities such as drawing for extended periods painful for her dominant right (R) hand, particularly around the first carpometacarpal (CMC), distal interphalangeal (DIP) and proximal interphalangeal (PIP) joints on the second and third digits. She found that her hands swelled the following morning, which resulted in her taking time each morning to work on being able to move her hand and fingers before her morning classes. Melanie also had developed a severe back pain; using an NRS, she rated her back pain when drawing for extended periods as 8.
Household Management (e.g. cleaning, laundry, cooking)	Melanie struggled to perform her duties such as laundry and cooking on the days when she was symptomatic, but normally she was independent.
Play/School (e.g. play skills, homework)	Melanie wanted to undertake some additional courses for her continuous professional development but was unable to do so because of pain and fatigue she experienced during work.

STEP 1C: Leisure

Quiet Recreation (e.g. hobbies, crafts, reading)	She used to like reading in the evenings to unwind but was finding that she was too tired to do so, and when she did she quickly fell asleep. However, her sleep was not refreshing as she fell in and out of sleep all through the night, starting on the sofa, while watching the evening news, then later in bed. She tended to wake up early, around 5 a.m., and then tried to perform housekeeping duties before starting to get ready for work.
Active Recreation (e.g. sports, outing, travel)	Melanie used to enjoy walking her dog regularly, up to 3 miles a day before her diagnosis, and practising yoga but was unable to do so due to pain and fatigue.
Socialisation (e.g. visiting, phone calls, parties, correspondence)	She kept socialising at the weekends to minimum as she tried to rest and recover from work during the week.

COPM Scoring

As a result of the COPM assessment Melanie identified her top five concerns and rated each concern according to her level of performance and satisfaction with her performance on a 1 to 10 scale (1 = poor performance no satisfies to 10 = great performance/extremely satisfied) (Table 35.5). She then rated each concern based on the importance of this concern for her. This importance rating acted as a weighting factor in the scoring of Melanie's performance and satisfaction for each activity (Law et al., 1990) (Table 35.6).

FOLLOW-UP WORKPLACE ASSESSMENT

A workplace assessment was conducted 2 weeks after the initial assessment to acquire an objective view of Melanie's work situation. Through this assessment it became apparent that being a secondary school teacher involved working in a very busy, noisy and stressful environment. She undertook a variety of tasks that were multifaceted. She spent long periods on her feet, with no time to rest in between these high-energy tasks. Most of these required bilateral upper-extremity strength and fine hand function.

Continued on following page

PRACTICE STORY 35.1

Melanie Turner: Therapeutic Work Rehabilitation Programme Using COPM (Continued)

TABLE 35.5
Melanie Turner's Baseline COPM Score

		INITIAL ASSESSMENT	
		Performance	Satisfaction
1	Unable to draw for extended periods	2	1
2	Unable to sit or stand for the length of a class period when teaching	3	2
3	Unable to drive to and from school during rush hours	4	2
4	Unable to perform her tasks to the best of her ability when working long hours with no regular rests	2	1
5	Unable to continue to run extra curriculum activities because of inability to work extended hours	2	2
Total		13	8
Number of problems		5	5
Score (Total score/No. of problems)		2.6	1.6

- Classroom duties: Prolonged walking in and around the class, periodic stationary standing during the class with no longer than 5 minutes rest before attending the next class to set the room up for students, which involved repetitive bending and reaching between chest and shoulder height, bending and reaching to hip height, repetitive lifting of boxes with art materials (weight of these boxes ranged from 2 to 6 kg per box).

- Office duties: Prolonged sitting while using a computer; 'hot-desking' with others, so did not have an ergonomically positioned desk, chair or desktop computer. She used a small mouse with click buttons on each side using the first and third digits of her right hand, and her forearm was positioned in pronation.

- Environment: A large, modern, well-insulated building with laminated flooring and good light. The school is well heated from 8.30 a.m. onwards, but cold in the early hours of the mornings (i.e. 7.00–8.30 a.m.) when Melanie tended to arrive to prepare for the day. She worked with a friendly and supportive team of colleagues.

GOAL SETTING

Long-term Goal

Melanie to be able to stay at full-time employment (job retention) and participate in social activities.

Short-term SMART Goals

Goal 1. To be able to draw at each class with support from the teacher assistant by 6 weeks.

Goal 2. To be able to drive to and from work independently during off-peak time by working flexibly at the end of week 2.

Goal 3. To be able to tolerate sitting/standing supported by ergonomic equipment when necessary by 12 weeks.

Goal 4. To be able to participate fully in desired social activities in the evenings and the weekends by planning ahead to conserve energy by the end of 6 weeks.

Goal 5. To stop running after school and holiday clubs for students with the help of a teacher assistant by the end of week 2.

Goal 6. To be able to continue to work full time and perform to the best of her ability as an art teacher at a school using self-management strategies at the end of a 12-week treatment.

TABLE 35.6
Melanie Turner's Weighted COPM Score Summary at Baseline

Problems	Importance	Performance	Satisfaction	Importance × Performance	Importance × Satisfaction
1	9	2	1	18	9
2	7	3	2	21	14
3	7	4	2	28	14
4	6	2	1	12	6
5	7	2	2	14	14
Total Scores	36	13	8	93	57
Score	7.2	2.6	1.6	**18.6**	**11.4**
Weighted Performance Score[a]: 18.6			**Weighted Satisfaction Score[a]: 11.4**		

COPM, Canadian Occupational Performance Measure.

[a]The weighted scores for performance and satisfaction are added separately to create two summative scores. These scores are divided by the number of rated activities to provide scores that can be used for comparisons across time (Law et al., 1990).

Melanie Turner: Therapeutic Work Rehabilitation Programme Using COPM *(Continued)*

WORK REHABILITATION PROGRAMME

Work-specific Interventions

Negotiation of working hours (pacing/energy conservation):

- Recommended disclosing condition to employer and discuss obtaining support/assistance in class (e.g. in the United Kingdom this is funded based on the Access to Work legislation) [Goal 1].

- Recommended Melanie discuss with her employer the possibility of adopting flexible hours to allow a later start and finish (i.e. 10.00 a.m. to 6.00 p.m. instead of 07.00 a.m. to 17.00 p.m.) to ensure that Melanie was not having to travel in rush-hour traffic, which would reduce her travel time by half [Goal 1].

- As a result of new, flexible hours, the number of hours Melanie worked were also reduced; however, she was still able to work full time (i.e. 37.5 hours/week) and she performed better as her feelings of fatigue were reduced [Goal 6].

- Wrote a letter to the head of school with the workplace assessment report, kindly recommending to make reasonable adjustments, such as the following:

  - Provision of a trolley for Melanie to move art equipment/teaching materials to/from the car and in between classes

  - Provision of personal desk, chair with a lumbar support and desktop computer and ergonomic assessment of working station by the school's health and safety department [Goal 3]

  - Provision of a dedicated teaching assistant to help Melanie to support students during classes (e.g. walking around the class to check their progress with the artwork and address issues) [Goals 1, 5 and 6]

These requests were met by the school and Melanie was provided with a dedicated teacher assistant to help and assist her with her classes. This included the following:

- The teaching assistant setting up each classroom while Melanie had a 10- to 15-minute break in between each class

- The teaching assistant taking over Melanie's after-school and holiday club duties and Melanie performing her duties within the official working hours/days to help her conserve her energy and manage her fatigue levels [Goal 4]

Health-specific Interventions

Splinting and exercise:

- Fit Melanie with Isotoner gloves (medium) to be worn on both hands during the night to provide compression to relieve hand pain at night and morning stiffness (Hammond et al., 2016) [Goal 1].

- Teach hand exercises and joint protection techniques to increase range of movement and decrease swelling and stiffness (Hammond, 2008; Hammond & Freeman, 2001) [Goal 1].

- Demonstrate how to adopt correct posture for back care.

- Recommend the use of antiinflammatory gels on hands and knees when symptomatic [Goals 1 and 3].

- Make a referral to rheumatology physiotherapy for assessment and treatment of the knee and back pain [Goals 2 and 3].

Dealing with fatigue:

- Encourage the use of a fatigue diary to identify the patterns and causes of fatigue (Hegarty, Conner, Stebbings, & Treharne, 2015) [Goals 4 and 5].

- Introduce a good sleep hygiene routine (i.e. maintain a regular wake and sleep pattern 7 days a week; avoid napping watching the television in the evenings; avoid stimulants such caffeine and alcohol too close to bedtime; do not consume large amount of food close to bedtime; establish a regular relaxing bedtime routine) to have normal, quality night-time sleep and full daytime alertness [Goals 4 and 5].

- Recommend that Melanie incorporates a gentle, graded exercise regimen such as walking her dog daily and taking up t'ai chi classes for arthritis to increase energy levels and maintain muscle tone (Callahan, Cleveland, Altpeter, & Hackney, 2016) [Goals 4 and 5].

Social/psychological support:

- Teach relaxation techniques to deal with pain and fatigue (e.g. use of visualisation, guided meditation, mindfulness); demonstrate how to challenge negative thought patterns through the use of cognitive behavioural therapy techniques; explain the importance of self-compassion as a way of enabling her to be more realistic in the standards she sets herself and in her workload (Davis, Zautra, Wolf, Tennen, & Yeung, 2015) [Goals 4 and 5].

- Encourage limiting work activities strictly to working days and hours and teach to pace herself when performing work activities by taking structured breaks to conserve energy and make time to participate in family and social activities at the weekend (Sverker et al., 2015) [Goals 4 and 5].

REASSESSMENT

Melanie was provided with 3 months of treatment and was reassessed at 6 months to decide whether to have a longer follow-up (e.g. 12 months) or discharge her from the occupational therapy work rehabilitation programme. A new COPM form was administered to reassess Melanie to evaluate the

Continued on following page

PRACTICE STORY 35.1

Melanie Turner: Therapeutic Work Rehabilitation Programme Using COPM (Continued)

outcome of the interventions and to identify any other occupational performance difficulties that may have emerged. No further problems were reported. Melanie was asked to rate her performance and satisfaction of the concerns she raised during the initial COPM assessment as a means of evaluating the impact of the work rehabilitation programme delivered (Table 35.7). This showed that Melanie's weighted Performance Score was improved by 31.2 points, from 18.6 to 49.8, and her Satisfaction Score was increased by 42.6 points, from 11.4 to 54, demonstrating an excellent improvement of her outcomes (Table 35.8).

As Melanie's current occupational performance issues were resolved and she was able to self-manage her RA while continuing to work full time, she was discharged from the occupational therapy. However, Melanie was informed that she should continuously monitor and take into account the impact of RA on her working life and she may have to return for therapy or adjust the strategies depending on the progress of the RA in the long term.

TABLE 35.7
Melanie's COPM Scores at the End of the Work Rehabilitation Programme

		REASSESSMENT	
		Performance	Satisfaction
1	Unable to draw for extended periods	6	7
2	Unable to sit or stand for the length of a class period when teaching	7	6
3	Unable to drive to and from school during rush hours	6	5
4	Unable to perform her tasks to the best of her ability when working long hours with no regular rests	8	10
5	Unable to continue to run extra curriculum activities because of inability to work extended hours	8	10
Total		**35**	**38**
Number of problems		**5**	**5**
Score (Total score / No. of problems)		**7**	**7.6**

COPM, Canadian Occupational Performance Measure.

TABLE 35.8
Melanie's Weighted COPM Scores After the Work Rehabilitation Programme

Problems	Importance	Performance	Satisfaction	Importance × Performance	Importance × Satisfaction
1	9	6	7	54	63
2	7	7	6	49	42
3	7	6	5	42	35
4	6	8	10	48	60
5	7	8	10	56	70
Total Scores	36	35	38	249	270
Score	7.2	2.6	1.6	49.8[a]	54[a]
Change in Performance[b]: 49.8 − 18.6 = **31.2**			**Change in Satisfaction[b]:** 54 − 11.4 = **42.6**		

COPM, Canadian Occupational Performance Measure.
[a]The weighted scores for performance and satisfaction are added separately to create two summative scores. These scores are divided by the number of rated activities to provide scores that can be used for comparisons across time (Law et al., 1990).
[b]Change in Performance and Satisfaction Scores = (Performance or Satisfaction Score 2 − Performance or Satisfaction Score 1 [from Table 35.6]).

COPM, Canadian Occupational Performance Measure.

David Cook: Therapeutic Work Rehabilitation Programme Using MOHOST

BACKGROUND

Referral

Diagnosis of major left hemisphere cerebrovascular accident (CVA) 6 months ago. Already received a period of rehabilitative interventions from a physiotherapist and speech therapist. Consultant referred Mr Cook for occupational therapy for graded return-to-work intervention.

History of Present Condition

Mr Cook was a 56-year-old gentleman recovering from a major left hemisphere CVA. He had no sensory/motor response from his right hand with deficits in spatial orientation to the right of his body (unilateral neglect) and had a slightly delayed speech. He was independent in performing basic activities of daily living (ADL) (i.e. eating, toileting, dressing, grooming, maintaining continence, bathing, walking and transferring) but had very low energy levels and struggled with some instrumental ADL, specifically with transportation (e.g. driving and using public transport), shopping and preparing meals. He was able to manage his finances, use the telephone and other communication devices and do light housework (e.g. dusting, making the bed, washing the dishes). Having been an active and successful businessman before his injury, he appeared frustrated with his inability to use his right hand and his delayed speech and was anxious about his potential to return to work.

Domestic/Social Situation

Mr Cook was divorced. He had two children, Matt, age 13, and Freya, age 12, who were in full-time education. Although he was not the children's main carer he saw them regularly, and every other weekend they stayed with him at his house, where he lived alone. He also had a financial responsibility to pay monthly child maintenance to his ex-wife.

Occupation (Work)

Mr Cook had a 21-year history as a senior management consultant in a large financial company where he worked full time. He had a long commute to work (1.5 hours each way) and used to work from home on Fridays before his injury to save time on travelling.

INITIAL ASSESSMENT

Mr Cook successfully completed a multidisciplinary rehabilitation programme initially in the hospital and later in the community. He was discharged from rehabilitation as his Medical Outcomes Study (MOS) Short Form-36 (SF-36) Physical Functioning Score (PFS) was 68 (Ware & Sherbourne, 1992) (SF-36 PF scores range 1–100, with higher scores indicating less disability). A score of 68 indicated that he had an above average PFS compared with the general population of adults and he was positive about his progress and rehabilitation outcome at the time of reassessment, which was 3 months after his CVA. However, his progress since his discharge slowed, and he became less hopeful about his recovery, realising that he may never regain the use of his right hand and have as much energy and stamina as he had before the CVA. He began having a sustained low mood and increased levels of anxiety; when the Hospital Anxiety and Depression Scale (HADS) was administered he scored 21, indicating he was at high risk of depression (HADS scores range from 0–7 = normal; 8–10 = borderline abnormal; 11–21 = abnormal (Zigmond & Snaith, 1983)). He lacked confidence in returning to full-time employment and taking on the same level of responsibilities he had before the CVA.

HOME-OFFICE ASSESSMENT VISIT

As Mr Cook appeared to have low self-esteem and confidence and was anxious about his return to work, he declined the option of a workplace assessment at his company office. However, as he worked from home 1 day a week he had a home office and suggested that the work assessment could take place at his home office instead. He demonstrated the tasks he would normally perform, explaining the pattern of activities he would do if he was working full time as a management consultant (e.g. travelling to work and meetings outside of work, accessing his office on the 19th floor in a tower block, using complex financial software for accounting, using various communication technologies at work (i.e. smart phone, electronic diary, scientific calculator, Skype, Macbook Air, iPad) and communicating with his personal assistant (PA) through email, text messaging and telephone throughout the day).

During this assessment he was able to perform the activities he deemed routine and adapt an activity when he struggled to conduct it the way he used to do it (e.g. as he was unable to speak on the phone and take notes at the same time using one hand, he put the telephone on the speaker and took notes with his left hand, as over the last 6 months he had taught himself to write using his nondominant left hand). Being a senior manager also helped to facilitate task management as he had a PA and autonomy to set his own targets and plan his own workload. He had the option to delegate some of his responsibilities (e.g. data entry using complex software) if it was appropriate, so he could use his time more efficiently on management duties.

Mr Cook was an articulate, educated man with clear but delayed speech. He was still having speech therapy and had daily homework to further improve his speech. Performing work-related activities (e.g. writing emails, filing, and telephoning) was taking him longer than he wanted as he was doing these using one hand. As it was also more effort

Continued on following page

PRACTICE STORY 35.2

David Cook: Therapeutic Work Rehabilitation Programme Using MOHOST (Continued)

for him to do this, he began to feel tired after an hour demonstrating a typical day at work. Despite this, he had excellent process skills and a very well organised electronic filing system, which made it easier to perform certain tasks (e.g. finding correspondence from clients, using templates to issue standard letters) and was quick to come up with problem-solving ideas when needed (e.g. using voice recognition software to type texts on his phone, using a speaker phone to be able to take notes while on the telephone).

His poor posture and mobility as a result of impaired spatial awareness inhibited his occupational performance at times (e.g. when performing activities requiring physical multitasking like checking invoices from different folders to produce a spreadsheet, moving around the room to locate the things he needed). In addition, his fatigue also limited his efforts to get things done to the level he used to in the time he used to be able to do it (e.g. responding to the large number of emails, phone calls and texts he receives daily).

His working environment at his home office was a little chaotic, with boxes of files and various printed documents and stationery lying around on the floor and on his desk. His occupational demands were high; as a management consultant he worked with more than 50 large corporate businesses with multilevel management needs that required high levels of communication processing and fast-paced decision making.

MOHOST RATING FORM

After the initial occupational therapy and home-office assessment conducted by the therapist, Mr Cook completed a MOHOST Rating Form to self-assess his occupational performance using the FAIR approach (Table 35.9). The results of this assessment were as follows:

(a) *Motivation for occupation (volition):* Mr Cook rated his ability to perform, expectation of success and interest in return to work as 'Inhibits occupational participation' as he was anxious to be able to perform to his high expectations. He rated his choices as 'Restricts occupational participation' as having worked as a management consultant for 21 years he could not envisage himself working elsewhere, in another role.

(b) *Pattern of occupation (habituation):* Here Mr Cook appeared more positive, marking the routines and adaptability of his job as 'Allows occupational performance' and his roles and responsibilities as 'Facilitates occupational performance' as he recognised the flexible nature of his work.

(c) *Communication and interaction skills:* Because of his speech delay, Mr Cook appraised his nonverbal skills as 'Inhibits occupational participation', but he was more positive about his conversation skills, being able to express himself vocally and interacting with others as he appraised these as 'Allows occupational performance'.

TABLE 35.9

David's MOHOST Assessment Summary Ratings

Motivation for Occupation				
Appraisal of ability	F	A	(I)	R
Expectation of success	F	A	(I)	R
Interest	F	A	(I)	R
Choices	F	A	I	(R)
Pattern of Occupation				
Routine	F	(A)	I	R
Adaptability	F	(A)	I	R
Roles	(F)	A	I	R
Responsibility	(F)	A	I	R
Communication & Interaction Skills				
Nonverbal skills	F	A	(I)	R
Conversation	F	(A)	I	R
Vocal expression	F	(A)	I	R
Relationships	F	(A)	I	R
Process Skills				
Knowledge	(F)	A	I	R
Timing	(F)	A	I	R
Organisation	(F)	A	I	R
Problem solving	(F)	A	I	R
Motor Skills				
Posture & mobility	F	A	(I)	R
Coordination	F	(A)	I	R
Strength & efffort	(F)	A	I	R
Energy	F	A	I	(R)
Environment				
Physical space	F	A	(I)	R
Physical resources	(F)	A	I	R
Social groups	(F)	A	I	R
Occupational demands	F	A	I	(R)

MOHOST Assessment Rating Scale

FAIR   **Facilitates** occupational participation
          Allows occupational participation
          Inhibits occupational participation
          Restricts occupational participation

MOHOST, Model of Human Occupation Screening Tool.

David Cook: Therapeutic Work Rehabilitation Programme Using MOHOST *(Continued)*

(d) *Process skills:* Mr Cook had good process skills; he was able to apply his knowledge and experience and manage his time, using his excellent problem-solving skills to adapt his activities. Therefore Mr Cook rated his process skills as 'Facilitates occupational performance'.

(e) *Motor skills:* This section was perhaps the most difficult for Mr Cook as he had to reflect on his impaired posture and mobility, which he rated as 'Inhibits occupational participation', and his decreased energy levels, which he rated as 'Restricts occupational participation'. On the other hand he was more positive about his improved coordination, rating this as 'Allows occupational performance', and newfound strength and effort as a result of posttraumatic growth (i.e. newfound resilience), which he rated as 'Facilitates occupational performance' despite his limitations in physical functioning and continuing struggle with fatigue.

(f) *Environment:* In terms of physical space, Mr Cook rated his office (at workplace) as 'Inhibits occupational participation' because of the distance he needed to travel to get there and its open-plan nature making it difficult to move around the desks, while rating his physical resources and social groups as 'Facilitators', given the fact he had help and assistance at the work place and a supportive team, which he regularly socialised with outside of work. Nevertheless, he found his occupational demands to be 'Restricting his occupational performance' as he continued to be anxious about meeting the growing needs of his role.

GOAL SETTING

The results of the work assessment was discussed with Mr Cook, highlighting the strengths and weaknesses identified, and he was invited to take an active part in planning his return-to-work programme to motivate him to move forward in his rehabilitation programme (Strand et al., 2015).

Long-term Goal

Mr Cook to return to work in the same company, doing the same or an equivalent job full time.

Short-term Goals

Goal 1. To be able to return to work in part-time capacity (i.e. 50% full-time equivalent [FTE]), working flexibly within 6 weeks.

Goal 2. To be able to use public transport independently within 12 weeks.

Goal 3. To develop an enhanced awareness of his neuro-behavioural impairments and to manage his expectations during the first 3 weeks of the graded return-to-work programme.

Goal 4. To stop and think about task at hand if he starts to become anxious and be able to tolerate a certain amount of anxiety when managing his workload within 4 weeks.

Goal 5. To have increased energy levels and muscle tone, and minimised pain, associated with immobility or abnormal joint alignment at the end of 12 weeks.

Goal 6. To have increased range of movement in his right hand and improved activity performance of the left hand by the end of 12 weeks.

Goal 7. To be able to independently move around and perform his work activities within an open-plan office by the end of 12 weeks.

Goal 8. To be able to attend a social/leisure event outside of his home or work environment once a week at the end of 12 weeks.

WORK REHABILITATION PROGRAMME

Work-specific Interventions

Liaising with the employer for job accommodations:

■ After a discussion of his options, David took the responsibility to contact his employer to arrange that he return to work initially 2 half-days per week [Goal 1], slowly increasing his workload each week, working from home 1.5 days a week for 6 weeks. He proposed to use Skype to attend off-site meetings to save time and energy on extra travelling. After the first 6 weeks, he was able to increase his working days to 3 days a week for another 6 weeks, still working from home once a week.

■ As he was not able to drive because of his unilateral neglect, he practiced various public transport options with the help of his family but did not feel confident to be able to travel independently at the end of the therapy. Instead, Mr Cook was offered a car-share by a colleague for 2 days a week, which he happily accepted [Goal 2].

■ His employers agreed to provide him with voice recognition software to help him with replying to various emails and writing letters and reports [Goal 1].

■ His workstation was adapted to meet his needs (e.g. his keyboard and mouse were adapted for one-handed use, he was given a lumbar support chair with arms to

Continued on following page

promote good posture and he was provided with a foot rest) by the occupational health department at his company, and they also made some environmental modifications for his safety (e.g. moved his desk to the front of the large open-plan office and turned to face the door to help with his visual neglect) [Goal 7].

■ His PA helped to get him to and from other businesses and off-site meeting by accompanying him to these meetings and taking the minutes of these meetings for his records [Goals 2 and 7].

Health-specific Interventions

Educating Mr Cook and his family about the impact of CVA:

■ Mr Cook was provided with verbal and written information about the impact of CVA on his health and functioning and given the opportunity to ask questions about his prognosis.

■ His family (i.e. his parents, siblings, ex-wife and children) were also provided with information and advice on the CVA recovery process to facilitate a helpful environment to support his return to work, so they could help Mr Cook to manage his expectations and set realistic goals [Goals 1 and 3].

■ The importance of maintaining a good level of social activity and participation in physical exercise was emphasised to Mr Cook and his family to prevent inactivity, loss of social roles and depression [Goal 8].

Occupational therapist liaising with the MDT about the rehabilitation goals:

■ Mr Cook consented to be referred to a physiotherapist with experience in neurology to devise an exercise programme to increase his standing/walking tolerance, minimise pain associated with immobility or abnormal joint alignment and raise his energy levels [Goal 5].

■ Occupational therapist liaised with the speech therapist with regards to the reassessment and treatment of his word-finding difficulties to improve his delayed speech and increase his confidence [Goal 8].

Hand therapy:

■ To help Mr Cook to regain his full hand function, an individualised hand therapy programme was devised to integrate muscular, skeletal and neurological functions using small, precise, coordinated movements, which involved the following:

   ■ Performing structured hand exercises using the affected hand and repeating the tasks, such as putting pegs in a pegboard and taking them out and timing himself doing this; shooting marbles into a cardboard box every day; using a rubber band to exercise his fingers; and squeezing a therapeutic putty to strengthen the affected hand.

   ■ Practice making a fist with the affected hand.

   ■ Practice using the unaffected left hand to write clearly and faster, type on the computer and touch screen technologies, type text messages on the phone, and groom himself daily without the help of a person or tool [Goal 6].

Psychological interventions:

■ Mr Cook was supported using counselling skills such as active listening, motivational interviewing, focusing on strengths and encouraging purpose with systematic guidance (Whitcher, 2004) [Goal 4].

■ The occupational therapist provided him with day-to-day anxiety management techniques such as learning to use breathing to gain an internal locus of control, avoiding negative self-talk, and practicing relaxation using audio recordings [Goal 4].

■ Mr Cook was also provided with the details of a local CVA support group which met bimonthly to encourage spending time with people who had similar experiences, with a view to providing a platform to share his fears and difficulties without the feeling of being judged by 'healthy' individuals [Goal 4].

REASSESSMENT

After an intensive 12-week occupational therapy programme in the community and reassessment at 6 months, Mr Cook:

■ Tolerated standing/walking for up to 3 hours and attended a gym to do structured exercise 3 days a week for an hour under the guidance of a physiotherapist with neurology expertise.

■ Improved his affected hand functioning by 4 points from 2 (baseline) to 6 (discharge at 6 months) on the Numerical Rating Scale (NRS; 1–10, 1 = not able to do it, 10 = able to do extremely well) and significantly increased his nondominant hand functioning by 5 points on the NRS from 4 (baseline) to 9 (discharge at 6 months).

■ Incorporated relaxation into his daily routine by practicing mindfulness to manage his fatigue and anxiety.

■ Decided to remain working part time, 3 days a week, to manage his energy levels, rather than going back to full-time employment.

■ Volunteered half a day a week at the local Brain and Spinal Injury Centre (BASIC), where he attended the CVA support group meetings, to provide financial and management support.

■ Was able to use the rail network independently for long-distance journeys.

■ Started a blog on the Internet to share his rehabilitation tips, with particular reference to return to work and battling with low mood and anxiety for other people who had a CVA.

PRACTICE STORY 35.2

David Cook: Therapeutic Work Rehabilitation Programme Using MOHOST (Continued)

- Joined a photography group at the local community centre, where they regularly met and planned weekends away to interesting places to photograph landmarks, architecture and nature. As an aside, he met his new partner at this group.

- His HADS score was reduced to 7 (normal) from 21 (borderline abnormal), indicating currently he was not at risk of depression and anxiety.

MOHOST, Model of Human Occupation Screening Tool.

PRACTICE STORY 35.3

Evrim Hepari: Therapeutic Work Rehabilitation Programme Using the ICF Framework

BACKGROUND

Referral

A referral was made from the community intermediate care team to the occupational therapy for Ms Hepari as she had difficulty carrying out household activities, driving and returning to work after major abdominal surgery.

History of Present Condition

Evrim was 40 years old. When she was referred for occupational therapy assessment she was still recovering from a major abdominal hernia repair/abdominoplasty that she had 6 weeks previously. Her surgery involved a transverse lower abdominal incision and resection of excess skin. Evrim had discomfort in her groin, weakness of the lower extremities and trunk, limited mobility and decreased ability to work because of impaired tolerance.

Domestic/Social Situation

Evrim was a single mother living with her three children, two school aged and one preschool aged, and an au pair who helped her with childcare up to 20 hours per week. She was relatively independent in her basic activities of daily living (ADL) (i.e. eating, toileting, dressing, grooming, bathing, walking and transferring) with some help from the au pair with dressing. She did her grocery shopping online, and the au pair helped out with dropping off and picking up kids from the school and nursery and doing some light housework such as washing up and making the kids' beds, and she had a cleaner coming in once a week to do heavier housework such as vacuuming the living room and bedrooms and cleaning the bathroom.

Occupation (Work)

Evrim worked full time as a home-based mobile beauty therapist. She had a dedicated room to see her clients at her home and also visited some clients at their own homes to deliver certain beauty treatments. She wanted to return to work as soon as possible as she had no other sources of income or sick pay because she was self-employed.

INITIAL ASSESSMENT

Using the ICF as Framework

Health Conditions. Evrim had other comorbidities such as hypothyroidism, high blood pressure, hip and knee osteoarthritis (OA) and type 2 diabetes, which started during her last pregnancy and remained unresolved. She was also treated for depression and had been on an increasing dose of antidepressants for 2 years before her operation.

Body Functions and Structure. Evrim reported experiencing severe pain in her abdomen postoperatively, describing the pain as constant but varying in intensity (e.g. pain is intensified on physical activity and after eating). Her pain score on a Visual Analogue Scale (VAS) (10 cm) after walking from the waiting room to the treatment room (approximately 50 metres) was 8.4 (Fig. 35.2).

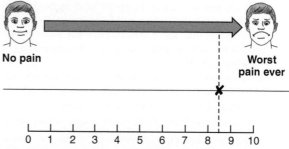

FIG. 35.2 ■ Evrim's Visual Analogue Scale (VAS) Pain Score for abdominal pain resting after walking around the room.

She also experienced chronic hip and knee pain because of the OA, which was exacerbated by her weight. She weighed 108 kg; at a height of 1.65 cm, she had a body mass index of 40.6, indicating that she was obese. The healthy weight range for her height was between 49.2 kg and 66.7 kgs.

Continued on following page

Evrim Hepari: Therapeutic Work Rehabilitation Programme Using the ICF Framework (Continued)

Evrim had significant reduction in upper body movement, as since the abdominoplasty she was unable to fully extend her upper body to stand upright and adopt a healthy posture. The severe pain and discomfort in her groin also affected her lower extremities, resulting in limited mobility and decreased tolerance for standing and walking.

Activities. She was independent with difficulty in self-care and needed help with the household tasks such as cooking, cleaning and shopping. She was unable to drive to visit clients' homes to provide mobile beauty treatments.

Participation. Evrim was unable to partake in leisure activities such as attending play groups with her youngest son as she was unable to drive and was not able to transfer her son to and from the car seat or buggy to be able to travel.

Contextual Factors.

■ Personal

Evrim was divorced 2 years ago and lived with her three children and a young female au pair from France. Her diagnosis of depression was made shortly after the divorce, as her marriage broke down after a series of particularly stressful events. Evrim was not in communication with her ex-husband, nor in receipt of maintenance payments or structured childcare support. At the time of the divorce she weighed 76 kg; although she was still overweight according to the recommended healthy weight range for her height, she was not obese. Her high blood pressure also developed during the last 2 years.

Evrim reported that she was experiencing some financial hardship and had to borrow large amount of monies to support herself and her family over the past 2 years. She was concerned as she had been unable to pay off her debts because she had not been able to work since her operation. Being self-employed meant that she did not receive any benefits such as annual leave, sick pay and employer pension contributions.

■ Environmental

Evrim lived in a four-bedroom detached house with large garden, which she privately rented, and was in receipt of Child Benefit, Housing Benefit and Working Tax Credit.

WORKPLACE ASSESSMENT – EVRIM'S USUAL WORK TASKS

As a beauty therapist Evrim performed a number of manual tasks such as manicure and pedicures, facials and laser hair removal. All tasks required bilateral or unilateral (right) hand and arm movements and many tasks involved repetitive fine motor activity. However, only a little upper-limb strength was required to execute these tasks, as she used wheeled trolleys to transport her equipment around the room and a portable battery-powered machine to file nails and remove hard skin. She only applied gentle massage to clients' face and upper body (mainly shoulders and arms) during facial treatments.

Evrim used her tablet and smart phone to accept bookings and record client information using the calendar function. The room she used for her work was of sufficient light, with wooden floors and good natural light through the south-facing French doors that opened to the back garden. She had an unbranded portable, lightweight massage table, a small fixed dresser with beauty products on shelves, and a chrome-based leather chair with padded seat, back support and wheels with adjustable height.

GOAL SETTING

Long-term Goal

Evrim to regain her mobility and range of movement and return to work as home-based/mobile beauty therapist within 8 weeks.

Short-term SMART Goals

Goal 1. To be able to move in and around the house within 2 weeks.

Goal 2. To be able to perform light cleaning and tidying around the house and beauty-therapy room by the end of 3 weeks.

Goal 3. To be able to move and transfer treatment box and therapist's stool in and out the car by 3 weeks.

Goal 4. To be able to resume driving by the end of 4 weeks.

Goal 5. To be able to work 3 days a week by the end of 4 weeks.

Goal 6. To be able to deal with stress and anxiety related to full-time work by the end of 8 weeks.

WORK REHABILITATION PROGRAMME

Work-specific Interventions

Graded activities to increase the level of physical functioning:

■ Tasks: Evrim was provided with a graded exposure to her work tasks, which involved starting with easier tasks such as checking her stocks for beauty products to identify what needed to be replenished, then slowly increasing task demands and intensity to activities requiring more strength and endurance to improve physical functioning, such as physically replacing treatment products on the shelves and refilling the treatment trolley (which required frequent changes between sitting, standing, and kneeling positions) [Goal 1, 2 & 3].

■ Time spent on tasks: Evrim's time spent on carrying out these tasks was gradually increased, with fewer breaks in between. Evrim was encouraged to conduct some ADLs around the house such as light cooking and cleaning, as well as the work activities [Goals 1, 2 and 3].

■ Organisation: Evrim was encouraged to return to work part time, initially working 1 day on and 1 day off and only taking on light treatments she could deliver while sitting on a stool at home, such as doing manicures

Evrim Hepari: Therapeutic Work Rehabilitation Programme Using the ICF Framework (Continued)

and pedicures, for the first 3 weeks, before starting to work full time and visit clients at their homes [Goal 5].

- Aids and adaptations: She was provided with a 'helping hand' (i.e. grabber) so that she could pick up items from the floor and help with reaching and grabbing distant objects, and a perching stool to be able to sit while a client was lying on the massage table to avoid standing for long periods. She was advised to use this equipment until she was fully recovered and able to do these activities comfortably [Goals 1, 2 and 3].
- Driving: Once Evrim was able to sit and stand comfortably and carry out light household activities, she started with driving short distances, such as to the nearest shop, and gradually increased the mileage. She was also able to move the trolley in and out of the car independently with no discomfort by 4 weeks [Goal 4].

Health-specific Interventions

Liaising with the members of the multidisciplinary team:

- Evrim had other health professionals involved in her care when the work rehabilitation programme started. She was visited by a district nurse at home to monitor the conservative management of her large wound (e.g. application of antibacterial and moisture-absorbing agents, topically applied skin barriers) twice a week as Evrim's scar was not healing quickly because of her diabetes. The occupational therapist liaised with the district nurse to understand how Evrim's scar was healing, so the intensity of the graded activities were planned to maximise the healing process [Goal 1].
- Community physiotherapists were also involved in Evrim's care, conducting an exercise programme for Evrim to perform hip flexor stretch in the half-kneeling position and treadmill exercises to improve walking tolerance (three times a week at the therapy gym) [Goal 4].
- After the occupational therapy assessment, Evrim was advised to visit her general practitioner (GP) for a referral for counselling and weight management as many of the issues surrounding her divorce remained unresolved to date, causing her anxiety and low mood [Goal 6].
- Evrim was recommended to seek advice from the Citizen Advice Bureau regarding debt management to reduce this stressor to help with the anxiety management [Goal 6].

Activities and participation:

- Evrim performed simulated tasks requiring repetitive and maximum lifting, stretching and bending using work simulation equipment (i.e. Valpar Component Work Samples System) (Hakkinen et al., 2003), reflecting the functional component of Evrim's job, to increase her strength and performance [Goals 1, 2 and 3].
- With advice from her GP, Evrim enrolled in a local weight loss club and subscribed to a lifestyle change through healthy eating with a goal to lose 1 kg a week, particularly to help with her hip and knee pain as obesity increases the likelihood of negative outcomes in OA (Canadian Agency for Drugs and Technologies in Health, 2014; Johns Hopkins Arthritis Center, 2015) [Goal 6].

Environmental factors:

- Her home environment was modified to optimise Evrim's independence and safety after discharge. This involved things like rearranging the shelves in the kitchen to bring cooking utilities to Evrim's chest level and to encourage her to start cooking and preparing meals for the family.
- Evrim was encouraged to hold a coffee morning at home for her friends with young children to engage her in leisure activities with friends and family and avoid social isolation, which is a precursor to anxiety and depression [Goal 6].

REASSESSMENT

At the end of an 8-week work rehabilitation programme, Evrim:

- Had a reduction in abdominal pain as noted by her VAS score of 3 of 10 when resting and moving around the house.
- Managed to lose 8 kg and wanted to adopt the healthy eating habits in the long-term to reach a healthy weight.
- Started contributing to household activities such as grocery shopping, cooking hot meals and doing light housework.
- Was able to stand up to an hour and walk 2 km independently.
- Reduced her intake of analgesic treatment to a therapeutic dose of NSAIDs as recommended by her GP.
- Resumed full-time work as a home-based and mobile beauty therapist at the end of 8 weeks.
- Was able to transfer her preschool-aged son to and from a car seat and do the school run as needed.

ICF, International Classification of Functional, Disability and Health; NSAIDs, nonsteroidal antiinflammatory drugs.

CONCLUSION

Work is an important occupation for health and well-being and predictive of increased levels of quality of life. Work instability and disability can occur after an illness, injury or impairment and can be the outcome of complex biopsychosocial factors rather than a direct consequence of health conditions. Occupational therapists play an important role in the early identification and treatment of work problems to retain employment, as well as facilitating return to work, because of their inherent knowledge of human occupation and holistic approach to assessment and work rehabilitation.

 http://evolve.elsevier.com/Curtin/OT

REFERENCES

Allaire, S., & Keysor, J. J. (2009). Development of a structured interview tool to help patients identify and solve rheumatic condition-related work barriers. *Arthritis Rheum, 61*, 988–995.

Allaire, S., Wolfe, F., Niu, J., & Lavalley, M. P. (2008). Contemporary prevalence and incidence of work disability associated with rheumatoid arthritis in the US. *Arthritis & Rheumatology, 59*, 474–480.

American Occupational Therapy Association (2011). Work rehabilitation. *American Journal of Occupational Therapy, 65*, S55–S64.

Backman, C., Village, J., & Lacaille, D. (2008). The Ergonomic Assessment Tool for Arthritis: development and pilot testing. *Arthritis Care Research, 59*, 1495–1503.

Baldwin, C., & Brusco, N. K. (2011). The effect of vocational rehabilitation on return-to-work rates post stroke: A systematic review. *Topics in Stroke Rehabilitation, 18*(5), 562–572.

Barnes, T., & Holmes, J. & College of Occupational Therapists Specialist Section: Work. (2009). *Occupational therapy in vocational rehabilitation: A brief guide to current practice in the UK.* Retrieved from London. https://www.cot.co.uk/sites/default/files/ss-work/public/OT-in-vocational-rehab.pdf.

Barrett, E. M., Scott, D. G., Wiles, N. J., & Symmons, D. P. (2000). The impact of rheumatoid arthritis on employment status in the early years of disease: A UK community-based study. *Rheumatology (Oxford), 39*(12), 1403–1409.

Black, C. (2008). *Working for a healthier tomorrow.* London: TSO. Retrieved from: https://www.gov.uk/government/uploads/system/uploads/attachment_data/file/209782/hwwb-working-for-a-healthier-tomorrow.pdf.

Braveman, B., & Page, J. J. (2012). *WORK: Promoting participation & productivity through occupational therapy.* Philadelphia: FA Davis.

Brey, J. K., & Wolf, T. J. (2015). Socioeconomic disparities in work performance following mild stroke. *Disability and Rehabilitation, 37*(2), 106–112.

Busch, M. A., Coshall, C., Heuschmann, P. U., McKevitt, C., & Wolfe, C. D. (2009). Sociodemographic differences in return to work after stroke: The South London Stroke Register (SLSR). *Journal of Neurology, Neurosurgery and Psychiatry, 80*(8), 888–893.

Callahan, L. F., Cleveland, R. J., Altpeter, M., & Hackney, B. (2016). Evaluation of tai chi program effectiveness for people with arthritis in the community: A randomized controlled trial. *Journal of Aging and Physical Activity, 24*(1), 101–110.

Christiansen, C. H., Baum, C. M., & Haugen, J. B. (2005). *Occupational therapy: Performance, participation, and well-being.* Thorofare, NJ: Slack.

Connelly, L. B., Woolf, A., & Brooks, P. (2006). *Cost-effectiveness of interventions for musculoskeletal conditions.* Washington, DC: World Bank.

Cook, C., & Lukersmith, S. (2010). Work rehabilitation. In M. Curtin, M. Molineux, & J. Supyk (Eds.), *Occupational therapy & physical dysfunction* (6th ed.). London: Churchill Livingstone.

College of Occupational Therapists. (2008). *Work matters: The College of Occupational Therapists' vocational rehabilitation strategy.* London: College of Occupational Therapists.

Davis, M. C., Zautra, A. J., Wolf, L. D., Tennen, H., & Yeung, E. W. (2015). Mindfulness and cognitive-behavioral interventions for chronic pain: Differential effects on daily pain reactivity and stress reactivity. *Journal of Consulting and Clinical Psychology, 83*(1), 24–35.

de Boer, A. G., Taskila, T., Ojajarvi, A., van Dijk, F. J., & Verbeek, J. H. (2009). Cancer survivors and unemployment: A meta-analysis and meta-regression. *Journal of the American Medical Association, 301*(7), 753–762.

Department for Work and Pensions. (2004). *Building capacity for work: A UK framework for vocational rehabilitation.* London: Department of Work and Pensions.

Eberhardt, K., Larsson, B. M., Nived, K., & Lindqvist, E. (2007). Work disability in rheumatoid arthritis – development over 15 years and evaluation of predictive factors over time. *Journal of Rheumatology, 34*(3), 481–487.

Engel, G. L. (1980). The clinical application of the biopsychosocial model. *American Journal of Psychiatry, 137*(5), 535–544.

Feldthusen, C., Bjork, M., Forsblad-d'Elia, H., & Mannerkorpi, K. (2013). Perception, consequences, communication, and strategies for handling fatigue in persons with rheumatoid arthritis of working age – a focus group study. *Clinical Rheumatology, 32*(5), 557–566.

Gaudreault, N., Maillette, P., Coutu, M. F., Durand, M. J., Hagemeister, N., & Hebert, L. J. (2014). Work disability among workers with osteoarthritis of the knee: Risks factors, assessment scales, and interventions. *International Journal of Rehabilitation Research, 37*(4), 290–296.

Gignac, M. A., Badley, E. M., Lacaille, D., et al. (2004). Managing arthritis and employment: making arthritis-related work changes as a means of adaptation. *Arthritis Rheum, 51*, 909–916.

Gilworth, G., Chamberlain, M. A., Harvey, A., et al. (2003). Development of a work instability scale for rheumatoid arthritis. *Arthritis & Rheumatology, 49*(3), 349–354.

Gjesdal, S., Bratberg, E., & Maeland, J. G. (2009). Musculoskeletal impairments in the Norwegian working population: The prognostic role of diagnoses and socioeconomic status: A prospective study of sickness absence and transition to disability pension. *Spine, 34*(14), 1519–1525.

Gordon, Lynch, B., Beesley, V., et al. (2011). The Working After Cancer Study (WACS): A population-based study of middle-aged workers diagnosed with colorectal cancer and their return to work experiences. *BMC Public Health, 11*, 604.

Gronning, K., Rodevand, E., & Steinsbekk, A. (2010). Paid work is associated with improved health-related quality of life in patients with rheumatoid arthritis. *Clinical Rheumatology*, *29*(11), 1317–1322.

Hakkinen, A., Sokka, T., Lietsalmi, A. M., Kautiainen, H., & Hannonen, P. (2003). Effects of dynamic strength training on physical function, Valpar 9 work sample test, and working capacity in patients with recent-onset rheumatoid arthritis. *Arthritis & Rheumatology*, *49*(1), 71–77.

Hallert, E., Husberg, M., & Bernfort, L. (2012). The incidence of permanent work disability in patients with rheumatoid arthritis in Sweden 1990-2010: Before and after introduction of biologic agents. *Rheumatology (Oxford)*, *51*(2), 338–346.

Hammond, A. (2008). Rehabilitation in musculoskeletal diseases. *Best Practice & Research Clinical Rheumatology*, *22*(3), 435–449.

Hammond, A., & Freeman, K. (2001). One-year outcomes of a randomized controlled trial of an educational-behavioural joint protection programme for people with rheumatoid arthritis. *Rheumatology (Oxford)*, *40*(9), 1044–1051.

Hammond, A., Jones, V., & Prior, Y. (2016). The effects of compression gloves on hand symptoms and hand function in rheumatoid arthritis and hand osteoarthritis: A systematic review. *Clinical Rehabilitation*, *30*(3), 213–224.

Harris, E. C., & Coggon, D. (2015). Hip osteoarthritis and work. *Best Practice & Research Clinical Rheumatology*, *29*(3), 462–482.

Hegarty, R. S., Conner, T. S., Stebbings, S., & Treharne, G. J. (2015). Feel the fatigue and be active anyway: Physical activity on high-fatigue days protects adults with arthritis from decrements in same-day positive mood. *Arthritis Care & Research (Hoboken)*,.

Holmes, J. (2007). *Vocational rehabilitation*. New York: John Wiley & Sons.

Hommel, M., Trabucco-Miguel, S., Joray, S., Naegele, B., Gonnet, N., & Jaillard, A. (2009). Social dysfunctioning after mild to moderate first-ever stroke at vocational age. *Journal of Neurology, Neurosurgery and Psychiatry*, *80*(4), 371–375.

Johns Hopkins Arthritis Center (2015). *Osteoarthritis: Role of body weight in osteoarthritis – weight management. Retrieved from*, http://www.hopkinsarthritis.org/patient-corner/disease-management/role-of-body-weight-in-osteoarthritis.

Joss, M. (2007). The importance of job analysis in occupational therapy. *British Journal of Occupational Therapy*, *70*(7), 301–303.

Kielhofner, G., & Burke, J. P. (1980). A model of human occupation, part 1. Conceptual framework and content. *American Journal of Occupational Therapy*, *34*(9), 572–581.

Laires, P. A., & Gouveia, M. (2014). Association of rheumatic diseases with early exit from paid employment in Portugal. *Rheumatology International*, *34*(4), 491–502.

Langley, P. C., Mu, R., Wu, M., Dong, P., & Tang, B. (2011). The impact of rheumatoid arthritis on the burden of disease in urban China. *Journal of Medical Economics*, *14*(6), 709–719.

Law, M., Baptiste, S., McColl, M., Carswell, A., Polatajko, H., & Pollock, N. (2005). *Canadian Occupational Performance Measure (COPM)* (4th ed.). Ottawa: Canadian Association of Occupational Therapists.

Law, M., Baptiste, S., McColl, M. A., Polatajko, H., & Pollock, N. (1990). The Canadian Occupational Performance Measure: An

outcome measure for occupational therapy. *Canadian Journal of Occupational Therapy*, *57*(2), 82–87.

Lerner, D., Amick, B. C., 3rd, Rogers, W. H., et al. (2001) The Work Limitations Questionnaire. *Med Care 39*, 72–85.

Lee, J., & Kielhofner, G. (2010). Vocational intervention based on the Model of Human Occupation: A review of evidence. *Scandinavian Journal of Occupational Therapy*, *17*(3), 177–190.

Maaijwee, N. A., Rutten-Jacobs, L. C., Arntz, R. M., et al. (2014). Long-term increased risk of unemployment after young stroke: A long-term follow-up study. *Neurology*, *83*(13), 1132–1138.

McArthur, M. A., Birt, L., & Goodacre, L. (2014). 'Better but not best': A qualitative exploration of the experiences of occupational gain for people with inflammatory arthritis receiving anti-TNFalpha treatment. *Disability and Rehabilitation*, 1–10.

McDonald, H. N., Dietrich, T., Townsend, A., Li, L. C., Cox, S., & Backman, C. L. (2012). Exploring occupational disruption among women after onset of rheumatoid arthritis. *Arthritis Care & Research (Hoboken)*, *64*(2), 197–205.

Mcfeely, G. (2012). Health at work: An analysis of Black's and Frost's independent review of sickness absence – what can occupational therapists offer? *British Journal of Occupational Therapy*, *75*(7), 343–345.

Mosey, A. C. (1980). A model for occupational therapy. *Occupational Therapy in Mental Health, Spring*, *1*, 11–31.

Neovius, M., Simard, J. F., & Askling, J. (2011). How large are the productivity losses in contemporary patients with RA, and how soon in relation to diagnosis do they develop? *Annals of Rheumatic Diseases*, *70*(6), 1010–1015.

Oxford Dictionaries. (2015). *Oxford Dictionary of English*. Oxford, UK: Oxford University Press.

Palmer, K. T., & Goodson, N. (2015). Ageing, musculoskeletal health and work. *Best Practice & Research Clinical Rheumatology*, *29*(3), 391–404.

Prior, Y., Bodell, S., Amanna, A., & Hammond, A. (2014). Rheumatoid arthritis patients' views of a vocational rehabilitation intervention provided by rheumatology occupational therapists. *Rheumatology (Oxford)*, *53*(Suppl 2), 125.

Prior, Y., Amanna, A., Bodell, S., et al. (2015). A qualitative evaluation of an occupational therapy-led work rehabilitation for people with inflammatory arthritis: perspectives of the therapists and their line managers. *British Journal of Occupational Therapy*, *78*, 465–466.

Rantalaiho, V. M., Kautiainen, H., Jarvenpaa, S., et al. (2013). Decline in work disability caused by early rheumatoid arthritis: Results from a nationwide Finnish register, 2000-8. *Annals of the Rheumatic Diseases*, *72*(5), 672–677.

Roessler, R. (1995). *The Work Experience Survey (WES) Manual: A Structured Interview for Identifying Barriers to Career Maintenance. A Service Provider's Guide*. USA: Arkansas University.

Roth, E. J., & Lovell, L. (2014). Employment after stroke: Report of a state of the science symposium. *Topics in Stroke Rehabilitation*, *21* (Suppl 1), S75–S86.

Schultz, P. N., Beck, M. L., Stava, C., & Sellin, R. V. (2002). Cancer survivors. Work related issues. *AAOHN Journal*, *50*(5), 220–226.

Shrey, D. E., & Mital, A. (2000). Accelerating the return to work (RTW) chances of coronary heart disease (CHD) patients: Part

2 – development and validation of a vocational rehabilitation programme. *Disability and Rehabilitation, 22*(13-14), 621–626.

Sokka, T., Kautiainen, H., Pincus, T., et al. (2010). Work disability remains a major problem in rheumatoid arthritis in the 2000s: Data from 32 countries in the QUEST-RA study. *Arthritis Research & Therapy, 12*(2), R42.

Spelten, E. R., Verbeek, J. H., Uitterhoeve, A. L., et al. (2003). Cancer, fatigue and the return of patients to work – a prospective cohort study. *European Journal of Cancer, 39*(11), 1562–1567.

Strand, V., Wright, G. C., Bergman, M. J., Tambiah, J., & Taylor, P. C. (2015). Patient expectations and perceptions of goal-setting strategies for disease management in rheumatoid arthritis. *Journal of Rheumatology, 42*(11), 2046–2054.

Sullivan, P. W., Ghushchyan, V., Huang, X. Y., & Globe, D. R. (2010). Influence of rheumatoid arthritis on employment, function, and productivity in a nationally representative sample in the United States. *Journal of Rheumatology, 37*(3), 544–549.

Sverker, A., Ostlund, G., Thyberg, M., Thyberg, I., Valtersson, E., & Bjork, M. (2015). Dilemmas of participation in everyday life in early rheumatoid arthritis: A qualitative interview study (the Swedish TIRA Project). *Disability and Rehabilitation, 37*(14), 1251–1259.

Symmons, D., Turner, G., Webb, R., et al. (2002). The prevalence of rheumatoid arthritis in the United Kingdom: New estimates for a new century. *Rheumatology (Oxford), 41*(7), 793–800.

Toussirot, E. (2010). Predictive factors for disability as evaluated by the health assessment questionnaire in rheumatoid arthritis: A literature review. *Inflammation & Allergy Drug Targets, 9*(1), 51–59.

Trygged, S., Ahacic, K., & Kareholt, I. (2011). Income and education as predictors of return to working life among younger stroke patients. *BMC Public Health, 11*, 742.

Uhlig, T. (2010). Which patients with rheumatoid arthritis are still working? *Arthritis Research & Therapy, 12*(2), 114.

Van der Meer, M., Hoving, J. L., Vermeulen, M. I., et al. (2011). Experiences and needs for work participation in employees with rheumatoid arthritis treated with anti-tumour necrosis factor therapy. *Disability and Rehabilitation, 33*(25-26), 2587–2595.

Verstappen, Boonen, A., Bijlsma, J. W., Buskens, E., et al. (2005). Working status among Dutch patients with rheumatoid arthritis: Work disability and working conditions. *Rheumatology (Oxford), 44*, 202–206.

Verstappen, S., Bijlsma, J., Verkleij, H., Buskens, E., Blaauw, A., ter Borg, E., & Jacobs, J. (2004). Overview of work disability in patients with rheumatoid arthritis as observed in transversal and longitudinal studies. *Annals of the Rheumatic Diseases, 51*(3), 488–497.

Waddell, G., & Aylward, M. (2005). *The scientific and conceptual basis of incapacity benefits.* London: Stationery Office Books.

Waddell, G., & Burton, A. K. (2004). *Concepts of rehabilitation for the management of common health problems.* London: Stationery Office Books.

Waddell, G., Burton, A. K., & Kendall, N. A. S. (2008). *Vocational rehabilitation: What works for whom and when?* London: The Stationary Office.

Ware, J. E., Jr., & Sherbourne, C. D. (1992). The MOS 36-item short-form health survey (SF-36). I. Conceptual framework and item selection. *Medical Care, 30*(6), 473–483.

Whitcher, K. (2004). Counselling skills in occupational therapy: A grounded theory approach to explain their use within mental health in New Zealand. *British Journal of Occupational Therapy, 67*(8), 361–368.

World Health Organization. (2001). *International classification of functioning, disability and health.* Geneva: WHO.

Wilkie, R., & Pransky, G. (2012). Improving work participation for adults with musculoskeletal conditions. *Best Practice & Research Clinical Rheumatology, 26*(5), 733–742.

Zigmond, A. S., & Snaith, R. P. (1983). The hospital anxiety and depression scale. *Acta Psychiatrica Scandinavica, 67*(6), 361–370.

36 BIOMECHANICAL STRATEGIES

HANIF FARHAN MOHD RASDI

Abstract

The use of biomechanical strategies became prevalent in occupational therapy in the 1960s, when the profession was seeking more objective and quantitative means of evaluating practice. However, a refocusing on the occupational nature of the profession from the 1980s led to the bottom-up and reductionist approach of biomechanical strategies being considered contrary to the top-down approach being championed by the profession. However, biomechanical strategies have a significant place in the assessment and intervention tools that occupational therapists use, even when working from an occupation-centred perspective. The use of biomechanical principles in occupational therapy to understand physical functions such as strength, endurance and range of movement complements the therapeutic value of occupation.

KEY POINTS

- Occupational therapists apply biomechanical strategies by integrating the principles of biomechanics such kinetics, kinematics and muscle activity into therapy.

- Basic knowledge of biomechanics informs the logic of biomechanical strategies to be used in occupational therapy.

- Biomechanical strategies may be applied to occupational therapy practice through three main approaches: (a) occupation-as-means, (b) occupation-as-end and (c) rehabilitative.

- Biomechanical strategies need to be conducted within occupation-based practice to ensure they have therapeutic value.

- As a unique skill of occupational therapists, activity analysis can guide how to evaluate in detail any activity or occupation within its context.

- The use of activities that are purposeful and meaningful is essential to achieve maximum therapeutic values.

INTRODUCTION

Biomechanical strategies are used almost exclusively by occupational therapists to improve the occupational performance of people who experience limitations in physical performance such as muscle weakness, inadequate range of motion or lack of endurance that can significantly affect their ability to perform daily occupation independently. The focus of this chapter is to explore and present how biomechanics is used by occupational therapists as a therapeutic method. Examples of two common biomechanical parameters, kinematics and kinetics, are included to inform the basics of biomechanics that further evolved into a therapeutic method. To carefully determine the therapeutic potential of an activity, a process called activity analysis is conducted by breaking down the activity into components. Furthermore, the importance of activity analysis as a framework for gradation and adaptation is also covered within this chapter. Biomechanical strategies are categorised into three main approaches: (a) occupation-as-means, (b) occupation-as-end and (c) rehabilitative. The assumptions that underlie each approach are also included. A practice story is included as an example on how to apply biomechanical strategies with people to maximise movement strategies to optimise function.

PARADIGM SHIFT: RATIONALE FOR BIOMECHANICAL STRATEGIES

The use of biomechanical strategies in occupational therapy has a strong theoretical basis from various disciplines. To classify the theory, the terms *paradigm, frame of reference* and *conceptual model of practice* are often used in the literature (Duncan, 2011). *Paradigm* refers to the common consensus concerning the most essential beliefs of occupational therapy. *Frame of reference (FOR)* is 'borrowed' theory from outside of the profession (e.g. engineering, psychology, art and architect) that is applicable within occupational therapy practice. The *conceptual models of practice (models)* are the occupation-focused theories that have been developed within the profession to explain the use of occupation as the therapeutic medium of practice.

According to Kielhofner (2009), paradigmatic development of occupational therapy profession can be divided into occupational paradigm (1900s–1940s), mechanistic paradigm (1950s–1970s) and contemporary paradigm (1980s onwards). During the occupational paradigm, the occupational therapy approach was based on the assumption that occupation is essential to life

and influences health and as such can be used to improve function. However, although this paradigm was thought to be holistic by focusing on personal motivation and the impact of the environment on performance, the approach and justification for occupational therapy services were subjective. As a result of the pressure from the medical profession, which sought objectivity to explain practice, the occupational therapy profession shifted from an occupational paradigm into the mechanistic paradigm. During the mechanistic paradigm, the biomechanical frame of reference became very prominent in the profession as therapists attempted to evaluate their practice using quantitative measurements.

However, because of the reductionist nature of the paradigm that separates mind from body, the profession entered a new era of professional crisis. According to International Classification of Functioning, Disabilities and Health (ICF), the impact of any illness, injury or impairment on a person can be categorised into body functions, body structures, activities and participation and environmental factors (Table 36.1) Wolf, Baum, & Connor, (2009). Through the use of bottom-up approaches (Table 36.2), the therapists were more likely to prioritise the impact of medical conditions on body function and structures (i.e. impairment) as the aim of the rehabilitation. This approach led to an uncertainty regarding whether or not the focus on the components of performance could affect a person's occupational issues. For instance, improving the range of motion (ROM) of the finger and thumb joints after a lesion of the flexor tendon muscles does not necessarily enable a person to be able to use the injured hand to engage in any activities of daily living (ADL). Focusing on the components of occupational performance (e.g. ROM) without holistically addressing the unique meaning and significance of the impact of the impairment from a person's perspective can compromise the therapeutic value of occupational therapy intervention. Therefore a call for the profession to return to the original impetus was initiated, and this development marked the rise of contemporary paradigm.

Within the contemporary paradigm, in contrast to the mechanistic paradigm, the profession regained its holistic view of occupational performance rather than concentrating on components of the performance. Although the paradigm had shifted, great achievements in mechanistic paradigm such as objective measurement and intervention in occupational therapy were retained and improved through a top-down approach. Within the contemporary paradigm, any issues of occupational performance were viewed based on the subjective experience of the person. The rise of the contemporary paradigm led to the development of models such as the Model of Human Occupation (Kielhofner, 2007) and the Canadian Model of Occupational Performance and Engagement (Polatajko & Townsend, 2007). These models have important roles in ensuring that biomechanical strategies were implemented using an 'occupational filter', underpinning the reductionist nature of these strategies with a focus on occupation-based practice.

TABLE 36.1
Common Illnesses, Injuries or Impairments Related to Biomechanical Strategies and Their Impact on Person's Life According to International Classification of Functioning, Disabilities and Health (ICF) Brief* Core Sets

Conditions	Definition	Impact on Person
Ankylosing spondylitis (Boonen, Braun, van der Horst Bruinsma, et al., 2010)	A form of chronic inflammation that predominantly affects the axial skeleton with inflammation of the sacroiliac joints and spine	**Body functions:** Mobility of joint functions, sensations related to muscles and movement functions, exercise tolerance functions **Body structures:** Structure of trunk, structures of pelvic region, additional musculoskeletal structures related to movement, and structure of lower extremity **Activities and participation:** Carrying out daily routine; changing basic body position; walking; acquiring, keeping and terminating a job; remunerative employment; recreation and leisure; driving **Environmental factors:** Products or substances for personal consumption, support and relationship
Hand conditions (Rudolf et al., 2012)	Any hand impairment from diseases or structural damages that limit and restrict daily activities	**Body functions:** Touch function, sensory functions related to temperature and other stimuli, sensation of pain, mobility of joint functions, stability of joint functions, muscle power functions, control of voluntary movement functions, protective functions of the skin **Body structures:** Spinal cord and related structures (e.g. peripheral nerves), structure of shoulder region, structure of upper extremity **Activities and participation:** Carrying out daily routine, lifting and carrying objects, fine hand use, hand and arm use, self-care, domestic life, work and employment **Environmental factors:** Products and technology
Low back pain (Cieza et al., 2004)	Pain, muscle tension, or stiffness localised below the costal margin and above the inferior gluteal folds, with or without sciatica	**Body functions:** Sensation of pain, muscle power functions, mobility of joint functions, exercise tolerance functions, muscle endurance functions, muscle tone functions, and stability of joint functions **Body structures:** Spinal cord and related structures, structure of trunk, and additional musculoskeletal structures related to movement **Activities and participation:** Maintaining a body position, lifting and carrying objects, changing basic body position, walking, remunerative employment, work and employment, other specified and unspecified, doing housework, dressing, toileting, acquiring, keeping and terminating a job **Environmental factors:** Design, construction and building products and technology of buildings for private use
Spinal cord injury (Cieza et al., 2010)	An injury at any level of the spinal cord resulting in a change of the cord's normal motor, sensory or autonomic function, either temporary or permanent.	**Body functions:** Muscle power functions, sensation of pain, muscle tone functions, mobility of joint functions **Body structures:** Spinal cord and related structures **Activities and participation:** Toileting, transferring oneself, carrying out daily routine, moving around, using equipment, changing basic body position, hand and arm use, using transportation, caring for body parts, and eating **Environmental factors:** Products and technology for personal indoor and outdoor mobility and transportation; products and technology for personal use in daily living; design, construction and building products and technology of buildings for public use; design, and construction and building products and technology of buildings for private use

*The brief ICF core sets were summarised by a group of experts in each study from comprehensive ICF core sets. The purpose of the comprehensive ICF core sets is to guide multidisciplinary assessments and facilitate research on functioning and health, whereas the purpose of the brief ICF core sets is to describe people with an injury, illness or impairment during clinical studies.

TABLE 36.2		
Bottom-Up Versus Top-Down Approaches		
	Bottom-Up	Top-Down
Focus	Impairment in body function and structure	Engagement in occupation
Approach	Emphasis on small and separate components of body function and structure (deductive)	Emphasis on daily occupation by incorporating the person's values, beliefs and spirituality (holistic)
Setting	Administered in artificial and standardised contexts	Administered according to the person's actual life contexts
Meaningfulness	Often secluded from relevant daily life contexts, thus may not be meaningful to the person	Integrates person's goal to determine tasks that are meaningful to the person's life

INTRODUCTION TO BIOMECHANICS

Originating from the engineering disciplines, biomechanics can be described as the study of motion and the effect of force on motion. The concept of biomechanics is often confused with kinesiology, which can be described as the study of functional anatomy, consisting of musculoskeletal systems, movement efficiency from the anatomical standpoint and the actions of joints and muscles during simple and complex movement (Hamill, Knutzen, & Derrick, 2015). Nowadays some aspects in kinesiology are incorporated into biomechanics curriculum to serve as a qualitative introduction to human movement, although biomechanics is generally quantitative in nature.

In occupational therapy, knowledge of biomechanics is important when describing how movement is executed, to ensure that appropriate assessments and interventions that suit the person's capabilities are selected. For instance, as a result of a transhumeral amputation of a dominant arm because of a motor vehicle accident, a teacher is unable to drive his car to school and states that this occupational issue is an utmost priority. To regain abilities and occupational performance, the therapist works with the teacher to enhance the function of the teacher's remaining arm (e.g. muscle power, muscle endurance, eye–hand coordination) through driving-related activities (e.g. steering manoeuvres, hand controls), as well as car modifications to suit the teacher's needs. In this case the application of biomechanical principles is crucial for safe driving, as well as to prevent any long-term health consequences as a result of improper body mechanics.

BIOMECHANICAL PARAMETERS

Kinetics

Kinetics is the study of the effect of force on motion. The current knowledge of kinetics is founded on Newton's three laws that describe how force can influence motion (Neumann, 2013). Newton's first law states that the body will remain in its current state unless acted upon by an external force (Law of Inertia). Newton's second law states that force will cause the body to accelerate in direct proportion to the magnitude of the force and in the same direction as the force (Law of Acceleration). Finally, Newton's third law states that when one body applies a force to another body, the second body applies an equal and opposite reaction force on the first body (Law of Reaction). In everyday situations, these three Newtonian laws are always applied. For instance, a shopping trolley will not move until a person pushes it (Law of Inertia). When kicking a ball, if the force applied to the ball is strong, the ball will move with speed and travel a long distance (Law of Acceleration). In order for a basketball player to jump, a sufficient amount of force must be exerted towards the ground so that the vertical ground reaction force will push the body upwards to a certain height (Law of Reaction).

In rehabilitation, there are some clinical measurements that are based on kinetics principles. For instance, electronic dynamometers and pinch gauges are designed based on the piezoelectric effect. This effect means that under mechanical loading, certain crystals (e.g. quartz) have the property to exhibit electrical charges. As raw mechanical signals, the electrical charges are then converted into digital output, which can easily be interpreted for clinical measurement. The concept of piezoelectric effect is also used in a force platform in balance-related studies. As explained in the Law of Reaction, whenever two objects are in contact with each other, an amount of force is exerted upon each object. A ground reaction force is one of the examples that represents the force exerted by the ground onto the body in contact with it (Fig. 36.1).

Kinematics

Kinematics is the study of movement regardless of the causes of the movement (e.g. mass, force). The characteristics of the movement can be described in terms of displacement (change in position), velocity (rate of change in displacement) and acceleration (rate of change in velocity) in linear and angular movements. From biomechanical perspective, body movement occurs in three planes of movements. Flexion–extension

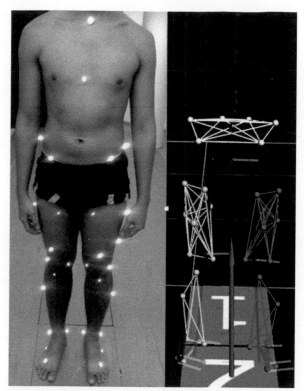

FIG. 36.1 ■ Ground reaction force in well-balanced static standing.

exists in the sagittal *(x)* plane, lateral flexion (bending to the right and left) exists in the frontal *(y)* plane and internal–external rotation exists in the transverse *(z)* plane. When a body is moving in a straight line (linear motion) in only one plane, the movement is described as one-dimensional (1D) (e.g. sitting (static) on a train that is moving on a straight direction). When a body is moving in a curved path, the movement is described as two-dimensional (2D) (e.g. bending and extending the trunk while sitting). Finally, when a body is moving in space (i.e. in all three planes), the movement is described as three-dimensional (3D) (e.g. swimming in a pool).

Occupational therapists use kinematic principles to observe and analyse how a person performs functional activities of daily living. An example of this is when an occupational therapist uses a goniometer to measure angular displacement (i.e. 2D) that occurs at each joint (range of motion). Motion analysis is an area of biomechanical studies that deals with comprehensive measurement of body movement. A common method of motion analysis is photogrammetry, which can be described as the study of motion, which includes recording, measuring and interpretation of the images (McGlone, Mikhail, & Bethel, 2004). Using the motion analysis technology, 3D kinematics of body movements can be analysed. In 3D motion analysis, the movements that occur during the activity can be viewed according to sagittal (flexion–extension), frontal (lateral flexion) and transverse (internal–external rotation) planes (Fig. 36.2). It is very unlikely that a 3D motion analysis will be used in the clinical setting because the instrumentation is complicated, expensive and time consuming. However, numerous research studies have applied the 3D motion analysis to described body movements associated with musculoskeletal problems such as low back pain (Gombatto et al., 2015), shoulder pain (Kijima et al., 2015), neck pain (Treleaven, Chen, & Bahat, 2015) and knee pain (Graci & Salsich, 2015).

Movement Production from Biomechanical Perspective

Electromyography is a specific technique that is used to record and evaluate the electrical activity that occurs within the muscle. Even during resting, about 90 millivolts (mV) of electrical potential have been found within muscle fibres (Kamen & Caldwell, 1996). When a skeletal muscle receives a stimulus from the central nervous system, muscle fibres generate tension to allow the muscle to shorten, lengthen or stay at the same length. Voluntary movement is initiated, maintained and terminated primarily via muscle contraction and regulated by the motor system. The motor system involves both the peripheral (i.e. muscles, motor nerve fibres and sensory nerve fibres) and central (cerebral cortex, basal ganglia, cerebellum, brainstem and spinal cord) nervous systems (Wise & Shadmehr, 2002). To perform a motor skill (e.g. reaching, bending and lifting), the motor system regulates muscle contraction to produce forces that cause movement.

In general, to explain the relationships among muscles in movement production, muscles can be divided into agonist and antagonist. The agonist muscles are the primary movers that produce the major force to execute primary movement. Simultaneously, an opposing force is commonly produced by the antagonist muscles without exceeding the forces from the agonist muscles in order to limit and control the movement. For instance, when flexing the trunk forward (e.g. when bending from a standing position to pick up a book from a table at knee level), the abdominal and back muscles are acting as agonist and antagonist, respectively. To pick up the object, the abdominal muscles perform concentric contraction (muscle shortening), while the back muscles may perform eccentric contraction (muscle lengthening) (Cresswell & Thorstensson, 1994). Both concentric and eccentric contractions are known as isotonic contractions because the muscle tension remains constant during contraction despite the change in muscle length.

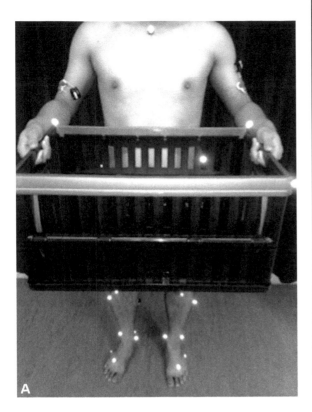
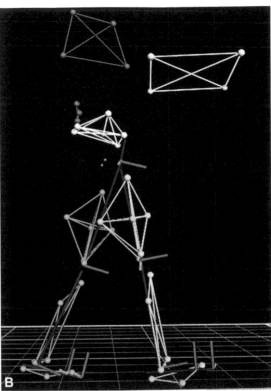

FIG. 36.2 ■ Movement as viewed in three dimensions (3D). (A) A person is holding an empty container to perform a carrying activity. (B) Carrying activity as viewed in sagittal *(x)* plane

(Continued)

Another type of muscle contraction is isometric, in which the muscle length is constant during the contraction. For instance, the Biering-Sorensen test is an isometric back-extension test that has been used to determine back muscle endurance for people who have low back pain (Biering-Sørensen, 1984; Demoulin, Vanderthommen, Duysens, & Crielaard, 2006). In the prone position, the upper edges of the iliac crests are positioned to be aligned with the edge of the examination table. The instruction is to maintain the unsupported upper body in horizontal position, and the holding time represents back muscle endurance.

When there is a constant velocity throughout the range of motion during muscle contraction, the muscle is performing an isokinetic contraction. A common example of isokinetic contraction is the action of the breaststroke during swimming, where the velocity of arm movement is constant because of water resistance. However, isokinetic contraction is rarely performed because only specific machines, which control the speed

of the movement throughout range of motion (e.g. isokinetic dynamometer), can allow such muscle contraction.

IMPLEMENTING BIOMECHANICAL STRATEGIES

From Theory to Practice

The theoretical foundation of biomechanical strategies is based on the biomechanical FOR. To provide sufficient professional reasoning to justify the practice within and outside the profession, theories can be used to underpin occupational therapy practice. Furthermore, the use of theories can assist in evidence-based practice because the theories are supported by empirical research. However, there is often confusion between the roles of different levels of theories (e.g. model and FOR) and a question of when is the right time to apply those theories in professional practice.

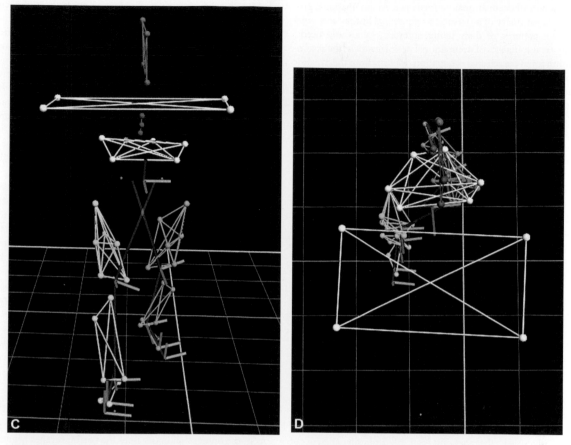

FIG. 36.2 Cont'd. (C) carrying activity as viewed in frontal *(y)* plane and (D) carrying activity as viewed in transverse *(z)* plane.

Biomechanical strategies start with a general idea of the person's occupational performance through the use of a model (Fig. 36.3). Usually an occupational therapist will choose only one model to conceptualise a person's occupation as a whole.

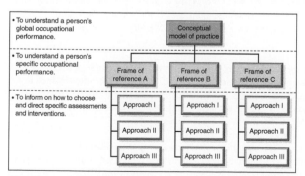

FIG. 36.3 ▪ Integrating conceptual model of practice, frames of reference and approaches.

Then, based on the person's occupational issues, more than one FOR can be selected. Each FOR has specific approaches; thus therapists have to use their professional reasoning to choose whichever intervention approaches are necessary to achieve the goals. In this chapter only the biomechanical FOR is discussed.

Once a person's occupational performance issues have been identified, the therapist may perform more specific assessments based on a biomechanical FOR (e.g. ROM, muscle strength, endurance). After the actual deficits have been identified, both the person and the therapist will establish a series of mutually agreed-on short- and long-term goals. During the intervention, the therapist may choose specific approaches to remediate or compensate the person's impairments.

Assessment

The evaluation stage of the occupational therapy process proposed by the American Occupational Therapy Association consists of developing an occupational profile and conducting an analysis of occupational performance. An occupational profile is 'a summary of a person's occupational history and experiences, patterns of daily living, interests, values and needs', whereas the analysis of occupational performance is 'the accomplishment of the selected occupation resulting from the dynamic transaction among the client, the context and environment and the activity or occupation' (American Occupational Therapy Association, 2014, pp. S14–S15).

During this period, any preferred model can be applied to investigate possible occupational performance issues that concern the person. Some models may lead the therapist to use specific assessments or methods developed to support or validate the practical use of the models. For instance, to obtain the occupational profile of a person, the therapist who uses the Model of Human Occupation may prefer to use the Occupational Performance History Interview II (Kielhofner, Mallinson, Forsyth, & Lai, 2001), whereas the therapist who is familiar with the Canadian Model of Occupational Performance and Engagement to guide practice may choose to use the Canadian Occupational Performance Measure (Law et al., 1998). The main difference between these assessments is that they were developed based on the core construct of their respective model. However, the use of any assessment under any specific model should not be limited just to that model. As long as the assessments can serve the purpose of gathering the required information, they can be used regardless of which model therapists are using.

When implementing occupation-based practice (i.e. a topdown approach), the occupational profile can be used to guide the selection of biomechanical assessments and interventions. For example, after the occupational performance issues have been identified, the therapist can perform the analysis of occupational performance. To conduct an analysis of occupational performance, the therapist can use specific assessments pertaining to the information that has been obtained regarding the person's primary concerns. Assessments can range from a qualitative observation while performing any activity (nonstandardised) to measuring the person's performance using validated assessments tools. Both types of evaluation methods can be complementary to each other because human occupation is unique. Assessment tools that incorporate biomechanical strategies are listed in Table 36.3.

For instance, the Modified Barthel Index (Shah et al., 1989) can be used to assess basic activities of daily living ADL such as personal hygiene, washing, eating, toileting, stair climbing, bowel and bladder control and chair/bed transfers. However, in some religious populations, such as people who follow the Islamic faith, prayer is valued as a basic activity of daily living (Margolis, Carter, Dunn, & Reed, 2003). A normal prayer involves repetitive movements such as standing, bending and sitting on knees and arms, hands and head movement. Therefore occupational therapists who have specific knowledge about prayer movements can briefly observe a person's physical abilities while performing those movements. As a result, occupational therapists may suggest training to remediate and improve the loss of skills or to adapt and modify the prayer task to suit the person's abilities accordingly.

Intervention

Intervention Continuum

The intervention continuum can be described as the period from the onset of an injury until the person reaches negotiated

---

TABLE 36.3

Examples of Assessment Tools That Are Relevant to Biomechanical Strategies

Assessment Components	Examples of Assessment Tools
Occupational profile	Canadian Occupational Performance Measure (COPM) (Law et al., 1999), the Model of Human Occupation Screening Tool (MOHOST) (Parkinson, Forsyth, & Kielhofner, 2006) and Occupational Performance History Interview – 2nd version (OPHI-II) (Kielhofner et al., 2001)
Analysis of occupational performance	
■ Occupations	Modified Barthel Index (Shah, Vanclay, & Cooper, 1989), Functional Independence Measure (Uniform Data System for Medical Rehabilitation, 1997) and Katz Index of Independence in Activity of Daily Living (Katz, Downs, Cash, & Grotz, 1970)
■ Performance skills	Assessment of Motor and Process Skills (Fisher & Jones, 1999), Functional Reach Test (Duncan, Weiner, Chandler, & Studenski, 1990) and Wolf Motor Function Test
■ Performance pattern	Activity checklist, occupational questionnaire, role checklist
■ Client factors	Berg Balance Test, dynamometry, goniometry, manual muscle testing, Minnesota Rate of Manipulation Test (Ziegler, 1939), O'Connor Finger Dexterity Test (Hines & O'Connor, 1926) and Tinetti's Balance and Gait Evaluation (Tinetti, Williams, & Mayewski, 1986)
■ Context and environments	Home assessment, wheelchair assessment and worksite assessment

occupational performance goals. According to Early (2013), the intervention continuum consists of four stages: adjunctive methods, enabling activity, purposeful activity and occupation. A description and examples of activities for each stage are summarised in Table 36.4. Although the stages can be manifested in a linear progression, it is not meant to be strictly interpreted as a step-by-step sequence. For instance, a person who survived an industrial injury that affects his body functions and structures (e.g. amputation, paralysis or visual loss) may not be able to resume his previous role as a worker. In a multidisciplinary rehabilitation team, adjunctive methods may be implemented by other professions to prepare the person's basic ability for functional tasks. In this instance the occupational therapist can help by directing the therapy towards more purposeful activity or occupational performance to help the person to reach his or her maximum level of independence.

Analysis, Gradation and Adaptation

The method of analysing the characteristics of a specific activity or occupation is called activity analysis. As one of the unique skills of occupational therapists, activity analysis can guide the professional reasoning that underpins the focus of occupation-based interventions. Activity analysis can help the therapist to ensure that any given interventions are still relevant to the person's occupational performance. An activity analysis can also be used to establish the parameters of the activity for the purpose of grading or adapting the activity. An example of an activity analysis can be found in Table 36.5. Grading an activity involves quantifiably increasing or decreasing the demands of an activity by changing the aspects of the activity, such as time, size, strength, repetition, or energy spent. *Adapting* an activity refers to modifying the contextual nature of the activity (e.g. physical, virtual) to improve the functional ability of a person. Both grading and adapting an activity follow the principles of biomechanics.

Specific Approaches in Biomechanical Strategies

In occupational therapy, biomechanical strategies can be used within the scope of occupation-based practice. It is important to ensure that people receiving occupational therapy services

---

TABLE 36.4

Intervention Continuum

Stages	Description	Examples
Adjunctive methods	■ To prepare for activity engagement ■ Target body functions and structures ■ Commonly seen in acute setting ■ May overlap with other health professions (e.g. physiotherapy, chiropractors or massage therapist)	Thermotherapy (e.g. fluidotherapy, hot packs, paraffin bath), cryotherapy (e.g. cold packs) and electrotherapy (e.g. transcutaneous electrical nerve stimulation)
Enabling activities	■ To prepare for purposeful activity ■ Target body functions and structures via motor and process skills ■ Person is more involved ■ Not considered purposeful because the goal of the enabling activities does not extend beyond the activities (i.e. no essential reason other than completing the activity)	Blocks, driving or work simulators, clothing-fastener practice boards, sanding boards, skateboards and stacking cones
Purposeful activities	■ Equivalent to occupation-as-means ■ Use common everyday activities ■ Target motor skills and process skills ■ Purposeful but not related to the person's context ■ Meaningfulness is immediate, does not extend to the person's occupational role	Crafts, dressing, feeding, games and sports
Occupational performance	■ Equivalent to occupation-as-end ■ Use everyday activities that are related to the person's context ■ Purposeful towards the person's context ■ Meaningfulness is long term and relevant to the person's occupational role (e.g. personal and community)	Any activities that are relevant to the person's areas of occupation (e.g. ADL, instrumental ADL, education, work, leisure and social participation)

	TABLE 36.5
	Example of Activity Analysis: Dry Cleaning
Demands	**Description**
Relevance and importance	Main responsibility as a dry cleaner.
Objects used	■ Dry cleaning machines
	■ Identification marker
	■ Ironing press
	■ Washing machines
Space demands	■ Dry and clear working space (e.g. from baskets, electricity cables and water outlets)
Social demands	■ Communicate with customers, supervisors, peers, or subordinates
Sequencing and timing	■ Load clothes into washers or dry cleaning machines
	■ Operate the machines
	■ Regulate the use of soap, detergent, water or bleach into specific machines
	■ Remove clothes from washers or dry cleaning machines
	■ Organise clothes removed from dryers
	■ Fold, hang, or wrap clothes
Required action and performance skills	■ Handling and moving objects
	■ Controlling machines and related processes
	■ Organising, planning, and prioritising work
	■ Performing manual activities (e.g. carrying, lifting, balancing, stooping)
Required body function	■ Good eye hand coordination
	■ Good hand dexterity
	■ Good visual functions (e.g. visual acuity, figure–ground discrimination)
	■ Verbal comprehension

have an optimum emphasis on their occupational performance issues. To achieve the goal, occupational therapists investigate the issues that hinder a person's ability to perform daily occupation and subsequently form a set of assumptions to guide the intervention accordingly. There are three main assumptions in occupational therapy that are mainly used to support biomechanical strategies (Table 36.6):

■ Assumption 1: The use of purposeful activity can maintain, improve or enhance occupational performance.
■ Assumption 2: The use of purposeful activity that is meaningful to a person's life roles has more impact on occupational performance.
■ Assumption 3: Modification and adaptation can compensate for the impact a person's loss of ability can have on occupational performance.

The aforementioned assumptions further shape the intervention approaches in biomechanical strategies. These approaches are occupation-as-means, occupation-as-end and rehabilitative. All approaches use the principle of *practice makes perfect* by repeating the activity. Occupational therapists can always use more than one approach according to the intervention goals.

An account of Madam Ruhani is included in Practice Story 36.1 to illustrate the application of the biomechanical approach.

Occupation-as-Means Approach. Occupation has unique therapeutic values that can assist in regaining a maximum level of occupational performance. Occupation-as-means can be described 'the use of occupation as a treatment to improve a person's impaired capacities and abilities to enable eventual occupational functioning' and 'is therapeutic when the activity has a purpose or goal that makes a challenging demand to the capacities and abilities that need to be improved' (Trombly, 2014, p. 345). Occupation-as-means involves the use of purposeful activity to remediate deficits involving (but not all-inclusive of) four interrelated aspects of physical impairment known as 4S. The concept of 4S includes strength, stamina, suppleness and stability and is used to summarise the focus of the occupation-as-means approach when working with people who have an illness, injury or impairment (Hagedorn, 2001):

■ *Strength* can be defined as the ability of a muscle or group of muscles to produce the maximum amount of force against some form of resistance (e.g. weight or gravity) in a single effort.
■ *Stamina* (or endurance) can be defined as the ability to remain active while maintaining the effort for a period.
■ *Suppleness* refers to joint range of motion – the flexibility of joint.
■ *Stability* can be defined as the ability to maintain a static or dynamic body equilibrium.

TABLE 36.6

Examples of Studies That Support the Assumptions in Biomechanical Strategies

Assumptions	Authors	Design	Main Aim	Main Results
Assumption 1 (occupation-as-means)	Thielman, Dean, and Gentile (2004)	Pre–post design (N = 12)	To evaluate the effectiveness of task-related training (TRT) versus progressive resistive exercise for improving paretic limb reaching in persons with chronic effects of stroke	Participants with low level of functioning (assessed using Motor Assessment Scale) in TRT group straightened hand paths, suggesting better coordination of elbow–shoulder motion, as well as improved Rivermead Motor Assessment score.
	Salbach et al. (2005)	Randomised controlled trial (N = 91)	To evaluate the efficacy of a task-oriented walking intervention versus upper extremity (UE) exercises in improving balance self-efficacy in persons with stroke	Task-oriented walking retraining enhances balance self-efficacy (assessed using Balance Confidence Scale) better compared to UE exercises.
Assumption 2 (occupation-as-ends)	Dobek, White, and Gunter (2007)	Pre–post design without control group (N = 14)	To determine the degree to which a novel ADL training programme would affect performance of ADL and physical fitness of older adults	After 10 weeks of intervention, significant improvements were found on outcomes measures including Physical Performance Test (testing both ADL and IADL), Physical Functional Performance – 10 (testing IADL) and three items in the Senior Fitness Test (testing physical fitness).
	Hagsten, Svensson, and Gardulf (2004)	Randomised controlled trial (N = 100)	To study the effects of an early, individualised and postoperative occupational therapy training programme on people with hip fracture	At discharge, the intervention group had better ability to dress, to take care of personal hygiene and bathing activities independently and to make toilet visits (ADL performance was measured using Klein-Bell ADL Scale).
Assumption 3 (rehabilitative)	Stark (2004)	Pre–post design without control group (N = 16)	To examine the effect of a home modification intervention programme (i.e. architectural modification and adaptive equipment) in a population of community-dwelling older adults with illness, injury or impairment	As measured by the Canadian Occupational Performance Measure, the satisfaction and performance in daily activities in the home were improved after the home modification.
	Rigby, Ryan, and Campbell (2009)	Baseline–intervention–baseline without control group (N = 30)	To evaluate the short-term impact of two adaptive seating devices on the activity performance and satisfaction with performance of children with cerebral palsy, as observed by their parents	Based on the parents' scores on the Canadian Occupational Performance Measure, seating intervention significantly improved performance and satisfaction scores overall and within self-care and play activity performance issues categories. Furthermore, three themes were derived from the Home Activity Log interviews with parents: (1) Adaptive seating can have an enabling influence on the child. (2) Caregivers and family find adaptive seating useful. (3) The adaptive seating devices did not meet every family's needs.

ADL, Activities of daily living; IADL, instrumental activities of daily living; OT, occupational therapy.

PRACTICE STORY 36.1

Madam Ruhani

BACKGROUND

Madam Ruhani was a 46-year-old housewife who lived with her husband and two school-age daughters in a two-bedroom apartment on the first floor. Six months ago she was diagnosed with rheumatoid arthritis and carpal tunnel syndrome. She was prescribed disease-modifying antirheumatic drugs and medication to relieve her pain. As a housewife, she took care of her household tasks such as cooking for her family, doing laundry and keeping the house clean. She also drove her own car to the grocery store twice a week. During her latest appointment with her rheumatologist, she complained about having pain in her hand, wrist and shoulder joints bilaterally while performing physical activities. She was then referred to occupational therapy department to improve her ability to perform her ADL.

ASSESSMENT

As preliminary assessments, the occupational therapist used the Disabilities of the Arm, Shoulder and Hand (DASH) questionnaire and Canadian Occupational Performance Measure (COPM) to understand Madam Ruhani's global occupational performance. Based on the results of the DASH, Madam Ruhani indicated that she had major difficulties in performing various activities. Furthermore, the results of COPM indicated that dressing and household managements (i.e. cleaning, laundry and cooking) were her most important occupational performance issues. To specifically analyse the impact of Madam Ruhani's problems on her occupational performance, the therapist performed a more detailed assessment, including the following:

- Using a goniometer to measure active range of motion
- Using a hand dynamometer to measure hand grip strength

- Visual analogue scale for pain to record her subjective experience of pain
- Jebsen-Taylor hand function test as an overall assessment of functional hand use

The assessment results indicated that Madam Ruhani had the following problems:

- Difficulty performing ADL such as buttoning a shirt, turning a car key, doing laundry and using kitchen utensils.
- Unable to continuously perform physical activities for more than 5 minutes.
- Pain in her hands, wrists and shoulders during movements.
- Weakness of her hand muscles.
- Decreased hand dexterity.
- Limited range of motion of the joints of her hands (i.e. limited grasp), wrists and shoulders as a result of pain.

FOCUS OF OCCUPATIONAL THERAPY INTERVENTION

Based on the outcome of the assessments, Madam Ruhani and the therapist agreed to focus on the following during intervention:

- Educate on joint protection, energy conservation and work simplification techniques.
- Educate on pain management.
- Educate on the use of adaptive devices.
- Fabricate wrist orthoses to protect the joint.
- Educate on median nerve gliding exercise.

INTERVENTIONS

Interventions for Madam Ruhani are presented in Table 36.7.

Although the activity may be purposeful and have an immediate effect, primarily during the activity, if it is not meaningful, the activity may not affect a person's occupational role and context. Therefore when using occupation-as-means approach, the therapist needs to ensure that the person understands the therapeutic purpose of performing the activity. It is very important that the person understands the relevance of implementing this approach, so that the activity will become meaningful and have relevance outside the clinical context, thus enhancing the true therapeutic value of the activity.

Occupation-as-End Approach. Whenever possible, the use of activity that relates to the person's role in daily life is highly recommended, so that the maximum therapeutic value of the activity can be achieved. Roles can be described as 'sets of

behaviours expected by society and shaped by culture and context' (American Occupational Therapy Association, 2014, p. S27). In most cultures, living independently is a very important role for a person in order to engage in his or her respective community. During an occupational therapy intervention session, the description of role is defined by the person. By continually engaging with activities that are meaningful, a person can directly face the actual challenges of doing the activity within his or her context. This approach is known as occupation-as-end, which can be described as 'the complex of activities and tasks that comprise roles' (Trombly, 2014, p. 342).

In the occupation-as-end approach, a therapist assesses an individual's limitation in engagement in occupational performance to maintain his or her life role. From there, the therapist assists the person by using the person's occupations that

TABLE 36.7

Preparatory, Occupation-as-Means, Occupation-as-Ends and Rehabilitative Interventions for Madam Ruhani

INTERVENTION

PREPARATORY STAGE	Physical agent modalities	■ Thermotherapy such hot packs and paraffin bath for pain relief ■ Cryotherapy such as cold pack to reduce inflammation ■ Electrotherapy such as transcutaneous electrical nerve stimulation (TENS) for pain relief

	Hand exercise	■ Median nerve gliding exercise that involves six positions (Rozmaryn et al., 1998):
		  1. Wrist in neutral while fingers and thumb are flexed
		  2. Wrist in neutral while fingers and thumb are extended
		  3. Wrist and fingers extended while thumb in neutral
		  4. Wrist, fingers and thumb extended
		  5. Wrist, fingers and thumb extended while forearm in supination
		  6. Wrist, fingers and thumb extended, forearm in supination and other hand gently stretches the thumb

OCCUPATION – AS – MEANS

■ Madam Ruhani will be instructed to perform any purposeful activities that remediate the loss of skills or impairments; for instance, to improve hand dexterity, Madam Ruhani may perform activities like putting beads in a bowl or placing pins on cribbage board.
■ Madam Ruhani and the therapist will work together on how to perform the activity in a safe, timely and productive manner.
■ Grade the activity:
➢ Simple to complex
➢ Slow to fast
➢ Limited to greater number of joints
➢ Lesser to greater ROM
➢ Short to long duration
➢ Low to high frequency
➢ Light to heavy loads
■ Activities are commonly conducted in a clinical setting.

OCCUPATION – AS – ENDS

■ Madam Ruhani will be instructed to demonstrate the actual activities that she had identified as problematic, such as cooking and cleaning.
■ Madam Ruhani and the therapist work together on how to perform the activity in a safe, timely and productive manner.
■ Grade the activity:
➢ Simple to complex
➢ Slow to fast
➢ Limited to greater number of joints
➢ Lesser to greater ROM
➢ Short to long duration
➢ Low to high frequency
➢ Light to heavy load
■ Activities can be conducted in either clinical or home-based settings.

REHABILITATIVE

	Adaptive devices	■ Wear a wrist splint while performing heavy household chores. ■ Use a long-handled reacher. ■ Use a button-hook. ■ Use built-up handles for kitchen utensils. ■ Use electric jar openers.
	Joint protection, energy conservation and work simplification techniques	■ Plan before starting any activity. ■ Balance between activity and rest. ■ Respect fatigue and pain. ■ Avoid activities that cannot be stopped. ■ Use larger joints. ■ Regularly change position. ■ Maintain good body mechanics in any activity.

he or she actually engages. Unlike occupation-as-means, the occupation-as-ends approach is both purposeful and meaningful and therefore enhances the therapeutic value of the intervention. Where possible the activities are performed within a person's actual context, and as a result the challenges that the person faces throughout the activity constitute real-life situations.

Rehabilitative Approach. The focus of the rehabilitative approach is to use a person's residual ability and modifying contextual factors (e.g. physical, environmental and virtual) to enable the person to engage and participate in daily occupations. Primarily this approach is used for those who have permanent illness, injury or impairment (e.g. paraplegia as a result of complete spinal cord injury, amputation). However, it is also applicable for people who have a temporary illness, injury or impairment while waiting for the body to undertake healing processes to recover the loss of body function or structures (e.g. fractures). A rehabilitative approach involves active teaching and learning for both therapist and person. For therapists, this approach requires them to revise the activity demand and analysis to ensure that any modifications or adaptations suit the person's capabilities and contexts. According to Dutton (1995), a rehabilitative approach consists of seven methods:

- Adaptive devices (e.g. long-handled utensils, universal cuff, stocking aid)
- Upper extremity orthotics (e.g. flexor hinge splint)
- Environmental modifications (e.g. ramps, grab rails next to the toilet)
- Wheelchair modifications (e.g. removable armrest, transfer board, heel strap at footrest)
- Ambulatory devices (e.g. crutches, cane, walker)
- Adapted procedures (e.g. energy conservation, work simplification)
- Safety education (e.g. safe transfer technique, lifting technique, joint protection technique)

Any modifications or adaptations will involve acquiring new skills and processes. Thus the therapist can apply appropriate learning theories, such as behaviourism, social-cognitive, constructivist, self-efficacy and motivational, to guide the rehabilitation process (Helfrich, 2014). During the learning process, the therapist needs to be aware of the person's ability and process of changing behaviour. Franche and Krause (2002) and Prochaska et al. (2008) identify five stages of change that occur within the person, and occupational therapists need to be cognisant and respectful of these stages to optimise mutually agreed goals of a rehabilitative approach.

- Precontemplation: Still have lack of awareness for change; good for the healing process.
- Contemplation: Starting to consider change; thinking about pros and cons.

- Preparation: Beginning to make plans for change; very responsive to external support.
- Action: Change is initiated and contributes to self-efficacy; still have risks of relapse.
- Maintenance: Able to cope and maintain tolerance for risks that can trigger relapse.

CONCLUSION

Occupational therapists apply biomechanical strategies by integrating the principles of biomechanics such as kinetics, kinematics and muscle activity into therapy. Occupational therapists should be able to communicate and justify the use of biomechanical strategies through professional reasoning. Activity analysis is one of the occupational therapy tools that helps identify and describe the components of activities according to their demands. After that, the therapists can decide on the use of specific occupation-based approaches that constitute the strategies. These approaches are occupation-as-means, occupation-as-end and rehabilitative. When working with people, the therapists will continue to iteratively analyse activities to grade or adapt them according to the approach being used.

 http://evolve.elsevier.com/Curtin/OT

REFERENCES

American Occupational Therapy Association (2014). *Occupational therapy practice framework: Domain & process.* American Occupational Therapy Association.

Biering-Sørensen, F. (1984). Physical measurements as risk indicators for low-back trouble over a one-year period. *Spine, 9* (2), 106.

Boonen, A., Braun, J., van der Horst Bruinsma, I. E., et al. (2010). ASAS/WHO ICF core sets for ankylosing spondylitis (AS): How to classify the impact of AS on functioning and health. *Annals of the Rheumatic Diseases, 69*(01), 102–107.

Cieza, A., Kirchberger, I., Biering-Sørensen, F., et al. (2010). ICF core sets for individuals with spinal cord injury in the long-term context. *Spinal Cord, 48*(4), 305–312.

Cieza, A., Stucki, G., Weigl, M., et al. (2004). ICF core sets for low back pain. *Journal of Rehabilitation Medicine, 36,* 69–74.

Cresswell, A., & Thorstensson, A. (1994). Changes in intra-abdominal pressure, trunk muscle activation and force during isokinetic lifting and lowering. *European Journal of Applied Physiology and Occupational Physiology, 68*(4), 315–321.

Demoulin, C., Vanderthommen, M., Duysens, C., & Crielaard, J.-M. (2006). Spinal muscle evaluation using the Sorensen test: A critical appraisal of the literature. *Joint, Bone, Spine, 73*(1), 43–50.

Dobek, J. C., White, K. N., & Gunter, K. B. (2007). The effect of a novel ADL-based training program on performance of activities of daily living and physical fitness. *Journal of Aging and Physical Activity, 15*(1), 13.

Duncan, E. A. (2011). *Foundations for practice in occupational therapy* (5th ed.). London: Churchill Livingstone Elsevier.

Duncan, P. W., Weiner, D. K., Chandler, J., & Studenski, S. (1990). Functional reach: A new clinical measure of balance. *Journal of Gerontology, 45*(6), M192–M197.

Dutton, R. (1995). Rehabilitation frame of reference. In *Cinical reasoning in occupational therapy*. Philadelphia: Lippincott Williams & Wilkins.

Early, M. B. (2013). Occupational therapy and physical disabilities: Scope, theory and approaches. In *Physical Dysfunction Practice Skills for the Occupational Therapy Assistant* (3rd ed.). St. Louis: Mosby Elsevier.

Fisher, A. G., & Jones, K. B. (1999). *Assessment of motor and process skills*. Fort Collins, CO: Three Star Press.

Franche, R.-L., & Krause, N. (2002). Readiness for return to work following injury or illness: Conceptualizing the interpersonal impact of health care, workplace, and insurance factors. *Journal of Occupational Rehabilitation, 12*(4), 233–256.

Gombatto, S. P., Brock, T., DeLork, A., Jones, G., Madden, E., & Rinere, C. (2015). Lumbar spine kinematics during walking in people with and people without low back pain. *Gait & Posture, 42*(4), 539–544.

Graci, V., & Salsich, G. B. (2015). Trunk and lower extremity segment kinematics and their relationship to pain following movement instruction during a single-leg squat in females with dynamic knee valgus and patellofemoral pain. *Journal of Science and Medicine in Sport, 18*(3), 343–347.

Hagedorn, R. (2001). *Foundations for practice in occupational therapy* (3rd ed.). Edinburgh: Churchill Livingstone.

Hagsten, B., Svensson, O., & Gardulf, A. (2004). Early individualized postoperative occupational therapy training in 100 patients improves ADL after hip fracture: A randomized trial. *Acta Orthopaedica, 75*(2), 177–183.

Hamill, J., Knutzen, K. M., & Derrick, T. R. (2015). *Biomechanical basis of human movement* (4th ed.). Philadelphia: Wolters Kluwer.

Helfrich, C. A. (2014). Principles of learning and behavior change. In B. A. B. Schell, G. Gillen, & M. E. Scaffa (Eds.), *Willard and Spackman's occupational therapy* (12th ed.). Philadelphia: Lippincott Williams & Wilkins.

Hines, M., & O'Connor, J. (1926). A measure of finger dexterity. *Journal of Personnel Research, 4,* 379–382.

Kamen, G., & Caldwell, G. E. (1996). Physiology and interpretation of the electromyogram. *Journal of Clinical Neurophysiology, 13*(5), 366–384.

Katz, S., Downs, T. D., Cash, H. R., & Grotz, R. C. (1970). Progress in development of the index of ADL. *The Gerontologist, 10*(1 Part 1), 20–30.

Kielhofner, G. (2007). *A model of human occupation: Theory and application*. Philadelphia: Lippincott Williams & Wilkins.

Kielhofner, G. (2009). *Conceptual foundations of occupational therapy practice*. Philadelphia: FA Davis.

Kielhofner, G., Mallinson, T., Forsyth, K., & Lai, J.-S. (2001). Psychometric properties of the second version of the Occupational Performance History Interview (OPHI-II). *American Journal of Occupational Therapy, 55*(3), 260–267.

Kijima, T., Matsuki, K., Ochiai, N., et al. (2015). In vivo 3-dimensional analysis of scapular and glenohumeral kinematics: Comparison of symptomatic or asymptomatic shoulders with rotator cuff tears and healthy shoulders. *Journal of Shoulder and Elbow Surgery, 24*(11), 1817–1826.

Law, M., Baptiste, S., Carswell, A., McColl, M. A., Polatajko, H., & Pollock, N. (1998). *Canadian occupational performance measure*. Ottawa: Canadian Association of Occupational Therapists.

Law, M., Baptiste, S., Carswell, A., McColl, M. A., Polatajko, H., & Pollock, N. (1999). *Canadian occupational performance measure (COPM)*. Ottawa: Canadian Association of Occupational Therapists.

Margolis, S. A., Carter, T., Dunn, E. V., & Reed, R. L. (2003). Validation of additional domains in activities of daily living, culturally appropriate for Muslims. *Gerontology, 49*(1), 61–65.

McGlone, C., Mikhail, E., & Bethel, J. (2004). *Manual of photogrammetry*. Bethesda, MD: American Society for Photogrammetry and Remote Sensing.

Neumann, D. A. (2013). *Kinesiology of the musculoskeletal system: Foundations for rehabilitation*. St. Louis: Mosby Elsevier.

Parkinson, S., Forsyth, K., & Kielhofner, G. (2006). *Model of human occupation screening tool (MOHOST) Version 2.0*. Chicago: University of Illinois at Chicago.

Polatajko, H., & Townsend, E. (2007). *Enabling occupation II: Advancing an occupational therapy vision for health, well-being & justice through occupation*. Ottawa: CAOT Publications ACE.

Prochaska, J. O., Butterworth, S., Redding, C. A., et al. (2008). Initial efficacy of MI, TTM tailoring and HRI's with multiple behaviors for employee health promotion. *Preventive Medicine, 46*(3), 226–231.

Rigby, P. J., Ryan, S. E., & Campbell, K. A. (2009). Effect of adaptive seating devices on the activity performance of children with cerebral palsy. *Archives of Physical Medicine and Rehabilitation, 90*(8), 1389–1395.

Rozmaryn, L. M., Dovelle, S., Rothman, E. R., Gorman, K., Olvey, K. M., & Bartko, J. J. (1998). Nerve and tendon gliding exercises and the conservative management of carpal tunnel syndrome. *Journal of Hand Therapy, 11*(3), 171–179.

Rudolf, K.-D., Kus, S., Chung, K. C., Johnston, M., LeBlanc, M., & Cieza, A. (2012). Development of the international classification of functioning, disability and health core sets for hand conditions: Results of the world health organization international consensus process. *Disability and Rehabilitation, 34*(8), 681–693.

Salbach, N. M., Mayo, N. E., Robichaud-Ekstrand, S., Hanley, J. A., Richards, C. L., & Wood-Dauphinee, S. (2005). The effect of a task-oriented walking intervention on improving balance self-efficacy poststroke: A randomized, controlled trial. *Journal of the American Geriatrics Society, 53*(4), 576–582.

Shah, S., Vanclay, F., & Cooper, B. (1989). Improving the sensitivity of the Barthel Index for stroke rehabilitation. *Journal of Clinical Epidemiology, 42*(8), 703–709.

Stark, S. (2004). Removing environmental barriers in the homes of older adults with disabilities improves occupational performance. *OTJR: Occupation, Participation and Health, 24*(1), 32–40.

Thielman, G. T., Dean, C. M., & Gentile, A. (2004). Rehabilitation of reaching after stroke: Task-related training versus progressive resistive exercise. *Archives of Physical Medicine and Rehabilitation, 85*(10), 1613–1618.

Tinetti, M. E., Williams, T. F., & Mayewski, R. (1986). Fall risk index for elderly patients based on number of chronic disabilities. *American Journal of Medicine, 80*(3), 429–434.

Treleaven, J., Chen, X., & Bahat, H. S. (2015). Factors associated with cervical kinematic impairments in patients with neck pain. *Manual Therapy,*.

Trombly, C. A. (2014). Occupation: Philosophy and concepts. In M. V. Radomski, & C. A. Trombly (Eds.), *Occupational therapy for physical dysfunction.* Philadelphia: Lippincott Williams & Wilkins.

Uniform Data System for Medical Rehabilitation (1997). *Guide for the uniform data set for medical rehabilitation (including the FIM™ instrument).* Buffalo: Uniform Data System for Medical Rehabilitation.

Wise, S., & Shadmehr, R. (2002). Motor control. In V. Ramachandran (Ed.), *Encyclopedia of the human brain.* Boston: Academic Press.

Wolf, T. J., Baum, C., & Connor, L. T. (2009). Changing face of stroke: Implications for occupational therapy practice. *American Journal of Occupational Therapy, 63*(5), 621–625.

Ziegler, W. (1939). *Minnesota rate of manipulation test.* New York: Educational Test Bureau.

HAND THERAPY

KATHY WHALLEY ■ SARAH BRADLEY ■ JO ADAMS

CHAPTER OUTLINE

Abstract

The role and importance of therapy delivered by occupational therapists for people with traumatic, inflammatory, degenerative and postoperative conditions affecting their hands is the focus of this chapter. The background and context of occupational therapy practice is presented. Examples for working alongside people with hand conditions are illustrated using the principles from the Canadian Practice Process Framework. Strategies to identify people's readiness to engage with hand therapy are documented, specific hand functional assessments are reviewed and collaborative intervention planning with individuals described. Approaches to implementing and monitoring occupational therapy intervention are included. Lastly, suggested options for review and evaluation of hand therapy effectiveness are detailed. A practice story is used within this chapter to provide additional contextual learning.

KEY POINTS

- Occupational therapists use a holistic approach to hand therapy that bases intervention and support on an individual's goals.

- Hand therapy intervention must be based on sound anatomical knowledge and an understanding of healing and inflammation.

- Standardised assessment and outcome measures provide important information to measure progress and effectiveness of interventions.

- People's engagement with hand therapy is facilitated if they are ready to change behaviour to incorporate self-management strategies into their daily routines.

- Although the degree of hand injury or disease is important to consider, it is more important to consider how the hand condition affects the individual's life; this consideration guides hand therapy intervention.

INTRODUCTION

The anatomy of the hand is intricate and complex and the functions of the hand are multifaceted. Integrity of the hand structures is essential for everyday functional living. Without efficient and effective coordination and movement of the different components of the hand, the management of basic tasks such as personal care, participation in leisure activities and performance of work tasks is compromised. The precise formation of the skeletal components of the hand, along with the complex soft tissue anatomy, allows the hand to perform sophisticated functions. Working with the thumb, the fingers manipulate objects with dexterity, with the thumb working with the index and middle fingers to form elements of the dynamic tripod grip for precision tasks; the addition of the ring and little fingers provides a power grip.

Occupational therapists have a unique perspective on understanding people within their social context and a holistic understanding of the impact illness, injury or impairment can have on individuals and their occupations. At the core of practice 'occupational therapists view people as occupational beings […] needing to engage in a balanced range of activities in their daily lives in order to sustain health and well-being' (College of Occupational Therapists (COT), 2015, p. 1). Thus disease or trauma affecting the hand can compromise people's independence and health and well-being. The role of the occupational therapist for people with hand conditions is to provide rehabilitation, practical support and guidance to facilitate recovery as well as to help empower individuals to live a fulfilled life. Understanding hand anatomy, biomechanics and movement performance is imperative to guide effective management and intervention for people with hand impairments.

Within many hand therapy services, occupational therapists and physiotherapists often work in collaboration to maximise people's occupational performance. There is usually a great deal of cross-disciplinary working, and the individual goals of people with hand conditions guide the approaches used. For example, occupational therapists as members of the hand therapy team may use transdisciplinary practice such as hand exercises creatively to restore hand impairment, which can then contribute to improvements in the recovery of functional movement (Lamb et al., 2015). The skill set required to deliver person-centred hand therapy intervention may not solely be the responsibility of one professional group. This merging of 'professional' skills has long been debated; recognition of the benefit occupational therapy skills bring to this area will future proof and sustain the valued professional contribution that occupational therapists provide within hand therapy services.

BACKGROUND TO HAND ANATOMY, INJURY HEALING AND REPAIR

Hand Anatomy

There are 29 bones in the hand and wrist. Small, intrinsic muscles are located within the hand, and larger, extrinsic muscles are located in the forearm. These muscles are inserted into the hand's skeleton by tendons. Three main nerves supply both sensory and motor components of the hand: median, ulnar and radial nerves. Arterial supply of blood is via the radial and ulnar arteries.

The skeletal structure of the hand is formed of carpal, metacarpal and phalange bones. There are eight carpal bones formed in two rows: the proximal and distal carpal rows. The proximal carpal row includes scaphoid, lunate, triquetrum, and pisiform. The distal carpal row includes trapezium, trapezoid, capitate, and hamate. The scaphoid forms a bridge between the two rows, and this position makes it vulnerable to fracture.

The distal carpal row articulates with the metacarpal bones by carpometacarpal (CMC) joints. The first CMC joint (base of the thumb) is formed by an articulation of the trapezium and first metacarpal bone by way of a saddle joint. This is the most mobile joint in the hand and allows the thumb to move on multidirectional planes, contributing significantly to the function of the human hand.

The metacarpal heads articulate distally with the base of the proximal phalanx of the respective digit. This articulation is called the metacarpophalangeal (MCP) joint. The fingers have two further interphalangeal joints: the proximal interphalangeal (PIP) joint and the distal interphalangeal (DIP) joint. The thumb only has one interphalangeal (IP) joint.

The hand has mobile, supple skin on the dorsal surface, allowing free mobility of the hand joints when the fingers move into a flexed position. In contrast the thick, anchored skin on the palmar surface of the hand is designed as both a resting and sensory surface. Flexion movement corresponds with the anatomical creases that form arches in the hand on the palmer surface of the hand. The arches run longitudinally along the fingers and metacarpals, transversely over the carpal bones (the proximal palmar crease) and distal ends of the metacarpal heads (the distal palmar crease) and obliquely from the thumb along to the little finger. These arches provide the basis for flexibility of the hand and enable the complex and versatile gripping, prehension and manipulation of objects.

An illustration of the anatomical features of the hand can be found in Fig. 37.1.

Hand Injury

Hand injuries account for 20% of presentations to accident and emergency departments (de Putter et al., 2012), the most common of which are fractures (Polinder et al., 2013), followed by soft tissue injuries, including cuts and lacerations (Saaqi, Ud-Din, Khan, & Chaudhery, 2009). Understanding

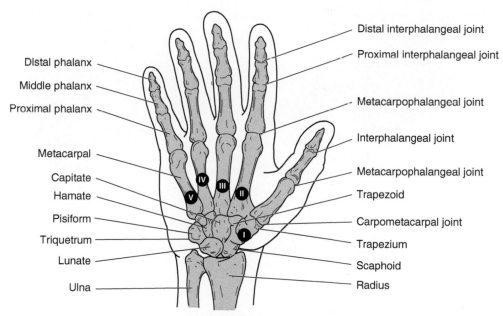

FIG. 37.1 ■ Anatomical features of the hand.

fracture, soft tissue and wound healing processes is fundamental to designing hand therapy intervention so as to improve the individual's condition while protecting the healing structures and promoting recovery. Stages of exercise and treatment modalities are guided by stages of healing, which are introduced next.

Fracture Healing

Primary fracture healing is completed within 6 to 8 weeks after injury, but bone remodelling continues for years. There are three phases to fracture healing (Sfeir, Ho, Doll, Azari, Hollinger, 2005):

1. Inflammatory: Peaking at 48 hours and completed within 1 week after injury, a fracture haematoma initiates the healing response.
2. Reparative: Within the first few days, often before the inflammatory phase has subsided, and lasting for several weeks, a reparative callus forms that will eventually be replaced by bone. Woven bone is deposited by osteoblasts, the cells responsible for building new bone.
3. Remodelling: This involves the replacement of the woven bone by plates of collagen fibre in the form of a mineralised matrix, known as lamella bone, and callus excess is reabsorbed to restore the normal cortical structure of the bone. This process takes years to be completed.

Wound Healing

Acute wounds normally heal in a very orderly and efficient manner characterised by four distinct but overlapping phases (Diegelmann & Evans, 2004):

1. Haemostasis: Blood components spill into the site of injury and platelets come into contact with exposed collagen, triggering the release of clotting factors.
2. Inflammation: Neutrophils enter the site and begin debriding injured tissue and bacteria.
3. Proliferation: Fibroblasts migrate in and deposit new extracellular matrix, causing new tissue growth. Granulation tissue is formed and the wound begins to contract.
4. Maturation: The collagen matrix becomes cross-linked and organised, increasing the strength of the scar. The acute healing usually takes place within 2 to 3 weeks, but the remodelling phase can continue for up to 2 years.

The inflammatory stage of wound healing is shown in Fig. 37.2A, and the later remodelling stage is illustrated in Fig. 37.2B.

Other soft tissues such as tendons and nerve tissue are subject to similar processes and timescales, and the healing processes of all structures are fragile and complex. Healing times are influenced by local and systemic factors including oedema, foreign bodies, infection, diabetes, immunosuppression and smoking. The normal cutaneous wound-healing processes are illustrated in Fig. 37.3

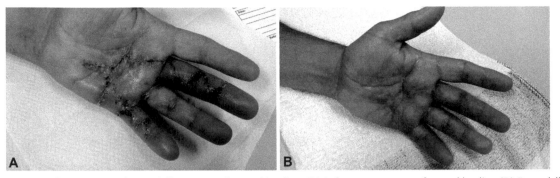

FIG. 37.2 ■ Inflammatory and remodelling stages of wound healing. (A) Inflammatory stage of wound healing (B) Remodelling stage of wound healing.

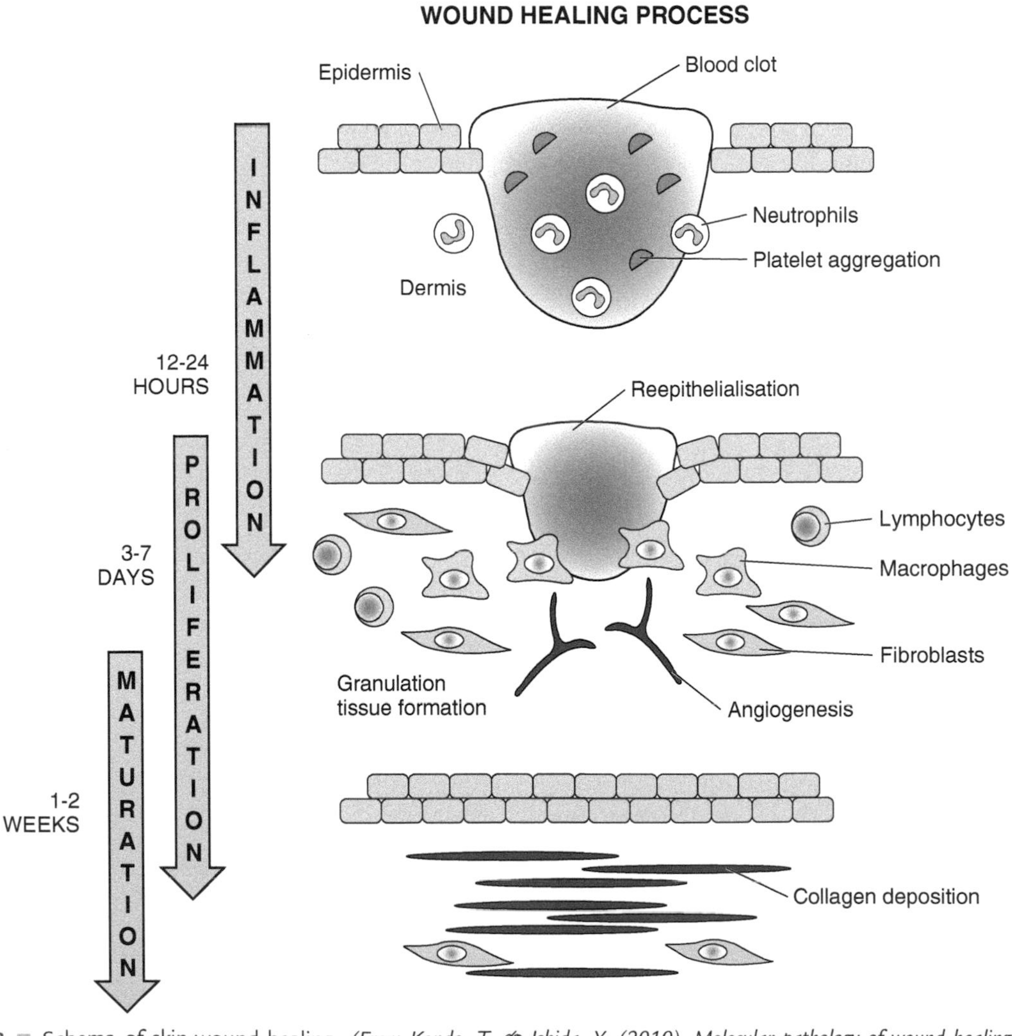

WOUND HEALING PROCESS

Epidermis

Blood clot

Neutrophils

Platelet aggregation

Dermis

12-24 HOURS

INFLAMMATION

Reepithelialisation

Lymphocytes

Macrophages

Fibroblasts

3-7 DAYS

PROLIFERATION

Granulation tissue formation

Angiogenesis

Collagen deposition

1-2 WEEKS

MATURATION

FIG. 37.3 ■ Schema of skin-wound healing. *(From Kondo, T, & Ishida, Y. (2010). Molecular pathology of wound healing.* Forensic Science International, 203(1-3), 93-98.)

SUPPORTING PEOPLE TO ENGAGE WITH HAND THERAPY

The process of supporting people with hand conditions and their expectations is complex. It is important to identify and negotiate each individual's goals and needs, and clear documentation should be kept regarding the professional reasoning that informed the occupational therapist's assessment, intervention and evaluation. Encouraging people to engage in hand therapy may, in part, be facilitated by their readiness to accept that their hand condition is important and that occupational therapy is relevant to achieve best outcomes. Most hand therapy approaches will advocate a self-management approach. Such an approach will encourage and support people to understand the relevance of education and advice provided relating to hand use and encourage the use and uptake of strategies to move and use the hands in an optimal way. This approach aims to mitigate the impact of disease or injury and to integrate the use of aids and equipment to facilitate occupational performance for people in their daily life. The use of graded activity where the complexity and difficulty of task is incrementally increased is a usual approach for the occupational therapist working alongside individuals with hand conditions.

Cooper (2013) stated that to ensure successful hand therapy outcomes occupational therapists should carefully consider what indicates success of intervention. This is important as it affects individuals' willingness to engage with hand therapy. Often people with hand injury, trauma or conditions do not use the same end points to define recovery and success as health professionals. Being perceptive and listening to individuals' narrative accounts of the impact of their hand condition can help occupational therapists understand each person's individual experience and not just focus on treating the hand injury. Understanding how the hand condition changes each individual's life will help facilitate engagement with hand therapy (Cooper, 2013).

People referred to occupational therapy for hand rehabilitation will vary in their readiness to adopt a self-management approach. Generally it has been reported that people who may have a low readiness to change may show more passive coping strategies and people who have higher levels may demonstrate more active coping strategies (Strand et al., 2007). It is important to consider such theories that acknowledge people's ability and readiness to change. Prochaska and DiClemente's (1984) Transtheoretical Model of Behaviour Change still provides a meaningful and useful guide for occupational therapists when engaging people to adopt self-management strategies to manage their hand condition. The Transtheoretical Model of Behaviour Change includes five different stages of change: precontemplation, contemplation, preparation, action, and maintenance (Prochaska & DiClemente, 1984). This remains a contemporaneous tool for current practice in optimising the development of self-management skills for individuals (Wegener

et al., 2014). Occupational therapists work to encourage people to take responsibility for their self-management and move from the precontemplation and contemplation stages to the preparation, action and maintenance stages to implement and maintain the hand therapy advised. Individuals will vary in the degree in which they are willing to make significant changes in areas of their daily life, especially after an illness or injury. When an individual is resistant to change and to self-management, motivational interviewing can be used to build the necessary intrinsic motivation to change and self-manage. Motivational interviewing is a person-centred approach that is designed to help facilitate behaviour change. The approach focuses on working with an individual to negotiate behaviour change rather than a static approach. Issues that may facilitate or hinder behaviour change are explored with an individual and time given to discuss how barriers to changing may be overcome (Flinn & Jones, 2011)

ASSESSMENT OF THE HAND

Assessment is a key part of the occupational therapy process. Assessment should be centred on occupational performance, engagement and participation in life roles (COT Code of Ethics and Professional Conduct, 2015). Careful assessment is critical to obtaining the information that the occupational therapist needs to appreciate the impact of the hand condition on the individual and the individual's roles and responsibilities. It should be undertaken responsibly, according to professional standards and with appropriate knowledge. This will then lead to effective and targeted intervention planning.

Assessment of people with hand trauma often follows a medical model; this is essential as early-stage interventions must be concordant with fracture and wound healing timelines and is grounded in a solid knowledge of hand anatomy. The occupational therapist needs to know and respect these timelines; for example, the focus of intervention during early fracture and wound healing will be on protecting healing structures with a splint until unrestrained functional rehabilitation can commence. In addition, the occupational therapist needs to be able to analyse what aspect of hand function is impaired in order to develop an intervention plan that meets the needs of the individual so that the individual's goals can be achieved. Assessment is unsurprisingly multidimensional and always starts with a history.

History Taking

The use of a narrative assessment is embedded in occupational therapy practice and is valuable during the initial history taking when a person is referred for hand therapy. Narrative assessment allows individuals to tell 'their story' of the injury or problem affecting their hands. Practice Story 37.1 illustrates how a narrative assessment is used. The initial history taking will shed light on the likely issues facing the occupational therapist with

Tammy: Integration of Narrative Assessment into the Occupational Therapy Process

Occupational therapist: So, Tammy, are you right or left handed?

Tammy: I'm right handed.

Occupational therapist: Thank you. It would be really helpful if you could tell how you hurt your wrist.

Tammy: I was ten-pin bowling with my family and slipped, falling forwards onto the bowling alley. I was in immediate pain in my wrist and it looked a strange shape, so my husband took me straight to the hospital.

Occupational therapist: What treatment did you have in the emergency department?

Tammy: They took an x-ray and told me I had a displaced fracture, which they then manipulated in the emergency department. They put me in a temporary cast for a week. Then I had a fracture clinic appointment where they changed the temporary cast for a fibreglass cast for 5 weeks. That was removed yesterday.

Occupational therapist: Thank you, that's really helpful. Tell me about home. You said you have a family?

Tammy: Yes, I have two young children. My husband works full time.

Occupational therapist: Do you work?

Tammy: Yes. I am a music teacher and professional violinist and pianist. I play in concerts regularly.

Occupational therapist: How is your wrist affecting your job work and your role as a mum?

Tammy: I can't work. I can't drive, so I couldn't get there, but there is no way I could teach the violin or piano. I'm even scared to try and hold my violin. I'm so worried I won't be able to play again. I am managing at home but relying heavily on my husband and friends to drive me and the boys around. I don't want them missing out on anything because of my wrist.

Occupational therapist: Do you have any hobbies or interests?

Tammy: I love performing. I play in an orchestra, and so when I'm not working or with the boys I'm usually practising.

From the discussions with Tammy the occupational therapist was able to identify hand dominance and the mechanism of the injury and appreciate the severity of the fracture. This was confirmed by looking at the x-rays taken before and after the manipulation. Most importantly it was identified that Tammy had a clear need to improve her hand function to enable her to return to work and hobbies.

---

regards to engaging an individual in therapy, the effects of the hand condition on the psychological status of the individual and the impact of the hand condition on the individuals' occupational status. The therapist should collect basic information that is common to all initial assessments, such as age, medical history, medications, social circumstances, occupation and interests. In addition, information specific to the hand should be collected, such as hand dominance, injury story (enabling the occupational therapist to appreciate the mechanism of the injury and speed at which it occurred to determine the likely impact on the tissues), and the impact of the hand condition on occupational performance. If the person referred for hand therapy has a chronic condition (e.g. arthritis), the occupational therapist should be able to ascertain what interventions have been delivered before and what was successful and unsuccessful.

The Assessment Procedure

In hand therapy the practical assessment of the hand is generally approached in three stages: look, touch/feel, and move. This sequential process enables the gathering of information in a way that is nonthreatening and informative; for example, watching the person walk from the waiting area, observing if, and how, the person is using their hands – the person may carry the injured hand in a protective manner that can suggest the person is experiencing pain or is fearful of movement. Based on the observations made in the look stage, proceeding to the touch/feel stage may need to be approached in a more considered, sensitive way if the person is to develop trust in the occupational therapist. The following outlines some of the key factors investigated at each stage of the assessment, and their clinical application is illustrated in Practice Story 37.2.

Look: Observe and note the individual's hand and limb resting posture and how the affected hand is carried and moved. In addition to these observations, look at skin colour of the hand and look for any swelling, wounds, scarring, nail changes and anatomical deformity.

Touch/feel: Check for skin moisture, sweating or dryness, hand sensation, pain, presence and type of oedema (acute/chronic), the origins of joint stiffness or laxity, presence of scarring and presence of adhesions.

Move: Carefully move the hand and if necessary the upper limb through supported range of movement to check for stiffness, pain, and the passive and active ranges of motion of the joints.

Tammy: Objective Assessment

Looking at Tammy's hand revealed that she had swelling in her wrist, hand and fingers, the skin was shinier and pinker than on the other hand and she rested her hand in a 'stiff' posture. There was no obvious deformity in the wrist, suggesting a good reduction of the fracture during manipulation.

On **touch**ing Tammy's hand her skin was smooth and warm. When touching the tips of the fingers, the sensation was slightly altered in the thumb, index and middle finger. There was no pain on touching the hand and wrist. On pressing into the skin on the back of the hand there was pitting, which demonstrated that the swelling had become organised and was contributing to her stiffness.

Tammy was then asked to **move** her fingers and wrist; she was unable to form a full fist and was stiff in her wrist and thumb. Extension of the wrist and supination of the forearm were especially reduced. She reported pain during wrist movement.

During the assessment process, Tammy demonstrated anxious behaviours, which appeared to be related to her concerns about not regaining enough movement to enable her to play her instruments.

The Use of Standardised Assessment/Outcome Measures

Once a clear history has been obtained, the occupational therapist may select outcome measures to more formally measure impairment dimensions (e.g. pain, oedema or functional impairment) and the impact of the hand condition on the life roles of an individual. The purpose of using outcome measures is to develop a baseline against which to measure change and to gain more in depth information about the nature of the problem.

There is an established collection of outcome measures available to occupational therapists working in hand therapy that provide robust, valid and reliable measurement properties to help guide and evaluate the effectiveness of interventions. For example, when working with a person whose functional capacity is restricted as a result of hand oedema, a volumeter can be used to measure the extent of oedema in the hand through the amount of water displaced at different stages of recovery to document whether the oedema is increasing or reducing in response to prescribed interventions. This will demonstrate objectively if there is a change in status and if the intervention has been effective. The outcome measures that were used with Tammy are described in Practice Story 37.3.

Appropriate selection of outcome measures when combined with a standardised approach can, when cross-referenced with the same measurements of other centres of hand therapy, add to the body of evidence of clinical effectiveness (Bucher &

Tammy: Outcome Measures

Having identified that Tammy had oedema and reduced motion and function, the following outcome measures were selected to objectively measure these impairments:

Range of motion: assessed using a goniometer, measuring range in the fingers, wrist and thumb.

As an example, the range of motion of Tammy's wrist on initial assessment was as follows:

- Extension/flexion = 22 degrees/24 degrees (NB: normal range = 70 degrees/75 degrees)
- Radial deviation/ulnar deviation = 10 degrees/12 degrees) (NB: normal range = 20 degrees/35 degrees)
- Pronation/supination = 70 degrees/0 degrees (NB: normal range = 70 degrees/85 degrees)

Quick Disability of the Arm, Shoulder and Hand (Quick DASH): (http://dash.iwh.on.ca/quickdash) a shortened version of the DASH, an assessment that measures the physical function and symptoms of people who have a musculoskeletal condition affecting the upper limbs. The standard DASH has 30 items and the Quick DASH has 11 items. It was selected for Tammy as a measure of her functional impairment (a score of 0 represents no disability and 100 represents maximum disability). Tammy's Quick DASH score was 68, suggesting that her hand injury had a moderate impact on her functional ability.

Hume, 2003). An example of a hand therapy assessment form is provided in Fig. 37.4.

Preoperative Assessment

In addition to assessment carried out to inform an intervention plan, assessment preoperatively can be beneficial for individuals awaiting hand surgery and for the therapist working with the individual. Benefits for individuals receiving preoperative assessment before hand surgery include the following:

- The expectations of intervention can be identified and communicated; for example, a PIP finger joint replacement may be indicated for pain relief but not improved motion, so this can be reinforced during preoperative discussions and education.
- Postoperative recovery and interventions can be explained.
- There is the opportunity for the individual to voice questions or concerns, and to have these addressed, to ensure that the pros and cons of surgery have been taken into consideration.
- There is the opportunity for the individual to consider postoperative functional status and plan ahead.

Poole Hospital NHS
NHS Trust

Right

Age:

Dominance:

Referrer:
Date:
Occupation:

Hobbies:

Affix addressograph here

Additional obs (tick if normal): sensation ☐ oedema ☐ T° ☐ colour ☐ deformity ☐ Ψ ☐

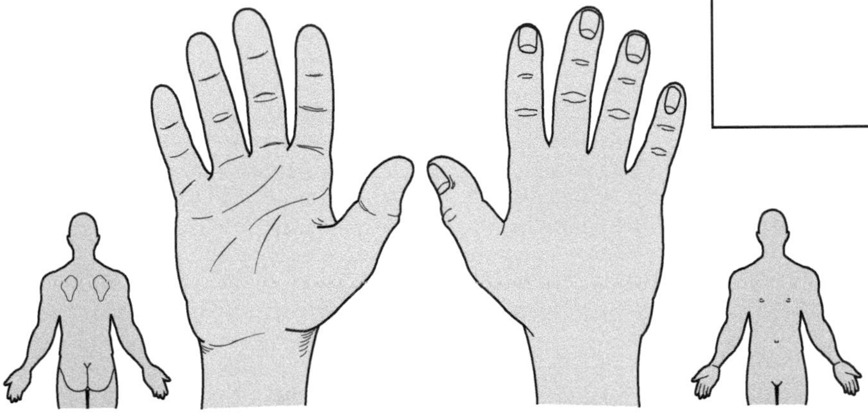

Diagnosis:

Injury date:	Op date:	/52:	/52:	/52:

HPC:

Subjective:

Function (personal/domestic ADL, work):

PMH:

DH:

FIG. 37.4 ■ An example of a hand therapy assessment form.

The benefits for the occupational therapist of conducting preoperative assessments include the following:

- The outcome of specific functional evaluation by the occupational therapist may guide the surgeon to select the most appropriate surgical procedure for the individual. For example, an individual with severe cognitive impairment and who lives in a residential home with limited support presenting with a tendon rupture in the thumb may be better managed with a taping method rather than tendon reconstruction surgery that carries with it a complex postoperative therapy regimen.

- Ensuring that bespoke postoperative care that is tailored for an individual is planned.
- Establishing a preoperative baseline measure against which change can be measured after the surgery has been completed.
- Postoperative outcome expectations can be discussed with the individual and the health care team. These expectations can be documented and can inform ongoing therapeutic discussion and support.
- Intervention goals can be discussed, agreed and communicated with the individual and the multidisciplinary team.

OBJECTIVE SETTING AND GOAL PLANNING

Occupational therapy intervention plans and recommendations should be shaped by the occupational needs of the service users, taking into account the cultures, background and contexts in which they engage in occupation on a daily basis. Needs are identified through assessment, and intervention is underpinned by evidence and research. The occupational therapist should work in partnership with the person in the planning process and in agreeing goals and priorities for intervention (COT, 2011).

By collecting information through assessment of the individual, and then classifying, analysing and identifying the physical, social and psychological factors that will affect intervention, the occupational therapist is able to collaborate with the individual, creating a problem list by which to agree on goals and objectives for intervention. This process is underpinned by professional reasoning (Chapparo & Ranka, 2008). For example, an individual who presents with swollen, stiff and painful fingers after a traumatic injury may, in addition, be unable to work, drive a car, walk the dog or participate in meaningful hobbies or activities. The individual may find doing self-care tasks difficult and be unable to fulfil the usual roles in caring for children and contributing to domestic activities in the home. The individual may begin to feel isolated, dependent on others and a sense of failure or guilt. The extent of the pain may cause the individual to have difficulty sleeping and lead to significant variations in mood.

These problems may form the basis of a discussion with the individual so that the individual and therapist can collaboratively identify realistic goals. These goals may be based on the professional reasoning of the occupational therapist but will need to be adjusted and graded to suit the individual needs of the person.

Basic goals for the individual described in the preceding paragraph may include the following:

- Improved hand function, sleep and mood within 2 weeks through the reduction of pain

- Improve the flexibility of the fingers within 3 weeks through reducing oedema
- Enable lifting of pans and shopping bags and control of manual care within 6 weeks through increasing grip strength.
- Improve finger dexterity to facilitate use of a keyboard and smart phone and development of an effective tripod grip for writing to enable return to work within 8 weeks.

Once the goals are agreed on, the occupational therapist will devise a therapeutic intervention plan to restore function and reduce the impact of impairment. A number of different modalities, interventions and activities may be used to achieve each goal. These should be from both a biomechanical and an occupational performance frame of reference. The application of problem list formulation and goal setting for Tammy is shown in Practice Story 37.4.

PRACTICE STORY 37.4

Tammy: Problem List

Based on the outcomes of the assessments used with Tammy the following problems were identified:

1. Oedema and stiffness has resulted in loss of functional ROM in the digits and wrist
2. Unable to perform specified activities of daily living and work tasks
3. Unable to play the violin or piano
4. Unable to drive the car

Through assessment and observation the therapist was able to highlight that one of the reasons for the loss of function in her hand and wrist was the established oedema. To increase Tammy's functional ROM, it was necessary to reduce the oedema and subsequently work on regaining the mobility she had lost.

The overall aim of therapy was for Tammy to participate fully in violin rehearsals by 6 weeks in preparation for a concert in 10 weeks.

Some specific goals for Tammy to achieve the overall aim were as follows:

- Reduce oedema to allow full finger range of motion at all MCP, PIP and DIP joints within 2 weeks.
- Improve supination by 70 degrees and ulnar deviation by 10 degrees in the wrist to enable Tammy to play simple pieces on the violin within 4 weeks.
- Drive the car within 2 weeks to allow return to work.

DIP, Distal interphalangeal; *MCP*, metacarpophalangeal; *PIP*, proximal interphalangeal; *ROM*, range of motion.

IMPLEMENTATION OF AN INTERVENTION PLAN

After assessment, formulation of a problem list and jointly agreed goals, the occupational therapist must decide how to address the impairments identified by the individual as important in order to deliver the expected outcomes. Hand therapy intervention usually focuses on five key target areas: manage and reduce swelling/oedema, prevent scar tissue formation, increase joint motion, manage and reduce pain, and increase hand function.

Manage and Reduce Swelling/Oedema

Oedema is a normal response to injury (Villeco, 2012) and caused by injury to the capillaries and lymphatics. It can also occur as a result of an acute inflammatory episode in a chronic condition such as rheumatoid arthritis. If left untreated, chronic oedema fills the dorsum of the hand, bringing the MCP joints into hyperextension and flattening the palmar arches (Cheema, 2014); if not controlled, persistent oedema can lead to delayed healing, pain, stiffness (Villeco, 2012) and a devastating loss of function as the hand posture for gripping is disrupted. Managing and reducing oedema in the hand is an important first goal of intervention and is the beginning of successful restoration of hand function (Warwick, Dunn, Melikyan, & Vadher, 2009). There are three common approaches to managing and reducing oedema: elevation, motion and compression.

> **Elevation:** For people with an acutely injured hand, elevation is required to reduce the interstitial pressure and thus should be the first approach to reducing oedema. Oedema is minimised by elevation (Cheema, 2014), so the individual should be encouraged to rest the hand in an elevated position and follow the principle of 'hand above heart' until the inflammatory phase of healing has passed.
>
> **Motion:** Active motion of an injured or affected hand after surgery may not be possible and as a result it is important that the proximal muscle groups (i.e. shoulder, upper arm, elbow and forearm muscles) are actively and regularly used to help disperse peripheral oedema. These proximal muscle groups are effective stimulators of the lymphatic system, which is responsible for redirecting the excess fluid into the circulatory system (Cheema, 2014).
>
> **Compression:** Compression of muscles facilitates the absorption of molecules by the venous and lymphatic systems, improving the flow of fluids in these systems and as a result reducing oedema (Artzberger, 2013). Compression to the hand may be provided simply by a compressive stockinette, such as Tubigrip, or by commercially available compression gloves. Gloves come in a variety of ready-made sizes or can be made to measure; for example, Jobskin manufactures custom-made compression garments. Compression of an individual digit can be achieved by

using an elastic, self-adherent wrap, such as Coban. This should be applied in a distal to proximal direction, with the fingertip exposed so that any changes in circulation can be observed. The wrapping should continue down the finger with a loose stretch applied. Commercially available finger sleeves are available in standard sizes – extra small to extra, extra large.

Compression of the hand or digit must not compromise the circulation in the extremity or hinder an individual's ability to move the affected area. Careful monitoring is required for allergic reactions, skin breakdown, and circulation or sensory impairments (Deshaies, 2013). Elevation and motion are preferable options for individuals with fragile skin, open wounds or unstable circulation

Prevent Scar Tissue Formation

Scarring is a normal physiological response to injury. Collagen is produced during the fibroblastic and remodelling phases of wound healing (Warwick et al., 2009), and wound contracture is an active and essential part of the repair process (Masson, 2003). In the hand, because of its complex anatomy, scarring can interfere with tendon-gliding structures and impair function. This is because scarring occurs both externally and internally. Soft tissue healing is not discriminate in terms of structure; that is, skin, tendon and ligament heal with the same cellular response, and consequently different tissues in the same area of the injury can get stuck together if motion is not maintained.

Because of the difficulty of measuring and quantifying external scar progression, evidence for the use of therapeutic techniques in this area is limited. However, there are three interventions used in both hand therapy and burns and plastics settings that are recognised for reducing scar tissue formation: massage, silicone gel and low-load prolonged stretch.

> **Massage:** Scar massage is anecdotally effective. However, there is currently scarce scientific data in the literature to support its effectiveness (Shin & Bordeaux, 2013). Scar massage appears to soften and flatten the scar on the skin surface, realign the collagen, and break down adhesions. Gentle but firm circular massage is performed over a healed scar using a basic, nonscented moisturising cream to hydrate the scar and reduce friction.
>
> **Silicone gel:** Silicone gel can be used in sheet form to line splints or be incorporated within compression garments to provide a firm, consistent pressure over the scar tissue, or in topical gel form. The mechanism of action of silicone on scars has not been completely determined (Mustoe, 2008), but it is thought to hydrate scars and reduce the local blood supply to prevent scar development from progressing. It is used primarily to improve the cosmetic appearance of scars but also helps keep them soft and pliable, which helps to facilitate movement. Cosmesis

is important as scars can cause psychological distress in some people (O'Brien & Jones, 2013). As silicone is used to facilitate scar maturation, it is unsuitable for use with open wounds.

Low-load prolonged stretch: Low-load prolonged stretch of a scar, which is usually achieved by splinting after hand surgery and trauma, can help reduce the contractures that can be caused by the formation of scar tissue and contribute to maintaining or improving range of motion (Larson & Jerosch-Herold, 2008).

Increase Joint Mobility

Stiffness and associated loss of joint range of motion is a major complication after hand injury and surgery. Stiffness alone may cause considerable functional loss and impairment. Persistent oedema, inactivity (immobilisation), soft tissue shortening (contracture), infection and underlying joint pathological conditions can all lead to the onset of stiffness (Villeco, 2012). Early management is essential in preventing the onset of stiffness and managing its presence. The following three interventions are often used to maintain and increase joint flexibility: exercises, splinting/orthotics, and functional activity.

Exercises: Exercises may be active, active assisted, passive and/or resistive and are used to improve motion, strength, dexterity, flexibility and control (Ehrman, Gordon, Visich, & Keteyian, 2013). The choice of exercise depends primarily on the structures involved and the stage of healing. The management of individuals after surgery will be directed by the postoperative protocol, which may differ from surgeon to surgeon. For occupational therapists, purposeful activity is core to practice; engaging the person in a home programme of exercises that mimic that person's usual daily living activities has been found to be more beneficial than standard nonfunctional exercises (Guzelkucuk, Duman, Taskaynatan, & Dincer, 2007). An example of this may be when the goal is to increase wrist extension range of motion combined with finger extension for an individual may be encourage to wipe down the surfaces in the kitchen at home with a cloth and progress the activity, as motion improves, to washing the windows. If the goal is to improve wrist extension combined with finger flexion, then a sponge may be used instead of a cloth, which encourages functional flexion of the digits. A recent study relating to the hand function of people who had rheumatoid arthritis found function to be improved in people who engaged in a regular graded exercise programme (Lamb et al., 2015). Active exercises of the wrist are illustrated in Fig. 37.5A and passive exercises to provide a stretch and improve range of motion are illustrated in Fig. 37.5B.

Splinting/Orthotics: Splints/orthotics may be used statically, dynamically or progressively to position or stretch a joint or soft tissue (Glasgow, Tooth, Fleming, & Peters, 2011).

Further explanation about the use and benefit of splints/orthotics orthotics are provided in the orthotics chapter in this book.

Functional activity: As range of motion returns it is important that the movements gained are translated into meaningful functional activity; therefore meaningful activity must be integrated into the intervention plan to facilitate functional motion and use of the hand (Guzelkucuk et al., 2007). Furthermore the use of purposeful activity has been found to increase adherence to rehabilitation programmes (Colaianni and Provident, 2010; Harte and Spencer, 2014). Some examples of how meaningful activities can facilitate restoration of function are shown in Fig. 37.6.

Manage and Reduce Pain

Pain presents as both an acute and chronic state. It is perceived through nociceptors located in skin, muscle, joints and viscera (Patel, 2010). Acute pain is generally of rapid onset, specifically localised and a normal physiological response to trauma to the tissues. It serves as a warning that signals the individual to withdraw from harm or seek medical help. Conversely, chronic pain is generally of longer duration and is often dull and poorly localised.

The classification of pain described by Nolan (1993) remains valid and useful for contemporary practice. Five components are identified:

1. Physiological: injury to the tissues
2. Perceptual: the sensations conveyed by the nociceptors to the ascending pain pathways of the spinal cord to the brain
3. Affective: an individual's emotional response to the pain
4. Cognitive: the individual's knowledge of the cause of the pain
5. Behavioural: the individual's expression of the pain experience

Recognising these components in individuals will help the occupational therapist understand how best to manage hand pain. Failure to manage pain will have a significant impact on an individual. Hand therapy interventions are therefore dependent on the type of pain and the individual's response. Occupational therapists can use a number of different strategies to facilitate the management of pain for people with hand conditions, including education, activity analysis and guidance, compression and splinting/orthotics.

Education: Occupational therapists need to explain and translate the medical terminology related to an individual's hand condition in simple and clear language. Occupational therapists are ideally placed to engage individuals in active learning about their pain experiences within the context of their injury or impairment. Time to respond to concerns will be required so that the expectations of an individual can then be identified, explored and supported. Education approaches can include specific advice and

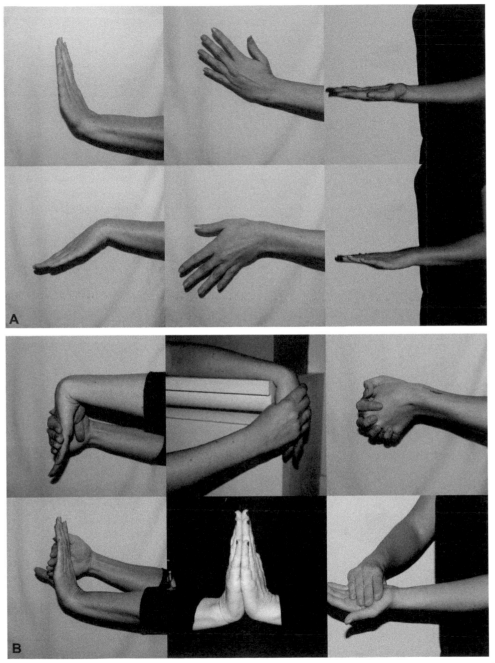

FIG. 37.5 ■ Active and passive exercises of the wrist. (A) Active exercise of the wrist. (B) Passive exercise to provide a stretch.

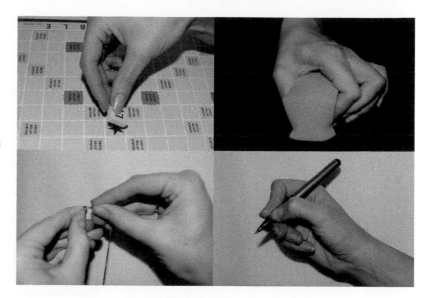

FIG. 37.6 ■ Meaningful activities can facilitate restoration of function.

guidance relating to joint protection and pain management strategies.

Activity analysis and guidance: Activity analysis, a core occupational therapy skill, is invaluable in hand therapy as the therapist can advise the individual on modifications to daily living activities so that the individual can carry out daily life roles while the injured or painful hand is protected. An assessment for daily living equipment to assist people to manage with their hand condition may also be useful.

Compression: Gentle pressure in the form of compression gloves, commonly used in oedema management, has also been found to reduce hand pain in rheumatoid arthritis. However, further robust evidence from high-quality trials on the clinical effectiveness of compression in controlling and reducing swelling and improving hand motion and function is required (Hammond, Jones, & Prior, 2016).

Splinting/Orthotics: Splinting/Orthotics may be applied as a means of managing and reducing the level of pain. These can be prescribed either off the shelf or tailor made by the occupational therapist to support structures that when moved produce a pain response. Further reading and details on orthotics are provided in the chapter on orthotics in this book.

Occupational therapists need to be watchful for development of pain states after hand injury as experience suggests that early identification and intervention reduce the risk of chronicity (Wertli, Bachmann, Weiner, & Brunner, 2013). Complex regional pain syndrome (CRPS) is a debilitating pain syndrome that occurs in approximately 7% of individuals who have a limb fracture, surgery or injury (Bruehl, 2015) and is associated with poor quality of life and large health care and socioeconomic costs (Goebel, 2011). Many cases resolve in the first year, with a subset progressing to chronic form (Bruehl, 2015). The characteristics of CRPS can include pain, disproportionate in time and degree to the usual course of known trauma or injury (Harden et al., 2013), sensory abnormality, abnormal regulation of blood flow, sweating, trophic changes, oedema of the skin and subcutaneous tissues and movement disorders (Binder & Baron, 2010). The cause remains unknown (Goebel, 2011). Diagnosis is made on the basis of clinical signs and symptoms (Bruehl, 2015), which are based on improved understanding, more effective treatments and significant scientific and clinical advancement over the last 15 years (Goebel, 2011). Treatment is challenging, but multidisciplinary care that centres on functionally focused therapies is recommended (Bruehl, 2015).

Increase Hand Function

The ultimate goal of the occupational therapist is to restore function to the hand and support the individual to participate in valued life roles and occupations. If therapeutic interventions address the preceding four key areas, the outcome should be increased hand function, except where there is permanent damage to the hand.

Hand function is complex and intricate. Purposeful hand function requires motion, strength, dexterity and motivation. Hand function has been analysed by many authors over the years, and classifications of grip formulated. Sollerman (1980) and Sollerman and Ejeskar (1995) identified and classified eight common handgrips: pulp pinch, lateral pinch, five-finger pinch, diagonal volar grip, transverse volar grip, tripod grip, spherical volar grip and extension grip. A classification system can be used as a way of capturing part of the dynamic quality of hand function and provide a useful tool to help communicate the intricacies of hand function to patients. These eight handgrips are illustrated in Fig. 37.7, in order of the frequency of their use in daily living.

Functional exercise groups are commonly used in hand therapy to facilitate the transition from formal exercise to function that is meaningful. Individuals with rehabilitation needs that do not require a one-to-one approach with the therapist can be effectively treated in a group setting. These groups generally provide an opportunity for individuals to practise, in a controlled and prescribed way, challenging functions of the hand. For example, restoration of pinch grip may be facilitated by asking the individual to practise doing an activity that requires use of the pinch grip, such as playing a board game picking up small pegs or placing pegs onto a line. These activities can provide the foundation for further developing daily hand function tasks such as manipulating a button, doing up a zip or fastening jewellery or more creative engagement with leisure activities such as sewing, gardening or painting.

Practically the individual will undertake warm-up exercises followed by a number of functional exercise stations that are selected to deliver the most appropriate movements to meet the goals of the individual.

Exercise can be delivered on a one-to-one basis with the occupational therapist or physiotherapist; however, compared with a home exercise programme, evidence supports the use of group-based exercise to deliver more positive health outcomes as the exercise is supervised by a professional therapist (Carmeli, Sheklow, & Coleman, 2006). The same study also highlighted the economic benefits of delivering treatment in groups versus individually.

A description of the implementation of Tammy's intervention plan can be found in Practice Story 37.5.

EVALUATION AND REVIEW

Occupational therapists have a duty, both to the individuals they are working with and to their employers, to ensure that their interventions are effective and their service is of a high quality.

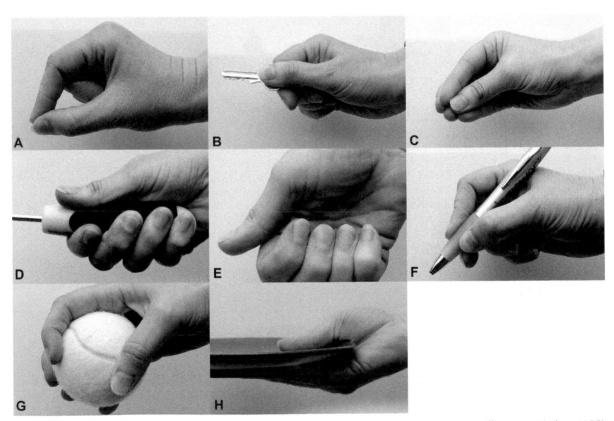

FIG. 37.7 ■ Eight handgrips in order of the frequency of their use in daily living (Sollerman 1980; Sollerman & Ejeskar, 1995). (A) Pulp pinch. (B) Lateral (key) pinch. (C) Five-finger pinch. (D) Diagonal volar grip. (E) Transverse volar grip. (F) Tripod grip. (G) Spherical volar grip. (H) Extension grip.

PRACTICE STORY 37.5

Tammy: Interventions

Before the commencement of interventions, time was taken to educate Tammy on the healing process of her fracture so that she could have confidence during the rehabilitation process, thus reducing her anxieties.

Oedema management: Tammy was not able to deal with her oedema solely with elevation at rest, and as a result she was supplied with an oedema/compression glove.

Reduced ROM in the fingers, thumb and wrist: Tammy was prescribed some functional exercises to improve the motion of her hand and the active and passive range of motion of wrist flexion, extension and, most importantly, supination. One of the exercises that she was given was to hold a half-filled water bottle at its neck and try to rotate the bottle from side to side, allowing the shifting of the water to facilitate the movement (Fig. 37.8). This exercise focused on functional supination and pronation combined with finger flexion.

ADL, Activity of daily living; *ROM,* range of motion.

Restoration of function: Using the process of activity analysis, light functional goals were set to facilitate the functional recovery of these motions. For example, Tammy was encouraged to use her affected hand every time she ate a meal. She was encouraged to use the hand as much as discomfort allowed in ADL.

Furthermore Tammy's musical skills were also used to facilitate the recovery of wrist movement. In particular, she was encouraged to play her piano for 10 minutes three times a day to encourage the combination of wrist extension with finger motion.

When ready, Tammy was encouraged to sit in the car and simulate the movement of her hand turning the steering wheel and using the handbrake. This allowed her to appreciate any remaining functional deficit. When she had done this she was asked to provide feedback about the experience to the occupational therapist. On review, if required, interventions could then be modified to increase the ROM needed for this activity.

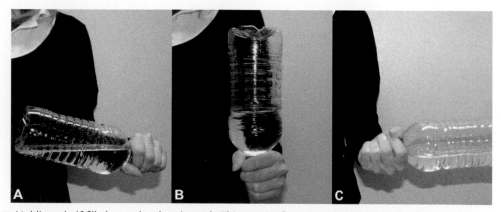

FIG. 37.8 ■ Holding a half-filled water bottle at its neck. This exercise focuses on functional supination and pronation combined with finger flexion. (A) Tip the water bottle in towards the body to encourage pronation of the forearm. (B) Hold the water bottle upright to obtain neutral forearm position. (C) Tip the water bottle away from body to encourage supination of the forearm.

It is therefore essential that throughout the occupational therapy process the individual is reevaluated. Reevaluation can reveal new findings by which to target interventions so that appropriate modifications and updates are made (Cooper, 2013). As an example, the initial goal of being able to hold a pen, using a functional tripod grip to enable an individual to write, may be reviewed a few weeks into the intervention programme. When revisited and reassessed, the individual may demonstrate the ability to attain the grip but remain unable to sustain the grip and manage effective handwriting. The goal is then revised to focus on pincer strength, enabling better control of the pen and improved endurance in handwriting. In the event that there remains a functional deficit after graded intervention, the occupational therapist, using a problem-solving approach, can advise the individual about assistive devices that may address the problem; for example, when osteoarthritis at the CMC joint of the thumb affects the ability of an individual to twist the lid off a jar, a jar-opening device may be suggested.

At the conclusion of the therapeutic process, evaluation of the whole approach must be considered to determine whether the individual's functional and therapeutic goals have been met and whether the interventions have been effective. Success looks different to different people and is dependent on many factors, including preexisting abilities, motivation, goals and performance demands of different tasks.

A description of the evaluation of Tammy's interventions can be found in Practice Story 37.6.

CONCLUSION

Studies have shown hand therapy to be effective in small subgroups: hand therapy techniques can improve pain and function in people with osteoarthritis and rheumatoid arthritis affecting their hands (Dziedzic et al., 2015; Lamb et al., 2015); group hand therapy that focuses on applying educational behavioural approaches are effective in improving self-management strategies and reducing pain for people with inflammatory arthritis (Hammond, 2003); and the most effective hand joint implant surgery is accompanied by hand therapy rehabilitation (Adams et al., 2012). Hand therapists have been leaders influencing postoperative splinting and exercise regimes that ultimately lead to fewer ruptures and better functional outcomes after tendon repair surgery (Peck et al., 2014). However, the full contribution that hand therapy provides after injury, disease and rehabilitation is still uncertain. To date, when predictors to individuals' self-reported satisfaction in hand outcomes are considered, the type and amount of hand therapy delivered by occupational therapists has not been included for

---

PRACTICE STORY 37.6

Tammy: Evaluation

Two weeks after commencing the interventions in Practice Story 37.5 Tammy was able to drive and had returned to work. She was playing the piano but was unable to hold her violin in position because of the ongoing restriction in her forearm supination ROM.

Reassessment of her ROM revealed an improvement in wrist movement:

- Wrist extension/flexion = 50 degrees/50 degrees)
- Supination = 75 degrees

At this stage, passive stretching exercises were added to her programme as well as resisted finger exercises to improve finger strength, dexterity and wrist stability.

Three weeks after commencing the interventions in Practice Story 37.5 Tammy was able to reach 13 out of the 16 notes she needed to play the violin. She identified that the problem in reaching the last few notes was that she was unable to flex her little finger across the neck of the violin to reach the fourth string when she was in full forearm supination.

At this stage exercises that focused on improving forearm supination with wrist and finger flexion were included. These exercises were done with a resistance sponge and low-resistance band (Fig. 37.9).

Six weeks after commencing the interventions in Practice Story 37.5 Tammy was able to participate in a music performance rehearsal but needed to take frequent breaks. She was able to reach all 16 notes in four of the seven positions on her violin. She still did not have enough forearm supination to reach the higher notes. She also indicated that she had not regained full arm and hand strength and noted that this affected her engagement in some aspects of her work, home and social life. The therapist indicated that her arm and hand

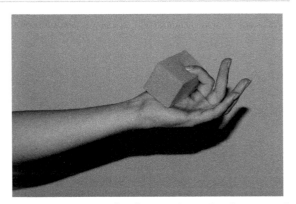

FIG. 37.9 ■ Exercises that focus on improving forearm supination with wrist and finger flexion. Exercises done with a resistance sponge.

strength would gradually improve as she continued to participate in her daily activities.

At this stage a reevaluation of her ROM, and DASH score indicated improvement compared with her initial scores. Her grip strength was also assessed at this stage, and compared with her unaffected side:

- Extension/flexion = 64 degrees/56 degrees
- Radial/ulnar deviation = 38 degrees/20 degrees
- Pronation/supination = 90 degrees/90 degrees
- Grip strength = 18 kg (24 kg on unaffected side)
- Quick DASH score = 9 (indicating that Tammy perceived that she had mild to no difficulties with her physical function)

DASH, Disability of the Arm, Shoulder and Hand; *ROM,* range of motion.

analysis (Marks, 2011). When research into hand therapy is reported, the predominant outcomes are often related to body functions and body structures, with less emphasis placed on activities, participation, and environmental factors (Winthrop Rose, Kasch, Aaron, & Stegink-Jansen, 2011), the overall focus of occupational therapy interventions. So much of the evidence that supports the effectiveness of hand therapy delivered by occupational therapists is considered 'low-level' evidence reporting on small-scale studies and with limited long-term follow-up (Huisstede et al., 2010). So, as with many other specialties, there is much more research work needed to establish a high-level evidence base for hand therapy delivered by occupational therapists.

In spite of this, occupational therapy core skills compliment the holistic and functional approach needed to enable individuals to reach their optimum function following hand injury or surgery or in the presence of disease. A good understanding of anatomy and healing underpins the therapists reasoning processes, and when teamed with individualised goals, hand therapy should aid recovery, reduce pain and improve function and wellbeing.

 http://evolve.elsevier.com/Curtin/OT

REFERENCES

Adams, J., Ryall, C., Pandyan, A., et al. (2012). Proximal interphalangeal joint replacement in patients with arthritis of the hand. A meta-analysis. *Journal of Bone and Joint Surgery, 94*(10), 1305–1312.

Artzberger, S. (2013). Edema reduction techniques: A biologic rationale for selection. In C. Cooper (Ed.), *Fundamentals of hand therapy – clinical reasoning and treatment guidelines for common diagnoses of the upper extremity* (pp. 36–40). St. Louis: Mosby Elsevier.

Binder, A., & Baron, R. (2010). Complex regional pain syndrome. In C. Stannard, E. Kalso, & J. Ballantyne (Eds.), *Evidence-based chronic pain management*. Oxford, UK: Blackwell Publishing.

Bruehl, S. (2015). Complex regional pain syndrome. *British Medical Journal, 351*, h2730.

Bucher, C., & Hume, K. I. (2003). A survey of current hand assessment practice in the UK. *Physiotherapy, 8*(3), 79–84.

Carmeli, E., Sheklow, S. L., & Coleman, R. A. (2006). A comparative study of organized class-based exercise programs versus individual home-based exercise programs for elderly patients following hip surgery. *Disability and Rehabilitation, 28*(16), 997–1005.

Chapparo, C., & Ranka, J. (2008). Clinical reasoning in occupational therapy. In J. Higgs, M. A. Jones, S. Loftus, & N. Christensen (Eds.), *Clinical reasoning in the health professions* (pp. 265–278). Oxford, UK: Butterworth Heinemann.

Cheema, T. A. (2014). Principles of treating complex hand injuries. In T. A. Cheema (Ed.), *Complex injuries of the hand*. London: JP Medical Ltd.

Colaianni, D., & Provident, I. (2010). The benefits of and challenges to the use of occupation in hand therapy. *Occupational Therapy in Health Care, 24*(2), 130–146.

College of Occupational Therapists (2011). *Professional standards for occupational therapy practice*. London: COT.

College of Occupational Therapists (2015). *Code of ethics and professional conduct*. London: COT.

Cooper, C. (2013). Fundamentals. In C. Cooper (Ed.), *Fundamentals of hand therapy: Clinical reasoning and treatment guidelines for common diagnoses of the upper extremity*. St. Louis: Mosby Elsevier.

De Putter, C. E., Selles, R. W., Polinder, S., Panneman, M. J. M., Hovius, S. E. R., & Van Beeck, E. F. (2012). Economic impact of hand and wrist injuries: Health care costs and productivity costs in a population based study. *Journal of Bone and Joint Surgery (American Volume), 94*(9), e56.

Deshaies, L. (2013). Burns. In C. Cooper (Ed.), *Fundamentals of hand therapy: Clinical reasoning and treatment guidelines for common diagnoses of the upper extremity*. St. Louis: Mosby Elsevier.

Diegelmann, R. F., & Evans, M. C. (2004). Wound healing: An overview of acute, fibrotic and delayed healing. *Frontiers in Bioscience, 9*(1), 283–289.

Dziedzic, K., Nicholls, E., Hill, S., et al. (2015). Self-management approaches for osteoarthritis in the hand: A 2 × 2 factorial randomised trial. *Annals of the Rheumatic Diseases, 74*, 108–118.

Ehrman, J. K., Gordon, P. M., Visich, P. S., & Keteyian, S. J. (2013). *Clinical exercise physiology*. Champaign, IL: Human Kinetics.

Flinn, S., & Jones, C. (2011). The use of motivational interviewing to manage behavioral changes in hand injured clients. *Hand Therapy, 24*(2), 140–146.

Glasgow, C., Tooth, L. R., Fleming, J., & Peters, S. (2011). Dynamic splinting for the stiff hand after trauma: Predictors of contracture resolution. *Journal of Hand Therapy, 24*(3), 195–205 quiz 206.

Goebel, A. (2011). Complex regional pain syndrome in adults. *Rheumatology, 50*(10), 1739–1750.

Guzelkucuk, U., Duman, I., Taskaynatan, M., & Dincer, K. (2007). Comparison of therapeutic activities with therapeutic exercises in the rehabilitation of young adult patients with hand injuries. *Journal of Hand Surgery American Volume, 32*, 1429–1435.

Hammond, A. (2003). Patient education in arthritis: Helping people change. *Musculoskeletal Care, 1*(2), 84–97.

Hammond, A., Jones, V., & Prior, Y. (2016). The effects of compression gloves on hand symptoms and hand function in rheumatoid arthritis and hand osteoarthritis: A systematic review. *Clinical Rehabilitation, 30*(3), 213–224.

Harden, R. N., Oaklander, A. L., Burton, A. W., et al. (2013). Complex Regional Pain Syndrome: Practical Diagnostic and Treatment Guidelines, 4th Edition. *Pain Medicine, 14*, 180–229.

Harte, D., & Spencer, K. (2014). Sleight of hand: Magic, therapy and motor performance. *Journal of Hand Therapy, 27*(1), 67–69.

Huisstede, B. M., Hoogvlict, P., Randsdorp, M. S., et al. (2010). Carpal tunnel syndrome. Part I: Effectiveness of nonsurgical treatments – a systematic review archives of physical medicine and rehabilitation. *Physical Medicine and Rehabilitation, 91*(7), 981–1004.

Lamb, S., Williamson, E. M., Heine, P. J., et al., on behalf of the Strengthening and Stretching for Rheumatoid Arthritis of the Hand Trial (SARAH) Trial Team. (2015). Exercises to improve function of the rheumatoid hand (SARAH): A randomised controlled trial. *The Lancet, 385*(9966), 421–429.

Larson, D., & Jerosch-Herald, C. (2008). Clinical effectiveness of post-operative splinting after surgical release of Dupuytren's contracture: A systematic review. *BMC Musculoskeletal Disorders, 9*, 104.

Marks, M. (2011). Determinants of patient satisfaction after orthopedic interventions to the hand: a review of the literature. *Journal of Hand Therapy, 24*(4), 303–312.

Masson, J. A. (2003). Wound and tissue healing. In R. Prosser, & W. B. Conolly (Eds.), *Rehabilitation of the hand and upper limb.* Butterworth Heinmann: Sydney.

Nolan, M. F. (1993). Contemporary perspectives on pain and discomfort. *Physical Therapy Practice, 2*, 14.

Mustoe, T. A. (2008). Evolution of silicone therapy and mechanism of action in scar management. *Aesthetic Plastic Surgery, 32*, 82–92.

O'Brien, L., & Jones, D. J. (2013). Silicone gel for preventing and treating hypertrophic and keloid scars. *Cochrane Database of Systematic Reviews, 2013*(9).

Patel, N. B. (2010). Physiology of pain. In A. Kopf, & N. B. Patel (Eds.), *Guide to pain management in low-resource settings* (pp. 13–18). Seatle: IASP Press.

Peck, F. H., Roe, A. E., Ng, C. Y., Duff, C., McGrouther, D. A., & Lees, V. C. (2014). The Manchester short splint: A change to splinting practice in the rehabilitation of zone II flexor tendon repairs. *Hand Therapy, 19*(2), 47–53.

Polinder, S., Iordens, G. I., Panneman, M. J., et al. (2013). Trends in incidence and costs of injuries to the shoulder, arm and wrist in the Netherlands between 1986 and 2008. *BMC Public Health, 13*, 531.

Prochaska, J. O., & DiClemente, C. C. (1984). *The transtheoretical approach: Crossing the traditional boundaries of therapy.* Melbourne, Florida: Krieger Publishing Company.

Saaqi, M., Ud-Din, H., Khan, M. I., & Chaudhery, S. M. (2009). Presentation and outcome of hand trauma in a plastic surgical unit. *Annals of the Pakistan Institute of Medical Science, 5*(3), 131–135.

Sfeir, C., Ho, L., Doll, B. A., Azari, K., & Hollinger, J. O. (2005). Fracture repair. In J. R. Liebermann, & G. E. Friedlander (Eds.), *Bone regeneration and repair: Biology and clinical applications.* Totowa, NJ: Humana Press.

Shin, T. M., & Bordeaux, J. S. (2013). The role of scar massage in scar management: A literature review. *Dermatological Surgery, 38*(3), 414–423.

Sollerman, C. (1980). *Assessment of Grip Function: Evaluation of a New Test Method.* Stockholm: Medical Innovation Technology (MITAB).

Sollerman, C., & Ejeskar, A. (1995). Sollerman Hand Function Test A standardised method and its use in tetraplegic patients. *Scandinavian Journal of Plastic and Reconstructive Surgery and Hand Surgery, 29*, 167–176.

Strand, E. B., Kerns, R., Christie, A., Haavik-Nilsen, K., Klokkerud, M., & Finset, A. (2007). Higher levels of pain readiness to change and more positive affect reduce pain reports – a weekly assessment study on arthritis patients. *Pain, 127*(3), 204–213.

Villeco, J. P. (2012). Edema: A silent but important factor. *Journal of Hand Therapy, 25*(2), 153–161 quiz 162.

Warwick, D., Dunn, R., Melikyan, E., & Vadher, J. (2009). *Hand surgery.* Oxford, UK: Oxford University Press.

Wegener, S. T., Castillo, R. C., Heins, S. E., et al. (2014). The development and validation of the Readiness to Engage in Self-Management after Acute Traumatic Injury Questionnaire. *Rehabilitation Psychology, 59*(2), 203–210.

Wertli, M., Bachmann, L. M., Weiner, S. S., & Brunner, F. (2013). Prognostic factors in complex regional pain syndrome 1: A systematic review. *Journal of Rehabilitation Medicine, 45*(3), 225–231.

Winthrop Rose, B., Kasch, M. C., Aaron, D. H., & Stegink-Jansen, C. W. (2011). Does hand therapy literature incorporate the holistic view of health and function promoted by the World Health Organization? *Journal of Hand Therapy, 24*(2), 84–88.

Trademark References

Coban 3 M, St. Paul, MN, USA

Jobskin, Nottingham, UK

Tubigrip Molnlycke Health Care, Gothenburg, Sweden

Hand Therapy Organisations Around the World

- American Society of Hand Therapists (ASHT): www.asht.org
- Australian Hand Therapy Association (AHTA): www.ahta.com.au
- British Association of Hand Therapists (BAHT): www.hand-therapy.co.uk
- British Health Professionals in Rheumatology (BHPR) integrated into the British Society for Rheumatology in April 2013. The whole organisation exists to unite and support members of the multidisciplinary team in delivering best quality care for patients: http://www.rheumatology.org.uk
- Canadian Society of Hand Therapists (CSHT): www.csht.org
- International Federation of Societies for Hand Therapy (IFSHT): www.ifsht.org
- European Federation of Societies for Hand Therapy (EFSHT): www.eurohandtherapy.org
- Federation of European Societies for Surgery of the Hand (FESSH): www.fessh.com
- International Federation of Societies for Surgery of the Hand (IFSSH): www.ifssh.info
- New Zealand Association of Hand Therapists (NZAHT): www.nzaht.org.nz

38 ORTHOTICS

NATASHA A. LANNIN ■ IONA NOVAK ■ MICHELLE JACKMAN

CHAPTER OUTLINE

Abstract
Orthotics is the practice of designing, fabricating, fitting and applying orthoses to restore or improve the occupational performance or structural characteristics of a body part. There are three types of orthoses: static, semidynamic and dynamic. These orthoses are used to facilitate occupational engagement and the attainment of occupational goals for people with a variety of hand and upper limb conditions. Orthoses are used for a wide range of reasons. These include immobilisation of the hand to promote joint protection, rest or wound healing; correction of deformity; prevention of scarring; improvement of hand use; reduction of pain; and reduction of oedema. Orthoses are only used when they contribute to the attainment of relevant and meaningful occupational outcomes for the person and his or her family. Every orthoses should be customised to achieve the unique occupational goals of each person; based on up-to-date information regarding efficacy, design, wearing protocol, materials and monitoring regimes; and relevant and practical in the person's life situation. Without careful attention to these three elements of orthoses prescription, even the most technically precise orthosis will not achieve occupational outcomes.

KEY POINTS

- Occupational therapists use orthoses to achieve occupational outcomes where equal attention is given to the scientific aspect of orthoses and to the person-centred aspect of practice.

- Orthoses are considered an adjunctive intervention as they are used to either 'establish or restore' a person's skills or prevent the occurrence or development of barriers to performance.

- Orthoses may be prescribed to immobilise or protect weak, painful or healing musculoskeletal structures;

prevent or correct developing deformities, including contractures and scarring; assist in providing improved abilities or serve as an attachment for assistive devices; and reduce pain by limiting motion or weight bearing.

■ There are three classes of orthoses: static, semidynamic and dynamic.

■ The type of orthosis, the position of the hand or arm, and the wearing protocol vary because each person is an individual, with unique occupational goals, unique injury or disease processes and unique rehabilitation goals.

■ Occupational therapists conduct a comprehensive occupation-focused assessment, which includes a review of relevant body structures and functions and consideration of environmental factors to determine whether an orthoses is appropriate.

■ Occupational therapists need to explicitly seek out and factor scientifically gained knowledge into their daily decision making, overcoming the inertia of practising within the 'comfort zones', and constantly remain abreast of scientific evidence.

INTRODUCTION

Orthoses are used in the treatment of hand and upper limb impairments by occupational therapists. Orthotics is the practice of designing, fabricating, fitting and applying orthoses to restore or improve performance or the structural characteristics of a person's hand or arm. Occupational therapists use orthoses to achieve occupational outcomes. As a consequence, occupational therapists who use orthotic strategies must be able to synthesise the technical aspects of orthoses prescription, design, fabrication and application, with the interpersonal dimensions of understanding a person's performance and life role goals. The focus on occupational outcomes taken in this chapter means that equal attention is given to the scientific aspect of orthoses and to the person-centred aspect of practice. Readers are encouraged to adopt an explicit attitude towards their reasoning when using orthoses in practice, so that the balance between the scientific and the personal occupation-focused dimension of therapy is maintained. Without this person-centred focus, the attainment of relevant, meaningful occupational outcomes through orthotics is unlikely.

This chapter does not aim to teach readers skills in splint or cast fabrication. There are specialist texts already available that meet this need and explain the biomechanical principles that underlie fabrication, and the reader can refer to the references at the end of this chapter (e.g. Coppard & Lohman, 2008; Goga-Eppenstien et al., 1999; Jacobs & Austin, 2014; Wilton, 2015). Rather, the chapter leads readers through foundation principles, provides examples and points out important issues that should be explicitly considered in the reasoning process.

For example, the Canadian Practice Process Framework can guide therapists in the prescription of orthotics. To meet the occupational goals of the person, orthoses should be thought of as an 'adjunctive' intervention (Copley & Kuipers, 2014); that is, they are always used in combination with other interventions designed to improve the person's occupational engagement.

WHAT ARE ORTHOSES?

Occupational therapists manufacture and prescribe orthoses as one specialised aspect of upper limb intervention. Upper limb orthoses are pieces of equipment that are applied externally to the body to restore or improve the functional and structural characteristics of the musculoskeletal and nervous systems. They can be splints, casts, garments or tape. Splints and garments are external devices designed to immobilise the limb in a position or stabilise joints to encourage a movement (Copley & Kuipers, 2014). Tape may be rigid or elastic, and applied to the limb to compensate for a lack of strength or provide stability to a joint (Appel, Perry, & Jones, 2014). Casts are made of plaster or fibreglass and are used to immobilise bones for fracture healing or to stretch muscles for reducing contractures (Lannin, Novak, & Cusick, 2007). The use of orthotics has developed largely from the experiences of therapists and is therefore predominantly based on expert opinion evidence (Kogler, 2002). This means that the scientific evidence base for the design, application and evaluation of orthoses is both recent and rapidly changing. It is vital, therefore, to maintain a working knowledge of developments and trends as a result of the dynamic nature of orthotic practice.

Orthoses can be made of a variety of materials, and the development of new orthotic products is increasing all the time as specialist companies search for improved product range and performance. There are also an increasing number of commercially available prefabricated orthoses. It is therefore important to seek out product information from local suppliers, benchmark this with recent evidence regarding performance of the material in professional investigations and choose the material that will best suit a person's needs, therapeutic goals and resource constraints. Applying skills in appraisal of evidence helps therapists select not only what type of orthosis design could be used but also what type of material may be most appropriate. The types of materials mentioned in this chapter are only indicative of the range that may be available. Newer materials are constantly being developed that address factors such as ease of application, cosmesis, comfort and durability.

WHO NEEDS ORTHOSES?

People who have a condition that affects the use of their hands may benefit from orthotic intervention. Occupational therapists use a range of information to determine whether orthotic intervention is appropriate. It is vital that the occupational goals of the person are clear before considering orthotic intervention.

Orthotics ought only to be considered after it is determined that an orthotic could address a factor limiting a person's goal achievement. Therapists conduct a comprehensive occupation focused assessment, which includes a review of relevant body structures and functions and consideration of environmental factors. Assessment may use a range of information sources including medical record review, standardised assessments, skilled observations, interview protocols, ecological measures and activity analysis (Dunn, 2000). People most likely to benefit from orthoses are those with musculoskeletal injury, neurological events such as stroke or spinal cord injury, and burn injuries, as well as degenerative conditions such as arthritis. The goal in all of these circumstances is to enhance occupational engagement through increased upper limb and hand use. Depending on the condition and the occupational goal, the person may require an orthosis that will support upper limb structures such as joints, muscles or skin or an orthosis that facilitates movement. The occupational goal always guides the selection of orthosis type and material – the same presenting condition may not require the same orthosis type as the occupational goals of the individual may vary. Unless the occupational goal is clear, the selection of orthosis type cannot be well informed and may not be appropriate.

Occupational therapists need to have an excellent understanding of the condition, the occupational goals of the person and the normal and abnormal structural properties of the upper limb and hand to inform the selection of orthoses as a suitable intervention strategy.

Julia's practice story (Practice Story 38.1) illustrates the professional practice of a certified hand therapist who maintains a person-centred, occupation-focus, and evidence-based practice.

The Condition

Any condition that adversely affects the use, comfort or cosmesis (aesthetic appearance) of the hand may indicate the need for an orthosis. Consideration of the disease process and pathology will allow the therapist to consider the extent to which the condition has affected normal structural features and processes and the likely course or prognosis of the disease. For example, rheumatoid arthritis generally passes through one of three disease phases: acute, subacute and chronic. The acute phase is characterised by inflamed, swollen and painful joints, whereas during the subacute phase the disease is less active. In the subacute phase the person's condition remains stable for longer periods, but joint deformity is progressing. By the chronic phase the disease is no longer active, but the residual mechanical problems in and around the joint produces pain, instability and stiffness, all resulting in a loss of performance. Being aware of the disease process allows the therapist to educate people about their condition and therapy goals and to predict how therapy goals will need to change in the future to meet each individual's occupational engagement goals. The type of orthosis selected for different phases of the condition, the wearing regimen recommended and the likely structural outcomes will vary according to the disease process characteristics and phases.

The Occupational Goals of the Person

The decision to use an orthoses will depend in part on the condition but also to a great extent on personal goals. The starting point for any relationship between therapists and the people with whom they work is establishing goals, which should emerge from a

---

PRACTICE STORY 38.1

Julia

Julia runs her own private hand therapy practice in Sydney, Australia, where she works with people who have hand injuries in addition to supervising junior staff. In her daily practice, she works with a wide variety of people who have been referred for hand therapy – some with a traumatic hand injury, some who have a musculoskeletal condition, some who have had a stroke and some who have had a brain injury. Being prepared to work with people who have a range of upper limb conditions requires Julia to have a sound understanding of anatomy, healing processes, underlying pathological conditions and, most of all, problem-solving strategies. Julia maintains that the most important skill for a hand therapist to develop is that of professional reasoning. She states that therapists have

to be able to assess everything that is going on for each individual person, not only their injury and its usual healing processes, but also their work, domestic and leisure tasks, in order to know what intervention will provide the best possible outcome.

Excellent professional reasoning skills not only allow Julia to choose interventions to meet individualised goals but also to be able to predict the time frame for healing, to advise each individual of potential complications and when to address them and to know that she will need to continually reassess her intervention plans. Julia's experience in hand therapy has taught her that providing a splint is never the complete therapy programme. It is important to acknowledge that the natural tissue-healing process means that the splint will require adjustments, changes or even prescription of a completely different splint to meet the ever-changing needs and goals of each individual. Experience has also taught Julia the benefits and limitations of different orthoses. She is flexible in her approach to splinting, which allows her to know how to modify a design to suit each person's unique occupational requirements. Expert therapists such as Julia employ professional reasoning to ensure their interventions are not only evidence-based, but that they are occupation-focused and tailored to meet each person's unique and individual needs.

collaborative rather than a prescriptive relationship. Although some therapists find open-ended discussion a useful way to identify occupational goals and evaluation criteria, others use semi-structured interviewing focused around development of goal attainment scales (Hurn, Kneebone, & Cropley, 2006; Ottenbacher & Cusick 1990), or structured approaches such as the Canadian Occupational Performance Measure (Law et al., 1990) to identify problems, priorities and impact measures. With or without structured instruments, the occupational therapist must identify how the altered hand performance is affecting the person's occupational engagement in self-care, productivity and leisure and the person's desired occupational outcomes. Goals relating to orthotic prescription may include changes in role performance, activity, particular desired movements, pain management, wound healing and cosmetic appearance. The occupational goals of the person are paramount for occupational therapists. Body structure problems, even when present, do not always translate to activities and participation impairments and therefore they may not need intervention (Copley & Kuipers, 2014; Wright, Rosenbaum, Goldsmith, Law, & Fehlings, 2008).

The Structural Properties of the Upper Limb and Hand

Occupational therapists need to have an excellent working knowledge of the anatomy and physiology of the upper limb and hand – it is the foundation to successful orthotic intervention. Therapists need to know how the 'normal' upper limb and hand is structured, how it works and the physiological processes that sustain it to be able to grasp the impact of disease or trauma and the likely mechanisms for recovery. As most orthoses use biomechanical principles in their design, a thorough understanding of biomechanical properties of the upper limb and hand is required. This is particularly important as biomechanical deficits are independent of specific disease processes that may be present in a condition.

Bone and joint injuries, infections, varying degrees of paralysis, joint diseases and trauma all have diverse causes and processes that may present similar biomechanical deficits. It is important to be mindful that biomechanical deficits do not necessarily translate to performance deficits and therefore comprehensive assessment that includes analysis of the individual's goals is necessary.

TYPES OF ORTHOSES

All orthoses are prescribed for one or more of the following purposes:

- To immobilise or protect weak, painful or healing musculoskeletal structures
- To prevent or correct developing deformities, including contractures and scarring
- To assist in providing improved abilities or serve as an attachment for assistive devices
- To reduce pain by limiting motion or weight bearing

The individual assessment will indicate what particular objectives will be pursued through the orthosis design, application and wearing regimen in support of the desired overarching occupational outcome.

There are three classes of orthoses: static, semidynamic and dynamic (American Society of Hand Therapists (ASHT), 1992). This classification is based on the key purpose of the orthosis. Static orthoses aim to prevent any movement by immobilising a joint. Semidynamic orthoses limit an aspect of movement in a joint while facilitating another movement in other joints. Dynamic orthoses are designed to mobilise joints, muscles and/or skin to facilitate a desired movement.

Static Orthoses

Static orthoses are also known as immobilisation splints (Fig. 38.1). These have no moving parts and aim to immobilise to help prevent further deformity or soft tissue contracture. Static orthoses immobilise a joint in a predetermined position selected on the basis of the occupational goal, features of the presenting condition and structural factors relating to the individual and the material used for fabrication. Static orthoses can rigidly support body structures, as in the case of fractures, inflammatory conditions and nerve injuries, where the body part must be stabilise and protected. Static orthoses can also apply a prolonged stretch to muscles or skin when stretch is required to achieve structural change, as in the case of neurological conditions or burns (Farmer & James, 2001; Fess, Gettle, Philips, & Janson, 2004; Lowe, 1995; Milazzo & Gillen, 2011; Wilton, 2015).

Examples of static orthoses include pressure splints (Taly, Nair, Murali, & Wankade, 2002), dorsal or volar wrist splints (Wilton, 2015), resting hand splints (Wilton, 2015), mallet splints (Handoll & Vaghela, 2004) and 'buddy' finger taping. The best known example is the resting splint (Fig. 38.2). A resting splint does what the name suggests, it immobilises the wrist, fingers and thumb in a 'resting' position. The position of 'rest' is carefully determined for each individual. Resting splints are usually made of thermoplastic material (although they could equally be constructed by any rigid material, such as plaster)

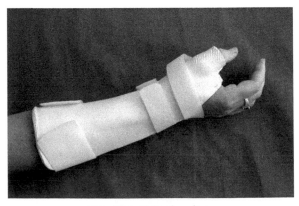

FIG. 38.1 ■ Static splint.

and are custom moulded and secured onto the upper limb by adjustable strapping.

Orthoses that immobilise may allow a therapist to immobilise skin (e.g. immediately after skin graft surgery), to protect joints (e.g. in arthritic conditions), to promote tissue healing (e.g. after hand trauma), to stretch skin (e.g. as in the case of burns or hand trauma after wound healing) or to stretch muscle (e.g. as in the case of neurological impairments).

Semidynamic Orthoses

Semidynamic orthoses (Fig. 38.3) restrict the force of a particular movement and facilitate another target movement using the intrinsic elastic property of the orthotic material. They can also substitute for loss of motor function by holding a joint in a position when the muscles do not have adequate strength or motor control. Materials such as Lycra, neoprene and rubber foam are used to manufacture semidynamic orthoses. Orthoses made from these materials are often named after the product, such as a 'neoprene splint' or 'Lycra garment'. Semidynamic orthoses are particularly useful for people with overuse injuries, burns

and neurological impairments. These orthoses tend to be circumferential in nature and either cover the target joint fully or run parallel to the line of desired muscle pull. An example of this is the tone and positioning (TAP) splint shown in Fig. 38.4.

Dynamic Orthoses

Dynamic orthoses are also known as mobilisation splints (Fig. 38.5). These have moving parts that promote, control or restore movement. They create an intermittent, gentle force on a segment of the upper limb resulting in motion of a joint or muscle. The force is created through the careful design of the orthoses so that the 'pull' of elastic bands, springs or mechanical devices will create the desired therapeutic effect. Dynamic splints allow a therapist to control the direction and amount of movement in joints, tendons and muscles. An example of a condition where dynamic splints are commonly used is in the rehabilitation phase after tendon repair. The therapist moulds a stable thermoplastic base splint from which they attach an 'outrigger', which pulls the target joint, tendons and muscles in a desired direction.

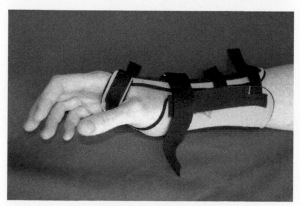

FIG. 38.2 ■ Resting splint.

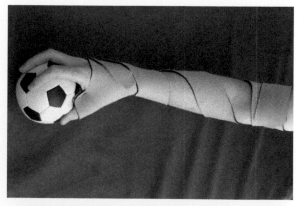

FIG. 38.4 ■ Tone and positioning (TAP) splint.

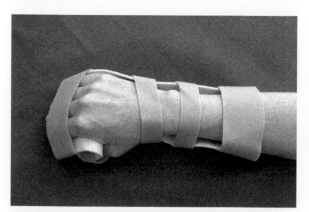

FIG. 38.3 ■ Semidynamic splint.

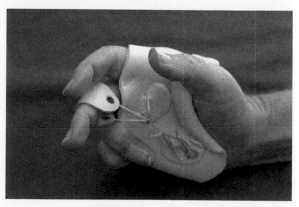

FIG. 38.5 ■ Dynamic splint.

HOW TO DESIGN ORTHOSES

Many possibilities exist for static, semidynamic and dynamic orthosis design and fabrication. The choice of design is informed by a good working knowledge of upper limb anatomy, a thorough assessment of the person that identifies problems limiting performance and, finally, understanding the capabilities and limitations of each type of orthosis. Extensive reference material exists on orthoses designs and their indications for use. Some of this material can be found in the Reference List at the end of the chapter.

The biomechanical approach provides a logical method of analysing presenting structural problems and considering corrective options. In the biomechanical approach, the therapist aims to maintain or increase movement by controlling adverse movements and preventing or addressing the structural changes to joints, muscles and soft issue caused by immobilisation and muscle imbalance (Copley & Kuipers, 2014). Although a range of information sources may be used to determine whether an orthotic intervention is potentially relevant, the actual design of the orthosis takes a particular approach. A biomechanical assessment is recommended as this explores all factors relevant to orthosis fabrication: a biomechanical examination (Table 38.1) typically includes assessment of range of motion, muscle strength, sensation and pain and analysis of the degree of voluntary movement possible (Wilton, 2015). The factors

TABLE 38.1
Biomechanical Orthotic Examination

Assessment	Rationale
Range of motion (ROM) assessment: ROM assessment is the numeric measurement of a joint's capability. Passive range of motion (PROM) is the movement available at a joint when it is moved by another person, and active range of motion (AROM) is the movement available at a joint when the person voluntarily moves the joint themselves. ROM is measured using a device called a 'goniometer'.	ROM is routinely taken when hypertonicity, injury causing immobilisation and joint conditions such as arthritis are present, because the risks of discomfort and joint contracture are elevated. ROM deficits can lead to a secondary loss of performance skills (Copley & Kuipers, 2014).
Muscle strength assessment: A muscle group's strength can be graded in relation to its ability to provide resistance to fundamental forces such as gravity and then to an external force such as an assessor or weighted objects. Various scales exist to describe strength classifications, in addition to devices called 'dynamometers', which is the preferred methodology where possible.	Muscle strength is an important element of AROM and endurance. Weakness affects movement and independence. Muscle weakness can be present as a primary impairment, for example, in muscle diseases and hypertonicity but also occurs as a secondary impairment from immobilisation and lack of limb use.
Pain assessment: Pain is assessed using a variety of tools. These include: visual analogue scale (VAS); self-report survey measures (Farrar, Young, LaMoreaux, Werth, & Michael, 2001); and the McGill Pain Questionnaire (Melzack, 1987).	The presence of pain will affect the self-selected use of the limb and available ROM. Use may exacerbate pain and inflammation and discontinued use may result in secondary impairments of loss of ROM and strength.
Voluntary movement assessment: The quantity and quality of voluntary movement available to the person is measured using numerous standardised assessments. The selection of an appropriate tool depends on the person's diagnostic group and age, the purpose for measurement and the instrument's psychometric properties. Taxonomies exist to assist therapists to select appropriate instruments (Unsworth, 2000).	The degree of voluntary movement possible affects the person's AROM, general limb use, quality of movement, compensatory movements adopted and success with tasks.
Person-centred self-assessment of upper limb movement: A number of standardised tools have been developed to help the therapist understand upper limb impairment from the person's perspective, such as the Duruoz Hand Index (DHI) (Poole, Cordova, & Brower, 2006) or the Disabilities of Arm, Shoulder and Hand (DASH) (Hudak, Amadio, & Bombardier, 1996).	The person may conceptualise his or her occupational role loss in a different way than the therapist and this can bring new and insightful information to the assessment process.

of interest are only those which are causing movement loss, pain or concern to the person as they relate to the occupational goal of orthotic intervention.

WHEN TO USE ORTHOSES

Orthoses may be used with people in whom joint immobilisation and protection are required. This may arise from the need to rest, to heal wounds or to facilitate performance. They may be required to correct deformities and prevent scarring or contractures. Orthoses may be used when there is a need to improve movement, reduce pain or decrease oedema. Each of these indications for orthotic intervention is now explored. In addition, a brief summary of which splints may be appropriate to achieve specific goals of therapy is provided in Table 38.2.

Immobilisation

Joint Protection

Perhaps the most common use for an orthosis is to immobilise a body part, such as during fracture healing. Immobilising orthoses can also be used to protect joints, minimise joint damage or joint deformity or help manage pain. Orthoses that are prescribed for joint protection may have wearing regimens governed by either presenting symptoms or features of the condition. For example, joint protection related to trauma may require an orthosis to be worn only when symptoms of pain are present, whereas joint protection related to the pathology of an arthritic joint requires a wearing regimen independent of symptoms for the protective goals to be achieved.

Immobilisation for Rest

Immobilisation may be undertaken to allow tissues to rest in a position that minimises complications associated with inflammation, contracture or pain (Wilton, 2015). Hand therapy literature maintains that at rest, the hand and wrist adopt a posture that allows a perfect balance of muscle and ligament tension (Wilton, 2015). Therapists often use static splints to mimic this position, known as the 'resting' or 'functional' position. The resting position is 10- to 20-degree wrist extension, 20- to 45-degree flexion of metacarpophalangeal (MCP) joints, and between 10 and 30 degrees of interphalangeal flexion (Wilton, 2015).

The evidence for the use of splints to immobilise the hand for rest is controversial in many diagnoses. When working with people with rheumatoid arthritis, splinting may not be beneficial (Adams, Burridge, Mullee, Hammond, & Cooper, 2008; Coppard & Lohman, 2008), particularly after steroid injection (Wallen & Gillies, 2006). There also continues to be limited evidence to support the use of night resting splints for adults with carpel tunnel syndrome (Page, Massey-Westdropp, O'Conner, & Pitt, 2012). Rest is seen by therapists to be beneficial; however, this must be carefully balanced with movement to guard against loss of motion (Pagnotta, Korner-Bitensky, Mazer, Baron, &

TABLE 38.2

Common Types of Splints to Achieve Specific Goals of Therapy

Goal of Therapy	Professional Reasoning for Selecting Common Types of Splints
Immobilisation	Static orthoses, such as a thermoplastic resting splint, may be used to protect a joint after a fracture, allow rest when there is inflammation or pain at a joint or allow for wound healing such as after a burn injury. Taping may be used to immobilise the joint when pain is present in a person with arthritis or carpel tunnel syndrome.
Preventing contractures	Static orthoses, such as a cast or resting splint, may be used to position joints so that stretch is maintained on soft tissues, such as in burns. Semidynamic splints, such as Lycra garments, may be used to provide stretch while allowing for some movement in burns, rheumatoid arthritis and neurological rehabilitation. Dynamic orthoses may be used after flexor tendon repair, to protect the joint while allowing motion at the joint to prevent contracture.
Scar management	Semidynamic splints, such as a pressure garment, may be combined with other therapies in an effort to reduce scar thickness.
Improving use of the hand	Dynamic, semidynamic and static splints may be used to improve an individual's use of the hand. The type of splint will be specific to the person's occupational goal. Static splints may include a wrist cock-up splint to position the wrist and compensate for weakness to facilitate grasp or a thumb post splint to stabilise the thumb MCP joint to allow a pincer grasp. Semidynamic orthoses, such as a supination splint, may facilitate supination to improve reach and grasp ability. Dynamic extensor bracing may be used to improve grip strength in lateral epicondylitis.
Pain management	Semidynamic orthoses may reduce pain in rheumatoid arthritis and carpel tunnel syndrome by providing support without compressing the carpal tunnel.
Decreasing oedema	Consistent circumferential pressure, through a pressure garment, may reduce oedema after a traumatic injury or peripheral or central nerve damage.

MCP, Metacarpophalangeal.

Wood-Dauphinee, 2005). For this reason taping (also known as kinesiology taping and by various trade names) has been studied as an alternative to static splinting. Taping has a lower profile and thus is less restrictive in terms of sustaining some use of the limb during the rest period. Systematic reviews and meta-analyses suggest that taping is at least as effective as other types of splinting, producing a marginal (but perhaps not meaningful) reduction in pain, and can be used as a reasonable alternative to more static orthoses (Montalvo, Cara, & Myer, 2014; Morris, Jones, Ryan, & Ryan, 2013).

Immobilisation for Wound Healing

Immobilisation may be undertaken to allow tissues to heal in a specific position, such as in the case of skin healing after skin graft surgery. Immobilising orthoses may be used for healing skin, bone and ligamentous structures, and also surgically released nerves. The position of the hand will be determined primarily by the damaged structures and the surgery (if any) performed. A balance is required between the immobilisation of damaged structures and the maintenance of movement in structures that have not been damaged. Injuries may also warrant different immobilising positions for day and night. Therapists should remain aware of such potential complications, which are all part of normal tissue-healing processes, and monitor the orthosis in order to make appropriate adjustments as required to ensure immobilisation (Fig. 38.6). For example, an orthosis applied in the first 72 hours after a traumatic injury may not fit the person shortly after application because of oedema. This is particularly the case with burn injuries as significant oedema in the initial phrases of treatment and recovery is often experienced.

The evidence for the effectiveness of immobilisation to facilitate wound healing is complex. Although immobilisation may facilitate wound closure, it can cause secondary impairments. Such is the case in microsurgical repair of the hand after a digital nerve injury. In this condition immobilisation splinting is used to protect against possible damage to the repaired nerve sheath. However, evidence suggests that people who wear these splints have more adverse outcomes than those who are not splinted; they take longer to return to work and the unwanted symptoms of pain and loss of range of motion take longer to recover from (Clare, & de Haviland Mee, & Belcher, 2004). The choice of orthosis materials is also important to successful outcomes. Research now suggests that immobilisation of fractures using splints rather than casts is better tolerated and results in better hand recovery at the completion of the immobilisation period (O'Connor et al., 2003; Plint, Perry, Correll, Gaboury, & Lawton, 2006).

Correcting Deformities and Preventing Contractures

If a body part is left immobile for a protracted period, joint capsule contraction and shortening of tendon and muscle groups that cross that joint occur. Such immobilisation occurs in many neurological conditions where the person loses the ability to activate the upper limb muscles. However, recovery from acute injury may also dictate immobilisation (e.g. immediately after skin graft surgery, tendon repairs or fracture). Loss of extensibility in muscles and soft tissues acting across a joint is a common sequela of immobilisation. Such losses in extensibility will result in imbalance between structures and can result in quite dramatic impairments (e.g. a small loss of extensibility of the wrist as a result of contracted structures such as flexor carpi radialis and ulnaris will dramatically impair grasps which require the wrist to be in midposition or greater wrist extension).

Biomechanical theory maintains that antideformity positioning and stretching is able to minimise shortening of tendons, collateral ligaments, joint capsules and muscle (Wilton, 2015). In many conditions, several predictable contractures occur in the upper limb; these contractures are generally associated with the flexed position of comfort. A key aspect to the reasoning process when aiming to prevent deformity is an understanding of the disease or condition processes coupled with a sound understanding of the available interventions that have good supporting research evidence. Although a strong history of practice supports the ability of an orthosis to correct deformity and prevent contracture, the evidence is less convincing (Harvey, deJong, Goehl, & Mardwedel, 2006; Harvey & Herbert, 2002; Katalinic et al., 2010).

Therapists may use static, semidynamic or dynamic orthoses to prevent the formation of, or to decrease, contracture (Fig. 38.7). However, the consistent aim is to provide a stretch. Static orthoses, such as casts or resting splints, are used to position joints so that a stretch is maintained on soft tissues. For example, for people with severe burns to the chest and upper limbs, axillary contractures are usually prevented by positioning the shoulders widely abducted with axillary splints, and elbow flexion contractures are minimized by statically splinting the elbow in extension. In the past, it was common for therapists to prevent contractures in the elbows of people after brain injury by using casts to maintain elbow extension and to increase range of motion in those people who had developed a contracture using serial casts. However, evidence now tells us that there is limited benefit to the use of stretch in preventing or improving contractures in the neurological population (Katalinic et al., 2010).

A semidynamic orthosis, such as a Lycra garment or tone-and-positioning splint (see Fig. 38.4), may also be used to provide a slow, low-force stretch while allowing some movement (Copley & Kuipers, 2014). Individually made Lycra garments are thought to produce continuous stretch of muscles for several hours. Such garments are more commonly used with children, although they are increasingly being used in rheumatoid arthritis, burn and neurological rehabilitation as well. A dynamic orthosis may also be applied for the purpose of preventing or treating contracture. A dynamic flexion splint after a flexor tendon repair provides controlled motion, protecting the healing tendon from excessive tension while allowing limited glide to prevent adherence of the tendon and the formation of a contracture.

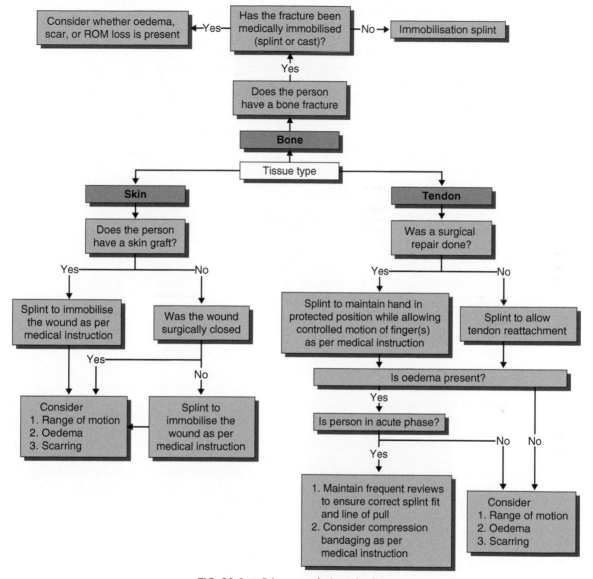

FIG. 38.6 ■ Primary goal: tissue healing.

The evidence to support splinting and casting for the management of contracture is limited, with the highest level of evidence suggesting stretch is not effective in preventing and improving contractures (Katalinic et al., 2010). In the adult neurological population, there is moderate- to high-quality evidence suggesting that stretch achieved using orthoses or alternative methods has little clinical benefit (Katalinic et al., 2010). There is less high-quality evidence to guide our practice in musculoskeletal conditions.

As a result of new evidence, occupational therapists have changed their practice when considering orthotic prescription with the aim of preventing contracture. The changing nature of evidence to guide our practice in the prescription of orthotics highlights the importance of therapists keeping abreast of current literature.

Correcting Deformities and Preventing Scarring

Wound healing from burns or open injuries is a multifaceted process, involving highly regulated cellular and chemical events intended to restore tissue integrity. Wound healing occurs

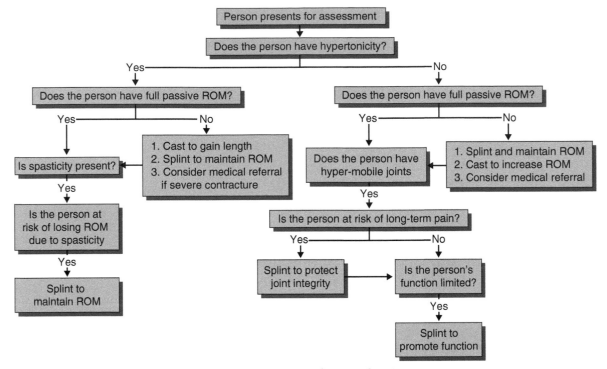

FIG. 38.7 ■ Primary goal: range of motion.

through scar formation. Scar tissue integrity is challenged if the new tissue structures are too weak, too strong or too abundant. This can result in hypertrophic scarring. Wounds are predisposed to hypertrophic scar formation when the healing process is prolonged, inflammation is present or the wound is scratched or if wound tension is excessive. Scar tissue is less elastic than normal soft tissue and thus can interfere with range of movement by preventing skin from moving adequately. Scar formation inside a wound can also cause adhesions that interfere with tendon gliding. Movement restrictions from lost skin elasticity or tendon glide can lead to further performance loss in the hand, affecting occupational role performance. Scar formation can also significantly affect the cosmesis of the hand and consequently the person's feeling about the limb's appearance and likely use (Kasch, 1998). Static splinting is common in burns management; however, there is no evidence to support the use of static splints and the need for randomised controlled trials in this area has been highlighted (Schouten, Nieuwehhuis, & van Zuijlen, 2012).

Intervention seeks to minimise scar formation, minimise scar adhesions and promote scar remodelling. Although an effective rehabilitation programme will also emphasise activity, stretch and exercise to prevent contracture development, therapy may additionally include the use of splints and compression to prevent scarring (Fig. 38.8). Mechanical pressure has long been advocated as a way to reduce or prevent scarring;

ever since research found that compression is able to rearrange the collagen in scars (Kischer, Shetlar, & Shetlar, 1975; Parks, Evans, & Larson, 1978). The reasoning behind using compression garments and splints on maturing scars is to apply perpendicular pressure that approximates capillary pressure (Carr-Collins, 1992). However, this theory has not been empirically tested. Despite this, a range of specialised scar management techniques are used, including scar compression garments which reduce the thickness of the resultant scar, massage to promote scar softening and extensibility, ultrasound, casts and splints with silicone gel sheet linings to promote scar elasticity and 'flattening'.

Scar management has been widely adopted in practice for reducing the performance and psychological effects of abnormal scar tissue. The evidence supporting the therapeutic approaches are inconclusive because of methodological weaknesses in the studies conducted (Mustoe et al., 2002; O'Brien & Pandit, 2006). Evidence-based guidelines recommend the use of silicone gel sheeting and intralesional corticosteroids for abnormal scar management (Mustoe et al., 2002), but a meta-analysis found no significant differences in efficacy between the varying approaches (Leventhal, Furr, & Reiter, 2006). New evidence is constantly being developed in this field. Weak evidence suggests that silicone gel sheeting reduces the incidence of scarring and improves scar elasticity (O'Brien & Pandit, 2006). Research also suggests that the wearing of burns compression garments

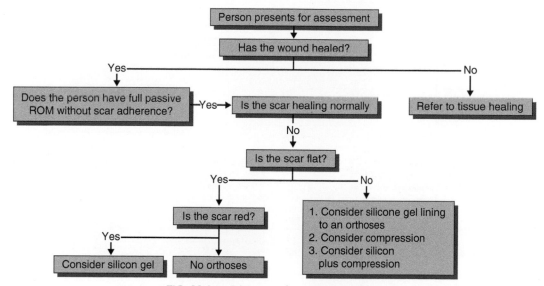

FIG. 38.8 ■ Primary goal: scar management.

reduces scar thickness (Van den Kerckhove et al., 2005). However, research data show that despite precise fitting techniques, pressure garments do not provide a consistent amount of pressure at the scar–garment interface (Macintyre & Baird, 2006). Reasoning must be applied in the treatment of scars; scientific evidence is inconclusive and the therapist must work with the person to determine the most appropriate intervention plan.

Improving Use of the Hand

Occupational therapists prescribe orthoses, in combination with adjunctive interventions, to facilitate attainment of occupational outcomes. Dynamic, semidynamic and static splints may be used to substitute for loss of movement (Fess et al., 2004). Consequently, an orthoses that aims to improve use of the hand will be one that takes into account not only the structural characteristics of the upper limb and hand but also the goals and preferences of the person who has the condition. As hand use is context and task specific, the selection, design and wearing protocol of a movement-enhancing orthoses must be based not only on the careful biomechanical assessment of upper limb and hand capacity and individual goals but also on the very best practice and research evidence available on the likely impact on recovery. Currently, much orthotic practice for the upper limb and hand is based on practice tradition, theoretical assumptions and a still emerging body of empirical evidence. Orthoses have, for example, been used for decades in practice to help 'position' a joint in a 'functional position' with the belief that use of the hand can then be more easily facilitated. Theoretical assumptions have also been made that

use of the hand will be improved with virtually all orthoses by diminishing pain, relieving movements and preventing deformity. These traditions and theoretical assumptions are being tested and there is a condition-specific evidence base under rapid development. Occupational therapists must keep up-to-date to ensure their selection, design and wearing protocol prescriptions for appropriate orthoses are evidence-based and relevant to varying conditions.

The types of hand movements that the therapist seeks to enhance through prescription of an orthoses include reach, grasp, release, carry, bimanual hand movements and in-hand manipulation. The application of an orthosis to improve hand use is likely to be a long-term therapy decision. Providing such orthoses therefore requires great care in assessment to ensure that the orthosis will correct biomechanical deficits and improve performance without causing secondary problems that can range from skin breakdown to social stigma. Central to long-term orthotic success is the wearer's willingness and ability to maintain appropriate wearing protocols. Consequently, comfort, observable change in either presenting symptoms or level of hand use, ease of application and cosmetic appearance are important user factors that could affect occupational outcomes.

Orthoses that improve hand use may be static, semidynamic or dynamic. The most common orthoses are static splints, which aim to immobilise either part or the whole of an upper limb or hand. Immobilisation can stabilise one component of the hand or arm to facilitate greater use of another aspect of the hand (Fig. 38.9).

The 'wrist cock-up splint' (Fig. 38.10) is such a splint and is seen commonly in practice and used with a wide variety of conditions. The rationale for the splint design is that if significant

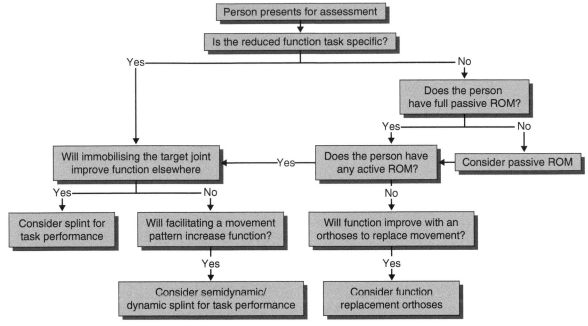

FIG. 38.9 ■ Primary goal: improving hand movement.

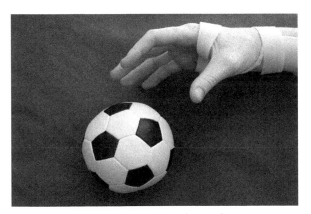

FIG. 38.10 ■ Wrist cock-up splint.

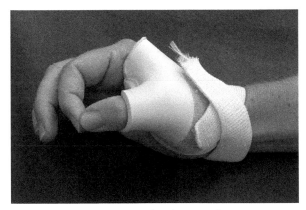

FIG. 38.11 ■ Thumb post splint.

weakness exists in finger extensors, the hand can compensate for the weakness by using an alternative movement pattern called 'tenodesis'. Tenodesis is when the person uses wrist flexion and extension, instead of finger extension, to open and close the fingers for grasp. If the occupational outcome of therapy requires finger extensor rather than tenodesis movement patterns, then an orthosis is required to prevent the unwanted pattern and facilitate the desired pattern. The wrist cock-up splint literally places the wrist at the desired angle, immobilises it to prevent wrist flexion and in doing so provides forced opportunities for active finger extension either as part of daily activity or as part of motor

training intervention. The wrist cock-up splint is thus commonly used when occupations requiring precise grasp and accurate hand aperture during prehension are therapy goals.

Another orthosis that operates on the basis of immobilising one joint to permit movement in another to achieve performance is the 'thumb post' splint (Fig. 38.11). Here the central biomechanical challenge being met by the splint is that of supporting an unstable metacarpal phalangeal joint (MCP) joint or blocking undesired thumb adduction and flexion movements. The orthotic material is figuratively moulded around the thumb, forming a type of 'post' to immobilise the MCP joint of the thumb into midrange flexion and abduction and at times aiming to block MCP hyperextension. The orthoses modifies or restores the position of the hand and thumb to externally facilitate desired thumb opposition movement for the pincer grasp.

Hand use can also be improved using dynamic or semidynamic orthoses. These are particularly useful when the occupational outcome requires weak movements to be assisted. The selection of material for fabrication is critical in these splints as it is the degree of active or passive force being applied that must match the biomechanical goal to support the occupational outcome. Common fabrication materials are Lycra or neoprene garments, or springs or elastic band components attached to thermoplastic base splints. An example of a common semidynamic orthosis used to promote a desired movement is the TAP splint (see Fig. 38.4). The TAP splint is made of neoprene. It helps the wearer to use supination and increase supination strength, as the splint wraps around the upper limb and is anchored at key joints in such a way to facilitate supination. It is the elastic properties of the neoprene that dynamically assist the movement.

Orthoses that improve hand use can also be developed to actually replace a movement that has been lost and is either unlikely to recover or is immediately needed by the person to achieve occupational goals. In these instances the orthosis replaces the upper limb or hand movement in the task. Common examples are splints designed to hold a pen, pencil or eating instrument, orthoses to allow wheel control while driving a car, and orthoses to type on a computer. In addition, neural stimulation devices can be inserted into orthoses to facilitate muscle contractions for hand use. These developing sophisticated devices usually require multidisciplinary expertise, including biomedical engineers or specialist prosthetic and orthotic professionals to devise safe and appropriate inclusions.

The literature researching the effectiveness of splinting in improving hand use is laden with methodological flaws. This is because the theoretical assumptions for orthotic intervention have changed so significantly over time, particularly in the field of hypertonicity management. Based on newer basic scientific evidence, no longer do occupational therapists believe that they reduce the muscle spasticity associated with hypertonicity using orthoses. A change in the focus of practice, from addressing underlying body functions and structures to now addressing activities and participation, has further enhanced our knowledge of how the hand should best be supported to maximise occupational outcomes. Rather than trying to position the hand in a 'typical' position for carrying out an occupation, we now know that supporting the hand in the position that best enables a person to use it is most effective. The evidence base for orthoses for improving hand use continues to lag behind, as research studies have included orthoses designed to simultaneously reduce spasticity and improve hand use, which confounds the interpretation of findings. In addition to major problems with orthosis design, most of the studies lack methodological rigor and appropriate outcome measures. There is a pressing need for more research in this area of practice, where newer studies employ appropriate methodologies and are underpinned by sound theory. To date,

the systematic review evidence about the efficacy of splinting people with hypertonicity to improve hand use is inconclusive. This is because orthoses need to be task specific (making clinical trial comparison difficult), which has resulted in few trials and a body of evidence built predominantly on studies of low methodological quality (Autti-Ramo, Anttila, Malmivaara. & Makela, 2006; Jackman, Novak, & Lannin, 2014; Teplicky, Law, & Russell, 2002). Randomized trials have been conducted in adults with stroke and brain injury, and results which showed limited effect of static splinting have changed the profession's clinical thinking (Lannin, Horsley, Herbert, McCluskey, & Cusick, 2003; Lannin, Cusick, McCluskey, & Herbert, 2007).

The evidence base for splinting to improve hand use in orthopaedic and trauma conditions is more robust. Positive evidence supports the use of dynamic extensor bracing for lateral epicondylitis to reduce pain while improving upper limb use and grip strength (Faes, van den Akker, de Lint, Kooloos, & Hopman, 2006). In addition, splinting the thumb joint of people with osteoarthritis leads to performance gain. These improvements are achieved no matter what thumb splint design is used (Wajon & Ada, 2005). However, the additional benefit of splinting is difficult to estimate when placebo controlled trials have yet to be conducted. Splinting is also useful for people with acute hand injuries. In this population, dynamic splinting initially produces the greatest rate of recovery, but by 6 months the performance outcomes of dynamic and static splints are equivalent (Mowlavi, Burns, & Brown, 2005).

Dynamic taping is another orthotic mechanism that is gaining popularity. Tape with elastic properties is applied to the limb with tension in an effort to compensate for weak or ineffective muscles. There is emergent evidence to support the use of dynamic taping for people with musculoskeletal conditions (Parreira, Costa, Hespnhol, Lopes, & Costa, 2014). Trial data suggest that taping improves both movement skills and activities of daily living performance in children with cerebral palsy, presumably by increasing proprioceptive feedback (Kaya Kara et al., 2015).

There is moderate-quality evidence to support splints improving hand use for people with inflammatory disorders, such as arthritis (Egan, Brosseau, Ouimet, Rees, Wells, & Tugwell, 2003). Evidence suggests that immobilisation of the wrist joint, in any variety of splint design, improves hand use and grip strength (Haskett, Backman, Porter, Goyert, & Palejko, 2004). These gains appear to be short-lived and applicable only to those with a more chronic or progressed inflammatory disease (Adams et al., 2008). It is important for occupational therapists to acknowledge that prescription of orthoses must have individualised benefits and fit with a person's occupational needs (Pagnotta, Korner-Bitensky, Mazer, Baron, & Wood-Dauphinee, 2005).

Reducing Pain

Orthoses may be appropriate when pain affects the attainment of occupational goals, and the provision of external structural support can help alleviate it. Occupational therapists should have a good understanding of pain mechanisms and the person's condition to determine whether or not the use of an orthoses will assist or whether there could be adverse consequences from continued use (in a dynamic or semidynamic splint or static orthosis) or disuse (with a static splint). The occupational therapist also needs to have a good understanding of the underlying pathology of different conditions to inform this decision.

Musculoskeletal pain may be as a result of stretch of a muscle, ligament or tendon, irritation of the synovial membrane, or abnormal movement in a joint, muscle or ligament. Joint pain may be caused by inflammation with resulting swelling and distension. Pain may be brought on by only the smallest amount of movement, or only at the extremes of range or upon actual stretching. When biomechanical factors and features of the condition are considered in the context of occupational goals, an orthosis will be only one of a range of pain management options. If an orthosis is required, the design will focus on positions, structures and support that prevent movements that must be avoided and permit stress or weight bearing where it is allowed and contraction of those muscles that are safe and required in specified uses (Fig. 38.12). In acute musculoskeletal conditions, or where pain is produced by overuse, fatigue or stretch, the choice of orthosis may be restricted to static immobilisation splints to enforce rest.

The evidence on the effectiveness of orthoses achieving pain reduction is mostly favourable but varies from one condition and joint to another. At the shoulder, the most effective treatments for reducing pain from subacromial impingement syndrome (SAIS) are not orthotics but rather other techniques such as exercise (Hanratty et al., 2012), joint mobilisation and laser therapy (Michner, Walsworth, & Burnet, 2004; Sauers,

2005). However, if the shoulder pain is secondary to cerebrovascular accident, the evidence to support pain reduction via orthoses such as shoulder slings is inconclusive because of poor methodological quality (Page & Lockwood, 2003), and alternative treatments, such as intramuscular electrical stimulation, may be more effective (Chae, Yu, Walder et al., 2005).

For the forearm, where pain is often associated with lateral epicondylosis ('tennis elbow'), orthoses are commonly prescribed to induce 'rest' by limiting movement, but the supporting scientific evidence is inconclusive (Borkholder, Hill, & Fess, 2004; Nimgade, Sullivan, & Goldman, 2005). Steroid injections during the first 3 months provide the most relief of all available interventions. Active therapies, such as acupuncture, exercise and ultrasound, are more effective than resting for reducing pain (Trudel et al., 2004).

To reduce the wrist pain associated with carpal tunnel syndrome (CTS), the following treatments are effective: splinting where wrist motion is immobilised without compressing the carpal tunnel, ultrasound, nerve gliding exercises, magnetic therapy and manual therapy (Muller et al., 2004). There continues to be limited evidence to support the use of night resting splints for carpel tunnel syndrome (Werner, Franzblau, & Gell, 2005; Page, Massy-Westropp, O'Connor, & Pitt, 2012). Splinting has been found to be equally as effective as steroid injections for reducing pain (Mishra, Prabhakar, Lal, & Modi, 2006) but is less effective than surgery (Gerritsen et al., 2002).

However, if the wrist pain is caused by rheumatoid arthritis, the scientific evidence depends on the type to orthosis. There does not appear to be any added benefit to prescribing rest in an orthosis after intraarticular steroid injections to reduce pain (Wallen & Gilles, 2006). Semidynamic orthoses have been found to reduce

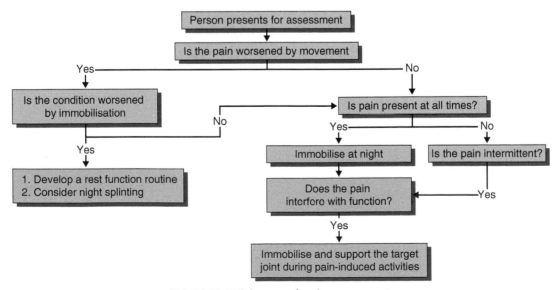

FIG. 38.12 ■ Primary goal: pain management.

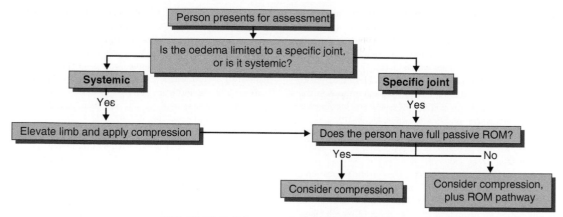

FIG. 38.13 ■ Primary goal: oedema management.

pain in rheumatoid arthritis, compared to wearing no orthosis (Veehof, Taal, Heijnsdijk-Rouwenhorst, & van de Laar, 2008).

Decreasing Oedema

When a person experiences burns, grafts, traumatic injury or conditions that result in immobilised and dependent limbs such as peripheral or central nerve damage, there is a risk of oedema. Oedema can contribute to joint stiffness and contracture, and reducing oedema is an important preventative and rehabilitative strategy (Fig. 38.13).

Although there is little scientific evidence to help inform therapists in this area of the best approach, there is no evidence that commonly used interventions are harmful if compression garments are worn correctly and safely; instead a systematic review (Geurts, Visschers, van Limbeek, & Ribbers, 2000) reported that no specific treatment has yet proven its advantage over other physical methods for reducing hand oedema that occurs after neurological damage (i.e. dependent oedema). The current approach to alleviating oedema is the provision of retrograde massage, with limb elevation and consistent limb pressure through circumferential orthoses (e.g. custom-fitted Lycra garments, tubular elastic dressings or elastic wrap bandaging). As there is a limited evidence base, occupational therapists who prescribe such orthoses must be alert to the safety aspects of splint and garment use: the impact that oedema has had on underlying structures and the line-of-pull of a splint; the person's ability to don a compression garment correctly and safely when supervised and unsupervised, with or without assistance; and the overall benefit for the person when fitting, purchasing and monitoring costs.

CONCLUSION

There is considerable variation in splinting practices. These variations include the design of the orthosis, critical period of orthotic use, wearing regimen, duration of use and theoretical rationale behind the orthosis. In practice, no simple design or type of orthosis exists that applies to all people who present with the same diagnosis. Selecting the orthosis, the position of the hand or arm and the wearing protocol will vary because each person is an individual, with unique occupational goals, unique injury or disease processes and unique rehabilitation goals.

The ability to professionally reason is based on the therapist's knowledge about the person's diagnosis, awareness of the person's occupational goals, motivation and compliance, an understanding of orthotic protocols and techniques, and practice experience. The reasoning of a therapist is informed by an ever-increasing evidence base. Key to improving outcomes is encouraging individual therapists to explicitly seek out and factor in scientifically gained knowledge into their daily decision making and involving end users (clinicians) in designing the very research on which we want to base our practices (Gooberman-Hill et al., 2013). Of course, this entails overcoming the inertia of practicing within the 'comfort zones' that occupational therapists have developed based on their training and constantly remaining abreast of scientific evidence.

Orthoses have historically been an integral part of the occupational therapy process when regaining performance or movement in the hand and upper limb. Each orthosis has a unique goal, and as the therapeutic goal changes, the design and use of the orthosis needs to be reconsidered in light of the person's occupational performance. As the occupational therapy body of research evidence evolves, so too must therapists' reasoning. In the future, it may be that therapists have more effective and efficient methods to produce better outcomes than those interventions currently used.

e http://evolve.elsevier.com/Curtin/OT

REFERENCES

Adams, J., Burridge, J., Mullee, M., Hammond, A., & Cooper, C. (2008). The clinical effectiveness of static resting splints in early rheumatoid arthritis: A randomised controlled trial. *Rheumatology, 47*, 1548–1553.

American Society of Hand Therapists (ASHT) (1992). *Splint classification system.* Chicago: ASHT.

Appel, C., Perry, L., & Jones, F. (2014). Shoulder strapping for stroke-related upper limb dysfunction and shoulder impairments: Systematic review. *NeuroRehabilitation, 35*(2), 191–204.

Autti-Ramo, I. S. J., Anttila, H., Malmivaara, A., & Makela, M. (2006). Effectiveness of upper and lower limb casting and orthoses in children with cerebral palsy: An overview of review articles. *American Journal Physical Medicine and Rehabilitation, 85,* 89–103.

Borkholder, C. D., Hill, V. A., & Fess, E. E. (2004). The efficacy of splinting for lateral epicondylitis: A systematic review. *Journal of Hand Therapy, 17*(2), 181–199.

Carr-Collins, J. A. (1992). Pressure techniques for the prevention of hypertrophic scar. *Clinics in Plastic Surgery, 19*(3), 733–743.

Chae, J., Yu, D. T., Walder, M. E., et al. (2005). Intramuscular electrical stimulation for hemiplegic should pain: A 12-month follow-up of a multiple-centre, randomized clinical trial. *American Journal of Physical Medicine & Rehabilitation, 84*(11), 832–842.

Clare, T. D., de Haviland Mee, S., & Belcher, H. J. C. R. (2004). Rehabilitation of digital nerve repair: Is splinting necessary? *Journal of Hand Surgery, 29B*(6), 552–556.

Copley, J., & Kuipers, K. (2014). *Neurorehabilitation of the upper limb across the lifespan: Managing hypertonicity for optimal function.* West Sussex: Wiley.

Coppard, B. M., & Lohman, H. (2008). *Introduction to splinting: A critical-thinking and problem-solving approach* (3rd ed.). St. Louis: Mosby.

Dunn, W. (2000). *Best practice occupational therapy.* Thorofare, NJ: Slack.

Egan, M., Brosseau, L., Ouimet, M. A., Rees, S., Wells, G., & Tugwell, P. (2003). Splints/orthoses in the treatment of rheumatoid arthritis. *Cochrane Database of Systematic Reviews, 1.*

Faes, M., van den Akker, B., de Lint, J. A., Kooloos, J. G., & Hopman, M. T. (2006). Dynamic extensor brace for lateral epicondylitis. *Clinical Orthopaedics and Related Research, 443,* 149–157.

Farmer, S. E., & James, M. (2001). Contractures in orthopaedic and neurological conditions: A review of causes and treatment. *Disability and Rehabilitation, 23,* 549–558.

Farrar, J. T., Young, J. P., LaMoreaux, L., Werth, J. L., & Michael, P. R. (2001). Clinical importance of changes in chronic pain intensity measured on an 11-point numerical pain rating scale. *Pain, 94,* 149–158.

Fess, E. E., Gettle, K., Philips, C. A., & Janson, R. (2004). *Hand and upper extremity splinting principles and methods* (3rd ed.). St. Louis: Mosby.

Gerritsen, A. A. M., de Vet, H. C. W., Scholten, R. J. P. M., Bertelsmann, F. W., de Krom, M. C. T. F. M., & Bouter, L. M. (2002). Splinting vs surgery in the treatment of carpal tunnel syndrome. *Journal of American Medical Association, 288*(10), 1245–1251.

Geurts, A. C., Visschers, B. A., van Limbeek, J., & Ribbers, G. M. (2000). Systematic review of aetiology and treatment of post-stroke hand oedema and shoulder-hand syndrome. *Scandinavian Journal of Rehabilitation Medicine, 32*(1), 4–10.

Gooberman-Hill, R., Jinks, C., Barbosa Boucas, S., et al. (2013). Designing a placebo device: Involving service users in clinical trial design. *Health Expectations, 16*(4), e100–e110.

Goga-Eppenstien, P., Hill, J. P., Philip, P. A., Philip, M., Seifert, T. M., & Yasukawa, A. M. (1999). *Casting protocols for the upper and lower extremities.* Gaithersburg: Aspen.

Handoll, H. H. G., & Vaghela, M. V. (2004). Interventions for treating mallet finger injuries. *Cochrane Database of Systematic Reviews, 3.*

Hanratty, C. E., McVeigh, J. G., Kerr, D. P., et al. (2012). The effectiveness of physiotherapy exercises in subacromial impingement syndrome: A systematic review and meta-analysis. *Seminars in Arthritis and Rheumatism, 42,* 297–316.

Harvey, L., de Jong, I., Goehl, G., & Mardwedel, S. (2006). Twelve weeks of nightly stretch does not reduce thumb web-space contractures in people with a neurological condition: A randomised controlled trial. *Australian Journal of Physiotherapy, 52*(4), 251–258.

Harvey, L. A., & Herbert, R. D. (2002). Muscle stretching for treatment and prevention of contracture in people with spinal cord injury. *Spinal Cord, 40*(1), 1–9.

Haskett, S., Backman, C., Porter, B., Goyert, J., & Palejko, G. (2004). A crossover trial of custom-made and commercially available wrist splints in adults with inflammatory arthritis. *Arthritis and Rheumatism, 15*(5), 792–799.

Hudak, P. L., Amadio, P. C., & Bombardier, C. (1996). Development of an upper extremity outcome measure: the DASH (disabilities of the arm, shoulder and hand) [corrected]. The Upper Extremity Collaborative Group (UECG). *American Journal of Industrial Medicine, 29*(6), 602–608.

Hurn, J., Kneebone, I., & Cropley, M. (2006). Goal setting as an outcome measure: A systematic review. *Clinical Rehabilitation, 20*(9), 756–772.

Jackman, M., Novak, I., & Lannin, N. (2014). Effectiveness of hand splint in children with cerebral palsy: A systematic review with meta-analysis. *Developmental Medicine & Child Neurology, 56*(2), 138–147.

Jacobs, M., & Austin, N. (2014). *Orthotic intervention for the hand and upper extremity: Splinting principles and processes* (2nd ed.). Philadelphia: Wolters Kluwer Health/Lippincott Williams and Wilkins.

Kaya Kara, O., Atasavun Uysal, S., Turker, D., Karayazgan, S., Gunel, M. K., & Baltaci, G. (2015). The effects of Kinesio Taping on body functions and activity in unilateral spastic cerebral palsy: A single-blind randomized controlled trial. *Developmental Medicine & Child Neurology, 57*(1), 81–88.

Kasch, M. A. (1998). Clinical management of scar tissue. In F. S. Cromwell, & J. Bear-Lehman (Eds.), *Hand rehabilitation in occupational therapy* (pp. 37–52). Philadelphia: Haworth Press.

Katalinic, O. M., Harvey, L. A., Herbert, R. D., Moseley, A. M., Lannin, N. A., & Schurr, K. (2010). Stretch for the treatment and prevention of contractures. *Cochrane Database of Systematic Reviews, 9.*

Kischer, C. W., Shetlar, M. R., & Shetlar, C. L. (1975). Alteration of hypertrophic scars induced by mechanical pressure. *Archives of Dermatology, 111,* 60–64.

Kogler, G. F. (2002). Orthotic management. In D. A. Gelber, & D. R. Jeffery (Eds.), *Clinical evaluation and management of spasticity* (pp. 67–91). Totowa, NJ: Humana.

Lannin, N., Horsley, S., Herbert, R., McCluskey, A., & Cusick, A. (2003). Splinting the hand in the functional position after brain impairment: A randomized controlled trial. *Archives of Physical Medicine and Rehabilitation, 84,* 297–302.

Lannin, N. A., Cusick, A., McCluskey, A., & Herbert, R. D. (2007). Effects of splinting on wrist contracture after stroke: A randomized controlled trial. *Stroke, 38*(1), 111–116.

Lannin, N. A., Novak, I., & Cusick, A. (2007). A systematic review of upper extremity casting for children and adults with central nervous system motor disorders. *Clinical Rehabilitation, 21*, 963–976.

Law, M., Baptiste, S., McColl, M., Opzoomer, A., Polatajko, H., & Pollock, N. (1990). The Canadian Occupational Performance Measure: An outcome measure for occupational therapy. *Canadian Journal of Occupational Therapy, 57*(2), 82–87.

Leventhal, D., Furr, M., & Reiter, D. (2006). Treatment of keloids and hypertrophic scars: A meta-analysis and review of the literature. *Archives of Facial and Plastic Surgery, 8*(6), 362–368.

Lowe, C. T. (1995). Construction of hand splints. In C. A. Trombly (Ed.), *Occupational therapy for physical dysfunction* Baltimore: Williams & Wilkins.

Macintyre, L., & Baird, M. (2006). Pressure garments for use in the treatment of hypertrophic scars—a review of the problems associated with their use. *Burns, 32*(1), 10–15.

Melzack, R. (1987). The short-form McGill pain questionnaire. *Pain, 30*, 193.

Michner, L. A., Walsworth, M. K., & Burnet, E. N. (2004). Effectiveness of rehabilitation for patients with subacromial impingement syndrome: A systematic review. *Journal of Hand Therapy, 17*, 152–164.

Milazzo, S., & Gillen, G. (2011). Splinting applications. In G. Gillen, & A. Burkhardt (Eds.), *Stroke rehabilitation: A function-based approach* St. Louis: Mosby.

Mishra, S., Prabhakar, S., Lal, V., & Modi, M. (2006). Efficacy of splinting and oral steroids in the treatment of carpal tunnel syndrome: A prospective randomized clinical and electrophysiological study. *Neurology India, 54*(3), 286–290.

Montalvo, A. M., Cara, E. L., & Myer, G. D. (2014). Effect of kinesiology taping on pain in individuals with musculoskeletal injuries: Systematic review and meta-analysis. *Physician and Sportsmedicine, 42*(2), 48–57.

Morris, D., Jones, D., Ryan, H., & Ryan, C. G. (2013). The clinical effects of Kinesio® Tex taping: A systematic review. *Physiotherapy Theory and Practice, 29*(4), 259–270.

Mowlavi, A., Burns, M., & Brown, R. E. (2005). Dynamic versus static splinting of simple zone V and zone IV extensor tendon repairs: A prospective, randomized, controlled study. *Plastic and Reconstructive Surgery, 115*(2), 482–487.

Muller, M., Tsui, D., Schnurr, R., Biddulph-Deisroth, L., Hard, J., & MacDermid, J. C. (2004). Effectiveness of hand therapy interventions in primary management of carpal tunnel syndrome: A systematic review. *Journal of Hand Therapy, 17*, 210–228.

Mustoe, T. A., Cooter, R. D., Gold, M. H., et al., International Advisory Panel on Scar Management. (2002). International clinical recommendations on scar management. *Plastic and Reconstructive Surgery, 110*(2), 560–571.

Nimgade, A., Sullivan, M., & Goldman, R. (2005). Physiotherapy, steroid injections, or rest for lateral epicondylosis? What the evidence suggests. *World Institute of Pain, 5*(3), 203–215.

O'Brien, L., & Pandit, A. (2006). Silicone gel sheeting for preventing and treating hypertrophic and keloid scars. *Cochrane Database of Systematic Reviews, 25*(1).

O'Connor, D., Mullett, H., Doyle, M., Mofidi, A., Kutty, S., & O'Sullivan, M. (2003). Minimally displaced Colles' fractures: A prospective randomized trial of treatment with a wrist splint or a plaster cast. *Journal of Hand Surgery, 28*(1), 50–53.

Ottenbacher, K. J., & Cusick, A. (1990). Goal attainment scaling as a method of clinical service evaluation. *American Journal of Occupational Therapy, 44*(6), 519–525.

Page, T., & Lockwood, C. (2003). Systematic review: Prevention and management of shoulder pain in the hemiplegic patient. *Joanna Briggs Institute Reports, 1*, 149–165.

Page, M. J., Massy-Westropp, N., O'Connor, D., & Pitt, V. (2012). Splinting for carpal tunnel syndrome. *Cochrane Database of Systematic Reviews, 7*.

Pagnotta, A., Korner-Bitensky, N., Mazer, B., Baron, M., & Wood-Dauphinee, S. (2005). Static wrist splint use in the performance of daily activities by individuals with rheumatoid arthritis. *Journal of Rheumatology, 32*, 2136–2143.

Parreira, P. C. S., Costa, L. C. M., Hespnhol, L. C., Lopes, A. D., & Costa, L. O. P. (2014). Current evidence does not support the use of Kinesio Taping in clinical practice: A systematic review. *Journal of Physiotherapy, 60*(1), 31–39.

Parks, D. H., Evans, E. B., & Larson, D. L. (1978). Prevention and correction of deformity after severe burns. *The Surgery Clinics of North America, 58*(6), 1279–1289.

Plint, A. C., Perry, J. J., Correll, R., Gaboury, I., & Lawton, L. (2006). A randomized, controlled trial of removable splinting versus casting for wrist buckle fractures in children. *Pediatrics, 117*(3), 691–697.

Poole, J. L., Cordova, K. J., & Brower, L. M. (2006). Reliability and validity of a self-report of hand function in persons with rheumatoid arthritis. *Journal of Hand Therapy, 19*(1), 12–16.

Sauers, E. L. (2005). Effectiveness of rehabilitation for patients with subacromial impingement syndrome. *Journal of Athletic Training, 40*(3), 221–223.

Schouten, H. J., Nieuwenhuis, M. K., & van Zuijlen, P. P. M. (2012). A review on static splinting theapy to prevent burn scar contracture: Do clinical and experimental data warrant it's clinical application? *Burns, 38*(1), 19–25.

Taly, A. B., Nair, K. P., Murali, T., & Wankade, M. (2002). Pneumatic splints: Fabrication and use in neurorehabilitation. *Neurology India, 50*, 68–70.

Teplicky, R., Law, M., & Russell, D. (2002). The effectiveness of casts, orthoses, and splints for children with neurological disorders. *Infants and Young Children, 15*, 42–50.

Trudel, D., Duley, J., Zastrow, I., Kerr, E. W., Davidson, R., & MacDermid, J. C. (2004). Rehabilitation for patients with lateral epicondylitis: A systematic review. *Journal of Hand Therapy, 17*(2), 243–266.

Unsworth, C. (2000). Measuring the outcome of occupational therapy: Tools and resources. *Australian Occupational Therapy Journal, 47*, 147–158.

Van den Kerckhove, E., Stappaerts, K., Fieuws, S., et al. (2005). The assessment of erythema and thickness on burn related scars during pressure garment therapy as a preventative measure for hypertrophic scarring. *Burns, 31*(6), 696–702.

Veehof, M. M., Taal, I., Heijnsdijk-Rouwenhorst, L. M., & van de Laar, M. A. F. J. (2008). Efficacy of wrist working splints in patients with rheumatoid arthritis: A randomised controlled study. *Arthritis and Rheumatism, 59*(12), 1698–1704.

Wajon, A., & Ada, L. (2005). No difference between two splint and exercise regimens for people with osteoarthritis of the thumb: A randomized controlled trial. *Australian Journal of Physiotherapy, 52*(1), 60.

Wallen, M., & Gilles, D. (2006). Intra-articular steroids and splints/restfor children with juvenile idiopathic arthritis and adults with rheumatoid arthritis. *Cochrane Database of Systematic Reviews, 1.*

Werner, R. A., Franzblau, A., & Gell, N. (2005). Randomized controlled trail of nocturnal splinting for active workers with symptoms of carpal tunnel syndrome. *Archives of Physical Medicine and Rehabilitation, 86*(1), 1–7.

Wilton, J. C. (2015). *Hand splinting / orthotic intervention: Principles of design and fabrication* (Revised ed.). Fremantle: Vivid Publishing.

Wright, F. V., Rosenbaum, P. L., Goldsmith, C. H., Law, M., & Fehlings, D. L. (2008). How do changes in body functions and strutures, activity, and participation relate in children with cerebral palsy? *Developmental Medicine & Child Neurology, 50,* 621–629.

39

WORKING WITH PEOPLE LIVING WITH VISION IMPAIRMENT

ALEXANDRA LONSDALE ■ CARLIA RIX ■ KIRSTY STEWART

CHAPTER OUTLINE

Abstract
Promoting and enabling independence for people living with vision impairment is a primary role of occupational therapy across a broad spectrum of specialist and general practice settings. People living with vision impairment require adaptive strategies and techniques to achieve their goals, aiming to promote health and well-being through social integration, meaningful engagement and participation at home, at work and in the community. Occupational therapy plays a fundamental role in fostering people's self-efficacy to attain occupational goals and independence. Specialist assessments and enabling strategies focus on light adaptation, contrast, magnification and developing compensatory skills by enhancing touch, smell, hearing and taste senses and visual memory. By incorporating specialist techniques and adaptive technologies based on brighter, bigger, bolder principles, therapists work to promote occupational performance by maximising functional vision in occupational environments and performance contexts.

KEY POINTS

- Occupational therapists have a fundamental role in promoting independence, self-efficacy and meaningful engagement in occupations for people living with vision impairment at home and in the community through adaptation and compensatory strategies.

- Occupational therapy assessment and enabling strategies for people living with vision impairment are based on brighter, bigger, bolder principles.

- Many occupational therapists have the opportunity to address vision impairment in general practice.

- Practical strategies guiding occupational practice in vision impairment are transferable to a variety of settings.

- There are a range of readily accessible resources to guide occupational therapy practice.

■ Occupational therapists working with an aging population will face increased prevalence of people requiring support to adapt to living with vision impairment.

INTRODUCTION

Vision is a primary part of the sensory system responsible for processing sensory information. Vision and visual perception involve motor, cognitive, communicative and emotive functions that allow for the rapid assimilation of details from the environment to enable decision making (Zolton, 2007). Vision enables people to see the beauty of the world, such as a sunset across the ocean; observe body language, such as making eye contact and nodding to indicate interest during a conversation; and to notice hazards in the environment, such as overhanging branches at head height or objects on a path.

It is estimated that more than 285 million people worldwide have a visual impairment; 39 million of these people are legally visually blind and 246 million have low vision. Approximately 90% of people with vision impairment live in low-income settings, with cataracts and uncorrected refractive errors being the main cause of vision loss within these populations. Approximately 82% of all people who are visually impaired are older than 50 years (World Health Organization, 2012). With an increasingly elderly population in many countries, greater numbers of people will be at risk of visual impairment as a result of chronic eye diseases and the aging process.

There are many reasons why a person's vision can be compromised, including congenital conditions, aging, disease, trauma and infections. The impact of living with vision impairment can be devastating as vision is a major physiological factor that enables a person to engage in occupation (Baum & Christiansen, 2005). It is because of the impact that vision has on a person's ability to engage in occupation that occupational therapists have a role in assisting people with vision impairment to engage in meaningful occupations by maximising their functional vision by using compensatory or rehabilitative techniques.

Occupational therapists* work to ensure that people with vision impairment are able to participate and engage in their chosen occupations and local communities. Therapists assess and develop intervention strategies for individuals with functional difficulties associated with vision loss. Often this work is carried out by a multidisciplinary team in a hospital, clinic or community setting, to ensure a holistic service is delivered to meet the needs of the individual. Visual impairment may affect a person's occupational performance in a number of ways, including the following:

■ Personal care activities, such as showering, dressing, grooming, eating, medication management and care of children
■ Domestic activities, such as meal preparation, cooking tasks, use of appliances, home maintenance tasks, laundry tasks, functional use of technology, writing and reading tasks, telephone use and time management
■ Community-based activities, such as money handling, banking and shopping
■ Recreational activities, such as craftwork, sports and hobbies
■ Accessing the home environment, including the bathroom, kitchen, lighting, front and back entrances
■ Accessing the work or educational environment, including functional and ergonomic use of technology

This chapter aims to introduce the functional difficulties people with a vision impairment may have and provide a platform for occupational therapists to assist these people to engage in personally meaningful occupation. Common themes around assessment, strategies and equipment are explored and resources for gaining further information are included.

VISION IMPAIRMENT

The World Health Organization (WHO) uses the term *visual impairment* to collectively describe low vision (moderate and severe visual impairment) and blindness (Resnikoff, Pascolini, Mariotti, & Pokharel, 2008). WHO defines low vision as vision equal to or less than 6/18 in visual acuity and blindness as vision equal to or less than 3/60 visual acuity. In practical terms, *low vision* refers to a level of vision that cannot be corrected to a visual acuity close to 6/6 with glasses, contact lenses or medical treatment.

Vision impairment can present as a reduction in visual acuity, visual field loss or a combination of both. It may remain stable or deteriorate over time. There are a number of conditions that cause vision impairment that a person can be born with, acquire or develop later in life; for the most common conditions that therapists may encounter when working with older adults in Western populations, refer to Table 39.1.

The Visual System

To understand the many reasons why vision loss can occur, it is important to understand the basic anatomy and physiology of the eye and visual system (Fig. 39.1). The visual pathway begins

---

Postgraduate Training: Postgraduate training for occupational therapists within this area of practice varies from country to country. For example, the United States of America has established the first graduate certificate in low-vision rehabilitation (also available to international students). This training is designed for occupational therapists already working in low-vision rehabilitation, those interested in starting low-vision rehabilitation programmes, and those just interested in expanding their practice skill (Warren, n.d.). In the United Kingdom, therapists can complete a degree in rehabilitation for people with visual impairment (Birmingham City University, 2015). Occupational therapists are encouraged to seek opportunities for additional professional development through tertiary providers and professional development courses provided by organisations and institutions.

TABLE 39.1

Common Vision Conditions in Adults (Western Population)

Condition	Definition	Functional Implications
Albinism	A hereditary condition in which there is a lack of pigment (melanin), either throughout the entire body or within the eyes. Lack of pigment does not allow the vision to develop fully.	Reduced visual acuity Nystagmus (involuntary movement of both eyes) Sensitive to glare
Cataracts	Occurs when the lens of the eye becomes cloudy, blocking the passage of light to the retina. Cataracts may be congenital or develop later in life.	Blurred vision (i.e. seeing any detail may be difficult) Depth perception issues Colour vision dulled May be sensitive to glare
Charles Bonnet syndrome	A term used to describe the situation when people with vision problems see things that they know are not real. Sometimes called visual hallucinations, the things people see can take all kinds of forms, from simple patterns of straight lines to detailed pictures of people or buildings.	May cause emotional distress, resulting in anxiety and social isolation
Diabetic retinopathy	Changes in the blood vessels within the retina, such as bleeding or blocking up, cause vision loss; can accompany long-term diabetes. The amount of vision loss depends on the extent of the damage. Blindness may result.	Dependant on extent and location of damage to vision
Glaucoma	Caused by an imbalance in the internal pressure within the eye relative to the ability of the nerve tissue to resist pressure. Total blindness may occur if not detected and treated. Drops, tablets or surgery are used to control the pressure and prevent further sight loss.	Progressive vision loss Peripheral vision loss that can lead to orientation and mobility difficulties May be sensitive to glare (i.e. bright environments may cause difficulty seeing) Reduced contrast perception
Hemianopia	The absence of half of the visual field, occurring on opposite sides or on the same side in one or both eyes. This is commonly associated with an interruption to the blood supply or an obstruction along the optic pathway between the optic chiasm and occipital lobe of the brain.	Location of the obstruction will determine type of hemianopia Difficulty with orientation and mobility (i.e. bumping into door frames, not seeing hazards when crossing a road, bumping into other people) May not see objects placed on the affected side
Keratoconus	An eye condition in which there is a bulging forward of the central cornea (clear front surface of the eye) with thinning and scarring as a result. Treated by way of hard contact lenses, which aim to reduce the growth of the cornea as well as provide clearer vision. In extreme cases, a corneal transplant may be performed.	Progressive vision loss May be sensitive to glare Distorted vision makes seeing detail difficult (i.e. when reading, seeing faces)
Macular degeneration	A condition causing the deterioration of the central vision. Peripheral (side) vision remains. Treatments in the form of antiangiogenic drugs and laser therapy are available that may slow or pause the progression of the degeneration.	Progressive vision loss Increasing difficulty viewing detail (i.e. reading, writing, seeing faces) Colour vision becomes dulled Issues with depth perception and reduced contrast sensitivity (i.e. stairs, uneven surfaces and liquid levels may be difficulty to perceive)
Nystagmus	Nystagmus is fine, continual and involuntary movement of both eyes. The nystagmus eye movement is controlled by brain centres, and all movements are nonintentional. Effects	Reduced visual acuity and difficulty finding a focal point Possible difficulty seeing details with distance vision, near vision or both

Continued on following page

TABLE 39.1		
Common Vision Conditions in Adults (Western Population) *(Continued)*		
Condition	Definition	Functional Implications
	of nystagmus may be reduced by the adoption of a compensatory head posture.	Possible neck/shoulder issues because of adoption of awkward postures to stabilise eye movement
Quadrantanopia	Visual field loss where there is a loss of one quarter of the visual field in one or both eyes.	Difficulty with orientation and mobility (i.e. items overhead or below knees dependant on quadrant field loss location).
Retinitis pigmentosa	A hereditary eye condition that causes a degeneration of the light sensitive cells and pigment layer of the retina. The field of vision becomes restricted (i.e. tunnel vision) and visual acuity decreases. Total blindness may result in later years.	Progressive vision loss Peripheral vision loss (i.e. difficulty with orientation and mobility) Loss of night vision

Modified from American Foundation for the Blind (2015).

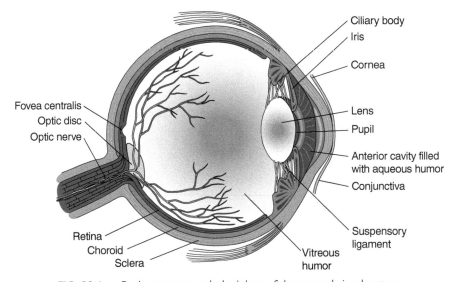

FIG. 39.1 ■ Basic anatomy and physiology of the eye and visual system.

with light rays reflecting from an object and entering the eye through the clear, outer layer known as the cornea. The light rays pass through the pupil and lens, which is behind the iris (coloured part of the eye). The cornea and the lens focus the light rays onto the retina at the back of the eye. The photoreceptor cells in the retina consist of rods and cones. Rods are located in the periphery of the retina and offer high sensitivity in low-light situations, although the acuity is poor. Cones are concentrated in the macula, the area responsible for detailed and colour vision, and are active in light providing good visual acuity. Photoreceptor cells in the retina pick up the light signals, change them into nerve impulses and convey these to the brain via the optic nerve and optic chiasm (the junction where nerve fibres cross to join other nerve fibres), where they can be perceived and understood as a visual image in the occipital lobe by the visual cortex (Fig. 39.2).

Measuring Vision

The degree of vision impairment is determined by a person's visual acuity, visual field loss or both. Visual acuity determines how well the central retina is functioning and refers to the ability to see fine detail up close (near visual acuity) and at a distance (distance visual acuity). Near visual acuity is measured using modified charts made of letters, words, numbers or shapes to determine a comfortable level for reading. It is often referred to as N with a number (e.g. N12). Distance visual acuity is often assessed by measuring the smallest letters a person is able to see on a standardised eye chart from a distance of 6 metres (20 feet).

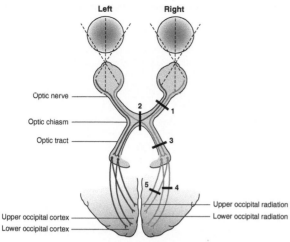

FIG. 39.2 ■ Visual pathway: optic nerve, optic chasm, optic tract.

TABLE 39.3	
Terms Used to Indicate That Vision Is Too Reduced to See a Chart	
Term	**Description**
Count fingers (CF)	Count fingers at distance specified
Hand movements (HM)	Can see a hand moving at a close distance in front of the eyes
Light perception (LP)	Can perceive light and dark but no detail
No light perception (NLP)	Totally blind

Modified from Vision Australia (2012a).

Normal visual acuity is recorded as 6/6 (20/20), meaning a person with normal vision can see the letters on the standardised chart from 6 metres. The larger the bottom number of the fraction, the more impaired is a person's visual acuity. For example, if a person's visual acuity were 6/24, the person would be able to see a line of letters on the chart at 6 metres that a person without visual impairment would be able to see at 24 metres. The number indicates the size of the objects that can be seen comfortably. Tables 39.2 and 39.3 provide examples of the terms given to measure visual acuity levels.

The visual field is the total area a person sees in a single view without turning the head or eyes. A full visual field with both eyes open is approximately 190 degrees horizontally and 135 degrees vertically. A central visual field loss includes the area immediately surrounding the spot on which the person is focusing as opposed to a peripheral field loss beyond and surrounding the central field. Visual field loss can be a result of damage anywhere along the visual pathway from the retina to the visual cortex and is described functionally as what cannot be seen. Visual field loss can be described in halves (and quarters) using anatomical reference points – for example, binasal hemianopia (half field loss on both sides of the nasal side of the eye), bitemporal hemianopia (half field loss on both sides of the temporal side of the eye), or right homonymous hemianopia (half field loss on the right side of each eye) (Fig. 39.3).

A total peripheral visual field loss with central field maintained will result in tunnel vision. If the central field is lost and the peripheral field maintained, vision requiring detail, such as reading, is lost. A visual field of less than 60 degrees will start to significantly affect a person's ability to move about within the environment. A person usually requires at least 120 degrees of visual field horizontally to drive a vehicle. A visual field of less than 20 degrees in the least affected eye will result in a person being deemed legally blind.

TABLE 39.2	
Impact of Visual Acuity Levels	
Visual Acuity Level	**Description**
6/6	Normal vision
6/12	Reduced vision (Australian legal driving limit)
6/18	Low vision (World Health Organization definition)
<6/60	Legal blindness (eligible for various entitlements)

Modified from Vision Australia (2012a).

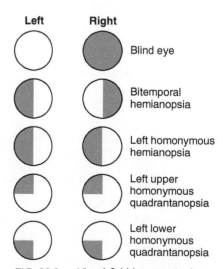

FIG. 39.3 ■ Visual field loss terminology.

Vision Perception

It may become clear during an assessment that neither a person's visual acuity nor visual field is the reason for the visual difficulties; rather the visual difficulties may be a result of a perceptual issue. Visual perception is the process whereby a person's eyes and brain take a raw image and organise, associate and provide a context from use of memory as to what is being seen. The visual image therefore becomes understandable and meaningful to the person.

Visual perceptual processing or visual information processing is a set of higher cognitive skills used to gather visual information and integrate it with other senses to create understanding and meaning from what is being experienced. This process allows the development of schemes to derive meaning from what is seen. Broadly, these skills can be divided into three groups: visual spatial skills, visual analysis skills and visual integration skills (Table 39.4).

For additional information on the assessment and intervention of visual perception deficits, review *Hierarchy of Vision Perception* by Mary Warren (1993a; 1993b). Warren provides a developmental framework to illustrate that higher levels of vision cognition and adaptation are built upon the lower levels of oculomotor control, visual fields and visual acuity.

TABLE 39.4
Visual Perceptual Processing Skills

Visuospatial Skills — OBSERVING AN OBJECT, THEN ACCURATELY REPORTING ITS RELATIONSHIP IN SPACE RELATIVE TO THE PERSON VIEWING THE OBJECT

Visuospatial Skill	Difficulties with Reduced Visuospatial Skill
Dyspraxia	Poor coordination and balance
Left/right discrimination	Inability to determine left and right direction and the difference between the two
Bilateral integration	Inability to cross the midline; inability to use both hands at the same time
Dysgraphia	Reversing numbers or letters when writing
Spatial integration/scanning	Difficulties reading horizontally or vertically
Position in space/spatial awareness	Difficulties observing an object, then accurately reporting its relationship in space relative to the person viewing the object

Visual Analysis Skills — IDENTIFY, SORT, ORGANISE, STORE AND RECALL INFORMATION

Visual Analysis Skill	Difficulties with Reduced Visual Analysis Skill
Figure ground	Difficulty attending to or searching for a specific form or item while ignoring irrelevant information
Form constancy	Difficulty discriminating the differences and consistencies in forms including shape, size, colour and orientation
Visual closure	Difficulty using clues to determine the appearance of the final image or object
Visuospatial memory	Difficulty recalling the spatial location of an object
Visual sequential memory	Difficulty viewing and then recalling a sequence of letters/numbers/objects in order
Visual agnosia	Difficulties recognising objects visually despite object being familiar to them; objects may be recognised using other senses

Visual Integration — COMBINE INFORMATION WITH OTHER SENSES OR WITH OTHER VISUAL INFORMATION

Visual Integration Skill	Difficulties with Reduced Visual Integrations Skill
Visualisation or visual-visual integration	Difficulties matching a written word with an image in the mind or vice versa
Visual-motor integration	Inability to coordinate visual information with gross motor and fine motor (e.g. threading a needle, catching a ball)
Visual-auditory integration	Inability to coordinate visual information with auditory information (e.g. seeing a word and saying it out loud)

Modified from Zolton (2007).

MULTIDISCIPLINARY TEAM MEMBERS IN VISION REHABILITATION

The provision of services for people with vision impairment varies between countries; there is no standard model of service delivery and funding. In addition, the funding available will differ among health, social and voluntary sectors. Occupational therapists specialising in vision impairment will usually work within coordinated teams of vision rehabilitation professionals. As well as an occupational therapist, the multidisciplinary vision rehabilitation team may include the following professionals:

■ Ophthalmologists (also known as eye specialists, eye surgeons, or eye doctors) who diagnose and provide medical/surgical treatments for eye conditions.
■ Optometrists who prescribe glasses (refraction) and contact lenses and diagnose, screen and monitor eye disease.
■ Orthoptists/low-vision optometrist who assess functional vision such as distance vision, near vision, contrast sensitivity, ocular movements, visual fields, depth perception, and colour vision and provide information and strategies to maximise the effective use of remaining vision.
■ Orientation and mobility specialists who equip people with vision impairment to have the necessary skills and concepts to move safely, efficiently, confidently and independently around an environment. They also assess and train people with vision impairment in the use of mobility aids (such as a white cane) and development of sensory awareness.
■ Adaptive technology consultants/trainers who provide advice on the most suitable technology solutions to meet individual circumstances. They can also install adaptive technology, provide basic technical support and offer training in computer skills, including touch typing; word processing, spreadsheet, database, presentation, email and Internet browsing applications; and using screen reading or screen magnification software.
■ Rehabilitation psychologists and counsellors who assist the person with vision impairment and families cope with the psychosocial issues related to vision impairment.
■ Case managers/social workers who coordinate services internal and external to the multidisciplinary team and often provide incidental counselling to the person with vision impairment and families.

Considerations of how members of the rehabilitation team communicate and guide a person with vision impairment can be found in Box 39.1.

ASSESSMENT OF PERSON WITH VISION IMPAIRMENT

To develop appropriate and effective intervention, it is important for occupational therapists to understand the nature of the person's diagnosis and level of functional vision. *Functional vision,* or *residual vision,* refers to the way in which a person uses their remaining vision to perform routine tasks.

An initial evaluation is performed by a low-vision specialist (either optometrist or orthoptist) and includes a number of assessments to determine visual acuity, contrast sensitivity, visual fields and neurological functions. For further information on visual functions and the most common tests used, refer to Meyers and Wilcox's (2011) chapter in the textbook *Occupational Therapy Interventions for Adults with Low Vision.*

The primary objective of evaluation is to measure the ability of the person with vision impairment to perform occupations and assist in determining interventions that will improve the person's ability to perform these occupations. Occupational therapists must complete a holistic evaluation to identify the unique factors that affect a person's engagement with the environment (physical, social, emotional). To assist therapists in achieving this, Scheiman, Scheiman, & Whittaker, (2007) set out four components of occupational therapy low-vision evaluation:

1. *Occupational profile/case history:* The evaluation process begins by gathering information about a person's ocular and health history. Therapists require an understanding of the person's pre- and post-morbid occupational performance and history to effect appropriate interventions. To facilitate this Scheiman et al. (2007) recommend the use of a low-vision visual functioning questionnaire such as the Veterans Affairs Low-Vision Visual Functioning Questionnaire (VA LV VFQ-48). This evaluation is designed to measure performance ability and establish the occupational performance goals. The Self-Report Assessment of Functional Visual Performance (Warren, Bachelder, Velozo, & Hicks, 2008) is an occupational profile tool that contains a self-report questionnaire and an observation assessment component. Recent updates to the assessment form include using smartphones and tablets as performance areas and a revision to the ratings to make it more useful for therapists to report a person's progress as required by federal regulations in the United States of America.

2. *Evaluation of visual factors:* Understanding of a person's visual status is gained from a low-vision evaluation. An effective evaluation obtains information on visual acuity (near and distance), visual field loss, contrast sensitivity, glare sensitivity, refraction/magnification outcomes. This provides therapists with information on the factors that act as a barrier to a person's performance. This is illustrated in Marj's practice story at the end of this chapter with details of the visual factors relevant to Marj provided in Practice Story 39.1. Occupational therapists who do not directly work with eye care professionals may be required to perform their own testing to understand a person's visual status. For example, with regards to

BOX 39.1
CONSIDERATIONS FOR WORKING WITH A PERSON WITH VISUAL IMPAIRMENT

GUIDING A PERSON WITH VISION IMPAIRMENT

People with vision impairment may find it helpful to be guided by another person, particularly in an unfamiliar environment. To do this safely, respectfully and efficiently, the following sighted guide techniques can be used (Vision Australia, 2012b):

- Ask the person if assistance is required. The person with vision impairment may hold the elbow of the person guiding. The person guiding should have a relaxed, slightly bent arm and describe the environmental landmarks and general travel direction to the person with vision impairment. Not all people with little or no sight will use this method, so it is important to ask what specific assistance they require.
- If the person with vision impairment uses a mobility aid (e.g. a walking stick), then encourage the person to use this aid. In addition, encourage the use of grab rails where available.
- Walk at a comfortable pace for the person with vision impairment, who should be approximately one pace behind the guide.
- Offer to guide the hand of the person with vision impairment, when required, to the grab rail, car door or other object to hold or manipulate.
- If the guide must leave, ensure that the person with vision impairment is aware of the location (verbally describe) and, if required, is either seated or positioned against a wall for stability and balance.

COMMUNICATING EFFECTIVELY WITH A PERSON WITH VISION IMPAIRMENT

Some strategies to assist communicating effectively include the following (Vision Australia, 2012c):

- Address the person with vision impairment by name and introduce yourself before commencing a conversation.
- Use accurate and specific language when giving directions; for example, 'The door is on your left' rather than 'The door is over there'.
- Use specific language when describing the person's surroundings; for example, specify the features of a building, such as the waiting area drink fountain, and identify the people present when entering a room.
- Identify what is making a particular sound when required, such as a meal cart travelling down a corridor.
- Inform the person with vision impairment when you are leaving and when other people have left the room or conversation.

NB: It is generally acceptable to use the words such as 'blind', 'look', 'see', and 'watch' in the course of normal conversation with a person with vision impairment. These concepts and words are part of normal language and do not need to be adjusted when communicating with a person vision impairment.

---

understanding visual field deficits after a neurological event, a basic confrontational visual field screening test that can be completed to evaluate visual factors is provided in Box 39.2.

3. *Evaluation of environmental factors:* The environment has a large impact on a person's ability to perform meaningful activities. It is therefore important that occupational therapists evaluate the environment surrounding the person's activities and interactions. Scheiman et al. (2007) state that careful consideration should be given to the following:

- Environmental lighting and glare
- Environmental organisation, including placement and storage of devices
- The ergonomics of performing tasks, including the positioning of reading stands and tables to maximise functional vision
- Escape and emergency responses to hazards

There are a small number of assessments that can be used to identify the visibility of space in a person's home. These assessments might identify such factors as light source type, wattage, light positioning, switch access and window coverings (Barstow, Bennett, & Vogtle, 2011). The Low Vision Home Assessment (Barstow, 2015; Bennett, Mainer, Westbrook, Barstow, & Vogtle, 2014) and the Home Environment Lighting Assessment (Perlmutter, 2013; Perlmutter et al., 2013) provide examples of assessments to guide therapists working to improve environmental conditions in existing homes. A component within these assessments is a light meter assessment. A light metre or lux metre is a device that measures the illumination levels within an area; measurements are provided in *lux* (Perlmutter et al., 2013). The advantage of a light metre assessment is that an objective measurement before and after lighting modification can be obtained (Barstow, 2015). Another advantage is that quantifiable measurements of lighting are a helpful platform to compare measurements with the minimum standards specified within the national building codes. Information may be used to justify recommendations for modifications in formal reports to funding bodies, landlords, employers, public building owners/designers. In Australia,

BOX 39.2
CONFRONTATIONAL VISUAL FIELD TEST

A basic confrontational field test can be used by therapists to screen if a person has a visual field loss. This test requires minimal equipment and sound observations (Zolton, 2007).

NB: Therapists conducting a confrontational visual field test will be testing their own visual field at the same time as the person with vision impairment in order to have a direct comparison of a normal visual field. If the therapist does not have a normal visual field, this test will not be appropriate.

In the explanation given here the therapist is a woman and the person with vision impairment is a man.

1. The therapist should be positioned 50 cm away from and facing the person with vision impairment. The therapist then asks the person to close/cover one eye; once the person has selected which eye to close/cover, the therapist closes/covers the opposite eye (i.e. if the person closes/covers his left eye, then the therapist should cover/close her right eye). The therapist then asks the person to stare at the therapist's open eye, and the therapist stares at the person's open eye.

2. Starting in the top outer quadrant the therapist slowly moves a finger/pen/object into her visual field, asking the person to indicate when he sees the finger/pen/object. The therapist compares where the person indicated the finger/pen/object was seen to when she saw the finger/pen/object entering her visual field.

3. The therapist repeats this process with each quadrant, ensuring that she starts from outside her own visual field.

4. Once all four quadrants have been assessed for one eye, the therapist assesses the person's other eye in the same manner.

5. If the therapist detects a visual field loss (i.e. the person's visual field does not match the therapist's visual field), the person should be referred on for formal testing by an orthoptist and optometrist.

---

the Australian Standard for interior lighting (Standards Australia/New Zealand Standard, 2009) outlines the minimum levels of illumination required by the general population in a variety of environments. However, it is important to note that the lux levels provided in this standard are minimums only and often do not meet the needs of people with low vision.

4. *Evaluation of occupational performance:* The final component of evaluation is an assessment of the multiple factors that underpin occupational performance. The therapist may ask a person to engage in usual daily tasks to observe activity demands, performance skills and performance patterns. Information obtained can then be used to develop a plan that endeavours to address the barriers to performance. Within Marj's practice story at the end of this chapter, an example of activity analysis for meal preparation to investigate the performance strengths and barriers is provided.

ENABLING STRATEGIES AND INTERVENTIONS

The central goal of occupational therapy is to promote health and participation through engagement in occupations (Warren & Nobles, 2011). Implementing strategies to support engagement when working with people who have a vision impairment follow the same frameworks, models, professional reasoning and evidence-based practice as other areas of occupational therapy practice. The therapist will identify the occupational performance components and consider ways to maximise functional vision, modifying the environment to suit the visual needs,

introducing visual aids or equipment and adapting the occupation. The unique aspects of interventions for people with vision impairment include the focus on decreasing the visual demands of a desired activity, increasing the visibility of the environment and developing the other senses to restore or promote occupational engagement (Gilbert & Baker, 2011).

In a systematic review by Arbesman, Lieberman, & Berlanstein, (2013), strong evidence was found that multicomponent occupational therapy programmes improve occupational performance for older adults with low vision. Multicomponent interventions were those that included education and exchange of information about low vision, training in problem-solving skills, relaxation techniques and instruction in the use of low-vision assistive technologies. Using a multidisciplinary approach to focus on personal goals and allowing multiple training sessions were also found to facilitate the development of independence in daily activities.

When working with people with vision impairment, occupational therapists should consider the principles of 'brighter, bigger, bolder.' Additionally, occupational therapists need to determine whether a person's other senses could be used to compensate for the vision loss. These strategies can often make a task easier, capitalising on functional vision and other senses, and should be implemented before including more complex solutions.

Brighter: Is There Enough Light

The visual system depends on light to operate; therefore appropriate lighting is the most important aid to vision. Contrast sensitivity and dark and light adaptation unfortunately diminish as people age. This is because less light reaches the retina in an aging eye. It is also difficult for an aging visual system to adapt quickly to dramatic changes in brightness. Recommending lighting changes in response to vision impairment is individual and there is no single lighting solution. The general approaches described next have been found to be effective in maximising functional vision (Thomas Pocklington Trust, 2010).

There are two types of lighting to consider: general and task lighting. *General lighting* refers to both artificial light and daylight. This improves distance vision tasks such as negotiating safely around the home. Recommendations to maximise general lighting include the following:

- Keep windows as clean as possible to allow the greatest amount of light into a room.
- Ensure window shades are up and shutters are open.
- Clear trees and shrubs away from windows.
- Curtains should be drawn away from the window so they do not obstruct light. If privacy is required, a very light net curtain may be sufficient.
- In most cases it is advisable to sit to the side of a window. This will provide even light on reading material or near tasks, while eliminating glare. It will also stop the person's body from blocking the light.
- Complete tasks by choosing the time of day when there is the best available light for the task, and reduce the impact of glare.
- Turn on available ceiling and other lights in the environment.
- Consider using brighter light fittings or additional lighting.

Task lighting is light focused on a particular area where a task is being performed (such as reading, sewing or using the telephone). By moving the light source closer to the viewed object, the intensity of light is increased. When you reduce the distance of the light source from the viewed object by half, the intensity of light on the object is increased four times. The light can be placed as close as 15 cm from the item the person is looking at. If the light is too bright or glare is reflecting into the person's eyes, the lamp should be repositioned or wattage decreased. The best position for an adjustable lamp is between the person and the item being looked at, directed at the task and below eye level. This positioning ensures that excess light shines away from the person's eyes; therefore reflections will not be a problem and the close proximity of the light source on the page will provide maximum illumination (Fig. 39.4).

For most people with low vision, lighting is a very useful tool for enhancing functional vision. However, it is equally important to remember that not all people benefit from additional lighting because of glare sensitivity (e.g. people diagnosed with cataracts, keratoconus, etc.). The challenge is to provide enough light without creating glare or shadows. If glare is a problem, venetian blinds, vertical blinds, curtains or tinted windows could be used to reduce discomfort from glare. Reflective glare can be reduced by placing a dark-coloured cloth or tea towel on the shiny object, sink, bench or table that is causing the reflection.

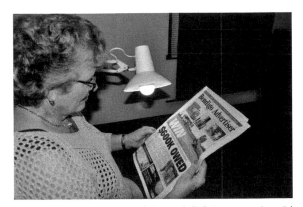

FIG. 39.4 ■ A woman applying task lighting to assist with reading the newspaper. The lamp is angled at approximately 45 degrees to, and is approximately 20 cm away from, the paper. She is also using her reading glasses at the working distance of 30 cm.

Bigger: Can the Detail Be Made Bigger?

Big objects are generally easier to see than small objects for most people. This can be achieved in many ways, both simple and complex, depending on individual needs. The process of enlarging an image on retina is known as magnification (Freeman, 2007). Magnification can be achieved using four different methods: relative size magnification, relative distance magnification, angular magnification and electronic magnification.

- *Relative size magnification* refers to enlarging the object. Doubling the size of the object makes the image on the retina twice as large. For example, accessing large-print calendars, clocks, phones (Fig. 39.5), books, crosswords, sheet music and cooking recipes can make these objects visually easier to see and read.

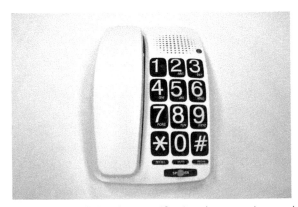

FIG. 39.5 ■ Relative size magnification: large numbers and buttons on a telephone; a tactile marker inserted on the speaker function is also illustrated.

■ *Relative distance magnification* refers to moving the object closer or moving closer to the object. This means as the distance from the object decreases, the object the retinal image of the object becomes larger. For example, when a person moves the lounge chair closer to the television or brings a book closer to the eyes, the retinal image of the television or book becomes larger, making it visually easier to see. It is important to note that eyestrain and discomfort can occur after a short period when a person is focusing on an object held at a close working distance (Freeman, 2007). When this occurs, a magnifier or optical lens should be considered to achieve maximum capacity of optimal functional vision.

Magnification devices come in many shapes, forms and strengths, including hand magnifiers (Fig. 39.6), stand magnifiers and pocket magnifiers. Some magnifiers have built-in lights to enhance illumination of the text. It is helpful to think of magnification devices as tools for a specific use, such as reading mail, seeing menus at a restaurant, watching a football game or reading street signs. Training to use magnification aids correctly is essential for success. It is important for therapists to be aware that the magnification device does not replace the vision that has already deteriorated; however, it will maximise a person's remaining vision when engaging in specific tasks.

■ *Angular magnification* is the magnification experience when a person looks through an optical device (e.g. telescope or a binocular) that creates an image which is larger than the actual object. This method is effective in producing magnification for distance objects while allowing the person to stay at his or her chosen distance from the object. For example, viewing a theatre production with a binocular or using a binocular to read the signs within the supermarket aisle will magnify the object of interest.

■ *Electronic magnification* refers to the use of electronic equipment with usage considerations of both relative size and distance magnification methods. Refer to the Adaptive

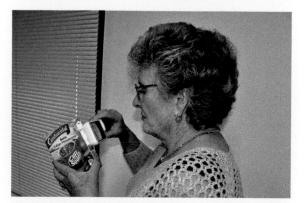

FIG. 39.6 ■ Relative distance magnification: handheld illuminated magnifier to read a jar label.

Technology and Vision Impairment section later in this chapter for details on equipment options available.

Bolder: Is There Enough Contrast?

Light/dark contrast is created by the amount of light that is reflected from different surfaces. The greater the contrast between the object and the object's background, the easier it is to see the differences. Black-on-white or white-on-black produces the best contrast for many people, but sometimes just putting light colours against dark backgrounds is enough to see objects more clearly. Possible examples for using colour contrast to assist people with vision impairment include the following:

■ Using a black felt-tipped pen for writing, instead of a ballpoint pen or pencil
■ Using a white plate on a dark-coloured placemat
■ Using contrasting electrical tape around light switches and power sockets
■ Painting the edge of stairs with a wide strip of contrasting paint

Incorporating the Use of Other Senses

Techniques that promote the use of sensory functions such as hearing, touch, smell and taste can provide people with visual impairments with additional information about the environment and the performance of a task. Often the information provided by the senses supplements and supports information being received visually (Gilbert & Baker, 2011). Sensory exercises can help people increase their overall sensitivity and abilities and assist them to gain trust in the information they receive from their remaining senses.

Hearing

Hearing can provide auditory awareness of a person's environment, such as the sound of a door being opened, a car driving past, a cup being filled, water boiling and the click of switches as appliances are turned on and off. For people with vision impairment, the use of audible devices such as clocks and kitchen scales, as well as audio screen readers or books, can assist in accessing information and reduce unnecessary visual fatigue.

Touch

Touch is an extremely important means for a person with visual impairment to receive information about the environment. For example, a person with vision impairment may rely on touch to identify coins by their individual shape, size and milling or the orientation of clothes when dressing.

The 'bolder' contrast principle can be transferred to incorporate tactile components by creating a tactile marker to make an item or object (e.g. a button on a microwave) stand out from its background by it feeling different. As an example, a tactile marker has been attached to the speaker button on the phone in Fig. 39.5 to assist a person to identify this button on the phone. Tactile markings such as Polymark paint or Velcro can be put onto appliances to assist with determining the various settings. Tactile symbol systems and braille have also been designed to assist with communication and literacy.

Touch is also critical in techniques used for travel. When using a mobility cane or other mobility device, the person will learn to identify the differences in surfaces and obstacles. People also may use a travel technique called trailing, in which they lightly touch the walls using the back of their hand as they walk, in order to receive tactile information of their route.

Smell and Taste

Using the senses of smell and taste can provide information on the freshness of fruit and vegetables or if food is burning in the oven. These senses can assist in differentiating between different flavours such as salt or sugar, herbs and spices. Aromas can also provide useful clues in orientation, such as the scent of flowers in the living room, baking aromas in the kitchen and detergent odours in the laundry room.

Using Visual Memory

In addition to the senses, a person can use visual memory to consciously form accurate mental pictures of people, places and everyday objects. A person can create an accurate mental picture of a space or object by recalling the vast storehouse of visual memories accumulated throughout a lifetime. This is part of the reason why most people can find the toilet at night without turning on the light.

Adaptive Technology and Vision Impairment

Only a very small proportion of written material is available in alternative formats for people with vision impairments or who have a print disability such as dyslexia. Often the alternative format consists of braille or audiobooks and excludes other written information such as street signs, pamphlets, information booklets, maps and documents sent via regular mail. Adaptive technology used to address this is becoming more accessible (both physically and financially) and more compatible with mainstream devices such as computers, smartphones and tablets (Table 39.5).

In choosing adaptive technology options for a person consideration should be given to the usability of the technology. Comprehensive training and support for the technology is also required to ensure successful integration of the technology into the everyday life of the person with vision impairment.

Ergonomics and Vision Impairment

Visual ergonomics is a significant consideration for therapists when adaptive technology and assistive aids are prescribed. The use of devices may require a person to adopt a forward leaning posture to create a specific working distance in order to maximise functional vision. It is essential for therapists to review how the prescribed aid is used in the environment. For example,

for a person who has been prescribed a magnifier and enjoys reading in his or her favourite lounge chair there is a need to assess the use of the magnifier (focal distance) and the person's posture when in the lounge chair. A lap tray or reading tilt table may be introduced to minimise muscle strain and to ensure the person is comfortable when using the magnifier for reading (Long, 2014).

Falls Prevention and Vision Impairment

Occupational therapists play a key role in assisting people with vision impairment to remain safe and independent in their home and community. Falls prevention education and techniques are essential for people with vision impairment as they are twice as likely to fall compared with a person without a vision impairment (Riddering, 2011). They are also likely to limit their participation in activity because of a fear of falling as a result of the perceived risk with reduced vision (Wang et al., 2012). Visual information received is used to balance and coordinate movement and avoid obstacles and hazards. Visual field loss, reduced contrast sensitivity, diplopia, multifocal optical lenses and a general fear of falling all increase the risk of falls (Martin, 2013). There are many factors that can place people with vision impairment at risk of a fall; some of these include their general health, balance and proprioception, vision loss, medications and the physical environment (Wood et al., 2011). Preventive strategies associated the factors that affect the risk of falls are summarised in Table 39.6.

CONCLUSION

Working with people living with vision impairment is a specialised and complex area of occupational therapy practice. Where possible, referral to low-vision specialist services will lead to improved outcomes for people who have low vision or blindness. However, the basic principles of assessment and intervention can be incorporated into practice easily when access to specialised services is limited. The assessment of a person with vision impairment can be both formal and informal; however, it should ultimately involve a multidisciplinary team in order to understand the full functional impact of vision loss for an individual. Understanding the functional difficulties of a person with vision loss will lead to effective interventions to assist the person to participate in meaningful occupation, aiming to promote health and well-being. Enabling strategies can be simple (bigger, bolder, brighter) or complex (adaptive technology, equipment and intensive therapy focusing on developing compensatory skills by enhancing touch, smell, hearing, taste senses and visual memory). Always at the centre of therapy is the person and the person's individual goals. For people with blindness and low vision, occupational therapy intervention can assist them to lead independent, meaningful and fulfilling lives.

Marj's practice story illustrates many of the points covered in this chapter (Practice Story 39.1).

TABLE 39.5
A Selection of Adaptive Technology Options for People with Vision Impairment

Type of Technology	Function
Video magnifiers (closed circuit televisions (CCTV))	These magnifiers can enlarge print between 2 to 60 times. There are portable and desktop models available. Print is placed under a camera and the document is displayed on a screen where the colour contrast and size can be manipulated. A woman using a CCTV to read her mail is shown in Fig. 39.7.

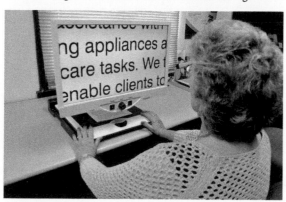

FIG. 39.7 ■ Electronic magnification: a desktop closed circuit television vision (CCTV).

Type of Technology	Function
Video magnifiers with speech	Some of the newer video magnifiers on the market also have the option for speech output, allowing the document to be read out.
Screen reader software	Converts text on a computer screen and synthesises it to voice output.
Optical character recognition (OCR) software	Scanned or photographed text is synthesised to a voice output. Software is available for traditional computers in addition to mobile devices.
Magnification software	Increases the size of text and images on a computer screen with minimal distortion of the image. Available within Windows and Apple operating platforms and as separate software depending on need.
Electronic location devices and Global Positioning System (GPS)	Used in conjunction with a white cane or a dog guide to provide additional information about the environment (including obstacles in the person's path) and assistance with directions.
Mobile technology (tablets and mobile telephones)	Screen magnification and screen reader software available for smartphones and tablets. There is a wide range of mobile software applications to enhance independence such as money identification, colour identifier and talking GPS.
e-Readers	Screen magnification and text manipulation available on e-reader devices such as Kindle and Kobo. Some e-reader devices are compatible with screen readers on Android and Apple operating platforms.
Digital Accessible Information System (DAISY) playback devices	Audio file format that is easier to navigate than a standard CD or audio file for books and written media. Dedicated playback devices are required; however, software is also available to allow content to be heard on mobile devices, web-based platforms and computers.
Braille notetakers	Portable devices with braille keyboards for entering information and use a speech synthesiser or braille display for information output. Allows the user to complete word processing, emails and basic Web browsing.
Braille embossers	Devices that can print braille document from an electronic document.
Refreshable braille displays	Portable devices that allow computer displays to be converted to an electronic braille display live. These devices can have either braille or QWERTY keyboard input. May or may not have a visual display.
Talking bar code scanner	Enables people to identify household and supermarket items using the existing barcode on the packaging.

TABLE 39.6

Falls Prevention Strategies for People with Vision Impairment

Performance Area Identified	Functional Observations	Strategies
Inability to visually identify obstacles in path of travel	Walking with hands outstretched to test for hazards Walking slowly and using feet to test for hazards Bumping into or tripping over items	Educate regarding visual loss to increase self-awareness. Use visual scanning techniques. Use mobility aid (e.g. long cane). Use sighted guide by a support person (refer to Box 39.1, Considerations for Working with a Person with Vision Impairment). Remove tripping hazards such as loose mats, electrical cords and hoses. Ensure that pathways are clear and that furniture remains in the same place.
Inability to identify changes in surfaces and gradients	Reduced contrast sensitivity Difficulty identifying edges of steps Walking slowly and using feet to test for depth of gradient change Tripping over or falling down declines	Make sure that lighting is adequate and consistent throughout the home and outdoor paths. Consider motion sensor lighting that automatically turns on and off when individuals enter or exit a room or area. Highlight the edges of steps with colour contrast (see Fig. 39.8). Apply contrast between furniture and flooring; for example, paint door frames in bright solid colours, add contrasting colour to legs of furniture near floor level. Modify home environment to allow zero-step entrance with flush or low-profile thresholds in bathrooms and entrances. Insert tactile ground surface indicators to indicate an approaching hazard (Standards Australia/New Zealand Standard, 2002) (see Fig. 39.8).
Inability to coordinate eye movement between different focal lengths of optical lenses (e.g. bifocal or multifocal glasses)	Difficulty changing focus from near vision to distance vision when wearing glasses Falling over when having to make sudden movements (sit to stand/walk) as unable to change focus and identify hazards Cervical spine in flexion when looking through near vision lens, and extension when looking through distance lens as opposed to moving eyes; may affect balance	Replace multifocal or bifocal glasses with single-vision glasses for specific tasks; for example, single-lens glasses for reading, and single-lens glasses for distance viewing
Avoidance of activities because of fear of falling	Reduced engagement in meaningful activities (e.g. gardening or walking a pet) Reduced community engagement and social activities outside of the home	Refer to an orientation and mobility specialist to assess for an appropriate mobility aid, mobility training and safe travel routes. Refer to a falls and balance clinic to improve balance and confidence. Use contrast colours or tactile markers to identify hazards (e.g. garden edges, bright-coloured dog leash). Report uneven surfaces to your local council for repair. Wear safe and comfortable footwear (i.e. firm-fitting shoes, low broad heels, nonslip sole).

	TABLE 39.6	
	Falls Prevention Strategies for People with Vision Impairment (*Continued*)	
Performance Area Identified	**Functional Observations**	**Strategies**
Inability to adapt vision to changing light conditions quickly	Reports discomfort in the presence of bright lights (directed or reflected sunlight or artificial light) Eye squinting or using hands to shield eyes Reports eyes take time to adapt to the changes in lighting levels (e.g. when coming indoors after being outdoors on a sunny day)	Wear a hat with a wide brim to reduce glare. Wear sunglass or 'fitover' sunglasses to reduce directed or reflected sunlight. Sunglasses will also reduce the amount of time needed to adapt from bright light to low light. Allow time for the eyes to adjust to changes in lighting conditions before moving around. If suitable, use a torch at night to direct the light on a path (e.g. to the toilet) rather than turning on a light as this reduces the amount of light adjustment required.

PRACTICE STORY 39.1

Marj

Marj, a 71-year-old lady, lived at home with her husband; she had two daughters and five grandchildren. Marj was the matriarch of the family and hosted Sunday roasts for her family. She was passionate about helping others and volunteered at a local charity shop. Every week she enjoyed driving her car out and meeting her girlfriends for a coffee at a local cafe.

Four months ago while volunteering at her local charity shop, Marj had some difficulty reading the clothes labels and gave the wrong change to a customer. Marj was embarrassed and decided it was time she went to visit her local optometrist to review her bifocal glasses. Her local optometrist immediately located abnormal blood vessels leaking into the region of the macula and referred Marj to an ophthalmologist. Marj was diagnosed with wet age-related macular degeneration.

For the next several weeks, Marj underwent eye injections to prevent further damage and to reduce the swelling. She was advised that she no longer met the standard for her to drive a car and that it was not possible to adjust her glasses to help her do things such as read the labels on clothes. The ophthalmologist provided Marj with a referral letter to the local blindness and low-vision community service. Marj returned home from that appointment devastated that she could no longer drive and that nothing further could be done. She did not return to her duties at the charity shop and declined invitations to go out with friends for a coffee.

Feeling miserable, Marj eventually found the courage to visit the local blindness and low-vision community service. She was initially hesitant in visiting the centre as she believed nothing could be done to improve her vision; she was worried that she would be given a white cane and labelled as blind.

Marj dropped in to the centre and advised the receptionist that her ophthalmologist had referred her to the service. She did not know how the service could help her and could not identify what services she required. She was invited to take a seat and was seen by an intake worker. Marj was introduced to the services available, and it was identified that Marj required support with reading, identifying money, accessing the community and daily tasks around the home. She was then referred to an orthoptist, occupational therapist and orientation and mobility specialist.

Sally was Marj's occupational therapist. She worked for the blindness and low-vision community service.

Some information related to Marj and Sally's social, practice and frame of reference context are presented in Table 39.7.

The seven stages of the Canadian Practice Process Framework (Polatajko, Craik, & Davis, 2007) are used to structure the interactions between Marj and Sally.

STAGE 1. ENTER/INITIATE

Sally reviewed Marj's notes that were recorded during the intake process and the initial referral letter. Sally called Marj to clarify the reason for the referral and to inform her about the occupational therapy role. During this conversation, Sally listened to the occupational narrative as Marj was prompted to share her hopes and expectations for services. From this first point of contact, Sally began to create an occupational profile for Marj and took note of Marj's support networks and daily occupations. Sally scheduled an initial centre-based appointment, the preferred means of contact and preferred format for information. Initial goals were defined and agreed upon by Sally and Marj.

Continued on following page

TABLE 39.7
Social, Practice and Frame of Reference Contexts Related to Marj

Societal Context:	Societal Context – Marj:	Societal Context – Sally:
Driving laws: The legal limit for holding a private driver licence in Australia is that a person's visual acuity must be 6/12 or better (using both eyes). *Stigma:* The prevalence of negative stereotypes and inaccurate myths in society that influence a person's attitudes; for example, being label as 'blind' and as a result being thought of as 'not normal'.	Volunteering provides Marj with a sense of community and purpose. She wants to be part of her community. She enjoys going out to catch up with friends. She believes that she is no longer helpful to anyone. She lives with her supportive husband and is a loving mother. She has had many life experiences.	Licensed to practice by national standards, current registration. Community therapist for a nonprofit agency that provides services to people with vision impairments. Believes all individuals have the right to successfully engage in their chosen occupations.

Practical Context

Sally's role with Marj is to promote engagement and independence in her daily occupations.

Sally can provide services to Marj at the centre or in Marj's home.

Sally is able to provide up to eight sessions with each client as per organisational policy.

Sally's role is funded by the Home and Community Care (HACC) Programme, which is the principal source of funding for services that support frail aged people, younger people with disabilities and carers in Victoria, Australia.

Frame of Reference

Sally will use the Occupational Performance Model (Australia) (Ranka & Chapparo, 2011) to organise information collected throughout her assessments.

Sally is guided by the Active Service Model (Victorian State Government, 2015) to build capacity for people to self-manage the activities of their daily life.

Sally will use a rehabilitation frame of reference to finalise therapeutic interventions.

STAGE 2. SET THE STAGE

During the initial centre-based appointment, Sally defined the working relationship between therapist and Marj and provided information on the policies of the organisation, which included information on privacy and confidentiality, complaints and suggestions for improvement, rights and responsibilities, and the use of an advocate. Consent was obtained to authorise an agency file be created for the purposes of retaining any relevant information and giving consent for the agency to obtain and exchange relevant information to and from other professionals, such as Marj's ophthalmologist and optometrist.

Sally began a directed interview to gather information on Marj's occupational experiences and life course narrative to further develop her occupational profile. Sally organised the information she collected using the Occupational Performance Model (Australia) (Ranka & Chapparo, 2011). Sally completed the Canadian Occupational Performance Measure (COPM) (Law et al., 1998) with Marj to identify her occupational strengths and challenges. Marj listed the following five occupational performance problems as the most important for her:

1. Preparing Sunday roast dinner for the family
2. Volunteering at the local charity shop
3. Reading the mail
4. Travelling independently to meet friends at the local coffee shop
5. Matching colours of clothing

It was agreed that Sally would complete a functional cooking assessment at Marj's home. Before conducting the cooking assessment Sally completed the home risk assessment according to her organisation's policy to assess potential hazards and risks for visiting the property. This assessment identified that Marj had two small indoor dogs. On Sally's request, it was agreed the dogs were to be restrained in the laundry during the home visit.

After the initial session with Marj, Sally scheduled a meeting with the orientation and mobility specialist and orthoptist to inform them of the outcomes of her initial session with Marj. As Marj had already seen both these professionals, the three professionals exchanged their assessment findings to assist with planning interventions.

The orthoptist provided a summary of Marj's recent orthoptic assessment (Table 39.8), which identified the need for good

PRACTICE STORY 39.1

Marj (Continued)

TABLE 39.8				
Marj's Orthoptic Assessment Results				
Vision Distance (with correction)	**Vision Near (with correction)**	**Refraction**	**Magnification**	**Contrast Sensitivity – Melbourne Edge Test**
RE 6/95+(EF) LE 6/18	N12 at 25 cm with focal light	RE+1.00/−0.50×70 LE −0.50 DS Add: +4.00 for reading	N6 with a 3.5× LED handheld magnifier (This device was purchased during the assessment.)	10 dB (with refraction correction and focal lighting)

DS, diopter sphere; *EF,* eccentric fixation; *LE,* left eye; *RE,* right eye.

lighting as she presented with reduced contrast sensitivity; Marj was also prescribed a 3.5× LED handheld magnifier to assist with reading small print. The orientation and mobility specialist advised she had prescribed Marj with an ID cane to assist with depth perception when negotiating steps in unfamiliar environments (Fig. 39.8). The orientation and mobility specialist recommended Sally assesses the risk of falls at Marj's front steps, as Marj is requiring additional supports to transfer up and down.

STAGE 3. ASSESS/EVALUATE

Sally reviewed Marj's orthoptic assessment results (see Table 39.8) to help with preparing for the functional cooking assessment.

The functional cooking assessment, involving an activity analysis, was completed in Marj's kitchen to assess her performance in a familiar environment. This assessment was conducted to determine how to address Marj's goal to be able to prepare Sunday roast dinner for her family. The results of the activity analysis are presented in Table 39.9.

STAGE 4. AGREE ON OBJECTIVES AND PLAN

In this practice story the focus is on Marj's wish to host Sunday roast lunch for the family. Sally would also be focusing on implementing strategies to assist Marj to manage coins and identify colours of clothes, both of which Marj would need to return to volunteering at the charity shop.

In relation to being able to prepare a Sunday roast: Sally spent time with Marj after her assessment to reflect upon the occupational challenges and the environmental factors impacting on her performance. Sally discussed a number of possible solutions to enhance her performance. Sally and Marj agreed upon the following objectives to achieve the goal of hosting Sunday roast for the family:

■ Enhance lighting and contrast to increase viability of all near tasks
■ Use a magnifier for a number of tasks
■ Reduce clutter
■ Educate her family on organisational strategies
■ Explore adaptive techniques and/or equipment to compensate for low vision

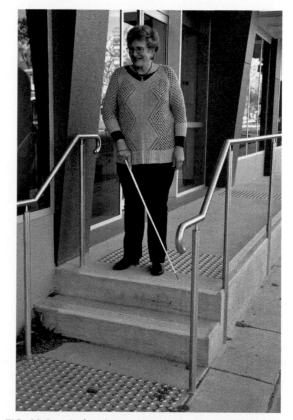

FIG. 39.8 ■ Lady using an ID cane to identify hazards and depth perception; tactile ground surface indicators (TGSIs) and contrast marking are also presented in this figure.

STAGE 5. IMPLEMENT THE PLAN

Sally scheduled another home visit to implement the agreed objectives within meal preparation. Outcomes for this session are listed in Table 39.10.

Continued on following page

PRACTICE STORY 39.1

Marj (Continued)

<table>
<tr><td colspan="5" align="center">**TABLE 39.9**</td></tr>
<tr><td colspan="5" align="center">**Marj's Kitchen Skills Assessment**</td></tr>
<tr><th>Task Analysis</th><th>I</th><th>A</th><th>D</th><th>Observations</th></tr>
<tr><td colspan="5">***Food Collection and Reading***</td></tr>
<tr><td>Collecting food items</td><td></td><td>A</td><td></td><td>Difficulty locating items in cupboards and drawers. Reduced contrast within pantry between shelving and products. Food items stored inconsistently within pantry and fridge.</td></tr>
<tr><td>Reading food labels/use-by date/ directions on packaging</td><td></td><td>A</td><td></td><td>Incorrectly identified spice jars and salt/pepper, condiments.</td></tr>
<tr><td>Reading recipes</td><td></td><td></td><td>D</td><td>Unable to read recipe book wearing glasses.</td></tr>
<tr><td colspan="5">***Food Preparation***</td></tr>
<tr><td>Chopping, slicing, peeling techniques</td><td></td><td>A</td><td></td><td>Cutting self when collecting knives from drawer. Difficulty slicing vegetables in even portions; unable to identify the skin when peeling vegetables. When Marj is positioned at bench, the central light casts a shadow at this area. Marj felt frustrated with excess of time taken.</td></tr>
<tr><td>Pouring techniques</td><td></td><td>A</td><td></td><td>Difficulty identifying water level in mug. Kettle positioned on opposite side of sink. Excess spillage on bench after task.</td></tr>
<tr><td>Use of utensils (e.g. can opener)</td><td></td><td>A</td><td></td><td>Difficulty locating utensils and bowls as numerous items stored on top of one another. No issues using can opener.</td></tr>
<tr><td>Measurement of ingredients</td><td></td><td>A</td><td></td><td>Difficulty identifying the correct measuring cups; unable to read measurement on scales with glasses, difficulty managing pouring from packets and scooping from narrow-mouthed containers.</td></tr>
<tr><td colspan="5">***Appliance use***</td></tr>
<tr><td>Use of stovetop (gas or electric)</td><td></td><td>A</td><td></td><td>Electric: Independent setting low-high temperature. Set and adjusted temperature accordingly throughout task. Difficulty locating the dial indicator to identify when stove off. When Marj is positioned at stove, the central light casts a shadow, inhibiting ability to read the dials and controls.</td></tr>
<tr><td>Use of oven (gas or electric)</td><td></td><td></td><td>D</td><td>Unable to identify temperature settings on oven dial, relied on memory.</td></tr>
<tr><td>Use of other appliances (toaster, sandwich makers, rice cooker, etc.)</td><td></td><td>A</td><td></td><td>Difficulty locating numbers on microwave.</td></tr>
<tr><td>Monitoring cooking process</td><td>I</td><td></td><td></td><td>Used wall clock in lounge room to monitor time, unable to read watch.</td></tr>
<tr><td>Identifying cooked food</td><td></td><td>A</td><td></td><td>Difficulty identifying sautéed garlic/onions. Cooked vegetables and meat accordingly to time specifications. Fearful of transferring hot items from the oven.</td></tr>
<tr><td colspan="5">***Clean-up***</td></tr>
<tr><td>Washing dishes/using dishwasher</td><td></td><td>A</td><td></td><td>Missed grime on plate when washing plates. Experiences glare in the late afternoon. Window faces west. Marj was required to pull down block-out blind, which prevented natural light from entering.</td></tr>
<tr><td>Cleaning sink, bench</td><td>I</td><td></td><td></td><td>Careful to wipe down bench.</td></tr>
</table>

Additional Comments

Lighting levels were recorded between 92 lux at sink and 85 lux at stove area with one central illuminare (15-watt compact fluorescent, 3000 k – warm light). When Marj is positioned at stove, the central light casts a shadow, inhibiting ability to read the dials and controls. Measurements of illumination (lux) levels were taken using a light metre with the lights switched on and daylight blocked out as much as

PRACTICE STORY 39.1

Marj (Continued)

TABLE 39.9			
Marj's Kitchen Skills Assessment *(Continued)*			
Task Analysis	I	A	D	Observations

possible in order to experience lighting levels that Marj would regularly be exposed to. Australian Standards recommend that illumination levels should be around 550–600 lux for task lighting in kitchens.

Hypotheses/Plausible Explanation

Reduced ability to read fine detail without appropriate levels of magnification and lighting. Increased clutter is causing visual confusion and increasing time delay.

Legend:
I = Independent
A = Assistance required (supervision, verbal prompts, hands-on assistance)
D = Dependent

TABLE 39.10	
Intervention outcomes	
Take Analysis	Intervention

Food Collection and Reading

Collecting food items	Education provided on increasing overall kitchen organisation and reduce clutter, such as the following:
	▪ Decide where items belong and return the items to the same place.
	▪ Insert frequently used items in the most accessible cupboards and drawers.
	▪ Group similar items together in small plastic baskets; when you need an item from a group, you can take the storage container and place it on a bench in good light for easier selection.
	Marj successfully trialled using a torch when locating items in dark pantry. Sally, the occupational therapist, provided the alternative option of painting the insides of cupboards white to maximise the brightness and contrast so that items are easier to find.
	Sally encouraged Marj to continue using sensory modalities and proprioceptive feedback when collecting food items, such as using touch, size/weight, shape, texture and smell.
	Sally recommended Marj stick to the same brands so that she becomes familiar with their features.
Reading food labels/use-by date/ directions on packaging	Trialled using her prescribed magnifier to read labels on food items. Marj felt frustrated picking up her magnifier to read each product. Large-print labels were then created and attached to items, enabling Marj to read the labels just wearing her glasses.
	Marj inserted a rubber band round the salt condiments to assist identifying using sense of touch.
Reading recipes	Trialled using her prescribed magnifier to read recipes. Marj found this to be comfortable as the magnifier was positioned in the same place as her recipe books.

Food Preparation

Chopping, slicing, peeling techniques	Knives stored separately in a knife block. It was recommended that knives were washed simultaneously after completion of tasks and returned.
	Sally demonstrated slicing techniques to apply. These included the following:
	▪ Use a contrast chopping board when preparing vegetables; for example, use a dark board when slicing light-coloured onions and potatoes.
	▪ Remove or cut a section of food to provide a flat surface for stability when cutting or slicing.
	▪ Throughout task, reorientate the food continually to provide a flat, stable base for cutting.

Continued on following page

PRACTICE STORY 39.1

Marj (Continued)

TABLE 39.10	
Intervention outcomes (Continued)	
Take Analysis	**Intervention**
	■ Where possible, maintain contact of the knife blade tip with the board when slicing.
	■ Once a section is sliced, do not remove the knife blade from the 'main' food source but continue to slice the next piece.
	■ Use the index finger of opposing hand to judge slice thickness (this finger can also be used to butt knife edge against before slicing).
	■ Sally suggested Marj also considers using a food processors and peeler as an alternative; vegetable peelers work well for slicing cheese/shaving chocolate.
	Sally demonstrated peeling techniques to apply. These included the following:
	■ Avoid washing vegetables before peeling so that the different surface texture changes can be used as a guide.
	■ Use a chopping board to stabilise 'long' food such as carrots, courgette and cucumber and peel downwards toward the board.
	■ Peel using a systematic method, such as top to bottom, left to right.
	■ Peel over a sink to contain peelings to avoid mess.
	■ Use unwashed potatoes, as the dirt and dark skin make recognising missed patches easier (do not wash potatoes beforehand).
	Focal lighting was successfully trialled during these tasks. This resulted in Marj installing an undercabinet fluorescent light to illuminate the counter area.
Pouring techniques	Sally demonstrated pouring techniques to apply. These included the following:
	■ Use adequate lighting to highlight the cup as much as possible; the undercabinet fluorescent light provided Marj with efficient lighting.
	■ Pour liquid over a sink area to ensure any spills are contained in the sink area.
	■ Connect the lip of the kettle or jug with the cup to ensure that water flows into the centre of the cup.
	■ Detect the level of the liquid being poured into the cup by listening for changes in water pitch as the cup fills.
	■ Use a white or lightly coloured cup to provide colour contrast to dark liquids such as tea or coffee and assist in determining the level of liquid. Add the milk last.
	■ Marj successfully trialled a liquid level indicator and purchased this to assist in preparing a cup of coffee.
Use of utensils (e.g. can opener)	Sally suggested that objects be stored only one row deep (not stacked) to reduce visual clutter. Marj concluded it was easier to group similar items together with a rubber band.
Measurement of ingredients	Sally labelled individual measuring cups with Polymark paint to assist in identifying ¼, ⅓, ½, ¾ and 1 cup. Sally discussed the option of using a chart that converts liquid measurements into cups, which Marj agreed to try. Sally recommended Marj used her magnifier to assist in reading the kitchen scales. Sally also demonstrated the option of talking scales to consider as desired. Marj transferred packets of dry foods into the available wide-mouthed storage containers, which allowed her to scoop contents out using measuring cups with greater stability and ease.
Use of Appliances	
Use of stovetop (gas or electric)	Sally inserted Polymark paint onto dial indicators with contrasting colours, enabling Marj to easily identify the dials. An additional undercabinet fluorescent light was installed to illuminate the dials and food cooking on the stove. Sally recommended to turn off dials before removing food as a safety precaution.

TABLE 39.10
Intervention outcomes (Continued)

Take Analysis	Intervention
Use of oven (gas or electric)	Sally applied tactile paint in contrasting colour onto dial indicators and frequently used temperature settings.
Use of other appliances	Marj successfully trialled large-print number stickers.
Monitoring cooking process	Sally trialled large-print watches and timers to assist Marj in monitoring cooking time. Marj purchased a large-print watch as she felt this had multiple uses.
Identifying cooked food	Sally demonstrated safe techniques to remove hot items from oven, which included the following: ■ Prepare area on bench to rest hot items near the oven. ■ Consider wearing elbow-length oven mitts to prevent injuries on forearm. These mitts were purchased by Marj. ■ As Marj is right-handed, it was suggested she stands at the left side of the oven, placing her nondominant hand on the counter next to the oven for balance support. Then she could use her right hand to find the oven door handle and open the oven door. ■ Locate the oven rack and pull it out a little. ■ With two hands, place the item to be baked on the oven rack and push the rack back in. ■ With her right hand, close the oven door. To determine whether the chopped onions had sautéed, it was suggested Marj uses a sensory approach to smell and hear the changes in cooking progress. Marj also thought timing this process helped, as well as a talking thermometer to be certain roast meat was cooked through.
Clean-up	
Washing dishes/using dishwasher	Sally suggested placing a tea towel over one shoulder to allow Marj to easily dry her hands and wipe spillages. To assist with the clean-up, it was recommended Marj fills her sink for cleaning hands and placing dirty dishes in as they are used. To reduce the impact of glare at the kitchen sink it was suggested Marj limited tasks completed when the glare was most intense or consider inserting translucent blinds to enable her to maximise the natural light entering while also controlling the impact of glare. Within the increased amount of natural light, Marj found washing dishes easier. Sally also recommended Marj run her fingertips lightly over object surfaces to locate food residue or areas requiring special attention and use her spare hand to locate a free/open space before placing dishes in the rack.
Cleaning sink, bench	Sally suggested using a systematic approach when wiping down the bench; for example, begin in the far right corner of the table surface, working from the far edge to the front edge using small circular movements and overlapping strokes.

STAGE 6. MONITOR AND MODIFY

The next session held at Marj's home reviewed her cooking ability using the purchased adaptations and modifications completed by the family.

STAGE 7. EVALUATE THE OUTCOME

After the completion of the previous intervention (along with interventions to assist Marj to achieve her other goals), Sally had a centre-based appointment with Marj to review her goals and readminister the COPM. It was concluded that there were no other occupational performance issues at this time.

STAGE 8. CONCLUDE/EXIT

During the centre-based meeting, Sally acknowledged with Marj that her condition was degenerative and that she would require further occupational therapy services in the future. Sally was provided with information about accessing these services as required.

http://evolve.elsevier.com/Curtin/OT

RESOURCES

Globally there are many agencies that provide support to people in the low-vision and blind community. These services often coordinate specialist rehabilitation professionals to work with people with vision loss. Linking vision-impaired people with low-vision services has been found to improve clinical and functional ability outcomes (Binns et al., 2012). The following list of agencies are an initial step to seeking further information when working with a person who has a vision impairment.

- American Foundation for the Blind (AFB): www.afb. orghttp://www.afb.org
- Blind Foundation: http://blindfoundation.org.nzhttp://blindfoundation.org.nz
- Guide Dogs Australia: http://www.guidedogsaustralia.comhttp://www.guidedogsaustralia.com
- National Federation of the Blind: https://nfb.orghttps://nfb.org
- Royal Blind: www.royalblind.orghttp://www.royalblind.org
- Royal National Institute of Blind People (RNIB): http://www.rnib.org.ukhttp://www.rnib.org.uk
- Royal London Society for Blind People (RLSB): http://www.rlsb.org.ukhttp://www.rlsb.org.uk
- Royal Society for the Blind: http://www.rsb.org.auhttp://www.rsb.org.au
- Texas School for the Blind and Visually Impaired: http://www.tsbvi.eduhttp://www.tsbvi.edu
- Thomas Pocklington Trust: http://www.pocklington-trust.org.uk
- VisAbility: http://www.visability.com.auhttp://www.visability.com.au
- Vision Australia: www.visionaustralia.org

YouTube Channels

Professionals and agencies also use YouTube as a platform to deliver information. The following YouTube channels provide additional learning, including assessments and the application of low-vision principles:

- AFB channel: https://www.youtube.com/user/afb1921/videos
- Guide Dogs (UK): https://www.youtube.com/user/GuideDogsUK/videos
- Optometry Today: https://www.youtube.com/user/OTMultimedia
- Perkins Vision: https://www.youtube.com/user/PSB1829/videos
- RNIB: https://www.youtube.com/user/rnibuk/videos

REFERENCES

American Foundation for the Blind. (2015). *Glossary of eye conditions.* Retrieved from, http://www.afb.org/info/living-with-vision-loss/eye-conditions/12.

Arbesman, M., Lieberman, D., & Berlanstein, D. R. (2013). Methodology for the systematic reviews on occupational therapy interventions for older adults with low vision. *American Journal of Occupational Therapy, 67*(3), 272–278.

Barstow, B. (2015). *Home environment evaluation for individuals with vision loss. In: Paper presented to the American Occupational Therapy Association (AOTA) 95th Annual Conference, Nashville, Tennessee.* Retrieved from, http://files.abstractsonline.com/CTRL/27/e/28e/c0a/5be/40a/9b3/66c/40b/a59/f35/8e/a2190_1. pdf.

Barstow, B. A., Bennett, D. K., & Vogtle, L. K. (2011). Perspectives on home safety: Do home safety assessments address the concerns of clients with vision loss? *American Journal of Occupational Therapy, 65*(6), 635–642.

Baum, C. M., & Christiansen, C. (2005). Person-Environment-Occupation-Performance Model: An occupation based framework for practice. In C. Christiansen, C. Baum, & J. Bass-Haugen (Eds.), *Occupational therapy performance, participation and well-being* (pp. 244–266). Thorofare, NJ: Slack.

Bennett, D., Mainer, K., Westbrook, J., Barstow, B., & Vogtle, J. (2014). *The low vision home evaluation.* Birmingham, AL and Gainesville, FL: Occupational Therapy Departments, University of Alabama at Birmingham and University of Florida at Gainesville.

Binns, A., Bunce, C., Dickinson, C., et al. (2012). How effective is low vision service provision? A systematic review. *Survey of Ophthalmology, 57*(1), 34–65.

Birmingham City University. (2015). *Rehabilitation work (visual impairment).* Retrieved from, http://www.bcu.ac.uk/courses/rehabilitation-work-visual-impairment-top-up.

Freeman, P. (2007). Overview and review of low vision evaluation. In M. Scheiman, M. Scheiman, & W. Whittaker (Eds.), *Low vision rehabilitation: A practical guide for occupational therapists* (pp. 94–102). Thorofare, NJ: Slack.

Gilbert, M., & Baker, S. (2011). Evaluation and intervention for basic and instrumental activities of daily living. In M. Warren, & E. Bartow (Eds.), *Occupational therapy interventions for adults with low vision* (pp. 227–268). Bethesda, MD: Bethesda American Occupational Therapy Association.

Law, M., Baptiste, S., Carswell, A., McColl, M. A., Polatajko, H., & Pollock, N. (Eds.), (1998). *Canadian occupational performance measure* (2nd ed.). Ottawa: CAOT Publications ACE.

Long, J. (2014). What is vision ergonomics. *Work, 47,* 287–2890.

Martin, M. (2013). *Falls in older people with sight loss: A review of emerging research and key action points. Research Discussion Paper 12.* London: Thomas Pocklington Trust. Retrieved from, http://www.pocklingtontrust.org.uk/Resources/Thomas%20Pocklington/Documents/PDF/Research%20Publications/RDP%2012_final.pdf.

Meyers, J., & Wilcox, D. (2011). Low vision evaluation. In M. Warren & E. Bartow (Eds.), *Occupational therapy interventions for adults with low vision* (pp. 47–74). Bethesda, MD: American Occupational Therapy Association.

Perlmutter, S. (2013). *Home environment lighting assessment (HELA).* St. Louis: Program in Occupational Therapy, Washington University School of Medicine. Retrieved from, https://www.ot.wustl.edu/mm/files/Home-Environment-Lighting-Assessment-(HELA).docx.

Perlmutter, M., Bhorade, A., Gordon, M., Hollingsworth, H., Engsberg, J. E., & Baum, C. M. (2013). Home lighting assessment for clients with low vision. *American Journal of Occupational Therapy, 67*(6), 674–681.

Polatajko, H. J., Craik, J., & Davis, J. (2007). Introducing the Canadian practice process framework (CPPF): Amplifying the context. In E. A. Townsend & H. J. Polatajko (Eds.), *Enabling occupation II: Advancing an occupational therapy vision for health, well-being, & justice through occupation* (pp. 229–246). Ottawa: CAOT Publications ACE.

Ranka, J., & Chapparo, C. (2011). Model illustration. *Occupational performance model (Australia)*. Retrieved from, http://www.occupationalperformance.com/model-illustration.

Resnikoff, S., Pascolini, D., Mariotti, S. P., & Pokharel, G. P. (2008). Global magnitude of visual impairment caused by uncorrected refractive errors in 2004. *Bulletin of the World Health Organization, 86*(1), 1–80. Retrieved from, http://www.who.int/bulletin/volumes/86/1/07-041210/en.

Riddering, A. (2011). Evaluation and Intervention for deficits in home and community mobility. In M. Warren & E. Bartow (Eds.), *Occupational therapy interventions for adults with low vision* (pp. 269–300). Bethesda, MD: American Occupational Therapy Association.

Scheiman, M., Scheiman, M., & Whittaker, W. (Eds.), (2007). *Low vision rehabilitation: A practical guide for occupational therapists.* Thorofare, NJ: Slack.

Standards Australia/New Zealand Standard. (2002). *Design for access and mobility. Part 4: Tactile indicators. 1428.4:2002.* Sydney: Standards Australia.

Standards Australia/New Zealand Standard. (2009). *Interior lighting: Safe movement. AS/NZS 1680.0:2009.* Sydney: Standards Australia.

Thomas Pocklington Trust. (2010). *Good housing design – lighting: A practice guide to improve lighting in existing homes.* London: Thomas Pocklington Trust. Retrieved from, *http://www.pocklingtontrust.org.uk/Resources/Thomas%20Pocklington/Documents/PDF/Research%20Publications/GPG5.pdf.*

Victorian State Government. (2015). *Active service model.* Retrieved from, http://www.health.vic.gov.au/hacc/projects/asm_project.htm#principles.

Vision Australia. (2012a). *Vision tests.* Retrieved from, http://www.visionaustralia.org/eye-health/assessing-vision-loss/vision-tests.

Vision Australia. (2012b). *Guiding a person who is blind or has low vision.* Retrieved from, http:/www.visionaustralia.org/living-with-low-vision/learning-to-live-independently/in-the-community/useful-tips-and-mobility-fact-sheets/guiding-a-person-who-is-blind-or-has-low-vision.

Vision Australia. (2012c). *Communicating effectively with people who are blind or vision impaired.* Retrieved from, http://www.visionaustralia.org/living-with-low-vision/family-friends-and-carers/communicating-effectively-with-people-who-are-blind-or-vision-impaired.

Wang, M. Y., Rousseau, J., Boisjoly, H., et al. (2012). Activity limitation due to a fear of falling in older adults with eye disease. *Investigative Ophthalmology & Visual Science, 53*(13), 7967–7972.

Warren, M. (n.d.). *Low Vision Rehabilitation Graduate Certificate, UAB School of Health Professionals.* Retrieved from, http://www.uab.edu/elearning/degrees-certificates/graduate/academic-certificates/low-vision-rehabilitation.

Warren, M., & Nobles, L. (2011). *Occupational therapy services for persons with visual impairment.* Bethesda, MD: American Occupational Therapy Association. Retrieved from, *http://www.aota.org/media/Corporate/Files/AboutOT/Professionals/WhatIsOT/PA/Facts/Low%20Vision%20fact%20sheet.pdf.*

Warren, M. (1993a). A hierarchical model for evaluation and treatment of visual perceptual dysfunction in adult acquired brain injury, part 1. *American Journal of Occupational Therapy, 47*(1), 42–54.

Warren, M. (1993b). A hierarchical model for evaluation and treatment of visual perceptual dysfunction in adult acquired brain injury, part 2. *American Journal of Occupational Therapy, 47*(2), 55–66.

Warren, M., Bachelder, J., Velozo, C., & Hicks, E. (2008). *The self-report assessment of functional visual performance.* Birmingham, AL & Gainesville, FL: Occupational Therapy Departments, University of Alabama at Birmingham and University of Florida at Gainesville. Retrieved from, *http://files.abstractsonline.com/CTRL/C4/1/5C4/97D/533/428/980/27B/657/EA4/C7C/82/a3260_2.pdf.*

Wood, J. M., Lacherez, P., Black, A. A., Cole, M. H., Boon, M. Y., & Kerr, G. K. (2011). Risk of falls, injurious falls, and other injuries resulting from visual impairment among older adults with age-related macular degeneration. *Investigative Ophthalmology & Visual Science, 52*(8), 5088–5092.

World Health Organization. (2012). *Vision impairment and blindness.* Retrieved from, http://www.who.int/mediacentre/factsheets/fs282/en.

Zolton, B. (Ed.), (2007). *Vision, perception and cognition. A manual for the evaluation and treatment of the adult with acquired brain injury.* Thorofare, NJ: Slack Incorporated.

40

OPTIMISING MOTOR PERFORMANCE AND SENSATION AFTER BRAIN IMPAIRMENT

ANNIE McCLUSKEY ■ NATASHA A. LANNIN ■ KARL SCHURR ■ SIMONE DORSCH

CHAPTER OUTLINE

Abstract

This chapter provides a framework for optimising motor performance and sensation in adults with brain impairment. Conditions such as stroke and traumatic brain injury are the main focus; however, the chapter content can apply to adults with other neurological conditions. The tasks of eating and drinking are used as examples throughout the chapter. Skills and knowledge required by graduates are identified, including knowledge of motor behaviour, the essential components of reaching to grasp and reaching in sitting, and how to identify compensatory strategies and develop and test movement hypotheses. Factors that enhance skill acquisition are discussed, including task specificity, practice intensity and timely feedback, with implications for therapists' teaching skills. Finally, a summary is provided of evidence-based interventions to improve motor performance and sensation, including high-intensity, task-specific training, mirror therapy, mental practice, electrical stimulation and constraint therapy.

KEY POINTS

- Essential knowledge in neurological rehabilitation includes an understanding of normal motor behaviour, muscle biology and skill acquisition.

- Abnormal motor performance can be observed during a task such as reaching for a cup and compared with expected performance. Hypotheses about the causes of observed movement differences can then be made and tested.

- Paralysis, weakness and loss of coordination affect upper limb motor performance. To improve performance after brain impairment, therapists should primarily focus on improving strength and coordination.

- Many people with brain impairment have difficulty understanding instructions, goals and feedback, and consequently may not practice well. To teach people to practice well and learn skills, therapists need to be good coaches.

- Motor performance and sensation can be improved using low-cost, evidence-based strategies such as high-intensity, repetitive, task-specific training, mirror therapy, mental practice, electrical stimulation and constraint-induced movement therapy.

INTRODUCTION

Upper motor neuron lesions typically cause impairments such as paralysis, muscle weakness and loss of sensation. These impairments can limit participation in everyday tasks such as eating a meal. *Motor control* is a term commonly used in rehabilitation (Shumway-Cook, 2012; van Vliet, Pelton, Hollands, Carey, & Wing, 2013) and refers to control of movements such as reaching to grasp a cup and standing up. Occupational therapists and physiotherapists retrain motor and sensory impairments that interfere with tasks such as grasping a cup and sitting safely on the toilet. The aim of this chapter is to provide a framework that helps therapists to systematically observe, analyse and measure motor and sensory impairments. Targeted evidence-based interventions will be described that can drive neuroplasticity. Therapists need to proactively seek muscle activity and sensation. It is not enough to teach a person how to compensate using one-handed techniques or to wait for recovery to possibly occur.

ESSENTIAL SKILLS, KNOWLEDGE AND ATTITUDES FOR IMPROVING MOTOR PERFORMANCE

Therapists should think of themselves as 'movement scientists' (Carr, Shepherd, Gordon Gentile, & Held, 1987; Refshauge, Ada,

& Ellis, 2005). A movement scientist uses specialist knowledge from basic science (e.g. neuroplasticity, muscle biology), applied science (e.g. biomechanics of normal movement and motor control), education and adult learning (e.g. coaching strategies, feedback and practice) to inform analysis and training. Valid reliable instruments are used to measure change in performance and evaluate the effectiveness of intervention. Systematic reviews and randomised controlled trials are critically appraised and their clinical implications used to guide treatment. The first step in this process involves movement analysis, where therapists identify missing or decreased essential components. Next, therapists can hypothesise about which impairments may be the cause of the movement problems and compensatory strategies, and make these impairments the focus of intervention. It is essential for therapists to understand the impairments that contribute to movement problems after stroke or brain injury.

ANALYSING MOVEMENT

Movement analysis involves observing a person as he or she attempts a task, then comparing the attempt with 'normal' movement. Therefore therapists need to understand the essential components and biomechanics of normal movement, including kinematics and kinetics. The biomechanics of reaching to grasp a glass or cup will be described to illustrate the process of movement analysis.

Normal Reaching to Grasp

The kinematics and kinetics of reaching to grasp have been described elsewhere (Alt Murphy & Häger, 2015). *Kinematics* refers to what can be seen (i.e. angular displacements, velocity and acceleration). For example, when a person reaches for a glass or cup, as shown in Fig. 40.1, shoulder flexion and thumb abduction movements can be seen. The *kinetics* (or forces) that cause these displacements can be inferred but not directly observed. In the example shown, the anterior deltoid, and thumb abductor muscles, respectively, cause the angular displacements that we observe.

It is helpful to have a framework when analysing reaching to grasp. Normal reaching to grasp can be divided into three phases: transport, preshaping and grasp (Table 40.1). Each phase involves essential components that are necessary for efficient performance (Carr & Shepherd, 2010). These essential components will be described in turn.

Transport refers to movement (trajectory) of the arm and hand forwards to the cup. Essential components include shoulder flexion, protraction and external rotation to move the arm forwards, with varying degrees of elbow flexion and extension, depending on reach height and distance. When adults reach for a cup that is close (e.g. within 60% of arm's length), there is minimal hip flexion or trunk movement (Dean, Shepherd, & Adam, 1999a). When reaching for a cup that is equal to or greater than an arm's length away (e.g. 100% or 140% of arm's length), the hips also flex to transport the trunk and arm towards the cup.

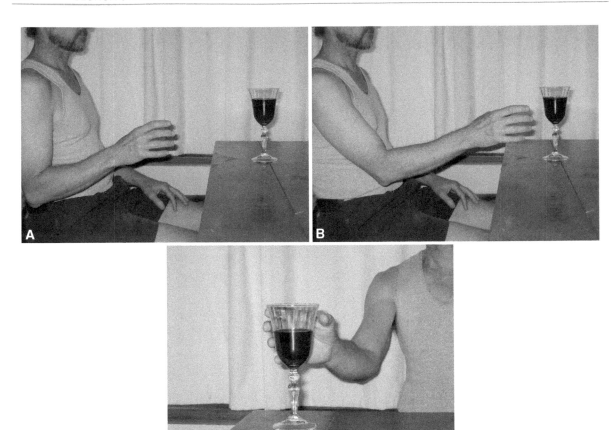

FIG. 40.1 ■ Transport and preshaping of the hand when reaching to grasp a glass. These illustrations present the kinematics of reaching (i.e. what can be seen). (A and B) The trajectory of the arm (the transport phase) and preshaping of the fingers and thumb. As the hand is transported forwards, the shoulder moves into forward flexion, external rotation (enabling the hand and thumb to reach the glass), elbow flexion and then elbow extension. (C) Wrist extension and the forearm held midway between pronation and supination. As preshaping occurs, the fingers are slightly flexed and rotated (at the metacarpal joints), producing pad-to-pad opposition in preparation for contact with the glass. The thumb is abducted to make a space for the glass but also rotated at the base of the thumb, allowing pad-to-pad opposition.

TABLE 40.1		
Phases and Essential Components of Reaching to Grasp a Glass: A Framework for Analysis		
Phase	**Essential components**	**Primary Muscles**
Transport:	External rotation	■ Infraspinatus, supraspinatus, teres minor, posterior deltoid
	Shoulder flexion	■ Anterior deltoid, pectoralis major and minor, coracobrachialis, biceps brachii
	Protraction	■ Serratus anterior, pectoralis major
	Elbow flexion and extension	■ Biceps brachii, brachialis, triceps brachii, brachioradialis
Preshaping:	Ulnar or radial deviation	■ Flexor and extensor ulnaris, flexor and extensor carpi radialis
	Supination	■ Supinator, biceps brachii
	Wrist extension	■ Extensor carpi radialis longus, extensor ulnaris
	Thumb abduction	■ Abductor pollicus longus and brevis

TABLE 40.1

Phases and Essential Components of Reaching to Grasp a Glass: A Framework for Analysis *(Continued)*

Phase	Essential components	Primary Muscles
	Thumb conjunct rotation (opposition)	■ Opponens pollicus; thumb abduction and flexion at the carpometacarpal thumb joint enabling pulp-to-pulp opposition of the thumb to the fingers
	Metacarpophalangeal extension	■ Extensor digitorum communis, extensor indicus (index finger), extensor digiti minimi (little finger)
	Interphalangeal flexion	■ Interossei, lumbricals, flexor digiti superficialis, flexor digiti profundus
	Finger abduction	■ Palmar interossei
Grasp:	Metacarpophalangeal flexion	■ Interossei; lumbricals
	Interphalangeal flexion	■ Interossei; lumbricals; flexor digiti superficialis, flexor digiti profundus
	Adduction and flexion of thumb	■ Adductor pollicus, first dorsal interossei, flexor pollicus longus and brevis, opponens pollicus

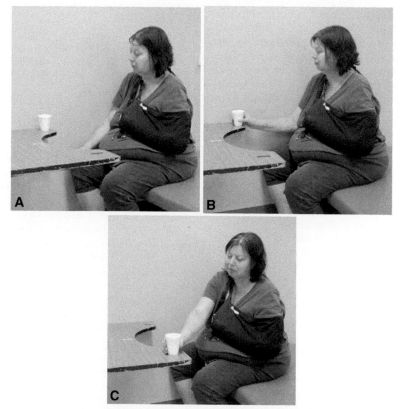

FIG. 40.2 ■ Reaching in sitting (cup within arm's length, then at 100% of arm's length). (A and B) There is minimal hip flexion and trunk displacement when this lady reaches for a cup which is close and within arm's length. Her elbow remains flexed even when grasping the cup. (C) The cup has been placed at arm's length and on her affected side. Hip and shoulder flexion and elbow extension all help this lady to successfully transport her hand forwards.

Trunk displacement via hip flexion is observed earlier in the movement sequence when people reach for objects farther away. The elbow may not fully extend at the end of reach (see Figs. 40.1B and 40.1C), unless that is the only way the object can be reached (Fig. 40.2).

Preshaping of the hand, fingers and thumb begins almost simultaneously with transport of the arm. Preshaping involves anticipating and making the shape and size of the cup. The forearm in Fig. 40.1 is midway between supination and pronation; the wrist is extended and the thumb abducted, with sufficient metacarpophalangeal (MCP) extension for the fingers to fit around the object. The interphalangeal joints of the fingers remain curved, replicating the shape of the wineglass shown. The fingers may also be slightly abducted to conform to the shape of the object.

Grasp begins when the fingers and thumb touch the object. MCP and finger flexion, thumb adduction, and conjunct rotation of the thumb and fingers enable grasp and apply an equal force from either side of the cup, keeping the cup upright in preparation for drinking. If any of these essential components are missing, a person will need to use compensatory strategies to reach, preshape and grasp. Compensatory strategies are discussed later in this chapter.

When reaching for an object, the brain automatically selects the most appropriate hand trajectory, decides when to begin forming the appropriate shape and anticipates how much grip force to use based on experience and visual input. There is initial acceleration of the hand followed by deceleration before grasp. The proportion of time allocated to acceleration and deceleration will vary depending on the nature of the object (e.g. a delicate wine glass vs. a pottery coffee mug) and the intent of the person (e.g. picking up a knife to cut food or place the knife in the sink). In addition, adaptations to these anticipated forces may need to be made at the point of grasp.

This process of normal reach occurs with little or no conscious thought. Grasp is based on the *intrinsic* properties of the object, such as the shape, size and perceived fragility (e.g. a plastic cup vs. a wineglass) as well as *extrinsic* factors, such as distance from the object and whether the person is sitting or standing.

This timing and the synchronisation of reaching requires careful, systematic observation if differences are to be recognised, compared with the expected essential components. For example, in healthy adults, transport of the arm and hand preshaping begin almost simultaneously (van Vliet, 1998), although the arm begins to move slightly before the thumb and fingers open.

Reaching to grasp in children has been investigated (e.g. Zoia et al., 2006) and compared with adults' reaching. If object size and distance reached are varied, adults and 5-year-old children show very similar reaching strategies. The major differences are longer movement duration and deceleration times and a larger hand aperture in 5-year-old children. People with sensory impairments who are uncertain about their grasp may also reach with a larger than necessary aperture.

In summary, when reaching forwards for a cup, the arm begins to move slightly before the hand opens. When reaching for close objects the elbow typically remains flexed, with shoulder flexion and external rotation helping to transport the hand forwards. When reaching for distant objects, trunk and hip flexion help transport the hand forwards together with shoulder flexion, external rotation and elbow extension. These features are often referred to as 'essential' components of reaching (Carr & Shepherd, 2010).

Postural Adjustments in Sitting

In the next section, a summary is provided of the adjustments needed to maintain sitting when reaching for a cup and what features to observe when analysing sitting. The focus is on analysing and training sitting and leg extensor activation, not upper limb reaching. The focus is on the leg muscles as they are essential for sitting, and are more likely to be affected by an upper motor lesion than the trunk muscles. It is primarily the leg, and not the trunk muscles, that prevent falling when a person reaches forwards or to the side. Other features, including *base of support, reaching distance* and *direction,* will be discussed. These features can be manipulated during analysis and training to make seated reaching easier or more challenging.

When reaching for a cup in sitting, it is intuitively known and anticipated what will happen when reaching forwards, sideways or towards the floor in response to the effect of gravity. The motor control system anticipates which muscles are necessary to maintain balance and avoid falling. These postural adjustments are required, for example, during dressing and toileting. The base of support and the direction and speed of reaching all influence the muscle activity required when reaching in sitting (Dean et al., 1999a, 1999b).

The *base of support* comprises the feet and thighs when sitting with both feet on the floor (see Figs. 40.2A–C). When reaching forwards beyond that base of support, the leg muscles are critical for maintaining sitting (Dean et al., 1999a, 1999b). For example, when reaching for a cup at 140% of arm's length, tibialis anterior contracts before anterior deltoid in the arm. Soleus, quadriceps and biceps femoris and quadriceps muscles contract soon after, to control the forwards movement of our body mass (Crosbie et al., 1995; Dean et al., 1999a) (Fig. 40.3).

If thigh support is reduced when reaching forwards, the contribution of the leg muscles also increases (Dean, Shepherd, & Adam, 1999b). If both feet are off the floor, the base of support now comprises only the thighs (see Fig. 40.3F). Consequently postural adjustments cannot be made using the large muscles that cross the knees and ankles and the feet cannot be stabilised on the floor. Instead, with this smaller base of support, only the muscles around the hip maintain sitting and prevent falling. Therefore reaching distance is significantly reduced when both feet are off the ground.

Reaching direction also influences leg muscle activity. Reaching for a cup on the right side results in increased right leg extensor activation (Dean et al., 1999b). As a result, if a person has a leg amputation, this will reduce the distance a person can reach to the amputated side when not wearing a prosthesis (Chari & Kirby, 1986).

Research on normal reaching in sitting can be applied during analysis and when training people who have difficulty staying upright while reaching. For example, if a person is unable to generate sufficient leg extensor force to prevent falling while reaching forwards, the person will need to learn to activate the leg extensor muscles. Reaching forwards will be easiest when

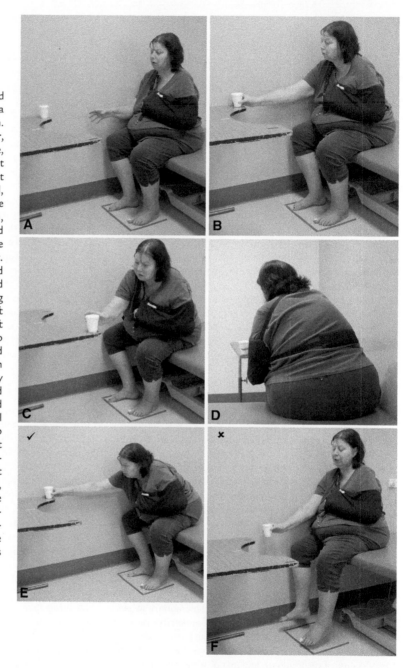

FIG. 40.3 ■ Postural adjustments required to stay upright in sitting, when reaching for a cup at distances greater than arm's length. (A) This lady has been asked to reach for, and pick up, a cup on her unaffected side, beyond arm's length. Her thighs and feet form her base of support. (B) She looks at the object, begins to preshape her hand, anticipates the effect that gravity will have on her base of support as she lifts her arm, then transports her arm forwards. To avoid falling forwards when lifting her arm, she pushes down on the ground with her feet. (C) This lady is reaching for a cup placed beyond arm's length and on her affected side. This task is difficult for her, requiring greater leg extensor activity from her left leg. If she does not push through her left leg and foot, she will fall forwards and to her left. (D) Her weight shifts forwards and to her left side. (E) A training session which involves practice of seated reaching. This lady is practising reaching for a cup placed beyond arm's length and to her unaffected side. When her skill and motor control improves, she will practise placing the cup across to the left side of the table. Her feet are on the floor and her thighs well supported. Electrical tape marks correct foot position. (F) The seat height has been raised, and this lady's feet are now off the floor. She cannot push down through her feet. Consequently, she is unable to reach as far forwards. To optimise successful reaching, the base of support available to a person needs to be carefully considered and planned.

there is maximal thigh support and the feet are on the floor. The person will be more successful if he or she is first asked to reach to a target within arm's reach. This practice will allow the person to learn to control hip flexion and forwards movement of the trunk as he or she reaches, before being expected to reach beyond arm's length.

Less muscle activity is required from the affected leg extensors if a person reaches to the unaffected side. Therefore during analysis and training, it will be easier for a person to first reach for a cup on the unaffected side. Task difficulty can be progressed by reaching farther, first to the unaffected side, then to the front, then to the affected side. As the person becomes more successful, the amount of thigh support can be reduced to increase the force required from the legs.

Feedback also helps to increase learning. If a person is unable to generate sufficient extensor force on the affected leg, he or she may need specific feedback about whether the leg muscles are working. Bathroom scales can give feedback about the force being generated through the affected leg (e.g. weight in kilograms). Bathroom scales can also indicate whether the leg muscles are pushing at the appropriate time (i.e. anticipating the transfer of weight forwards) to prevent the person falling. Systematic and persistent practice of reaching in this way can improve reaching ability in sitting in stroke survivors in acute hospital (Dean, Channon, & Hall, 2007) and community settings (Dean & Shepherd, 1997).

Before concluding this section, it is important to emphasise the problems that result from 'facilitating' or manually guiding a person to move. Training postural adjustments and sitting balance by moving a person will result in very different muscle activation patterns compared with self-generated movement. The person cannot anticipate when disturbances to movement will occur, nor the direction or force. Manual guidance is unlikely to help the person activate the muscles necessary for self-generated movement (e.g. when cleaning himself or herself on the toilet). Such 'training' strategies are unhelpful and may cause the person to become fearful of moving during therapy.

Strategies used during analysis and training should aim to mimic the normal sequence of muscle activity specific to the task (see Table 40.2 for examples). If a person is unable to sit, the therapist will need to analyse the reasons why the person cannot sit and then develop training strategies specific to those difficulties.

In summary, seated reach can be progressed by gradually increasing the distance and changing the direction of reach (i.e. to the unaffected side, then forwards, then to the affected side) and decreasing the amount of thigh support.

Focus on Positive Versus Negative Impairments

Impairments after a stroke or brain injury can be classified as either *positive* or *negative* (Ada & Canning, 2005). *Positive* impairments are 'added' features and include abnormal postures and exaggerated reflexes producing spasticity. *Negative* impairments are the loss of body functions and include paralysis (inability to activate muscles), weakness (loss of muscle strength), loss of coordination and loss of sensation. These negative impairments, particularly weakness, limit people with neurological conditions more than the positive impairments. Negative impairments after a stroke or brain injury have shown a clear association with activity limitations, whereas positive impairments have shown no consistent association (Ada, O'Dwyer, & O'Neill, 2006b; Harris & Eng, 2007; Zackowski, Dromerick, Sahrmann, Thach, & Bastian, 2004).

Therapy textbooks (e.g. Brashear & Elovic, 2011) and many experienced therapists focus on the diagnosis and management of spasticity (a positive impairment) but provide less guidance on strength or coordination training. Yet addressing the positive impairments after stroke and brain injury is unlikely to improve activity. While acknowledging the possible presence of spasticity and contracture, we question the emphasis placed on these impairments. In this chapter, examples are provided of intervention strategies that focus on loss of strength and coordination (the negative impairments) along with the evidence for these strategies. A focus on the negative impairments is more likely to improve outcomes.

A final note about analysing and labelling motor impairments: therapists sometimes use the terms *spasticity* or *high tone* to refer to stiff or tight muscles or stiff joints. Often what therapists describe as spasticity or high tone is a shortening of muscles (a contracture). Therapists need to learn how to distinguish between contracture and spasticity in order to plan appropriate intervention. Commonly used assessments such as the Modified Ashworth Scale do not distinguish between contracture and spasticity, whereas the Tardieu Scale does (Patrick & Ada, 2006). The Tardieu Scale assesses the response of a muscle to a fast or slow stretch. A reduction in range of movement in response to a slow stretch is due to contracture, whereas a reduction in movement in response to a fast stretch is due to spasticity.

Recognising Contractures

Changes in the mechanical-elastic properties of muscles and connective tissue limit joint range of movement after stroke (Vattanasilp, Ada, & Crosbie, 2000) and other neurological conditions. When analysing movement, a contracture can be recognised by loss of joint range and increased resistance to passive movement at a joint (Ada & Canning, 2005). Resistance is typically due to peripheral changes in muscle fibres and connective tissue (O'Dwyer, Ada, & Neilson, 1996; Pandyan et al., 2003), not to central nervous system changes or spasticity. Animal studies have found that muscles shorten and lengthen in response to immobilisation. Animal muscles decrease in length when immobilised in a shortened position, such as in a plaster cast (Tabary et al., 1972; Williams & Goldspink, 1978).

Contractures are undesirable for many reasons, including the effect they can have on a person's performance. The incidence of contractures after a stroke is surprisingly high. A recent study of 200 consecutive stroke survivors found that 52% had developed a contracture at one or more joints by their 6-month follow-up (Kwah, Harvey, Diong, & Herbert, 2012). A person with contractures of pectoralis major, biceps brachii, wrist or finger flexor muscles may be unable to reach forwards and pre-shape their hand to achieve normal grasp. Efforts are required to actively prevent muscle contractures using motor retraining, because there are no effective treatments for contractures once they develop (Katalinic et al., 2010). Short duration stretch methods such as passive ranging of joints and external devices

TABLE 40.2
Summary of Seated Reaching without Back Support

Reaching Forwards in Sitting without Back Support, Feet on the Floor	Anticipatory Muscle Activity Leg/Trunk	Implications for Intervention	Possible Training Strategies
Within arm's length	Back extensors Hip extensors	■ Begin to train reaching within arm's length if person is unable to activate hip extensors ■ Sit with back support to minimise initial task difficulty ■ Provide trunk support if unable to sit without assistance	**Practice Set-up** ■ Sitting with back support: practice moving forwards (hip flexors) and back (hip extensors) towards the back support ■ Provide vertical cue for sitting alignment (i.e. if the person is falling towards the **left,** position the person with a wall on the **right** side to provide a close vertical cue and feedback when the person begins to fall ■ Provide visual cue (e.g. line on wall for appropriate shoulder position)
Greater than arm's length	Hip extensors Knee extensors Plantar flexors	■ Practise sitting on a stable surface ■ Specific training of hip and knee extensor strength and endurance on affected side ■ Sitting on lower surface and maximising thigh support to decrease extensor force required ■ Feet well supported on the floor	**Feedback:** 1. How long can the person maintain vertical alignment? (i.e. keep shoulder next to the wall or next to the line on the wall) 2. How much weight has the person put through the affected leg? Place bathroom scales under affected foot for feedback about weight bearing
Reaching to the side	Ipsilateral hip, knee and ankle extensors	■ Train reaching to nonaffected side and to the front initially if person is unable to reach to the affected side ■ Gradually increase distance the person is attempting to reach ■ Gradually introduce reaching across the midline towards the affected side ■ Ensure appropriate alignment of weight-bearing leg (i.e. knee over foot, leg not abducted) ■ Ensure person begins to use leg extensors in anticipation of weight transference to affected side	**Progression** Progress difficulty by: ■ Increasing time in sitting ■ Increasing distance from wall ■ Decreasing thigh support ■ Increasing height of surface ■ Increasing distance reached ■ Increasing distance reached to affected side

such as handsplints do not reverse contractures (Lannin, Cusick, McCluskey, & Herbert, 2007). Therefore strategies to elicit muscle contractions and initiate movement are required. These are discussed later in this chapter.

In summary, muscles adapt quickly to altered positions and immobilisation. Sarcomeres and connective tissue can undergo structural changes resulting in loss of joint range of motion and resistance to movement which can be felt during analysis. As yet there are no demonstrated interventions that prevent or reverse contractures.

Recognising Compensatory Strategies

When analysing performance, therapists need to recognise the compensatory strategies that a person may use resulting from loss of normal muscle activity (Carr & Shepherd, 2010). Compensations may be caused by a muscle contracture, muscle weakness or both. For example, a person who cannot successfully reach forwards to grasp a cup may use hip flexion and/or shoulder abduction to compensate for poor shoulder flexion. In previous years, these patterns of muscle contraction were called 'abnormal synergies' and believed to be part of the normal stages of recovery. However, there is no neurophysiological explanation for these synergies. Rather, this compensatory muscle activity is used as the best biomechanical option available to the person who cannot activate the required muscles appropriately (Carr & Shepherd, 2010).

The more a person practices using compensations, the more he or she learns these neural pathways, which then become difficult to change. Therefore therapists need to help people to contract their muscles more appropriately. When observing a person reach to grasp a cup, the kinematics of this movement should be compared with normal movement. For example, when a person is preshaping his or her hand to reach for a cup within arm's reach, is the person opening the hand and abducting the thumb at the beginning of reaching? Thumb abduction and MCP extension of the fingers are essential and result in a grasp aperture large enough to accommodate the cup. Typically, people who have difficulty abducting their thumb and/or extending their fingers and wrist may compensate by extending their thumb, pronating their forearm and/or abducting their shoulder (Carr & Shepherd, 2010) (Fig. 40.4). These strategies may lead to successful contact with a cup, but like all compensations, they are inefficient and inflexible in the long term.

When a person transports his or her arm towards a cup that is nearby (i.e. within arm's reach), observe whether or not the person is using the shoulder flexors and external rotators without using excessive shoulder elevation, internal rotation or abduction. The latter three compensatory movements may suggest weakness or paralysis of the person's shoulder flexors and/or external rotators. Alternatively, these shoulder movements may be a strategy to compensate for poor control of forearm, wrist, thumb or finger muscles. For example, if thumb abduction is missing but the person is able to extend the thumb, the person may pronate the forearm and abduct and internally rotate the shoulder to enable the altered aperture between the thumb and index finger to approach the cup, as shown in Fig. 40.4B. For a full discussion and analysis, see Carr and Shepherd (2010).

When reaching in sitting, it is normal to flex at the hips to reach distances at arm's length or greater (Dean et al., 1999a). However, it is not normal to use hip flexion when reaching for an object that is close. In this case hip flexion and trunk movement may be compensations for weak shoulder flexors and/or external rotators.

In summary, compensatory strategies are common but should be minimised because they can prevent the learning of normal movement. Therapists need to analyse performance, identify missing essential components, hypothesise about the causes of observed compensations and then test these hypotheses.

Hypothesising about Compensatory Strategies

The final step in the process of analysing movement is to develop and test hypotheses about the causes of missing essential components in order to plan interventions. One hypothesis might be that a person's shoulder muscles are paralysed or too weak to lift

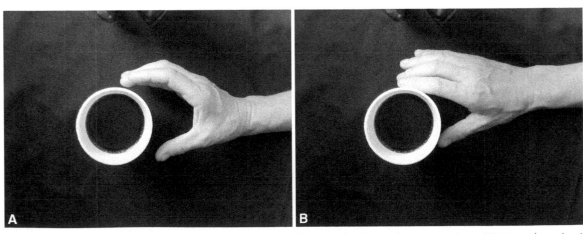

FIG. 40.4 ■ Normal preshaping while reaching for a cup and commonly observed compensations. (A) Normal preshaping during reaching, with the thumb abducted and opposed and the person's wrist extended ready to grasp the cup. (B) This person is pronating the forearm during reaching to compensate for poor control of thumb abduction (a missing essential component). Instead of abducting the thumb, the person is extending the thumb and pronating the forearm (two compensations), to try and grasp the cup.

the limb up against gravity to reach for a cup. That hypothesis can be tested by assessing muscle strength (i.e. conducting a manual muscle test or palpating the muscle belly during a movement attempt). If a person cannot easily reach forwards, two key muscles to check are anterior deltoid (a shoulder flexor) and infraspinatus (an external rotator). If these muscles are weak, strengthening will be required.

A second hypothesis might be that muscles such as the internal rotators, elbow, wrist and finger flexors are short or stiff due to contractures. The opposing muscles may be incapable of generating the necessary force to lift the arm, extend the wrist or open the hand. This hypothesis can be tested by manually checking the passive range of external rotation, forward flexion, elbow, wrist and finger extension and thumb abduction. Loss of range at any one of these joints will change the person's ability to reach for an object such as a cup.

A third possible hypothesis might be that the person is using excessive muscle force to achieve the task (i.e. to pick up the cup). The person may be using too many muscles, too much force, or both. A group of muscles such as the finger and wrist flexors may contract with excessive force when movement is attempted. Overactivity may occur, where most muscles in the arm switch on with effort to help compensate for weakness in particular muscle groups, such as the shoulder flexors. This hypothesis can be tested by setting up the practice task so that effort is minimised. For example, the person could practice reaching with the arm supported on a table and a sheet of paper or cloth under the hand to reduce friction during reaching.

A fourth hypothesis might be that the task or environmental set-up is too challenging given the person's current functional abilities. The cup may be positioned too far in front or to the side for the person to grasp without compensating, or the table may be too high. These hypotheses can be tested by placing the cup closer or lowering the table. Taping a light polystyrene cup into the hand will also decrease task demands and eliminate the need for preshaping. The person can then concentrate on transporting the cup and not preshaping. Each movement hypothesis can be tested in turn.

Assuming the person's movement problems have been correctly analysed, the missing essential components and compensations identified and hypotheses tested, the next step is to design a programme to improve performance. This programme will need to address motor learning.

TEACHING MOTOR SKILLS

People with brain impairment often have difficulty understanding instructions, using feedback, remembering their practice and learning motor skills. Therefore therapists need to develop critical teaching skills and become effective coaches. Therapists need to understand motor learning, provide training that is task specific and give useful, timely feedback. Each of these factors will influence motor learning.

The Stages of Motor Learning

There is considerable literature on motor learning. The three stages originally described by Fitts and Posner (1967) are often used to inform rehabilitation practice: These stages are (1) the verbal-cognitive stage, (2) the motor stage, and (3) the autonomous stage. In the first stage, learners rely on verbal feedback and external environmental information to achieve goals and understand the demands of a task. In the second stage, the focus is on the quality of movement, mass practice (Mastos et al., 2007) and decreasing mistakes. Finally, in the third stage the learner is able to perform the task with less cognitive effort, cope more effectively with distractions and draw on his or her problem-solving skills when performing the task in novel situations. At each stage, learners need timely feedback about performance and goal achievement (Magill, 2011; Schmidt & Lee, 2005).

Using the previous training example of reaching for a cup while sitting, a goal might be for the person to sit upright for 30 seconds without falling to the affected side. In the first stage of learning, the person may require continual feedback about pushing through the affected leg to avoid falling to the affected side. In the second stage the person may recognise when he or she is beginning to fall, make an attempt to prevent this but require occasional assistance or prompting. In the third stage, the person can sit without assistance, conduct a conversation and reach forwards to pick up an object without falling to the affected side. If practice tasks are too demanding in the early stages of learning, the person may be unable to achieve the goal. For example, asking the person to reach to the affected side before he or she can sit upright for 5 seconds would be unrealistic.

Making Training Task Specific

The terms *task-specific training, task-related practice* and *specificity of training* are used in the literature (e.g. Hubbard, Parsons, Neilson, & Carey, 2009; Michaelsen, Dannenbaum, & Levin, 2006). These terms refer to therapy involving intentional practice of a specific movement, action or task, versus repetition of nonspecific tasks (Bayona, Bitensky, Salter, & Teasell, 2005) such as lifting the arm up high for no reason, touching the head or nose or stacking cones instead of practicing reaching for a cup. Examples of task-specific training include practice of pen or cutlery manipulation to improve writing and eating, respectively, or picking up a cup to improve drinking. In the early stages of motor recovery, when a person cannot hold objects, implements can be taped into the affected hand or placed in front to encourage task-specific reaching.

Studies also demonstrate the importance of using real-life tasks for motor training. People with a brain injury produced more movement and improved coordination when reaching to control a computer game (Sietsema et al., 1993) and while engaging in kitchen activities (Neistadt, 1994) compared with simulating the tasks.

The bottom line is that people learn what they practise. If a person wants to improve drinking from a cup, they should practise reaching for and transporting a cup, not a plastic shape or cone that vaguely resembles a cup. Early training might involve sliding or placing a lightweight plastic cup forwards on a low table, with the cup taped into the person's hand if the person does not have active hand movement. Advanced coordination training might involve moving and manipulating objects of interest, such as garments, eyeglasses, cutlery and writing implements, not beans or plastic counters. Training should replicate the skill or task that a person wants to learn. Valuable time should not be wasted on nonspecific practice.

Maximising Practice and Repetitions

More time spent practising leads to improved performance across many skill areas, including leisure tasks (such as chess and golf), work tasks (such as typing) and playing musical instruments (Ericsson, 2014). In a study involving 20-year-old violinists (Ericsson, 2004) the best performers, as judged by conservatory teachers, averaged 10,000 hours of practice during their lives. The second-best performers averaged 7500 hours, the next-best, 5000 hours and so forth.

A similar commitment to practice is required by learners with brain impairment and therapists if motor performance is to improve. In a randomised controlled trial that demonstrated significant improvements in sitting ability (Dean & Shepherd, 1997), people who had a stroke each performed 2970 reaches beyond arm's length during a 2-week training period. Carey, Macdonell, & Matyas, (2002) found that 1200 repetitions of a finger-tracking task resulted in neuroplasticity as observed on functional magnetic resonance imaging scans. These changes in the brain also correlated with improved motor performance on the Box and Block test.

Massed practice and multiple repetitions are also features of constraint-induced movement therapy (CIMT; Taub et al., 2013). CIMT involves intensive practice of tasks using the affected arm while the unimpaired arm is restrained. CIMT studies require participants to practise for 3 to 6 hours a day, aiming for at least 250 repetitions per hour. The number of repetitions required to improve performance after brain impairment remains unknown but thousands of repetitions are likely to be required.

Setting a repetition target can dramatically increase practice. In one study (Waddell, Birkenmeier, Moore, Hornby, & Lang, 2014), 15 participants who had a stroke completed an average of 2956 repetitions of upper limb tasks during their hospital admission and averaged 289 repetitions per hour (95% CI, 280–299). Active practice during each therapy session averaged 47 minutes (95% CI, 46.1–48.0). Action Research Arm Test scores improved by a mean of 10 points, from 25/57 at baseline up to 35/57 at discharge and 40/57 1 month later. In a companion study (Birkenmeier, Prager, & Lang, 2010), 15 outpatients who had had a stroke completed an average of 5476 repetitions over 6 weeks, with an average of 322 repetitions of upper limb tasks per hour (95% CI, 285–358). Time spent actively practising

during each therapy session averaged 47 minutes, and Action Research Arm Test scores improved by a mean of 8 points (95% CI, 4–12) from 21/57 at baseline, up to 29/57 6 weeks later and 29/57 1 month later.

Finally, practice that involves many repetitions but no transfer of learning may limit skill development. For example, using a fork with a built-up handle to repeatedly pick up pieces of soft bread will not enable a person to eat a meal successfully in a restaurant with a normal fork. People improve their performance by practising in a variety of situations and experiencing errors during learning. People need to practise in different settings, with different movement parameters (e.g. forks with different handles and different foods). Increasing demands in this way helps learners to problem solve and fathom the rules underlying task performance (Magill, 2011).

Giving Feedback

Accurate feedback is critical to the teaching and learning of motor skills. Feedback can be provided by the task itself (intrinsic feedback), or by an outside source such as the therapist, biofeedback device or timer (extrinsic feedback). Extrinsic feedback has been further classified into two types: knowledge of performance and knowledge of results (Kilduski & Rice, 2003).

Knowledge of performance refers to information about the movement process or attempt – for example, 'You kept your elbow too close to your body'. Extrinsic feedback can be very helpful to learners, particularly concerning corrections that need to be made and features to focus on during subsequent attempts (Kernodle & Carlton, 1992). *Knowledge of results* refers to information about the movement outcome – for example, 'You picked up the cup 10 times in 20 seconds'. Knowledge of results within a training session (i.e. how long it took to complete a task or the number of successful attempts to complete a task) can be used to set short-term goals that are meaningful to the learner and related to the task being practised. See Fig. 40.5 for an example of a practice task involving feedback.

The amount and timing of feedback are important. Too much feedback can negatively influence learning (van Vliet & Wulf, 2006). Intermittent feedback is more effective than constant feedback (Winstein & Schmidt, 1990). Concurrent knowledge of results – that is, feedback provided during performance – may also negatively influence learning. Providing summary or average feedback after task completion is more likely to benefit learning (van Vliet & Wulf, 2006).

In summary, therapists should aim to provide auditory and visual feedback and encourage self-monitoring during sessions. Although it is not known exactly what feedback schedule produces the best outcomes in rehabilitation, therapists can help people to monitor their own performance and generate their own feedback. Only then will learners be able to effectively practice unsupervised and maximise their rehabilitation outcomes.

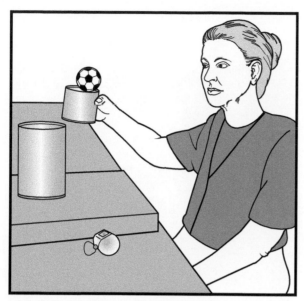

FIG. 40.5 ■ Practice with feedback. This lady's practice has been set up so that she receives feedback about her reaching. The mini football will roll off the tin if she uses insufficient external rotation, forearm supination and wrist extension. Knowledge of performance provided by the therapist might include stating that 'You are moving your body forward. You need to keep your back against the chair and lift your arm higher'. Knowledge of results might include the number of successful attempts out of 10 repetitions or time taken to complete 10 repetitions.

EVALUATING CHANGES IN MOTOR PERFORMANCE

Therapists need to reevaluate motor (and occupational) performance by using objective measures before and during training. Ideally a review of performance and goals will occur at every session. Performance can be measured using simple equipment. For example, to determine whether a person with sitting balance problems is bearing weight equally through both legs, bathroom scales may be used. Other simple measures of performance include the number of correctly performed movements versus those performed with compensations, or the distance reached.

If performance is not changing, the problem may lie with the therapist rather than the learner. Common reasons for lack of improvement include unclear instructions, feedback and goals. If instructions are unclear, the learner may not understand the expected goal. Similarly, if feedback is unclear (or absent), the person may not understand how to change the next movement attempt to achieve success.

In addition to considering the words therapists use to explain and correct movement attempts, the task chosen to elicit a movement attempt is also important. If the task is too difficult (or too easy), progress may not be seen. When remeasurement of performance shows little or no progress, it is vital to reflect on the possible reasons. If the movement hypotheses are correct, therapists can then critically appraise their teaching skills. Alternatively, if a different movement hypothesis is made, new training strategies will be needed. Therapists should not underestimate the importance of remeasuring performance, reflecting on their teaching skills and, above all, persisting and expecting to see improved motor performance in every session.

Practice Story 40.1 shows how one occupational therapist developed his teaching and analysis skills and applied evidence-based practice in rehabilitation.

EVIDENCE-BASED INTERVENTION TO IMPROVE UPPER LIMB MOTOR PERFORMANCE AND SENSATION

There are several reasons why a person may be unable to reach for, grasp and drink from a cup, or dress without overbalancing. Different causes will require different interventions. Many therapy interventions have been tested in randomised trials and the collective findings synthesised in systematic reviews. Interventions found to be effective in randomised controlled trials and systematic reviews are referred to in this section (see also Table 40.3). It will be noted if interventions and training strategies have not been rigorously tested and rely on lower level evidence or personal experience.

In adult rehabilitation, interventions found to improve performance of upper limb motor control commonly involve greater intensity of practice and repetitions and task-specific training strategies to improve strength (Pollock et al., 2014; Veerbeek et al., 2014). By definition, more intense practice and repetitions require the active involvement of the learner. One of the biggest challenges in rehabilitation is increasing the amount of practice. People need to spend as much time as possible actually practising. One hour of therapy doing 100 repetitions is better than 1 hour of therapy doing 10 or 20 repetitions. Setting a target, such as 300 repetitions per session, recording and reviewing repetitions helps to increase practice intensity (Birkenmeier et al., 2010; Waddell et al., 2014).

With greater recognition that intensive practice can improve outcomes, many therapists prescribe homework. In hospital, homework can be tailored to the individual and may involve use of 'off-the-shelf' programmes such as the Graded Repetitive Arm Supplementary Program (GRASP; Harris, Eng, Miller, & Dawson, 2009), available at http://neurorehab.med.ubc.ca/grasp. Use of GRASP exercises in hospital significantly improved arm recovery compared with usual therapy in the trial by Harris et al. (2009). GRASP represents a low-cost, efficient mode of delivery, which can be family-assisted. Programmes such as GRASP may be helpful for students and novice therapists who are learning how to prescribe task-specific motor training.

PRACTICE STORY 40.1

Leo and Mary

Leo is an occupational therapist in a large district hospital in rural Australia. He has more than 10 years' experience in adult neurological rehabilitation. Leo is dedicated to developing his skills. He has attended upper limb motor training workshops, videotaped clients and discussed his training programmes with peers. He has organised fortnightly peer review sessions where staff observe each other conducting a therapy session and provide feedback about analysis and teaching skills. Leo regularly attends rehabilitation conferences because 'They are a great pick-me-up'. Leo increased his knowledge and skills by conducting a randomised controlled trial of task-specific training as part of a master's degree (Ross, Harvey, & Lannin, 2009).

Here, Leo gives an example of Mary, whom he saw after her stroke. He describes her motor control problems and compensations and the upper limb training programme provided over several months. This lady could not use her affected arm much when engaging in daily tasks. She could not hold or transport objects such as a cup or a knife during meals.

MARY

> *I saw Mary recently who had recovery of some muscles in her arm, but a lot of overactivity, many compensations and little control in her hand. For example, when attempting to reach forwards to grasp a cup, she elevated her shoulder and abducted her arm, clenched her fingers, flexed her elbow and moved her whole body forwards instead of just her arm and hand. She compensated for poor shoulder flexion, loss of external rotation and thumb adduction by using every muscle possible in her arm. It was hard work.*

> *Training sessions targeted her shoulder flexors in a lying position, which reduced the effect of gravity. We focused on the anterior deltoid muscle. This lady was asked to rest her hand on her forehead with the elbow flexed, and control her anterior deltoid in that position. When she could hold her arm there, she started sliding her hand back from her forehead (in a lying position) to the pillow and the crown of her head, to control anterior deltoid in lying, then reaching higher to the wall to touch a marker. It was too difficult for her in sitting. She couldn't lift her arm up against gravity without compensating. Other practice tasks focused on her shoulder external rotation, elbow, wrist and finger extension and thumb abduction. We pieced each component together, then eventually began working on functional reaching in a seated position [Fig. 40.6].*

> *Mary practiced for about 2 hours a day for 3 months (unsupervised for some of the time), then 1 hour daily for another 3 months, then about 3 hours a week for the last 3 months. It took 36 weeks or 6 months before she had a functional grasp and release. In the first 6 weeks she completed 12,810 repetitions, with an average of 427 reps per session or 85 per exercise. After 36 weeks, she achieved a score of 16/57 on the Action Research Arm Test, compared with 2/57 at the beginning, representing a 14-point change. With a combination of task-specific training, persistence on both our parts, objective measurement, intensive practice and feedback, Mary achieved improved hand function. Without this persistence and practice, I don't think she would have achieved this outcome.*

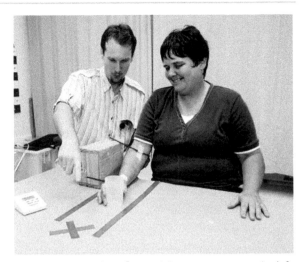

FIG. 40.6 ■ Practice of essential components required for reaching (forward flexion and external rotation) and drinking from a cup. Since having a stroke, Mary has had limited opportunities to engage in occupations such as drinking from a cup with her dominant right hand. She has weak shoulder flexors and external rotators and cannot open her thumb or fingers to preshape correctly. The occupational therapist is helping her to practice shoulder flexion and external rotation – essential components of reaching – while also maintaining wrist extension and forearm supination. In this photograph, she is sliding the cup forwards while staying inside the lines (electrical tape stuck to the table). The practice environment encourages external rotation, wrist extension and supination and discourages compensations such as internal rotation and abduction.

Two drinking straws have been applied to her arm, one to the inner elbow and another on to the back of her wrist. These straws act as visual cues, reminding her to maintain shoulder external rotation (the straw stays in contact with the wooden block) and wrist extension (her knuckles stay in contact with the flexible straw). She is also learning to monitor her own performance, so that she can practise alone outside of therapy sessions. Notice the timer near the therapist's right hand, to record practice time and repetitions.

Ensuring enough practice by people who have had a stroke or brain injury is a challenge: to help ensure individuals spend plenty of time each day practising, Leo uses typed practice records with imported digital photographs. The rehabilitation team runs a cross-disciplinary upper limb group several times a week, where people who have had stroke or brain injury follow their own practice programme with co-learners and supervision from therapists. Therapy assistants and relatives also help supervise individual practice after this has been documented with instructions, goals and illustrations by the therapist. Family members are involved in helping with practice as early as possible, because of the limited time available for one-to-one therapy.

TABLE 40.3
Summary of Motor Control and Sensory Problems Affecting the Upper Limb, and Possible Interventions for People with Neurological Conditions

Problem	Possible Interventions and Evidence from Key Studies
Eliciting contractions in paralysed muscles	■ Repetitive contractions and practise of shoulder protraction in sitting 'rocking chair therapy' (Feys et al., 1998, 2004) ■ Cyclical electrical stimulation (Nascimento et al., 2014) ■ Mental practice (Braun et al., 2013) ■ Mirror therapy (Thieme et al., 2012; Wu et al., 2013)
Increasing strength in weak muscles	■ Robotic therapy (Hayward et al., 2010) ■ SMART arm device (Barker et al., 2008; Hayward et al., 2010) ■ Electrical stimulation (Howlett et al., 2015; Nascimento et al., 2014) ■ Triggered electrical stimulation (Hayward et al., 2010; Thrasher et al., 2008)
Decreasing force in overactive muscles	■ Repetitive contractions and practice, wrist and forearm muscles (Bütefisch, Hummelsheim, Denzler, & Mauritz, 1995)
Increasing coordination, speed and control	■ Constraint-induced movement therapy (Kwakkel et al., 2015; Nijland et al., 2011; Stevenson et al., 2012) ■ Task-related training in groups (Blennerhassett et al., 2006)
Improving sensation	■ Mirror therapy (Doyle et al., 2010; Wu et al., 2013) ■ Electrical stimulation (Conforto et al., 2010; Fleming et al., 2015). ■ Task-orientated sensory training (Carey et al., 2011)

Strength Training for Paralysed and Very Weak Muscles

Some individuals may be unable to elicit a muscle contraction because of paralysis or produce adequate muscle force as a result of weakness. They need coaching to first elicit a muscle contraction, then increase the duration and strength of that contraction. Muscle strength training that involves effortful, repetitive practice improves strength and function and, importantly, does not increase spasticity as many therapists believe (Ada, Dorsch, & Canning, 2006a; Harris & Eng, 2010; Morris, Dodd, & Morris, 2004).

A systematic review of interventions for severe upper limb paresis (Hayward, Barker, & Brauer, 2010) evaluated the evidence for robotic therapy, electromyographic or position-triggered electrical stimulation, rocking chair therapy and the SMART arm device. There was strong evidence that robotic therapy improves the strength and activity of the upper arm but not the hand. There was limited evidence for the effect of other interventions on strength and activity.

One of the few randomised controlled trials targeting very weak muscles was conducted by Feys et al. (1998). These researchers recruited 100 people early after having a stroke and seated them in a rocking chair with their affected arm in a full-arm airsplint and resting on a table. The airsplint held their arm in elbow extension and enabled repetitive practice of shoulder protraction and retraction for 30 minutes daily over 6 weeks. The experimental group improved significantly more than the control group, and gains were maintained after 5 years. Greater gains were found in people who had severe deficits at baseline. In a trial of the SMART arm, a mechanical device that provides a near frictionless surface to enable reaching movements and continuous visual feedback, greater gains were also found in people who had severe motor deficits at baseline (Barker, Brauer, & Carson, 2008). The implications of these studies are that providing a practice environment that allows high-intensity, active, repetitive practice can make a difference to outcomes for people with severe motor deficits in the affected arm.

Examples of practice tasks aimed at increasing muscle strength are shown in Figs. 40.7 to 40.12.

Electrical Stimulation

For people who are unable to elicit a muscle contraction (i.e. the very weak), electrical stimulation will produce muscle contractions. Nascimento, Michaelsen, Ada, Polese, & Teixeira-Salmela, (2014) examined the effect of cyclical electrical stimulation on strength and activity after a stroke in a systematic review of the literature. A total of 11 randomised controlled trials were included in the pooled analysis of the effect of electrical stimulation on *strength*. There was a moderate effect size in favour of cyclical electrical stimulation. Six trials were included in the pooled analysis of the effect of cyclical electrical stimulation on *activity*. There was a small effect size in favour of cyclical electrical stimulation. Overall, Nascimento et al. (2014) concluded that electrical stimulation increased arm movement more than conventional therapy.

Howlett, Lannin, Ada, & McKinstry, (2015) later synthesised the findings from published trials that evaluated the efficacy of electrical stimulation applied *during* activity (i.e. functional electrical stimulation, or FES). Subgroup analyses found that FES had a large effect on upper limb activity (standardised mean difference 0.69, 95% CI, 0.33–1.05). In summary, electrical stimulation is being used increasingly in adult stroke survivors. Further research is needed to determine the most effective protocols for electrical stimulation.

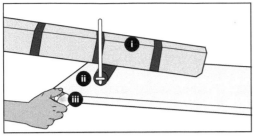

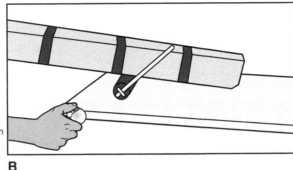

(i) Cardboard cylinder secured with tape, to hold the elbow in extension

(ii) Small plastic or wooden cylinder, which rolls easily on the table

(iii) Metal counter or clicker in the right hand, to record repetitions

B

A

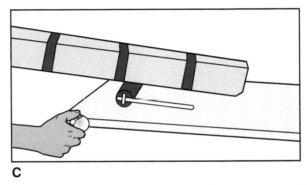

C

FIG. 40.7 ■ Eliciting shoulder protraction. When a person is very weak and cannot move the affected arm, this protraction exercise can sometimes elicit movement. Figure 40.7A demonstrates the physical setup. The table is positioned close to the person's body, with the shoulder a little below 90 degrees. The left elbow is held in extension by a cylinder made from a dismantled cardboard box, held together with tape. The cylinder is supported on a smaller cylinder or wooden dowel, providing a friction-free surface. There is a straw attached to the dowel with adhesive tape. The goal is for the person to protract the left shoulder, to move the straw from a vertical position to touch a mark on the table. Notice that this man has been given the responsibility of counting his practice and repetitions using the metal clicker in his right hand. (i) Cardboard cylinder secured with tape, to hold the elbow in extension. (ii) Small plastic or wooden cylinder, which rolls easily on the table. (iii) Metal counter or clicker in the right hand, to record repetitions. (B) Halfway towards achieving the goal. (C) The straw touches the table. Goal achieved.

Mirror Therapy

Mirror therapy uses visual illusion to trick the brain and promote motor recovery. The person watches a mirror reflection of his or her intact hand while performing repetitive movements. The mirror gives an illusion that the affected arm can move. This therapy is used with people who have moderate to severe weakness, to improve motor and sensory function and reduce neglect (i.e. where a person does not attend to the limb or environment on the affected side and may collide with doorways or ignore food on one side of his or her plate). Most trials provided 30 to 60 minutes of supervised mirror therapy daily for 4 weeks. The most recent Cochrane review included 14 trials published up to June 2011 (Thieme, Mehrholz, Pohl, Behrens, & Dohle, 2012). They concluded that mirror therapy can improve motor function and activity performance but has

less effect on neglect. More recent randomised controlled trials have broadly confirmed these findings (Invernizzi et al., 2013; Lee, Cho, & Song, 2012), with additional benefits reported for sensation (Wu, Huang, Chen, Lin, & Yang, 2013) and neglect (Thieme et al., 2013). Although improvements in some trials were small, mirror therapy is inexpensive to deliver, can be completed in hospital or at home and is suitable for people with moderate to severe weakness.

Reducing Muscle Force During Grasp

Some individuals contract too many muscles, or the wrong muscles, when reaching for and grasping objects. This behaviour is characteristic of early skill acquisition (and is not spasticity). Until learners have mastered a new skill, they recruit too many muscles. Therefore one aim of therapy is to reduce effort and

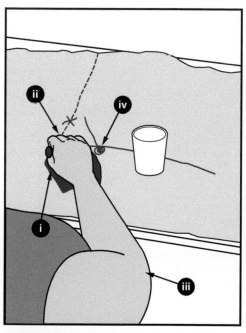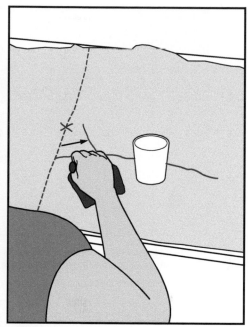

(i) Cloth placed under her hand to reduce friction

(ii) Dotted line drawn on the paper, showing the starting position

(iii) A small cylinder is held between her right elbow and her body (not visible),
     for example a light plastic cup

(iv) The goal

FIG. 40.8 ■ Eliciting external rotation – a home practice setup.
    This lady is practising external rotation in preparation for forwards reaching. (A) The physical setup of the exercise. There is a large sheet of paper on the table, with pen marks showing the start position for her right hand (the dotted line, placed directly in front of her navel). Her hand and forearm are supported on the table to reduce the effect of gravity and make practice easier. The cloth under her right hand reduces friction when she moves. She places a small cylinder between her right elbow and her body, to reduce abduction and extension of her shoulder (which are compensations). The goal is to cover the pen mark by sliding her hand to the right, following the arc drawn on the paper, without abducting her arm. (i) Cloth placed under her hand to reduce friction; (ii) dotted line drawn on the paper, showing the starting position; (iii) a small cylinder is held between her right elbow and her body (not visible), such as a light plastic cup; (iv) the goal: a pen mark or line. (B) The lady has externally rotated her shoulder and covered the pen mark on the paper without dropping the cylinder into her chair. As she becomes more proficient, she will slide her hand farther across the arc to her right, towards the cup.

help the person focus on the muscle actions required for task performance.

    Changing the demands of a task and the environment can reduce effort. For example, asking a person to lift a light plastic cup off the table instead of a glass, or slide rather than lift a cup along the table, will help to reduce effort. If a person is unable to grasp while reaching, taping a cup into his or her hand will reduce task demands and help the person concentrate on reaching. If too much force is applied, using a disposable polystyrene cup that deforms easily when grasped will give the person feedback about his or her force production

(Figs. 40.13 and 40.14). No trials of these interventions have been published to date.

    Different instructions may also help a person to become more self-aware and learn to control some muscles more, and others with less force. For example:

*When you next reach forwards for the cup, **slide** rather than lift your hand. Watch your hand and keep it the same shape as the cup. Notice if your fingers and thumb are closing as you reach. If they start to close, see if you can keep your fingers and thumb 'soft' as you reach.*

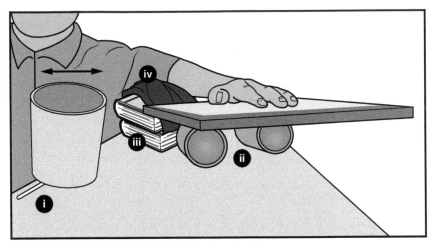

(i) Straw taped underneath the container, and to the table, to allow the container to rock when touched (in the direction of the arrows)

(ii) Cans or cylinders beneath the board, to minimise friction

(iii) Books to raise the shoulder to a horizontal position

(iv) Slide sheet to reduce friction

FIG. 40.9 ■ Eliciting elbow flexion and extension. This man's elbow and upper arm are supported on a high table and firm surface such as telephone directories or a box, so that elbow flexion and extension are possible in the horizontal plane. A slidesheet has also been placed under his forearm to minimise friction. His hand rests on a flat board, which rolls on top of two cylindrical tins, which minimises friction. The plastic container in front of his body has a straw taped underneath, which is taped to the table. When the container is touched, it tips to his right but returns to the start position thereafter. This setup allows him to practise without a therapist present. The goal is for him to slide the board across to tip the lightweight plastic container 10 times by flexing his elbow, each time returning to the start position. (i) Straw taped to the base of the container and to the table, to allow the container to rock when touched (in the direction of the arrows); (ii) cans or cylinders beneath the board, to minimise friction; (iii) books used to raise the shoulder to a horizontal position; (iv) slide sheet used under the upper arm and elbow to reduce friction.

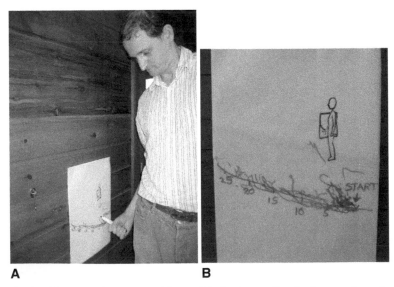

A   **B**

FIG. 40.10 ■ Practice for shoulder external rotation and forward flexion in standing. Both external rotation and shoulder forward flexion are essential for transporting the arm and hand forwards to reach for a cup or telephone.

Continued

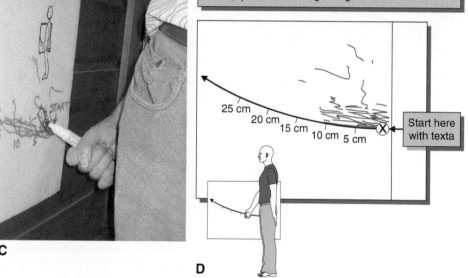

Goal one: Keep texta pentip touching the X mark for
5 seconds x 3 times in a row
Goal two: Draw a line with the texta 5 cm up the wall
x 3 times in a row

Instructions
1. Stick the paper onto the wall with tape (X mark at hip height).
2. Stand beside the poster with texta in hand.
3. Rotate the texta out so the felt tip touches the X mark. Keep shoulder rotated out.
4. Hold for 5 seconds, rest and repeat.
5. Try drawing a line up the wall – no further than 5 cm initially

Check
• Look ahead – don't turn inwards, towards the wall or bend your trunk.
• Remember to breathe while practicing.
• Keep your elbow straight/lengthened.

25 cm   20 cm   15 cm   10 cm   5 cm   Start here with texta

C

D

FIG. 40.10, CONT'D   While this man is using extra muscle force to hold the pen (increased finger flexion), his response is typical of new skill acquisition and is not a major concern to the therapist at this stage. (D) This man's practice sheet illustrates the short- and medium-term goals and instructions to help minimise compensations.

The first goal (Goal 1: Keep the Texta felt tip touching the X mark on the paper for 5 seconds) demands a sustained contraction of his external rotators combined with full supination. Without some external rotation, the goal cannot be achieved (except by trunk rotation). The second goal (Goal 2: Draw a line 5 cm up the wall) demands sustained external rotation and shoulder flexion.

or

This time, when you close your fingers around the polystyrene cup, don't press so hard. Try not to squash or deform the cup. If you press too hard, the water will come up above the marked line. Use light pressure on the sides of the cup.

Coordination Training

Some individuals can grasp and pick up but not manipulate objects such as a cup, knife or fork. Training of advanced hand function involves more than cutting up slices of bread or copying lines of writing. Careful analysis enables therapists to

Goal one: To lift your wrist back to straight. Hold for 10 seconds x 20 repeats/day

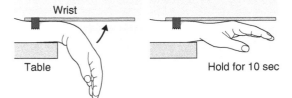

Wrist

Table

Hold for 10 sec

Instructions
1. Tape straw on forearm
2. Hand on table; elbow straight
3. Let wrist drop down so fingers hang over edge of table
4. Keep fingers **straight**
5. Bring your hand back to straight by moving your wrist

Critical features
- Wrist back **evenly**
- Fingers straight throughout
- Thumb does not move outwards away from hand

* Record number correct/number of attempts

Date	No. correct
17/7	14/20
17/7	15/20
26/7	21/25
30/7	9/10
	7/10
02/8	20/25
03/8	22/25

FIG. 40.11 ■ Wrist extension. Wrist extension is essential for most activities involving reaching, such as picking up a cup to drink. The page shown from a practice book illustrates the wrist extension exercise, the goal (to lift the wrist back to the 'straight' position and hold for 10 seconds, for 20 repetitions), extra instructions and a place to record practice attempts (date, number of correct attempts).

determine which essential components of skilled performance are missing or altered. This stage of analysis and training demands careful observation and problem solving. Tasks requiring advanced skill performance (and analysis) include handwriting, use of cutlery and chopsticks.

With small objects, training of grip force during lift-off and manipulation will be required, with repetitions and feedback. Healthy adults typically apply a force slightly higher than the minimum required, to prevent object slippage (Nowak & Hermsdorfer, 2003). However, people with chronic stroke and intact sensation ($n = 10$) often apply significantly greater mean grip forces ($\geq 39\%$) at lift-off compared with healthy adults

Goal: After 10 minutes stretch, to move your forearm over so that the cup touches the pink 'blob', hold for 10 seconds x 30 repeats

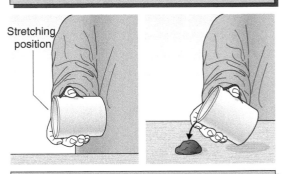

Stretching position

Instructions
1. Sitting with your right arm supported on a table, elbow straight
2. Tape a cup into your hand so that your thumb web space is stretched
3. Use your left hand to take your arm over and hold it in a stretch
4. Take your left hand off, hold the cup on the 'blob' for 10 seconds
5. Come back so that the cup is upright
6. Move the cup back so that the lip touches the 'blob'

Date	No. correct
10/7	0/30
21/7	0/30
27/7	0/20
30/7	3/30
03/8	5/30

FIG. 40.12 ■ Supination practice. Practice book showing the exercise (forearm supination) and goal, in the learners own words: 'After 10 minutes stretch, to move your forearm over so that the cup touches the pink 'blob', hold for 10 seconds'. Additional instructions have also been added and a section for recording practice attempts.

(Quaney, Perera, Maletsky, Luchies, & Nudo, 2005). Blennerhassett, Carey, & Matyas, (2006) reported different findings for 45 people with stroke and 45 healthy adults, who were able to pick up a pen lid concealed from view, using a pinch grip. They reported prolonged time and excessive grip force before commencing the lift in half the people with stroke, as well as fluctuating forces and extreme slowness. However, excessive safety margins were not present in all cases.

The message for therapists from these studies is that people who have had a stroke typically have difficulty preparing a suitable grip force and using the normal feed-forward mechanisms. Impaired sensation is likely to compound these problems. However, training strategies are likely to be similar for people with and without sensory impairment. Training needs to involve

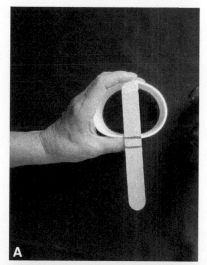

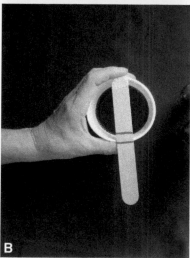

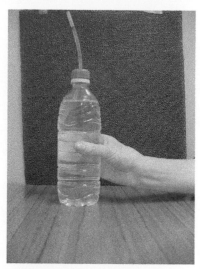

FIG. 40.14 ■ Practice to modulate finger and thumb flexion force while holding a plastic bottle which deforms easily. The person has been asked to gently press the sides of the plastic bottle and control the water levels between the two black lines on the tube. Too much pressure causes a jet of water to shoot out the top, which gives immediate feedback to the learner about the amount of force being generated. The practice demands attention for successful performance.

To construct the training device, first drill a hole in the top of a plastic bottle cap. The hole should be just large enough to accommodate the suction tubing. Insert tubing down through the hole, fill the bottle with water and seal the unit tightly with the screw top. If necessary, seal the unit with tape to prevent air escaping.

Short-Term Goal: In sitting, push water up and down between the two black lines five times, without water escaping from the tube.

Medium-Term Goal: In sitting, keep the water level at the upper black line and lift the bottle up onto a 5-cm box, five times, without water escaping from the tube.

FIG. 40.13 ■ Practice to decrease finger and wrist flexion force while transporting a cup to drink or while carrying liquid. The person has been asked to gently press the side of the polystyrene cup and move the cup edge between the two lines on the wooden stick (A). When the short-term goal has been achieved, the person can progress to transporting the cup of liquid up onto a box, stand up while holding the cup and finally walk while carrying the cup.

Short-Term Goal: Press the cup inwards 1 cm to the second pen mark, release and repeat three times.

Medium-Term Goal: In sitting, maintain the round shape of the cup (B) and lift onto a 5-cm box.

Medium-Term Goal: Maintain the round shape of the cup (B) while standing up and sitting down five times from a 45-cm chair.

Long-Term Goal: Carry a full cup of water three times, from the kitchen to the dining room table, without spilling any liquid.

task-specific practice, with numerous repetitions and frequent feedback. If a person has difficulty using a knife, fork or pen, the person needs to engage in part-practice with these utensils. Picking up an object precisely without spinning or rotating the handle, cutting food and writing all require appropriate force production and accurate opposition of the forces of the thumb and fingers to be successful. See Figs. 40.15 and 40.16 for two examples.

Mental Practice

Mental practice and imagery have been used to promote motor recovery. This type of practice is used routinely in sports training to improve skill acquisition. In rehabilitation, a person can, for example, mentally rehearse the task of picking up a cup and imagine the transport and preshaping actions without physically

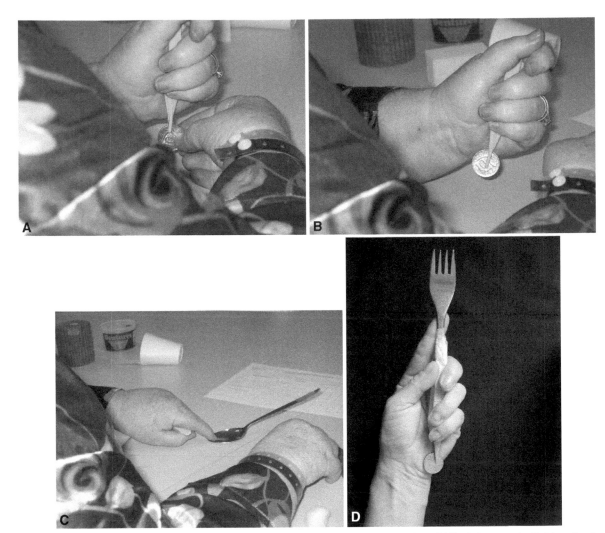

FIG. 40.15 ■ Practice to improve fork control. This lady cannot sustain flexion of her fourth and fifth digits around a fork handle when trying to pick up food. When she tries to use her fork, the handle rotates and she loses her grasp. Part-practice has been devised to help improve flexion of her ring and little fingers around a fork handle. (A and B) Setting up the practice. She has been asked to hold a coin between plastic tweezers for 5 seconds. This task sustains her attention. She gets feedback instantly if her grasp weakens, because the coin drops onto the table.

(C) Holding the tweezers and coin (coin no longer visible), then turning the hand over, flexing the wrist and pressing the index finger down on the end of a spoon. She finds it much more challenging to keep her fourth and fifth digits flexed in this position while her index finger is extended, as it needs to be while using a fork. Again, she receives instant feedback if her grasp weakens because the coin drops out of the tweezers – feedback which would not be provided by a standard fork. (D) Illustration of how the tweezers and fork handle can be taped together, to enable fork practice to progress. This lady can continue her practice with the coin held between plastic tweezers and learn to transport small pieces of soft vegetable or bread squares from plate to plate, without dropping the coin.

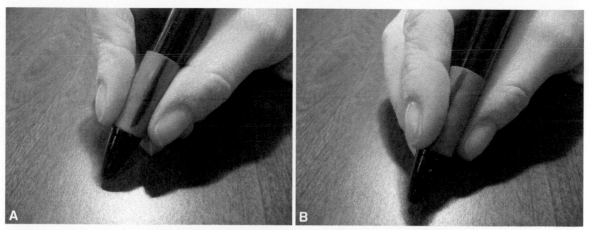

FIG. 40.16 ■ Part-practice of pen rotation. This practice aims to improve pen control and handwriting. The short-term goal is to rotate the pen or pencil 10 times in 30 seconds by the end of 1 week. The medium-term goal is to rotate the pen or pencil 10 times in 20 seconds by the end of 2 weeks.

Instructions remind the person to do the following:

- Roll the pen or pencil a half turn in each direction.
- Aim to cover and then uncover a pen mark along the barrel of the pen (see arrows).
- Allow the pen or pencil to rest against the web space while practising.
- Use the middle finger to readjust pen position when necessary.
- Avoid using the other hand to help.
- Aim to practice for 5 minutes three times daily (15 minutes daily).
- Try not to hold the pen tightly.
- Practise with different pens or pencils to help generalise this skill.

attempting the actions. This therapy is not used with people who are paralysed or who have significant cognitive or communication difficulties. Participants need to be able to concentrate, plan and physically attempt a movement when unsupervised.

A recent systematic review of mental practice (Braun et al., 2013) summarised the effects of 16 studies, 14 of which involved people who had a stroke. Positive short-term effects were reported for arm and hand function; activities of daily living; and cognition, including attention, planning and route finding and arousal. Longer-term outcomes have not been reported to date. There was large variability in the type and dose of therapy provided in the trials. This therapy requires discipline and has some similarities with meditation. Mental practice is not expensive or harmful and has the potential to improve arm function in stroke participants who can engage with the therapy.

Constraint-induced Movement Therapy

Constraint-induced movement therapy (CIMT) improves movement and use of the affected hand and promotes neuroplasticity of the brain. CIMT involves four active components delivered intensively over 2 weeks: (1) task-specific repetitive practice, for between 3 and 6 hours per day; (2) one-to-one

shaping or coaching, with feedback and progression of task practice; (3) a restraint such as a mitt, or splint and sling, worn for 90% of the waking day; and (4) a transfer-of-training package involving home practice (Taub et al., 2013). The restraint is used to discourage physical use of the unaffected hand and greater use of the affected hand, but the restraint does not appear to be essential (Brogårdh, Vestling, & Sjölund, 2009; Brogårdh & Lexell, 2010; Krawczyk et al., 2012). It is probably the intensive task-specific practice and coaching that promote neuroplasticity and change arm function. For a detailed description of CIMT eligibility criteria and procedures, see Taub et al. (2013).

The collective research in stroke rehabilitation (more than 50 randomised trials and six systematic reviews) has found a moderate effect of CIMT on upper limb motor performance, measured using instruments such as the Action Research Arm Test (Nijland et al., 2011; Stevenson, Thalman, Christie, & Poluh, 2012). Eligible participants in trials typically have active wrist and finger extension at study commencement. Most studies have used a modified CIMT programme (44/51 trials; see Kwakkel, Veerbeek, van Wegen, & Wolf, 2015). It is not yet known if CIMT can drive recovery in people with a very weak or paralysed arm, who have no hand function. A systematic review by Nijland and colleagues (2010) suggested that lower intensity CIMT in hospital, for up to 3 hours per day, is feasible and improves outcomes more than standard upper limb therapy. A Norwegian trial (Thrane et al., 2015) provided CIMT early after stroke, for 3 hours daily over 10 days. The researchers found significant improvements at discharge, but differences between experimental and control groups were not maintained after 1 month.

Sensory Retraining

Therapists can use active and passive approaches to address sensory impairments. Active approaches involve the person exploring and discriminating between stimuli, such as the shape, weight and texture of a lightweight plastic cup versus a pottery coffee mug. Passive approaches include use of electrical stimulation, thermal stimulation (heat or cold), pressure or movement by a therapist to increase sensory awareness of the limb, such as intermittent pneumatic compression, but typically with little or no active exploration by the person.

A Cochrane review highlighted preliminary evidence for the effect of one active approach, mirror therapy, and two passive approaches, thermal stimulation and intermittent pneumatic compression (Doyle, Bennett, & McKenna, 2010). Since that time, other studies have confirmed small effects from mirror therapy on sensation (Internizzi et al., 2013). Fleming et al. (2015) found immediate benefits in arm and hand function after 12 sessions of electrical stimulation to the three upper limb nerves, administered immediately before a task-specific motor training session. Although benefits were recorded after 2 days, these gains were lost after 3 and 6 months. Conforto et al. (2010) also applied electrical stimulation to the median nerve of stroke survivors immediately before motor training and found immediate changes in function, but differences between control and experimental groups had reduced after 2 months. Therefore electrical stimulation to a person's affected arm may help to improve return of movement and sensation.

Finally, sensory discrimination training of the affected upper limb has had positive results in one trial compared with nonspecific exposure to sensory stimuli (Carey et al., 2011). In that study, 50 people who had a stroke and were living in the community were randomly assigned to either an experimental or control group. The 25 experimental group participants received 10 training sessions of generalised sensory discrimination training, with one third of each session divided equally between training of texture discrimination (discriminating between different plastic grids and fabrics), limb position sense (wrist angle) and tactile object recognition (exploring and manipulating objects such as a cup, cutlery or coins). Training involved graded progression of discriminations from easy to difficult, provision of feedback and intensive training. After 4 weeks, changes in the Standardised Somatosensory Deficit (SSD) index were significantly greater for the experimental versus control group (19.1 vs. 8.0, respectively) with a mean between-group change of 11.1 SSD points (95% CI, 3.0–19.2) in favour of the experimental

group. Improved sensation was maintained at the 6-week and 6-month follow-ups. Although that study and intervention still need to be replicated, the sensory training programme can be implemented by therapists with fidelity using the manual and DVD (Carey, 2012; available at http://www.florey.edu.au/research/new-tools-for-a-new-era-in-sensory-training).

PREVENTING AND MANAGING SECONDARY IMPAIRMENTS

Contractures

Loss of shoulder external rotation range of movement is common after stroke. In one study (N = 52), the majority of people with stroke experienced a loss of external rotation range greater than 60 degrees (Lindgren et al., 2012), with some participants unable to attain neutral (0 degrees) or mid-range between internal and external rotation. This loss of range correlated with shoulder pain (Lindgren et al., 2012) and will affect performance of self-care tasks. Therefore it is important for therapists to anticipate and prevent contractures.

Muscle stretching has become a popular intervention for managing muscle length changes and contracture, in addition to strengthening opposing muscles. Some years ago, animal studies suggested that stretches of 30 minutes prevented the development of contractures in otherwise immobilised mice soleus muscles (Goldspink & Williams, 1990; Williams, 1990). Unfortunately the changes observed in animal muscles were not reproduced in human stretching studies. For a complete review of stretching research, see Katalinic et al. (2010). Disappointingly, high-quality randomised controlled trials have not found statistically or clinically worthwhile benefits from prolonged stretches in people who have had a stroke, traumatic brain injury or spinal cord injury. One study involving people who had had a stroke provided shoulder, arm and hand positioning for 30 minutes 5 days a week for a month in conjunction with task-specific motor training; that study demonstrated a small benefit, which was maintained when stretches stopped (Horsley, Herbert, & Ada, 2007).

Sustained stretches have also been applied using serial casts to immobilise muscles in their stretched positions. Serial casts produce transient changes in range of motion at the elbow in adults with traumatic brain injury; however, these improvements were not sustained after cast removal (Moseley et al., 2008).

Studies investigating the effect of hand splinting to prevent contracture after stroke and brain injury have found no difference in wrist extensibility compared with controls (no splint), even when splints were worn overnight for 4 weeks (Lannin, Cusick, McCluskey, & Herbert, 2007) and overnight for 3 months for thumb web-space contractures (Harvey, de Jong, Goehl, & Mardwedel, 2006).

To conclude, there is uncertainty about whether stretch interventions are effective in the long term, and if they are, it is not known for how long stretches should be held or how often stretches should be administered. The current evidence strongly suggests that therapists should not be routinely applying stretches or splints while people are participating in active rehabilitation.

Shoulder Pain

Shoulder pain can limit a person's participation in activities. Therefore therapists often aim to reduce pain. The causes of shoulder pain are still uncertain but may include impingement of tissues around the shoulder joint, trauma from pulling on the arm and loss of external rotation. A Cochrane systematic review (Ada, & Foongchomcheay, & Canning, 2005a) found that shoulder strapping with adhesive tape delayed the onset of shoulder pain but did not reduce pain once it had developed, nor did strapping improve function. Since that review, other randomised controlled trials have confirmed the benefits of strapping for preventing and delaying the onset of shoulder pain after a stroke (Appel, Mayston, & Perry, 2011; Griffin & Bernhardt, 2006; Pandian et al., 2013). For example, Griffin and Bernhardt (2006) reported a mean of 26 pain-free days for the intervention group, compared with 19 pain-free days in a placebo-controlled group and 16 pain-free days in the control group.

Electrical stimulation can also reduce shoulder pain when applied to the supraspinatus, posterior and middle deltoid and trapezius muscles (Koog, Jin, Yoon, & Min, 2010; Viana, Pereira, Mehta, Miller, & Teasell, 2012).

Shoulder Subluxation

Shoulder slings and supports have not been well researched despite their frequent use in practice (Ada et al., 2005a). Current expert opinion is that external supports such as wheelchair and chair attachments are needed to support the weight of the arm (Foongchomcheay et al., 2005). Triangular slings can reduce a shoulder subluxation, but slings that do not support the arm will probably not reduce a subluxation (Ada et al., 2005b).

Electrical stimulation shows more promise as an intervention by stimulating muscles around the shoulder joint. Electrical stimulation is typically used with people who have little or no muscle activity. Ada and Foongchomcheay (2002) conducted a meta-analysis involving four trials of electrical stimulation to prevent subluxation early after a stroke (average 17 days poststroke). Electrical stimulation reduced subluxation by an average of 6.5 mm but had no worthwhile effect on reducing pain or improving functional recovery. No clinically important differences were found when stimulation was applied later (60 days or more poststroke), based on meta-analysis of data from three randomised trials. Ultimately individuals need active training to help strengthen paralysed and very weak muscles around the shoulder and upper arm.

Improving Movement in People with Spasticity

There is growing evidence that therapists overestimate the number of people with clinical spasticity (e.g. O'Dwyer et al., 1996).

Research has also demonstrated that when spasticity is reduced using botulinum toxin (type A), this intervention does not improve active use of the hand or arm (Shaw et al., 2010; Sheean et al., 2010). Taken together, these findings suggest that routine interventions to reduce spasticity in adults with a neurological condition are not indicated and therapists should focus on addressing negative impairments, loss of strength and motor control.

For people with spasticity that interferes with function, the most common medical intervention is chemodenervation using botulinum toxin type A (BoNT-A). Results from a meta-analysis show that BoNT-A can reduce spasticity compared with placebo treatment (Cardoso et al., 2005). However, BoNT-A does not improve dexterity or functional outcomes. The BoTULS study (Shaw et al., 2010) was a large trial that evaluated the addition of BoNT-A to an upper limb therapy programme. No between-group differences were reported in upper limb function when measured by the Action Research Arm Test. So, although BoNT-A can temporarily reduce spasticity, it has not been found to lead to improved functional use of the hand.

In summary, people affected by a stroke or brain injury usually want improved use of their hand, not just less spasticity. The evidence-based interventions recommended in this chapter have been found to improve function and may be a better focus for therapists than BoNT-A.

FUTURE DIRECTIONS

The earlier rehabilitation begins, the better the recovery from conditions such as stroke and brain injury. Greater intensity of treatment translates into better outcomes. Gains in motor control and sensory recovery continue for many years. Many therapists are moving away from 'hands-on' therapies towards evidence-informed interventions that apply motor learning theory and promote neuroplasticity. One-on-one therapy is being supplemented with homework and group programmes where people practice together. Family-assisted programmes such as GRASP (Harris et al., 2009) are also being implemented more in hospitals to increase practice opportunities.

Telerehabilitation is one mode of delivery that can increase practice and reduce travel time and costs, with some sessions provided with therapists and some by distance using telephone and the Internet (Chumbler et al., 2012). However, evidence of improved upper limb outcomes after stroke using telerehabilitation was still limited at the time of the most recent Cochrane review (Laver et al., 2013).

The need for increased intensity of practice has led to the testing of novel rehabilitation techniques such as virtual reality and robotic therapy. Virtual reality, including interactive low-cost videogames such as the Wii, enable people to practice independently or semisupervised, helping to increase practice dosage. A systematic review was recently conducted of studies involving virtual reality and interactive videogames and adults with stroke (Laver, George, Thomas, Deutsch, & Crotty, 2015). Virtual reality significantly improved upper limb function (standardised mean difference 0.28, 95% CI, 0.08–0.49) based on 12 studies with 397 participants. Robotic therapy allows some of the labour-intensive training to be performed by automated devices, increasing repetitions, upper limb function and activities of daily living post stroke (Mehrholz, Hadrich, Platz, Kugler, & Pohl, 2012; Pollock et al., 2014). Although improvements are similar to those achieved with dose-matched intensive task-specific training (Norouzi-Gheidari, Archambault, & Fung, 2012), a robotic device allows individuals to practise semisupervised. The cost of robotics will hopefully decrease in future, allowing more services to offer this intervention to people with neurological conditions.

As the evidence grows in support of more intensive therapy, interventions such as constraint therapy, virtual reality and robotics will be used more often because they increase practice and improve arm recovery. With technologies improving continuously, it is not possible to predict what advances will become routine practice in the future. The important message is therefore to remain abreast of current scientific evidence.

CONCLUSIONS

This chapter has focused on the process of analysing and retraining motor performance and sensation in adults with brain impairment. The content is necessarily impairment-focused because much of upper limb rehabilitation, particularly in hospital settings, focuses on eliciting muscle activity and strength training before return of functional grasp. Therapists need to remind themselves and the people they are working with of the occupational goals of training – for example, eating a meal with family members using cutlery in both hands. Once a person can grasp and manipulate objects, tasks and goals are more obvious. Although the overall goal may be to increase engagement in occupations, therapists should not ignore impairment-focused interventions.

 http://evolve.elsevier.com/Curtin/OT

REFERENCES

Ada, L., & Canning, C. (2005). Changing the way we view the contribution of motor impairments to physical disability after stroke. In K. Refshauge, L. Ada, & E. Ellis (Eds.), *Science-based rehabilitation: Theories into practice* (pp. 87–106). Edinburgh: Elsevier Butterworth Heinemann.

Ada, L., Dorsch, S., & Canning, C. (2006a). Strengthening interventions to increase strength and improve activity after stroke: A systematic review. *Australian Journal of Physiotherapy, 52,* 241–248.

Ada, L., O'Dwyer, N., & O'Neill, E. (2006b). Relation between spasticity, weakness and contracture of the elbow flexors and upper limb activity after stroke: An observational study. *Disability & Rehabilitation, 28,* 891–897.

Ada, L., & Foongchomcheay, A. (2002). Efficacy of electrical stimulation in preventing or reducing subluxation of the shoulder after stroke: A meta-analysis. *Australian Journal of Physiotherapy, 48,* 257–267.

Ada, L., Foongchomcheay, A., & Canning, C. (2005a). Supportive devices for preventing and treating subluxation of the shoulder after stroke. *Cochrane Database of Systematic Reviews, 1.*

Ada, L., Foongchomcheay, A., & Canning, C. (2005b). Use of devices to prevent subluxation of the shoulder after stroke. *Physiotherapy Research International, 10,* 134–145.

Alt Murphy, M. A., & Häger, C. K. (2015). Kinematic analysis of the upper extremity after stroke: How far have we reached and what have we grasped? *Physical Therapy Reviews, 20*(3), 137–155.

Appel, C., Mayston, M., & Perry, L. (2011). Feasibility study of a randomized controlled trial protocol to examine clinical effectiveness of shoulder strapping in acute stroke patients. *Clinical Rehabilitation, 29*(9), 833–843.

Barker, R., Brauer, S., & Carson, R. (2008). Training of reaching in stroke survivors with severe and chronic upper limb paresis using a novel non-robotic device: A randomized clinical trial. *Stroke, 29,* 1800–1807.

Bayona, N. A., Bitensky, J., Salter, K., & Teasell, R. (2005). The role of task-specific training in rehabilitation therapies. *Topics in Stroke Rehabilitation, 12,* 58–65.

Birkenmeier, R. L., Prager, E. M., & Lang, C. E. (2010). Translating animal doses of task-specific training to people with chronic stroke in 1-hour therapy sessions: A proof-of-concept study. *Neurorehabilitation and Neural Repair, 24*(7), 620–635.

Blennerhassett, J. M., Carey, L. M., & Matyas, T. A. (2006). Grip force regulation during pinch grip lifts under somatosensory guidance: Comparison between people with stroke and healthy controls. *Archives of Physical Medicine and Rehabilitation, 87,* 418–429.

Brashear, A., & Elovic, E. P. (Eds.). (2011). *Spasticity diagnosis and management.* New York: Demos Medical.

Braun, S., Kleynen, M., van Heel, T., Kruithof, N., Wade, D., & Beurkens, A. (2013). The effects of mental practice in neurological rehabilitation: A systematic review and meta-analysis. *Frontiers in Human Neuroscience, 7*(390), 1–23.

Brogårdh, C., & Lexell, J. (2010). A 1-year follow-up after shortened constraint-induced movement therapy with and without mitt poststroke. *Archives of Physical Medicine and Rehabilitation, 91*(3), 460–464.

Brogårdh, C., Vestling, M., & Sjölund, B. H. (2009). Shortened constraint-induced movement therapy in subacute stroke—no effect of using a restraint: A randomized controlled study with independent observers. *Journal of Rehabilitation Medicine, 41,* 231–236.

Bütefisch, C., Hummelsheim, H., Denzler, P., & Mauritz, K. (1995). Repetitive training of isolated movements improves the outcome of motor rehabilitation of the centrally paretic hand. *Journal of the Neurological Sciences, 130*(1), 59–68.

Cardoso, E., Rodrigues, B., Lucena, R., Oliveira, I. R., Pedreira, G., & Melo, A. (2005). Botulinum toxin type A for the treatment of the upper limb spasticity after stroke. *Arquivos de Neuro-Psiquiatria, 91,* 30–33.

Carey, L., Macdonell, R., & Matyas, T. A. (2011). SENSe: Study of the effectiveness of Neurorehabilitation on Sensation: A randomized controlled trial. *Neurorehabilitation and Neural Repair, 25*(4), 304–313.

Carey, L. (2012). *SENSe: Helping stroke survivors regain a sense of touch. A manual for therapists.* Heidelberg, Australia: Florey Neuroscience Institute.

Carey, J. R., Kimberley, T. J., Lewis, S. M., et al. (2002). Analysis of fMRI and finger tracking training in subjects with chronic stroke. *Brain, 125*(4), 773–788.

Carr, J. H., Shepherd, R. B., Gordon, J., Gentile, A. M., & Held, J. M. (1987). *Movement science: Foundations for physical therapy in rehabilitation.* Rockville, MD: Aspen.

Carr, J. H., & Shepherd, R. B. (2010). Reaching and manipulation. In *Neurological rehabilitation: Optimizing motor performance* (2nd ed., pp. 123–162). Edinburgh: Churchill Livingstone Elsevier.

Chari, V. R., & Kirby, R. L. (1986). Lower-limb influence on sitting balance while reaching forward. *Archives of Physical Medicine and Rehabilitation, 67*, 73–733.

Chumbler, N., Quigley, P., Li, X., et al. (2012). Effects of telerehabilitation on physical function and disability for stroke patients. A randomized controlled trial. *Stroke, 43*(8), 2168–2174.

Conforto, A. B., Ferreiro, K. N., Tomasi, C., et al. (2010). Effects of somatosensory stimulation on motor function after subacute stroke. *Neurorehabilitation and Neural Repair, 24*(3), 263–272.

Crosbie, J., Shepherd, R., & Squire, T. (1995). Postural and voluntary movement during reaching in sitting: The role of the lower limbs. *Journal of Human Movement Studies, 28*, 103–126.

Dean, C., Channon, E., & Hall, J. (2007). Sitting training early after stroke improves sitting ability and quality and carries over to standing up but not to walking: A randomised controlled trial. *Australian Journal of Physiotherapy, 53*, 97–102.

Dean, C., & Shepherd, R. (1997). Task related training improves performance of seated reaching tasks after stroke: A randomised controlled trial. *Stroke, 28*, 722–728.

Dean, C., Shepherd, R., & Adam, R. (1999a). Sitting balance 1: Trunk and arm coordination and the contribution of the lower limbs during self-paced reaching in sitting. *Gait and Posture, 10*, 135–146.

Dean, C., Shepherd, R., & Adam, R. (1999b). Sitting balance 11: Reach direction and thigh support affect the contribution of the lower limbs when reaching beyond arm's length in sitting. *Gait and Posture, 10*, 147–153.

Doyle, S., Bennett, S. E., & McKenna, K. T. (2010). Interventions for sensory impairment in the upper limb after stroke. *Cochrane Database of Systematic Reviews, 6*.

Ericsson, K. A. (2004). Deliberate practice and the acquisition and maintenance of expert performance in medicine and related domains. *Academic Medicine, 79*, S70–S81.

Ericsson, K. A. (2014). *The road to excellence: The acquisition of expert performance in the arts and sciences, sports and games.* New York: Psychology Press.

Feys, H. M., de Weerdt, W. J., Selz, B. E., et al. (1998). Effect of a therapeutic intervention for the hemiplegic upper limb in the acute phase after stroke: A single-blind randomized multicentre trial. *Stroke, 29*, 785–792.

Feys, H. M., de Weerdt, W. J., Verbeke, G., et al. (2004). Early and repetitive stimulation of the arm can substantially improve the long-term outcome after stroke: A 5-year follow-up study of a randomized trial. *Stroke, 35*, 924–929.

Fitts, P. M., & Posner, M. I. (1967). *Human performance.* Belmont, CA: Brooks/Cole.

Fleming, M. K., Sorinola, I. O., Roberts Lewis, S. F., Wolfe, C. D., Wellwood, I., & Newham, D. J. (2015). The effect of combined somatosensory stimulation and task-specific training on upper limb function in chronic stroke: A double-blind randomized controlled trial. *Neurorehabilitation and Neural Repair, 29*(2), 143–152.

Foongchomcheay, A., Ada, L., & Canning, C. (2005). Use of devices to prevent subluxation of the shoulder after stroke. *Physiotherapy Research International, 10*, 134–145.

Goldspink, G., & Williams, P. (1990). Muscle fibre and connective tissue changes associated with use and disuse. In L. Ada, & C. Canning (Eds.), *Key issues in neurological physiotherapy* (pp. 197–218). Oxford, UK: Butterworth Heinemann.

Griffin, A., & Bernhardt, J. (2006). Strapping the hemiplegic shoulder prevents development of pain during rehabilitation: A randomized controlled trial. *Clinical Rehabilitation, 20*, 287–295.

Hayward, K., Barker, R., & Brauer, S. (2010). Interventions to promote motor recovery in stroke survivors with severe paresis: A systematic review. *Disability and Rehabilitation, 32*, 1973–1986.

Harris, J. E., & Eng, J. J. (2007). Paretic upper-limb strength best explains arm activity in people with stroke. *Physical Therapy, 87*, 88–97.

Harris, J. E., Eng, J. J., Miller, W. C., & Dawson, A. S. (2009). A self-administered Graded Repetitive Arm Supplementary Program (GRASP) improves arm function during inpatient stroke rehabilitation: A multi-site randomized controlled trial. *Stroke, 40*, 2123–2128.

Harris, J. E., & Eng, J. J. (2010). Strength training improves upper limb function in people with stroke. A meta-analysis. *Stroke, 41*, 136–140.

Harvey, L., de Jong, I., Goehl, G., & Mardwedel, S. (2006). Twelve weeks of nightly stretch does not reduce thumb web-space contractures in people with a neurological condition: A randomised controlled trial. *Australian Journal of Physiotherapy, 52*, 251–258.

Horsley, S., Herbert, R., & Ada, L. (2007). Four weeks of daily stretch has little or no effect on wrist contracture after stroke: A randomised controlled trial. *Australian Journal of Physiotherapy, 53*(4), 239–245.

Howlett, O. A., Lannin, N. A., Ada, L., & McKinstry, C. A. (2015). Functional electrical stimulation improves activity after stroke: A systematic review with meta-analysis. *Archives of Physical Medicine & Rehabilitation, 96*(5), 934–943.

Hubbard, I. J., Parsons, M. W., Neilson, C., & Carey, L. M. (2009). Task-specific training: Evidence for and translation to clinical practice. *Occupational Therapy International, 16*(3-4), 175–189.

Internizzi, M., Negrini, S., Da, S. C., Lanzotti, L., Cisari, C., & Baricich, A. (2013). The value of adding mirror therapy for upper limb motor recovery of subacute stroke patients: A randomized controlled trial. *European Journal of Physical and Rehabilitation Medicine, 49*(3), 311–317.

Katalinic, O. M., Harvey, L. A., Herbert, R. D., Moseley, A. M., Lannin, N. A., & Schurr, K. (2010). Stretch for the treatment and prevention of contractures. *Cochrane Database of Systematic Reviews, 9*.

Kernodle, M. W., & Carlton, L. G. (1992). Information feedback and the learning of multiple-degree-of-freedom activities. *Journal of Motor Behaviour, 24*, 187–196.

Kilduski, N. C., & Rice, M. S. (2003). Qualitative and quantitative knowledge of results: Effects on motor learning. *American Journal of Occupational Therapy, 57,* 329–336.

Koog, Y. H., Jin, S. S., Yoon, K., & Min, B. (2010). Interventions for hemiplegic shoulder pain: Systematic review of RCTs. *Disability and Rehabilitation, 32*(4), 282–291.

Krawczyk, M., Sidaway, M., Radwańska, A., Zaborska, J., Ujma, R., & Cztonkowska, A. (2012). Effects of sling and voluntary constraint during constraint-induced movement therapy for the arm after stroke: A randomized, prospective, single-centre, blinded observer rater study. *Clinical Rehabilitation, 26,* 990–998.

Kwah, K. L., Harvey, L. A., Diong, J. H., & Herbert, R. D. (2012). Half of the adults who present to hospital with stroke develop at least one contracture within six months: An observational study. *Journal of Physiotherapy, 58,* 41–47.

Kwakkel, G., Veerbeek, J. M., van Wegen, E. H., & Wolf, S. L. (2015). Constraint induced movement therapy after stroke. *Lancet Neurology, 14,* 224–234.

Lannin, N. A., Cusick, A., McCluskey, A., & Herbert, R. D. (2007). Effects of splinting on wrist contracture after stroke: A randomized controlled trial. *Stroke, 38,* 111–116.

Laver, K. F., Schoene, D., Crotty, M., George, S., Lannin, N. A., & Sherrington, C. (2013). Telerehabilitation services for stroke. *Cochrane Database of Systematic Reviews, 12.*

Laver, K. E., George, S., Thomas, S., Deutsch, J. E., & Crotty, M. (2015). Virtual reality for stroke rehabilitation. *Cochrane Database of Systematic Reviews, 2.*

Lee, M. M., Cho, H. Y., & Song, C. H. (2012). The mirror therapy program enhances upper limb motor recovery and motor function in acute stroke patients. *American Journal of Occupational Therapy, 91*(8), 689–696.

Lindgren, I., Lexell, J., Jönsson, A. C., & Brogardh, C. (2012). Left-sided hemiparesis, pain frequency, and decreased passive shoulder range of abduction are predictors of long-lasting poststroke shoulder pain. *Physical Medicine and Rehabilitation, 4,* 561–568.

Magill, R. A. (2011). *Motor learning and control: Concepts and applications* (9th ed.). New York: McGraw-Hill.

Mastos, M., Miller, K., Eliasson, A. C., et al. (2007). Goal-directed training: Linking theories of treatment to clinical practice for improved functional activities in daily life. *Clinical Rehabilitation, 21,* 47–55.

Mehrholz, J., Hadrich, A., Platz, T., Kugler, J., & Pohl, M. (2012). Electromechanical and robot-assisted arm training for improving generic activities of daily living, arm function and arm muscle strength after stroke. *Cochrane Database of Systematic Reviews, 6.*

Michaelsen, S. M., Dannenbaum, R., & Levin, M. F. (2006). Task-specific training with trunk restraint on arm recovery in stroke. *Stroke, 27,* 186–192.

Morris, S. L., Dodd, K. J., & Morris, M. E. (2004). Outcomes of progressive resistance strength training following stroke: A systematic review. *Clinical Rehabilitation, 18,* 27–39.

Moseley, A. M., Hassett, L. M., Leung, J., Clare, J. S., Herbert, R. D., & Harvey, L. A. (2008). Serial casting versus positioning for the treatment of elbow contractures in adults with traumatic brain injury: A randomized controlled trial. *Clinical Rehabilitation, 22*(5), 406–417.

Nascimento, R., Michaelsen, S. M., Ada, L., Polese, J. C., & Teixeira-Salmela, L. F. (2014). Cyclical electrical stimulation increases strength and improves activity after stroke: A systematic review. *Journal of Physiotherapy, 60,* 22–30.

Neistadt, M. (1994). The effect of different treatment activities on functional fine motor coordination in adults with brain injury. *American Journal of Occupational Therapy, 48*(10), 877–882.

Nijland, R., Kwakkel, G., Bakers, J., & van Wegen, E. (2011). Constraint-induced movement therapy for the upper paretic limb in acute or sub-acute stroke: A systematic review. *International Journal of Stroke, 6,* 425–433.

Norouzi-Gheidari, N., Archambault, P. S., & Fung, J. (2012). Effects of robot-assisted therapy on stroke rehabilitation in upper limbs: Systematic reviews and meta-analysis of the literature. *Journal of Rehabilitation Research and Development, 49*(4), 479–496.

Nowak, D. A., & Hermsdorfer, J. (2003). Selective deficits of grip force during object manipulation in patients with reduced sensibility of the grasping digits. *Neuroscience Research, 47,* 65–72.

O'Dwyer, N. J., Ada, L., & Neilson, P. D. (1996). Spasticity and muscle contracture following stroke. *Brain, 119,* 1737–1749.

Pandian, J. D., Kaur, P., Arora, R., et al. (2013). Shoulder taping reduces injury and pain in stroke patients. *Neurology, 80,* 528–532.

Pandyan, A. D., Cameron, M., Powell, J., et al. (2003). Contractures in the post-stroke wrist: A pilot study of its time course of development and its association with upper limb recovery. *Clinical Rehabilitation, 17*(1), 88–95.

Patrick, E., & Ada, L. (2006). The Tardieu Scale differentiates contracture from spasticity whereas the Ashworth Scale is confounded by it. *Clinical Rehabilitation, 20,* 173–182.

Pollock, A., Farmer, S. E., Brady, M. E., et al. (2014). Interventions for improving upper limb function after stroke. *Cochrane Database of Systematic Reviews, 11.*

Quaney, B. M., Perera, S., Maletsky, R., Luchies, C. W., & Nudo, R. J. (2005). Impaired grip force modulation in the ipsilesional hand after unilateral middle cerebral artery stroke. *Neurorehabilitation and Neural Repair, 19,* 338–349.

Refshauge, K. M., Ada, L., & Ellis, E. (Eds.), (2005). *Science-based rehabilitation: Theories into practice.* Edinburgh: Elsevier Butterworth-Heinemann.

Ross, L. F., Harvey, L. A., & Lannin, N. A. (2009). Do people with acquired brain impairment benefit from additional therapy specifically directed at the hand? A randomized controlled trial. *Clinical Rehabilitation, 23*(6), 492–503.

Schmidt, R. A., & Lee, T. D. (2005). *Motor control and learning: A behavioural emphasis* (4th ed.). Champaign, IL: Human Kinetics.

Shaw, L., Rodgers, H., Rice, C., et al. (2010). BoTULS: A multicentre randomised controlled trial to evaluate the clinical effectiveness and cost effectiveness of treating upper limb spasticity due to stroke with botulinum toxin type A. *Health Technology Assessment, 14*(26), 1–113.

Sheean, G., Lannin, N. A., Turner-Stokes, L., et al. (2010). Botulinum toxin assessment, intervention and aftercare for upper limb hypertonicity in adults: International consensus statement. *European Journal of Neurology, 17,* 74–93.

Shumway-Cook, A. (2012). *Motor control: Translating research into clinical practice.* Philadelphia: Wolters Kluwer Health/Lippincott Williams & Wilkins.

Sietsema, J. M., Nelson, D. L., Mulder, R. M., et al. (1993). The use of a game to promote arm reach in persons with traumatic brain injury. *American Journal of Occupational Therapy, 47*(1), 19–24.

Stevenson, T., Thalman, L., Christie, H., & Poluh, W. (2012). Constraint-induced movement therapy compared to dose-matched interventions for upper-limb dysfunction in adult survivors of stroke: A systematic review with meta-analysis. *Physiotherapy Canada, 64*, 397–413.

Tabary, J. C., Tabary, J. C., Tardieu, C., et al. (1972). Physiological and structural changes in the cat's soleus muscle due to immobilization at different lengths by plaster case. *Journal of Physiology (London), 224*, 231–244.

Taub, E., Uswatte, G., Mark, V. W., et al. (2013). Method for enhancing real-world use of a more affected arm in chronic stroke: Transfer package of constraint-induced movement therapy. *Stroke, 44*, 1383–1388.

Thieme, H., Mehrholz, J., Pohl, J. M., Behrens, J., & Dohle, C. (2012). Mirror therapy for improving motor function after stroke. *Cochrane Database of Systematic Reviews, 3*.

Thieme, H., Bayn, M., Wurg, M., Zange, C., Pohl, M., & Behrens, J. (2013). Mirror therapy for patients with severe arm paresis after stroke: A randomized controlled trial. *Clinical Rehabilitation, 27*(4), 314–324.

Thrane, G., Askim, T., Stock, R., et al. (2015). Efficacy of constraint induced movement therapy in early stroke rehabilitation: A randomized controlled multisite trial. *Neurorehabilitation & Neural Repair, 29*(6), 517–525.

Thrasher, A., Zivanovic, V., McIlroy, W., & Popovic, M. (2008). Rehabilitation of reaching and grasping function in severe hemiplegic patients using functional electrical stimulation therapy. *Neurorehabilitation and Neural Repair, 22*, 706–714.

van Vliet, P. M., & Wulf, G. (2006). Extrinsic feedback for motor learning after stroke: What is the evidence? *Disability and Rehabilitation, 28*, 831–840.

van Vliet, P. M. (1998). *An investigation of reaching movements following stroke.* Nottingham. University of Nottingham PhD thesis.

van Vliet, P., Pelton, T. A., Hollands, K. L., Carey, L., & Wing, A. M. (2013). Neuroscience findings on coordination of reaching to grasp and object: Implications for research. *Neurorehabilitation and Neural Repair, 27*(7), 622–635.

Vattanasilp, W., Ada, L., & Crosbie, J. (2000). Contribution of thixotropy, spasticity and contracture to ankle stiffness after stroke. *Journal of Neurology Neurosurgery and Psychiatry, 69*, 34–39.

Veerbeek, J. M., van Wegen, E., van Peppen, R., et al. (2014). What is the evidence for physical therapy post-stroke? A systematic review and meta-analysis. *PLoS One, 9*(2).

Viana, R., Pereira, S., Mehta, T., Miller, T., & Teasell, R. (2012). Evidence for therapeutic interventions for hemiplegic shoulder pain during the chronic stage of stroke: A review. *Topics in Stroke Rehabilitation, 19*(6), 514–522.

Waddell, K. J., Birkenmeier, R. L., Moore, J. L., Hornby, T. G., & Lang, C. E. (2014). Feasibility of high-repetition, task-specific training for individuals with upper-extremity paresis. *American Journal of Occupational Therapy, 68*, 444–453.

Williams, P. (1990). Use of intermittent stretch in the prevention of serial sarcomere loss in immobilised muscle. *Annals of Rheumatological Disease, 49*, 316–317.

Williams, P. E., & Goldspink, G. (1978). Changes in sarcomere length and physiological properties in immobilized muscle. *Journal of Anatomy, 127*, 459–468.

Winstein, C. J., & Schmidt, R. A. (1990). Reduced frequency of knowledge of result enhances motor skill learning. *Journal of Experimental Psychology, 16*, 677–691.

Wu, C. Y., Huang, P. C., Chen, Y. T., Lin, K. C., & Yang, H. W. (2013). Effects of mirror therapy on motor and sensory recovery in chronic stroke: A randomized controlled trial. *Archives of Physical Medicine and Rehabilitation, 94*, 1023–1030.

Zackowski, K. M., Dromerick, A. W., Sahrmann, S. A., Thach, W. T., & Bastian, A. J. (2004). How do strength, sensation, spasticity and joint individuation relate to the reaching deficits of people with chronic hemipareis? *Brain, 127*, 1035–1046.

Zoia, S., Pezzetta, E., Blason, L., et al. (2006). A comparison of the reach-to-grasp movement between children and adults: a kinematic study. *Developmental Neuropsychology, 30*(2), 719–738.

41 COGNITIVE AND PERCEPTUAL STRATEGIES

CAROLYN ANNE UNSWORTH

CHAPTER OUTLINE

Abstract

At some point during their career, nearly all occupational therapists will work with a person who has a cognitive or perceptual impairment that produces difficulties in occupational engagement. This person may be a child, teenager, adult or older person, and the occupational therapist may be working in a hospital, community centre, school or residential care facility. The purpose of this chapter is to provide an overview of different types of cognitive and perceptual problems, a range of evaluation strategies that an occupational therapist may use, and ideas for implementing and evaluating therapy. The chapter is illustrated with the story of Jill and Vivian to provide detailed information on how an occupational therapist may work with an individual who is experiencing occupational performance problems as a result of cognitive and perceptual problems. An occupational perspective is taken, so the chapter focuses on practical ideas for occupation-based assessment and intervention. However, the chapter draws on the work of neuropsychologists, speech therapists and occupational therapists (Árnadóttir, 1990; Bradshaw & Mattingley, 1995; Katz; 2011; Lezak, 1995; Ponsford, 2004; Unsworth, 1999).

KEY POINTS

- After acquired brain damage, problems with thinking (cognition) and making sense of the world (perception) are relatively common.

- A variety of cognitive and perceptual problems can affect people's ability to perform the occupations they want or need to do.

- People may have problems with attention and concentration, memory, executive functions, apraxia, unilateral neglect, agnosias and complex perceptual problems.

- Occupational therapists who work with people who have cognitive and perceptual problems use a variety of theoretical approaches such as theories of occupation and models of cognitive and perceptual rehabilitation to guide therapy.

- There is a growing body of evidence to support a variety of interventions for people with cognitive and perceptual problems.

INTRODUCTION: WHAT ARE COGNITION AND PERCEPTION?

Cognition and perception are capacities that are often taken for granted. Being able to think, remember, learn and make sense of the world are fundamental to carrying out all daily occupations. However, when disease, trauma, tumours, toxins or infection affect these abilities, the consequences can be devastating. While some degree of habilitation or rehabilitation is often possible, many people with cognitive and perceptual problems are not able to live alone, hold down paid employment or sustain a family life and relationships. These problems can produce great personal difficulties, hardships and burden for family and considerable financial cost to the individual, his or her family and the community (Unsworth, 1999). Cognitive and perceptual problems are also very puzzling, and individuals and their families may be very confused about why, for example, the individual:

- Can 'see' the breakfast tray on some occasions but not others;
- Cannot put clothes on the correct body parts;

- Cannot brush teeth despite intact motor skills and a perfect description of what to do; and/or
- Does not seem to be able to learn to use the walking aid.

Occupational therapists are well placed to assist individuals who experience cognitive and perceptual problems to minimise or overcome the occupational impact of these problems and continue to lead meaningful lives.

Cognition is usually defined as the capacities that enable people to think, which includes concentrating or paying attention, reasoning, remembering and learning. Executive functions are sometimes discussed under this heading as well. Executive functions include the capacity to plan, manipulate information, initiate and terminate activities, recognise errors, problem-solve and think abstractly. Perception is the dynamic process of receiving the environment through sensory impulses (e.g. visual, auditory, tactile) and translating those impulses into meaning based on previous environmental experience/learning (Árnadóttir, 1990; Grieve, 1993). The resulting awareness of objects and experiences within the environment enables the individual to make sense out of a complex and constantly changing internal and external sensory environment (Sharpless, 1982).

Why Do People Have Problems with Cognition and Perception?

Occupational therapists work with individuals across the lifespan. People with mental health disorders such as schizophrenia or chronic depression, neurological conditions such as Parkinson's disease or multiple sclerosis, and other degenerative diseases such as Alzheimer's disease may experience cognitive and perceptual problems. Although the information contained in this chapter may be relevant to working with individuals who have these problems, the focus of this chapter is on working with adults who have acquired brain damage through the following mechanisms:

- Tumours that are benign or malignant
- Trauma resulting from motor vehicle accidents, falls or violent incidents (e.g. sport or gunshot)
- Infections such as encephalitis
- Anoxia as may occur after near drowning, cardiopulmonary arrest or carbon monoxide poisoning
- Toxins such as alcohol or substance abuse
- Vascular disease, which may produce an infarct or haemorrhagic stroke

The largest two groups of people who acquire cognitive and perceptual problems are people who experience stroke and traumatic brain injury (TBI). Figures from the United States of America, United Kingdom and Australia are all similar, with Australian data provided here. After coronary heart disease, stroke is the second largest cause of death and a leading cause of disability among Australians (Australian Institute of Health and Welfare (AIHW), 2012). It has been estimated that in 2014, approximately 51,000 Australians experienced a new or recurrent stroke and around 437,000 people were living with the effects of stroke. Data concerning the incidence and prevalence of traumatic brain injury are more difficult to gather. Data for the period 2006 to 2007 indicated that there were 75,000 hospital separations for 'injuries to the head' with an average stay of 2.8 days (Australian Institute of Wealth and Welfare (AIHW), 2008). Community-based surveys provide further evidence that the lifetime prevalence of TBI is between 5% and 10% (Butterworth, Anstey, & Jorm, 2004).

How People Make Sense of the World: Normal and Abnormal Cognition and Perception

People make sense of the world by taking in information through their senses and combining it with what they already know and think. When these capacities are interrupted, the individual needs to learn new ways to understand the world or adapt to it. Therapists must have a good understanding of the capacities normal individuals possess in order to work with individuals who are having problems. This section of the chapter provides an overview of some of the main kinds of cognitive and perceptual capacities and problems.

Attention and Concentration

After brain damage, problems with attention and concentration are the most commonly reported deficits (Cicerone, 1996; van Zomeren & Brouwer, 1994). Even individuals with mild brain damage often complain of slowed thinking, being more easily distracted and having trouble doing more than one thing at a time (Cicerone, 1996). Attention and concentration are generally referred to as existing in three forms: sustained, focused (selective), and divided/alternating.

Sometimes referred to as a concentration span, sustained concentration is the capacity to attend to relevant information during occupations. A person who has problems with this kind of concentration may report that they start to read the newspaper and then 'just drift off'.

Problems with focused attention or concentration are often referred to as distractibility. The capacity to selectively attend or concentrate requires the individual to disregard irrelevant environmental visual or auditory stimuli.

Alternating attention or concentration is the capacity to move flexibly between tasks and respond appropriately to the demands of each task. Divided attention is the capacity to respond simultaneously to two or more tasks. Divided attention is required when more than one response is required or more than one stimulus needs to be monitored (Mateer, Kerns, & Eso, 1996). Individuals who have difficulty with alternating and divided forms of attention and concentration may also have great difficulties with more complex daily living activities such as cooking a meal or driving.

Memory and Learning

Memory may be broadly defined as the capacity to store experiences and perceptions for recall and recognition. Memory comprises acquisition or learning, storage or retention, and retrieval or recall (Abreu, 1999).

Learning has been described as a relatively permanent change in the capacity for responding which, resulting from practice and experience, persists with time, resists environmental changes and can be generalised in response to new tasks and situations (Schmidt, 1988). Learning is crucial in rehabilitation.

Using a temporal taxonomy, three levels of memory are often described: immediate recall, short-term memory and long-term memory (Atkinson & Shiffrin, 1968). Immediate recall involves retention of information that has been stored for a few seconds. Short-term memory mediates retention of events or learning that has taken place within a few minutes, hours or days (Lezak, 1995). Long-term memory consists of early experiences and information acquired over a period of years. Individuals who do not have long-term memory are often described as having amnesia.

Metacognition and Executive Functions

Metacognition is generally the term used to describe an individual's knowledge about his or her ability to think, whereas executive functions are often referred to as an individual's ability to start and stop a behaviour, persist at a task or switch as needed, plan, be flexible, self-monitor and think abstractly (Winegardner, 1993; Zinn, Bosworth, Hoenig, & Swartzwelder, 2007). Problems with executive functions are common after acquired brain injury. Wolf, Barbee, and White, (2011) report mild-to-moderate executive functions problems in 27% to 68% of people who experience mild stroke, and Holmqvist, Ivarsson, & Holmefur, (2014) found these problems were a focus for occupational therapy interventions for people with traumatic brain injury.

Lezak (1995) proposed that executive functions consist of four overlapping components: volition (the capacity to determine what one needs and wants to do and conceptualise a future realisation of one's needs and wants); planning (identifying and organising the steps and elements such as skills, material or other people needed to do something or achieve a goal); purposive action (capacities for productivity and self-regulation, including the ability to structure an effective and fluent course of action by initiating, maintaining, switching and stopping complex action sequences in an orderly manner to realise a goal); and effective performance (capacity for quality control, including the ability to self-monitor and self-correct one's behaviour). In a recent study of occupational therapy practice patterns for individuals after TBI, Holmqvist et al. (2014) noted that Swedish occupational therapists focused on occupational performance, with particular attention paid to executive functions.

Perception of a Whole World – Unilateral Neglect

Intact perception enables people to perceive the whole world and attend to all the information in it. After acquired brain damage, difficulties with attending to the body or space in one hemisphere is termed unilateral neglect. Unilateral neglect (sometimes referred to as hemi inattention, unilateral visual inattention or visual neglect) is most often seen after damage to the right cerebral hemisphere (Vallar, 1993).

Persons with neglect may appear not to perceive or to ignore auditory, visual or tactile stimuli coming from the opposite (contralesional) side of space, despite intact sensory abilities. Paradoxically, such persons may be overattentive to and distracted by stimuli coming from the ipsilesional side.

Perhaps the most perplexing aspect of the phenomenon of neglect is that individuals can be unaware of this deficit. It seems as though half of the world has ceased to exist. In some cases, this may extend to the point where a person may deny any dysfunction or the presence of paresis. This particular problem is referred to as anosognosia (Gialanella, Monguzzi, Santoro, & Rocchi, 2005; Halligan & Marshall, 1993).

Simple and Complex Perception

Disorders of perception are often classified as either simple or complex. Individuals with simple perceptual problems are often described as having an agnosia or an inability to recognise or make sense of incoming information despite intact sensory capacities (Bauer & Rubens, 1993).

Agnosias are often classified according to the sensory modality that is affected, such as vision, audition or taste, and specific things such as face, sounds or colours. The main types of agnosias are alexia, or 'word blindness' (an acquired inability to comprehend written language) (Friedman, Ween, & Albert, 1993); auditory agnosia (the inability to distinguish between sounds or to recognise familiar sounds); colour agnosia (the inability to associate objects with particular colours); prosopagnosia (the inability to recognise familiar faces despite intact sensory abilities (Bauer & Rubens, 1993)), simultanagnosia (difficulty in recognising the elements of a visual array) (Ellis & Young, 1988); tactile agnosia, or astereognosis (the inability to recognise objects by touch alone with vision occluded); and visual object agnosia (the inability to recognise objects by looking at them, despite intact vision).

Complex perceptual functions include body scheme abilities and visuospatial functioning. Body scheme abilities are defined as perception of body position, including and involving relation of body parts to each other. Unilateral neglect, as stated earlier, is often described as a difficulty with complex perception. Visuospatial abilities are defined as the ability to relate objects to each other or to the self. This includes spatial perceptions, object relationships (sometimes combined and referred to as spatial relations), constructional abilities, figure–ground discrimination, form discrimination, perception of depth and unilateral spatial attention, as well as topographical orientation.

Praxis

Praxis is the capacity to carry out learned skilled movements. Apraxia, then, is an inability to perform purposeful movements,

and these difficulties cannot be accounted for by inadequate strength, loss of coordination, impaired sensation, attentional difficulties, abnormal tone, movement disorders, intellectual deterioration, poor comprehension or uncooperativeness (Croce, 1993; Kirshner, 1991; Tate & McDonald, 1995). Apraxia is more common after left hemisphere damage, and so may individuals with this problem also present with aphasia (Lezak, 1995). Two main forms of apraxia discussed in the literature are ideomotor and ideational apraxia. A third form, buccofacial or oral apraxia, is actually a type of ideomotor apraxia and is characterised by difficulties with performing the purposeful movements that involve facial muscles related to the mouth (Bradshaw & Mattingley, 1995).

Ideomotor apraxia refers to a breakdown between the concept of what to do and the actual performance. An individual with ideomotor apraxia may be able to carry out habitual tasks automatically and describe how they are done but is unable to imitate gestures or perform on command (Mozaz, Marti, Carrera, & de la Puente, 1990; Raade, Gonzalez Rothi, & Heilman, 1991). Individuals with ideomotor apraxia are unable to perform tasks on request that require use of many implements and that have many steps. For example, an individual will usually be unable to 'blow' on command. However, if presented with a bubble wand, the individual can spontaneously blow bubbles (Mozaz et al., 1990; Raade et al., 1991). Movements are observed to be clumsy and awkward, with impairment in the timing, sequencing and spatial organisation of movement (Tate & McDonald, 1995).

On the other hand, ideational apraxia is a failure to conceptualise what is to be done. The individual is unable to perform a purposeful movement either automatically or on command. In many cases, the individual can perform isolated components of a task but is unable to combine them into a complete act. Finally, the person cannot verbally describe the process of performing an activity (Mayer, Reed, Schwartz, Montgomery, & Palmer, 1990).

FRAMEWORKS FOR OCCUPATIONAL THERAPY WHEN PEOPLE HAVE COGNITIVE AND PERCEPTUAL PROBLEMS

In 2001 the World Health Organization (WHO) revised its classification of health states and proposed the International Classification of Function, Disability, and Health (ICF). This system has been adopted widely by health care professionals and provides an ideal foundation for occupational therapists to organise practice and describe it to others (see e.g. AIHW, 2003; College of Occupational Therapists, 2004). When using ICF terminology for individuals who have cognitive and perceptual problems, *impairment* (or problems with body structure and function) is the term used to describe memory problems, apraxia or perceptual problems, for example. These impairments produce activity limitations, which are the resulting problems an individual may experience when performing daily occupations such as dressing, driving, or typing on the computer. Depending on how the individual is able to interact with society, activity limitations may lead to participation restrictions, or handicap. Once impairments have been identified, the emphasis for occupational therapists is on assessing and treating the individual's activity limitations or occupational performance and assisting the individual to minimise the participation restrictions that may result. The ICF domains of impairment, activity and participation are also mitigated by barriers and facilitators and the environment.

In addition to using an ICF framework, an occupational therapist will select an overarching occupational therapy theory to guide practice, such as the Canadian Model of Occupational Performance and Engagement (Townsend & Polatajko, 2013, or the Model of Human Occupation (Kielhofner, 2008), and a practice model specific to working with people who have cognitive and perceptual problems. This is sometimes referred to as an umbrella framework as practice models sit under the overarching theories (Unsworth, 2004). The selection of a practice model is particularly crucial as this will guide the kinds of evaluations and interventions that the therapist will undertake (Unsworth, 1999). One of the main differences between practice models is whether they adopt a remedial and adaptive approach to therapy.

The main practice models that a therapist could use when working with individuals who have cognitive and perceptual problems have been comprehensively reviewed (Katz, 2011; Unsworth, 1999) and include the Dynamic Interaction Approach (Toglia, 1992) and the Retraining Approach (Averbuch & Katz, 1992), which are remedial; the Neurofunctional Approach (Giles & Wilson, 1992) and Compensatory/Rehabilitation Approach (Fisher, 1997a), which are adaptive or compensatory; and the Quadraphonic Approach (Abreu, 1990), which combines aspects that are both remedial and adaptive or compensatory.

The practice story of Vivian and her occupational therapist, Jill, is used to illustrate this chapter. After an introduction to Vivian and Jill, the theoretical frameworks adopted by Jill are described (Practice Story 41.1). Because Jill uses the Canadian Practice Process Framework (Townsend & Polatajko, 2013) the practice story follows the eight action points of the model (Table 41.1). These action points are identified throughout the practice story.

ASSESSMENT STRATEGIES

Once the therapist has selected an appropriate theoretical orientation, the assessments and interventions that follow are logically linked to that approach. Hence, a therapist using a remedial retraining approach will probably select assessments such as the Lowenstein Occupational Therapy Cognitive Assessment (Averbuch & Katz, 1992) or the Rivermead Behavioural Memory Test (Wilson et al., 2008). Conversely, a therapist using a compensatory rehabilitative approach may consider the

Assessment of Motor and Process Skills (AMPS) (Fisher, 1997b) as the assessment of choice.

The purpose of administering an assessment may include one or more of the following: identify the individual's problem areas, establish a baseline for intervention, provide information for intervention planning or predict performance in activities of daily living. The assessments described in this chapter will assist the therapist to determine which cognitive and perceptual abilities are intact and which are limited. The importance of accurate and thorough assessment cannot be overemphasised. Hence, this section of the chapter describes the importance of screening the person for motor and sensory problems before assessment of cognitive and perceptual problems and discusses some of the noncognitive or perceptual related issues that may influence assessment results and therefore must be factored in to the evaluation process. Finally, a selection of standardised assessments are presented, and a hypothesis testing approach to identifying an individual's cognitive and perceptual problems is outlined.

Preassessment Considerations

Before assessing an individual for the presence of cognitive or perceptual problems, the therapist must have initially determined whether the person has any sensory or physical deficits such as a sensory loss, language impairment, hearing loss, motor loss (weakness, spasticity, incoordination), visual disturbance (poor eyesight, homonymous hemianopia), disorientation, or lack of comprehension. The therapist needs to be able to distinguish between these kinds of physical and sensory problems and problems that are of a cognitive or perceptual nature. For example, if the therapist has not completed a sensory assessment, she will be unable to determine whether a person who has had a stroke wearing a blindfold cannot recognise the item before them because of a tactile sensory loss or an agnosia.

Assessment should also not commence until the individual is medically stable, not in a state of posttraumatic amnesia (i.e. a period of confusion and disorientation that follows traumatic brain injury, but not stroke, during which a person does not have the capacity to form new memories), and is psychologically and emotionally ready for assessment. The therapist needs to be aware of behaviours that reflect a person's psychological response to illness rather than particular cognitive or perceptual abilities. Anxiety over capabilities may inhibit a person's optimal performance during assessment and therapy, and therapists should spend time reassuring individuals of a positive outcome, regardless of assessment results. Finally, depression, fatigue and medication can also reduce an individual's performance during assessment and the therapist should try to take these factors into account when interpreting assessment results. For example, after a stroke, 31% of people experience depression, and these symptoms can easily be mistaken for cognitive or perceptual problems (Hackett & Pickles, 2014).

Finally, it should be noted that not all areas of performance loss are typically detected within the hospital setting. It is not uncommon for the person to perform adequately in self-care skills after therapy in the hospital but to fail on the same tasks in other environmental contexts, such as the home. Higher-level tasks, such as driving, banking or planning a meal, may only emerge as areas of difficulty once the person is discharged home. When appropriate, the person's competence in these areas should be considered within the context of an instrumental activity of daily living (ADL) assessment.

Standardised Assessments

A standardised assessment has a uniform procedure to administer and score the assessment so that the tester can be confident that every time the assessment is administered, it is done so in the same way. Standardised assessments also have a method for referencing an individual's scores, or determining the person's level of performance (Anastasi, 1988; de Clive-Lowe, 1996) using normative data (a norm-referenced assessment) (de Clive-Lowe, 1996) or a predetermined criteria (criterion-referenced assessment).

When selecting a standardised assessment the therapist must consider many factors, such as what the therapist wants to learn about the person and what the assessment can potentially reveal (Unsworth, 1999). In many cases a single assessment will not provide all the information required by a therapist to plan intervention, so several assessments may have to be administered. Several screening or battery assessments that are commonly used by occupational therapists to assess an individual's cognitive and perceptual status are listed in Table 41.2.

Several other global measures could also be used to measure the outcome of a person's rehabilitation, such as the Medical Outcomes Study Short Form Health Survey (Ware & Sherbourne, 1992); Australian Therapy Outcome Measures (Unsworth, 2005; Unsworth & Duncombe, 2014); Canadian Occupational Performance Measure (Law et al., 1998); Rivermead Rehabilitation Centre Life Goals Questionnaire (Davis et al., 1992); Reintegration to Normal Living Index (Wood-Dauphinee, Opzoomer, Williams, Marchand, & Spitzer, 1988); or the Functional Independence Measure (Adult FIM SM) (*Guide for the Uniform Data Set for Medical Rehabilitation*, 1999). Some of these assessments also incorporate items that measure cognition and perception. For example, the FIM includes three cognition-related items: memory, problem solving and social interaction.

Observation of Performance (Hypothesis Testing)

Gathering information about an individual's cognitive and perceptual problems while engaged in everyday occupations can be another useful way to assess a person. Referred to as hypothesis testing, this is a systematic approach to observing an individual's performance and considering the kinds of cognitive and perceptual impairments that may be present. A detailed description of this process is documented in Unsworth (1999) and an overview is presented here.

This approach has many similarities to the dynamic interaction approach to assessment developed by Toglia (1992). In both of these assessment procedures, the therapist selects an activity to undertake with the person and proposes a hypothesis, which is then tested. Although the hypothesis testing approach cannot replace standardised assessments, the approach remains useful for therapists who are not trained to use assessments such as the Árnadóttir Occupational Therapy Neurobehavioural Evaluation (A-ONE) or AMPS, or for students and less experienced therapists to use in conjunction with other standardised assessments. The steps in the hypothesis testing approach include the following:

1. Observe the person performing an occupation (such as dressing or grooming or making a snack) and identify problem areas.
2. Consider the person's strengths and difficulties that are known at this stage.
3. Generate a single or multiple hypotheses that explain the difficulties.
4. Select an occupation of daily living to test the hypotheses.
5. The therapist structures the occupation in order to control some of the variables present and manipulate or alter the relative presence or absence of others. In this way, changes can be introduced that allow the therapist to exclude alternative or competing explanations or hypotheses for the person's difficulties. This will lead to confirmation or rejection of the hypotheses.
6. The therapist examines the data and accepts or rejects each hypothesis, or may return to the first step to redefine the problem and generate new hypotheses. The information gained during hypothesis testing supplements information gained during standardised assessment.

Jill describes the processes of assessing Vivian in the second part of the practice story (Practice Story 41.2).

INTERVENTION STRATEGIES

Once a particular theoretical orientation has been decided upon, therapists can confidently direct therapy towards remedial or compensatory interventions. However, many therapists who commence intervention using a remedial approach may introduce compensatory ideas and strategies with an individual once progress has plateaued, or when discharge is imminent. The following section of the chapter introduces a variety of remedial and compensatory intervention ideas and strategies when working with individuals who have cognitive and perceptual dysfunction. Although there is research evidence to support some of these techniques, a great deal more research is required to support occupational therapy practice in this area.

TABLE 41.1
The Eight Action Points of the Canadian Practice Process Framework (Townsend & Polatajko, 2013)

Action points	Key enablement and actions – With occupational therapist working within frames of reference/theoretical models – With person participating and power sharing as much as possible
1. Enter/initiate	The occupational therapist is the first point of contact with the person. Establish why the person has come to be in occupational therapy. Detail any requirements for service such as disclosure.
2. Set the stage	Work with client to clarify beliefs, assumptions, expectations and desires. Build rapport. Establish any ground rules. Through reading case notes and collaborating with the person, identify possible priority occupations and possible occupational goals.
3. Assess/evaluate	Assess/evaluate client occupational status, dreams and potential for change. Consult with the client and other specialists, and use specialist evaluations where appropriate.
4. Agree on objectives and plan	Collaborate to identify priority occupations, in light of evaluation. Collaborate to negotiate and plan goals/objectives.
5. Implement the plan	Occupational therapy programme is implemented. Person is engaged through occupation. Techniques and strategies used to effect or prevent change as appropriate.
6. Monitor and modify	Monitor occupational therapy programme to enable success: consult, collaborate, advocate and educate.
7. Evaluate outcome	Reassess and evaluate and compare to initial findings. Make recommendations for next steps.
8. Conclude/exit	Communicate conclusion of occupational therapy with person. Ensure coordinated transfer to other services or reentry to occupational therapy.

Interventions for Problems with Attention and Concentration

Although attention and concentration, as defined earlier in the chapter, were divided into the categories of sustained, focused (selective) and divided/alternating, there is limited empirical evidence to support interventions with these specific forms. Hence, the interventions described next may be tried with different presentations of the problem.

Remedial Approach

The purpose of therapy is to increase the individual's attention to appropriate stimuli and disregard inappropriate stimuli. Individuals can be trained to scan the visual environment in a slow and systematic manner. It may also be useful to set time or speed limits, amplify critical stimuli, and make the crucial stimuli salient (noticeable) to the individual (Diller & Weinberg, 1972). A Cochrane review (Loetscher & Lincoln, 2013) revealed six controlled trials of attention training for people who had a stroke. The review found that training improved alertness and sustained attention on measures of these capacities, but there was no evidence to support or refute the use of cognitive rehabilitation for attention deficits to improve independence. Couillet et al. (2010) conducted a randomised clinical trial with 12 people to investigate the effect of training on divided attention. Participants undertook two computer-based or pen-and-paper tasks simultaneously, and a positive training effect was found. However, the benefits of training were not transferred to everyday activities.

Compensatory Approach

The inability to attend to significant stimuli is compounded for many individuals by distraction as a result of extraneous stimuli in the environment such as noise. Therefore the environment can be controlled to maximise the individual's ability to concentrate (Ponsford, Sloan, & Snow, 2012). Fasotti, Kovacs, Eling, & Brouwer, (2000) have reported successfully teaching people with head injury to compensate for slowed information processing by using time pressure management, and Sohlberg, McLaughlin, Pavese, Heidrich, & Posner, (2000) documented the effectiveness of attention process training.

Problems with Memory and Learning
Remedial Approach

The aim of memory retraining is to enable the individual to effectively encode and recall information so that learning can occur. One of the foundation skills for this is to be able to attend and concentrate. Therefore, when working on memory skill, therapists should also be working with individuals to improve attention (Abreu, 1999). When working with the individual to effectively code information, it is important to teach the person strategies to organise material to be remembered and make logical associations. A determination should be made of how the individual used to remember information so that the therapist can help to build on these past strategies. Although there is little evidence to support the use of computers games in the rehabilitation of memory skills, the therapist may be able to help

Introducing Vivian and Her Occupational Therapist, Jill

ACTION POINTS FROM THE CPPF

1. Enter/Initiate and 2. Set the Stage

Vivian was assigned to Jill's caseload. Jill is a senior therapist and has worked on the neurological rehabilitation team for 17 years. Jill consulted Vivian's medical record where some notes had been made by the admission team. Vivian is a 65-year-old divorced woman who was admitted to an acute care facility after a right parietal infarct (stroke). After 4 days, she was discharged to a specialist rehabilitation facility. On admission to the facility, she showed signs of mild, resolving hemiparesis of the left upper and lower limbs and some reduced coordination. Jill read that Vivian had been previously in good health although she had been involved in a minor car accident 5 years ago in which her right leg was broken and as a result she experiences ongoing stiffness and minor pain, which seems to be aggravated by cold weather.

Jill conducted an interview with Vivian. Jill gathered information about Vivian's family and family commitments, daily life routines, habits, work, home life and interests and began to form a profile of Vivian as a person and what she wanted to achieve. Jill learned that Vivian retired a year ago from her job as a secondary school teacher of Spanish and history and lived with one of her three sons in a single level home that she rents. She also had a 36-year-old son who lived interstate and a 40-year-old son with schizophrenia and an intellectual disability who recently moved from living with Jill to residential care. Vivian disclosed that her financial situation was adequate and that she did not have any worries about this hospital stay. Vivian stated that she enjoyed lawn bowls, reading the daily papers, painting and drawing and often went to the local community centre where there was a Spanish club and discussion group.

Through administering the Canadian Occupational Performance Measure (COPM) (Law et al., 1998) with Vivian, Jill found that Vivian did not think her problems were very severe and that she would be able to return home in a few days. Vivian identified that what she most looked forward to doing on her return home was being able to attend her Spanish group, where she has many friends, visit her son in the residential care facility and return to her usual home jobs such as caring for the house and cooking evening meals for her son. Vivian previously drove to Spanish group and to visit her son and thought that there would be no problems with doing this when she returned home.

During the interview Jill became concerned that Vivian seemed to focus just on the right side of her body and that her clothing was falling off on her left. When Jill moved to a chair on the left of Vivian, Vivian seemed to think Jill had left the room. This information indicated to Jill that Vivian might be experiencing a unilateral neglect. Jill considered that this was consistent with the site of Vivian's stroke in the right parietal lobe.

Jill used the Canadian Practice Process Framework from the Canadian Model of Occupational Performance and Engagement (Townsend & Polatajko, 2013) to guide her therapy and adopted the retraining approach (Averbuch & Katz, 1992) as a practice model. When a person's performance in daily occupations has plateaued and she worked towards a home discharge, Jill often turned to a rehabilitation frame of reference (Trombly, 1995) to finalise her therapeutic interventions. Hence, Jill believed in neural plasticity of the brain and that skills taught in one environment can be generalise to other environments. However, when an individual person's performance had plateaued and discharge was imminent, Jill became more pragmatic in her approach and began to modify the environment and arrange for home service to do the tasks the person was unable to complete.

Consistent with these theoretical approaches, Jill usually administered standardised cognitive and perceptual assessments such as those identified in Table 41.2 during Action Point 3 of the CPPF and the COPM (Law et al., 1998). Because many people with cognitive and perceptual problems can have limited insight into the nature and extent of their impairments, Jill searched for research articles, such as the one by Hobson (1996), that discussed enhancing person-centred practice when a person has cognitive and perceptual problems to help guide her practice.

CPPF, Canadian Practice Process Framework.

---

the individual identify skills gained and reinforce these during everyday occupations. A recent Cochrane review (das Nair & Lincoln, 2007) found only two controlled trials exploring mnemonic memory training after a stroke. The trial by Doornheim and De Haan (1998) found that memory training had no significant effect on memory impairment or subjective memory complaints. The study by Kaschel (2002) reported the use of imagery mnemonics improved delayed recall of material on some of the outcome measures. The Cochrane reviewers concluded that there was insufficient evidence to support or refute the effectiveness of rehabilitation for memory problems after stroke. Although errorless learning has been used in rehabilitation for some time, there is increasing evidence that this approach may be beneficial for retraining memory. For example,

TABLE 41.2

Summary of Key Features of Standardised Assessments Used with People Who Have Cognitive and Perceptual Problems

Assessment	Purpose/Content	Developed by an OT	Used with Remedial, Adaptive or Both Approaches	Training Required	Uses ADL	Is Partial Administration Recommended	Evidence of Test-Retest Reliability, Interrater Reliability	Evidence of Content Validity, Criterion Validity, and Construct Validity	Time to Administer (mins)
A-ONE (Árnadóttir, 1990)	Developed to measure a person's neurobehaviour through daily living tasks (dressing, grooming, hygiene, transfer and mobility, feeding and communication). A wide variety of cognitive and perceptual impairments can be detected with this assessment.	Yes	Both	Yes	Yes	Yes	Preliminary data Yes	Yes No Yes	30–40
SOTOF (Laver & Powell, 1995)	Designed to assess older persons' level of occupational performance and neuropsychological functioning after neurological damage of cortical origin. Consists of a screening assessment, neuropsychological checklist, and four ADL scales (eating from a bowl, pouring a drink and drinking, putting on an upper body garment, and washing and drying hands).	Yes	Both	No	Yes	No	Yes Yes	Yes Yes Preliminary	45
AMPS (Fisher, 1997a)	A structured, observational evaluation of a person's performance in daily living activities. The therapist observes the person's performance on two or three familiar personal or	Yes	Both	Yes	Yes	No	Yes Yes	Yes Yes Yes	30–60

Assessment	Description												Time (min)
	instrumental activities of daily living of their choice and then rates the quality of this performance in terms of how effortless, efficient, safe or independent the person's ADL motor and ADL process skills are in the context of the task performance (the dynamic interaction of the person with the environment).												
RPAB (Whiting et al., 1985)	Assesses visual perceptual deficits in people after head injury or stroke. Consists of 16 performance tests that assess form discrimination, colour constancy, sequencing, object completion, figure–ground discrimination, body image and inattention and spatial awareness.	Yes	Both	No	No	No	Yes	Yes	Yes	Yes	Yes	60
BIT (Wilson et al., 1987)	Assesses individuals for the presence of unilateral visual neglect and provides the therapist with information concerning how the neglect affects the person's ability to perform everyday occupations. The BIT consists of nine activity-based subtests and six pen-and-paper subtests.	No	Both	No	No	Yes	Yes	Yes	Preliminary	Yes	No	60
LOTCA (Itzkovich et al., 1990)	Battery-style assessment composed of 20 subtests that assess four areas: orientation, visual and spatial perception, visuomotor organisation and thinking operations.	Yes	Both	No	No	No	No	Yes	Yes	Yes	Yes	30–45
RBMT-3 (Wilson et al., 2008)	Assesses a person's everyday memory abilities. It offers the therapist an initial assessment of the individual's memory	No	Both	No	No	No	Yes	Yes	Yes	Yes	Yes	30

Continued on following page

TABLE 41.2

Summary of Key Features of Standardised Assessments Used with People Who Have Cognitive and Perceptual Problems *(Continued)*

Assessment	Purpose/Content	Developed by an OT	Used with Remedial, Adaptive or Both Approaches	Training Required	Uses ADL	Is Partial Administration Recommended	Evidence of Test-Retest Reliability, Interrater Reliability	Evidence of Content Validity, Criterion Validity, and Construct Validity	Time to Administer (mins)
	function and an indication of appropriate areas for treatment, and enables the therapist to monitor memory skills throughout the treatment programme.								
BADS (Wilson et al., 1996)	Measures everyday executive function and higher-level cognitive functions. Includes six subtests and a 20-item questionnaire.	No	Remedial	No	Some	No	Yes Yes	Yes Yes Yes	30–45
TEA (Robertson et al., 1994b)	Measures selective attention, sustained attention and attentional switching. Includes eight ADL-based subtests such as elevator counting, map and telephone book searching and lottery tickets.	No	Remedial	No	Some	No	Yes Preliminary	Yes Yes Yes	45–60
COGNISTAT (Kiernan et al., 1987)	Cognitive screening assessment. Items include measures of attention, level of consciousness and orientation, language, memory, calculations and reasoning.	No	Remedial	No	No	No	Yes Yes	Yes Yes Yes	10–30
OT-APST (Cook, 2005)	Visual perception screening assessment of 25 items in the areas of agnosia, visuospatial skill (including awareness of body scheme and unilateral neglect), constructional skill, apraxia and acalculia.	Yes	Both	No	No	No	Yes Yes	Yes Yes Yes	20–25

Test	Description											Time (min)
MoCA (Nasreddine et al., 2005)	Comprehensive cognitive screening test including memory, attention, abstraction, language, orientation and visuospatial skills.	No	Remedial	No	No	No	Yes	Yes	Yes	Yes	Yes	10
CAM (Rustad, 1993)	Provide an overview of cognitive functioning in adults. Seventeen subtests cover attention, memory, visual neglect, auditory memory, simple maths, problem solving and safety.	Yes	Both	No	No	No	Yes	Yes	Yes	Yes	Yes	20–30
CAMCOG (Roth et al., 1986)	This is the cognitive component of the CAMDEX. There are 67 items to measure cognitive impairment including language, memory, praxis, attention and abstract thinking	Yes	Both	No	No	No	Preliminary	Preliminary	Yes	Preliminary	Yes	20–25
Kettle Test (Hartman-Maeir et al., 2009)	A performance test where the individual is scored when preparing two hot drinks.	Yes	Both	No	Yes	No	Yes	Yes	Yes	Yes	No	5–20
EFPT (Baum et al., 2008)	Evaluates five executive function constructs: initiation, organisation, sequencing, safety and judgement and completion of four ADL tasks.	Yes	Both	No	Yes	No	No	Yes	Yes	Yes	Yes	30–45

ADL, Activity of daily living; A-ONE, Árnadóttir Occupational Therapy Neurobehavioural Evaluation; AMPS, Assessment of Motor and Process Skills; BADS, Behavioural Assessment of Dysexecutive Syndrome; BIT, the Behavioural Inattention Test; CAM, Cognitive Assessment of Minnesota; CAMCOG, Cambridge Cognition Examination; COGNISTAT, Neurobehavioural Cognitive Status Screening Examination; EFPT, Executive Function Performance Test; LOTCA, Loewenstein Occupational Therapy Cognitive Assessment; MoCA, Montreal Cognitive Assessment; OT-APST, Occupational Therapy Adult Perceptual Screening Test; RPAB, Rivermead Perceptual Assessment Battery; RBMT-3, Rivermead Behavioural Memory Test; SOTOF, Structured Observational Test of Function; TEA, Test of Everyday Attention.

Fish et al. (2014) reported significant improvements with 14 people with impaired event-based prospective memory problems. These authors concluded that an errorless learning approach may be valuable in completing day-to-day event-based prospective memory tasks.

Compensatory Approach

The use of a diary or notebook system (memory log) can help many individuals to manage their daily living activities (Ownsworth & McFarland, 1999). Environmental prompts such as a beeper or a wall calendar can be useful to assist individuals to remember their routine or to look at their diary. Mnemonics training may be successful with some individuals (Kaschel et al., 2002). In 2014 Lannin et al. conducted a randomised controlled trial to investigate the effectiveness of handheld computers against standard rehabilitation for improving everyday memory functioning in people with acquired brain impairment.

The standard rehabilitation included general occupational therapy and the use of nonelectronic memory aids, and the intervention group received general occupational therapy and an 8-week training programme in using a personal digital assistant with an occupational therapist. The authors reported statistically significant improvements in achieving functional memory goals and in memory scores on a standardised subtest of a memory scale.

Problems with Metacognition and Executive Functions

Remedial Approach

The provision of a structured environment, feedback and routine can enable a person to reduce the impact of their problems with executive functions (e.g., providing the individual with steps to follow, assisting the task to become routine by repeated practice, or providing immediate feedback about

---

PRACTICE STORY 41.2

Assessing Vivian

ACTION POINTS FROM THE CPPF

3. Assess/Evaluate

Given the issues noted by Jill during the initial interview, she decided to conduct a Visual Confrontation Test (Gainotti, D'Erme, & Bartolomeo, 1991; Unsworth, 1999) and Extinction Test (as developed by Lynn Robertson and cited in Rafal, 1994), a Behavioural Inattention Test (BIT) (Wilson, Cockburn, & Halligan, 1987) (Fig. 41.1) and hypothesis testing assessment of Vivian making a cup of tea (Fig. 41.2 and Table 41.3).

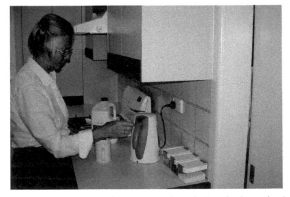

FIG. 41.2 ■ Vivian making a cup of tea during the hypothesis testing procedure.

The first three steps in the hypothesis identification process are outlined in Table 41.3.

In Table 41.3, the hypotheses that Jill thought were the best at this stage are underlined in the third column. After this, Jill selected a new activity and tested her hypotheses. For example, Jill could test out these hypotheses during grooming. Jill needed to manipulate task demands in order to test her hypotheses. Because Jill has hypothesised that Vivian may have some short-term memory problems, she could test this out by asking Vivian the steps she needed to follow for grooming and then provide a written or pictorial list of these steps. If Vivian's performance improved when following the written or pictorial list, this would support Jill's hypothesis that Vivian had a short-term memory impairment.

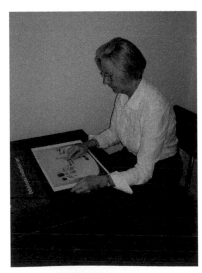

FIG. 41.1 ■ Vivian undertaking the Behavioural Inattention Test (Wilson et al., 1987).

TABLE 41.3
Findings from Hypothesis Testing Activity of Making a Cup of Tea

Problem Occupation	Observations	Hypotheses
Vivian chose to make a cup of tea with milk and sugar in the occupational therapy kitchen.	Jill showed Vivian where the tea-making items are located in the occupational therapy kitchen. Vivian talked about liking tea and how she took it (white with half a teaspoon of sugar). She said she needed to get a tea bag, sugar and spoon and milk, and commented that the tea bags and sugar were on the bench.	Good planning skills
	Vivian then turned on the jug, Jill reminded her to check if it was full first.	Unfamiliar kitchen – Vivian probably has her jug full at home Problem-solving difficulties
	Vivian turned jug off, opened the lid and stated that it was sufficiently full.	Shows some problem-solving skills
	Vivian found the tea bags and sugar containers on the right side of the bench and opened these. Stated 'I'm just waiting for the jug to boil.'	No difficulty locating objects on the right side
	Jill asked if she needed anything else. Vivian stated, 'Oh yes, I need milk'.	Short-term memory problem
	Vivian turned around and seemed to look around the kitchen. She asked Jill where the fridge was (the fridge was on Vivian's left side). Jill prompted Vivian to look at each object around the kitchen and she then located the fridge.	Unilateral neglect Visual object agnosia
	Vivian opened the fridge with her right hand. The fridge handle was at waist height on the right side of the fridge, and the door opened to the left. The milk was on the door on Vivian's left. Vivian spent several minutes looking in the fridge and moved several objects on her right side to look behind them.	Unilateral neglect Visual object agnosia
	On hearing the kettle boil, splutter and turn off, Vivian shut the fridge, and walked back to the jug, saying, 'The water's ready now'.	Concentration problem (selective) Short-term memory problem
	Vivian then asked the therapist for a cup. The therapist told her the location and Vivian found one easily in the cupboard above. The therapist prompted Vivian by asking if she had everything she needed. With prompting, Vivian eventually replied she needed milk.	Unilateral neglect Short-term memory problem
	Vivian found the fridge again, and with prompting and positioning of Vivian's hand on the top of the fridge door, Vivian took several minutes to locate the milk. Vivian and Jill walked back to the bench. Vivian placed the large milk container in the middle of the bench and Jill moved it to the left.	
	Vivian then took out a tea bag and placed it in the cup, poured in water, and then asked where the milk had gone. Jill stood on Vivian's left and tapped the bench next to the milk and asked Vivian to draw her attention to that side of the bench. Vivian stated again that she could not find the milk, and Jill guided Vivian's right hand over to it. Jill stated, 'Oh! There it is.'	Unilateral neglect
	Jill then asked Vivian for a spoon for the sugar, and Jill directed Vivian to the drawers on Vivian's right. The spoon was located on the left side of the drawer. Vivian stated this must be the wrong drawer. She turned to Jill and then when she turned back to the drawer, she saw the spoon, which was now on her right side. Vivian placed the sugar in the cup, stirred and drank the tea. She used her right hand throughout the task.	Unilateral neglect

Continued on following page

Assessing Vivian (Continued)

Jill could also test her competing hypotheses of whether Vivian had a unilateral neglect or visual object agnosia by laying out three objects on Vivian's right side (e.g. toothpaste, lipstick and deodorant) and three different objects on her left side (e.g. brush, comb, soap). Jill could then ask Vivian to name all the items in front of her. If Vivian could name the three items on her right, this negates the hypothesis of visual object agnosia and supports the hypothesis of unilateral neglect.

When administering the Visual Confrontation Test, Jill looked to see if Vivian had a left homonymous hemianopia (HH) as well as a left unilateral neglect (UN). When a person has a homonymous hemianopia, the person has a sensory-based visual problem, meaning that she is not able to see. However, in a unilateral neglect, the person can 'see' but cannot attend to this information. Other differences between an HH and a UN are that individuals with HH often have insight into the visual loss and people with UN, like Vivian, do not.

Another way to distinguish between individuals with HH and UN is whether the phenomenon of extinction is present. Extinction is evident when the person can attend to isolated stimuli coming from either side as presented during the confrontation test. However, when presented with simultaneous stimuli (i.e. stimuli simultaneously from both sides) the individual may respond only to the stimulus on the non-neglected side, thus 'extinguishing' stimuli on the neglected side. It has also been noted that extinction may be more subtle and resilient than a unilateral neglect (Robertson & Eglin, 1993). In people with HH, simultaneous extinction is not present because individuals will never see stimuli on the left side. Finally, during ADLs, a consistent loss is noted in individuals with HH. However, people with UN show an inconsistent performance as they are able to respond appropriately to some stimuli but not others.

Jill also conducted a brief physical and sensory evaluation with Vivian and found Vivian's right body side had normal sensation and motor control (although some stiffness resulting from the orthopaedic injuries sustained in the car accident were present). Although Vivian had full passive and active range of motion in her left arm, her strength was reduced. She also demonstrated some reduced coordination and fine motor skills and altered sensation on the left. Jill also worked on these issues with Vivian; however, it is beyond the scope of this chapter to include discussions on assessment and intervention of Vivian's physical and sensory problems.

After all assessments (initial interview, Canadian Outcome Performance Measure, the BIT, Extinction Test, Visual Confrontation Test and hypothesis testing) Jill reasoned that although Vivian did have a neglect with extinction, there was no evidence of homonymous hemianopia. The assessments also revealed some difficulties with divided attention and concentration, mild short-term memory problems and difficulties with insight to her problems. Jill felt confident in identifying these problems and decided to pursue goal setting rather than conduct further standardised tests such as the Rivermead Behavioural Memory Test (Wilson et al., 2008).

In summary, Jill drew up the information presented in Table 41.4 as a summary of Vivian's strengths and problems to work on during therapy (please note that this table omits sensory and physical problems).

TABLE 41.4

Vivian's Strength and Problem List Drawn from Hypothesis Testing and Standardised Assessments – Using ICF Framework

Impairments	Capacities
■ Unilateral neglect (with extinction) ■ Decreased concentration/attention (some distractibility) ■ Limited short-term memory	■ Communication (expressive and receptive) ■ Walks independently ■ Intact vision
Activity Limitations (Disabilities)	**Activity Strengths (Abilities)**
■ Personal activities of daily living (ADLs) (e.g. showering, grooming, dressing, eating) ■ Instrumental ADLs (e.g. domestic activities such as cooking, telephone use and cleaning the house and community activities such as driving, shopping and banking)	■ Aspects of personal ADL, such as toileting
Participation/Participation Restrictions	**Environmental Resources (Family, Community and Organisational Supports)**
■ Unknown at this stage and require examination closer to the time of discharge	■ Spanish group members (have visited) ■ Son (with whom Vivian lives) ■ Vivian's son is being cared for in a residential care facility (Vivian is very happy with the care provided)

ADL, Activity of daily living; CPPF, Canadian Practice Process Framework.

the individual's behaviour and the effect it has on others). The therapist initially acts as the individual's frontal lobes and gradually transfers these responsibilities to the person. However, unless the person has some awareness of the problems (insight), a remedial approach will not be particularly successful (Ponsford et al., 2012). Honda (1999) reported a study with three individuals who were provided with self-instructional training, a problem-solving procedure and physical-set changing exercises over a 6-month period. Although two of the participants had improvements on the neuropsychological test used as an outcome measure, all participants improved in personal and instrumental activities of daily living. Limitations of this study include the small sample size and lack of control participants, because it could be expected that these individuals would make spontaneous recovery over the 6-month study period. Hewitt, Evans, & Dritschel, (2006) investigated whether a 30-minute training session that aimed to prompt retrieval of memories in people after TBI could support planning skills. The researchers found the technique to be effective, but larger trials are needed that track retention of learning over time.

Compensatory Approach

When using a compensatory approach, intervention focuses on working with the individual to use other intact cognitive functions or modify the environment in order to complete the occupation. For example, the therapist might ask the person to perform a task in a room with minimal distractions or change the demands of the person's work, home or community to diminish the need to employ executive functions. A beeper or alarm clock, along with a range of other compensatory techniques, may be used to assist a person overcome poor initiation (Duran & Fisher, 1999; Ponsford et al., 2012). In 2007 Zinn et al. reported development of compensatory rehabilitation techniques for use with people who have problems with executive functions after stroke. However, literature detailing these techniques has not yet been published.

Problems with Unilateral Neglect

Remedial Approach

Unlike some of the other cognitive and perceptual impairments, a great deal of research has been conducted to identify interventions for unilateral neglect. In particular, the reader is referred to two excellent reviews by Bowen, Hazelton, Pollock, & Lincoln, (2013) and Luaute, Halligan, Rode, Rossetti, & Boisson, (2006) which describe and evaluate the effectiveness of several of the interventions outlined here. Asking the individual with unilateral neglect to move the left body side (hemispheric activation approaches), such as simply clenching and unclenching the fist, can improve attention to the left body side and hemispace (Eskes, Butler, McDonald, Harrison, & Phillips, 2003). In one of the first studies using this technique, Robertson,

Tegnér, Goodrich, & Wilson, (1994a) carried out a study with six individuals who were asked to walk through a doorway. Each of the individuals' walking trajectory (pathway) was measured, and it was found that all trajectories were significantly deviated to the right of centre. Participants were then asked to clench and unclench their left hands before, and during, walking through the doorway. The researchers found that this procedure significantly assisted participants to centre their walking trajectories.

Other techniques that have been used successfully with individuals with unilateral neglect include eye-patching (Tsang, Sze, & Fong, 2009), prism glasses (Jacquin-Courtois et al., 2010; Keane, Turner, Sherrington, & Beard, 2006), neck vibration therapy (Karnath, Christ, & Hartje, 1993), phasic alerting (Robertson, Mattingley, Rorden, & Driver, 1998), constraint induced therapy (Taub, 1999), and caloric stimulation (where cold water is irrigated contralesionally and warm water ipsilesionally into the external ear canal) (Rode, Perenin, Honore, & Boisson, 1998). However, these techniques are not yet common in occupational therapy and further research to support their effectiveness is required. For example, a recent randomised controlled trial by Machner, Konemund, Sprenger, von der Gablentz, & Helmchen, (2014) reported no additional benefits of eye patching and optokinetic stimulation over regular therapy in a sample of 21 individuals after stroke. It is also suggested that the use of verbal instructions should be minimised with individuals who experience neglect, and simple verbal instructions should be used to encourage the person to turn the head to the left to anchor his or her attention to that side of space (Herman, 1992).

Compensatory Approach

Initially, therapists educate individuals and carers about the condition, and then strategies to manage everyday activities are devised. For example, when reading a book or newspaper, a red ribbon may be placed on the left margin and the person is taught to scan back to this point after completing each line (Van Deusen, 1993). The environment may also be adapted to facilitate left turn-taking. Hospital staff can place the person's call button, telephone, and other essential items on the unaffected side so the person is able to easily use them. A mirror may be placed in front of the person while he or she is dressing or ambulating to draw attention to the neglected side.

Problems with Simple and Complex Perception

A Cochrane review investigated nonpharmacological interventions for perceptual disorders for people with acquired brain injuries (Bowen, Knapp, Gillespie, Nicolson, & Vail, 2011). They reported on six trials that included 338 participants who underwent a variety of interventions including sensory stimulation. However, there was no evidence to support the effectiveness of interventions provided. In the absence of evidence, therapists are advised to continue to provide a variety of neurorehabilitation interventions. Some of the intervention ideas used to address simple perceptual problems (the agnosias) are presented before techniques used with individuals who have complex perceptual problems (spatial-relations disorder). These ideas are not exhaustive, and a mixture of both remedial and compensatory techniques is suggested.

Visual Object Agnosia

Individuals are usually able to compensate for visual object agnosia automatically by using information from other senses such as touch, audition and smell to recognise the object.

Anosognosia

Anosognosia is not a particularly common condition and often resolves spontaneously in the first 3 months after stroke (Maeshima et al., 1997). However, until the condition resolves, it seriously hampers rehabilitation (Maeshima et al., 1997). It is extremely difficult to compensate for if the condition persists long-term. Safety is of paramount importance in intervention and discharge planning, because individuals typically do not acknowledge that they have a disability and will therefore refuse to take care during potentially dangerous daily occupations such as cooking, or even adjusting water temperature when showering (Sharpless, 1982).

Somatoagnosia

Using a remedial approach the therapist aims for the individual with somatoagnosia to associate sensory input with an adaptive motor response. Facilitation of body awareness is accomplished through sensory stimulation to the body part affected. For example, the individual can rub the affected body side with a rough cloth as the therapist names it or points to it (Fisher, Murray, & Bundy, 1991).

Right and Left Discrimination

If using a compensatory approach for people with right–left discrimination problems, the words *right* and *left* should be avoided. Instead, pointing or providing cues using distinguishing features of the limb are more effective (e.g. 'the arm with the watch'). These guidelines are particularly salient for the therapist teaching locomotion or transfers, where confusing instructions may have dangerous consequences. The right side of all common objects such as shoes and clothing can be marked with red tape or seam binding.

Figure–Ground Disorder

If using a remedial approach to address figure–ground disorder, the therapist can arrange for practice in visually locating objects in a simple array (such as three very different objects) and progress to more complex arrays (four or five dissimilar objects and three similar ones). If using a compensatory approach, the person can be taught to use other, intact senses (e.g. touch) when searching for items such as clothing or grooming items. When learning to lock a wheelchair, the person can be advised to locate the brake levers by touch rather than by searching for them visually. Brightly coloured tape can be used to mark the edges on stairs.

Form Discrimination

In a remedial approach, the person with form discrimination difficulties can practise describing, identifying, and demonstrating the use of similarly shaped and sized objects. The individual can sort like objects and should be assisted to focus on differentiating cues. When using a compensatory approach with individuals who can read, frequently used and confused objects can be labelled. The individual can be encouraged to use vision, touch, and self-verbalisation in combination when objects are confused.

Problems with Praxis

Therapists tend to use similar interventions whether the person has an ideomotor or ideational apraxia. A systematic review by Lindsten-McQueen et al. (2014) provides an excellent overview of the interventions available and the limited evidence to support these.

Remedial Approach

The therapist needs to speak slowly and provide one-step commands only. When teaching a new task, it should be broken down into its component parts. In one approach, the person is taught one component at a time, with the therapist physically guiding the person through the task if necessary. It should be completed in precisely the same manner each time. When all the individual units are mastered, an attempt to combine them should be made. A great deal of repetition may be necessary (Wall, 1982). Family members can be advised to use the same approach. An example of a young woman relearning how to drink from a cup using this technique is provided by Butler (1999). Using the sensorimotor approach, multiple sensory inputs are used on the affected body parts to enhance the production of appropriate motor responses. A Cochrane review investigated if therapy is effective to reduce ideomotor apraxia after stroke (West, Bowen, Hesketh, & Vail, 2008). Three trials with 132 participants were included, and a small, short-lived therapeutic effect was noted in two trials supporting change in ADL status. However, the change was not clinically significant and did not remain at long-term follow-up.

Compensatory Approach

A randomised controlled study by Donkervoort, Dekker, Stehmann-Saris, & Deelman, (2001) reported that occupational therapy 'strategy training' was an effective intervention with people who have apraxia. In strategy training, the individual is taught compensatory techniques to overcome the apraxia in ADLs such as the use of pictures in the correct sequence to support everyday occupations. Further trials have investigated if there is transfer of training techniques taught, with modest but promising results (Geusgens, van Heugten, Cooijmans, Jolles, & van den Heuvel, 2006, 2007).

In the third and final part of the practice story of Vivian and Jill, the interventions are described and the approach to documenting therapy outcomes are provided (Practice Story 41.3).

Intervention and Evaluation of Therapy Outcomes with Vivian

ACTION POINTS FROM THE CPPF

4. Agree on Objectives and Plan, 5. Implement the Plan, 6. Monitor and Modify, 7. Evaluate Outcome, 8. Conclude/Exit

Based on her problem list and the findings from administering the Canadian Occupational Performance Measure (COPM) (Law et al., 1998), Jill and Vivian began to set goals and map out intervention activities. Jill and Vivian set long-term goals in relation to performing ADLs (both personal and instrumental).

Initially, Jill found she needed to set quite simple goals such as getting dressed, because Vivian was not able to understand how the unilateral neglect affected her activities of daily living. Once Vivian became more involved and Jill was able to provide video feedback of her performance, Vivian became more insightful of the nature of her difficulties. As Vivian gained insight and understood that she would need to stay in rehabilitation for several weeks, Jill was able to work with Vivian to develop goals that were more closely related to her abilities.

Intervention Occupations. Vivian and Jill began to work on a variety of personal and domestic activities of daily living during therapy. Jill and Vivian also talked of her wish to visit her son and to be able to attend her weekly Spanish group. In this practice story, one intervention session has been written in detail to provide an idea of the kinds of techniques and strategies Jill used with Vivian.

RATIONALE: Selection of an Intervention Occupation. Jill and the medical rehabilitation consultant explained to Vivian that she could not drive when she returned home and that she would require a specialised driving assessment with an occupational therapist to determine whether she would be able to resume driving. This specialist assessment was scheduled for 6 months after her stroke so that Jill was aware of the process and to make it clear that she would have to arrange alternative transport in the meantime. The rehabilitation consultant told Jill that he expected Vivian's unilateral neglect would not resolve. Therefore although Vivian wanted to be able to use public transport in the short term, Jill was making sure that Vivian was as independent as possible so that she would be able to manage in the short term and long term as a public transport user. Jill also spoke to the son who lived with Vivian. Vivian's son explained that although he could help with shopping, he was not able to drive Vivian to her Spanish group, as he was at work at this time, and that it was better for Vivian to visit the residential care facility during the day rather than in the evenings, because her son in residential care was better able to cope with visitors during the day. Vivian and Jill planned to purchase a 6-month local ticket just before her discharge so that Vivian would only need to validate rather than purchase a ticket for each journey.

In addition to the fact that Vivian wanted to be a competent public transport user to access the community (visit her son and attend her Spanish group), Jill reasoned that Vivian would also need to be able to use public transport to shop. Jill also thought

that this was an ideal activity as it provided plenty of opportunity to determine how Vivian's unilateral neglect affected her performance and to develop strategies to overcome these problems. In addition to working on Vivian attending to both hemispaces, peripersonal spaces and both her body sides, this activity required many other cognitive and perceptual skills such as concentration (Vivian needed to sustain concentration when she was using public transport so that she was able to follow directions and knew when to alight the bus), executive function (planning, problem solving and judgement to determine the route and what to do when a bus did not arrive), memory (names of suburbs and addresses of where she needed to go), and complex perceptual skills (route finding and map use).

Therefore one long-term goal and one short-term objective documented by Jill in consultation with Vivian were as follows:

Long-Term Goal. For Vivian to be able to use the local public bus (to attend Spanish group, to shop and to visit her son in residential care).

Short-Term Objective.

WHO:	Vivian
GIVEN WHAT:	Precursor activity of bean bag toss game using left upper limb (this limb activation promotes attention to the left hemispace during this and subsequent activities (Robertson et al., 1994a), use of a perceptual anchor and red ribbon and all necessary equipment (street directory, bus maps and timetable, pen and pencil).
DOES WHAT:	Plans the buses to take and understands the timetables for taking public transport to visit her son.
HOW WELL:	Vivian will have prepared a written daily schedule of suitable buses and times to visit her son and be able to follow the route on a map. Before discharge, Jill and Vivian will try out these plans on a day outing.
BY WHEN:	The end of a 60-minute therapy session.

Information on the kinds of therapy activities that Jill and Vivian undertook during her 4-week stay are provided in Table 41.5. Included in this table are details about a home visit and a family meeting so that Vivian's sons had a chance to talk with Vivian and the whole team about her progress, discharge plans, the ongoing difficulties Vivian may experience, and supports that may assist her.

In addition, details of one therapy session are provided in Table 41.6 to demonstrate the kinds of strategies and grading processes that might be used with Vivian. In this table, the steps for the activity are detailed in the first column. The second column describes the problems that Vivian might have with this activity. The third column provides details of the interventions used to address Vivian's cognitive and perceptual difficulties at each step.

Continued on following page

PRACTICE STORY 41.3

Intervention and Evaluation of Therapy Outcomes with Vivian (Continued)

TABLE 41.5

Example of a 4-week Occupational Therapy Programme for Vivian; Jill Also Spent Time with Vivian Each Morning Working on Dressing and Grooming

Day	Week 1	Week 2	Week 3	Week 4
MON Session 1	Initial interview assessment	Instrumental ADL session Simple meal preparation (sandwich and cold drink)	Drawing session	Feedback with Vivian from home visit Practice skills related to any problems from home visit
MON Session 2	Visual Confrontation Test BIT assessment	Cooking activity with scanning (Vivian to choose a type of biscuit or scones with opportunity for spacing on the baking tray)	Money management session (role play shopping and check money handling) Preparation for outing to use public transport	Indoor lawn bowls and reassessment using Visual Confrontation Test
TUE Session 1	Breakfast time – Hypothesis testing making tea and toast	Newspaper reading Video recording of session with play-back to gain insight to neglect	Indoor lawn bowls Video recording of session with play-back to gain insight to neglect	Morning outing to test out use of public transport to visit her son (as developed in Table 41.6)
TUE Session 2	COPM and goal setting	Indoor lawn bowls Video-record and play back to increase Vivian's insight to her neglect	Variety of simple games such as balloon tennis, bean bag throwing, floor maze challenge	As earlier
WED Session 1	Scanning board game of Vivian's choice (e.g. Scrabble, Monopoly)	Bean bag toss activity (limb activation on left side as precursor activity for Session 2)	Instrumental ADL session Telephone use	Newspaper reading
WED Session 2	Drawing session (layout of equipment/attending to the whole drawing, such as a vase of flowers) (Fig. 41.3)	Planning to use public transport to visit her son (see detailed notes in practice story and Table 41.6)	Newspaper reading, and planning to use public transport to shop and go to Spanish group	Reassessment using COPM
THU Session 1	Indoor lawn bowls (also serves as a precursor activity for newspaper reading)	Drawing session (this is one of Vivian's hobbies and provides opportunity to attend to both halves of the page	Instrumental ADL session Main meal preparation	Family meeting with Vivian and her sons to plan discharge
THU Session 2	Newspaper reading Video-record and play back to increase Vivian's insight to her neglect	Variety of simple games such as balloon tennis, bean bag throwing, floor maze challenge to encourage left turn taking Video-recording of session with play-back to gain insight to neglect	Scanning board game of Vivian's choice (e.g. Scrabble, Monopoly)	Discharge planning session, including linking with follow-up outpatient services
FRI Session 1	Extension of goal-setting activity using video feedback to increase Vivian's insight	Drawing session	Home visit	Reassessment using BIT
FRI Session 2	Review of progress Video-recording of a game of memory cards and play-back to gain insight to neglect	Instrumental ADL session Main mean preparation, and eat this for evening meal	Home visit	Cake-baking activity to take a cake home on discharge

ADL, Activity of daily living; *BIT,* Behavioural Inattention Test; *COPM,* Canadian Outcome Performance Measure.

Intervention and Evaluation of Therapy Outcomes with Vivian (Continued)

TABLE 41.6

Outline of a Session to Enable Vivian to Use a Bus to Visit her Son: Activity Steps, Difficulties Vivian May Have, Strategies and Grading Used to Facilitate Performance (Focus on Unilateral Neglect), Using Remedial and Some Compensatory Strategies

Activity Steps (What Is To Be Done/Achieved)	Possible Problems the Person Will Have with this Step	Strategies or Grading to Overcome the Problem or Facilitate Performance
1. Precursor activity to stimulate left limb activation (Robertson et al., 1994a). Bean bag toss: Vivian throws the beanbags with her left arm onto a scoreboard on the floor (there are circles with points written inside, and the highest points are on the left of the board).	Vivian tries to throw with her right hand. Vivian misses throwing to the left of the board.	Offer verbal prompting to use left hand, and to throw to the higher scores on the left of the board. Place a wide red strip of card or ribbon on the left of the scoreboard on the floor and prompt Vivian to scan for this before throwing a bean bag. The use of this precursor activity (which stimulates motor circuits on the left) should also lead to improved performance in the main activity for the session, which is planning to use public transport. Upgrade and downgrade the activity during the whole session by manipulating variables related to the environment, the therapist and the task. Some examples have been provided next, although these are not exhaustive.
2. Plan the activity with Vivian and gather all the necessary equipment. Start by discussing the objective for the session: Vivian, given a precursor activity of bean bag toss game, use of a perceptual anchor and red ribbon and all necessary equipment, will plan the buses to take and the timetables for taking public transport to visit her son, so that Vivian will have prepared a written daily schedule of suitable buses and times to visit her son, and be able to follow the route on a map, by the end of the 60-minute therapy session.	Jill and Vivian have agreed on the objective for the session, so this should be a straightforward discussion on what the session will involve. Vivian may forget the objective is to plan transport to visit her son (e.g. another session will also need to plan transport to get to Spanish group). Vivian needs to gather relevant materials for the activity (street directory, bus maps and timetable, pen and pencil), and some of these are placed in the left side of the cupboard, or in a cupboard on the left side of the room, which she may not attend to. Additionally, she may forget to gather some of these items.	Provide verbal prompts to gather items and where they are located. Verbal prompts can be downgraded to provide Vivian with a written checklist of things she needs to gather for the activity or the goal and steps of the activity. Because Vivian may have difficulty locating cupboards on the left, or items in the left side of the cupboard, Jill can assist by guiding Vivian to the relevant cupboards and then prompting Vivian to scan for all edges of the cupboard before locating the equipment. The activity can be downgraded by Jill gathering all the items for Vivian or by placing the items in cupboards on the right side of the room and the middle or right side of the cupboard.
3. Use the street directory and find Vivian's street and house and the street and the residential care facility where her son lives. Make a colour photocopy of this page of the map. Vivian's home is on the right side of the double map page, and the residential facility is on the far left.	Vivian may have difficulty locating the index pages on the left side to find her street and the residential care facility. Vivian may forget the grid reference for her street and the residential care facility.	Perceptual 'anchoring' can be used, and Vivian can place her left arm at edge of the page and be prompted to scan across to her arm at each step. This can be used when finding the street names in the index and also when finding the streets on the actual map.

Continued on following page

PRACTICE STORY 41.3

Intervention and Evaluation of Therapy Outcomes with Vivian (Continued)

TABLE 41.6
Outline of a Session to Enable Vivian to Use a Bus to Visit her Son: Activity Steps, Difficulties Vivian May Have, Strategies and Grading Used to Facilitate Performance (Focus on Unilateral Neglect), Using Remedial and Some Compensatory Strategies (Continued)

Activity Steps (What Is To Be Done/Achieved)	Possible Problems the Person Will Have with this Step	Strategies or Grading to Overcome the Problem or Facilitate Performance
		Verbally prompt Vivian to write the grid reference for the maps she needs. Use a highlighter pen to mark her house (street) and the residential care facility (and street). If Vivian is managing well, walk down to the administration office of the facility and make a colour copy of the map. Downgrade: Jill to have a copy that she made earlier ready for use.
4. Use the notes on the street directory to determine which bus line and number operates in the area. Trace the bus route onto a photocopy of the street directory. The bus leaves from the end of Vivian's street, and there is a bus stop at the entrance to the residential care facility. Do activity seated at table with all equipment (map, ruler, highlighter pen, bus timetable, pen and paper).	Vivian may have difficulty locating the residential care facility on the left of the map, and the bus numbers. Vivian may have difficulty with tracing from her home (on the right) towards the residential care facility (on the left of the map).	Jill to sit at the table on Vivian's left side. Provide verbal prompts to locate the bus symbols and bus numbers in blue on the map. As earlier, use perceptual anchor to the left of the street directory map. Prompt Vivian to place her left index finger on the care facility, and she can trace towards this when highlighting the route with a pen. Downgrade by adding red ribbon to the left margin of the page if needed.
5. Look up the bus number in the Bus Timetable booklet and decide on the bus times that best suit Vivian's routine and suitable visiting times at the residential care facility.	The bus timetable book is quite small and therefore is quite central in Vivian's spatial field. However, Vivian may have some difficulty in scanning the columns and locating the right bus and reading the times.	Verbally prompt Vivian to locate the left side of the schedule and use her left hand as a perceptual anchor to hold the book open, then place a clear ruler over the page and hold with left hand, and use right finger to point to relevant bus times. Vivian to identify suitable times, and Jill to write these down (days, departure times and arrival times). Upgrade by asking Vivian to look up the schedule and record the details on paper. Downgrade by having another preprepared bus timetable with the relevant bus and times highlighted.
7. Vivian can practice tracing out the bus route on the map using her finger. Identify landmarks that will be on the right (library, park and large house with two palm trees at the entrance) and left (police station, three shops together, post box and house with the high green fence) of the bus on the journey. Plan a strategy to prompt looking to the left.	Vivian may have difficulty tracing her finger over the map all the way to the residential care facility. It may be difficult for Vivian to identify landmarks on the left of the bus and then recognise when she arrives at the residential facility, which will also be on the left of the bus. When she returns home, her home will be on the right of the bus, so she should not have difficulty with this.	Place left arm as a perceptual anchor and verbally prompt Vivian to scan to her arm as she traces with her right index finger along the bus route. Verbally prompt Vivian to look to the residential care facility as marked on the map as she commences the task. Downgrade by placing the map on a cork board and sticking coloured pins at the site of her home and the residential care facility.

PRACTICE STORY 41.3

Intervention and Evaluation of Therapy Outcomes with Vivian (Continued)

	TABLE 41.6	
	Outline of a Session to Enable Vivian to Use a Bus to Visit her Son: Activity Steps, Difficulties Vivian May Have, Strategies and Grading Used to Facilitate Performance (Focus on Unilateral Neglect), Using Remedial and Some Compensatory Strategies (Continued)	
Activity Steps (What Is To Be Done/Achieved)	**Possible Problems the Person Will Have** with this Step	**Strategies or Grading to Overcome the** Problem or Facilitate Performance
8. Evaluate the session by reviewing if the objective has been met. Plan for the outing in the final week to test out using the bus.		If Vivian is able to monitor the progress of the bus as they drive, then she will be able to practise 'Look Left' and search specifically for the landmarks she has identified with Jill. Downgrade: If Vivian is unable to locate the residential care facility on the left side, she will need to ask the bus driver to tell her they are at the residential care facility bus stop. Downgrade. If Vivian is unable to catch the bus independently, arrange for half-price taxi voucher so that Vivian has an alternative means of transport.

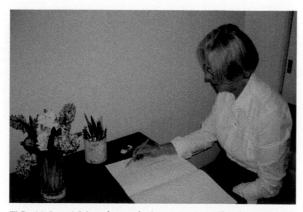

FIG. 41.3 ■ Vivian draws during a session. The therapist will ask Vivian to place her left arm on the left edge of the page to serve as a perceptual anchor.

The final stage of the intervention process is to evaluate outcomes with the individual and determine what the individual would like and benefit from follow-up services such as outpatient therapy or community links. Jill evaluated the outcome of each session with Vivian. For example, after the first bus route finding session, Jill and Vivian concluded that although Vivian had successfully completed the task (thus meeting the objective), they would repeat this session in a few days to refine Vivian's skills and continue to work on attending to the left hemispace. Although insight was initially a problem, as Vivian progressed, her insight into her problems increased. However, as Vivian became more aware of her problems, she also became more depressed.

Jill also evaluated the programme at the time of Vivian's discharge by talking with Vivian, her sons and other therapy colleagues to determine whether they thought Vivian had improved and documenting whether generalisation of skills learned in occupational therapy had transferred to other aspects of Vivian's life. In addition, Jill readministered the standardised assessments used on Vivian's admission (the BIT and COPM) and nonstandardised assessments (interview, Extinction Test and Visual Confrontation Test) to document improvements made. Finally, Jill examined the long-term goals she had set with Vivian and determined which had been met.

Vivian wanted to continue some outpatient therapy at the centre and Jill supported an outpatient programme of two visits per week for a month with a review and possible extension of this. With Vivian's approval, Jill also arranged for Vivian to receive home help from the local council to assist with cleaning, and a half-price taxi voucher so that Vivian would have access to affordable taxi transport in the evenings or if she chose not to use the bus.

ADL, Activity of daily living; *CPPF,* Canadian Practice Process Framework.

COMMUNITY INTEGRATION: THE ULTIMATE GOAL OF COGNITIVE AND PERCEPTUAL REHABILITATION

Occupational therapists work with individuals to improve cognitive and perceptual function so that people can return to their community and lead fulfilling lives through occupational engagement. Therefore therapists are increasingly focused on community integration as the ultimate outcome of rehabilitation in this field (Doig, Fleming, & Tooth, 2001; Kim & Colantonio, 2010; Willer, Rosenthal, Kreutzer, Gordon, & Rempel, 1993; Williams, Rapport, Millis, & Hanks, 2014). Community integration may be defined as the following:

- Comprising assimilation, or being able to fit in with other people, knowing the environment and being accepted (McColl et al., 1998, 2001)
- Occupation that includes meaningful and productive activity to be involved in as well as having things to do for fun (McColl et al., 1998, 2001; Willer et al., 1993)
- Independent living, including making everyday decisions and life choices (McColl et al., 1998, 2001)
- Having social support, or being part of a network of family, friends and acquaintances (McColl et al., 1998, 2001; Willer et al., 1993)

Increasingly, community integration is seen as the best outcome measure of rehabilitation for people, particularly after head injury. However, a great deal more research is required to examine whether people with cognitive and perceptual impairments manage their home and community living activities, and whether they are satisfied with their lives and their ability to engage in these activities (Kim & Colantonio, 2010; Willer et al., 1993). Specifically, research is required to identify and measure the types of community integration difficulties people face and factors that predict community integration. The findings of such studies will assist occupational therapists to develop interventions that will promote long-term community integration.

CONCLUSION

Occupational therapists work with individuals to improve cognitive and perceptual capacities so they can engage in the occupations they want or need to do and thus lead fulfilling lives as part of the community. This chapter provided an overview of a range of cognitive and perceptual problems, the kinds of diseases or accidents that can lead to such problems, theories that guide an occupational therapist when working with individuals who experience problems in this area, ways therapists can evaluate these problems and, finally, the kinds of evidence-based interventions that can be used to assist individuals overcome these problems. The chapter has been illustrated with the detailed practice story of Vivian. This practice story outlines aspects of therapy undertaken by the occupational therapist and provides the reader with clear guidelines for the use of the Canadian Practice Process

Framework (Townsend & Polatajko, 2013) to structure therapy. The chapter also provides extensive references and resources so the reader can pursue excellence in practice when working with people who have cognitive and perceptual problems.

 http://evolve.elsevier.com/Curtin/OT

REFERENCES

Abreu, B. C. (1990). *The quadraphonic approach: Management of cognitive and postural dysfunction.* New York: Therapeutic Service Systems.

Abreu, B. C. (1999). Evaluation and intervention with memory and learning impairment. In C. A. Unsworth (Ed.), *Cognitive and perceptual dysfunction: a clinical reasoning approach to evaluation and intervention* (pp. 163–208). Philadelphia: FA Davis.

Anastasi, A. (1988). *Psychological testing* (6th ed.). New York: Macmillan.

Árnadóttir, G. (1990). *The brain and behavior: Assessing cortical dysfunction through activities of daily living.* St Louis: Mosby.

Atkinson, R. C., & Shiffrin, R. M. (1968). Human memory: A proposed system and its control processes. In K. W. Spence & J. T. Spence (Eds.), *The psychology of learning and motivation (Volume 2)* (pp. 89–195). New York: Academic Press.

Australian Institute of Health and Welfare. (2003). *ICF Australian user guide. Version 1.* Canberra: Australian Institute of Health and Welfare.

Australian Institute of Health and Welfare. (2008). *Australian hospital statistics 2006-7. Health Services Series no. 31, Cat. N. HSE55.* Canberra: Australian Institute of Health and Welfare.

Australian Institute of Health and Welfare. (2012). *Australia's health, 2012.* Canberra: Australian Institute of Health and Welfare.

Averbuch, S., & Katz, N. (1992). Cognitive rehabilitation: A retraining approach for brain-injured adults. In N. Katz (Ed.), *Cognitive rehabilitation: Models for intervention in occupational therapy* (pp. 219–239). Boston: Andover Medical.

Bauer, R. M., & Rubens, A. B. (1993). Agnosia. In K. M. Heilman. & E. Valenstein (Eds.), Clinical neuropsychology (3rd ed., pp. 215–278). Oxford, UK: Oxford University Press.

Baum, C. M., Connor, L. T., Morrison, T., Hahn, M., Dromerick, A. W., & Edwards, D. F. (2008). Reliability, validity, and clinical utility of the Executive Function Performance Test: A measure of executive function in a sample of people with stroke. *American Journal of Occupational Therapy, 62,* 445–455.

Bowen, A., Hazelton, C., Pollock, A., & Lincoln, N. B. (2013). Cognitive rehabilitation for spatial neglect following stroke. *Cochrane Database of Systematic Reviews, 7.*

Bowen, A., Knapp, P., Gillespie, D., Nicolson, D. J., & Vail, A. (2011). Non-pharmacological interventions for perceptual disorders following stroke and other adult-acquired, non-progressive brain injury. *Cochrane Database of Systematic Reviews, 4.*

Bradshaw, J. L., & Mattingley, J. B. (1995). *Clinical neuropsychology: Behavioral and brain science.* San Diego: Academic Press.

Butler, J. (1999). Evaluation and intervention with apraxia. In C. A. Unsworth (Ed.), *Cognitive and perceptual dysfunction: A clinical reasoning approach to evaluation and intervention* (pp. 257–297). Philadelphia: FA Davis.

Butterworth, P., Anstey, K., & Jorm, A. F. (2004). A community survey demonstrated cohort differences in lifetime prevalence of self-reported head injury. *Journal of Clinical Epidemiology, 57*, 742–748.

Cicerone, K. D. (1996). Attention deficits and dual task demands after mild traumatic brain injury. *Brain Injury, 10*, 79–89.

College of Occupational Therapists. (2004). *Guidance on the use of the International Classification of Functioning, Disability and Health (ICF) and the Ottawa Charter for Health Promotion in occupational therapy services.* London: College of Occupational Therapists.

Cook, D. M. (2005). *Occupational Therapy – Adult Perceptual Screening Test (OT-APST).* Brisbane: Function for Life.

Couillet, J., Soury, S., Lebornec, G., et al. (2010). Rehabilitation of divided attention after severe traumatic brain injury: A randomized trial. *Neuropsychological Rehabilitation, 20*(3), 321–339.

Croce, R. (1993). A review of the neural basis of apractic disorders with implications for remediation. *Adapted Physical Activity Quarterly, 10*(173), 1993.

das Nair, R., & Lincoln, N. B. (2007). Cognitive rehabilitation for memory deficits following stroke. *Cochrane Database of Systematic Reviews, 3*, CD002293.

Davis, A., Davis, S., Moss, N., et al. (1992). First steps towards an interdisciplinary approach to rehabilitation. *Clinical Rehabilitation, 6*, 237–244.

de Clive-Lowe, S. (1996). Outcome measurement, cost-effectiveness and clinical audit: The importance of standardised assessment to occupational therapists in meeting these new demands. *British Journal of Occupational Therapy, 59*, 357–362.

Diller, L., & Weinberg, J. (1972). Differential aspects of attention in brain-damaged persons. *Perceptual and Motor Skills, 35*, 71–80.

Doig, E., Fleming, J., & Tooth, L. (2001). Patterns of community integration 2-5 years post-discharge from brain injury rehabilitation. *Brain Injury, 15*, 747–762.

Donkervoort, M., Dekker, J., Stehmann-Saris, F. C., & Deelman, B. G. (2001). Efficacy of strategy training in left hemisphere stroke patients with apraxia: A randomized clinical trial. *Neuropsychological Rehabilitation, 11*, 549–566.

Doornheim, K., & De Haan, E. H. F. (1998). Cognitive training for memory deficits in stroke patients. *Neuropsychological Rehabilitation, 8*, 393.

Duran, L., & Fisher, A. G. (1999). Evaluation and intervention with executive functions impairment. In C. A. Unsworth (Ed.), *Cognitive and perceptual dysfunction: A Clinical reasoning approach to evaluation and intervention* (pp. 209–254). Philadelphia: FA Davis.

Ellis, A. W., & Young, A. W. (1988). *Human cognitive neuropsychology.* Hillsdale, NJ: Lawrence Erlbaum Associates.

Eskes, G. A., Butler, B., McDonald, A., Harrison, E. R., & Phillips, S. J. (2003). Limb activation effects in hemispatial neglect. *Archives of Physical Medicine and Rehabilitation, 84*, 323–328.

Fasotti, L., Kovacs, F., Eling, P. A., & Brouwer, W. H. (2000). Time pressure management as a compensatory strategy training after closed head injury. *Neuropsychological Rehabilitation, 10*, 47–65.

Fisher, A. G. (1997a). An expanded rehabilitative model of practice. In A. G. Fisher (Ed.), *Assessment of motor and process skills* (2nd ed., pp. 73–85). Fort Collins, CO: Three Star Press.

Fisher, A. G. (1997b). *Assessment of motor and process skills* (2nd ed.). Fort Collins, CO: Three Star Press.

Fisher, A. G., Murray, E. A., & Bundy, A. C. (1991). *Sensory integration: Theory and practice.* Philadelphia: FA Davis.

Friedman, R. B., Ween, J. E., & Albert, M. L. (1993). Alexia. In K. M. Heilman, & E. Valenstein (Eds.), *Clinical neuropsychology* (3rd ed., pp. 37–62). Oxford, UK: Oxford University Press.

Gainotti, G., D'Erme, P., & Bartolomeo, P. (1991). Early orientation of attention toward the half space ipsilateral to the lesion in patients with unilateral brain damage. *Journal of Neurology, Neurosurgery and Psychiatry, 54*, 1082–1089.

Geusgens, C., van Heugten, C., Cooijmans, J. P. J., Jolles, J., & van den Heuvel, W. (2007). Transfer effects of a cognitive strategy training for stroke patients with apraxia. *Journal of Clinical and Experimental Neuropsychology, 29*(8), 831–841.

Geusgens, C., van Heugten, C., Donkervoort, M., van den Ende, E., Jolles, J., & van den Heuvel, W. (2006). Transfer of training effects in stroke patients with apraxia: An exploratory study. *Neuropsychological Rehabilitation, 16*(2), 213–229.

Gialanella, B., Monguzzi, V., Santoro, R., & Rocchi, S. (2005). Functional recovery after hemiplegia in patients with neglect: The rehabilitative role of anosognosia. *Stroke, 36*, 2687–2690.

Giles, G. M., & Wilson, J. C. (1992). *Occupational therapy for the brain injured adult: A neurofunctional approach.* London: Chapman and Hall.

Grieve, J. (1993). *Neuropsychology for occupational therapists: Assessment of perception and cognition.* Oxford, UK: Blackwell Scientific Publications.

Guide for the Uniform Data Set for Medical Rehabilitation (Adult FIM SM). (1999). Version 5.0. Buffalo: State University of New York at Buffalo.

Hackett, M. L., & Pickles, K. (2014). Part 1: Frequency of depression after stroke: An updated systematic review and meta-analysis of observational studies. *International Journal on Stroke, 9*(8), 1017–1025.

Halligan, P. W., & Marshall, J. C. (1993). The history and clinical presentation of neglect. In I. H. Robertson & J. C. Marshall (Eds.), *Unilateral neglect: Clinical and experimental studies* (pp. 3–25). Hove: Lawrence Erlbaum Associates Ltd.

Hartman-Maeir, A., Harel, H., & Katz, N. (2009). Kettle test-a brief measure of cognitive functional performance. Reliability and validity in stroke rehabilitation. *American Journal of Occupational Therapy, 63*(5), 592–599.

Herman, E. W. M. (1992). Spatial neglect: New issues and their implications for occupational therapy practice. *American Journal of Occupational Therapy, 46*, 207–212.

Hewitt, J., Evans, J. J., & Dritschel, B. (2006). Theory driven rehabilitation of executive function: Improving planning skills in people with traumatic brain injury through the use of an autobiographical episodic memory cueing procedure. *Neuropsychologia, 44*(8), 1468–1474.

Hobson, S. (1996). Reflections on being client-centred when the client is cognitively impaired. *Canadian Journal of Occupational Therapy, 63*(2), 133–137.

Holmqvist, K., Ivarsson, A., & Holmefur, M. (2014). Occupational therapist practice patterns in relation to clients with cognitive impairment following acquired brain injury. *Brain Injury, 28*(11), 1365–1373.

Honda, T. (1999). Rehabilitation of executive function impairment after stroke. *Topics in Stroke Rehabilitation*, 6, 15–22.

Itzkovich, M., Elazar, B., Averbuch, S., & Katz, N. (1990). *The Loewenstein Occupational Therapy Assessment (LOTCA)*. Pequannock, NJ: Maddak.

Jacquin-Courtois, S., Rode, G., Pavani, F., et al.(2010). Effect of prism adaptation on left dichotic listening deficit in neglect patients: Glasses to hear better? *Brain*, 133(3), 895–909.

Karnath, H. O., Christ, K., & Hartje, W. (1993). Decrease of contralesional neglect by neck muscle vibration and spatial orientation of trunk midline. *Brain*, 116, 383–396.

Kaschel, R., Della Sala, S., Cantagallo, A., Fahlbock, A., Laaksonen, R., & Kazen, M. (2002). Imagery mnemonics for the rehabilitation of memory: A randomised group controlled trial. *Neuropsychological Rehabilitation*, 12, 127–153.

Katz, N. (Ed.), (2011). *Cognition and occupation and participation across the lifespan* (3rd ed.). Bethesda, MD: American Association of Occupational Therapy.

Keane, S., Turner, C., Sherrington, C., & Beard, J. R. (2006). Use of Fresnel Prism glasses to treat stroke patients with hemispatial neglect. *Archives of Physical Medicine and Rehabilitation*, 87, 1668–1672.

Kim, H., & Colantonio, A. (2010). Effectiveness of rehabilitation in enhancing community integration after acute traumatic brain injury: A systematic review. *American Journal of Occupational Therapy*, 64, 709–719.

Kielhofner, G. (2008). *A model of human occupation: Theory and application* (4th ed.). Baltimore: Williams & Wilkins.

Kiernan, R. J., Mueller, J., Langston, J. W., & Van Dyke, C. (1987). The Neurobehavioral Cognitive Status Examination: A brief but differentiated approach to cognitive assessment. *Annals of Internal Medicine*, 107, 481–485.

Kirshner, H. (1991). The apraxias. In W. Bradley, R. Daroff, G. Fenichel, & C. Marsden (Eds.), *Neurology in clinical practice: Principles of diagnosis and management: Vol. 1*. London: Butterworth-Heinmann.

Lannin, N. A., Carr, B., Allaous, J., Mackenzie, B., Falcon, A., & Tate, R. (2014). A randomized controlled trial of the effectiveness of handheld computers for improving everyday memory functioning in patients with memory impairments after acquired brain injury. *Clinical Rehabilitation*, 28(5), 470–481.

Laver, A. J., & Powell, G. E. (1995). *The Structured Observational Test of Function (SOTOF)*. Windsor, England: NFER–NELSON.

Law, M., Baptiste, S., Carswell, A., McColl, M., Polatajko, H., & Pollock, N. (1998). *The Canadian Occupational Performance Measure* (3rd ed.). Toronto: Canadian Association of Occupational Therapy.

Lezak, M. D. (1995). *Neuropsychological assessment* (3rd ed.). New York: Oxford University Press.

Lindsten-McQueen, K., Williamson Weiner, N., Wang, H.-Y., Josman, N., & Tabor Connor, L. (2014). Systematic review of apraxia treatments to improve occupational performance outcomes. *OTJR Occupation, Participation and Health*, 34(4), 183–192.

Loetscher, T., & Lincoln, N. B. (2013). Cognitive rehabilitation for attention deficits following stroke. *Cochrane Database of Systematic Reviews*, 5.

Luaute, J., Halligan, P., Rode, G., Rossetti, Y., & Boisson, D. (2006). Visuo-spatial neglect: A systematic review of current interventions and their effectiveness. *Neuroscience and Behavioral Reviews*, 30(7). 961-862.

Machner, B., Konemund, I., Sprenger, A., von der Gablentz, J., & Helmchen, C. (2014). Randomized controlled trial on hemifield eye patching and optokinetic stimulation in acute spatial neglect. *Stroke*, 45, 2465–2468.

Maeshima, S., Dohi, N., Funahashi, K., Nakai, K., Itakura, T., & Komai, N. (1997). Rehabilitation of patients with anosognosia for hemiplegia due to intracerebral haemorrhage. *Brain Injury*, 11, 691–706.

Mateer, C. A., Kerns, K. A., & Eso, K. L. (1996). Management of attention and memory disorders following traumatic brain injury. *Journal of Learning Disabilities*, 29, 618–632.

Mayer, N. H., Reed, E., Schwartz, M. F., Montgomery, C., & Palmer, C. (1990). Buttering a hot cup of coffee: An approach to the study of errors of action in patients with brain damage. In D. E. Tupper & K. D. Cicerone (Eds.), *The neuropsychology of everyday life: Assessment and basic competencies* (pp. 94–295). London: Kluwer.

McColl, M. A., Carlson, P., Johnston, J., et al.(1998). The definition of community integration: Perspectives of people with brain injuries. *Brain Injury*, 12, 15–30.

McColl, M. A., Davies, D., Carlson, P., Johnston, J., & Minnes, P. (2001). The community integration measure: Development and preliminary validation. *Archives of Physical Medicine and Rehabilitation*, 82, 429–434.

Mozaz, M., Marti, J., Carrera, E., & de la Puente, E. (1990). Apraxia in a patient with lesion located in right sub-cortical area: Analysis of errors. *Cortex*, 26, 651–655.

Nasreddine, Z. S., Phillips, N. A., Bédirian, V. , et al.(2005). The Montreal Cognitive Assessment, MoCA: A brief screening tool for mild cognitive impairment. *Journal of the American Geriatrics Society*, 53, 695–699.

Ownsworth, T. L., & McFarland, K. (1999). Memory remediation in long-term acquired brain injury: Two approaches in diary training. *Brain Injury*, 13, 605–626.

Ponsford, J. (2004). *Cognitive and behavioral rehabilitation*. New York: The Guilford Press.

Ponsford, J., Sloan, S., & Snow, P. (2012). *Traumatic brain injury: Rehabilitation for everyday adaptive living* (2nd ed.). Hove: Lawrence Erlbaum.

Raade, A. S., Gonzalez Rothi, L. J., & Heilman, K. M. (1991). The relationship between buccofacial and limb apraxia. *Brain and Cognition*, 16, 130–146.

Rafal, R. (1994). Neglect. *Current Opinion in Neurobiology*, 4, 321–326.

Robertson, I. H., Mattingley, J. B., Rorden, C., & Driver, J. (1998). Phasic alerting of neglect patients overcomes their spatial deficits in visual awareness. *Nature*, 395, 169–172.

Robertson, I. H., Tegnér, R., Goodrich, S. J., & Wilson, C. (1994a). Walking trajectory and hand movements in unilateral left neglect: A vestibular hypothesis. *Neuropsychologia*, 32, 1495–1502.

Robertson, I., Ward, T., Ridgeway, Y., & Nimmo-Smith, I. (1994b). *The test of everyday attention*. Bury St Edwards: Thames Valley Test Co.

Robertson, L. C., & Eglin, M. (1993). Attentional search in unilateral visual neglect. In I. H. Robertson & J. C. Marshall (Eds.), *Unilateral neglect: Clinical and experimental studies* (pp. 169–192). Hove: Lawrence Erlbaum Associates.

Rode, G., Perenin, M. T., Honore, J., & Boisson, D. (1998). Improvements of the motor deficit of neglect patients through vestibular stimulation: Evidence for a motor neglect component. *Cortex, 34,* 253–261.

Roth, M., Tym, E., Mountjoy, C. Q., et al. (1986). CAMDEX. A standardised instrument for the diagnosis of mental disorder in the elderly with special reference to the early detection of dementia. *British Journal of Psychiatry, 149,* 698–709.

Rustad, R. A. (1993). *The Cognitive Assessment of Minnesota.* San Antonio, TX: Therapy Skill Builders.

Schmidt, R. A. (1988). *Motor control and learning: A behavioral emphasis* (2nd ed.). Champaign, IL: Human Kinetics.

Sharpless, J. W. (1982). *Mossman's a problem oriented approach to stroke rehabilitation* (2nd ed.). Springfield, IL: Charles C Thomas.

Sohlberg, M. M., McLaughlin, K. A., Pavese, A., Heidrich, A., & Posner, M. I. (2000). Evaluation of attention process training and brain injury education in persons with acquired brain injury. *Journal of Clinical Experimental Neuropsychology, 22,* 656–676.

Tsang, M. H. M., Sze, K. H., & Fong, K. N. K. (2009). Occupational therapy treatment with right half-field eye-patching for patients with subacute stroke and unilateral neglect: A randomized controlled trial. *Disability and Rehabilitation, 31*(8), 630–637.

Tate, R., & McDonald, S. (1995). What is apraxia? The clinician's dilemma. *Neuropsychological Rehabilitation, 5,* 273–297.

Taub, E. (1999). New discovery equals change in clinical practice. *Journal of Rehabilitation Research Development, 36,* vii–viii.

Toglia, J. P. (1992). A dynamic interactional approach to cognitive retraining. In N. Katz (Ed.), *Cognitive rehabilitation: Models for intervention in occupational therapy* (pp. 104–143). Boston: Andover Medical Publishers.

Townsend, E. A., & Polatajko, H. J. (2013). *Enabling occupation II: Advancing an occupational therapy vision for health, well-being, and justice through occupation* (2nd ed.). Ottawa: Canadian Association of Occupational Therapists.

Unsworth, C. A. (1999). *Cognitive and perceptual dysfunction: A clinical reasoning approach to evaluation and intervention.* Philadelphia: FA Davis.

Unsworth, C. A. (2004). How therapists think: Exploring therapists' reasoning when working with patients who have cognitive and perceptual problems following stroke. In G. Gillen, & A. Burkhardt (Eds.), *Stroke rehabilitation: A function-based approach* (2nd ed., pp. 358–375). St. Louis: Mosby.

Unsworth, C. A. (2005). Measuring outcomes using the Australian Therapy Outcome Measures for Occupational Therapy (AusTOMs-OT): Data description and tool sensitivity. *British Journal of Occupational Therapy, 68*(8), 354–366.

Unsworth, C. A., & Duncombe, D. (2014). *AusTOMs for occupational therapy* (3rd ed.). Melbourne: La Trobe University.

Vallar, G. (1993). The anatomical basis of spatial hemineglect in humans. In I. H. Robertson & J. C. Marshall (Eds.), *Unilateral neglect: Clinical and experimental studies* (pp. 27–59). Hove: Lawrence Erlbaum Associates.

Van Deusen, J. (1993). *Body image and perceptual dysfunction in adults.* Philadelphia: Saunders.

van Zomeren, A. H., & Brouwer, W. H. (1994). *The clinical neuropsychology of attention.* New York: Oxford University Press.

Wall, N. (1982). Stroke rehabilitation. In M. K. Logigian (Ed.), *Adult rehabilitation: A team approach for therapists* (pp. 225–240). Boston: Little Brown.

Ware, J. E., & Sherbourne, C. D. (1992). The MOS 36 item short-form health survey (SF36): Conceptual framework and item selection. *Medical Care, 30,* 473–483.

West, C., Bowen, A., Hesketh, A., & Vail, A. (2008). Interventions for motor apraxia following stroke. *Cochrane Database of Systematic Reviews, 1.*

Whiting, S., Lincoln, N., Bhavnani, G., & Cockburn, J. (1985). *RPAB-Rivermead Perceptual Assessment Battery.* Windsor, England: NFER-NELSON.

Willer, B., Rosenthal, M., Kreutzer, J., Gordon, W., & Rempel, R. (1993). Assessment of community integration following rehabilitation for TBI. *Journal of Head Trauma Rehabilitation, 8,* 11–23.

Williams, M. W., Rapport, L. J., Millis, S. R., & Hanks, R. A. (2014). Psychosocial outcomes after traumatic brain injury: Life satisfaction, community integration and distress. *Rehabilitation Psychology, 59*(3), 298–305.

Wilson, B., Alderman, N., Burgess, P., Emslie, H., & Evans, S. S. (1996). *Behavioural assessment of dysexecutive syndrome.* Bury St Edmunds: Thames Valley Test Company.

Wilson, B., Cockburn, J., & Halligan, P. W. (1987). *Behavioural Inattention Test.* Bury St Edmunds: Thames Valley Test Company.

Wilson, B., Greenfield, E., Clare, L., et al.(2008). *The Rivermead Behavioural Memory Test (RBMT-3)* (3rd ed.). Bury St Edmunds: Thames Valley Test Company.

Winegardner, J. (1993). Executive functions. In H. Cohen (Ed.), *Neuroscience for rehabilitation* (pp. 346–353). Philadelphia: Lippincott.

Wolf, T.J., Barbee, A.R., & White, D. (2011). Executive dysfunction immediately after mild stroke. *OTJR Occupation, Participation and Health, 31*(S1), S23–S29.

Wood-Dauphinee, S. L., Opzoomer, M. A., Williams, J. L., Marchand, B., & Spitzer, W. O. (1988). Assessment of global function: The Reintegration to Normal Living Index. *Archives of Physical Medicine and Rehabilitation, 69,* 583–590.

World Health Organization. (2001). *International Classification of Functioning, Disability, and Health.* Geneva: World Health Organization.

Zinn, S., Bosworth, H. B., Hoenig, H. M., & Swartzwelder, S. (2007). Executive function deficits after stroke. *Archives of Physical Medicine and Rehabilitation, 88,* 173–180.

42

COGNITIVE ORIENTATION TO DAILY OCCUPATIONAL PERFORMANCE

HELENE J. POLATAJKO ■ SARA E. MCEWEN
DEIRDRE R. DAWSON ■ ELIZABETH R. SKIDMORE

Abstract
CO-OP, which stands for Cognitive Orientation to daily Occupational Performance and is now formally referred to as the CO-OP Approach, is a performance-based, problem-solving intervention that has the use of a global problem-solving strategy at its core. Rather than focusing on problems related to performance components, CO-OP helps individuals to develop cognitive strategies to solve occupational performance problems. This chapter describes how cognitive strategies can improve occupational performance by providing an overview of cognitive strategy use, a description of the CO-OP Approach, and illustrations of cognitive strategy use with practice stories. Finally, the chapter provides a summary of evidence that supports cognitive strategy use with adults who have experienced cerebrovascular or traumatic brain injury, as well as lessons learned from several studies.

KEY POINTS

- CO-OP Approach is:
  - an occupation-based intervention that directly works on improving occupational performance;
  - embedded in a learning paradigm and is focused on performance, NOT performance components;
  - a task-oriented approach that enables occupational performance through a process of dynamic performance analysis and guided discovery;
  - an approach that uses cognitive strategies to change performance;
  - an evidence-based approach;
  - an approach that was first introduced for use with children with motor-based performance problems; and
  - now used with a number of populations including adults who have experienced a cerebrovascular accident or traumatic brain injury.
- Numerous peer-reviewed publications investigating CO-OP Approach with adults who have experienced a cerebrovascular accident or traumatic brain injury suggest that this approach improves performance on trained and untrained self-selected goals and may also positively influence participation in these populations.

INTRODUCTION

CO-OP, which stands for Cognitive Orientation to daily Occupational Performance and is now formally referred to as the CO-OP Approach, is a performance-based, problem-solving intervention that has the use of a global problem-solving strategy at its core. Drawing on knowledge from cognitive science and human movement science, the CO-OP Approach guides people in the discovery of strategies that are specific to their individual occupational performance needs. Rather than focusing on problems related to performance components, CO-OP stimulates individuals to develop cognitive strategies to solve occupational performance problems. Emerging evidence demonstrates that this approach leads to better occupational performance, as well as improved motor and cognitive performance.

Occupational performance is understood to result from the interaction of person, environment and occupation. Although interventions can address performance issues by enabling a change in the person, the environment or the occupation, traditionally the primary focus of occupational therapy has been to change the person (Townsend & Polatajko, 2013). The underlying idea was that the most effective way to change a person's occupational performance was to address the physical, cognitive or affective problems related to performance issues (Polatajko et al., 2013). Although such impairment-focused therapies may have led to improvements in the specific impairments targeted, they did not lead to changes in meaningful occupations, inspiring the continued search for effective alternatives.

Over the last two decades, across a number of rehabilitation professions, task-specific training has emerged as an attractive alternative to impairment-focused therapy (Chua, Ng, Yap, & Bok, 2007; French et al., 2008; Hubbard, Parsons, Neilson, & Carey, 2009). Task-specific training uses repetitive practice of the targeted task, such as catching a ball, dressing an effected limb or using a walker, with specific techniques to improve motor learning (such as mnemonics, incremental increases in difficulty, backward chaining). These approaches have been found to have better outcomes compared with impairment reduction techniques. However, improvement does not generally transfer to other tasks or occupations. For example, improvement in dressing the upper body has not necessarily lead to improvements in using a knife and fork during eating. A growing body of evidence suggests that these limitations can be overcome by adding global cognitive strategy training to a task-specific approach (Dawson et al., 2009; Dawson, Binns, Hunt, Lemsky, & Polatajko, 2013b; Geusgens, Winkens, van Heugten, Jolles, & van den Heuvel, 2007; Liu, Chan, Lee, & Hui-Chan, 2004; McEwen, Polatajko, Huijbregts, & Ryan, 2010, McEwen et al., 2015b; Skidmore et al., 2015). Much of this evidence is drawn from the CO-OP Approach.

There is mounting evidence that the CO-OP Approach not only supports performance during therapy but also, more importantly, enables people to generalise what is learned in therapy to their own environments and transfer to learning to other occupations. Notably, evidence is also building to indicate the approach has effects at the level of impairment, in some cases reducing component motor and cognitive impairment even in individuals who have entered the chronic phase of their illness, injury or impairment. The purpose of this chapter is to draw on the findings from research investigating the CO-OP Approach to describe how cognitive strategies can improve occupational performance. The chapter begins with an overview of cognitive strategy use, followed by a description of the CO-OP Approach. Next, use of the CO-OP Approach with adults with neurological impairments is presented and illustrated with two practice stories. Finally, the evidence to support its use with adults who have experienced a cerebrovascular accident (CVA) or traumatic brain injury (TBI) and lessons learned conclude the chapter.

COGNITIVE STRATEGY USE: AN OVERVIEW

Cognitive strategies are conscious, goal-directed plans of action (Toglia, Rodger, & Polatajko, 2012). Effective goal-directed behaviour tends to rely on higher-level cognitive functions (Luria, 1966). For the purposes of CO-OP, Polatajko and Mandich (2004) identified two types of cognitive strategies: global and domain specific.

Global cognitive strategies, also referred to as executive or metacognitive strategies, are evaluative or regulatory in nature and include processes to make decisions about which actions to take or which domain-specific strategies to use if a goal has not been reached. Global cognitive strategies make use of executive cognitive functions, those 'integrative cognitive processes that determine goal-directed and purposeful behaviour and are superordinate in the orderly execution of daily life functions ... includ[ing]: the ability to formulate goals; to initiate behaviour; to anticipate the consequences of actions; to plan and organise behaviour according to spatial, temporal, topical or logical sequences; and to monitor and adapt behaviour to fit a particular task or context' (Cicerone et al., 2000, p. 1605).

In the last 10 years, considerable research has been directed at understanding the various components of these high-level functions, which are largely mediated by systems and networks involving the frontal lobes. Cicerone, Levin, Malec, Stuss, & Whyte, (2006) describe four broad areas of executive or 'frontal' functions:

1. Executive cognitive functions that are control functions involved in planning, monitoring, switching and inhibiting subordinate cognitive functions.
2. Behavioural self-regulation that is involved in controlling emotional and behavioural responses in order to produce a more adaptive response.
3. Activation or energising behaviours that allow people to persist in working towards a goal.
4. Metacognitive processes that are thought to further link the first three functions.

Metacognition refers to a person thinking about how he or she is thinking in the context of being self-aware and being able to evaluate these thoughts. For example, when planning a complex activity such as a summer vacation not only does a person think about what needs to be done (choose dates, choose a destination, etc.) but also about organising and sequencing plans to attain the goal (e.g. need to know if accommodation is available on specific dates before booking air travel), forming intentions about when things need to be done (e.g. awareness of the date by which balance must be paid in full and making a plan to execute payment before that date), making decisions about potential behaviour changes if a specific outcome cannot be achieved (e.g. travel partner is not responding to emails about potential destinations, therefore make a decision to try communication by telephone) and making conscious changes to plans (e.g. preferred destination is not available during current vacation dates, so make arrangements to switch vacation dates or look at other destinations). Clearly, metacognition is necessary for problem solving and goal attainment.

Research into metacognitive strategy training became prevalent in the 1970s particularly in education and psychology. Donald Meichenbaum (1977, 1991), a prominent psychologist considered a founder of cognitive behavioural modification therapy, adopted the rubric *goal, plan, do, and check*, introduced by Bash and Camp (1986), as part of his approach to using a problem-solving strategy to support behavioural change. This paved the way for occupational therapists and researchers to begin to use this and similar rubrics as a 'cognitive scaffold' to address executive difficulties among people with neurological problems. Table 42.1 shows a sample of various problem-solving rubrics used in different global problem-solving approaches.

In contrast to global strategies, domain-specific strategies are generated to solve specific problems that occur while working through a particular occupational performance problem (Mandich, Polatajko, Missiuna, & Miller, 2001). Toglia, Rodger, & Polatajko, (2012) refer to domain-specific strategies as 'mind tools' and developed a classification system that places them in three broad groupings: modality-specific strategies (sensory cues or prompts provided by the person themselves), mental or self-verbalisation strategies, and task modification strategies (modifying or adapting the task or environment). As described by Mandich et al. (2001), CO-OP uses both a global strategy and domain-specific strategies.

THE CO-OP APPROACH

The CO-OP Approach is 'a client-centred, performance-based, problem solving, approach that enables skill acquisition through

---

*Although the term *person-centred* is the preferred term for this book, the term *client-centred* is used in this chapter when referring to a key feature of the CO-OP Approach.

TABLE 42.1

Examples of Global Strategies Used in a Variety of Strategy Training Approaches

Authors	Global Strategy
Bash & Camp (1986) Adopted by Meichenbaum (1991); by Polatajko et al. (2001)	GPDC: Goal; Plan; Do; Check
Lawson & Rice (1989)	WSTC: What should I be doing?; Select a strategy; Try the strategy; Check the strategy
van Heugten, Dekker, Deelman, Stehmann-Saris, & Kinebanian, (1998)	Initiation; Execution; Controlling
Ylvisaker, Feeney, & Szekeres, (1998)	Goal; Plan; Predict; Do; Review
von Cramon, Matthes-von Cramon, & Mai, 1991	Problem-Solving Therapy (PST): Orient to problem; Define problem; Generate alternatives; Make a decision; Do it; Verify the solution
Levine et al. (2000)	Stop; Define; List; Learn; Do; Check
Levine et al. (2011)	Stop; Be in the present; State; Split; Check

a process of strategy use and guided discovery' (Polatajko & Mandich, 2004, p. 2). The approach is designed to achieve four goals: skill acquisition, cognitive strategy use, skill and strategy generalisation, and skill and strategy transfer. It comprises seven key features: client-centred*, occupation-based goal setting; dynamic performance analysis; cognitive strategy use; guided discovery; enabling principles; significant other involvement; and intervention format. In this section, an overview of the CO-OP Approach's development is provided, followed by a detailed description of the seven key features.

Development

The CO-OP Approach was developed in response to an identified need for a new approach for helping children diagnosed with developmental coordination disorder (DCD) meet occupational performance goals. Previously, the majority of intervention approaches were impairment focused, derived from a neurodevelopmental perspective on motor performance. Polatajko et al., (2001) decided to adopt a learning paradigm – to consider skilled motor performance as the outcome of skill learning rather than neuromotor development. An intervention was created that was modelled after the Meichenbaum's cognitive behaviour modification approach where, as mentioned earlier, children were taught to use verbal self-guidance for problem solving with a *global* cognitive strategy, GOAL-PLAN-DO-CHECK, to learn new skills.

Meichenbaum's approach was adapted to fit within an occupation-based, client-centred framework and augmented by principles taken from motor learning. The approach focused on the acquisition of client-chosen occupational goals through a collaborative process of using the GOAL-PLAN-DO-CHECK global strategy to solve performance problems. The role of the therapist was to guide the child to test out potential strategies to improve performance, evaluate the results and ultimately acquire the desired skill.

Original investigations of the approach, then called Verbal Self-guidance (VSG), indicated that the approach did indeed support motor skill acquisition through a process of cognitive strategy use and therapist verbal guidance and verbal self-guidance (Polatajko et al., 2001). The approach was called VSG to emphasise the importance of verbal guidance to the approach; however, careful analysis of videotapes of VSG intervention sessions revealed that cognitive strategy use was essential to the approach. Hence, the name was changed to Cognitive Orientation to daily Occupational Performance (CO-OP).

From the videotaped analysis it also became clear that during the sessions the children used not only the global cognitive strategy GOAL-PLAN-DO-CHECK but also a number of domain-specific strategies (Mandich et al., 2001). These domain-specific strategies, derived from a process of dynamic performance analysis and guided discovery, were found to be specific to the child and the task. In addition, as skill performance improved, specific strategies were used less and less and then not at all once the skill was well established. In contrast, children learned and continued to use the global strategy over time within the same task and across different tasks.

Subsequent studies have continued to provide evidence of the effectiveness of cognitive strategies, identified through a client-centred problem-solving approach, in supporting skill acquisition. Studies now reveal that the CO-OP Approach is not only effective with children with DCD but can also be used with adult populations, including individuals with neurological impairments that result from CVA or TBI (Scammels, Bates, Houldin, & Polatajko, 2016).

The CO-OP Approach: The Seven Key Features

As originally described by Polatajko et al. (2001), CO-OP Approach comprises seven key features: client-chosen goals, dynamic performance analysis, cognitive strategy use, guided discovery, enabling principles, parent or significant other involvement and intervention format. In 2011 an international invitational meeting of CO-OP Approach scholars was held to consider, among other things, the essential elements of the approach. In particular, the scholars examined the relevance of the original seven key features. Based on current evidence and the collective experience with administering and teaching others to administer the approach, they determined that the seven key features should be maintained but their relevance should be

further specified. Accordingly, the original seven key features were specified as either essential or structural elements. Essential elements are key features that must be present for the intervention to be considered CO-OP Approach. Structural elements are key features that are preferred or suggested elements but may be altered to meet the specific needs of the person or practice setting. An overview of the refined key features, now divided into essential and structural elements, is presented in Table 42.2.

In the CO-OP Approach, through these key features, the cognitive, affective and physical components of performance are addressed simultaneously, as are the occupational and environmental contributions to performance. *Goals* must be identified through collaboration with the person and must address occupation-based needs identified by the person. The Canadian Occupational Performance Measure (Law et al., 2014) is used to support the identification of priority occupational performance issues to be addressed using CO-OP. After identification of these issues, *dynamic performance analysis (DPA)* is used to investigate current performance. DPA is an active, iterative process through which therapists and those receiving therapy services examine person, occupation and environmental aspects to identify performance breakdowns (Polatajko, Mandich, & Martini, 2000). DPA typically occurs while observing performance.

TABLE 42.2

The CO-OP Approach Seven Key Features – the Essential and Structural Elements

Seven Key Features Essential Elements	Critical Attributes
Occupation-focused Goals	Collaborative, client-centred, occupation-based
Dynamic Performance Analysis (DPA)	Active, iterative process, evoked initially by therapist; becomes a collaborative process with both therapist and client; in many cases, client eventually conducts DPA spontaneously and independently
Cognitive Strategy Use	Global (metacognitive) or domain specific
Guided Discovery	Optimises client's role in learning
Enabling Principles	Promotes learning, generalisation, transfer

Structural Elements	Variable Attributes
Parent or Significant Other Involvement	May be critical for children; may or may not be necessary for adults, depending on the client
Intervention Format	May vary in session sequence, format, length, frequency, duration or materials needed

Cognition is explicitly brought into play in the CO-OP Approach through the key feature *cognitive strategy use*. The CO-OP Approach global strategy, GOAL-PLAN-DO-CHECK, provides the cognitive scaffold for performance and is applicable to all goals. It is a metacognitive strategy as it provides a mechanism for a person to think about his or her thinking. It also provides a structure for self-monitoring with CHECK, a built-in evaluation of performance. The complementary domain-specific strategies support task-specific performance. Domain-specific strategies are sometimes but not always transferable across tasks. For example, developing a domain-specific strategy of using a timer for cooking may be transferable to using a timer for remembering to move the washing to the dryer or leave in time to make an appointment. On the other hand, a domain-specific strategy of using a specialised cutting board for one-handed cutting during meal preparation is specific to this task and is therefore less likely to be useful with another goal.

Guided discovery is the method of instruction in the CO-OP Approach. It supports self-discovery by the person, as he or she is guided to 'discover' solutions to performance problems with guidance from the therapist. The person's self-discovery ensures that cognition is used; the therapist's guidance ensures the person does not become overly frustrated with repeated unsuccessful performance attempts using the same ineffective strategy.

Supporting the guided discovery process are the *enabling principles*. This key feature comprises a group of instructional and feedback methods designed to optimise learning, generalisation and transfer of skills.

Two of the key features, *significant other involvement* and *intervention format*, are considered structural rather than essential elements; that is, they are considered important to the CO-OP Approach but are modifiable based on the needs of the person, practice setting and other factors. *Significant other involvement* is recommended so that important people in the person's life are aware of the approach, know the global cognitive strategy, GOAL-PLAN-DO-CHECK, and can enable generalisation and transfer of achievements in therapy to the person's real-world environment. Although the setting and number of sessions can vary based on the person's needs, the *intervention format* should include a preintervention assessment phase, an intervention phase with homework, and a postintervention assessment phase.

In terms of pre- and postintervention, typically subjective and objective measures are used. The Canadian Occupational Performance Measure (Law et al., 2014) is used to measure the person's own judgement of their pre- and postintervention performance and satisfaction with performance of the targeted tasks. The Performance Quality Rating Scale (PQRS; Martini, Rios, Polatajko, Wolf, & McEwen, 2015) is a reliable and responsive tool to be used by the therapist to evaluate pre- and postintervention performance of client-selected goals objectively. The PQRS is a 10-point scale, designed for use in the CO-OP Approach, to rate performance quality of the targeted tasks, with 1 indicating that the activity is not done at all and 10 indicating that the activity is done very well.

THE CO-OP APPROACH AND ADULTS WITH NEUROLOGICAL IMPAIRMENTS

As mentioned earlier, CO-OP Approach was originally designed for use with children with DCD as an alternative to traditional neurodevelopmental approaches that lacked evidence of efficacy. Around the same time, researchers working with other populations, including adults with neurological impairments, were also seeking to replace impairment-focused neurodevelopmental techniques. Evidence emerged to support the use of task-specific training (see e.g. French et al., 2008). However, over time it became apparent that although these approaches were associated with improvements in the activities trained, they were not followed by long-term change in the performance of the trained tasks, and transfer to other activities did not occur.

Although task-specific training clearly had promise, additional intervention components were needed to optimise outcomes. Early testing of CO-OP, which combines cognitive strategy use with task-specific training, demonstrated that it can help adults with neurological injury improve their performance in client-chosen tasks (Dawson et al., 2009; Henshaw, Polatajko, McEwen, Ryan, & Baum, 2011; McEwen, Polatajko, Huijbregts, & Ryan, 2009). In addition, this approach appeared to promote longer-term change in performance. Importantly, once people had learned the method, they seemed to be able to apply it to improve their performance in other tasks (McEwen et al., 2010, 2015b; Skidmore et al., 2014, 2015). The use of CO-OP Approach to improve occupational performance of two people who have experienced neurological impairment as a result of CVA or head injury is illustrated through Practice Stories 42.1 and 42.2.

Evidence for the CO-OP Approach with Individuals with Neurological Injuries

Combined, the evidence to date suggests that for individuals who have experienced CVA or TBI, the CO-OP Approach can be expected to improve performance on trained self-selected goals and have transfer effects for improved performance on untrained self-selected goals. The CO-OP Approach may also yield improvements in selected impairments and behaviours, as well as positively influence participation. At present, there are several additional clinical trials examining the use of the CO-OP Approach, or some derivation, for improving outcomes after CVA and TBI (e.g. Dawson et al., 2013a; McEwen et al., 2015a). These trials should be monitored for additional evidence regarding the expected outcomes for CO-OP Approach after CVA and TBI.

Impact on Occupational Performance Goals

The primary expected outcome of the CO-OP Approach is improvement in occupational performance. Evidence from several studies with people who have experienced CVA or TBI provides support for this expected outcome. Evidence from

Addressing Occupational Performance Issues after CVA – Ms Fine

Ms Fine was a 56-year-old teacher, living with her husband, who experienced a right middle cerebral artery cerebrovascular accident (CVA). This resulted in moderate hemiparesis of her left arm and leg, sensory loss throughout her left side, and issues with initiation, planning and spatial perceptual judgement. Ms Fine spent 1 week in an acute care hospital and was then transferred to an inpatient rehabilitation programme. Her occupational therapist, Genevieve, conducted an extensive assessment that began with a goal-setting interview.

During this interview, Ms Fine discussed her valued occupations with Genevieve and reflected on the occupations she most wanted to work on during her rehabilitation. She decided that her priority occupational performance issues were difficulty getting around with the wheelchair (including transfers), reading books and eating 'properly'. Together Ms Fine and Genevieve identified four goals: (1) that she would be able to transfer from the bed to the wheelchair and back again; (2) that she be able to propel the wheelchair to the door of her bathroom; (3) that she would be able to hold a book with two hands; and (4) that she would be able to cut and eat food 'properly' (which she defined as neatly and with a knife and fork).

As a starting point for intervention Genevieve then conducted an analysis of Ms Fine's pre-intervention performance of her identified goals. She asked Ms Fine to demonstrate transferring to the bed from the wheelchair, propelling her wheelchair, holding and reading a book, and cutting food and eating. During these demonstrations, Genevieve ensured Ms Fine was safe but did not provide any verbal or physical assistance to help her complete the tasks. Genevieve used the Performance Quality Rating Scale (PQRS) to evaluate initial performance in these tasks. Ms Fine scored a 2/10 on wheelchair transfer, 4/10 on wheelchair propulsion, 5/10 on holding and reading a book and 2/10 on using both hands to cut and eat food.

While observing Ms Fine perform these activities, Genevieve carried out a dynamic performance analysis. She noticed that while Ms Fine had motor limitations, this was not the only problem limiting her ability to perform the tasks. Ms Fine also did not seem to know all the steps in the activities or mixed up the sequence of the steps. For example, while attempting to perform a transfer from bed to wheelchair, she started to try to get up before ensuring the wheelchair was located beside the bed and before having moved herself forwards into a position to best facilitate standing up. As a result, her performance of the task broke down at several steps.

After the baseline assessment, Genevieve taught Ms Fine the global cognitive strategy GOAL-PLAN-DO-CHECK. Ms Fine's specific GOAL was to be able to transfer from her bed to her wheelchair and back again, safely and without physical assistance. Over the next two intervention sessions, Genevieve guided her to discover a PLAN. Through multiple small

experiments carrying out potential plans (PLAN, DO and CHECK), Ms Fine solved multiple problems related to a good angle for the wheelchair to be positioned beside the bed and the best height of the bed to facilitate standing up and discovered that standing up was easier if her heels were a little bit behind her knees. Learning through discovery took more time than it would have taken for Genevieve to simply tell Ms Fine what to do. However, this would not have optimally engaged Ms Fine in the problem-solving process. That is, it would not have drawn on her cognitive skills, and it may not have resulted in domain-specific strategies that worked particular well for her.

In this specific situation, Genevieve found that the GOAL-PLAN-DO-CHECK process took longer than it generally does when she works with people who have had a CVA. This was because initially Ms Fine seemed to have difficulty responding to open-ended questions. For example, when Genevieve said, 'Where do you think the wheelchair should be positioned to make the transfer easier?' Ms Fine did not respond. Eventually Ms Fine replied that she did not know.

To avoid frustrating Ms Fine, Genevieve switched to a closed form of questioning. While still encouraging her to think through the problem, Genevieve provided Ms Fine with options to try in solving the problems presented in each step of the task. For example, at the step of positioning the wheelchair Genevieve asked, 'Do you think it would be easier to transfer if the wheelchair was directly in front of you, or angled at the side of the bed?' 'Should we put it on the left or the right?' 'Once you are standing up, will it be easier to turn to the left or the right?' By the end of the third session, Ms Fine was problem solving more, responding to open-ended questions and engaging in discussions with Genevieve about possible strategies. Through this process, Ms Fine discovered a strategy that helped her to remember the sequence of steps 'chair, feet, up', and her PQRS score for transferring became a 7/10.

As she was now feeling very confident in her abilities, she added a new goal of propelling her wheelchair to the dining room to eat her meals. She and Genevieve worked on this together and accomplished the goal in a single session. After 3 weeks on the inpatient rehabilitation unit, Ms Fine had accomplished her goals with PQRS scores of 10/10, except for eating with a knife and fork, for which she scored a 6/10. She had added additional goals during her stay, including a tub transfer, a car transfer, dressing and walking to the toilet independently with her four-point cane.

Genevieve encouraged Ms Fine to apply the process to new challenges she would meet at home. Once she was home, these activities included unloading the dishwasher, folding laundry and taking her dog out on a leash. She was able to confidently apply the global cognitive strategy GOAL-PLAN-DO-CHECK to learn these activities to her satisfaction.

Addressing Occupational Performance Issues After Traumatic Brain Injury – Ms Role

Ms Role sustained a severe traumatic brain injury (TBI) in a motor vehicle crash at age 28, emerged from a coma after 9 days and then spent about 2 months on an inpatient rehabilitation unit. On discharge home she received community-based therapy (occupational therapy, physiotherapy, speech therapy) for 9 months. More than 20 years later, at age 50, she enrolled in a research study on the CO-OP Approach. She had never been competitively employed since her TBI but did participate in several hours of community volunteer work each month.

Because of the length of time since her injury, details about her immediate postinjury impairments were not available. Her research pretest, administered by a trained research assistant, included a test that allowed her premorbid IQ to be estimated to have been in the superior range. During this assessment she complained of mood difficulties, pain (headaches) and fatigue, noting that the latter interfered with her day-to-day activities more than half the time. In addition, she complained of significant difficulties with organisation, memory and distraction.

Further assessments (Table 42.3), also carried out for research purposes, suggested that Ms Role was mildly to moderately depressed and moderately anxious. In terms of executive functioning, she scored in the impaired range on a standardised measure (the Behaviour Rating Inventory of Executive Function – Adult Version (Roth, Isquith, & Gioia, 2005)). At pretest she also indicated on the Mayo-Portland Adaptability Inventory Participation Index (www.tbims.org/combi/) that her ability to participate in leisure and social activities was substantially limited.

A research occupational therapist administered the Canadian Occupational Performance Measure (Law et al., 2014), during which Ms Role identified five areas of difficulties. From these difficulties, related goals that she wanted to address during her therapy were identified. As per the research protocol (Dawson et al., 2013b), she was able to select one of these to address during therapy: the other four were randomised such that two were addressed in therapy and two remained untrained (Table 42.4).

The therapist, Mary, identified baseline performance on the three trained goals through conversation, as observation was not possible. Once Mary felt she had a good understanding of the situation she began the process of guiding Ms Role to develop plans that would facilitate her goal attainment.

TABLE 42.3
Pre-test, Post-test and Follow-up Scores for Ms Role

Executive Function Measure	Pre-test Score	Post-test Score	Follow-up Score
Depression: PHQ-9 (lower better)	9	4	10
Anxiety: GAD-7 (lower better)	12	8	14
DKEFS Letter Fluency (higher better) (scaled score)	9	12	11
DKEFS Tower Test – first move time (scaled score)	9	14	14
BRIEF-A (t-score) (lower better)	77	68	77
MPAI Participation Index (lower better)	16	10	14

BRIEF-A, Behaviour Rating Inventory of Executive Function – Adult Version; DKEFS, Delis-Kaplan Executive Function System; GAD-7, Generalised Anxiety Disorder 7-item Questionnaire; MPAI, Mayo-Portland Adaptability Inventory; PHQ-9, Patient Health Questionnaire.

TABLE 42.4
COPM Scores

COPM–PERFORMANCE	Pre-test score	Post-test score	Follow-up score
To get funding to pay for online course	4	9	10
To stick to budget while grocery shopping	1	10	7
To organise finances using a specific software program	1	6	8
To plan menus and cook meals (untrained)	6	8	10
To organise day in order to manage fatigue (untrained)	1	8	8

COPM–SATISFACTION	Pre-test score	Post-test score	Follow-up score
To get funding to pay for online course	1	9	10
To stick to budget while grocery shopping	1	10	9
To organise finances using a specific software program	1	6	5
To plan menus and cook meals (untrained)	5	6	10
To organise day in order to manage fatigue (untrained)	1	6	8

Addressing Occupational Performance Issues After Traumatic Brain Injury – Ms Role *(Continued)*

Mary found the first several sessions with Ms Role particularly difficult, as Ms Role would move from topic to topic in conversation very quickly. Mary shared this observation with Ms Role, stating, 'I'm getting quite confused during our sessions – I lose track of what is happening. Is that something you are experiencing?' Ms Role immediately confirmed that she was also having this experience and so a plan was generated that when either of them started to feel confused they would stop the session and ask themselves what goal they were working on. This plan worked well and was used throughout the intervention.

As per the research protocol, Mary provided Ms Role with goal sheets in a binder. These sheets included columns for plans, the desired outcome for the plan, whether the plan was executed and whether the plan worked. For example, in working on the goal of organising her finances using a commercial software program, Ms Role made a plan to watch the instructional video so that she could learn how to synchronise her bank account with the program. Part of her plan included the domain-specific strategy of paying attention to her fatigue level and stopping to rest as needed through the activity.

Ms Role watched the video but was not able to synchronise her bank account with the program. In analysing her performance with Mary, she realised that she had not set enough time aside to fully understand the video and then do the synchronisation. Her next plan was to take more time. She did this but was still not able to accomplish the synchronisation. She then made a plan to call the help line. She used the domain-specific strategy of writing relevant information (e.g., account number) on Post-It notes and putting these on the computer screen. In this way, she was ultimately able to accomplish her goal.

As shown in Tables 42.3 and 42.4, Ms Role received considerable benefit from the CO-OP Approach intervention. Her performance and satisfaction with performance improved substantially on all of her goals (trained and untrained) and her gains were maintained 3 months after the invention was finished. These findings suggest that Ms Role had learned strategy use and was transferring it to new situations. This is considered far transfer – that is, transfer of learning to a context and task that is different from where the original learning occurred (Barnett & Ceci, 2002).

---

12 single-case experimental design participants (Dawson et al., 2009; McEwen et al. 2009, 2010; Ng, Polatajko, Marziali, Hunt, & Dawson, 2013), three single-case studies (Henshaw et al., 2011; Skidmore et al., 2011), and five pilot randomised controlled trials (Dawson et al., 2013b; McEwen et al., 2015b; Polatajko, McEwen, Ryan, & Baum, 2012; Poulin, Korner-Bitensky, Bherer, Lussier, & Dawson, 2016; Skidmore et al., 2015) suggests that the CO-OP Approach leads to improvement in performance in self-selected goals.

Furthermore, CO-OP intervention has been associated with larger improvements in the objectively rated PQRS scores compared with usual care occupational therapy, with one study demonstrating a medium effect of between-group differences immediately after treatment and a large effect on between-group differences 3 months later (McEwen et al., 2015b). These data provide convincing evidence that CO-OP intervention is associated with improved performance in self-selected goals.

Perhaps more important is the evidence that addresses some of the transfer effects of the CO-OP Approach. These transfer effects have been demonstrated in performance improvements on untrained goals, as measured by the self- and significant other–reported Canadian Occupational Performance Measure (COPM) and the observer-rated PQRS (Dawson et al., 2009, 2013b; McEwen et al., 2010, 2015b; Ng, Polatajko, Marziali, Hunt, & Dawson, 2013; Poulin et al., 2016). Of note, transfer effects have also been noted in measures of impairments and behaviours that were not the direct target of CO-OP Approach intervention. For

example, two separate pilot randomised controlled trials demonstrated significantly greater improvements in measures of executive functions compared with an attention control condition in acute CVA (Skidmore et al., 2015) and compared with usual care in subacute CVA (Wolf, et al., 2016). Additional evidence suggests that CO-OP intervention has an effect on self-efficacy (McEwen et al., 2015b; Poulin et al., 2016) and sustained goal-directed behaviour (i.e. low levels of apathy symptoms) (Skidmore et al., 2014).

Impact on Participation

Perhaps the best measure of the overall impact of a CVA and TBI rehabilitation intervention is the effect of the intervention on participation. Evidence from pilot randomised controlled trials suggests that CO-OP intervention is associated with a moderate effect on participation, as measured by the Stroke Impact Scale and the Community Participation Index, compared with usual care (McEwen et al., 2015b) and with improvements on the Mayo Portland Adaptability Inventory Participation Index (Dawson et al., 2013b).

Impact on Impairment

Recent evidence suggests that metacognitive strategy training, based heavily on the CO-OP Approach, is feasible to administer during acute inpatient rehabilitation (Skidmore et al., 2011, 2014) and is associated with significantly greater reductions in disability (measured with the Functional Independence

Measure) and improvement in executive cognitive functions (measured with selected indices of the Delis Kaplan Executive Functioning System) among adults with cognitive impairments after acute CVA (Skidmore et al., 2015). A separate research group found similar results for people in the subacute phase after a CVA (Wolf et al., 2016). Further, Wolf and colleagues reported a moderate effect of CO-OP compared with contemporary therapy on arm and hand capacity using the Action Research Arm Test. These changes came after an average of 12 45-minute intervention sessions, about 9 hours of treatment.

LESSONS LEARNED FROM THE CO-OP APPROACH: USE WITH CEREBROVASCULAR ACCIDENT AND TRAUMATIC BRAIN INJURY

From the experience of using the CO-OP Approach with individuals after CVA or TBI a number of important lessons were learned regarding whether a person might benefit from the CO-OP Approach, session structure and strategy specifics.

Who Will Benefit from the CO-OP Approach?

To benefit from the use of CO-OP, the person must have occupational performance goals and sufficient language ability to participate in the GOAL-PLAN-DO-CHECK process, which includes problem-solving discussions with the therapist.

In terms of physical or cognitive capacity, nature of the injury or length of time since the injury, boundaries are still being tested. The CO-OP Approach or a very similar strategy training approach has been used successfully with people as early as 3 days after a neurological event and as long as decades later. CO-OP Approach has been used with people with very limited motor recovery, including people with Chedoke-McMaster Stroke Assessment Impairment Inventory (Miller, et al., 2008) scores as low as 2/7 for arm, hand and foot (indicating spasticity present but no voluntary movement) and 3/7 for leg (indicating marked spasticity present and voluntary movement only within synergistic patterns). It has been used with people with moderate cognitive impairment, scoring as low as 21 on the Montreal Cognitive Assessment (Nasreddine, et al., 2005), and with people with moderate to severe executive function impairments after TBI (Dawson et al., 2009). Although these scores describe minimum levels of physical and cognitive function of previous CO-OP Approach participants, the minimum physical and cognitive capabilities required to benefit from the CO-OP Approach have not yet been established. However, it is likely that insight into, or awareness of, deficits is not necessarily a prerequisite, as the focus on occupation in combination with a problem solving strategy may lead to an awareness of, performance problems and the identification of effective strategies to solve the problems. Thus if a person has occupational goals and wishes to try a cognitive strategy-based approach, then implementing CO-OP Approach may be a possibility.

Facilitating Goal Setting

In the original CO-OP Approach format with children, a daily activity log and the Canadian Occupational Performance Measure (COPM) were used to facilitate goal setting. With adults with neurological injuries, it is recommended that, if time permits, they complete the daily activity log over a week, to provide a fuller idea of the activities in which they are engaged. Other methods to help with the identification of valued occupations before administering the COPM that might be considered include the Activity Card Sort (Baum & Edwards, 2008) and the elucidation module of Personal Projects Analysis (Egan, Scott-Lowery, De Serres Larose, Gallant, & Jaillet, 2016; Little, 2011).

Evaluating Performance Before and After Intervention

Many people living with the effects of neurological injury, particularly those who have lived with the effects of the injury for longer periods, have complex participation goals, such as planning a wedding or obtaining a job interview. For these goals, it may not be possible to administer the PQRS as part of the baseline assessment, as the related activities stretch out over time and over environments. In these cases, the person's self-report of performance and satisfaction with performance using the COPM is relied upon for preintervention and postintervention evaluation. If an additional perspective on the person's performance is desired or required, it is sometimes possible to also ask a significant other to rate the person's performance using, for example, the COPM.

Significant Other Involvement

The involvement of significant others in the CO-OP Approach is a structural key feature. It is recommended that they attend the first few sessions so that they have an understanding of GOAL-PLAN-DO-CHECK and the process within which it is used. This involvement is believed to be an important facilitator of generalisation and transfer. However, with adults, it may be difficult for family members to attend sessions and should not be considered as a prerequisite for the person's participation.

Intervention Format

The CO-OP Approach key feature *intervention format* is considered a structural feature rather than an essential element. All iterations of the CO-OP Approach should include a preintervention assessment phase, an intervention phase, which includes teaching the global cognitive strategy in the first session and using it in subsequent sessions, and homework, and a postintervention assessment phase. The specific details of each of these phases can vary depending on the characteristics of the population, the setting and the individual's needs. Some of the alterations from the classic intervention format described in 2004 (Polatajko & Mandich, 2004) include using scripts and presentations to teach the global cognitive strategy and maintaining flexibility regarding the number of intervention sessions.

Adults with neurological injuries are far from a homogeneous group in terms of type or severity of their impairments. Those with more severe impairments may require more than the originally suggested 10 intervention sessions. Adults with subacute CVA have required, on average, about 12 sessions (McEwen et al., 2015b). Adults with TBI with identified executive dysfunction have been trialed with both 20 and 15 sessions, with 15 sessions seeming to work for most. Some people with relatively minor impairments and relatively intact cognition may require only 5 or 6 sessions.

CONCLUSION

Since 2009, numerous peer-reviewed publications investigating CO-OP Approach with adults with CVA and TBI have suggested that CO-OP Approach improves performance on trained and untrained self-selected goals and may also positively influence participation in these populations. Using CO-OP Approach with adults with neurological injuries requires that therapists focus on occupational performance rather than occupational performance components during assessment and treatment, that they embrace client-centred, occupation-based goal setting, and that they give up a degree of control to people receiving their services by using guided discovery as the instructional method and enabling people to self-discover their own strategies. Although implementing CO-OP Approach may at first present some challenges, occupational therapists can expect to be rewarded by long-term significant improvements in the occupational performance of people who are receiving their services.

 http://evolve.elsevier.com/Curtin/OT

REFERENCES

Barnett, S. M., & Ceci, S. J. (2002). When and where do we apply what we learn? A taxonomy for far transfer. *Psychological Bulletin, 128*(4), 612–637.

Bash, M. A., & Camp, B. W. (1986). Training teachers in the think aloud classroom program. In G. Cartledge & J. F. Milburn (Eds.), *Teaching social skills to children: Innovative approaches* (2nd ed.). New York, NY: Pergamon Press.

Baum, C., & Edwards, D. F. (2008). *The activity card sort* (2nd ed.). Bethesda, MD: American Association of Occupational Therapy.

Chua, K. S., Ng, Y. S., Yap, S. G., & Bok, C. W. (2007). A brief review of traumatic brain injury rehabilitation. *Annals of the Academy of Medicine, Singapore, 36*(1), 31–42.

Cicerone, K. D., Dahlberg, C., Kalmar, K., Langenbahn, D. M., Malec, J. F., Bergquist, T. F., … Morse, P. A. (2000). Evidence-based cognitive rehabilitation: Recommendations for clinical practice. *Archives of Physical Medicine and Rehabilitation, 81*(12), 1596–1615.

Cicerone, K., Levin, H., Malec, J., Stuss, D., & Whyte, J. (2006). Cognitive rehabilitation interventions for executive function: Moving from bench to bedside in patients with traumatic brain injury. *Journal of Cognitive Neuroscience, 18*(7), 1212–1222.

Dawson, D. R., Anderson, N. D., Binns, M. A., Bottari, C., Damianakis, T., Hunt, A., … Zwarenstein, M. (2013a). Managing executive dysfunction following acquired brain injury and stroke using an ecologically valid rehabilitation approach: A study protocol for a randomized, controlled trial. *Trials, 14.* 306-6215-14-306.

Dawson, D. R., Binns, M. A., Hunt, A., Lemsky, C., & Polatajko, H. J. (2013b). Occupation-based strategy training for adults with traumatic brain injury: A pilot study. *Archives of Physical Medicine and Rehabilitation, 94*(10), 1959–1963.

Dawson, D. R., Gaya, A., Hunt, A., Levine, B., Lemsky, C., & Polatajko, H. J. (2009). Using the cognitive orientation to occupational performance (CO-OP) with adults with executive dysfunction following traumatic brain injury. *Canadian Journal of Occupational Therapy, 76*(2), 115–127.

Egan, M., Scott-Lowery, L., De Serres Larose, C., Gallant, L., & Jaillet, C. (2016). The use of personal projects analysis to enhance occupational therapy goal identification. *The Open Journal of Occupational Therapy, 4*(1), 4.

French, B., Leathley, M., Sutton, C., McAdam, J., Thomas, L., Forster, A., … Watkins, C. (2008). A systematic review of repetitive functional task practice with modelling of resource use, costs and effectiveness. *Health Technology Assessment, 12*(30). Retrieved from http://dx.doi.org/10.3310/hta12300.

Geusgens, C. A., Winkens, I., van Heugten, C. M., Jolles, J., & van den Heuvel, W. J. (2007). Occurrence and measurement of transfer in cognitive rehabilitation: A critical review. *Journal of Rehabilitation Medicine, 39*(6), 425–439.

Henshaw, E., Polatajko, H. J., McEwen, S. E., Ryan, J. D., & Baum, C. M. (2011). Cognitive approach to improving participation after stroke: Two case studies. *The American Journal of Occupational Therapy, 65*(1), 55–63.

Hubbard, I. J., Parsons, M. W., Neilson, C., & Carey, L. M. (2009). Task-specific training: Evidence for and translation to clinical practice. *Occupational Therapy International, 16*(3-4), 175–189.

Law, M., Babtiste, S., Carswell, A., McColl, M. A., Polatajko, H. J., & Pollock, N. (2014). *Canadian occupational performance measure* (5th ed.). Ottawa, ON: CAOT Publications ACE.

Lawson, M. J., & Rice, D. N. (1989). Effects of training in use of executive strategies on a verbal memory problem resulting from closed head injury. *Journal of Clinical and Experimental Neuropsychology, 11*(6), 842–854.

Levine, B., Robertson, I. H., Clare, L., Carter, G., Hong, J., Wilson, B. A. , … Stuss, D. T. (2000). Rehabilitation of executive functioning: An experimental-clinical validation of goal management training. *Journal of the International Neuropsychological Society, 6*(3), 299–312.

Levine, B., Schweizer, T. A., O'Connor, C., Turner, G., Gillingham, S., Stuss, D. T., … Robertson, I. H. (2011). Rehabilitation of executive functioning in patients with frontal lobe brain damage with goal management training. *Frontiers in Human Neuroscience, 5*(9), 1–9.

Little, B. R. (2011). *Personal Project Analysis [Workbook]*. Retrieved from http://www.brianrlittle.com/Topics/research/assessment-tools/.

Liu, K. P., Chan, C. C., Lee, T. M., & Hui-Chan, C. W. (2004). Mental imagery for promoting relearning for people after stroke: A randomized controlled trial. *Archives of Physical Medicine and Rehabilitation, 85*(9), 1403–1408.

Luria, A. R. (1966). *Higher cortical functions in man (B. Haigh Trans.).* New York: Basic Books.

Mandich, A. D., Polatajko, H. J., Missiuna, C., & Miller, L. T. (2001). Cognitive strategies and motor performance in children with developmental coordination disorder. *Physical & Occupational Therapy in Pediatrics, 20*(2/3), 125–143.

Martini, R., Rios, J., Polatajko, H. J., Wolf, T., & McEwen, S. E. (2015). The performance quality rating scale (PQRS): Reliability, convergent validity, and internal responsiveness for two scoring systems. *Disability and Rehabilitation, 37*(3), 231–238.

McEwen, S. E., Donald, M., Dawson, D. R., Egan, M. Y., Hunt, A., Quant, S., … Linkewich, E. (2015a). A multi-faceted knowledge translation approach to support persons with stroke and cognitive impairment: Evaluation protocol. *Implementation Science, 10* (157), 1–11.

McEwen, S. E., Polatajko, H. J., Baum, C., Rios, J., Cirone, D., Doherty, M., & Wolf, T. (2015b). Combined cognitive-strategy and task-specific training improve transfer to untrained activities in subacute stroke: An exploratory randomized controlled trial. *Neurorehabilitation and Neural Repair, 29*(6), 526–536.

McEwen, S. E., Polatajko, H. J., Huijbregts, M. P., & Ryan, J. D. (2009). Exploring a cognitive-based treatment approach to improve motor-based skill performance in chronic stroke: Results of three single case experiments. *Brain Injury, 23*(13-14), 1041–1053.

McEwen, S. E., Polatajko, H. J., Huijbregts, M. P., & Ryan, J. D. (2010). Inter-task transfer of meaningful, functional skills following a cognitive-based treatment: Results of three multiple baseline design experiments in adults with chronic stroke. *Neuropsychological Rehabilitation, 20*(4), 541–561.

Meichenbaum, D. (1977). *Cognitive-behavior modification: An integrative approach.* New York: Plenum Press.

Meichenbaum, D. (1991). *Cognitive behavior modification.* London, Ontario, Canada: Workshop presented at Child and Parent Research Institute Symposium.

Miller, P., Huijbregts, M., Gowland, C., Barreca, S., Torresin, W., Moreland, J., … Barclay-Goddard, R. (2008). *Chedoke-McMaster stroke assessment development, validation and administration manual.* Hamilton, Ontario: McMaster University and Hamilton Health Sciences.

Nasreddine, Z. S., Phillips, N. A., Bedirian, V., Charbonneau, S., Whitehead, V., Collin, I., … Chertkow, H. (2005). The Montreal Cognitive Assessment, MoCA: A brief screening tool for mild cognitive impairment. *Journal of the American Geriatrics Society, 53* (4), 695–699.

Ng, E. M., Polatajko, H. J., Marziali, E., Hunt, A., & Dawson, D. R. (2013). Telerehabilitation for addressing executive dysfunction after traumatic brain injury. *Brain Injury, 27*(5), 548–564.

Polatajko, H. J., Cantin, N., Amoroso, B., McKee, P., Rivard, A., Kirsh, B., … Lin, N. (2013). Occupation-based enablement: A practice mosaic. In E. A. Townsend & H. J. Polatajko (Eds.), *Enabling occupation II: Advancing an occupational therapy vision for health, well-being, & justice through occupation* (2nd ed., pp. 177–201).

Polatajko, H. J., & Mandich, A. D. (2004). *Enabling occupation in children: The cognitive orientation to daily occupational performance (CO-OP) approach* (1st ed.). Ottawa, Canada: CAOT Publications ACE.

Polatajko, H. J., Mandich, A. D., & Martini, R. (2000). Dynamic performance analysis: A framework for understanding occupational performance. *The American Journal of Occupational Therapy: Official Publication of the American Occupational Therapy Association, 54*(1), 65–72.

Polatajko, H. J., Mandich, A. D., Missiuna, C., Miller, L. T., Macnab, J. J., Malloy-Miller, T. , et al. (2001). Cognitive orientation to daily occupational performance (CO-OP): Part III - the protocol in brief. *Physical & Occupational Therapy in Pediatrics, 20*(2/3), 107–123.

Polatajko, H. J., McEwen, S. E., Ryan, J. D., & Baum, C. M. (2012). Pilot randomized controlled trial investigating cognitive strategy use to improve goal performance after stroke. *The American Journal of Occupational Therapy, 66*(1), 104–109.

Poulin, V., Korner-Bitensky, N., Bherer, L., Lussier, M., & Dawson, D. R. (2016). Comparison of two cognitive interventions for adults experiencing executive dysfunction post-stroke: A pilot study. *Disability and Rehabilitation.* (Epub ahead of print).

Roth, R. M., Isquith, P. K., & Gioia, G. A. (2005). *Behavioral rating inventory of executive function - adult version (BRIEF-A).* Lutz, Florida: Psychological Assessment Resources, Inc.

Scammels, E., Bates, S., Houldin, A., & Polatajko, H. J. (2016). The cognitive orientation to daily occupational performance: A scoping review. *Canadian Journal of Occupational Therapy.* (Epub ahead of print).

Skidmore, E. R., Dawson, D. R., Butters, M. A., Grattan, E. S., Juengst, S. B., Whyte, E. M., … Becker, J. T. (2015). Strategy training shows promise for addressing disability in the first 6 months after stroke. *Neurorehabilitation and Neural Repair, 29*(7), 668–676.

Skidmore, E. R., Dawson, D. R., Whyte, E. M., Butters, M. A., Dew, M. A., Grattan, E. S., … Holm, M. B. (2014). Developing complex interventions: Lessons learned from a pilot study examining strategy training in acute stroke rehabilitation. *Clinical Rehabilitation, 28*(4), 378–387.

Skidmore, E. R., Holm, M. B., Whyte, E. M., Dew, M. A., Dawson, D. R., & Becker, J. T. (2011). The feasibility of meta-cognitive strategy training in acute inpatient stroke rehabilitation: Case report. *Neuropsychological Rehabilitation, 21*(2), 208–223.

Toglia, J. P., Rodger, S. A., & Polatajko, H. J. (2012). Anatomy of cognitive strategies: A therapist's primer for enabling occupational performance. *Canadian Journal of Occupational Therapy, 79*(4), 225–236.

Townsend, E. A., & Polatajko, H. J. (2013). *Enabling occupation II: Advancing an occupational therapy vision for health, well-being & justice through occupation* (2nd ed.). Ottawa, ON: CAOT Publication ACE.

van Heugten, C. M., Dekker, J., Deelman, B. G., Stehmann-Saris, J. C., & Kinebanian, A. (1998). Outcome of strategy training in stroke patients with apraxia: A phase II study. *Clinical Rehabilitation, 12* (4), 294–303.

von Cramon, D. Y., Matthes-von Cramon, G., & Mai, N. (1991). Problem-solving deficits in brain-injured patients: A therapeutic approach. *Neuropsychological Rehabilitation, 1*(1), 45–64.

Wolf, T. J., Polatajko, H. J., Baum, C., Rios, J., Cirone, D., Doherty, M., & McEwen, S. E. (2016). Combined cognitive-strategy and task-specific training impacts cognition and upper extremity function in sub-acute stroke: An exploratory randomized controlled trial. *American Journal of Occupational Therapy.* (Epub ahead of print).

Ylvisaker, M., Feeney, T., & Szekeres, F. (1998). Traumatic brain injury rehabilitation: Children and adolescents. In M. Ylvisaker (Ed.), (2nd ed). Boston: Butterworth-Heinemann.

43

ASSISTIVE TECHNOLOGY

NATASHA A. LAYTON

Abstract

The focus of this chapter is on the role of technologies, in particular assistive technology (AT) devices, in enabling occupation. Assistive technology is one of a number of interventions used to enhance the person–environment–occupation fit. Using the Canadian Practice Process Framework (CPPF), the role of the occupational therapist in assistive technology provision is reviewed. The societal and practice contexts in which occupational therapists recommend assistive technologies are discussed, as well as the challenges of balancing pragmatic concerns against person-focused outcome delivery. A range of contemporary issues affect AT provision; discourses of disability and stigma and the realities of policy and funding concerns influence what is possible. The dynamic pace of technology innovation and design movements, such as the universal and inclusive design movements, are altering perspectives of technology and the idea of 'normal' and 'specialised' AT devices. The chapter presents good practice principles from the perspective of AT users and AT literature and provides a contemporary frame of reference as a way forward to realise the potential of AT to meet people's occupational goals. These principles are described and illustrated by three people who use AT.

KEY POINTS

- Assistive technology (AT) and accessible environments form a 'technology chain' used by all humans on the spectrum of human variation.

- AT is an effective intervention to enable participation and engagement, when tailored to the person, environment and occupation.

- Effective matching of person, environment and AT device to enable occupation often requires skilled service provision.

- Professional reasoning and person-empowerment are critical to AT provision.

- International good practice principles for AT provision exist and can be linked to the Canadian Practice Process Framework.
- The availability, selection and uptake of AT are influenced by sociopolitical factors.
- Systemic/political practice of occupational therapy may be indicated where there are societal barriers to realising good practice.

INTRODUCTION

Occupational therapists engage with consumers to promote and enable participation and engagement in life tasks. Assistive technology (AT) is one key strategy or intervention to enable this to happen. The best contemporary framework through which to introduce the role of occupational therapists and enabling strategies in context is the International Classification of Functioning, Disability and Health (ICF) (World Health Organization (WHO), 2001). Providing a comprehensive framework for human participation, which is applicable to all, the ICF proposes that health and well-being are a function of the interaction between numerous factors. The ICF framework proposes that participation is dependent on the complex interaction among personal factors, environmental factors, health condition, body functions and structures and activities in which a person engages. Any of these elements can act as barriers or facilitators to a person's overall performance and can contribute to experiences of disability.

Occupational therapists have an identified role at every level of the ICF framework. Occupational therapists do the following:

- Use remediation techniques at the body structure and function level
- Address health conditions through education, health promotion and compensatory strategies
- Address the impact of personal factors using therapeutic strategies to mediate and strengthen a person's responses
- Adapt and transform environmental barriers into facilitators
- Analyse, adapt and modify activities as the building blocks of occupation
- Facilitate participation through collaborative practice and goal setting, and matching person, environment and activity.

Within the ICF framework, activity and participation can be grouped into three broad categories: foundation activities, activities and participation (Table 43.1). All human occupations fit into these broad categories. Occupational therapists may work with people from the bottom up, focusing on foundation skills and activities, or from the top down, focusing on participation. Occupational therapists also understand that occupational performance is an outcome of the transaction among the person, environment and occupation (Law, Cooper, Stewart, Rigby, & Letts, 1996).

TABLE 43.1	
ICF Categories of Human Occupation with Examples	
ICF Category	**Examples of Human Occupations**
Participation	■ Major life areas (e.g. education, work) ■ Community, social and civic life (e.g. cultural, religious, recreational and political)
Activities	■ Self-care ■ Domestic life ■ General tasks and demands ■ Mobility
Foundation activities	■ Interpersonal interactions and relationships ■ Communication ■ Learning and applying knowledge

ICF, International Classification of Disability, Function, and Health.

This chapter introduces the role of the occupational therapist in the context of human functioning and capability and explores the intervention of technology within the context of environment. A range of theoretical approaches to design, outcomes measurement and consumer coproduction are provided. Three practice stories illustrate the role of the occupational therapist when implementing AT strategies and interventions.

THE CAPABILITY APPROACH

The view of health and well-being provided in the ICF is well accepted, yet resource allocation in many practice contexts is still bound to a diagnostic view of need. For example, people must *qualify* as *sufficiently disabled* to be eligible for many publicly funded AT devices and services. One contemporary theory that addresses human need in a human rights paradigm is the capability approach (Nussbaum, 2011; Sen, 1999). The capability approach identifies what is needed for people, given their capabilities and the limitations of their environments, to achieve outcomes. The capability approach is congruent with occupational therapy models. It relocates problems or deficits away from the individual, allowing for the social model of disability's notion of *disablement by the environment*, and embraces the *political practice of occupational therapy* (Pollard, Sakellariou, & Kronenberg, 2008). This approach is explained next from the perspective of person, environment, and occupation.

Person: To engage in occupation and to reach goals and aspirations, individuals call upon their capabilities. Human capabilities consist of abilities (capacities) and personal factors. Abilities include body structures and functions as well as capacities such as personality and resilience. Personal factors include such things as demographics, circles of support and socioeconomic situation. The full set of capabilities for each person depends on three interrelated elements: innate skills and capacity to function; agency or freedom to choose to engage in valued occupations; and whether the environment enables or inhibits the person to flourish (e.g. whether the person is affected by, for example, poverty or discrimination) (Whalley Hammell, 2015).

Environment: As well as using capabilities to engage in tasks and to reach desired outcomes, people use a range of accommodations and supports. Examples include a continuous path of travel making it possible to get from home to work or an elevator to get to the 20th floor of a building for a meeting. Some people require more accommodations and supports than others, to mediate or fill the 'gap' between aspiration and capability. The concept of a *capability gap* (Nussbaum, 2011) is powerful in that it opens space for the idea of occupational *fit*.

Occupation: Occupational performance will naturally be influenced by the congruence – or lack of it – between a person's capabilities and occupational goals – that is, the occupations that a person wishes to participate in and the tasks or activities the person must master to achieve this involvement. Professor Stephen Hawking, a world-renowned Cambridge-based physicist, participates in an active educational and economic life. His particular capability gap is significant, as his only reliable motor response is a blink or eye gaze. This capability gap is mediated with a sophisticated AT solution including specialised seating system, head-controlled wheelchair and eye-gaze operated communication system. The occupational goal of an economic and educational

life, given the accommodations in place, is achieved. In contrast, a person with vision impairment in the urban city of Bangalore, India, wishes to learn a trade. His capability gap requires several relatively straightforward accommodations, including tactile indicators, education and resources in Braille and a reliable path of travel. Although he is able to move around his home through tactile sensing, he is unable to rely on environmental supports outside his front door, no tactile indicators are present on the unmade roads, and he has no safe access to transport or Braille supports at school. Further, poverty and his position in the caste system represents an additional barrier to the goal of a trade qualification and a job. In his case the capability gap remains unfilled, his potential unrealised and the occupational goals of education and work unmet. The capability approach is illustrated in Fig. 43.1. In this figure the capability gap of three different people can be seen to affect their capacity to overcome barriers (depicted by a fence) and achieve outcomes (depicted as balloons). The capability gap can be expressed in terms of activity limitations or participation restrictions. The capability gap can be bridged or filled through the use of supports such as AT, environmental interventions, and personal support. Although each person has an equal set of supports (the boxes upon which they stand), this is not adequate to provide equal outcomes. Reallocating supports according to individual capability gaps enables equal outcomes to occur.

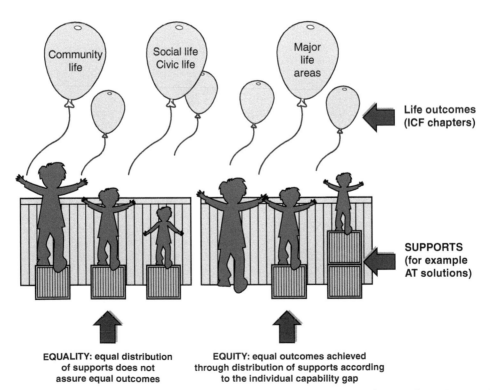

FIG. 43.1 ■ The capability gap using the World Health Organization's International Classification of Functioning, Disability and Health language.

Disability is a term used to describe impairment and/or the presence of barriers to functioning. Usually this is applied to people living with the effects of congenital or acquired impairment or people ageing into functional limitation. Many people with an impairment note that the term *disability* is stigmatising and represents a focus on a person's limitations rather than strengths.

A more holistic view, in line with the ICF, is that impairments are part of *universal human variation* (Bickenbach, Chatterji, Bradley, & Ustun, 1999; Patston, 2007). In other words, having strengths and challenges is a feature of being human, and, taking a lifespan view, will be experienced by all humans at some stage in their life. In this view, mediating the capability gap is an ongoing, relational and human interaction and exchange. An example would be the personal support that a frail elderly person may receive from a neighbour. Many mediators have profound impacts and are seen as entirely common and not unusual. These mediators include such things as glasses and hearing aids used to augment body functions and fill sensory capability gaps.

Disability scholars also observe that the experience of disability has a lot to do with barriers within the environment and low expectations from the *nondisabled* world. This social model of disability (Shakespeare, 2008) approach argues that the environment plays a key role in disablement, and as a result issues of person/environment fit should not be perceived as problems within an individual.

The United Nations Convention on the Rights of Persons with Disabilities (United Nations, 2006) supports the right of *all* people to engage in *all* occupations and identifies a role for member states to make this happen. This 'rights-based' approach indicates that health workers, including occupational therapists, have a responsibility to address the systemic causes of capability gaps. These ideas will be picked up later, after the focus on technology.

HUMANS AND TECHNOLOGY

From the time early human beings fashioned tools, technology has been a critical enabler of occupation. Technology use is ubiquitous and in many ways a seamless element of identity. Possessing the newest smartphone, for example, can be experienced as a marker of status. The same is rarely said for assistive technologies (Hocking, 1999). The assistive technologies developed over the nineteenth and twentieth centuries were characteristically medically focused and institutionalised in intent and appearance (Albrecht, Seelman, & Bury, 2001). In line with the medical model lens, products focused on managing basic activities such as self-care and mobility. The resulting *independent living market*, although certainly providing necessary AT devices, has dominated perceptions of what people living with impairment can and should aspire to and use and in some ways has contributed to the othering, or problematic identity, of disability.

An example of identity related to AT devices is that of hiking poles versus a walking stick: both provide a point of support for walking, but one presents an image of outdoor recreation, whereas the other is more likely to be associated with age or infirmity. Historical images of assistive technology devices (variously termed equipment, invalid aids, or appliances) include leather and buckle callipers (Fig. 43.2), medical implements and specially adapted homes. Current and future developments include robotics, innovative designs such as the Segway, and exoskeletal products. Effectively, then, AT represents a strategy that can either *enable* or *disable*. It is interesting therefore to consider the phenomenon of AT users' 'reluctance to use compensatory and assistive technology' (Hansson, 2007, p. 264). Probably this speaks to the fact that AT devices are seen as markers of illness and loss, identity and stigma (Cook & Hussey, 2008; Hocking, 1999). AT devices have typically been designed, manufactured and marketed by niche suppliers for the *disabled other* (Hobbs, Close, Downing, Reynolds, & Walker, 2009), and the resulting lack of consultation and consideration regarding the views, attitudes and tastes of individuals correlates with AT nonuse and abandonment (Wessels, Djicks, Soede, Gelderblom, & Witte, 2003).

A range of ethical issues has emerged in the wake of new inventions. *Nonhuman* designs such as prosthetic cheetah legs are no longer replacing or augmenting human functioning; they in fact provide *superhuman* capabilities (Fig. 43.3). A range of technologies such as robots to replace personal care from other humans, such as to perform the functions of a mobile hoist, or electronic responsive soft toys to simulate nurturing, introduce the risk that technology will replace human contact. Critical writings from the disability perspective note the danger that the needs and autonomy of people living with impairment become subordinated to the technologies in use. The rapid

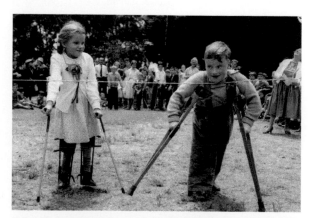

FIG. 43.2 ■ Children using callipers and crutches at the Yooralla Sports Day in Victoria, Australia, 1958. *(Reproduced courtesy of Rosslyn Pickhaver and Polio Australia.)*

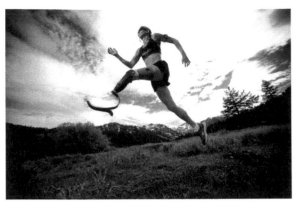

FIG. 43.3 ■ Participation in running using nonhuman design. *(From Chabner, D.-E. (2012). Medical terminology: A short course (6th ed.). St. Louis: Saunders Elsevier.)*

diversification of enabling technologies holds significant implications for AT users and for the practitioners who prescribed and provide these technologies.

There are many definitions of AT, and it is important to understand where they come from and how they are used. Definitional differences greatly affect what governments and private AT insurance will provide, and are often based upon custom and practice (Masso, Owen, Stevermuer, Williams, & Eager, 2008). Obtaining AT devices often involves a transaction mediated through professionals as gatekeepers of equipment funds (Barbara & Curtin, 2008). In this transaction, individuals with impairments are in a position of requiring the appropriate *label* to match the device, effectively reducing the person to a disability identity (Rioux, Basser, & Jones, 2011). The scope of AT, as defined by AT funders and health insurers, is often restricted to items that are 'medically necessary' – a criterion itself subject to interpretation based upon the 'narrowest administrative definition of clinical need' (Barbara & Curtin, 2008, p. 58). AT is defined by many funding systems as a *medical device*. This becomes problematic because it perpetuates the medical model view of disability, rather than the alternate conceptualisations of disability, and may prevent recognition of AT as technology that supports inclusion through participation in life occupations (Ripat & Booth, 2005).

The key concepts outlined next summarise some directions to address the human–technology interface issues described earlier.

KEY CONCEPTS: ASSISTIVE, UNIVERSAL, AND INCLUSIVE DESIGN

As technology is all about augmenting human functioning, it is difficult to think of any technology that is not *assistive*. However,

there are many examples of devices that require effort or adaptation on the part of the human user, such as complex mobile phone interfaces, poor colour contrast and tiny symbols on TV remote controls, and can openers that require two hands to operate. Design has typically focused upon the *archetypal user*, usually understood to be an adult male. As a consequence, many products such as seating, workbench height, and reach range are designed using anthropometric measurements which do not match the user requirements of the population as a whole (Imrie & Hall, 2001).

The first wave of user-focused design came to be known as the universal design movement. Universal design focused on accommodating the needs of the majority of users through the application of universal design principles (equitable use, flexibility in use, simple and intuitive use, perceptible information, tolerance for error, low physical effort and size and space for approach and use) (Steinfeld & Danford, 2006). The *majority of users* is usually taken to mean a majority percentage of the population bell curve, up to the 80th or 90th decile. This is depicted in Fig. 43.4a and b. The universal design approach therefore endeavours to meet the needs of 80% to 90% of users but is unlikely to cater for the needs of the outliers or last deciles on the curve.

Universal design tenets have shifted towards an inclusive view of the population (Steinfeld, 2010) and address the needs of *most* but not *all*. Inclusive design uses a 'deep understanding of diversity' (Dong, 2007, p. 70) to move beyond norms and outliers. From an inclusive design perspective, the traditional bell curve population is now characterised as a circular entirety with a series of segments that capture the ergonomic diversity of the population (Dong, 2007) (Fig. 43.4c). An inclusive design perspective can be illustrated by a common kitchen aid such as a potato peeler: a small moulded pistol-grip potato peeler suits both adolescent hand size and older people with weakened grip caused by arthritic conditions; a heavier cylindrical-grip potato peeler suits adults with large hands but poor dexterity as well as people with athetoid upper limb and hand movements. These examples illustrate that differently tailored designs can meet the diverse needs of the whole population, where a single design might only meet the needs of a proportion (albeit a large proportion) of that population. The *special* aspects of the designs are marketed in a way that does not distinguish disability but rather distinguishes particular design features. Such inclusivity has the potential for a paradigm shift from 'designing special aids and equipment for disabled people (an assistive technology approach), to designing mainstream products for as many people as possible (a universal design approach)' (Dong, 2007, p. 67).

As design becomes democratised, as 3D printers become within reach and consumer empowerment increases, the role of AT users should also extend into the design and testing of AT products, a strategy that will address a long history of exclusion from research, design and development. Such

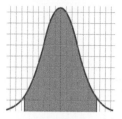 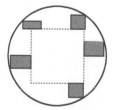 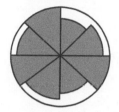

a) Frequency distribution Bell curve

Locating the human population as norms or outliers

b) Specialist disability design

Does not address the population as a whole

c) Designed for diversity

Design for diversity removes disable/able bias

FIG. 43.4 ■ Contrasting conceptualisations of the human population in ergonomics, universal design and inclusive design (Acknowledgement of these inclusive design concepts is made to Dong (2007) and Wijk (2001, pp.1–28)).

inclusion strategies have the potential to ameliorate, in part, the abandonment and nonuse of AT devices and to normalise and universalise *disability* technologies (Scherer & Gluekauf, 2005; Wessels et al., 2003).

THE TECHNOLOGY CHAIN

A parallel reconceptualisation of AT in relation to the world around it is the *technology chain*. AT devices are always used in an environmental context, and the substantial relationship between AT and environmental interventions has been conceptualised as a technology chain (Association for the Advancement of Assistive Technology in Europe (AAATE), 2012). For example, the provision of AT devices such as a bathseat will not be required if the shower-overbath is replaced with a stepless recess and a built in propping ledge; in other words, the barriers or facilitators of environments create or remove the need for a specific AT device or aspect of personal support.

ASSISTIVE TECHNOLOGY IN THE CONTEXT OF OTHER INTERVENTIONS

Occupational therapists have a range of interventions available to them. A useful tool to understand the provision of assistive devices in relation to other interventions, and to outcomes, is the IMPACT 2 Model developed by Roger Smith and colleagues (Smith, 2002) (Fig. 43.5). The model demonstrates that outcomes of interventions can be described by considering the following six stages: (1) Preintervention, (2) Context, (3) Baseline, (4) Intervention Approaches, (5) Outcome Covariates, and (6) Outcomes. A left-to-right bold arrow indicates the direction. The applications of universal design and health promotion are delineated in the lower left hand corner as 'Preintervention',

which are two methods to improve functional performance. An arrow connects the preintervention approaches to the Context stage, consisting of person–task–environment. The Context stage is represented as the person using assistive technology to perform a task within an environment. The Context stage is connected by an arrow to the next stage of Function, which is composed of an evaluation of performance, quality of life, and participation. The fourth stage, the Intervention Approaches, has six components, which represent six methods available to improve functional performance. These are: (1) Reduce the Impairment, (2) Compensate for the Impairment, (3) Use Assistive Technology Devices and Services, (4) Redesign the Activity, (5) Redesign the Environment, and (6) Use Personal Assistance. The next stage is the Outcome Covariates, which identifies potential precursor variables of satisfaction of devices and services, dissatisfaction of device or services, and use and discontinuance of assistive technologies. The final stage, Outcomes, involves reevaluation of the individual's performance, quality of life and participation to determine the outcomes of the intervention. It is important to understand that the preintervention and the person–task–environment context must be considered throughout the process. It is also important to isolate an intervention from other concurrent interventions to understand the outcome of that particular intervention. Dollar signs are located next to the Preintervention stage, the Baseline measurement of function, the Intervention Approaches, and the Outcomes measurement of function to show where cost needs to be considered (Smith, 2002).

To illustrate these various strategies, Smith and Benge (2004) provide an example of a person with cerebral palsy and a motor speech impairment (dysarthria) engaged in the task of ordering food in a restaurant. In this situation:

■ *reducing the impairment* entails providing remedial activities to speak more clearly to achieve functional vocalisation;

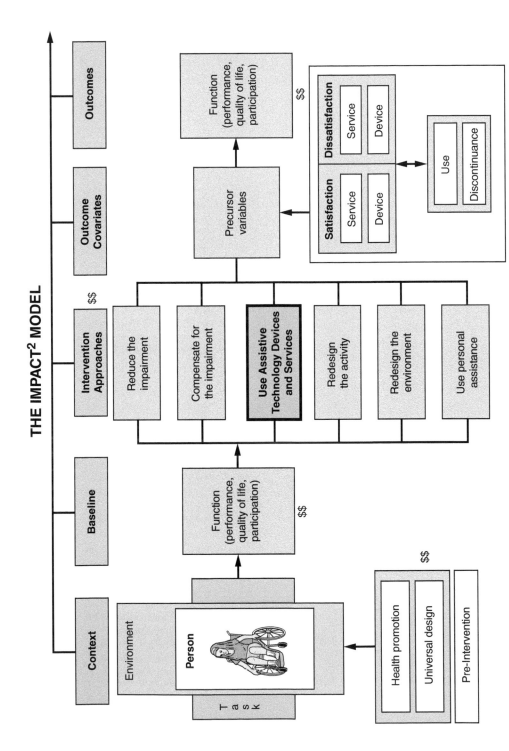

FIG. 43.5 ■ IMPACT model. (© 2004 Rehabilitation Research Design & Disability (R₂D₂) Center, UW-Milwaukee, www.r2d2.uwm.edu.)

- *compensating for the impairment* may involve bypassing the speech impairment by pointing to items on a menu and using gestures;
- *redesigning the activity* might entail using a set menu;
- *using AT devices* might involve the use of a speech synthesiser or communication board;
- *redesigning the environment* could be going to a cafeteria-style restaurant; and
- *using personal assistance* would have an attendant order the food or perhaps interpret the vocalisation.

Occupational therapists will often use one or more interventions in collaboration with the people they work with to tailor effective solutions to meet each person's self-determined goals. A study of 100 AT users found that, on average, 13 elements were used to form an AT solution, where a solution was defined as including AT, elements of environmental modification and personal support (Layton, Wilson, & Andrews, 2010). When *soft technologies* such as occupational analysis, task simplification and adaptation and work hardening are added to these interventions, it is evident that individualised interventions will be multiple in nature.

DEFINING ASSISTIVE TECHNOLOGY

A range of terms is used to delineate those assistive technologies that mediate the effects of impairment or minimise barriers within the environment. These include rehabilitation technology, everyday technologies, adapted technologies, health care technologies, assistive technology and assistive products and ergonomics (Scherer, 2012). WHO defines *AT* as 'An umbrella term for any device or system that allows individuals to perform tasks they would otherwise be unable to do or increases the ease and safety with which tasks can be performed' (WHO, 2001, p. 10). The International Organization for Standardization (ISO) publishes the international taxonomy *Assistive Products for Persons with Disability*, or ISO 9999, which provides standards for assistive technologies for persons with disability and defines AT as 'Any product (including devices, equipment, instruments and software), especially produced or generally available, used by or for persons with disability' (ISO, 2016, p. 2).

These definitions offer a critical departure from previous approaches in line with current approaches to inclusive design, as the definitions include commonly available devices and everyday technologies when these provide assistance to people living with impairment to participate and engage in occupations (ISO, 2016). How assistive technologies are defined is important as the definition can affect whether a particular technology will be funded. For example, when having an impairment is seen to require *special* devices, this led to policies where, for example, mainstream devices such as a digital tablet (e.g. iPad) were not eligible for funding, even if this could replace a more costly communication device.

Currently, the international taxonomy enables any AT device to be theoretically classified. The ISO 9999 classification system offers 650 device categories across 11 classes, which are listed in Table 43.2. The nonconsecutive numbering of the classes allows space for future technologies and categories to be added. Within each class, three levels of classification are offered: for example, class 12 denotes assistive products for personal mobility, with 14 subclasses including walking products, cars, cycles, wheelchairs and transferring and turning products, with additional divisions for powered wheelchairs, foot-driven wheelchairs, and so on.

Within most of these broad classes, a range of complexity is evident. Some AT devices (e.g. an angled comb) may be categorised as *straightforward, noncomplex* or *low tech* (Cook & Polgar, 2008). Some AT devices have inherent technological complexity yet are relatively straightforward in terms of a therapy recommendation (e.g. noise-cancelling headphones). Other simple AT devices become complex in terms of their application and utility: a palmar pocket and pointer to maximise hand function for someone with tetraplegia may be

TABLE 43.2
ISO Classification

Class	Description
04	Assistive products for measuring, supporting, training or replacing body functions
05	Assistive products for education and for training in skills
06	Assistive products attached to body for supporting neuromusculoskeletal or movement related functions (orthoses) and replacing anatomical structures (prostheses)
09	Assistive products for self-care activities and participation in self-care
12	Assistive products for activities and participation relating to personal mobility and transportation
15	Assistive products for domestic activities and participation in domestic life
18	Furnishings, fixtures and other assistive products for supporting activities in the indoor and outdoor human-made environments
22	Assistive products for communication and information management
24	Assistive products for controlling, carrying, moving and handling objects and devices
27	Assistive products for controlling, adapting or measuring elements of the physical environment
28	Assistive products for work activities and participation in employment
30	Assistive products for recreation and leisure

ISO, International Organization for Standardization.

adapted for a range of small aids (spoon, toothbrush) and even digital devices. In this last example, *straightforward* technologies deliver significant outcomes if planned with a full spectrum of occupational goals in mind. The ability to envision the potential of AT mapped to a person's occupational goals, and implemented based on a thorough knowledge of AT devices and environmental factors, is dependent on the skill of the therapist; the involvement of a therapist in the assessment and prescription of AT brings into play the *human factors*.

Hard and Soft Technologies

AT devices are considered *hard technologies,* and practitioner activities such as assessment, education and advice, customising and training are considered *soft technologies.* The terms *hard technologies* and *soft technologies* were first used to describe AT by Odor (1983, cited by Cook and Hussey, 2008) and are a useful way of identifying the interrelated nature of therapist or practitioner support and actual devices. The effectiveness of any hard technologies depends on the therapist employing appropriate soft technologies to ensure a fit between the AT and the person, occupation and environment. Lack of appropriate soft technologies can lead to poor prescription, abandonment and nonuse of AT (Wessels et al., 2003), as evident in the example of a nonambulant person being provided with a wheelchair to move around the home and community. However, when using the wheelchair, the person was unable to reach bench tops, manoeuvre through doorways and transport the wheelchair in a car. As a result the person was not able to achieve meaningful occupational outcomes and ceased using the wheelchair. Hence, soft technologies are critical to ensuring that AT devices meet the needs of the users (Scherer & Sax, 2009).

Soft Technology Skills and Processes

At the core of any intervention is the therapeutic alliance between therapists and the people they work with. Therapeutic alliances have been demonstrated to positively contribute to outcomes (Kayes & McPherson, 2012, p. 190).

A valuable set of indicators of the effective use of soft technologies has emerged from research on the motivations and incentives of a range of AT stakeholders in Australia (De Jonge, Layton, Vicary, & Steel, 2015). An overview of what users want from assistive technology services is in Box 43.1. For AT users, an effective soft technology approach must include person-centred, relational and holistic features. A range of professionals (usually allied health or rehabilitation engineering), specialised AT suppliers and expert AT users may provide one or many of these elements. Occupational therapists have relevant expertise across a large range of AT devices.

Good practice steps for AT provision have been published internationally (AAATE, 2012; Fagerberg, 2011) and adapted

---

BOX 43.1
WHAT AT USERS WANT FROM AT SERVICES

Determination of the best combination of devices, personal care and environmental design.

Access to sufficient funding for good quality and long-lasting devices.

Funding to meet AT needs in every area of life.

Holistic assessment of needs, so that each device works well and does not interfere with other supports.

Consideration of AT needs across the lifespan and as needs change.

Support throughout the process of getting AT, including device trial, training and maintenance.

Access to resources when needed.

Active involvement in decision making.

Consideration of personal preferences and identity so that AT is chosen to suit lifestyle and participation.

AT, Assistive technology.

---

for use in Australia (Australian Rehabilitation and Assistive Technology Association (ARATA), 2012). The broad steps applicable to assessing and matching the AT device to the person, occupation and environment are presented in Fig. 43.6. Implementing the good practice steps requires access to both hard and soft technologies, adapted to a user's own skillset and support needs. For example, successful matching of AT devices such as environmental controls or wheelchairs to an individual requires a comprehensive understanding of the hard technology (the device) and a systematic application of the needs assessment, setup, trial, training and follow-up (soft technology) for optimal outcomes (Cook & Hussey, 2008; McDonald, 2010).

Pragmatic Constraints on Good Practice

Occupational therapists may find themselves working in situations where it is difficult to follow good practice steps because of the design of AT policy and therefore of AT service delivery. *Pragmatic reasoning* is the term used in the professional reasoning literature to describe practical considerations within the practice context of the occupational therapist, which may influence decision making (Unsworth, 2004). Occupational therapists may therefore need to engage in a range of systemic advocacy activities identifying shortfalls in policy or service provision guidelines, against benchmarks such as practice guidelines (where available) or good practice steps. Common scenarios and potential pragmatic actions to address these can be found in Table 43.3.

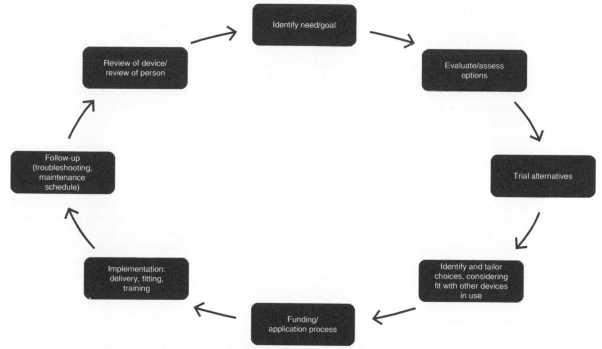

FIG. 43.6 ■ Best practice steps for assistive technology provision.

TABLE 43.3	
Examples of Pragmatic Constraints and Possible Actions	
Pragmatic Constraint	**Possible Actions**
The AT funding scheme generally funds the AT device (the hard technology) yet does not fund soft technology supports.	Occupational therapists may need to articulate to managers and to policymakers that, to follow evidence-based practice principles, good practice steps should be adhered to. Informing and partnering with consumers and consumer advocates to argue for rights to support under the CRPD (United Nations, 2006) is changing policy in many countries.
The AT funding scheme provides a limited subsidy for a limited range of AT device.	Occupational therapists who present a limited range of options to the consumer, in line with funding constraints, are operating pragmatically but not ethically. A more empowering approach would be to collaboratively discuss the full range of options and support the consumer to making a decision taking into account factors such as funding constraints. This may include seeking alternate funds, making representation as a self-advocate for consideration, or providing data on undermet need to funders and policymakers to develop improved policy.
AT recommendations, particularly for AT devices seen as complex, are often mediated by an occupational therapist or other AT practitioner; however, there is an assumption that 'straightforward' AT can be identified and readily provided without supports.	Evidence demonstrates that devolving practice-based tasks to support workers, as a way around the shortage of occupational therapy community services, may result in a partial response to complex needs and compromise the right to, and quality of, services (Carrier et al., 2010). A study of access to everyday assistive technologies by frail older people in West Australia found consumers experienced great difficulty identifying and obtaining AT devices even where these were readily commercially available, and that generic staff such as home care workers and nurses 'missed' unmet need for AT devices. In this study, even where AT devices had been introduced, a lack of consideration of the occupation and environment led to a range of difficulties, such as mobility aids being difficult or impossible to use in a home environment which had not been assessed or adapted (Layton et al., 2014). Researching peer-reviewed literature and identifying pertinent evidence can support occupational therapists in making the case for the complexity that arises among person, occupation and environment, even where one is deemed *straightforward*.
Service delivery triage systems attempt to define noncomplex users.	Several studies have also looked at indicators of complexity in the person as a strategy to determine when an occupational therapist may be required (Guay et al., 2012).

AT, Assistive technology; *CRPD,* Convention on the Rights of Persons with Disabilities.

ASSISTIVE TECHNOLOGY AND OUTCOMES

There are some methodological complexities in researching the effectiveness of AT. One difficulty with AT outcomes research is separating AT from other interventions as the use of AT is pervasive. Conducting controlled trials where one cohort of people is denied AT is ethically problematic, and it can be difficult to identify and remove ubiquitous technologies from a person's life in order to evaluate effectiveness. For example, in a commonly used rehabilitation measure, the Functional Independence Measure (FIM) (Uniform Data System, 1999), people are scored a 7 for *full independent performance* and a 6 for *independence with aids*. Occupational therapists administering this measure before and after rehabilitation may identify, for example, the shower stool and handrails as necessary *aids* which enable a person to be fully independent as no assistance is required from another person. However, according to the FIM scoring guidelines, a score of 6 would be assigned, as independence is only possible because of the shower stool and handrail. It is not clear how preexisting AT such as glasses, or technology chain facilitators such as a stepless shower entrance and bannister rail, are accounted for in the scoring. In reviewing the literature and noting these inconsistencies, Rust and Smith (2005) suggest that the full effectiveness of AT is significantly underestimated because of this difficulty in identifying 'naked' performance.

In spite of the difficulties with researching the outcomes of AT, there is moderate to strong evidence (Cook & Polgar, 2008; Layton, 2014) that AT are effective in doing the following:

- Preserving independence, decreasing functional decline and reducing hospital admission rates
- Preventing secondary complications
- Preventing falls
- Maintaining occupational roles
- Alleviating carer burden
- Reducing residential care placement
- Enabling activity and participation in specific life domains
- Maintaining health and community involvement
- Improving quality of life

This set of outcomes identifies a further conceptual issue with AT outcomes research. The outcomes listed here relate largely to costs and cost minimisation and are of great interest to stakeholders, such as funding agencies and insurers. However, AT users describe valuing a wider and more nuanced set of outcomes. As the evidence base is generally governed by professionals, researchers and funders rather than AT users themselves, AT users warn that the full effects and outcomes of AT from the perspectives of AT users are not known. Scherer (2002) suggests that the AT users' perspectives can be obtained using an idiographic approach. In this approach the person is the unit of analysis, proposing that individuals

> [...] prioritize their own desired outcomes and then rate over time the progress in achieving them [...] in this way, outcomes are measured in terms of changes in the person's satisfaction in being able to get to where he/she wants to go, whether by walking or some other means, rather than just by the functional capability to do so. (2002b, p. 171)

This proposal for 'pre and post' case methodology is congruent with occupational therapists' use of the Canadian Occupational Performance Measure (Polatajko et al., 2007) as well as a range of AT-specific outcome measures that focus on evaluating the impact of AT devices, including the Quebec User Evaluation of satisfaction with Assistive Technology (Demers et al., 2002); Psychosocial Impact of Assistive Devices (Jutai & Day, 2002); Individually Prioritized Problem Assessment (Wessels et al., 2002); the Social Cost Analysis Inventory (Andrich, 2002); Milieu–Person–Technology Model (Scherer, 1998); and the AT Device Predisposition Assessment (Scherer & Sax, 2009).

However, when it comes to demonstrating outcomes of meaning to all stakeholders, the ICF offers a common language. In contrast to FIM, the ICF attempts to separate out the components of the technology chain and can be used to rate *naked* compared with *contextualised* performance. Some examples of outcomes of AT devices expressed in ICF terms can be found in Table 43.4.

PRACTICE STORIES: OCCUPATIONAL THERAPY PRACTICE IN AT PROVISION AND THE IMPACT OF CONTEXT

To illustrate occupational therapy practice in AT provision, the practice stories of three AT users, Heather, Ricky and Peter, are included in this chapter (Practice Stories 43.1 to 43.3). These individuals are introduced using ICF language, and examples of AT interventions are given using the Canadian Practice Process Framework. The impact of societal and practice contexts are addressed at the conclusion of the examples.

The Impact of Societal Context

Ricky, Heather and Peter live in urban or regional areas of Australia. The social contract that exists between individuals and the state differs according to country (e.g. the limited health safety net in the United States for those people who are uninsured compared with the national health scheme in the United Kingdom). The social contract also changes over time, with Australia and many countries moving from charitable approaches to social justice and human rights approaches, as enshrined in the Convention on the Rights of Persons with Disabilities (United Nations, 2006). The

TABLE 43.4	
Examples Linking AT Devices to Outcomes in ICF Terms	
Outcomes Expressed in ICF Language	**Examples**
Maintaining or improving functioning and independence	A wheeled walker enables ambulatory mobility while carrying shopping.
Facilitating participation	A child uses a Jellybean switch to engage in a Wii game with her nondisabled siblings.
Enhancing well-being	Communication at a family meal is enabled with an electronic communication device.
Protecting, supporting, training, measuring or substituting for body functions, structures and activities	Continence is managed with a range of continence products.
Preventing avoidable impairments, activity limitations and participation restrictions	Skin integrity is maximised with a pressure cushion and mattress.

AT, Assistive technology; *ICF,* International Classification of Functioning, Disability, and Health.

Convention advocates the following general principles (United Nations, 2006, Article 3):

- Respect for inherent dignity, individual autonomy including the freedom for individuals to make own choices, and independence of persons
- Nondiscrimination
- Full and effective participation and inclusion in society
- Respect for difference and acceptance of persons with disabilities as part of human diversity and humanity
- Equality of opportunity
- Accessibility
- Equality between men and women
- Respect for the evolving capacities of children with disabilities and respect for the right of children with disabilities to preserve their identities

The Convention can be viewed as a tool for social justice and social change. Just as disabled persons organisations write 'shadow reports' to inform the UN as to how countries that are signatories to the Convention are delivering on their commitment, occupational therapists and the people receiving their services may choose to document the achievement of occupational goals, or failure to achieve goals, using the Convention as a blueprint. Occupational therapists and the people receiving their services can use many of the Articles that specifically relate to access to AT and accessible environments to demonstrate whether outcomes are realised or unrealised, as part of the argument for resourcing.

For example, in relation to the three practice stories:

- Ricky is dependent on government social security (pensions), rental accommodation (housing), health care (medicines and monitoring) and disability supports (personal care, AT, environmental modifications). The difficulties she experiences coordinating all these supports can be examined in relation to Article 25 (Health), Article 26 (Habilitation & rehabilitation) and Article 28 (Adequate standard of living and social protection).

- Limited access to information and communication technology means Heather cannot participate in further education, get around her neighbourhood or engage in community activities. Heather's rights to do so are called up in the following articles: Article 19 (Living independently and being included in the community), Article 21 (Freedom of expression and opinion, and access to information), and Article 24 (Education).
- Peter finds he is unable to access Parliament House through the main entrance as there are steps and the rear ramped entrance is closed because of renovations. This situation is addressed in Article 9 (Accessibility), Article 20 (Personal mobility) and Article 29 (Participation in political and public life).

In these examples, Ricky, Heather and Peter and their occupational therapists can identify that policy systems 'lag behind' policy rhetoric and that available programmes have not yet realised the human right to fulfilment of capability gaps and therefore to equal outcomes. Thus the idea of systemic advocacy to influence societal and practice context is of relevance to occupational therapists (Pollard et al., 2008).

The Impact of Practice Context

A good starting point is for occupational therapists to consider the practice context in which they are working. Practice contexts will vary in terms of resourcing and a range of other pragmatic constraints. For example, private and insurance-based facilities have caps on bed days and limit potential postdischarge follow-up, and specific-purpose clinics may not be set up to enable occupational therapists to follow through on aspects of a person's life that are not related to the clinic's purpose. A range of other implicit or hidden motivations and incentives can affect practice and professional reasoning. These may include departmental 'rewards' for statistics, prompt discharges and coming in on budget (De Jonge et al., 2015). In other words, the lens of the practitioner will be influenced by the practice context in which the practitioner works.

In the past, the rehabilitation approach, underpinned by a normative agenda, with its focus on achieving independence and remediating impairment, was an approach of choice when assessing for and providing AT. However, this approach has been severely critiqued by individuals living with impairment as it locates the problem with the individual (Swain, French, Barnes, & Thomas, 2004), privileges professional priorities (Rist, Freas, Maislin, & Stineman, 2008) and lacks appreciation of the diverse engagements with diversity (Shakespeare, 2008). The use of person-focused occupational performance measures and tools such as the Canadian Practice Process Framework ensure that the aspirations and capabilities of the person are foregrounded, even when working in settings with acute, rehabilitative or other foci. At times therapeutic work requires the occupational therapist to seek out approaches of specific relevance to the worldview of the consumer. For example, the Kawa Model (Iwama, Thomson, & Macdonald, 2009) conceptualises life as a flowing river and impairments and barriers as elements to be negotiated which may influence the river's flow and direction over the lifespan. This view of health and adversity may be more congruent with the universalising, life-course experience of individuals with, for example, mental health or relapsing–remitting conditions.

Selecting Frames of Reference

Person-centred practice means that occupational therapists must start from the conceptualisation of person, occupation and environment. Astute practitioners will also recognise the impact of societal context and practice context as important influences. Occupational therapists can select models, theories and approaches that deliver person-centred practice and manage the pragmatic constraints that societal and practice contexts may create. When occupational therapists choose one or more theories, models or approaches, they are constructing *a frame of reference* or lens through which to view and work with the consumer. For Ricky, Heather and Peter, the following frames of reference were considered:

- Ricky describes many negative experiences with medical or rehabilitation approaches. In Ricky's experience, professionals value recovery and 'trying harder', and this is problematic when the trajectory of chronic illness does

not fit with the linear progression that is often the focus in many rehabilitation services. She also noted a tension between independence (as valued by health professionals) and her own version of independence, which she referred to as, 'My bossing, and someone else's hands'. Ricky based her service decisions around whether she was supported in her decisions around independence versus energy conservation in self-care activities. A frame of reference comprising approaches which supports individual autonomy and self-efficacy, such as chronic disease self-management and self-direction, are more likely to meet Ricky's needs.

- Heather greatly values her independence and control, yet a feature of deafblindness is the lack of experiential knowledge of what is possible without direction from practitioners and others. Useful theoretical constructs for Heather then include occupational deprivation theory, to guide and inform a rights-based plan for occupational enrichment, as well as adult learner approaches to build iterative knowledge capital for Heather to make informed choices and decisions.

- The experience of Peter and others who have had polio is embedded in the medical model. However, the postpolio community have been cautious regarding the rehabilitation approaches as they consider these approaches to be inappropriate for people with postpolio syndrome. Peter explains his experience and his preferred approach: 'My experience of the late effects of polio (LEoP) is that physical deterioration is from overuse, not a sedentary lifestyle. For many polio patients, a program of healthy movement may have far greater and longer benefits than load bearing or repetitive movement. This has been my experience. My use of bracing, sticks, powered wheels and respiratory support has lessened the load on weakened muscles, reduced pain, and enabled me to become more active. I believe more permanent benefits are likely to be a result of healthy weight management, supported movement, use of assistive technology, an accessible environment and avoiding fatigue from overuse'. Useful theoretical lenses for working with Peter include life course approaches and the collaborative application of daily living skills, including self-help–based work simplification, energy conservation, occupational balance and relaxation strategies.

PRACTICE STORY 43.1

Ricky

Ricky is a young blogger, and web designer and has a chronic illness. Ricky is a systemic advocate, that is, a self-advocate who also works towards improving systems for others.

Body structures and functions: Ricky has several severe metabolic/systemic disorders that became incapacitating

during her university years. Orthostatic intolerance and hyper-mobile joints mean Ricky spends most of her time in bed in a supine position and makes some short trips in her reclined power wheelchair. Ricky experiences severe fatigue, sensory sensitivity (vision and hearing) and fluctuating

PRACTICE STORY 43.1

Ricky (Continued)

cognitive issues, such as word finding and concentration difficulties. Her hand dexterity is unaffected but her fluctuating systemic functioning means she fatigues quickly and experiences overuse symptoms when typing on her computer keyboard or hand sewing for moderate periods.

Activities and participation: Ricky actively seeks opportunities, within her limited physical capacity and occupationally deprived environment, to engage with the world. Ricky fosters cats in need of socialising and enjoys growing and tending many climbing plants. She builds meaning through her online contacts and takes every opportunity to read, learn and engage with the world via small engagements and projects (e.g. craft projects and organising feed for the birds outside her window). Before her illness Ricky studied computer science. Ricky retains strong interests in artificial intelligence research, languages and assistive technology (AT). She actively engages in online dialogue and system advocacy regarding disability and human rights issues.

Environments: After a period of homelessness, Ricky was placed on the ground floor of an inner city Ministry of Housing flat, 45 minutes from her family and far from the semirural, outer suburban area in which she grew up. Her physical environment comprises an electrically adjustable bed in the living room, with a view of the hallway and living room window. The flat is wheelchair accessible but circulation spaces are too narrow for the bed to be moved into any other rooms. A wall between the living room and the kitchen prevents Ricky from viewing the kitchen or participating in kitchen-related activities, including supervising her support workers. Ricky runs her part-time web design business from her bed and is an active member of virtual communities using a combination of mainstream technologies, such as an Apple Mac computer, iPhone and large high-definition computer screen, and assistive technologies, such as a computer monitor stand attached to the hospital bed and foam postural supports for positioning. (Fig. 43.7)

OCCUPATIONAL GOALS

Ricky wishes to maintain and extend her participation in virtual communities. She wants to spend less time and energy negotiating and navigating through different funding bodies and services and to participate in more formal education. She wishes to have some choice over where she lives and to be in closer proximity to family and friends to increase the ease with which they can visit. The Canadian Practice Process Framework (CPPF) example shown here outlines occupational therapy intervention for the goal of information and communication technology performance.

The application of the CPPF with Ricky can be found in Table 43.5.

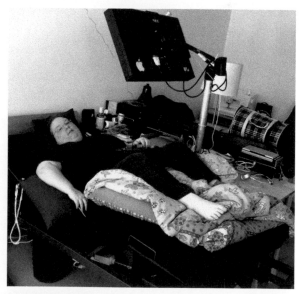

FIG. 43.7 ■ Ricky with her information and communication technology set up around her bed.

TABLE 43.5	
Application of the Canadian Practice Process Framework with Ricky	
Action Stages of the Canadian Practice Process Framework	**Application of the CPPF to Address Ricky's Assistive Technology Requirements**
Action Point 1: Enter/initiate and	Ricky was referred to ComTEC Yooralla (an independent nonprofit assistive technology consultancy service).
Action Point 2: Set the stage	In addition to completing the standard information form required by ComTEC, Ricky provided a comprehensive written summary of her AT system and vision for what was needed. This demonstrated her depth of knowledge of technology and spoke from the outset of her right to seek equality and respect from the relationship between her and the consultant occupational therapist.

Continued on following page

PRACTICE STORY 43.1

Ricky (Continued)

TABLE 43.5
Application of the Canadian Practice Process Framework with Ricky (Continued)

Action Stages of the Canadian Practice Process Framework	Application of the CPPF to Address Ricky's Assistive Technology Requirements
	The occupational therapist conducted the initial session on site at Ricky's unit, as Ricky's sitting tolerance, fatigue and postural hypotension meant travelling to ComTEC was not possible. Ricky was informed of the basic structure of the session (discussion, trial and formulate a plan) and informed that she could take a pause or even reschedule if she felt unwell at any point.
	Having the session at Ricky's home further established equality and allowed the occupational therapist to observe the context for Ricky's home-based technology-related occupations.
	Initial active listening and validation by the occupational therapist led to a shared awareness and appreciation of Ricky's unique requirements as an expert user of AT, and her desire to collaborate on equal terms was established. As evidence of emerging trust, Ricky disclosed instances of prior discrimination by health professionals, attributing these to the lack of a formal diagnosis of her condition. She also shared her frustration at the lack of technical knowledge of some health professionals and her experiences of inequality arising out of hospital-based services.
Action Point 3: Assess/evaluate	Information in the referral was reviewed together and feedback sought as to its perceived currency and accuracy. Ricky demonstrated her AT use to the occupational therapist.
	Initial consideration was given to the possibility of integrating system components (i.e. integrated AT where one device can encompass multiple purposes to enhance efficiency of access ('reward for effort' equation) and potentially reduce costs of the system over the longer term.
	New AT options that the occupational therapist brought to the session were explored and trialled briefly. Key features of the AT options were highlighted in language appropriate to Ricky's level of experience and expertise and level of alertness at the time. Task analysis encompassed Ricky's physical, sensory and cognitive interactions with the equipment in the proposed environment of use (Ricky's bedroom/living area), and Ricky's observations as she explored each AT option were sought and noted.
	The occupational therapist talked through his observations of relevant environmental influencers and constraints and sought confirmation of these with Ricky. The availability of support to assist with the setup of the system, as well as potential requirements for maintenance and troubleshooting (technical support), were identified as key considerations.
Action Point 4: Agree on objectives, plan	Based on the assessment outcomes, Ricky and the occupational therapist determined the following objectives and priorities of Ricky's proposed system requirements:
	■ Maintain and develop online relationships with friends, colleagues and health and other professionals via efficient and effective computer access (keyboard and mouse option that permits Ricky to work comfortably for required duration).
	■ Independently set and edit alarms, voice reminders, and calendar entries on computer and phone as these can assist in compensating for intermittent difficulties with recall and information retention.
	■ Take notes during phone conversations.
	■ Use phone in speaker phone mode (possibility of portable voice amplification system).
	■ Access to entertainment (stored locally on disc & drive; online via streaming services).
	■ Establish home automation control of lights, TV, stereo and DVD.
	An action plan was developed that focused on trialling AT systems to meet the objectives and priorities.
	One option included trialling alternative ergonomic keyboards. The occupational therapist discussed funding options for the AT along with the time frame involved in arranging the trial of the options.

PRACTICE STORY 43.1

Ricky (Continued)

TABLE 43.5

Application of the Canadian Practice Process Framework with Ricky (Continued)

Action Stages of the Canadian Practice Process Framework	Application of the CPPF to Address Ricky's Assistive Technology Requirements
	Ricky and the occupational therapist also determined an evaluation criteria of equipment trial that took into account the variability in Ricky's symptoms. It was decided that AT options would need to be on loan for at least 1 month for Ricky to be able to decide if they were suitable. It was also decided that as the various components were to be used as part of a system, the trial equipment was to be used concurrently rather than sequentially, even though at times it might have been preferred to trial AT options individually.
	The occupational therapist investigated funding options for the AT options (e.g. an Apple trackpad and X-Keys software and the ergonomic keyboard) assuming a successful trial is attained.
	The occupational therapist also further explored and evaluated both mainstream and purpose-built smart device–based reminder and calendaring apps and shared his findings with Ricky.
Action Point 5: Implement plan	The occupational therapist facilitated the trial of ergonomic keyboard, programmable number pad and portable voice amplifier by liaising with known specialist equipment suppliers, while respecting Ricky's rights to privacy and confidentiality and only disclosing the minimum required information to allow the trials to proceed.
	Once the equipment arrived, training was provided for Ricky and regular visiting support staff of her choice in the operational features of the system, including setup and positioning of trial items. The use of photographs and written instructions were employed to supplement verbal instructions. Ricky and staff were encouraged to call or email the occupational therapist with concerns or queries should they arise during the trial period.
	Ricky was encouraged to maintain a log of her comfort levels and duration of use when interacting with the equipment during the trial phase. Ricky used her smartphone to take notes and record observations.
Action Point 6: Monitor/modify and Action Point 7: Evaluate outcome	A 1-month trial of options was completed and a follow-up call was made to evaluate progress.
	Ricky reported that she found the split keyboard heavy when she was fatigued and that moving it in and out of the position of use (over her abdomen) caused pain in her left thumb. She provided a digital image via email of the thumb position when she relocated the keyboard and it was visibly hyperextended at the CMC joint. An alternative fully split tethered keyboard was suggested as this was lighter and could also allow her to type with her arms fully supported by her sides in bed. A trial of this was proposed to Ricky and she agreed to continue the exploration process.
	Ricky reported that she found setting up the voice amplifier cumbersome. She had independently located a simple and inexpensive phone mount online that positioned her phone close enough so the speaker on the phone could be used. An update to the operating system of the phone allowed her to use full hands-free mode for voice dialling of her contacts, which further reduced the effort involved in operating her phone.
	A programmable number pad was effective in allowing her to activate frequently required functions with prestored shortcuts, and Ricky reported she had already added to those initially programmed, demonstrating her competence and ownership of this component of her computer access system.
Action Point 8: Conclude/exit	During a subsequent planned follow-up call, Ricky reported that the second keyboard trial was successful.

Continued on following page

PRACTICE STORY 43.1

Ricky (Continued)

TABLE 43.5
Application of the Canadian Practice Process Framework with Ricky (Continued)

Action Stages of the Canadian Practice Process Framework	Application of the CPPF to Address Ricky's Assistive Technology Requirements
	Funding for the system components was obtained from a philanthropic grant. The components were purchased and provided under a long-term loan scheme. Several months later Ricky reported that an operating system update on her Apple computer caused an issue with the keyboard. ComTEC Technical Support Officer contacted the manufacturer and a firmware update was issued and installed to fix the issue.
	Ricky and the occupational therapist agreed that this phase of the process was complete.

AT, Assistive Technology; *CPPF,* Canadian Practice Process Framework.
This practice story was provided by Ricky Buchanan and David Harraway, an occupational therapist with ComTEC Yooralla at the time of writing.

PRACTICE STORY 43.2

Heather

Activities and participation: Heather is independent, artistic and a lover of cats. Living alone without hearing or sight, Heather is an active self-advocate in the deafblind community.

Body structures and functions: Heather is a woman in her 50s who has Ushers syndrome, a genetic disorder affecting her hearing and sight. She has lived with complete deafness all her life, and lost her sight in her 20s. Heather explains, 'Being Deafblind is very difficult and isolating and I am always determined to make my life the best as I can'.

Participation: Heather's ability to participate in most activities is facilitated through computer-based communication or tactile communication with another person. She works hard to structure her days and her weeks. Heather requires support workers or *communication guides* to be skilled in tactile communication techniques. Heather elects to use some of her limited personal support hours to enable her to swim and she feels 'fantastic after that'. She also uses her support worker hours for more basic needs; she provides the example of using her support worker to 'cancel swimming, to make contact calls [and to read] snail mail if it doesn't come through email'.

Environment: Heather receives approximately 25 hours per week of specialised support and 5 hours per week of council home care and lives independently in the company of her cat, in a house purchased with support through a housing association. Heather's combination of mainstream and adaptive technology, as well as extensive soft technology (training across environments), enables her to meet a range of life goals (mapped across education, community, civic and social areas of the ICF). Simple labelling procedures at home such as Hi Mark (a tube

of quick-hardening raised putty) on the microwave and washing machine and Dymo Braille tape or magnets on food ingredients, enable Heather to manage her domestic life. As the world around is tangible only through touch and smell, vibrating alerts (e.g. clock, doorbell, smoke alarm, vibrating pager with four different alerts for phone) and tactile input via human or via computer, are the ways in which Heather can receive and impart communication. Emerging technologies such as the use of an iPhone with a Braille app connected to a refreshable Braille device enables Heather to, for example, use Facebook to connect with others. The known environs are easily managed by Heather, who is familiar with her dwelling, able to walk around the block with a white cane and perform transactions at known shops, and able to take the train to the city independently. Crossroads and unfamiliar terrain, especially if uneven and with poor tactile signage, present barriers. AT such as the Mini-Guide (a vibrating alert which detects objects in vicinity) helps Heather to identify barriers such as traffic but does not help her to negotiate these barriers.

Occupational goals: Heather values 'regularity and personal activity; in her life and longs to be more active, stating 'I don't need any help for showers or things like that [...] I have my shower, eat my breakfast, open the computer to see if I've received any emails [...,] go outside and check the weather. All though the day [...] sometimes I'm quite bored, I put the computer on and I'm backwards and forwards checking for emails, I play with the cat, I do many laps of the block with my white cane'. The application of the Canadian Practice Process Framework with Heather's use of AT to enhance leisure and creativity options can be found in Table 43.6.

PRACTICE STORY 43.2

Heather (Continued)

	TABLE 43.6
	Application of the Canadian Practice Process Framework with Heather

Action Stages of the Canadian Practice Process Framework	Application of the CPPF to Address Heather's Leisure Objectives
Action Point 1: Enter/initiate and Action Point 2: Set the stage	Heather identified herself as a creative person and wished to enrich and fill her time. Heather essentially lived in a state of occupational deprivation because of her profound sensory losses. The primary absence of visual and auditory inputs was compounded by the secondary loss of incidental communication and environmental feedback. These losses resulted in significant activity and participation restrictions. A key strategy for Heather was her involvement in the deafblind self-advocacy movement. As well as teaching the community about deafblindness, this group met regularly for leisure activities. It was in this context that Heather sought to engage in art and craft.
Action Point 3: Assess/evaluate	Heather had successfully constructed and given characters and backstories to a range of hand puppets for use in video storytelling. Heather wished to extend her repertoire and described her passions for animals and her childhood love of drawing and creating.
Action Point 4: Agree on objectives, plan	Heather's objective was to reengage with drawing as a meaningful recreation. Heather described how she used to draw despite her vision loss, using her fingers to track her drawing progress, but being unable to see the final result. To achieve this objective, activity analysis and task adaptation was undertaken so that the occupation of drawing could occur in a way that used Heather's capabilities despite her sensory losses.
Action Point 5: Implement plan	As Heather and her colleagues within the deafblind advocacy group met regularly, enjoyed socialising and had similar needs and objectives, several sessions were planned for the group in a sunny courtyard with tables and seating, as well as a wet area. Clay tablets with a range of stylus tools were introduced. Carving into the tablets was demonstrated with hand-over-hand techniques, and participants were encouraged to experiment with the material and the effect of the different stylus tools (Fig. 43.8). They were also encouraged to share their results through tactile contact with each other's work.
Action Point 6: Monitor/modify and Action Point 7: Evaluate outcome	Mastery was gained over several sessions. Heather created two key pieces: one was a profile of a dog, and another, the interlinking images of hands. Heather explained the strong visual image she had of the dog which she had drawn, and her delight in being able to feel the outline she had created in the clay. The interlinking hands were a strong symbol of tactile communication and connectivity; other group members used similar image metaphors, such as fences and linked chains. In addition to producing artworks, the occupational engagement enjoyed by Heather and the group was significantly enriched as a shared experience and provided opportunities for deep and important connection to themes that mattered to these individuals.

AT, Assistive Technology; *CPPF,* Canadian Practice Process Framework.

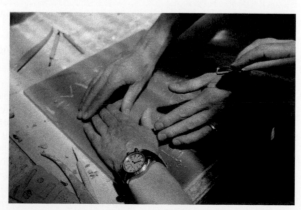

FIG. 43.8 ■ Heather learning to draw in clay. *(Image courtesy Self-Advocacy Resource Unit.)*

PRACTICE STORY 43.3

Peter

Peter is a retired bookseller, parent and highly dedicated volunteer who has lived with the effects of polio since he was 4 years old.

Body structures and functions: Peter is 65 years of age. He is a tall man who is approaching 100 kg in weight. He recently retired from work because of the effects of postpolio syndrome. Peter states that his capacity is limited by shortness of breath, difficulty exhaling, fatigue, loss of muscle strength in arms and legs, and previous back and left shoulder injuries. He can walk around his home and garden with bilateral knee-ankle-foot orthoses and a single-point stick. However, if he walks for more than 5 minutes he is severely affected by fatigue, twitching or fasciculation and cognitive difficulties.

Activities and participation: Peter is a writer. He is currently researching postpolio syndrome and its management from a consumer perspective. He is active in systemic advocacy through consumer groups. For 6 months Peter attended counselling to come to terms with his life changes; currently Peter describes a high level of reward from his community visits to people in nursing homes, and running the local polio network. He has applied for a disability support pension and self-funded his scooter last year.

Environment: Peter lives in an unrenovated brick single-storey dwelling in need of some maintenance, with his wife and young adult children. Only minimal modifications have been performed on Peter's home. Peter stated, 'When I knew this was happening I put the bricks out the back [forming level access around the house to the back entrance], and a single handrail adjacent to shower-overbath, but no alteration to the single step at front patio'. Peter is not in a position to purchase many of the major items of assistive technology that would minimise his capability gap, including improved respiratory equipment and an extensive home renovation. Peter currently uses AT such as a pickup stick around the house and a continuous positive airways pressure machine overnight.

Occupational goals: Peter is planning to demolish his home and build two smaller units on the block, both accessible, one for resale and one as the family home. He has found that the powered scooter does not provide the flexibility to traverse indoor areas and cannot be transported easily in a vehicle. As Peter's walking speed, endurance and balance change, he wishes to find a better way to mobilise and replace his walking.

The application of the Canadian Practice Process Framework with Peter can be found in Table 43.7.

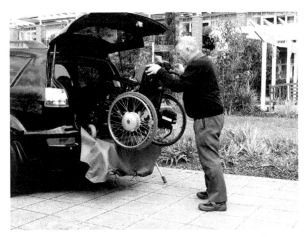

FIG. 43.9 ■ Peter putting his lightweight powerchair in the car.

TABLE 43.7	
Application of the Canadian Practice Process Framework with Peter	
Action Stages of the Canadian Practice Process Framework	**Application of the CPPF to Address Peter's Assistive Technology Requirements**
Action Point 1: Enter/initiate and Action Point 2: Set the stage	As a retiree living with the late effects of polio, Peter was planning for a likely change from ambulation with bilateral callipers to powered mobility. Peter researched his options online, with the local Independent Living Centre and with several AT suppliers. Through these actions Peter became informed as to what options were on the market, and he was able to identify that a powered wheelchair rather than a scooter or any other type of wheeled mobility device would meet his needs. Peter was aware that he was the 'expert in his own condition', but identified a need for professional input regarding fitting an AT device to his current and future physical capacities and his lifestyle as well as impartial advice as to AT device performance in his environments of use – in other words, he was seeking advice on ensuring a fit between the powered wheelchair and the person–environment–occupation.

PRACTICE STORY 43.3

Peter (Continued)

TABLE 43.7

Application of the Canadian Practice Process Framework with Peter *(Continued)*

Action Stages of the Canadian Practice Process Framework	Application of the CPPF to Address Peter's Assistive Technology Requirements
Action Point 3: Assess/evaluate	Peter elected to collaborate with an occupational therapist specialising in polio, who was familiar with the progressive nature of his impairment as well as its contraindications. The occupational therapist met with Peter at his home, and evaluated his home environment, using person-centred planning principles to elicit Peter's occupational goals. Peter wanted to be able to move around his home and neighbourhood and continue his community visits to residents in a nursing home. He wanted the powered wheelchair to be able to manage gutters, tram tracks and some grassy terrain and to have a range of at least 10 km. As Peter was currently writing a book and intended to visit a range of libraries and archives, he also required the powered wheelchair to be taken on public transport. Finally, Peter intended to be able to transport the AT device in the boot of his car when he travelled.
	The occupational therapist's lens was influenced by her knowledge of the difficulty of obtaining funding and the need for the recommended device to meet Peter's needs for 3–5 years. The occupational therapist was also mindful of the progressive nature of postpolio syndrome and hence of the need to ensure the wheelchair would be still be suitable for Peter in 3–5 years (e.g. it was possible that Peter would require postural trunk supports, and the occupational therapist felt that it was important that these supports could be added to the wheelchair in the future if required).
	Peter's perspective was somewhat different. He still drove a car and had been using a powered scooter; thus he envisaged a wheelchair that was flexible enough to be pushed, dismantled, travel over unknown terrain and be used on public transport.
Action Point 4: Agree on objectives, plan	In light of Peter's extensive community mobility goals (travelling to archives and libraries where access is unsure, and using public transport as well as driving), Peter and the occupational therapist explored the compromise between seating integrity and the option to dismantle the wheelchair. This resulted in the selection of a folding powerchair that was able to be transported in vehicles.
Action Point 5: Implement plan	The occupational therapist discussed the options Peter had previously found during his research and did some additional research to establish which of the available powered wheelchairs that had suitable features would be eligible for funding. The number of wheelchairs trialled, and the schedule of trials, was influenced by Peter's fatigue (one per week, in the mornings) and the availability of the occupational therapist. Appointments were made with AT suppliers who provided powerchairs for trials. Each device was set up and Peter was trained in its use. Peter and the occupational therapist evaluated the performance of the powered wheelchairs on a similar 'circuit' for comparison. Peter then trialled each chair for a few days.
	After the trial periods, the preferred options were discussed by telephone, and the occupational therapist put in a funding application. A wait list of 18 months was experienced. Once Peter reached the top of the list, a further occupational therapy home assessment was conducted to ensure the features of the powered wheelchair remained suitable and reviewed the newer models that have become available. The powered wheelchair was then purchased and delivered.
Action Point 6: Monitor/modify and Action Point 7: Evaluate outcome	Peter was delighted to take delivery of the powerchair. Over the next 3 weeks, Peter identified that the castors provided were too small to cope with train track crossings. Peter discussed this with the occupational therapist over the phone, and they decided to trial a larger set, mindful that this would affect the size of the turning circle. Peter funded this alteration himself, as it was quicker than waiting for the funding body to consider and approve this change.

Continued on following page

PRACTICE STORY 43.3

Peter (Continued)

TABLE 43.7	
Application of the Canadian Practice Process Framework with Peter (Continued)	
Action Stages of the Canadian Practice Process Framework	**Application of the CPPF to Address Peter's Assistive Technology Requirements**
	To tailor the situation still further, Peter wanted to explore alternatives to dismantling the power wheelchair to lift into the boot, which, although feasible, was physically tiring and time consuming. Although Peter was still physically able to dismantle and lift the wheelchair components into the boot of his car, the 18-month wait had seen deterioration in his physical capacity and endurance. Peter reviewed alternative vehicle apertures and found that a second-hand stationwagon enabled him to merely fold the backrest, tilt the front wheels off the ground and push the chair in (Fig. 43.9).
Action Point 8: Conclude/exit	Peter was satisfied that he had a device that met his self-identified occupational performance outcome.
	The occupational therapist anticipated that the folding powerchair offered less stability and suspension than a rigid-framed wheelchair and noted that a rigid wheelchair with folding accessories, along with an appropriate vehicle, may have been a better selection. The occupational therapist reflected that at the time of the assessment Peter was not prepared to alter his goals and change the car that he was driving, particularly as vehicle choices such as vans were not 'family friendly'. The occupational therapist felt that Peter had been supported in his choice and that this choice was made after a thorough assessment and trial.
	After Peter had received the powered wheelchair, the occupational therapist did recommend a drop-in postural seat and backrest that would provide Peter with better support than the standard seat and backrest that came with the wheelchair, and Peter accepted this recommendation.

AT, Assistive Technology; *CPPF*, Canadian Practice Process Framework.

CONCLUSION

The assessment and prescription of assistive technologies are a key intervention used by occupational therapists to enable occupation. Occupational therapists are uniquely placed to deliver AT interventions because of their professional reasoning capabilities and their understanding of the person–environment–occupation fit. The challenges for practitioners working with AT include keeping up with the rapid diversification of AT devices and design paradigms and managing the sociopolitical factors that influence AT supply and practice. Occupational therapists working in the field of assistive technology, as in many other fields of practice, are encouraged to enact systemic advocacy roles in achieving the best possible outcomes with and for people with impairment. Strategies to do this include adhering to best practice principles for occupational therapy practice and AT service delivery, using key frameworks such as the WHO ICF and the UN Convention on the Rights of Persons with Disabilities to articulate and document practice, and contributing to the evidence base for AT as an intervention.

 http://evolve.elsevier.com/Curtin/OT

REFERENCES

Association for the Advancement of Assistive Technology in Europe. (2012). *Service delivery systems for assistive technology in Europe: Position paper.* Retrieved from, http://www.atis4all.eu/news/detail.aspx?id=406&tipo=1.

Albrecht, G., Seelman, K., & Bury, M. (Eds.). (2001). *Handbook of disability studies.* Thousand Oaks, CA: SAGE.

Andrich, R. (2002). The SCAI instrument: Measuring costs of individual assistive technology programmes. *Technology and Disability,* 14, 95–99.

Australian Rehabilitation and Assistive Technology Association. (2012). *The ARATA 'Making a difference with AT' papers. Silvan: Australian Rehabilitation and Assistive Technology Association.* Retrieved from https://www.arata.org.au/download/NDIS/fullbkgndpapers_v10int.pdf.

Barbara, A., & Curtin, M. (2008). Gatekeepers or advocates? Occupational therapists and equipment funding schemes. *Australian Occupational Therapy Journal,* 55(1), 57–60.

Bickenbach, J., Chatterji, S., Bradley, E., & Ustun, T. (1999). Models of Disablement, Universalism and the International Classification of Impairments, Disabilities and Handicaps. *Social Science and Medicine,* 48, 1173–1187.

Carrier, A., Levasseur, M., & Mullins, G. (2010). Accessibility of occupational therapy community services: A legal, ethical, and clinical analysis. *Occupational Therapy in Health Care, 24*(4), 360–376.

Cook, A., & Hussey, S. (Eds.). (2008). *Assistive technologies: Principles and practice.* St. Louis: Mosby Elsevier. Vol. 3.

Cook, A., & Polgar, J. (2008). *Cook & Hussey's assistive technologies: Principles and practice* (3rd ed.). St. Louis: Mosby.

De Jonge, D., Layton, N., Vicary, F., & Steel, E. (2015). Motivations and incentives: exploring assistive technology service delivery from the perspectives of multiple stakeholders. Paper presented at the RESNA 2015: New Frontiers in Assistive Technology, Arlington, VA.

Demers, L., Weiss-Lambrou, R., & Ska, B. (2002). The Quebec User Evaluation of Satisfaction with Assistive Technology (QUEST 2.0): An overview and recent progress. *Technology and Disability, 14.*

Dong, H. (2007). Shifting paradigms in universal design. In C. Stephanidis (Ed.), *Universal access in human computer interaction: Coping with diversity* (pp. 66–74). Berlin: Springer-Verlag.

Fagerberg, G. (2011). From HEART to date. *Technology and Disability, 23,* 183–189.

Guay, M., Dubois, M., Desrosiers, J., & Robitaille, J. (2012). Identifying characteristics of 'straightforward cases' for which support personnel could recommend home bathing equipment. *British Journal of Occupational Therapy, 75*(12), 563–569.

Hansson, S. O. (2007). The ethics of enabling technology. *Cambridge Quarterly of Healthcare Ethics, 16,* 257–267.

Hobbs, D., Close, J., Downing, A., Reynolds, K., & Walker, L. (2009). Developing a national research and development centre in assistive technologies for independent living. *Australian Health Review, 33*(1), 152–160.

Hocking, C. (1999). Function or feelings: Factors in abandonment of assistive devices. *Technology and Disability, 11,* 3–11.

Imrie, R., & Hall, P. (2001). *Inclusive design: Designing and developing accessible environments.* London & New York: Spon Press.

International Organization for Standardization. (2016). *Assistive products for persons with disability — Classification and terminology.* Geneva: International Organisation for Standardisation.

Iwama, M., Thomson, N., & Macdonald, R. (2009). The Kawa model: The power of culturally responsive occupational therapy. *Disability and Rehabilitation, 31*(14), 1125–1135.

Jutai, J., & Day, H. (2002). Psychosocial Impact of Assistive Devices Scale (PIADS). *Technology and Disability, 14,* 107–111.

Kayes, N., & McPherson, K. (2012). Human technologies in rehabilitation: 'Who' and 'how' we are with our clients. *Disability & Rehabilitation, 34*(22), 1907–1911.

Law, M., Cooper, B., Stewart, D., Rigby, P., & Letts, L. (1996). The Person-Environment-Occupation Model: A transactive approach to occupational performance. *Canadian Journal of Occupational Therapy, 63,* 9–23.

Layton, N. (2014). *Assistive technology solutions as mediators of equal outcomes for people living with disability* (Doctor of Philosophy). Burwood, Victoria: Deakin University. Retrieved from, *http://dro. deakin.edu.au/eserv/DU:30067351/layton-assistive-2014A.pdf.*

Layton, N., Wilson, E., & Andrews, A. (2014). *Pathways to non complex assistive technology for HACC clients in WA.* Perth: Independent Living Centre of WA. *Retrieved from,* http://ilc.com.au/wp-content/uploads/2009/08/Full-Report-Pathways-to-Non-Complex-Assistive-Technology-for-HACC-Clients1.pdf.

Layton, N., Wilson, E., Colgan, S., Moodie, M., & Carter, R. (2010). *The equipping inclusion studies: Assistive technology use and outcomes in Victoria.* Burwood: Deakin University. *Retrieved from,* http://dro.deakin.edu.au/view/DU:30030938.

Masso, M., Owen, A., Stevermuer, T., Williams, K., & Eager, K. (2008). Assessment of need and capacity to benefit for people with a disability requiring aids, appliances and equipment. *Australian Occupational Therapy Journal, 56*(5), 315–323.

McDonald, R. (2010). Wheelchairs: posture and mobility. In M. M. Curtin, J. Supyk-Melton (Eds.), *Occupational Therapy and Physical Dysfunction* (6 ed., pp. 472–473). Elsevier.

Nussbaum, M. (2011). *Creating capabilities: The human development approach.* Boston: Harvard University Press.

Odor, P. (1984). Hard and soft technology for education and communication for disabled people. *Proceedings International Computer Conference.* Perth, Australia.

Patston, P. (2007). Constructive functional diversity. A new paradigm beyond disability and impairment. *Disability & Rehabilitation, 29*(20-21), 1625–1633.

Polatajko, H. J., Townsend, E. A., & Craik, J. (2007). The Canadian Model of Occupational Performance and Engagement (CMOP-E). In E. A. Townsend, & H. J. Polatajko (Eds.), *Enabling Occupation II: Advancing an occupational therapy vision of health, well-being, & justice through occupation* (pp. 22–36). Ottawa: CAOT Publications ACE.

Pollard, N., Sakellariou, D., & Kronenberg, F. (Eds.), (2008). *A political practice of occupational therapy.* Philadelphia: Churchill Livingstone Elsevier.

Rioux, M., Basser, L. A., & Jones, M. (Eds.), (2011). *Critical perspectives on human rights and disability law.* Leiden, Boston: Martinus Nijhoff Publishers.

Ripat, J., & Booth, A. (2005). Characteristics of assistive technology service delivery models: Stakeholder perspectives and preferences. *Disability and Rehabilitation, 27*(24), 1461–1470.

Rist, P., Freas, D., Maislin, G., & Stineman, M. (2008). Recovery from Disablement: What functional abilities to rehabilitation professionals value the most? *Archives of Physical Medicine and Rehabilitation, 89,* 1600–1606.

Rust, K., & Smith, R. (2005). Assistive technology in the measurement of rehabilitation and health outcomes: A review and analysis of instruments. *American Journal of Physical Medicine and Rehabilitation, 84*(10), 780–793.

Scherer, M. (1998). *The Scherer Milieu-Person-Technology Model: Matching people with technologies.* New York: Webster.

Scherer, M. (2002). *Policy issues in evaluating and selecting assistive technology and other resources for persons with disabilities.* Paper presented at the Bridging Gaps: Refining the Disability Research Agenda for Rehabilitation and the Social Sciences. Washington: DC.

Scherer, M. (2012). *Assistive technologies and other supports for people with brain impairment.* New York: Springer.

Scherer, M., & Gluekauf, R. (2005). Assessing the benefits of assistive technologies for activities and participation. *Rehabilitation Psychology, 50*(2), 132–141.

Scherer, M., & Sax, C. (2009). Measures of assistive technology predisposition and use. In E. Mpofu, & T. Oakland (Eds.), *Rehabilitation and health assessment.* New York: Springer.

Sen, A. (1999). *Development as freedom.* Oxford, UK: Oxford University Press.

Shakespeare, T. (2008). Disability: Suffering, social oppression, or complex predicament? In D. M. C. Rehmann-Sutter, & D. Mieth (Eds.), *The contingent nature of life: Bioethics and limits of human existence* (pp. 235–246). Netherlands: Springer.

Smith, R. O. (2002). *IMPACT 2 MODEL. Retrieved from,* http://www.r2d2.uwm.edu/archive/impact2model.html.

Smith, R. O., & Benge, M. (2004). Using assistive technology to enable better living. In C. H. Christiansen, & K. M. Matuska (Eds.), *Ways of living: Adaptive strategies for special needs* (3rd ed., pp. 397–421). Bethesda, MD: AOTA Press.

Steinfeld, E. (2010). Advancing universal design. In J. L. Maisel (Ed.), *The state of the science in universal design: Emerging research and developments* (pp. 1–19). Buffalo, NY: State University of New York at Buffalo, Bentham Sciences Publishers.

Steinfeld, E., & Danford, S. (2006). *Universal design and the ICF. In: Living in Our Environment: The Promise of ICF Conference in Vancouver, June 4-5, 2006.* Retrieved from, http://www.icfconference.com/New%20Presentations/ICF%20Presentation%20Notes.pdf.

Swain, J., French, S., Barnes, C., & Thomas, C. (Eds.). (2004). *Disabling barriers Enabling environments* (2nd ed.). London: SAGE Publications.

Uniform Data System (1999). *About the FIM system. Retrieved from,* http://www.udsmr.org/WebModules/FIM/Fim_About.aspx.

United Nations. (2006). *Convention on the rights of persons with disabilities and optional protocol. Retrieved from,* http://www.un.org/disabilities/convention/conventionfull.shtml.

Unsworth, C. (2004). Clinical reasoning: How do pragmatic reasoning, worldview and client-centredness fit? *British Journal of Occupational Therapy, 67*(1), 10–19.

Wessels, R., Djicks, B., Soede, M., Gelderblom, G. J., & Witte, L. D. (2003). Non-use of provided assistive technology devices, a literature overview. *Technology and Disability, 15,* .

Wessels, R., Persson, J., Lorentsen, O., et al. (2002). IPPA: Individually prioritised problem assessment. *Technology and Disability, 14,* 141–145.

Whalley Hammell, K. (2015). Quality of life, participation and occupational rights: A capabilities perspective. *Australian Occupational Therapy Journal, 62,* 78–85.

Wijk, M. (2001). The Dutch struggle for accessibility awareness. In W. F. Preiser, & E. Ostroff (Eds.), *Universal design handbook.* New York: McGraw-Hill.

World Health Organization. (2001). *International classification of functioning, disability and health: ICF.* Geneva: World Health Organization.

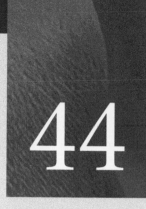

44 UNIVERSAL DESIGN

SHARON JOINES ■ ANDREW PAYNE

CHAPTER OUTLINE

Abstract
Universal design is a paradigm in which products, buildings
and outdoors spaces are created to be usable by all people.
Ultimately products and spaces that are universally designed
will support social integration of all people regardless of their
size, age or conditions affecting sight, hearing, cognition or
physical ability. Applications of universal design address personal needs in the home, in public and at work; the best
examples of universal design become invisible as a result
of their benefit and acceptance by all individuals. Universal
design is framed around seven principles: equitable use, flexibility in use, simple and intuitive use, perceptible information, tolerance for error, low physical effort and size and
space for approach and use. As a result of their training in
ability assessment, occupational therapists are strong candidates for home and work design modification consultants
and may benefit from implementing the universal design
principles in their daily practice.

KEY POINTS

- Universal design supports individuals with varied abilities and those in their social sphere with the need for

adaptation or special equipment. Universal design
promotes solutions that are useable, useful and desirable for all people.

- There are seven principles of universal design: equitable
use, flexibility in use, simple and intuitive use, perceptible information, tolerance for error, low physical effort
and size and space for approach and use.

- Universal design benefits individuals in private and
public spaces, using transportation, at work, at school,
during communications, and while travelling. Within
the home entrances, kitchens, and bathrooms are
considered the most critical areas in which principles
of universal design can be applied.

- Although universal design solutions evolve with
technology, are time sensitive and may be context
dependent, the best examples of universal design are
often invisible.

- Occupational therapists can play a major role in environment adaptation and product selection to support
individuals and those in their social sphere by considering the principles of universal design when making
recommendations.

671

INTRODUCTION

The concept of universal design has worldwide recognition and offers significant benefit to the occupational therapy profession. Universal design is a broad conceptual revision to traditional design practice where much of the environment and products contained therein are designed to the specifications of an 'average male' in the prime of life. This paradigm suggests it is possible to design products, buildings and exterior spaces intended to be usable by all, acknowledging that in specific cases some additional modifications may be necessary.

History of Universal Design

Universal design was defined by architect Ron Mace* as 'the design of products and environments to be usable by all people, to the greatest extent possible, without the need for adaptation or specialised design' (Mace, 1985). This paradigm of including people of all abilities in the intended population of users (Herwig, 2008; Jordan, 2008; Mace, 1985; Ostroff, 2011; Null, 2014; Story, 2011; U.S. Forest Service, 2007) of a product or environment is known by many names around the globe – inclusive design (Clarkson & Coleman, 2015; Nussbaumer, 2012), design for all (Bühler & Stephanidis, 2004), lifespan design (AIPatHome Staff, 2015; Beran, 2007) or barrier-free design (Herwig, 2008). Regardless of the term, universal design benefits people of all ages and abilities. At the Center for Universal Design (CUD), a group comprised of architects, product designers, engineers and environmental design researchers collaborated to establish a set of principles of universal design. The seven principles (Box 44.1) were intended to guide a wide range of design disciplines including those focused on environments, products and communications in order to make products and environments more usable (Connell et al., 1997).

As the global population experiences unprecedented and rapid aging (United Nations, 2001), the need for designs that accommodate a wide range of abilities continues to grow. This is underscored by the statistics documenting the increase in individuals living with age-related impairments and having difficulty with everyday tasks (Centers for Disease Control, National Center for Health Statistics, 2015; Erickson, Lees, & von Schrader, 2014). Thus universal design is more important than ever before and will remain relevant to good design in the coming decades.

Many designers and consumers have difficulty distinguishing between universal design and accessibility and are left wondering, if the law required accessible designs, why is universal design required? To understand the benefit of universal design beyond accessibility it is helpful to understand the difference between the two.

---

*Ron Mace was the founder and programme director of the Center for Universal Design at the College of Design at NC State University.

Differences Between Universal Design and Accessibility

The Americans with Disabilities Act (ADA) prohibits discrimination against people with disabilities in employment, transportation, public accommodation, communications, and governmental activities as well as establishing requirements for telecommunications relay services. Modelled after earlier laws prohibiting discrimination based on race and gender, the ADA focuses on requirement to meet the needs of individuals with disabilities in areas including mobility, stamina, sight, hearing, communication and learning. Five separate areas are addressed (Titles I–V, respectively): the workplace, state and local government services, public and commercial facilities, phone companies and miscellaneous instructions to federal law enforcement agencies. Clarification and reiteration of who is covered by the ADA was signed into law 28 September 2008 as an amendment and became effective 1 January 2009. Although the Architectural and Transportation Barriers Compliance Board, also known as the Access Board, issues guidelines to ensure that buildings, facilities and transit vehicles are accessible and usable by people with disabilities, enforcement of the ADA is spread across five federal agencies (U.S. Department of Labor, 2015):

■ Two agencies within the Department of Labor enforce portions of the ADA. The Office of Federal Contract Compliance Programs has coordinating authority under the employment-related provisions of the ADA. The Civil Rights Center is responsible for enforcing Title II of the ADA as it applies to the labour- and workforce-related practices of state and local governments and other public entities.

■ The Equal Employment Opportunity Commission enforces regulations covering employment.

■ The Department of Transportation enforces regulations governing transit.

■ The Federal Communications Commission enforces regulations covering telecommunication services.

■ The Department of Justice enforces regulations governing public accommodations and state and local government services.

Thus accessibility refers to and the ADA (and associated guidelines) defines the minimum requirements in order to not legally discriminate against those with disabilities. Universal design, focusing on including all people, is not codified, legislated or enforced. Universal design is pursued, the principles deployed and thought processes expanded to make designs usable by all people – to the extent possible. Thus a building designed with the entrance 60 cm above the ground level using a combination of steps and ramps provides ADA-compliant access to the building. The building is accessible; the building is not universally designed. A building designed with an entrance at ground level provides the same access to people who use wheelchairs as to those who can ambulate – this is universal design.

One of the challenges of the unobtrusive, inclusive nature of universal design is that the best examples become invisible and

BOX 44.1

THE PRINCIPLES OF UNIVERSAL DESIGN VERSION 2.0 – 4/1/97

PRINCIPLE ONE: EQUITABLE USE

The design is useful and marketable to people with diverse abilities.

Guidelines:
1a. Provide the same means of use for all users: identical whenever possible; equivalent when not.
1b. Avoid segregating or stigmatising any users.
1c. Provisions for privacy, security, and safety should be equally available to all users.
1d. Make the design appealing to all users.

PRINCIPLE TWO: FLEXIBILITY IN USE

The design accommodates a wide range of individual preferences and abilities.

Guidelines:
2a. Provide choice in methods of use.
2b. Accommodate right- or left-handed access and use.
2c. Facilitate the user's accuracy and precision.
2d. Provide adaptability to the user's pace.

PRINCIPLE THREE: SIMPLE AND INTUITIVE USE

Use of the design is easy to understand, regardless of the user's experience, knowledge, language skills, or current concentration level.

Guidelines:
3a. Eliminate unnecessary complexity.
3b. Be consistent with user expectations and intuition.
3c. Accommodate a wide range of literacy and language skills.
3d. Arrange information consistent with its importance.
3e. Provide effective prompting and feedback during and after task completion.

PRINCIPLE FOUR: PERCEPTIBLE INFORMATION

The design communicates necessary information effectively to the user, regardless of ambient conditions or the user's sensory abilities.

Guidelines:
4a. Use different modes (pictorial, verbal, tactile) for redundant presentation of essential information.
4b. Provide adequate contrast between essential information and its surroundings.
4c. Maximise 'legibility' of essential information.
4d. Differentiate elements in ways that can be described (i.e. make it easy to give instructions or directions).
4e. Provide compatibility with a variety of techniques or devices used by people with sensory limitations.

PRINCIPLE FIVE: TOLERANCE FOR ERROR

The design minimises hazards and the adverse consequences of accidental or unintended actions.

Guidelines:
5a. Arrange elements to minimise hazards and errors: most used elements, most accessible; hazardous elements eliminated, isolated, or shielded.
5b. Provide warnings of hazards and errors.
5c. Provide fail safe features.
5d. Discourage unconscious action in tasks that require vigilance.

PRINCIPLE SIX: LOW PHYSICAL EFFORT

The design can be used efficiently and comfortably and with a minimum of fatigue.

Guidelines:
6a. Allow user to maintain a neutral body position.
6b. Use reasonable operating forces.
6c. Minimise repetitive actions.
6d. Minimise sustained physical effort.

PRINCIPLE SEVEN: SIZE AND SPACE FOR APPROACH AND USE

Appropriate size and space is provided for approach, reach, manipulation, and use regardless of user's body size, posture, or mobility.

Guidelines:
7a. Provide a clear line of sight to important elements for any seated or standing user.
7b. Make reach to all components comfortable for any seated or standing user.
7c. Accommodate variations in hand and grip size.
7d. Provide adequate space for the use of assistive devices or personal assistance.

taken for granted, as illustrated by automatic doors. A ramp or curb cut is just as welcoming to a person pushing a baby stroller or rolling a briefcase as it is to someone using a wheelchair. In addition to being useful for those of varied levels of mobility, universal designs are intuitive and provide no difference in experience for individuals regardless of literacy level, first language or hearing ability. No one is stigmatised or inconvenienced by their use.

Although an individual's capabilities do not change as a result of the design, the person's abilities do. By redefining problems, changing environments and selecting different products, the quality of life of people experiencing illness, injury or impairment, and those in their social sphere, may be enhanced. An individual's social sphere is composed of family (parents, spouses, children, and siblings), caregivers, friends, therapists, doctors and close community members. The environment and products available can ease burdens, facilitate relationships and reduce stress during activities for all members of the social sphere. Selecting universal design products and environments enables individuals to use their capabilities (senses, strength, coordination, reflexes and sensation) to accomplish tasks (Joines, 2009). This chapter is written for occupational therapists, as they help people throughout their lifespan to accomplish everyday tasks, learn new skills, adapt to permanent losses, and participate fully in life.

UNIVERSAL DESIGN ENVIRONMENTS

Universal design requires thoughtful assessment of the current wants and needs of a user and projection of the potential changes in the capabilities of the user or the needs of secondary users. Rapid changes in technology make previously impossible tasks realistic, even ubiquitous. The following outlines some of the features of universally designed environment.

Site Conditions

Site conditions may offer an opportunity to use landscaped earth pathways for a more natural and blended solution than other options. This approach may include a retaining wall, an earth berm and sometimes a bridge. A safe path with a gentle slope of 1:20 (rise to length) can be built without railings (unless there are abrupt drop-offs on either side or if users need them), thereby avoiding the cost and intrusive appearance of railings. Landscaped options may be more expensive than a functionally equivalent ramp solution but usually have a longer lifespan and require less maintenance. Integrated site solutions are generally more aesthetic and usually generate a more universally designed solution (Figs. 44.1 and 44.2).

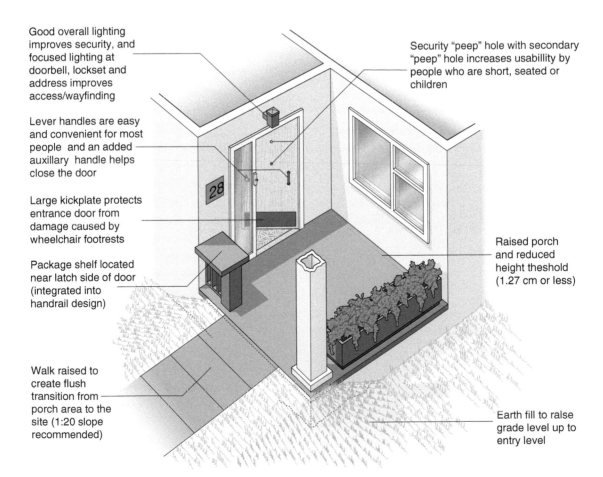

Good overall lighting improves security, and focused lighting at doorbell, lockset and address improves access/wayfinding

Lever handles are easy and convenient for most people and an added auxillary handle helps close the door

Large kickplate protects entrance door from damage caused by wheelchair footrests

Package shelf located near latch side of door (integrated into handrail design)

Walk raised to create flush transition from porch area to the site (1:20 slope recommended)

Security "peep" hole with secondary "peep" hole increases usabillity by people who are short, seated or children

Raised porch and reduced height theshold (1.27 cm or less)

Earth fill to raise grade level up to entry level

FIG. 44.1 ■ Earth, cut and fill at entrance.

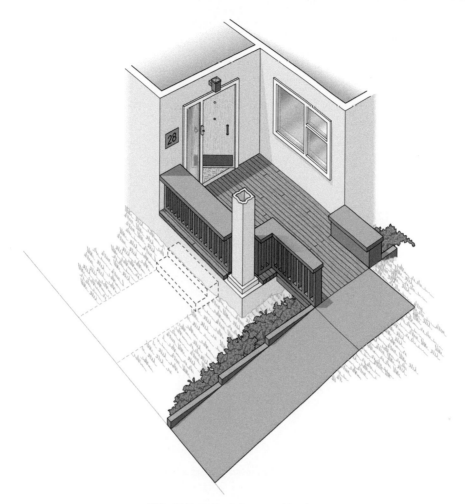

FIG. 44.2 ■ Earth berm and bridge.

Recent notable universally designed public landscape projects include landscape architect Michael Van Valkenburgh Associates' Brooklyn Bridge Park in New York, Olin Studio's redesign of the Washington Monument's grounds in Washington, DC, and the Crown Fountain at Millennium Park in Chicago, Illinois, designed by artist Jaume Plensa. All of these projects incorporate several universal design principles by eliminating steps, ramp slopes less than 5%, contrasting material colours, and opportunities to be active or to rest.

Building Entries and Exits

There are common barriers to gaining entry into various types of buildings. Be it entering a residence, arriving to a place of employment or participating in recreational and leisure pursuits, entries to public and private spaces share similar challenges. Uneven ground, sloping landscapes, stairs, inadequately identified points of entry, thresholds and narrow doorways impede an individual's ability to unlock, open, enter and close the entry door (Fig. 44.3). The solutions critical to a person with a temporary or permanent impairment, an older adult or a person with a gait impairment also benefit the young professional with a rolling briefcase, luggage or bags of groceries, children with overstuffed book bags and sporting equipment, parents with strollers and movers delivering heavy appliances.

A universal entrance is composed of many features that allow use by a person with impairment, including approaching the entrance at the same level as the door, without steps or excessive

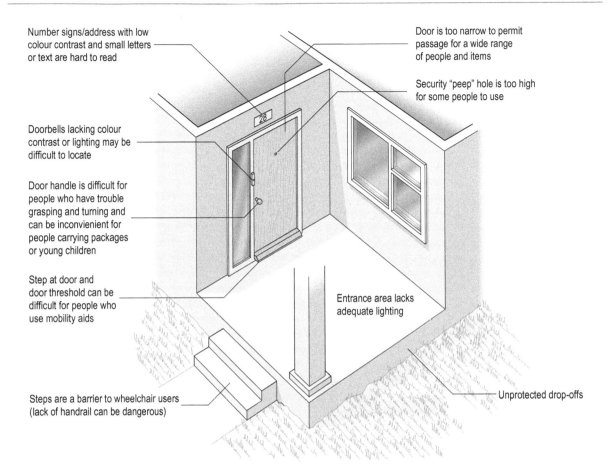

Number signs/address with low colour contrast and small letters or text are hard to read

Door is too narrow to permit passage for a wide range of people and items

Security "peep" hole is too high for some people to use

Doorbells lacking colour contrast or lighting may be difficult to locate

Door handle is difficult for people who have trouble grasping and turning and can be inconvienient for people carrying packages or young children

Step at door and door threshold can be difficult for people who use mobility aids

Entrance area lacks adequate lighting

Steps are a barrier to wheelchair users (lack of handrail can be dangerous)

Unprotected drop-offs

FIG. 44.3 ■ Common barriers at entrances.

slopes. Additional elements include parking close to the entry, a gently sloping walk, a minimum 1.52 m × 1.52 m manoeuvring space at the entrance, and a door with a minimum clear width of 86.5 to 91.5 cm. Additional features, when incorporated, result in a truly universal entrance providing safe and *equitable use* by all people. Examples of additional features include a cover over the entrance to provide protection from the outdoor environment, a movement/motion sensor to automatically turn on an overhead light when someone approaches, or ambient and focused lighting at the keyhole and high-visibility address numbers (Fig. 44.4).

An ideal entrance would allow a person with a walker, cane, wheelchair or other mobility device enough room to manoeuvre while opening the door. Reducing the threshold minimises tripping hazards and is an advantage to small children, people with vision loss, older adults who may have difficulty walking and others. The space on either side of the door should be uncluttered and have a bench to place packages or sit and rest. In

residential construction, providing a place to rest objects while closing and locking the door after entering will also provide a similar staging area when leaving the home. When considering building modifications, the typical factors of style, characteristics of the site and type of construction cannot be as easily manipulated as they can in new construction. When modifying an existing entrance, options to create a stepless entrance include ramps, vertical platform lifts and landscaping. An often overlooked solution, provided land is available, is to reposition the entrance as shown in Fig. 44.5. The advantages and disadvantages for each option must be carefully considered. Mats and area rugs designed to minimise the transmission of dirt into the building can pose additional barriers and may pose trip hazards to individuals using crutches or walkers or those with balance issues.

Ramps are the most familiar accessible entrance modification. They can be built relatively quickly and inexpensively and even be temporary. Ramps accommodating excessive

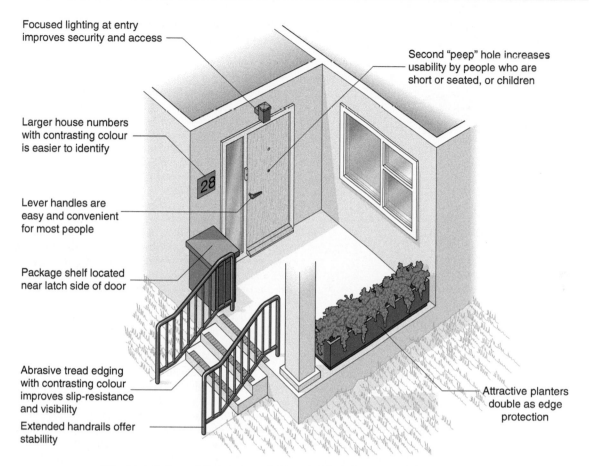

Focused lighting at entry
improves security and access

Second "peep" hole increases
usability by people who are
short or seated, or children

Larger house numbers
with contrasting colour
is easier to identify

Lever handles are
easy and convenient
for most people

Package shelf located
near latch side of door

Abrasive tread edging
with contrasting colour
improves slip-resistance
and visibility

Extended handrails offer
stabillity

Attractive planters
double as edge
protection

FIG. 44.4 ■ Remodelled entrance (with stairs) includes universal design features.

heights may require extensive construction, be very long and quite expensive, and require maintenance. Ramps should be thoughtfully planned so they are constructed in a style and material compatible with the building to avoid stigmatising the occupants. A universal benefit of adding ramps to existing inaccessible buildings is the added access provided to those who find steps inconvenient, such as delivery persons or a person pushing a cart.

Lobbies and Waiting Areas

For buildings with an ante space, lobby, or waiting area where congestion or the gathering of people may occur, there are many opportunities to avoid issues before they arise. In addition to entry solutions identified earlier, considerations should be given to providing comfort and security, public and private communications and ease of navigation through way-finding. Access in and around lobby and waiting areas should accommodate

potential users in wheelchairs, pushing shopping carts and using a walker and those who are obese. Furniture should be movable, not fixed, and available in a wide range of size and sitting positions. The floor materials should be nonglare, antireflective, and slip resistant. If entry mats are warranted, they should be recessed flush with the floor and have a firm, level surface. The mat should remove rainwater from the soles of shoes and from the wheels of prams, pushchairs, trollies and wheelchairs.

Kitchens

For many contemporary households the kitchen is the centre of home activities, including food preparation, cooking, socialisation and experience sharing. It is for all these activities that a kitchen should be universally designed. Universal design features affording improved usability to individuals with limited reach and people who use wheelchairs include lower cabinets

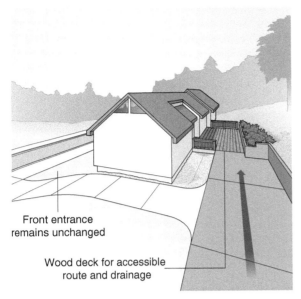

Front entrance
remains unchanged

Wood deck for accessible
route and drainage

FIG. 44.5 ■ Repositioned entrance.

with adequate toe room, drawers rather than shelves and shallow sinks coupled with cabinets with swing away doors (Fig. 44.6). Upper cabinets' usability can be improved for individuals with limited reach by mounting the cabinets lower than standard or on adjustable track.

Universal design solutions that afford increased participation in kitchen activities are highlighted in Table 44.1. Careful selection and installation of appliances reduces reliance on reach and strength. Purchasing universally designed containers and forgiving cookware and surfaces minimises the impact of impairments. Similarly, a well-designed visual management system supports the members of the household equally, both mentally and emotionally.

Central to a universally designed kitchen is the sink. Faucet controls have a strong impact on the ease of use for a sink. Levered faucets (Fig. 44.7A and B) allow individuals the ability to control the water flow without requiring gripping capability. Although not controlling water flow rate or temperature, touch and motion-sensitive technologies allow faucets to be turned on and off by individuals without the need to grasp. These faucet designs also have the potential to reduce germ transmission. Reach requirements can be reduced by installing faucets and placing soap on the side of the sink. Selecting easy-plunge (Fig. 44.7C) or motion-activated soap dispensers (Fig. 44.7D) are inexpensive universal design choices. To limit scalding (especially for individuals with decreased tactile sensitivity), temperature controls should be installed in plumbing systems. To minimise contact burns (for wheelchair users), hot and cold water supply lines should be concealed below wall-mounted, pedestal and cantilevered sinks to prevent injury. These

universal design sink-related solutions should also be applied in the bathroom, laundry and mud rooms.

Bathrooms

Common problems in the bathroom include narrow doorways, insufficient turning space, lack of knee room under the sink, insufficient transfer area for the bath and toilet, and lack of reinforced walls for grab bars. There are three primary opportunities for application of the universal design principles in the bathroom (Dobkin & Peterson, 1999) (Fig. 44.8): (1) the shower/bath, (2) the toilet area, and (3) the sink.

One of the difficulties with traditional showers and baths is the effort needed and fear associated with entering and exiting the shower and bath for individuals with mobility and strength challenges. In addition to the step required to enter most showers or baths, individuals are also entering or exiting a wet area. The addition of water to slick floor coverings makes for a hazardous combination. One universal design solution is the installation of curbless showers, which use a 5- to 10-cm threshold/trench drain instead of a centre drain (Fig. 44.9).

Two other universal design alternatives for bathing are also popular. The first is the installation of a new walk-in tub designed with half-doors that seal watertight. Traditional deep soaking tubs often force caregivers to adopt awkward postures while assisting an individual with bathing. The extreme postures put both the individual being assisted and the caregiver at risk of injury. The second approach is to provide an oversized flat surface flush with the top of the bath to allow individuals to transfer or simply sit before lowering themselves into the bath. This solution requires greater upper body strength if the individual lifts and lowers himself or herself into and out of the tub. If the bath surface is wide enough, the individual may choose to be showered while seated, reducing the effort for the individual bathing and his or her caregiver.

Strategically located support bars (either traditional grab bars or new towel racks and toilet paper holders) can aid when transferring on and off the toilet and transitioning in and out of the shower or simply provide stability while standing to be towelled off or while putting on clothes. Such support bars can be helpful to an individual working with a person who has had a stroke. Although support bars are traditionally installed horizontally to aid seated transfers, a vertical installation may maximise an individual's ability to support weight or maintain balance while standing or stepping.

Design standards for accessibility contain many details describing toilet height, clear floor space, distance from a wall or adjacent fixture, location of flush valve and so on. One of the key features for designing a universally usable bathroom is adequate clear floor space for approach and use of the toilet. A modest change in the wall at the back of the toilet combined with additional space to the side of the toilet greatly increases the independent, as well as assisted, use of the fixture. Offsetting the toilet wall 25.4 to 30.5 cm provides extra space for the

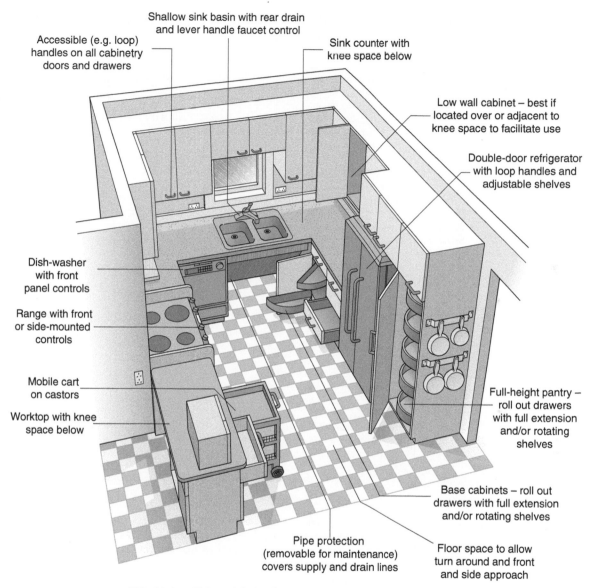

Accessible (e.g. loop) handles on all cabinetry doors and drawers

Shallow sink basin with rear drain and lever handle faucet control

Sink counter with knee space below

Low wall cabinet – best if located over or adjacent to knee space to facilitate use

Double-door refrigerator with loop handles and adjustable shelves

Dish-washer with front panel controls

Range with front or side-mounted controls

Mobile cart on castors

Worktop with knee space below

Full-height pantry – roll out drawers with full extension and/or rotating shelves

Base cabinets – roll out drawers with full extension and/or rotating shelves

Pipe protection (removable for maintenance) covers supply and drain lines

Floor space to allow turn around and front and side approach

FIG. 44.6 ■ Universal design features improve usability in the kitchen.

user to position the wheelchair seat parallel to the toilet seat. A safer and easier parallel transfer can then be made (Fig. 44.10).

Although new lower or taller toilets (Fig. 44.11) may be purchased and installed, this may not be feasible within a residence. A standard height or taller toilet used in combination with a stool has multiple benefits. Use of stools may help individuals obtain a squat posture which facilitates bowel evacuation. A stool may also help shorter individuals ascend the toilet without

aid and prevent their legs from dangling, which results in decreased circulation in the lower extremities if extended time on the toilet is necessary. This benefits older individuals with problems sitting and rising, short-stature adults and adults having recently had surgery, delivered babies, prone to constipation or lacking bowel control as a result of a neurological disorder. Another universal design solution in toileting is the installation of a lid with dual diameters for the seat opening (Fig. 44.12) to mitigate small bottoms from 'falling into the potty'.

TABLE 44.1
Universal Design Solutions in the Kitchen

Reducing Reliance on	UD Solutions
Reach	▪ Select separate stovetops and built-in ovens (install such that cooked items are placed and retrieved at approximately counter height). ▪ Select ovens with side-swing doors. ▪ Select controls that require two steps for activation, located towards the front of the appliance to address competing concerns for usability and minimisation of accidental activation. ▪ Controls should have clear indicators of position with asymmetrical shapes or clear, high-contrast labels. ▪ Select refrigerators with handles that extend the height of the machine door. ▪ Create multiple-height work and eating surfaces. ▪ Consider under-the-counter cutting boards and nonslip cutting boards. ▪ Install faucets and place soap on the side of the sink.
Strength and Coordination	▪ Support large and hot items. ▪ Select placemats with antiskid textures to keep plates and mixing bowls in place. ▪ Select food storage containers that provide a grip along the length of the package and control the direction and flow of materials. ▪ Select plates and counter surfaces that are chip resistant and forgiving (shock absorbing). ▪ Consider levers, touch, or motion-sensitive technology for faucet control. ▪ Select easy-plunge or motion-activated soap dispensers.
Memory	To aid in cooking and food preparation: ▪ Group task-related items together in drawers, in bins or in sight (e.g. hang insulated gloves adjacent and within sight of the oven rather than placing them in the drawer for storage). ▪ Augment a written recipe, an old fashioned memory aid and process guide, with photos of the items needed and the process. To aid in daily and household management tasks: ▪ Use a visual management system (VMS). This expands the traditional idea of posting the shopping list on the refrigerator to using a whiteboard or corkboard in a central location (e.g. in the kitchen or by the back door). ▪ Include information on the VMS for emergency/frequent contacts, daily or weekly schedules (including medical/therapy appointments), event reminders, shopping lists, assignment of responsibilities (such as who is driving whom), and recognition for accomplishments and notes of encouragement.

UD, Universal design.

Some problems and universal design solutions in the bathroom are similar to those previously discussed for the kitchen (including sink shape and clearance, faucet selection and location, cabinet door swings, toe room and water temperature control). Universal design solutions may also focus on organisation; grouping task-related items together for personal hygiene, grooming, dressing and cleaning using a combination of under-counter drawers and baskets on shallow shelves with heights ranging from 76.2 to 114.3 cm to promote independence and efficiency. Such universal design solutions allow individuals to retrieve stored materials without the increased effort associated with bending, twisting or stooping to reach under cabinets behind closed doors. Although a bathroom may have adequate floor space and other universal design features, if a person is unable to enter the bathroom those features are of no value. Narrow doorways should be avoided in new designs. In existing designs, additional clearance may be gained with modest effort by replacing traditional door hinges with swing-clear hinges. If the

space and budget allow, a sliding or pocket door or a new door and frame might be considered. This will be discussed in greater detail in the next section on living spaces.

Living Spaces

Although a great deal of modern living occurs in the kitchen, the creation of universally designed living spaces throughout the home will improve the quality of life for everyone living in and visiting the house. Attention must be paid to universal design principles when selecting furniture, flooring materials, interior doors and lighting as well as being mindful of archways, halls, and clear space within a room.

Design characteristics, such as the apron, arms and seat pan height and depth, affect an individual's experience with furniture. A couch with a low apron inhibits an individual from sliding his or her feet under the couch (and therefore under his or her centre of gravity), making it more difficult for individuals

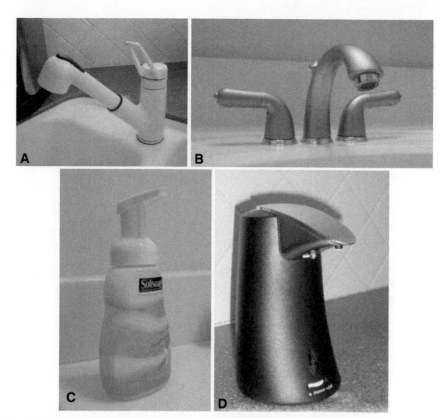

FIG. 44.7 ■ (A) Single-lever faucets allow individuals the ability to control the water flow and temperature without requiring gripping capability. (B) Double-lever faucets allow individuals the ability to control the water flow and temperature without requiring gripping capability. (C) Selecting easy-plunge soap dispensers activated by pushing down. (D) Automatic soap dispenser activated by motion sensor.

with decreased lower extremity strength or joint problems to stand up from the couch without assistance. Furniture without armrests facilitate an individual's ability to transfer from the side of the piece of furniture; however, armless chairs reduce a person's ability to use upper body strength to augment the lower body strength when standing up and sitting down. Although chairs that have low seat pans can fit the popliteal height of a person of shorter stature, people using these chairs may require additional effort (e.g. strength in the quadriceps) when standing up. Deep seat pans afford curling up and reading a book, but they also require weaker, smaller individuals to scoot forward multiple times to gain purchase on the edge of the seat in order to stand up. This may be embarrassing for an adult to do in front of peers or family. Although not all needs can be met with one piece of furniture, purchasing coordinating pieces with design characteristics supporting a range of abilities will make the living space useful and desirable for the multiple individuals and needs present in a social sphere.

The selection of floor materials affects the mobility of people by creating concerns of tripping, slipping, falling and fatigue. This results ultimately in a sedentary lifestyle by limiting their movement between multiple spaces (Dobkin & Peterson, 1999). Trade-offs must be considered based on the potential competing needs of the different members within the social sphere. Hard floors are easier for users of wheelchairs, crutches and canes; however, those with degenerative joints and altered joint angles benefit from the cushion associated with a thick carpet. Trip hazards and impediments to movement can be created by change to floor materials, unsecured edges, creases or buckles in rugs.

Another consideration to promote movement throughout the house is the transition space between rooms, including doorways, archways and halls. These transition spaces should be at least 81.3 cm wide, preferably 91.5 cm. Although archways separate spaces without requiring the effort associated with opening and closing doors, they do not control noise or provide privacy. There are several items to be considered in the selection and installation of interior doors: traffic patterns and room layout, path of door motion, hinge mechanisms, door handles and visibility. Traffic patterns in transition spaces can be complicated

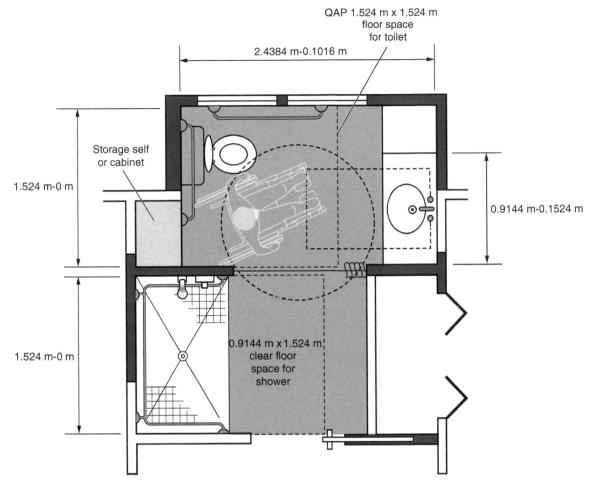

FIG. 44.8 ■ Universally designed bathroom with curbless shower. NB: This design affords transfer from the side or front of the-toilet. The reaches required for and usability of all fixtures are good and there is generous unobstructed turning space. The lavatory counter width affords easy retrieval and storage of frequently used personal hygiene items or those of multiple users. This design also includes a linen closet, base cabinet and windows. In order to afford greater privacy and the opportunity for simultaneous users, moisture-resistant (shower) curtains are located in front of the 'curbless' roll-in shower and between the wet area and the toilet/sink area. A pocket door minimises the use of the clear space for door swing into the bathroom or the hall.

by interior walls, the path through which a door moves when it opens and closes, the location of electrical outlets and built-in features such as hearths and towel racks. The width of doorway opening can be maximised by using swing-clear hinges on traditional doors or choosing pocket doors (which are also of benefit in confined spaces where multiple rooms come together) where the door slides into the adjacent wall. Although pocket doors do not require individuals to change direction to accommodate a door swing, both pocket and traditional interior doors require the use of a hand to open and close them. A swinging door hung to stay open once pushed out of the way affords the privacy of a door without requiring the use of a hand to open or close it. If a door's swing path travels into two spaces, being able to see through the door at multiple heights will help avoid colliding with an individual approaching from the opposite direction. Doors with lever handles do not require the user to have the same strength or range of motion necessary to grip and turn traditional, round door knobs.

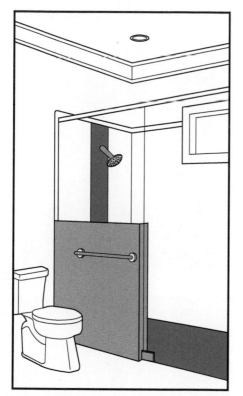

FIG. 44.9 ■ Curbless shower with threshold/trench drain.

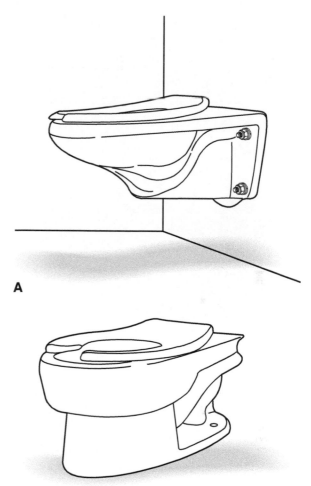

A

B

FIG. 44.11 ■ (A) Higher-height wall-mounted toilet alternative. (B) Lower-height toilet alternative.

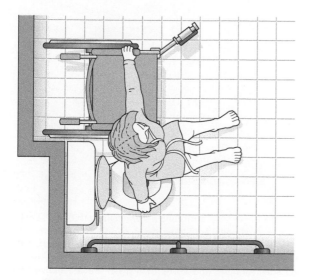

FIG. 44.10 ■ Toilet offset for parallel transfer.

In addition to selecting universally designed furnishings, providing clear space within the living space will afford a person room to enter and move within a room without bumping into or knocking over objects (Dobkin & Peterson, 1999). Clear space is created by thoughtfully placing furniture, ensuring cords are out of the way and identifying storage to avoid clutter; this is a case when less is more. Similar to a universally designed entrance into a building, the ability to move freely within a room is liberating and provides the sense that one fits and is welcome in this space.

The occupants' quality of the experience within a space, sense of well-being, and ability to engage in varied activities can be affected by lighting. In addition to providing

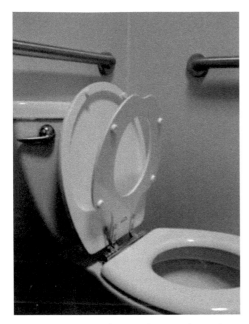

FIG. 44.12 ▪ Dual-rim toilet seat alternative.

illumination, natural lighting positively affects mood (Day, Theodorson, & Van Den Wymelenberg, 2012; Joines, 2009; Van Den Wymelenberg, 2015) but needs to be well controlled and directed (McKeown, 2008). Although blinds are popular for handling natural light, the operational mechanisms for blinds vary. Select long levers that may be used at multiple heights, avoiding small bobbles and cords that twist and are difficult to operate (Fig. 44.13).

The level of illumination, spectrum, direction and level of control for general room and task lighting are all important to consider when creating universally designed environments. Task lighting can benefit both an individual working alone and those working in a group of mixed visual capabilities. Individuals with low vision or performing precision tasks may require higher levels of illumination in a focused area. Because adequate lighting for one individual may produce glare for another, universal design lighting solutions include general room and task lighting preferably with dimming features. The ease of use of a light fixture is a function of controls and placement. A floor lamp, placed behind a chair, with a small thumb wheel control will be of little use to an individual with decreased pinch grip strength, tactile sensitivity, range of motion or limited reach or mobility challenges. Light fixtures placed within reach could be controlled using pull chains descending below lamp shades or touch sensitivity. Lights positioned behind or adjacent to furniture should be controlled by portable or wall switches with wide toggles or sliding dimmers.

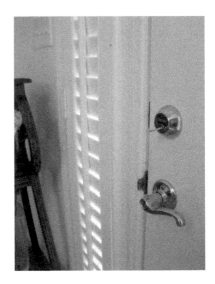

A

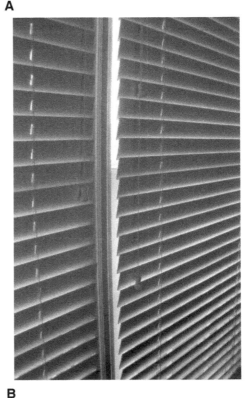

B

FIG. 44.13 ▪ (A) Controlling natural light with blinds: Long-handle on blinds and lever door handle. (B) Controlling natural light with blinds: Small fingertip pull on blinds. NB: Select long levers that may be used at multiple heights, avoiding small bobbles and cords that twist and are difficult to operate.

Parks and Recreations Spaces

One overly generalised argument may be that everyone should have equal experiences throughout the park, regardless of ability, age, or interest. More importantly, public park design should be aesthetically pleasing, inviting to all, having no special use equipment for differently abled users, including water features and play structures that offer interaction for people of all ages and athletic fields for adaptive sports. Public parks, by their nature, provide open spaces, free and usable by everyone. Therefore to achieve maximum enjoyment, activities and interactions should provide feedback through multiple means of perceptible information. Public services should be centralised and recognisable. The desire for a variety of experiences is understandable and experiencing a trail, activity, vista or destination should be made available to the most people when possible. Not all spaces have to be equally accessible or designed to the lowest common denominator of accessibility; instead there could be a number of options provided. If everyone has to participate the same way and the experiences are no different, then there is no excitement or exploration. When discussing the design process for the Forest Glen Park in Wheaton, Illinois, Mark Trieglaff (2014) said,

> One of the requirements of the Access to Recreation grant was to hold public meetings for input on the park design. A comment received from several parents was that their child enjoyed having more challenging play elements. It was determined to add higher-level play components that required a transfer platform for accessing these elevated areas. Adding this design feature offers the challenge some children are looking for. (p. 4)

When considering the design of public parks in the United States of America, the National Park Service (NPS) provides guidelines and an activities checklist to better identify the programmes to be provided. This checklist, NPS Universal Design and Accessibility Scoping Form for Outdoor Developed Areas (NPS, 2013) addresses campgrounds, picnic areas, overlooks, trailheads, trails and beach access routes and fishing/boating facilities. By incorporating a checklist or user survey in the initial design discussions, a design team can better identify opportunities for universal design. Again, designing to meet the ADA minimums will miss the opportunity to make the greatest impact.

APPLICATION TO PRACTICE

The universal design approach to solution development applied in the home environment can be extended into the workplace to support the needs and desires of people wishing to remain active and independent regardless of age or physical or sensory circumstance. Where individuals of 60 years old were once expected to begin retirement, today they often are starting second careers or downsizing and buying second homes. Universal design solutions afford the ability to participate in activities of daily living at home and to continue to contribute in the workplace without stigma. Practice Stories 44.1 to 44.4 highlight how universal design can be used to solve specific changes in ability.

PRACTICE STORY 44.1

Meredith

Meredith is 36 years old, lives in the suburbs and works in a large-sized downtown accounting firm. She is an up-and-coming leader in the company and is focused on her career. Between her 45-minute commute and 10-hour work schedule, her days are long. Meredith's job mainly consists of meetings and managing client accounts on her computer.

ISSUE

Meredith has chronic back pain as a result of a motor vehicle accident when she was a teen. Because of her duties at work she is often sitting for extended periods. The pain in combination with her static posture often limits her ability to focus.

SOLUTION

An electric height adjustable workstation (EHAW) and multi-positional chair were purchased for Meredith. The desk is adjustable from a seated height to a standing work height by way of an electric touch pad. The controls offer one-touch preset heights, which are programmable to multiple positions for different users. The ability for Meredith to alternate from sitting to standing while working relieves much of the pain associated with long-term sitting. Also, standing allows for improved blood circulation and mental acuity. The potential for benefits are even greater after a longer period using the EHAW (Hedge, 2004). The chair is fully adjustable in height, arm rests, seat tilt and lumbar support, making comfort even more achievable.

PRACTICE STORY 44.2

Scott

Scott is a recent high school graduate and has been accepted to a local university. Scott plans to live in the on-campus dormitory to gain the full college experience. He is registered as a full-time student but has yet to declare a major. Scott is very active socially and looks forward to moving away from home to attend college.

ISSUE

Because of an infection in the nervous system as an infant, Scott is paralysed from the waist down and uses a manual wheelchair. He has full use of his upper body and is very independent. Because of Scott's ability to care for himself, the biggest challenge with dorm life will be the daily personal hygiene tasks.

SOLUTION

The dorm room should be large enough to allow for movement around furniture and fixtures without needing assistance. This layout may also be more comfortable to his roommate and guests. The bathroom should provide a reasonable opportunity to wash. This can be accomplished by a roll-in (or curbless) shower or a bath with controls within reach from both inside and outside of the basin. The roll-in shower is preferred by many because it reduces the chance of a slip and fall from having to move over a curb.

PRACTICE STORY 44.3

Archer

Archer is retired and lives with his wife of 49 years. Archer's family, including his brother, sister, two daughters and three grandchildren, lives in the same county and often visit throughout the week and on weekends. Recently Archer was diagnosed with stage IV cancer after having experienced a series of mini-strokes and most recently a brain bleed. After receiving intensive inpatient therapy, Archer is being released to go home.

ISSUE

Archer's physical and cognitive abilities have changed. No longer able to control his left side, Archer will need his primary caregiver, his wife, to assist him with his activities of daily living. His 63-year-old wife needs help understanding what changes need to be made for Archer to be able to live at home, have visitors and maintain a good quality of life.

SOLUTION

Universal design is most easily and cost effectively achieved early in the design process. However, that does not mean that individuals cannot be informed by and benefit from universal design once an environment has been created. When individuals' abilities change, there is an opportunity to infuse universally designed solutions into the environment by thinking not just of what the capabilities and needs are of that one individual but of the needs and abilities of all the individuals in the space and those who come to visit.

Archer now uses a wheelchair, which is wider than the opening of the door width. After completing a walkthrough of the home simulating a day in Archer's life in order to identify potential areas of stress, and speaking with Archer, his wife and family, Archer's occupational therapist suggests that there are many ways to address the issue. First, Archer could be restricted from using that doorway and potentially limiting access to part of the home. This would require Archer to have a bed in the den, take sponge baths and use a bedside commode. Second, the doors could be removed, allowing access; however, the lack of privacy afforded by the doors (into the bathroom) may negatively affect his visitors. Third, swing-clear hinges could be installed, effectively making the doorway openings wider (by the thickness of the door) by moving the door out of the way when opened. Finally, new doors and frames could be installed to widen the openings. Because there was not enough space beside the doorframes to widen the doors in a cost-effective manner, Archer's son-in-law installed swing-clear hinges on the doors to the living room, the bedroom and both bathrooms.

Shelly

Shelly is a successful CEO of a software company that employs 15 individuals with diverse educational backgrounds supporting clients on six continents. Shelly recognises communication has been central to the success of the company.

ISSUE

The business has grown faster than the ability of the employees to provide documentation and training. With the release of a new product, Shelly is interested in pushing to launch documentation, training and communications that will support their diverse group of clients. This includes clients and their employees with impairments.

SOLUTION

Universal design should be an important part of any communication process. Providing suitable communications to people, including people with impairments, creates an inclusive, positive engagement from the beginning (Joines & Valenziano, 2015). Technology can support communication, and, although there are many resources for providing detailed universal design communication recommendations, one trend is that simpler methods almost always result in more universally designed materials. Shelly has recommendations for how her company will handle emails, info sheets in PDF and webpages, and images in documentation and communications.

Plain text is the only type of email processed the same by all email clients. If a web link to additional information is to be shared, a URL-shortening service is used to avoid mistyping of long addresses. Info sheets are provided in PDF files to preserve formatting, content, and accessibility (as long as the end-user has a free PDF viewer installed on his or her computer Internet access not required). Although PDFs are widely used, a webpage may be preferable because more people use web browsers than PDF readers. Instead of relying on viewing an image to understand the message, the image can be described for a user using alternative text (alt-text). Users can read or hear alt-text description of an image.

A BRIEF COMMENT ON THE IMPACT OF GLOBAL SOCIETY ON UNIVERSAL DESIGN EFFORTS

Universal design supports people travelling globally and companies selling products in multiple markets. With the increase in connectivity between people and countries, the needs, cultures and norms associated with multiple societies must be considered when seeking a single, universally designed solution. Foregrounded in the needs of multicultural regions and the development of products to be shipped around the globe using next-day delivery services, the universal design principles of simple and intuitive use (where the focus is on a design that is easy to understand, regardless of the user's experience, knowledge, language skills or current concentration level) and principle of tolerance for error (where the design minimises hazards and the adverse consequences of accidental or unintended actions) are paramount. The economic impact for a business of having a single product for multiple countries rather than country-specific versions of a product highlights the benefit of universal design from a business perspective. At the same time, global travellers waking in different time zones within a short period also benefit from a universally designed product that performs as well in Lubbock, Texas as it does in Kayseri, Turkey. With the pervasiveness of the Internet and associated connectivity, consumers' expectations have increased; tolerance for software, apps and products that are not easily portable across time zones and platforms is limited. Thus the focus on the user experience is inadvertently underscoring the continued relevance of universal design to the ever-increasing global society. The global citizen, regardless of ability, can travel to different cities and enjoy a range of experiences if the transportation and monetary systems, museums and lodging facilities have been informed by the principles of universal design.

CONCLUSION

Occupational therapists can affect the lives of the individuals they are working with by informing them and their caregivers about how to leverage universally designed products and approaches in their lives and living spaces. By discussing the activities of daily living performed throughout a residence or at work with a person, occupational therapists may identify areas of stress. In these areas of stress, occupational therapists can discuss home and work design modifications with the person. These discussions can highlight the opportunities to include universal design principles in daily activities through major and minor purchases, facilities modifications and changes to room layouts. By redefining problems, changing environments, and selecting universal design products and approaches, the quality of life of people and those in their social sphere may be greatly enhanced (Box 44.2).

BOX 44.2
IDENTIFYING OPPORTUNITIES FOR UNIVERSAL DESIGN SOLUTIONS

- Identify the obstacles to the person by performing a walkthrough of the person's day (preferably with the person). The occupational therapist should ask about how well the person can do the following:
  - Get out of bed, dress, and get to the bathroom
  - Move from the bathroom to the kitchen, prepare meals and eat
  - Perform activities of personal hygiene
  - Clean the house, and wash the dishes and laundry
  - Interact with family, friends and care assistants
- Consider the equitable and ease of use philosophy incorporated in the principles of universal design when visualising or observing the task being performed:
  - During each daily activity, is the person forced to exert extra effort or limited by the available products, fixtures or structures?
  - Ask questions pertaining to the principles such as the following:
    - Does the person have to reach or stretch to accomplish a task?
    - Can the person see and understand the information in the environment?

- Is text large enough, in the correct language, in an easy-to-understand word choice?
- Is there adequate lighting and good contrast?
- Are redundant channels of feedback available, such as auditory, tactile or haptic feedback?

- Consider the context in which the activity is normally performed. In addition to the simple activities such as turning a door knob, look at the person's ability to perform an entire sequence of tasks such as entering or exiting the house:
  - Can the person enter the house with groceries or enter quickly and safely, avoiding being a target for conflict?
  - Does the solution scream 'here lives someone with a disability' or does if afford most users a similar experience?
  - Can activities of daily living be improved significantly by the design of the built environment, not relying exclusively on adaptive aids?
  - Is this solution going to make someone feel an enhanced sense of competence?

---

 http://evolve.elsevier.com/Curtin/OT

REFERENCES

AIPatHome Staff (2015). *Universal design & lifespan design allow for people's changing needs over time.* Retrieved from, http://blog.aipathome.com/universal-desigin-lifespan-design-allow-for-peoples-changing-needs-over-time/.

Beran, M. (2007). Lifespan perspectives on the foreseeable use of consumer products. *Ergonomics in Design, 15,* 12.

Bühler, C., & Stephanidis, C. (2004). European co-operation activities promoting design for all in information society technologies. In International Conference on Computers for Handicapped Persons (pp. 80–87). Springer Berlin: Heidelberg.

Centers for Disease Control and Prevention, National Center for Health Statistics. (2015). *Health Data Interactive.* Atlanta: US Department of Health and Human Services. Retrieved from, http://www.cdc.gov/nchs/hdi.htm.

Clarkson, P., & Coleman, R. (2015). History of inclusive design in the UK. *Applied Ergonomics, 46*(B), 235–247.

Connell, B., Jones, M., & Mace, R., et al. (1997). *The principles of universal design: Version 2.0.* Raleigh. NC: The Center for Universal Design.

Day, J., Theodorson, J., & Van Den Wymelenberg, K. (2012). Understanding controls, behaviors and satisfaction in the daylit perimeter office: A daylight design case study. *Journal of Interior Design, 37*(1), 17–34.

Dobkin, I., & Peterson, M. (1999). *Gracious spaces: Universal interiors by design.* New York: McGraw-Hill.

Erickson, W., Lee, C., & von Schrader, S. (2014). *2012 Disability Status Report: United States.* Ithaca, NY: Cornell University Employment and Disability Institute (EDI). Retrieved from, http://www.disabilitystatistics.org/.

Hedge, A. (2004). *Effects of an Electric Height-Adjustable Worksurface on Self-assessed Musculoskeletal Discomfort and Productivity in Computer Workers.* Cornell University Human Factors and Ergonomics Research Laboratory. NY: Ithaca.

Herwig, O. (2008). *Universal design: Solutions for a barrier-free living.* Basel, Boston: Birkhèauser.

Joines, S. (2009). Enhancing quality of life through Universal Design. *NeuroRehabilitation, 25,* 313–326.

Joines, S., & Valenziano, S. (2015). Universally designed communications for researchers. *Submitted to Design Research and Methods Journal.*

Jordan, W. (2008). *Universal design for the home: Great looking, great living design for all ages, abilities, and circumstances.* Beverly, MA: Quarry Books.

Mace, R. (1985). Universal Design: Barrier Free Environments for Everyone. *Designers West, 33*(1), 147–152.

McKeown, C. (2008). *Office ergonomics: Practical applications.* Boca Raton, FL: CRC Press.

National Park Service, Universal Design Standards (2013). *NPS universal design and accessibility scoping form for ABAAS outdoor recreation facilities*. Retrieved from, https://www.nps.gov/dscw/ds-universal-design.htm#nps.

Nussbaumer, L. (2012). *Inclusive design: A universal need*. New York: Fairchild Books.

Null, R. (2014). *Universal design: Principles and models*. Boca Raton, FL: CRC Press.

Ostroff, E. (2011). Universal design: An evolving paradigm. In W. Preiser, & K. Smith (Eds.), *Universal design handbook* (2nd ed., pp. 1.3–1.11). New York: McGraw-Hill.

Story, M. (2011). The Principles of Universal Design. In W. Preiser, & K. Smith (Eds.), *Universal design handbook* (2nd ed.). New York: McGraw-Hill.

Trieglaff, M. (2014). *Forest Glen Park Design Case Study – universal design in a park and recreational setting*. Wheaton, IL: Accessibility Consultation and Training Services. Retrieved from, http://actservicesconsulting.com/images/FGPCaseStudyws.pdf.

United Nations. (2001). Population Ageing and Living Arrangements of Older Persons: Critical Issues and Policy Responses. Population Bulletin of the United Nations, Special Issue Nos. 42/43. Sales No. E.01.XIII.16. New York: United Nations. Retrieved from, http://www.un.org/esa/population/publications/bulletin42_43/Frontcover_note_preface.pdf.

U.S. Department of Labor. (2015). *Disability resources: Americans with Disabilities Act*. Washington, DC: U.S. Department of Labor. Retrieved from, http://www.dol.gov/dol/topic/disability/ada.htm.

U.S. Forest Service. Southwestern Region. (2007). *Whitewater Picnic Area and Catwalk National Recreation Trail: A unique universal design trail winding through a water filled canyon*. Albuquerque, NM: U.S. Dept. of Agriculture, Forest Service, Southwestern Region.

Van Den Wymelenberg, K. (2015). *The benefits of natural light: Research supports daylighting's positive effect on building performance and human health*. Washington, DC: Architectural Lighting. Retrieved from, http://www.archlighting.com/technology/the-benefits-of-natural-light_o.

45

HOME MODIFICATION

CATHERINE ELIZABETH BRIDGE ■ PHILLIPPA CARNEMOLLA

CHAPTER OUTLINE

Abstract

This chapter coalescences the beginning of an evidence base for effective home modification interventions with a person-centred approach and examines how occupational therapists can employ it to produce improved outcomes within the home of the person to whom they are providing an occupational therapy service. Rapid technological advances increase levels of specialisation, and this is no different with home modification, where the connected home of the future and the Internet of things will be the next frontier opening new possibilities and challenges. Person-centeredness, akin to the client-centeredness movement in medicine, has a long history in occupational therapy but can be difficult to implement as health care and rehabilitation practices have become more technical and are increasingly driven by impersonal standards, protocols and guidelines. In the home space the individual and the individual's preferred activities, rhythms and routines and support system are central, and personal preferences are critical to good outcomes. There is an increasing body of evidence that home modification and changes in the structural design and fabric of the dwelling can reduce care burden, improve quality of life and afford greater autonomy and independence across the lifespan. Ensuring a safe, accessible, affordable and secure home base enables people with an illness, injury or impairment to build on their abilities while maintaining function longer with greater dignity in a place of their choosing and with a degree of control over their daily activities and social participation.

KEY POINTS

- Policy changes, such as the move towards self-directed funding, make it critical to understand how a person's home and the objects within can best enable autonomy, control and life quality.

- Home modifications can be effective in reducing falls, improving engagement in activities of daily living, increasing social participation and reducing caregiving and disability-related expenses.

■ Access standards and building codes, although useful for general guidance, cannot account for individual need as they do not account for users' occupational habits and preferences and generally assume standardised mobility device usage or full upper-limb reach ranges.

■ Self, and informal and formal care, are correlated to how enabling or disabling an environment is for the occupations that need to be performed within it.

■ Detailed knowledge of a person's everyday tasks, such as entering, passing through, listening, viewing, toileting, feeding and bathing, are critical to effective home-modification intervention.

INTRODUCTION

The practice of home modifications as relevant to occupational therapy practice is the focus of this chapter. Key concepts in home modifications are presented along with a justification for why home modification should be considered as a practice area. This includes the necessary knowledge about home modification assessments and interventions that may be used by occupational therapists. The practice stories included in this chapter provide illustrations of how to approach home modification for people who have an illness, injury or impairment. The research evidence base in terms of what is known about home modification efficacy as an intervention strategy is presented.

KEY CONCEPTS IN HOME MODIFICATION*

The potential for change to the physical environment to reduce the impact of illness, injury or impairment has been well documented (Altman & Barnartt, 2014; Straton et al., 2003) and housing interventions that ameliorate dependence on home and community-based services are important because they help maintain independence and enable individuals to live in their own homes and communities. Further, home design and population well-being and health outcomes are linked (Bridge, Flatau, Whelan, Wood, & Yates, 2003; Thomson, Thomas, Sellstrom, & Petticrew, 2013).

Home modification refers to a type of housing intervention that includes structural changes to the home environment to help people experiencing illness, injury or impairment to be able to exercise greater autonomy and control.

Consequently there are a number of mainstream housing design approaches specific to increasing the availability of more accessible and liveable housing across the board. These are particularly associated with the advent of both population aging and deinstitutionalisation. All mainstream approaches seek to make new housing more flexible and adaptable to accommodate change over people's lifespans. These approaches include universal design (UD), visitable design, adaptable design and inclusive design. UD also ensures that the general layout and fabric of a building enables basic modifications to be undertaken at minimal cost – for example, bathroom walls that are able to take grab rails if required.

A major benefit of UD implementation in initial building construction is that it potentially decreases the need for, and cost of, home modifications, alterations or retrofits later on. Importantly, UD allows home modification (retrofit) to be primarily used for customising a home for a particular person or family depending on the particular illness, injury or impairment and occupational needs. This can contribute to such things as enabling people to live in their homes as long as possible. This is referred to as aging in place, which reduces pressure on health and aged care systems by reducing dependence on institutional care and is therefore a preferred option for government policy makers and providers (Tinker, 1997; Wiles, Leibing, Guberman, Reeve, & Allen, 2012). Increasing the practice of both more universal or inclusive home design as part of the practice of home modifications has dual societal and individual roles, as illustrated in Fig. 45.1.

Aging in place and deinstitutionalisation more generally are seen as having benefits to individuals, the community and government. On an individual level, the ability to remain in one's home while aging or experiencing illness, injury or

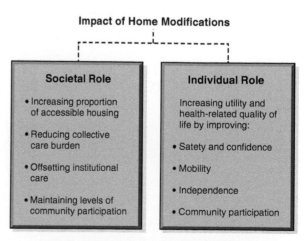

Impact of Home Modifications

Societal Role
- Increasing proportion of accessible housing
- Reducing collective care burden
- Offsetting institutional care
- Maintaining levels of community participation

Individual Role
Increasing utility and health-related quality of life by improving:
- Safety and confidence
- Mobility
- Independence
- Community participation

FIG. 45.1 ■ Dual role of home modifications.

impairment helps support and maintain independence, autonomy and social connections (Wiles et al., 2012). At a community level, having older people and people who have an illness, injury or impairment remain active members of the community can ensure that their civic contributions are maintained and that the greater community retains its diversity.

Nevertheless, international inclusive housing design standards or policies do not yet exist and in most countries where they do exist they are voluntary and differ significantly. Hence, current practice is haphazard at best and the majority of people who have an illness, injury or impairment often make do with very minor changes to their home often only in response to a functional crisis.

IMPORTANCE OF PERSON-CENTEREDNESS IN HOME MODIFICATIONS

Person-centred and self-funding approaches to disability and aging service provision call for more transparency and consistency of principles with practice. This can lead to individualised and occupationally appropriate intervention and facilitation, combined with a more person-focused purchasing and management approach. This service paradigm calls for greater individual, service sector and community knowledge and capacity building.

Additionally, many individuals and families continue to be presented with options that do not support occupational lifestyles of choice but instead demand that people stay indefinitely in the family home or move into more institutional environments. Importantly, living outside institutions and within communities and neighbourhoods does not mean people who have an illness, injury or impairment are truly 'at home'. This is because the autonomy, safety and emotional comfort afforded by being able to accomplish valued occupations may not be available.

SELF-DETERMINATION AS EXEMPLIFIED THROUGH PRACTICE STORIES

Internationally significant shifts in policy are underway towards a more personalised planning and support approach for home modification intervention that better promotes self-determination. A more personalised planning approach is increasingly part of a self-directed funding approach where public (government) monies (funds) are given to individuals rather than the older block funding model where funds were provided to services and the individual applied to the service to get the housing modification intervention done (Lynch & Findlay, 2007).

Technological advances, including simpler and easier-to-use hand tools and kits of parts that are widely available via hardware retailers, such as a handheld shower kit, have facilitated a get in and do it building and renovation culture that is actively promoted via the media, through lifestyle shows and publications. The technology that is available and the ways in which materials can be put together in an aesthetically pleasing manner are features of the *do-it-yourself* (DIY) phenomenon, whose origins and determinants are still not well known (Bogdon, 1996). This phenomenon is not just in mainstream renovation but in home modification for people who have an illness, injury or impairment as well. For instance, the British television programme 'Grand Designs' featured the house that Jon built (Grand Design, 2014). Jon lost both legs above the knee and his right arm at his elbow after active duty in Afghanistan. Learning on the job with mentoring and support during his own home build, he is now running a project management consultancy in building projects. Jon's story and many other DIY stories exemplify the importance of a shift in focus towards aspirations, goals and individual choices, not just apparent need. High home ownership and the move to self-managed funding in combination with the popularisation and growth of self-help media mean this is only likely to grow in coming years, especially as it is easy to obtain information, with the Internet and YouTube providing a growing plethora of 'how to' guidance (Bleasdale, McNamara, Zmudzki, & Bridge, 2014).

The four practice stories represent a diversity of issues covering a number of variables that have been identified as being of relevance to effective home modification practice (Practice Stories 45.1 to 45.4). The practice stories explore how aspirations, goals and individual experience shape home modification strategies and personal engagement. The stories include differences in how people who have an illness, injury or impairment may differ in terms of their context, knowledge, skill, self-efficacy and competence, and in such factors as the following:

- Age and life stage
- Profession/education level
- Impact of illness, injury or impairment on occupational performance
- Recency of illness, injury or impairment
- Urban or rural location
- Financial means
- Access to retail stores
- Help with installing products
- Uptake of smartphone technology
- Engagement with Internet technology

The key characteristics of the individuals in the practice stories in relation to five relatively simple home modification interventions are presented in Table 45.1. More detail can be obtained by reading the individual practice stories and watching the associated short videos.

The home I Designed and Built Myself – Chris's Story

In 2000 Chris moved from the United Kingdom to Australia to take up an information technology (IT) management position. After an accident that resulted in a complete T6 paraplegia, he met his wife, an occupational therapist, changed careers and now works in an access consultancy business in partnership with his wife.

Funded by accident compensation, Chris was able to design and purpose-build a house to accommodate his impairment and the needs of his growing family of four children under the age of 7. The house was 5 minutes from the consultancy business where he worked.

Chris and his wife had no family around for support, so they used order and routine to keep life running smoothly. Their children helped Chris to reach things when the floor became too cluttered with their toys. Chris designed things like an accessible pool filter, work bench and rubbish disposal system that allowed him to be independent and the opportunity to do as many of the 'boys jobs' as possible.

Before Chris's accident he worked in IT and so was familiar with computer-aided design software. He expanded on his ability to use this software to design his whole house. He became what he described as super 'teched up'.

Chris (Fig. 45.2) was incredibly well informed through a personal interest and work interest. He used universal and adaptable design principals when designing his house. His product choices were a result of rigorous research, mostly online but also through conversations with friends, visiting retailers, advice from builders and tradeworkers and some creative adaption of 'not for that purpose' products. Grab rails were the only do-it-yourself modification Chris did not incorporate, regarding them as not necessary for his needs.

To listen to Chris' home modification story, go to https://www.youtube.com/watch?v= GqdDZc_kH4M.

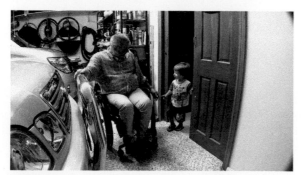

FIG. 45.2 ■ Chris in his garage. *(Photo by Shelley O'Neil, www.jumpthefence.com.)*

Once a Mechanic and a Doer, Always a Doer – Jack's Story

Jack lived on his own in the three-bedroom house he and his now deceased wife bought when he was 83 years old. Jack was very independent and capable despite his 93 years, back problems, pronounced stoop and loss of mobility in his right shoulder and the loss of purpose he had felt since his wife passed away at home a year ago.

Jack was able to drive and would regularly drive to visit family, the club and his exercise class. He did all his own shopping and cooking and would rather his son did not take over the lawn mowing, saying, 'You go stale if you just sit around'.

Jack's daughter and son Gary were very present in his life, and his adult grandchildren visited often. Jack served in New Guinea in the army and so had financial support from Veterans Affairs.

Jack had significant hearing loss and a timid German Shepherd. After he was burgled 2 years ago he had a four-camera video security system installed. Jack did not use a mobile phone or a computer and did not see that he had any need for these types of technologies.

An occupational therapist contracted to Veterans Affairs visited Jack every so often to advise him on his home modification needs. Over the years, handrails, chair stills, and grab rails were installed. A handheld shower was also installed, which Jack rejected.

Jack liked to potter and make things. He improved on the chair stills and put the old shower head back on. He built his first ramp soon after moving into the house, just before he 'had his knee done', using his building skills and found materials. He welded the handrails himself. Jack and his family more recently built a replacement ramp as the other was rotting and the handrails were not high enough (Fig. 45.3).

To listen to Jack's home modification story, go to https://www.youtube.com/watch?v= sIh8oEdU3mo.

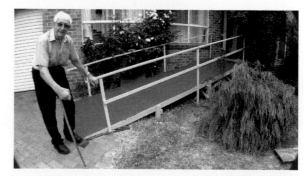

FIG. 45.3 ■ Jack and the ramp he built. *(Photo by Shelley O'Neil, www.jumpthefence.com.)*

PRACTICE STORY 45.3

Aging at Home in the Country – Paul's Story

Two years ago Paul and his wife, Robyn, 'sold up' their 100-acre 'retirement project' property and moved into a nearby country town because it was becoming too much for them. Paul had a fall 2 years before their move that brought on epilepsy, and a back operation left him with double incontinence and constant pain. Robyn was driving Paul the 200-km return trip to the nearest hospital at least once a week for his medical needs. More recently, Paul had a hip replacement that temporarily left him immobile.

Paul and Robyn's daughter was about to move to the United States of America with their 'one and only' grandson so that her American husband could fulfil his family obligations. Paul's son-in-law was an engineer and had installed many of Paul's do-it-yourself home modifications.

Robyn had an old mobile phone, but she did not like to use it. She had it when she worked at a pharmacy because she had a long drive home at night. They had a computer at home, which Paul used to write grant applications for the Lions Club they belonged to and Robyn used to find quilting patterns.

Paul felt the hospital staff were not very helpful in considering his housing needs and preferences and gave no advice about assistive technology and home modification. As a result he felt he and his family had to 'wing it'. Consequently Paul relied on word of mouth from their friends in regards to receiving community services such as the building service used for constructing his ramps. Paul used the Internet to find a special walker tall enough and retail assistants at their nearest hardware outlet to find a suitable handheld shower and grab rails (Fig. 45.4).

To listen to Paul's home modification story, go to https://www.youtube.com/watch?v= liiyitT3cJc.

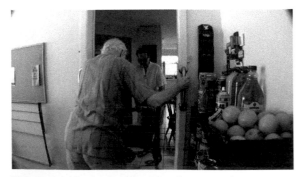

FIG. 45.4 ■ Paul using his grab rail to move down a step. *(Photo by Shelley O'Neil, www.jumpthefence.com.)*

PRACTICE STORY 45.4

Serial Renovation Experience – Toni's Story

After a few years in her apartment Toni felt the bathroom and laundry were too small, so she engaged a builder to remodel the space according to her vision. Toni referred to herself as a 'serial renovator' and loved keeping up with the latest products by looking online and in retail stores. Toni sourced most of her components through a local bathroom retailer (Fig. 45.5).

Toni worked part time as a disability consultant despite her sometimes very debilitating autoimmune disease. The disease affected all her joints and her mobility; when her condition was severe she required a wheelchair, and when her condition was less severe she could do most things around the house.

Toni lived alone with her two cats in a two-bedroom apartment in a modern block. Downstairs was a trendy café where she often caught up with friends. Toni had a strong friend network and had built relationships with her neighbours through mutual assistance arrangements such as child minding, looking after keys and sharing in potluck dinners. Toni paid a cleaner to come once a week to clean her apartment.

Toni's daughter lived locally and Toni regularly looked after her two grandchildren. Toni and her daughter's family also socialised at least twice a week. Toni was quite technically savvy; she had a smartphone and a new iMac for work and personal use.

To listen to Toni's home modification story, go to https://www.youtube.com/watch?v= TWIhSD-79Qo.

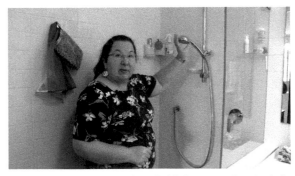

FIG. 45.5 ■ Toni and her handheld shower. *(Photo by Shelley O'Neil, www.jumpthefence.com.)*

TABLE 45.1

Overview of Home Modifications for Chris, Paul, Jack and Toni

Name and Brief Background	Handheld Shower	Grab Rail	Hand Rail	Level Access Shower	Ramps
Chris					
■ Middle aged ■ Access consultant ■ Married with four kids ■ Urban location	✓		✓	✓	✓
Jack					
■ Older person ■ Veteran ■ Retired mechanic ■ Widower					✓
Paul					
■ Older person ■ Husband ■ Grandparent ■ Retired pharmacist ■ Rural location	✓	✓	✓		✓
Toni					
■ Middle aged ■ Small business owner ■ Grandparent ■ Divorced	✓	✓		✓	

HOME MODIFICATION IN OCCUPATIONAL THERAPY PRACTICE

Where a person is at risk of losing the ability to live independently or safely in the home, home modification can be undertaken to improve the accessibility and enabling characteristics of that home. Thus where structural changes are made specifically to improve independence and safety, decisions about housing changes are made based on the existing structure and design of the existing dwelling and the health and well-being of the person living there. This is an expression of the interplay among location, structure, person and modification.

The term *home modification* is a composite of two words: *home* and *modification*. Housing studies indicate that the concept of home has a plethora of characteristics, some of which are not mutually exclusive (Booth, 1982; Fallis, 2014; Harvey, 2010). For instance, a home can be thought of as a commodity having the following key features, which make it, like a person, unique:

■ Heterogeneous in type, quality, space, age, upkeep
■ Spatially fixed (services such as water, power and waste cannot be easily moved)
■ A commodity that people cannot do without
■ Durable (lifespan of housing can be 200 years)
■ Changes ownership infrequently

■ Land is permanent and improvements have a long life expectancy
■ Changeable: ability to be retro-fitted, modified and updated
■ Various uses (e.g. shelter, privacy, status) that are not mutually exclusive

Historically the term *home modification* has been closely associated with the notion of home renovation or remodelling but was thought of as less extensive and is more associated with disability (Bridge, 2009). The term *modification* implicitly deemphasises fashion, aesthetic or stylistic concerns that are inherent in the notion of remodelling. More formally, in a programme or block funding sense, the term *home modification* typically refers to structural changes to a person's home to improve occupational performance, safety or accessibility.

Home modifications are not assistive technology, and they are not the act of moving a rug across a room. Home modifications do not include general repairs to the home or improvements designed for lifestyle, fashion or aesthetics alone. Home modification is often associated with other assistive technology interventions such as grab rails or bars, the dynamics of which have been described as 'complex' in a number of research studies (Johansson, Lilja, Petersson, & Borell, 2007; Lord, Menz, & Sherrington, 2006).

A grab bar is clearly a piece of assistive technology. Its correct placement and installation is not unlike assistive technology that sits with health and therapeutic good legislations and regulation. The installation of a grab rail is governed by building codes and requires, in addition, an understanding of the who, what, where and why specifications associated with the domain of building and construction. For this reason, home modification work typically involves working with builders and designers who may sit outside the health and social care services. Although legislation varies from country to country and region to region, there are typically a number of requirements, which apply everywhere (Bridge, 2009).

It is important to check relevant environmental legislation and regulations before making any home modification recommendation (Bridge, 2009), especially as zoning laws and development legislation may directly affect home modification options. Knowledge of accessibility guidelines, local and national building codes and other relevant legislation (i.e. negligence, product liability, trespass, etc.) is helpful. On one hand, building codes stipulate the minimum necessary standards to achieve health, safety, amenity and sustainability of the building; on the other hand, accessibility codes provide guidance on aspects of physical accessibility relevant to some if not all home modifications.

Yet the human experience of housing is highly individualised and each person's physical health and level of ability is unique, which directly affects what daily tasks they can perform within the person's home and the extent to which they can perform these tasks. Thus the practice of home modification, unlike universal design, is bespoke. This is similar to buying a garment off the rack that, even though it is the right size, may not fit perfectly compared with having a garment individually designed and tailored based on a person's specific measurements, requirements, preferences and intentions; the custom-made garment is much more likely to 'fit' perfectly.

EVIDENCE OF HOME MODIFICATIONS' EFFECTIVENESS

The increasing quantity of available research evidence since the 1990s is an encouraging trend towards improving the understanding of how home modifications effect caregiving, safety, health, well-being and social participation. A systematic review (Carnemolla & Bridge, 2015) commissioned by Home Modifications Australia (MOD.A), the peak organisation for home modification services within Australia, enabled a first-of-its-kind, bird's-eye overview or mud map of what is currently globally known about the effectiveness of home modifications as a practice area. Of the 77 studies included in the review, it is important to note that a large number of terms were used to refer to either home modifications or a multifactorial intervention that included home modifications. These terms ranged from the very specific (i.e. *bath grab bar*) to the very general (i.e. *environmental adaptation*).

Seven key themes have been identified within home modification publications. These themes provide an understanding of what home modifications might achieve for individuals. For instance, falls reduction research and activities of daily living

(ADLs) or function-related effects are strongly supported by high-quality studies, whereas home modifications' effects on physical health and well-being, caregiving, economic effectiveness, aging process and social participation are more weakly understood. The seven themes are illustrated as stacked bars in Fig. 45.6 and include falls, self-care and independence, physical health and well-being, caregiving, economics, aging and social participation.

Theme 1: Fall Prevention

The strongest evidence for home modification effectiveness has been associated with falls (Carnemolla & Bridge, 2015). Several systematic reviews found positive evidence that a home modification intervention can reduce the likelihood of a fall or injury occurring (Chang et al., 2004; Clemson, Mackenzie, Ballinger, Close, & Cumming, 2008; Tse, 2005; Turner et al., 2011). Despite some contradictory evidence (Wahl, Fänge, Oswald, Gitlin, & Iwarsson, 2009) on the effect of home modifications on falls prevention, five systematic reviews found home modifications effective in reducing the likelihood of a fall or injury occurring as a part of a *multifactorial intervention* (i.e. home modification in combination with assistive technology and exercise) (Chang et al., 2004; Clemson et al., 2008; Tse, 2005; Turner et al., 2011). Overall it was found that home modifications may have a positive effect by doing the following:

- Improving confidence and reducing fear of falling (Chase, Mann, Wasek, & Arbesman, 2012)
- Reducing injuries in older people living at home (i.e. those persons with osteoporotic changes and/or the loss of skeletal muscle mass and strength as a result of aging) (Plautz, Beck, Selmar, & Radetsky, 1995).

Theme 2: Self-care and Independence

Home modifications' effect on the autonomy and ability to carry out valued self-care activities without assistance was a focus of research as home modifications could either eliminate, change or reduce caregiving. Indeed, all systematic reviews (Chase et al., 2012; Wahl et al., 2009) and five randomised controlled trials (Gitlin, Corcoran, Winter, Boyce, & Hauck, 2001; Mann, Ottenbacher, Fraas, Tomita, & Granger, 1999; Szanton et al., 2014; Wilson, Mitchell, Kemp, Adkins, & Mann, 2009) found that home modifications led to an improvement in a person's function and/or a reduction in ADL difficulty. Additionally, others found improvements in the following:

- Feelings of self-efficacy (Gitlin et al., 1999, 2006; Ostensjo, Carlberg, & Vollestad, 2005; Petersson et al., 2012)
- Mobility (Berg, Hines, & Allen, 2002; Ostensjo et al., 2005)
- Cognitive function (Guo, Tsai, Liao, Tu, & Huang, 2014)

For people who have cognitive impairment, their homes act as a vessel of memories and a cue to action and can contribute to keeping people at home longer via sensitive modifications (Van Hoof, Kort, van Waarde, & Blom, 2010).

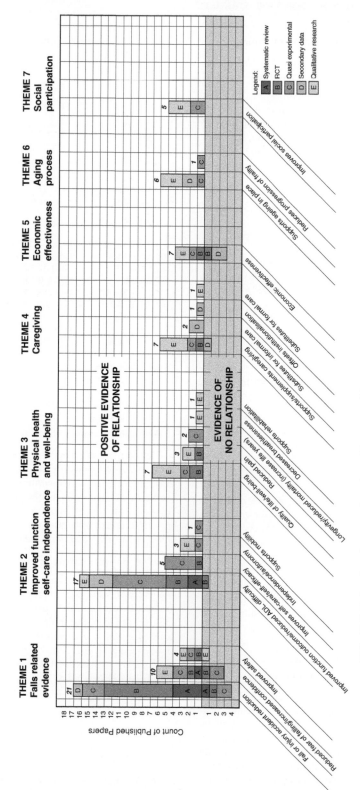

FIG. 45.6 ■ Results of systematic review of home modification impacts. *(From Carnemolla & Bridge, 2015.)*

Theme 3: Physical Health and Well-being

Physical health and well-being is part of 'quality of life' and life satisfaction research and in this category there were reported improvements in the following:

- Health, comfort and happiness by the person with an illness, injury or impairment – featured in two randomised controlled studies (Ahmad, Shakil-ur-Rehman, & Sibtain, 2013; Lin, Wolf, Hwang, Gong, & Chen, 2007).
- Breathing as a result of reducing moulds, pollens and pollutants, accommodating respirators and reducing steam build-up
- Reduction in pain as a result of less strain on joints and muscles

Theme 4: Caregiving

Caregiver impact can be best understood in terms of who provides the care. Three types of caring have been identified (Aronson & Neysmlth, 1997; Australian Bureau of Statistics, 2012):

- Care delivered by paid staff or trained volunteers (i.e. formal care)
- Care delivered by unpaid carers, usually family members (i.e. informal care)
- Self-care, or the capacity of a person to undertake tasks associated with showering or bathing, dressing, eating, toileting, and bladder or bowel control

Home modification has the potential to make caregiving easier, safer and more time efficient by ensuring adequate circulation space and by installation of mechanical lifters and so on (Agree, Freedman, Cornman, Wolf, & Marcotte, 2005; Anderson & Wiener, 2013; Newman, Struyk, Wright, & Rice, 1990). This is particularly important in the context of funding formal care and taking time out of paid work to provide informal care. Caregiver stress is exacerbated by workforce shortages in combination, leading to the demand for care exceeding its supply (Carnemolla & Bridge, 2011; Gray & Heinsch, 2009). Davy, Adams, & Bridge, (2014) found that home design and modification considerations needed to consider the perspectives and views of carers and other members of the household, as well as those of the person with an illness, injury or impairment, particularly in regards to how the proposed modification of the home could do the following:

- Assist carers in specific care activities
- Provide a private space to retreat to
- Facilitate activities of other household members

Carnemolla (2015) used a quasi-experimental mixed-methods research design to examine how 157 participants changed their care patterns after a home modification intervention. Results from quality-of-life scores and informal and formal care hours were compared before and after home modifications, and the key finding was that home modification directly substituted for care. Informal care was the most sensitive, with reductions in care as high as:

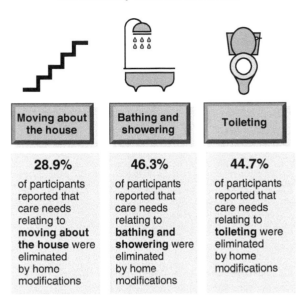

Where is care likely to be substituted by home modifications?

Moving about the house	Bathing and showering	Toileting
28.9%	**46.3%**	**44.7%**
of participants reported that care needs relating to **moving about the house** were eliminated by home modifications	of participants reported that care needs relating to **bathing and showering** were eliminated by home modifications	of participants reported that care needs relating to **toileting** were eliminated by home modifications

FIG. 45.7 ■ How home modifications substitute for care in the home. *(Adapted from Carnemolla, 2015)*

- 63% for bathing and showering;
- 47% for toileting; and
- 41.1% for moving about the house.

The greatest reduction in formal care occurred in moving about the house, followed by bathing and showering. These results clearly indicate that care is sensitive to home modifications, with a 47% overall reduction in the care provided. As shown in Fig. 45.7, home modifications may not only support caregiving but substitute for it, and this suggests a strong relationship between home modification and improved health-related quality of life.

Theme 5: Economic Effectiveness

Home modification is typically a large one-off cost compared with ongoing smaller costs such as providing a formal caregiver to assist someone in bathing. This large one-off cost has been shown to be effective as an economic strategy for reducing cost overall, but this depends on a number of factors, and perspectives vary depending on who pays over what period of time. Nevertheless, home modifications as a multifactorial intervention are generally viewed as cost effective (Heywood & Turner, 2007; Jutkowitz, Gitlin, Pizzi, Lee, & Dennis, 2012; Lansley et al., 2004; Mann et al., 1999).

Theme 6: Aging Process

There is a lack of strong experimental data that has focused on the impact of home modification on the aging process. However, home modifications has been linked to the following:

- Slower progression of frailty (Hwang et al., 2011; Mitoku, 2014; Safran-Norton, 2010)

■ Enhanced meaning of home for some people (Tanner, Tilse, & De Jonge, 2008), but not always (Ahn & Hegde, 2011)

Given the mixed finding about the emotive impact, it can be conjectured that nonaesthetic or stigmatising interventions such as ramps that take up most of the front yard could have a negative effect, whereas an intervention that improved value and home pride would have the opposite effect.

Theme 7: Social Participation

Studies on social participation, although scarce, suggest that home modifications may have a positive effect on social participation in the form of:

■ reduced effort, greater visit-ability and increased perceptions of competence and control (Heywood et al., 2001; Ostensjo et al., 2005; Pettersson, Löfqvist, & Malmgren Fänge, 2012; Randström, Asplund, & Svedlund, 2012; Vik, Nygard, & Lilja, 2007).

The fact that international policy and guidelines promote active aging and greater social participation (Cannuscio, Block,

& Kawachi, 2003; Noreau et al., 2004) is important as modifying the home environment appears to be one means of improving a person's ability to leave the home, entertain at home and add value to themselves and others.

HOME ASSESSMENT AND FOLLOW-UP

Occupational therapists receive some training in modification as part of their undergraduate training and during practice placements. However, this training is not comprehensive nor always in context. For example, the assessment of a domestic environment in the hospital context for a person who has a spinal cord injury is very different to that carried out for a person with dementia living in public housing.

Occupational therapy home assessors should consider the physical features and subfeatures, characteristics and subcharacteristics (relevant to the people receiving occupational therapy services) as outlined in Table 45.2. The items in Table 45.2 are indicative only but do demonstrate the level of analysis that the therapist should consider before making

			TABLE 45.2		
		Features and Subfeatures, Characteristics and Subcharacteristics Relevant to Assessment for Home Modification (Millikan, 2012)			
Feature	**Subfeature**	**Characteristics**	**Subcharacteristics**		**Impact on Function**
Access	■ Street frontage (or equivalent) ■ Driveway ■ Front access ■ Back access ■ Side access ■ Internal access	■ Gutter/kerbing ■ Stairs/steps ■ Ramp ■ Driveway ■ Lift/elevator ■ Lighting	■ Material (concrete, wood, tiles, etc.) ■ Slope/gradient ■ Ownership		■ Mobility
Bath	■ Main or en suite ■ Indoor or outdoor ■ Large/small ■ Upstairs/ downstairs	■ Shower ■ Bath ■ Hand shower ■ Sliding glass door ■ Shower enclosure ■ Flooring ■ Taps, faucet (single or double) ■ Storage ■ Drainage	■ Materials (tiled, linoleum, timber, concrete sheet, concrete slab) ■ Tap type, faucet type, tap control		■ Transfers ■ Mobility ■ Personal care
Toilet	■ Main or en suite ■ Indoor or outdoor ■ Size ■ Location	■ Style ■ Seat height ■ Seat position ■ Cistern location ■ Grab rails/assistive technology ■ Bidet	■ Materials ■ Floor covering, ■ Flush control mechanism ■ Toilet paper ■ Storage		■ Transfers ■ Personal care
Hallway	■ Size ■ Length ■ Purpose	■ Lighting ■ Access/egress	■ Floor surface/covering ■ Direction/prompts ■ Control of lighting		■ Mobility

Continued on following page

TABLE 45.2
Features and Subfeatures, Characteristics and Subcharacteristics Relevant to Assessment for Home Modification (Millikan, 2012) *(Continued)*

Feature	Subfeature	Characteristics	Subcharacteristics	Impact on Function
Bedroom	■ Location and access to room ■ Main/secondary/spare ■ Use/size ■ Upstairs/downstairs	■ Access/egress ■ Furniture ■ Users – shared, sole occupant, activity	■ Windows/window dressings and control thereof ■ Thermoregulation (passive) and temperature management tools and control thereof ■ Power sources and control thereof ■ Lighting and control of lighting	■ Transfer ■ Mobility ■ Personal care ■ Domestic tasks
Kitchen	■ Location ■ Size ■ Set out (galley, square, rectangle, open plan)	■ Access/egress ■ Users ■ Use of room (eating or preparation only)	■ Appliances: type of and location of: –fridge/freezer/kettle, etc. –stove type and controls –oven type and controls –microwave type and controls –direction of door opening ■ Source of drinking water	■ Transfer ■ Mobility ■ Eating/drinking ■ Domestic tasks
Lounge	■ Location ■ Size ■ Position/aspect	■ Access/egress ■ Seating ■ Furniture position and use	■ Thermoregulation (passive), and temperature management tools and control ■ Windows/window dressings ■ Power sources ■ Lighting ■ Appliances: –television –DVD/video player/stereo/remote control –fans/air conditioners ■ Seating – type and control (if relevant)	■ Transfer ■ Mobility ■ Eating/drinking ■ Domestic tasks
Garden	■ Location ■ Size ■ Position/aspect	■ Access/egress ■ Yard furniture position and use ■ Seating ■ Yard equipment (clothesline) ■ Verandah/pergola ■ Roofed area ■ Pool ■ Garden tap ■ Fencing	■ Materials (tiled, paving, timber, concrete sheet, concrete slab) ■ Tap type, faucet type, tap control, ■ Paths	■ Transfer ■ Mobility ■ Eating/drinking ■ Domestic tasks ■ Home maintenance ■ Yard care ■ Pet care ■ Security

a recommendation. Careful examination and analysis of the person and the person's abilities and environment is crucial before making recommendations about the modification of a person's home.

Basic task and activity analysis is the key to quality assessment of functional problems. However, as stated in Millikan (2012), the competent therapist needs to look more widely than just task analysis and observations when proposing home modification intervention. For example, in addition to a person's level of ability to clean his or her body, it is critical to reflect on the following:

■ Physical attributes and design of the room
■ Body cleansing tools available
■ Alternative body cleansing techniques, assistive products and technologies

Looking at each aspect of the tasks, including the environmental and tool-based requirements, the therapist may be able to identify additional issues, modifications, equipment or a change in the process should be considered. Looking at each aspect of the tasks enables the therapist to collect the evidence required to support the recommendations for an environmental modification.

As stated in Fishpool and Bridge (2012), most home modification interventions include some postassessment follow-up with people. Some form of postmodification follow-up is needed to gather information about the impact of the modification for the person, as modifications can be complex. Failure to follow up can risk missing important feedback necessary both for optimal outcomes and one's own personal learning (Sanford & Butterfield, 2005).

A variety of checklists, attention direction frameworks, surveys and observation techniques can be used to guide the assessment and follow-up process, measure the completion of recommendations (Cumming et al., 1999) and review changes to the person's ability and function. However, as Barras (2005) noted, no consistent and standardised assessment tool currently exists. Home modification follow-up, as distinct from initial assessment, requires additional specific attention to the following:

- Installation (i.e. asking if the modification has been correctly installed to specification by the agreed installer)
- Usage (i.e. to ascertain if the person is using the modification and if there are any questions about how to use the modification)

- Functionality (i.e. to determine that this modification has solved the functional issue satisfactorily)
- Safety (i.e. questioning regarding any risks or unintended consequences associated with the modification)

It is important to be aware that, although home modification service funders typically place the highest priority on functional outcomes, failure to factor in meaning and personalisation can lead people to reject the modifications (Bridge et al., 2007; Clemson, Cusick, & Fozzard, 1999). For instance, homes fulfil many needs for the occupants: they provide a place of self-expression, a vessel of memories, and a place of refuge from the outside world, in addition to affording a place to transact self-care and other care tasks.

BARRIERS TO HOME MODIFICATION INTERVENTION

There are a number of factors outside the person that may present barriers to home modification intervention. For instance, Bridge et al. (2007) suggest that there are seven barriers. These are included in Fig. 45.8.

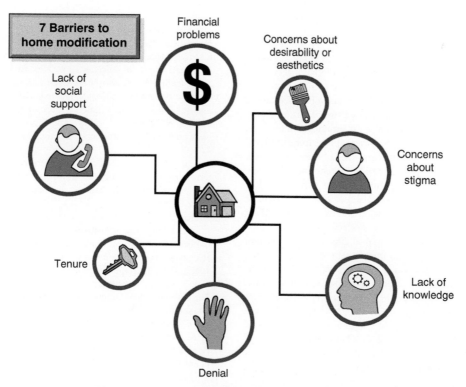

FIG. 45.8 ∎ Barriers to home modification interventions.

The seven barriers fall into two main categories: practical and psychological. Practical barriers include financial problems, lack of knowledge, aesthetics/desirability and tenure. Practical barriers can be significant; however, the psychological barriers to home modifications, which include concerns about stigma, lack of social support and perception of need, may be more problematic and are often underexplored by therapists.

Also as cited in Bridge et al. (2007), previous research has found that people with modification needs may often have a low socioeconomic status, high unemployment rates and are woman who tend to live alone and not own their dwellings. Significantly, many people with illness, injury or impairment are unaware of relevant existing services and funding that can be used for home modifications. For instance, general knowledge and acceptance of the formal service system are generally viewed as better predictors of home modification service usage than the demographics of functional capacity (Naik & Gill, 2005). Indeed, good information regarding what works, how much it will cost and the implications can be hard to locate as most governments and services have not systematically gathered or invested in these data and may erroneously believe that less information available to the general public may help cap modification services and associated government funding. Tenure is another significant issue, and if a person lacks a secure home base, or has to get building approval from others such as relatives, landlords or a body corporate, this can result in a clear pattern of significant differences in home modification rates even after controlling for age (ERMA et al., 2007).

Additionally, the stigma of being viewed by others as less capable and the need a person has to protect his or her self-image in the onset of traumatic change and loss of functional capacity often lead people to implement psychological strategies to help them cope with the anxiety associated with functional losses. These strategies preserve individuals' sense of self-worth during adjustment to the physical, functional and environmental limitations being experienced even though they may appear to be irrational from the perspective of outsiders (Katz, Fleming, Keren, Lightbody, & Hartman-Maeir, 2002). It is important to be aware that the psychological strategies may involve either a gradual psychological adaptation process (Calabro, 1990), brief defensive mechanisms such as denial, repression and rationalisation (Katz et al., 2002), or a mixture of the two strategies (Calabro, 1990).

Aside from lack of insight, denial can involve a belief system that considers the functional impairment to be temporary, views the residential situation as safe and comfortable, and/or perceives the financial implications as being too great. Further, any decision making entails predicting the future, and oftentimes people imagine how the outcomes of their choices will make them feel (emotional consequences), so it is not uncommon to avoid what they fear (Douglas & Jones, 2007). However, when the level of dysfunction tips from intermittent or moderate to severe, denial is typically replaced by action (Gitlin, 1995).

CONCLUSION

An overview of the importance of home modification has been presented in this chapter. With regards to home modifications, a better understanding of who, what, where and why is critical for occupational therapists in presenting information to the people they serve and for the people themselves in choosing to either accept or reject modifications to their homes that may improve their quality of life.

Home modification interventions are complex and are shaped by a variety of factors. Importantly, there is strong evidence that home modifications can reduce the likelihood of falls and injury, reduce fear of falling and improve confidence of those at risk of falls. Additionally, improvements in confidence and reduction of fear are also related to the well-being effects of improving a person's living space by modifying it.

 http://evolve.elsevier.com/Curtin/OT

REFERENCES

Agree, E., Freedman, V., Cornman, J., Wolf, D., & Marcotte (2005). Reconsidering substitution in long-term care: When does assistive technology take the place of personal care? *The Journals of Gerontology Series B: Psychological Sciences and Social Sciences, 60*(5), S272–S280.

Ahmad, J., Shakil-ur-Rehman, S., & Sibtain, F. (2013). Effectiveness of home modification on quality of life on wheelchair user paraplegic population. *Rawal Medical Journal, 38*(3), 263–265.

Ahn, M., & Hegde, A. (2011). Perceived aspects of home environment and home modifications by older people living in rural areas. *Journal of Housing for the Elderly, 25*(1), 18–30.

Altman, B., & Barnartt, S. (2014). *Environmental Contexts and Disability: (Vol. 8).* London: Emerald Group Publishing.

Anderson, W., & Wiener, J. (2013). The impact of assistive technologies on formal and informal home care. *The Gerontologist, 55*(3), 422–433.

Aronson, J., & Neysmlth, S. (1997). The retreat of the state and long-term care provision: Implications for frail elderly people, unpaid family carers and paid home care workers. *Studies in Political Economy, 53*, 37–66.

Australian Bureau of Statistics (2012). *Disability, Aging and Carers, Australia: Summary of Findings, 2012. (4430.0).* Retrieved from, Canberra Australia: Australian Bureau of Statistics. http://www.abs.gov.au/AUSSTATS/abs@.nsf/Lookup/4430.0Explanatory%20Notes5002012?OpenDocument.

Barras, S. (2005). A systematic and critical review of the literature: The effectiveness of Occupational Therapy Home Assessment on a range of outcome measures. *Australian Occupational Therapy Journal, 52*(4), 326–336.

Berg, K., Hines, M., & Allen, S. (2002). Wheelchair users at home: Few home modifications and many injurious falls. *American Journal of Public Health, 92*(1). 48.

Bleasdale, M., McNamara, N., Zmudzki, F., & Bridge, C. (2014). *Positioning paper: DIY home modifications: Point-of-sale support for people with disability and their carers.* Sydney: Home Modification Information Clearinghouse, UNSW Australia. Retrieved from, www.homemods.info.

Bogdon, A. S. (1996). Homeowner renovation and repair: The decision to hire someone else to do the project. *Journal of Housing Economics, 5*(4), 323–350.

Booth, P. (1982). Housing as a product: Design guidance and resident satisfaction in the private sector. *Built Environment,* 20–24.

Bridge, C. (2009). Home modification: Occupation as the basis for an effective practice. In M. Curtin, M. Molineaux, & J. Supyk J (Eds.), *Occupational therapy and physical dysfunction: Enabling occupation* (6th ed., pp. 409–430). Edinburgh: Churchill Livingstone Elsevier.

Bridge, C., Flatau, P., Whelan, S., Wood, G., & Yates, J. (2003). *Housing assistance and non-shelter outcomes: Australian Housing and Urban Research Institute.* Sydney: AHURI. Retrieved from, www.ahuri.edu.au/attachments/80188_final_housingassist.pdf.

Bridge, P. Phibbs, Gohar, N., & Chaudhary, K. (2007). *Evidence Based Research: Identifying barriers to home modifications.* Sydney: Home Modification Information Clearinghouse, UNSW Australia. Retrieved from, www.homemods.info.

Calabro, L. (1990). Adjustment to disability: A cognitive-behavioral analysis and clinical management. *Journal of Rational-Emotive and Cognitive-Behavior Therapy, 8*(2), 17–22.

Cannuscio, C., Block, J., & Kawachi, I. (2003). Social capital and successful aging: The role of senior housing. *Annals of Internal Medicine, 139*(5 Part 2), 395–399.

Carnemolla, P. (2015). *Measuring non-shelter effects of housing design: A mixed-methods exploration of home modifications, caregiving and health-related quality of life.* Unpublished PhD thesis.

Carnemolla, P., & Bridge, C. (2011). *Home modifications and their impact on waged care substitution.* Sydney: Home Modifications Information Clearinghouse.

Carnemolla, P., & Bridge, C. (2015). *Systematic review; evidence on home modifications.* Sydney: Home Modifications Information Clearinghouse.

Chang, J., Morton, S., Rubenstein, L., et al. (2004). Interventions for the prevention of falls in older adults: Systematic review and meta-analysis of randomised clinical trials. *BMJ, 328* (7441), 680.

Chase, C., Mann, K., Wasek, S., & Arbesman, M. (2012). Systematic review of the effect of home modification and fall prevention programs on falls and the performance of community-dwelling older adults. *American Journal of Occupational Therapy, 66*(3), 284–291.

Clemson, L., Cusick, A., & Fozzard, C. (1999). Managing risk and exerting control: Determining follow through with falls prevention. *Disability and Rehabilitation, 21,* 531–541.

Clemson, L., Mackenzie, L., Ballinger, C., Close, J., & Cumming, R. (2008). Environmental interventions to prevent falls in community-dwelling older people a meta-analysis of randomized trials. *Journal of Aging and Health, 20*(8), 954–971.

Cumming, R. G., Thomas, M., Szonyi, G. , et al. (1999). Home visits by an occupational therapist for assessment and modification of environmental hazards: A randomized trial of falls prevention. *Journal of the American Geriatrics Society, 47*(12), 1397–1402.

Davy, L., Adams, T., & Bridge, C. (2014). *Caring for the carer: Home design and modification for carers of young people with disability.* Sydney: Home Modification Information Clearinghouse, University of New South Wales Australia. Retrieved from, www.homemods.info.

Douglas, K., & Jones, D. (2007). How to make better choices. *New Scientist, 194*(2602), 35–43.

Environmental Resources Management Australia (ERMA), Phibbs, P., & Bridge, C. (2007). *Research into the nature of the need for home modification products and services in Queensland (final report).* Brisbane: Qld: Queensland Department of Housing and Public Works.

Fallis, G. (2014). *Housing economics.* Newmarket, ON: Butterworth-Heinemann.

Fishpool, J., & Bridge, C. (2012). *Follow-up efficacy post environmental modifications; a guide for clinical practice.* Sydney: Home Modification Information Clearinghouse, University of New South Wales. Retrieved from, www.homemods.info.

Gitlin, L. N. (1995). Why older people accept or reject assistive technology. *Generations, XIX*(1), 1–9.

Gitlin, L., Corcoran, M., Winter, L., Boyce, A., & Hauck, W. (2001). A randomized, controlled trial of a home environmental intervention: Effect on efficacy and upset in caregivers and on daily function of persons with dementia. *The Gerontologist, 41*(1), 4.

Gitlin, L., Hauck, W., Winter, L., Dennis, M., & Schulz, R. (2006). Effect of an in-home occupational and physical therapy intervention on reducing mortality in functionally vulnerable older people: Preliminary findings. *Journal of the American Geriatrics Society, 54*(6), 950–955.

Gitlin, L., Miller, K., & Boyce, A. (1999). Bathroom modifications for frail elderly renters: Outcomes of a community-based program. *Technology and Disability, 10*(3), 141–149.

Grand Designs (2014). *The Crooked Chocolate Box Cottage: Revisited. Series 13, Ep 4.* British Broadcasting: Commission. Retrieved from, http://docuwiki.net/index.php?title=Grand_designs:_series_14#The_Crooked_Chocolate_Box_Cottage_Revisited.

Gray, M., & Heinsch, M. (2009). Aging in Australia and the increased need for care. *Aging International, 34*(3), 102–118.

Guo, J., Tsai, Y., Liao, J., Tu, H., & Huang, C. (2014). Interventions to reduce the number of falls among older adults with/without cognitive impairment: An exploratory meta-analysis. *International Journal of Geriatric Psychiatry, 29*(7), 661–669.

Harvey, D. (2010). *Social justice and the city: (Vol. 1).* Athens, GA: University of Georgia Press.

Heywood, F., Oldman, J., & Means, R. (2001). *Housing and home in later life.* Buckingham: McGraw Hill Education.

Heywood, F., & Turner, L. (2007). *Better outcomes, lower costs. Implications for health and social care budgets of investment in housing* adaptations, improvements and equipment: review of the evidence London: Office for Disability Issues/Department of Work and Pensions.

Hwang, E., Cummings, L., Sixsmith, A., & Sixsmith, J. (2011). Impacts of home modifications on aging-in-place. *Journal of Housing for the Elderly, 25*(3), 246–257.

Johansson, K., Lilja, M., Petersson, I., & Borell, L. (2007). Performance of activities of daily living in a sample of applicants for home modification services. *Scandinavian Journal of Occupational Therapy, 14*(1), 44–53.

Jutkowitz, E., Gitlin, L., Pizzi, L., Lee, E., & Dennis, M. (2012). Cost effectiveness of a home based intervention that helps functionally vulnerable older adults age in place at home. *Journal of Aging Research, 2012,* 680265.

Katz, N., Fleming, J., Keren, N., Lightbody, S., & Hartman-Maeir, A. (2002). Unawareness and/or denial of disability: Implications for occupational therapy intervention. *Canadian Journal of Occupational Therapy, 69.5*(2002), 281–292.

Lansley, P., McCreadie, C., & Tinker, A. (2004). Can adapting the homes of older people and providing assistive technology pay its way? *Age and Aging, 33*(6), 571–576.

Lin, M., Wolf, S., Hwang, H., Gong, S., & Chen, C. (2007). A randomized, controlled trial of fall prevention programs and quality of life in older fallers. *Journal of the American Geriatrics Society, 55* (4), 499–506.

Lord, S., Menz, H., & Sherrington, C. (2006). Home environment risk factors for falls in older people and the efficacy of home modifications. *Age and Aging, 35*(2), ii55–ii59.

Lynch, K., & Findlay, I. (2007). *A new vision for Saskatchewan: Changing lives and systems through individualized funding for people with intellectual disabilities [a research report].* Saskatoon: Community-University Institute for Social Research and Centre for the Study of Co-operatives.

Mann, W., Ottenbacher, K., Fraas, L., Tomita, M., & Granger, C. (1999). Effectiveness of assistive technology and environmental interventions in maintaining independence and reducing home care costs for the frail elderly: A randomized controlled trial. *Archives of Family Medicine, 8,* 210–217.

Millikan, L. (2012). *Environmental assessment & modification for Australian occupational therapists.* Sydney: Home Modification Information Clearinghouse, University of New South Wales. Retrieved from, www.homemods.info.

Mitoku, K. (2014). Home modification and prevention of frailty progression in older adults: a Japanese prospective cohort study. *Journal of Gerontological Nursing, 40*(8), 40–47.

Naik, A. D., & Gill, T. M. (2005). Underutilisation of environmental adaptations for bathing in community-living older people. *Journal of the American Geriatric Society, 53,* 1497–1503.

Newman, S., Struyk, R., Wright, P., & Rice, M. (1990). Overwhelming odds: Care-giving and the risk of institutionalization. *Journal of Gerontology, 45*(5), S173–S183.

Noreau, L., Desrosiers, J., Robichaud, L., Fougeyrollas, P., Rochette, A., & Viscogliosi, C. (2004). Measuring social participation: Reliability of the LIFE-H in older adults with disabilities. *Disability & Rehabilitation, 26*(6), 346–352.

Ostensjo, S., Carlberg, E., & Vollestad, N. (2005). The use and impact of assistive devices and other environmental modifications on everyday activities and care in young children with cerebral palsy. *Disability & Rehabilitation, 27*(14), 849–861.

Petersson, I., Lilja, M., & Borell, L. (2012). To feel safe in everyday life at home a study of older adults after home modifications. *Ageing and Society, 32*(5), 791–811.

Pettersson, C., Löfqvist, C., & Malmgren Fänge, A. (2012). Clients' experiences of housing adaptations: A longitudinal mixed-methods study. *Disability and Rehabilitation, 34*(20), 1706–1715.

Plautz, B., Beck, D., Selmar, C., & Radetsky, M. (1995). Modifying the environment: A community-based injury-reduction program for elderly residents. *American Journal of Preventive Medicine, 12* (4 Suppl), 33–38.

Randström, K., Asplund, K., & Svedlund, M. (2012). Impact of environmental factors in home rehabilitation: A qualitative study from the perspective of older persons using the International Classification of Functioning, Disability and Health to describe facilitators and barriers. *Disability and Rehabilitation, 34*(9), 779–787.

Safran-Norton, C. (2010). Physical home environment as a determinant of aging in place for different types of elderly households. *Journal of Housing for the Elderly, 24*(2), 208–231.

Sanford, J., & Butterfield, T. (2005). Using remote assessment to provide home modification services to underserved elders. *Gerontologist, 45*(3), 389–398.

Straton, J., Saunders, N., Broe, T., Brown, W., Earle, L., & Gregory, B. (2003). *Promoting healthy ageing in Australia.* Retrieved from, http://www.dest.gov.au/science/pmseic/documents/promoting healthy aging report.doc.

Szanton, S. L., Wolff, J., Leff, B., et al. (2014). CAPABLE trial: A randomized controlled trial of nurse, occupational therapist and handyman to reduce disability among older adults: Rationale and design. *Contemporary Clinical Trials, 38*(1), 102–112.

Tanner, B., Tilse, C., & De Jonge, D. (2008). Restoring and sustaining home: The impact of home modifications on the meaning of home for older people. *Journal of Housing for the Elderly, 22*(3), 195–215.

Thomson, H., Thomas, S., Sellstrom, E., & Petticrew, M. (2013). Housing improvements for health and associated socio-economic outcomes. *Cochrane Database of Systematic Reviews, 2,* CD008657.

Tinker, A. (1997). Housing for elderly people. *Reviews in Clinical Gerontology, 7*(02), 171–176.

Tse, T. (2005). The environment and falls prevention: Do environmental modifications make a difference? *Australian Occupational Therapy Journal, 52*(4), 271–281.

Turner, S., Arthur, G., Lyons, R., et al. (2011). Modification of the home environment for the reduction of injuries. *Cochrane Database of Systematic Reviews, 2,* CD003600.

Van Hoof, J., Kort, H., van Waarde, H., & Blom, M. (2010). Environmental interventions and the design of homes for older adults with dementia: an overview. *American Journal of Alzheimer's Disease and Other Dementias, 25*(3), 202–232.

Vik, K., Nygard, L., & Lilja, M. (2007). Perceived environmental influence on participation among older adults after home-based rehabilitation. *Physical & Occupational Therapy in Geriatrics, 25* (4), 1–20.

Wahl, H., Fänge, A., Oswald, F., Gitlin, L., & Iwarsson, S. (2009). The home environment and disability-related outcomes in aging individuals: What is the empirical evidence? *The Gerontologist, 49*(3), 355–367.

Wiles, J. L., Leibing, A., Guberman, N., Reeve, J., & Allen, R. (2012). The meaning of 'ageing in place' to older people. *The Gerontologist, 52*(3), 357–366.

Wilson, D., Mitchell, J., Kemp, B., Adkins, R., & Mann, W. (2009). Effects of assistive technology on functional decline in people aging with a disability. *Assistive Technology, 21*(4), 208–217.

46 MOBILITY

KRISTY MAREE ROBSON

CHAPTER OUTLINE

Abstract

Mobility is key to healthy aging and is intimately linked to overall health status and quality of life (Webber, Porter, & Menec, 2010). With an aging population, mobility limitations are likely to have a significant impact on the individual, community and the health sector at large. Given mobility issues are common in the older population, addressing these issues can lead to improved function, safety, community participation and quality of life (Brown & Flood, 2013).

Falls in older people comprise the greatest contributors to mobility decline in this population group. Older people have increased susceptibility for injury given the increased prevalence of aged-related physiological changes, comorbidities and chronic disease and delayed functional recovery. These can all lead to musculoskeletal deconditioning, which further increases the risk of subsequent falling (Rubenstein & Josephson, 2002).

Mobility issues and fall-related risk can be challenging and complex to manage and require a comprehensive approach to work collaboratively with older people to maintain safe independence and community engagement. Occupational therapists have a significant role to play within the multidisciplinary team by facilitating the individual mobility goals and activities of the older person.

KEY POINTS

- Mobility issues in the adult population have a significant impact on a person's social participation, quality of life and physical well-being. As mobility issues are complex in nature, they require a holistic approach that encompasses both the individual and the physical and social environment in order to be managed.

- The ability to walk plays a significant role in mobility and independence. Evaluating a person's gait is an important strategy to determine where functional limitations are, so that targeted interventions can be implemented to reduce the risk of falls and improve mobility.

- Mobility limitations can be the result of chronic disease, psychological conditions or injury. However, as these three areas can be interrelated, issues arising in one area will often lead to increasing risk of developing limitations in the other two areas. When working with people to maintain or improve their mobility, considering all three areas is important.

- Falls in the older person are a significant public health issue across the world. Falling not only affects the individual but also family, friends, the community and the health sector. The role of a health professional is to identify older people who are at greatest risk of fall-related injury so that appropriate intervention strategies can be implemented.

- Fall-related injury can be related to a number of different risk factors. Commonly there are three general domains in which fall risk is categorised: extrinsic risk factors, intrinsic risk factors and behavioural risk factors. However, it is usually the interplay among multiple risk factors within all three domains, rather than just one or two, that poses the greatest threat to falling.

- Managing fall risk in older people is complex and challenging. A comprehensive multidisciplinary approach is needed to address all of the risk factors associated with fall risk to achieve effective intervention outcomes.

- Many older people are reluctant to admit to health professionals that they have fallen. This reduces the ability to address key risk factors before significant injury occurs. When interacting with older people, health professionals should be taking the opportunity to ask about a history of falls to assist in the identification and management of potential risk factors before an older person's risk status increases.

INTRODUCTION

The human body is designed for movement, and from a young age people are encouraged to develop the necessary skills to independently move around their environment. However, this ability to move around is often taken for granted. It is not until something happens as a result of illness, injury or impairment that people realise how important their mobility is to function effectively in their daily lives and community.

Usually people wish to have long, productive and independent lives without the consequences of illness, injury or impairment.

However, as people age there are greater threats to their mobility, with the most complex tasks, such as walking, being the first to be affected and signalling the first signs of declining mobility (Rantanen, 2013). One of the greatest contributors to mobility decline in the older population is fall-related injury. Falling has a significant impact not only on the individual but also on family and friends, the community and the health sector. Older people have greater susceptibility to injury given the increased prevalence of age-related physiological changes, comorbidities and chronic disease, combined with delayed functional recovery. These can all lead to musculoskeletal deconditioning, which further increases the risk of subsequent falling (Rubenstein & Josephson, 2002).

WHAT IS MOBILITY?

Mobility can be defined as the ability to move, either independently or with the use of an assistive device, within the home and community at large (Webber et al., 2010). Mobility is a key component in ensuring independence and enhancing health and quality of life (Oxley & Whelan, 2008). Limited mobility, which may or may not require the use of assistive devices, can encompass a range of mobility issues such as difficulties walking and climbing stairs, moving both inside and outside the home, using community transport and interacting with environmental infrastructure (Prohaska, Anderson, Hooker, Hughes, & Belza, 2011; Webber et al., 2010).

Alongside the physical element of mobility, it important to consider mobility limitations in the context of financial, psychosocial, environmental, cognitive, gender, cultural and biological factors (Webber et al., 2010). It is also useful to distinguish between an individual's current function and what capacity the individual has to achieve (Glass, 1998).

Mobility issues are very common among older people (Guralnik et al., 2000) and relatively common for adults in middle age (Melzer, Gardener, & Guralnik, 2005). Often the first sign of declining mobility starts in middle age, with an estimated 10% to 20% of middle-aged adults (50–65 years) reporting limitations in their mobility (Gardener, Huppert, Guralnik, & Melzer, 2006; Iezzoni, McCarthy, Davis, & Siebens, 2001; Melzer et al., 2005).

Mobility issues are complex to address across the adult population, requiring a multifaceted approach that considers the demographic, physiological, psychological and health status of the individual, as well as the health behaviours and living environment in order to successfully manage these issues (Stenholm, Shardell, Bandinelli, Guralnik, & Ferrucci, 2015).

WHY IS MOBILITY IMPORTANT?

When mobility is reduced or lost, it has significant impact on a person's social participation and quality of life and negative consequences on physical well-being. Alongside this, there are a number of public health burdens related to reduced or lost mobility in older populations (Satariano et al., 2012).

Problems associated with mobility can be linked to reduced access to goods and services, which can lead to poorer health outcomes (Oxley & Whelan, 2008). Mobility limitations increase sedentary behaviour, resulting in an increase in a number of chronic conditions (Lee & Buchner, 2008), these limitations may also restrict the instigation of preventative strategies in a timely manner (Fitzpatrick, Powe, Cooper, Ives, & Robbins, 2004), leading to further decline in health.

Commonly, multiple interrelating reasons for mobility problems can be identified rather than a single cause. For example, an adult who presents with osteoarthritis in a knee joint will likely have reduced range of movement available at this joint. This restriction can cause pain and a reduction of physical activity. This can lead to the person opting for a more sedentary lifestyle, potentially leading to increased risk of chronic conditions such as obesity, cardiovascular disease or diabetes, further affecting mobility (Fig. 46.1). A restriction in mobility limits opportunities to successfully manage chronic comorbidities, which can be improved with increases in physical activity. It also reduces the capacity for the individual to undertake these types of intervention strategies, possibly leading to poorer health outcomes in the long term.

Maintaining mobility is central to supporting a high quality of life and being able to undertake many of the activities required for independence, such as walking, shopping, attending appointments and generally engaging within the community (Shumway-Cook et al., 2003). Limited mobility is associated with multiple adverse outcomes and can lead to further functional decline, increased risk of comorbidities, increased financial costs in health care, institutionalisation and even death (Hardy, Kang, Studenski, & Degenholtz, 2011; Newman et al., 2006).

A number of studies that have shown the significant role that safe walking and mobility play in the quality of life of older adults (Hörder, Skoog, & Frändin, 2013; Verghese et al., 2006). Functional limitations and impairments can greatly affect the occupational engagement of people within their environment as well as their physical and mental well-being. However, just as poor health outcomes can be linked to impaired mobility, enhancing health and well-being through effective strategies to improve mobility is likely to be beneficial (Satariano et al., 2012).

Factors associated with mobility issues in adults can be challenging and need to be viewed in a holistic way to ensure that an individual's independence and quality of life are maintained (Meyer, Janke, & Beaujean, 2014). Health professionals need to view the complexity of mobility limitations through a comprehensive approach to successfully manage or prevent this important public health issue (Webber et al., 2010).

THE PRINCIPLES OF WALKING

As the ability to walk plays a significant role in mobility and independence, knowing the principles behind walking is useful for understanding how physical limitations can affect walking. Physiologically, walking involves the integration of functioning musculoskeletal, cardiorespiratory, sensory and neural systems (Rantanen, 2013). Alongside this, appropriate lower limb strength and postural balance are required to generate movement and maintain an upright position (Rantanen, Guralnik, Ferrucci, Leveille, & Fried, 1999). A deficit in any one of these systems is likely to affect a person's ability to walk and be mobile.

The skill of moving or walking requires a complicated process involving the brain, spinal cord, peripheral nerves, muscles, bones and joints (Whittle, 2002). It is important to understand the process of walking to appreciate what factors can influence mobility issues in the adult population.

Walking is defined as the ability of moving from one place to another through one's own mechanism or power (Whittle, 2002). There are four major elements essential to walking:

- **Equilibrium:** the ability to assume an upright posture and maintain balance.
- **Locomotion:** the ability to initiate and maintain rhythmic stepping.
- **Musculoskeletal integrity:** bone, joint and muscle function are needed.
- **Neurological control:** messages sent and received to inform the body how to move.

When there is a disruption in any of these four elements either by disease or injury, invariably mobility will be impaired.

What Are the Main Tasks Associated with Walking?

Three main tasks are associated with walking.

Weight acceptance: This is the most demanding task when walking. It involves transferring the body weight onto a lower limb that has just completed swinging forwards and is in unstable alignment. It also involves the ability to absorb shock when the foot hits the ground and allow for the forwards progression of the body.

Single leg support: This requires one lower limb to support the entire weight of the body. It also requires the same lower limb to provide trunk stability while the body continues progression.

Limb advancement: This requires the foot to clear the floor. The limb swings through three positions (behind the body, in

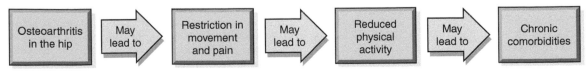

FIG. 46.1 ■ Interrelating causes for mobility limitations.

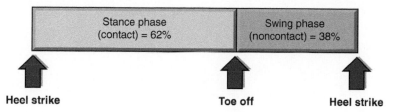

FIG. 46.2 ■ Phases of gait.

line with the body and in front of the body) as it travels through the swing phase.

Overview of the Gait Cycle

In a typical gait cycle there are two phases (Fig. 46.2):

- *Stance phase* (which takes up approximately 62% of the gait cycle)
- *Swing phase* (which takes the remaining 38% of the gait cycle)

The gait cycle is defined as the time from when the heel of one leg strikes the ground to the time when the same heel contacts the ground again. The stance phase is also known as the contact phase and is considered the time that the foot is in contact with the ground. The swing phase is also known as the noncontact phase and is the time when the foot is in the air.

During gait there are times when both feet are on the ground *(double support phase)* and other times when only one foot is on the ground *(single support phase)*. Double support phase occurs at heel strike when one foot is hitting the ground and the other leg is in toe-off. Single support phase occurs when one foot is in the middle of stance phase and the other leg is in swing phase.

During the single support phase the body is at its most unstable as all weight and balance must be achieved through one leg. Adults with mobility or balance problems are at the greatest risk of falling during the single support phase.

Joint Movement in Gait

Upper Body

During the gait cycle the upper body moves forwards with varying speed. It moves fastest during the double support phases and slowest when the body is in the middle of stance and swing phases (Whittle, 2002). The trunk twists around a vertical axis, with the shoulders rotating in opposite directions to the pelvis (Whittle, 2002). The arms will swing opposite to the corresponding leg so that the leg and pelvis can move forwards. That is when the right leg and pelvis are moving forwards, and so too are the left arm and left shoulder girdle (Whittle, 2002).

Hip

During the gait cycle the hip will flex and extend once. Maximum flexion is achieved around the middle of the swing phase, and it remains flexed until heel strike. Maximum extension is achieved before the end of stance phase and then the hip will begin to flex again (Whittle, 2002).

Knee

The knee will flex and extend twice during each gait cycle. It is extended before heel strike and then flexes during the early part of stance phase, extending again towards the end of stance phase and flexing again during early and middle parts of swing phase before extending again ready for heel strike (Whittle, 2002).

Ankle and Foot

At initial contact the ankle is around neutral (90 degrees); then it starts to plantarflex to bring the forefoot to the ground. As the lower leg moves forwards during contact phase, the ankle will start to dorsiflex and then just before toe-off the ankle will start planarflexing again and then move into a dorsiflexed position during swing phase in order to clear the ground, moving into a neutral position just before heel strike again (Whittle, 2002).

These joint movements during the gait cycle are illustrated in Fig. 46.3.

Changes in an adult's gait may be related to adaptions because of joint restrictions or other age-related alterations in the motor or sensory systems, in an attempt to improve or maintain stability (Salzman, 2010). Disorders associated with gait and balance are one of the main causes of falls (Ganz et al., 2007). Evaluation of a person's gait is important in order to determine where specific functional limitations are (Salzman, 2010) so that appropriate interventions can be instigated to minimise fall risk.

WHAT CAN AFFECT A PERSON'S MOBILITY?

Optimal mobility can be defined as the ability to safely and reliably walk from one area to another (Satariano et al., 2012), where reduced ability to walk can be defined as a limitation in a person's physical ability to navigate the environment (Marko, Neville, Prince, & Ploutz-Snyder, 2012). A report in the United States of America found that up to 30% of older adults had difficulty walking three city blocks or climbing one flight of stairs, with approximately 20% needing a mobility aid to assist them (Centers for Disease Control and Prevention, 2009).

As people age there are often signs that indicate they are having issues with their gait. These signs include increased stance

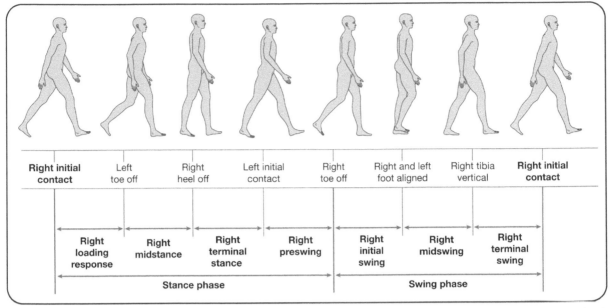

FIG. 46.3 ■ Overview of the gait cycle. *(From Braddom, R. L. (2011). Physical medicine and rehabilitation. Philadelphia: Saunders.)*

width, increased time spent in the double support phase, a bent posture and difficulty producing a smooth and effective toe-off movement (Salzman, 2010). A number of these changes can represent compensations as a result of problems with the sensory or motor systems in an attempt to produce a safer or more stable gait (Salzman, 2010).

There are a number of physical and sensory factors that can cause issues with gait, and as a result issues with mobility, in the adult population. Poor mobility and balance is commonly associated with an underlying neurological condition. Neurological gait abnormalities are a result of either focal or generalised lesions found in the neural pathways that link the cortical motor centres to the peripheral neuromuscular systems (Verghese et al., 2006) and are the most obvious cause of mobility limitations. However, there are also a number of nonneurological causes that can pose challenges to effective gait and mobility.

Musculoskeletal issues are common among the adult population. Any condition that affects the joint range of movement, whether it be a bone or joint deformity or restriction and issues associated with muscle or soft tissue function, can affect a person's mobility. The presence of generalised pain can also lead to compensations in walking that may cause instability.

Chronic diseases such as cardiovascular disease, obesity and diabetes, can limit a person's ability to stay mobile, as can issues related to vision. Mobility issues can be caused by a range of physical factors which have a neurological and nonneurological cause. Some examples of these causes are listed in Table 46.1.

In addition to the range of physical and sensory factors, a person's mobility can also be affected by a number of cognitive,

TABLE 46.1
Examples of Neurological and Nonneuro- logical Causes of Mobility Limitations

Physical Cause	Examples
Neurological	Parkinson's disease, multiple sclerosis, cerebrovascular accident (CVA), cerebral palsy, spina bifida, acquired brain injury, neuropathy
Nonneurological	Osteoarthritis, rheumatoid arthritis, joint restrictions caused by trauma, amputation, soft tissue restrictions, pain, foot deformity, cardiovascular disease, obesity, diabetes, vision impairment

psychological, environmental and financial factors (Webber et al., 2010). A number of these factors are listed in Table 46.2.

Life events affect mobility. For example, an older person diagnosed with Parkinson's disease who has walking difficulties may rely on a spouse to drive and to assist community mobility. If the person loses the spouse, then this is likely to have a significant effect on the person's ability to move around the community. Although a single element can limit a person's mobility, it is often the interrelationship of a number of these elements that can have the greatest impact on successful mobility (Brown & Flood, 2013; Inouye, Studenski, Tinetti, & Kuchel, 2007).

The key areas to think about when considering risk factors associated with limited mobility are illustrated in Fig. 46.4. Chronic

TABLE 46.2			
Cognitive, Psychological, Environmental and Financial Factors That Can Affect Mobility			
Cognitive Factors	**Psychological Factors**	**Environmental Factors**	**Financial Factors**
▪ Mental status ▪ Memory ▪ Speed of processing ▪ Executive functioning	▪ Self-efficacy ▪ Coping behaviours, especially around stigma ▪ Mental health issues (e.g. depression) ▪ Fear ▪ Motivation	▪ Physical obstacles ▪ Poor design or layout ▪ Inappropriate or challenging access	▪ Lower income is seen to be a risk factor for mobility impairment. ▪ Limited resources affect the ability to access assistance or make modifications to assist to compensate for mobility impairment.

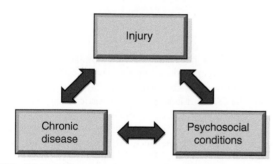

FIG. 46.4 ▪ Key areas that can affect mobility.

disease (e.g. diabetes, obesity, arthritis, cerebrovascular accident, Parkinson's disease) can significantly affect mobility (Brown & Flood, 2013; Gill, Murphy, Gahbauer, & Allore, 2013). Psychosocial conditions such as depression, cognitive impairment or fear of falling can also result in reduced mobility (Gill et al., 2013; Rivera, Fried, Weiss, & Simonsick, 2008). Injury as a result of a fall can also affect a person's mobility, not only directly as a result of the injury but also in the longer term if ongoing physical and psychological restrictions occur as a result of the injury.

Issues arising in one of these areas, whether chronic disease, psychosocial or injury, increase the risk of developing issues in the other two areas; that is, they are often interrelated, and it is important to address all key areas when working with people to maintain or improve their mobility. Alongside the consequences that reduced mobility have for the individual person, it is important to consider the impact on their family and the wider community.

FALL-RELATED INJURY IN OLDER PEOPLE

Falls in the older person are a significant public health issue across the world and represent the leading cause of unintentional injury in this population (Gelbard et al., 2014). It has

been reported that 1 in 3 older adults falls each year (Lord, Delbaere, Tiedeman, Smith, & Sturnieks, 2011; Watson, Clapperton, & Mitchell, 2011) with 20% to 30% suffering moderate to severe injuries as a result of their fall (Stevens, Corso, Finkelstein, & Miller, 2006). Falling has a significant impact not only on the individual, but also on family and friends, the community and the health sector.

The impact of falls can result in injury, impairment, loss of confidence and subsequent reduction in general activity as well as participation within the community (Close et al., 2012). Falling also significantly increases the chance of an older person being admitted into a residential aged care facility (Tinetti & Williams, 1997), with only about half of those hospitalised as a result of a fall-related fracture being able to return home (Moller, 2003).

When discussing a fall, health care providers commonly talk about the consequences of falling, such as the injury, health of the person and anatomical landing point (Zecevic, Salmoni, Speechley, & Vandervoort, 2006), whereas older people will often describe a fall as a loss of balance or unsteadiness (Haung et al., 2012). The World Health Organization (WHO) defines a fall as 'inadvertently coming to rest on the ground, floor or other lower level, excluding intentional change in position to rest in furniture, wall or other objects' (WHO, 2007, p. 1). However, the more commonly cited definition is from the Kellogg International Working Group on the Prevention of Falls in the Elderly, who defined a fall as 'unintentionally coming to ground, or some lower level not as a consequence of sustaining a violent blow, loss of consciousness, sudden onset of paralysis related to stroke or an epileptic seizure' (Gibson, Andres, Isaacs, Radebaugh, & Worm-Petersen, 1987, p. 4).

Given that falling poses significant risk to the older population, it is important that health professionals are clearly identifying older people who are at most risk of fall-related injury. Therefore health professionals should regularly ask older people about a fall history. The Prevention of Falls Network Europe (ProFaNE) suggest that health professionals ask older people, 'In the past month, have you had any fall including a slip or trip in which you lost your balance and landed on the floor or ground or lower level?' (Lamb, Jorstad-Stein, Hauer, & Becker, 2005).

RISK FACTORS ASSOCIATED WITH FALLS

A range of specific causes of falling are discussed in the literature. Commonly there are three general domains in which fall risk is categorised:

- Extrinsic risk factors
- Intrinsic risk factors
- Behavioural risk factors

Extrinsic risk factors can be defined as external or environmental factors that interact with the person. These types of risk factors include steps, vegetation such as leaves or seed pods on the ground, cracked footpaths or pavers, hoses, mats on the floor, pets, slippery floor surfaces, poor lighting, and bad footwear or long clothing (Ambrose, Geet, & Hausdorff, 2013; Grundstrom, Guse, & Layde, 2012; Rubenstein, 2006).

Intrinsic risk factors can be defined as relating to the individual person, such as chronic disease, vision impairment, muscle and balance limitations, multiple medications and types of medications, age, cognitive impairment, and incontinence (Ambrose et al., 2013; Grundstrom et al., 2012; Rubenstein, 2006).

Behavioural risk factors that have been cited in the literature include fear of falling or reduced physical activity (Painter et al., 2012), risk-taking behaviour linked to individual personality traits (Zhang, Ishikawa-Takata, Yamazaki, & Ohta, 2004), and hurrying when walking (Berg, Alessio, Mills, & Tong, 1997). More current research has found that risk-taking behaviour can be influenced by an older person's desire to maintain independence, which can result in older people knowingly undertaking high-risk activities (Robson, 2015).

It is important to understand that falling is usually the result of an interplay among multiple risk factors within all three domains, rather than just one risk factor (Fig. 46.5). Health professionals need to be mindful that facilitating the management of one or two risk factors does not necessarily mean that they have reduced an individual's risk. They may, in fact, inadvertently increase the risk for the older person if their health messages are focused on managing only some of the risk factors without considering the interplay of all three domains. This may result in older people perceiving they are no longer at risk because they have implemented the health professional's recommendations, and they continue to undertake high-risk activities because they perceive they are safe.

The concept of the interplay among the different domains can be demonstrated in Alfred's story. Alfred is in his 80s and lives with his wife, Beryl. Alfred had a mild stroke 5 years ago, which has resulted in a muscle weakness in his left leg. Since the stroke he has had three falls around the house, which have only resulted in minor injuries. After his last fall, Alfred's doctor

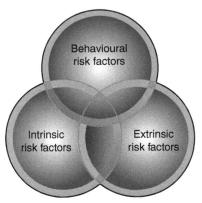

FIG. 46.5 ■ Interplay among the different domains of fall risk factors.

recommended that he attend a falls programme at the local hospital where he completed a strength and balance programme. He was also encouraged to keep active and exercise regularly. Recently he fell off a ladder when he was cleaning the leaves out of the gutters on his roof and broke his hip. Alfred and Beryl have no family close by so they have to undertake their own house and garden maintenance. Alfred believed it was safe because he was using a ladder he had used many times previously without incident. The story of Alfred can be used to identify the many elements involved in fall risk. These are listed in Table 46.3.

There are a lot of interplaying risks that could have contributed to Alfred's fall. The underpinning issue is that Alfred perceived that he was able to undertake this task successfully himself rather than organising someone to complete it for him. His behavioural decision to take the risk may have been influenced by the following:

- *The value he places on maintaining his independence.* By completing his own maintenance he demonstrates he is still independent.
- *His understanding of all of the possible risks.* If older people are not informed of the interplay between all domains, then they are unable to accurately determine whether a task is safe or not.
- *His experience doing the task.* If he successfully cleaned the gutters 12 months ago without incident, then he may perceive that he is still able to complete this task without appreciation that he has further aged.
- *Alfred's understanding of health messages.* He may misinterpret that getting up on a ladder is being active and that's how he can maintain his muscle strength.

The role of health professionals is not to limit an older person's ability to maintain his or her independence but rather to enable the person to safely and independently manage fall

TABLE 46.3

Risk Factors That Contributed to Alfred's Fall

Extrinsic Risk Factors	Intrinsic Risk Factors	Behavioural Risk Factors
■ The ladder may not have been well maintained, making it unstable. ■ The need to access all areas of the gutter may mean the ladder was placed on an uneven ground. ■ Alfred may have been wearing unsupportive shoes. ■ The time of day may have affected the amount of light available in all aspects of the house.	■ Alfred's muscle strength and his ability to get up and down the ladder successfully ■ Alfred's balance on the ladder and ability to reach outside his centre of gravity to clean the gutters ■ Any vision issues that may lead Alfred to not be able to adequately see the steps on the ladder ■ Possible comorbidities such as hypertension or the use of medications which may cause dizziness	■ Alfred's decision that he could successfully complete the task himself, rather than organising someone else to do it, without considering all the associated risks ■ Believing that by undertaking house maintenance, such as cleaning the gutters, was being active, which is what the health professionals wanted him to do ■ Alfred's perceiving that the ladder was safe because he had used it on numerous occasions previously and had not fallen off

risk. Awareness that a combination of multiple risks usually results in a fall is important for older people and the general community. When undertaking high-risk activities, consideration on the safest way to undertake the task should be encouraged. As health professionals it is important to increase the general understanding of the types of risks that can influence falling through using every opportunity to start the conversation with older people on fall risk. Health professionals' increasing discussion with older people on fall risk may help to reduce the number of injurious falls that occur in the community.

ASSESSING MOBILITY AND FALL RISK

There are a range of approaches for assessing mobility in adults. Performance-based measures can provide an objective measure to assess physical mobility issues within a practice setting (Patla & Shumway-Cook, 1999). However, it is important to appreciate that older people who may demonstrate adequate physical mobility may still be restricted in their ability to be successfully mobile as a result of other limitations such as cognitive, psychological or financial factors (Webber et al., 2010).

The International Classification of Functioning, Disability, and Health (ICF) is designed to enable practitioners to recognise that activities such as mobility can be influenced by existing health conditions, environmental elements and personal factors (Prohaska et al., 2011). The ICF also distinguishes mobility issues between performance and capacity. *Performance* refers to the activities that are observed, whereas *capacity* is concerned with a person's ability to undertake mobility tasks (Prohaska et al., 2011).

Commonly used performance-based tests for mobility in adults are shown in Table 46.4.

MANAGING FALL RISK IN OLDER PEOPLE

Managing fall risk in older people is complex and challenging. A comprehensive multidisciplinary approach is needed in order to achieve effective outcomes in reducing falls and fall-related injury among older people, depending on each older person's needs and identified risk factors. In the literature there are a wide range of interventions reported to manage fall risk. However, a Cochrane systematic review of randomised trials of interventions to reduce falls in older people living in the community (Gillespie et al., 2012) found the following areas demonstrated positive results in reducing falls:

■ Multifactorial interventions that assessed and managed the identified individual risk factors reduced the number of falls in older people but not the number of people falling.

■ Home modifications appear to be effective, especially in 'at risk' older people, when carried out by an occupational therapist.

■ Exercise programmes specifically aimed at reducing falls also appeared to reduce the number of fractures.

■ Group and home-based exercise programmes (containing some balance and strength).

■ Undertaking T'ai chi exercises.

■ Vitamin D supplementation for individuals with low levels of vitamin D may reduce falls.

■ Gradual withdrawal of drugs used to improve sleep, reduce anxiety and treat depression.

■ Cataract surgery in women having the operation on the first affected eye.

■ Insertion of a pacemaker in people with carotid sinus hypersensitivity who had been frequently falling.

TABLE 46.4
Performance-based Tests for Mobility

Performance Based Test	Description	Outcome Measure	Equipment Needed	References
Timed Up And Go Test (TUG)	Measures the time taken for a person to rise from a chair and walk 3 metres at a normal pace with his or her usual assistive device, turn, return to the chair, and sit down.	A time of 12 seconds or greater indicates an increased risk of falling.	■ Chair ■ Measured point of 3 metres ■ A watch with a minute hand or stopwatch	Rose et al. (2002); Close & Lord (2011); Alexandra et al. (2012)
Berg Balance Scale	Consists of 14 items that are scored on a scale of 0–4. A score of 0 is given if the person is unable to do the task and score of 4 if they are. The tasks include standing unsupported, sit-to-stand, transfers, single-leg stance, turning 360 degrees, etc.) Maximum score = 56.	Score of <45 indicates that older individuals may be at greater risk of falls (Berg et al., 1997). Score of ≤ 40 indicates almost a 100% fall risk (Shumway-Cook et al., 1997).	■ Stop watch ■ Chair with arm rests ■ Measuring tape ■ Object to pick up off the floor ■ Step stool	Berg et al. (1992); Thorbahn & Newton (1996) Shumway-Cook et al. (1997)
Figure-of-8 Walk Test (F8W)	Designed to measure walk skill, it requires a person to walk in a figure of 8 around two cones placed 1.5 m apart. Assesses time taken, the number of steps taken and accuracy in figure-of-8 formation.	A time > 10.49 seconds and >17.5 steps indicate walking difficulties.	■ A cleared area ■ Two cones or similar objects ■ Stopwatch ■ Tape measure	Hess et al. (2010)
Sit-to-Stand (STS)	Measures lower limb strength, speed and coordination through recording the time taken to complete five STS sequences as fast as possible from a chair.	A time of ≥12 seconds indicates increased risk of falling.	■ Chair of standard height (43 cm)	Tiedemann et al. (2008)
Modified Elderly Mobility Scale (MEMS)	Assesses motor function in older people with varying functional levels. Tasks include: lying to sitting, sitting to lying, sit-to-stand, standing, gait, walking 10 m, functional reach and stairs. Maximum score = 23.	Scoring is based on the level of assistance required to complete specific tasks as well as the time taken to complete the task. Higher scores indicate higher levels of function.	■ Measuring tape or metre ruler ■ Stopwatch ■ Access to a bed and chair ■ 10-m walkway ■ Steps	Kuys & Brauer (2006)
Functional Reach (FR)	Assesses the functional reach of an individual when positioned next to a wall with one arm raised to 90 degrees with fingers extended and a yardstick mounted on the wall at shoulder height.	Although there is some age-related variability, in general individuals should be able to reach >30 cm.	■ Yardstick mounted on a wall ■ Measuring tape	Duncan et al. (1990)

■ Assessment by a podiatrist providing review of footwear and management of foot pain and impairment reduced the number of falls but not the number of people falling.
■ Falls prevention education alone was inconclusive on whether it reduced falls in older people.

Occupational therapists working in a multidisciplinary team play a significant role in increasing or maintaining functional independence through addressing mobility concerns and fall-related risks (Steultjens et al., 2004) and supporting older people to remain safe in their environment (Chase, Mann, Wasek, & Arbesman, 2012). There is strong evidence to suggest that a reduction in fall-related injury can be achieved through a combination of education and home modifications, which can be expertly facilitated by occupational therapy practitioners (Chase et al., 2012).

Multifactorial Interventions

Multifactorial interventions that include a combination of approaches such as home modification, health and safety education, medication reviews, vision management, strength and balance training, and targeted exercise have been found to reduce the number of falls experienced by older people (Chase et al., 2012; Clemson et al., 2004; Gillespie et al., 2012). Programmes that include a combination of targeted strength and balance exercise and education sessions, such as the Stepping-On Program, have been found to be successful in reducing the risk of falls (Clemson et al., 2004).

Home Modifications

Home risk assessment and modifications are effective for older people who are at high risk of falls (Clemson, Mackenzie, Ballinger, Close, & Cumming, 2008; Karlsson, Vonschewelov, Karlsson, Coster, & Rosengen, 2013). Occupational therapists can review potential hazards in the home, such as mats, poor lighting and slippery floors, and unsafe behaviour, such as leaving clutter in high-traffic areas or wearing loose shoes or clothes that are too long. Understanding an older person's daily mobility challenges and providing appropriate education can lead to modifications made to reduce risk. However, it is unlikely that the removal of a home hazard alone is sufficient to reduce fall risk, because often it is the interaction between physical limitations of older person and the exposure of that person to a home hazard that creates the greatest risk (Lord et al., 2006). Therefore home assessment and modification should always be considered as part of a multifactorial approach towards managing fall risk (Tse, 2005).

Interestingly, Cumming et al. (2001) found that only about half of all older people who received home safety modifications adhered to the recommendations. They also found that if the older person understood that the modification could prevent his or her risk of falling, this increased the person's compliance in following the recommendations. Their study highlights that occupational therapists need to engage in a person-centred approach to facilitate collaborative discussion with older people about how their personal fall-related risk factors may interact with hazards within their environment, resulting in subsequent falls.

Education

Educating older people on how to safely navigate their environment and problem-solve solutions is an important element to assist in the prevention of fall-related injury (Clemson, Cusick, & Fozzard, 1999). The role of health professionals is to facilitate the independence of older people by enabling them to remain active while keeping safe or reducing the risk of injurious falls. Given that the home environment is the most common location for falls (Luukinen, Koski, Laippala, & Kivelä, 1995), education on potential risk factors is an important aspect of allowing older people to make decisions on how to undertake necessary tasks safely or determining that the task poses too great a risk, and external support is needed. Empowering older people to make appropriate decisions regarding risks using a person-centred approach is likely to have the greatest impact on managing the burden of fall-related injury.

Mobility Aids

Mobility aids, which are sometimes referred to as *ambulation devices* or *gait aids,* help people with temporary or permanent injury or impairment to move around their environment. Examples of mobility aids include crutches, canes, walking frames, manual and electric wheelchairs and motorised scooters (Gell, Wallace, Lacroix, Mroz, & Patel, 2015). These aids are designed to assist persons to walk or to move about their home and community, contributing to their independence (Bähr et al., 2014; Bateni & Maki, 2005). By providing greater support and balance, mobility aids such as canes and walkers can compensate for gait and mobility limitations (Bateni & Maki, 2005; Joyce & Kirby, 1991).

Biomechanically, mobility aids that assist with walking, such as crutches, canes and walking frames, can increase the base of support, which in turn provides greater stability when walking (Bateni & Maki, 2005). These aids can also provide a reduction in lower limb loading when muscle weakness, joint restriction or pain is present (Joyce & Kirby, 1991). Mobility aids also increase feelings of confidence and autonomy in older people (Smith, Quine, Anderson, & Black, 2002).

There are a range of different types of mobility aids for walking (Fig. 46.6), including the following:

■ Sticks (canes)
  ■ Single-point sticks
  ■ 4-point sticks
  ■ 3-point sticks
■ Crutches
  ■ Axillary crutches (underarm)
  ■ Elbow crutches
  ■ Gutter crutches

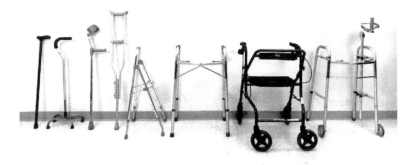

FIG. 46.6 ■ Mobility aids.

- Walking frames
  - Zimmer frames (nonwheeled standard pickup)
  - Folding pickup frames
  - Gutter frames (forearm support frames)
  - Wheeled pickup frames
  - Rollators (two wheels)
  - Wheelie walkers (four wheels)

As many factors can influence the outcome of the use of mobility aids for walking, when considering the use of these types of devices, it is important that an individualised assessment is undertaken so that the most suitable device is prescribed (O'Hare, Pryde, & Gracey, 2013).

Mobility aids for walking have been found to minimise pain, compensate for musculoskeletal and neurological deficits and improve confidence (Gooberman-Hill & Ebrahim, 2007). However, appreciation of how older people perceive these types of aids must be considered as this can affect their engagement with this type of intervention (Lupton & Seymour, 2000). Regular reassessment of the effectiveness of the mobility aid for walking is also essential to ensure ongoing suitability in the presence of physical and environment change (O'Hare et al., 2013).

UNDERSTANDING THE COMPLEXITY OF IDENTIFYING AND MANAGING FALL RISK IN THE COMMUNITY

Occupational therapists can play a role in the early identification of older people who may be at high risk of falling and facilitate appropriate intervention pathways. However, identifying at risk individuals can be challenging, as many older people are reluctant to admit to health professionals that they have fallen (Dollard, Braunack-Mayer, Horton, & Vanlint, 2014).

It is important that all health professionals, including occupational therapists, are actively engaged in communicating with older people about their fall history. Making the assumption that an older person will inform a health professional about his or her fall history may result in a considerable number of falls occurring in the community that health professionals are unaware of. This reduces the ability to address key risk factors before more significant injury occurs. It also poses significant challenges from an injury risk management perspective because without a systematic approach towards identifying at-risk older people, appropriate and timely falls interventions are unlikely to be implemented in this vulnerable population.

Even if older people are successfully identified and referred into fall-related interventions, there are still challenges associated with managing the fall risks. A number of factors can influence the uptake of fall-related interventions, such as the value older people place on independence, the level of understanding an older person has about risk and the willingness to accept support, which all influence behavioural decisions to undertake an activity or task. If the older person does not perceive there is a risk, even if the person has previously fallen, it is unlikely this person will engage with fall-related interventions (Delbaere, Close, Brodaty, Sachdev, & Lord, 2010). Even if older people do attend fall risk education programmes, it may not result in them taking on board advice given to reduce their risk (Hughes et al., 2008). It is important that health professionals do not assume that because an older person has been referred to a fall intervention programme everything will be fine. Adequate follow-up and ongoing communication with older people are essential. If an older person is reluctant to implement recommendations, such as home modifications, then an open dialogue as to why these are important should be facilitated to ensure the person is making an informed choice and that alternative options are considered.

Continual reassessment of older people's fall risk is also an important factor to consider because of comorbidities and the aging process. The consequences of a lack of routine follow-up may mean that any fall intervention strategies that were previously instigated may no longer be the most appropriate or may not address all of the current risk factors, leaving older people vulnerable for subsequent falls with more severe outcomes.

In all interactions with older people, health professionals should take the opportunity to ask whether they have fallen in the last 12 months, which is recommended by international guidelines (Close & Lord, 2011). By facilitating increased discussion with older people who are reluctant to self-report their falls history, health professionals may be able to identify potential risk factors early so that appropriately interventions can be instigated before the older person's risk status increases.

CONCLUSION

Evidence suggests that mobility issues, including falls, are complex to address in the older population and requires a multifaceted approach to consider the demographic, physiological, psychological and health status of the individual, as well as the health behaviours and living environment to successfully manage these issues (Stenholm et al., 2015). Without appropriately addressing the mobility concerns of older people, not only will preventable risk factors be poorly managed, potentially leading to further decline in the physical and emotional wellbeing of the older person, but it also has the flow-on effect of consuming a considerable sum of government health budgets, resulting in less resilient communities in the future.

 http://evolve.elsevier.com/Curtin/OT

REFERENCES

Ambrose, A. F., Geet, P., & Hausdorff, J. M. (2013). Risk factors for falls among older adults: A literature review. *Maturitas*, 75, 51–61.

Alexandra, T. S., Meira, D. M., Rico, N. C., & Mizuta, S. K. (2012). Accuracy of Timed Up and Go Test for screening risk of falls among community-dwelling elderly. *Brazilian Journal of Physical Therapy*, 16(5), 381–388.

Bähr, M., Klein, S., Diewald, S., et al. (2014). PASSAge: Personalized Mobility, Assistance and Service Systems in an Aging Society. In *Ambient assisted living* (pp. 109–119). Berlin: Springer.

Bateni, H., & Maki, B. E. (2005). Assistive devices for balance and mobility: Benefits, demands, and adverse consequences. *Archives of Physical Medicine and Rehabilitation*, 86(1), 134–145.

Berg, W. P., Alessio, H. M., Mills, E. M., & Tong, C. (1997). Circumstances and consequences of falls in independent community-dwelling older adults. *Age and Aging*, 26(4), 261–268.

Berg, K. O., Maki, B. E., Williams, J. I., Holliday, P. J., & Wood-Dauphinee, S. L. (1992). Clinical and laboratory measures of postural balance in an elderly population. *Archives of Physical Medicine and Rehabilitation*, 73(11), 1073–1080.

Brown, C., & Flood, K. (2013). Mobility limitation in the older patient. *Journal of the American Medical Association*, 310(11), 1168–1177.

Centers for Disease Control and Prevention. (2009). Prevalence and most common causes of disability among adults – United States, 2005. *MMWR Morbibity and Mortality Weekly Report*, 58(16), 421–426.

Chase, C. A., Mann, K., Wasek, S., & Arbesman, M. (2012). Systematic review of the effect of home modification and fall prevention programs on falls and the performance of community-dwelling older adults. *American Journal of Occupational Therapy*, 66(3), 284–291.

Clemson, L., Cumming, R. G., Kendig, H., Swann, M., Heard, R., & Taylor, K. (2004). The effectiveness of a community-based program for reducing the incidence of falls in the elderly: A randomized trial. *Journal of the American Geriatrics Society*, 52(9), 1487–1494.

Clemson, L., Cusick, A., & Fozzard, C. (1999). Managing risk and exerting control: Determining follow through with falls prevention. *Disability & Rehabilitation*, 21(12), 531–541.

Clemson, L., Mackenzie, L., Ballinger, C., Close, J. C., & Cumming, R. G. (2008). Environmental interventions to prevent falls in community-dwelling older people a meta-analysis of randomized trials. *Journal of Aging and Health*, 20(8), 954–971.

Close, J. C. T., & Lord, S. R. (2011). Fall assessment in older people. *British Medical Journal*, 343, d5153.

Close, J. C. T., Lord, S. R., Antonova, E., et al. (2012). Older people presenting to the emergency department after a fall: A population with substantial recurrent healthcare use. *Journal of Emergency Medicine*, 29, 742–747.

Cumming, R. G., Thomas, M., Szonyi, G., Frampton, G., Salkeld, G., & Clemson, L. (2001). Adherence to occupational therapist recommendations for home modifications for falls prevention. *American Journal of Occupational Therapy*, 55(6), 641–648.

Delbaere, K., Close, J. C. T., Brodaty, H., Sachdev, P., & Lord, S. R. (2010). Determinants of disparities between perceived and physiological risk of falling among elderly people: A cohort study. *British Medical Journal*, 341, c4165.

Dollard, J., Braunack-Mayer, A., Horton, K., & Vanlint, S. (2014). Why older women do or do not seek help from the GP after a fall: A qualitative study. *Family Practice*, 31(2), 22–228.

Duncan, P. W., Weiner, D. K., Chandler, J., & Studenski, S. (1990). Functional reach: A new clinical measure of balance. *Journal of Gerontology*, 45(6), M192–M197.

Fitzpatrick, A. L., Powe, N. R., Cooper, L. S., Ives, D. G., & Robbins, J. A. (2004). Barriers to health care access among the elderly and who perceives them. *America Journal of Public Health*, 94, 10.

Gardener, E. A., Huppert, F. A., Guralnik, J. M., & Melzer, D. (2006). Middle-aged and mobility-limited: Prevalence of disability and symptom attributions in a national survey. *Journal of General Internal Medicine*, 21(10), 1091–1096.

Ganz, D. A., Bao, Y., Shekelle, P. G., & Rubenstein, L. Z. (2007). Will my patient fall? *Journal of the American Medical Association*, 297(1), 77–86.

Gell, N. M., Wallace, R. B., Lacroix, A. Z., Mroz, T. M., & Patel, K. V. (2015). Mobility device use in older adults and incidence of falls and worry about falling: Findings from the 2011–2012 National Health and Aging Trends Study. *Journal of the American Geriatrics Society*, 63(5), 853–859.

Gelbard, R., Inaba, K., Okoye, O. T., et al. (2014). Falls in the elderly: A modern look at an old problem. *American Journal of Surgery*, 208(2), 249–253.

Gibson, M. J., Andres, R. O., Isaacs, B., Radebaugh, T., & Worm-Petersen, J. (1987). The prevention of falls in later life. A report of the Kellogg International Work Group on the Prevention of Falls by the Elderly. *Danish Medical Bulletin*, *43*(S4), 1–24.

Gill, T. M., Murphy, T. E., Gahbauer, E. A., & Allore, H. G. (2013). Association of injurious falls with disability outcomes and nursing home admissions in community-living older persons. *American Journal of Epidemiology*, *178*(3), 418–425.

Gillespie, L. D., Robertson, M. C., Gillespie, W. J., et al. (2012). Interventions for preventing falls in older people living in the community. *Cochrane Database of Systematic Reviews*, *9*.

Glass, T. A. (1998). Conjugating the 'tenses' of function: Discordance among hypothetical, experimental, and enacted function in older adults. *The Gerontologist*, *38*(1), 101–112.

Gooberman-Hill, R., & Ebrahim, S. (2007). Making decisions about simple interventions: Older people's use of walking aids. *Age and Ageing*, *36*(5), 569–573.

Grundstrom, A. C., Guse, C. E., & Layde, P. M. (2012). Risk factors for falls and fall-related injuries in adults 85 years of age and older. *Archives of Gerontology and Geriatrics*, *54*, 421–428.

Guralnik, J. M., Ferrucci, L., Pieper, C. F., et al. (2000). Lower extremity function and subsequent disability consistency across studies, predictive models, and value of gait speed alone compared with the Short Physical Performance Battery. *The Journals of Gerontology Series A: Biological Sciences and Medical Sciences*, *55*(4), M221–M231.

Hardy, S. E., Kang, Y., Studenski, S. A., & Degenholtz, H. B. (2011). Ability to walk 1/4 mile predicts subsequent disability, mortality, and health care costs. *Journal of General Internal Medicine*, *26*(2), 130–135.

Haung, A. R., Mallet, L., Rochefort, C. M., Eguale, T., Buckeridge, D. L., & Tamblyn, R. (2012). Medication-related falls in the elderly – causative factors and preventative strategies. *Drugs and Aging*, *29*(5), 259–376.

Hess, R. J., Brach, J. S., Piva, S. R., & VanSwearingen, J. M. (2010). Walking skill can be assessed in older adults: Validity of the Figure-of-8 Walk Test. *Physical Therapy*, *90*(1), 89–99.

Hörder, H., Skoog, I., & Frändin, K. (2013). Health-related quality of life in relation to walking habits and fitness: A population-based study of 75-year-olds. *Quality of Life Research*, *22*(6), 1213–1223.

Hughes, K., van Beurden, E., Eakin, E. G., et al. (2008). Older person's perception of risk of falling: Implications for fall-prevention campaigns. *American Journal of Public Health*, *98*(2), 351–357.

Iezzoni, L. I., McCarthy, E. P., Davis, R. B., & Siebens, H. (2001). Mobility difficulties are not only a problem of old age. *Journal of General Internal Medicine*, *16*(4), 235–243.

Inouye, S. K., Studenski, S., Tinetti, M. E., & Kuchel, G. A. (2007). Geriatric syndromes: Clinical, research, and policy implications of a core geriatric concept. *Journal of American Geriatrics Society*, *55*(5), 780–791.

Joyce, B. M., & Kirby, R. L. (1991). Canes, crutches and walkers. *American Family Physician*, *43*(2), 535–542.

Karlsson, M. K., Vonschewelov, T., Karlsson, C., Coster, M., & Rosengen, B. E. (2013). Prevention of falls in the elderly: A review. *Scandinavian Journal of Public Health*, *41*, 442–454.

Kuys, S. S., & Brauer, S. G. (2006). Validation and reliability of the modified elderly mobility scale. *Australasian Journal on Aging*, *25*(3), 140–144.

Lamb, S. E., Jorstad-Stein, E. C., Hauer, K., & Becker, C. (2005). Development of a common outcome data set for fall injury prevention trials: The prevention of Falls Network Europe Consensus. *Journal of American Geriatrics Society*, *53*, 1618–1622.

Lee, I., & Buchner, D. M. (2008). The importance of walking to public health. *Medicine & Science in Sports and Exercise*, *40*(7S), S512–S518.

Lord, S. R., Delbaere, K., Tiedeman, A., Smith, S. T., & Sturnieks, D. L. (2011). Implementing falls prevention research into policy and practice: An overview of a new National Health and Medical Research Council Partnership Grant. *NSW Public Health Bulletin*, *22*(3-4), 84–87.

Lord, S. R., Menz, H. B., & Sherrington, C. (2006). Home environment risk factors for falls in older people and the efficacy of home modifications. *Age and Aging*, *35*(S2), ii55–ii59.

Lupton, D., & Seymour, W. (2000). Technology, selfhood and physical disability. *Social Science & Medicine*, *50*(12), 1851–1862.

Luukinen, H., Koski, K., Laippala, P., & Kivelä, S. L. (1995). Predictors for recurrent falls among the home-dwelling elderly. *Scandinavian Journal of Primary Health Care*, *13*(4), 294–299.

Marko, M., Neville, C. G., Prince, M. A., & Ploutz-Snyder. (2012). *Journal of the American Physical Therapy Association*, *92*, 1148–1159.

Melzer, D., Gardener, E., & Guralnik, J. M. (2005). Mobility disability in the middle-aged: cross-sectional associations in the English Longitudinal Study of Aging. *Age and Aging*, *34*(6), 594–602.

Meyer, M. R. U., Janke, M. C., & Beaujean, A. A. (2014). Predictors of older adults' personal and community mobility: Using a comprehensive theoretical mobility framework. *The Gerontologist*, *54*(3), 398–408.

Moller, J. (2003). *Projected costs of fall-related injury to older persons due to demographic change in Australia*. Report to the Commonwealth Department of Health and Aging under the National Falls Prevention for Older People Initiative. Commonwealth of Australia.

Newman, A. B., Simonsick, E. M., Naydeck, B. L., et al. (2006). Association of long-distance corridor walk performance with mortality, cardiovascular disease, mobility limitation, and disability. *Journal of the American Medical Association*, *295*(17), 2018–2026.

O'Hare, M. P., Pryde, S. J., & Gracey, J. H. (2013). A systematic review of the evidence for the provision of walking frames for older people. *Physical Therapy Reviews*, *18*(1), 11–23.

Oxley, J., & Whelan, M. (2008). It cannot be all about safety: The benefits of prolonged mobility. *Traffic Injury Prevention*, *9*(4), 367–378.

Painter, J. A., Allison, L., Dhingra, P., Daughtery, J., Cogdill, K., & Trujillo, L. G. (2012). Fear of falling and its relationship with anxiety, depression, and activity engagement among, community-dwelling older adults. *American Journal of Occupational Therapy*, *66*(2), 169–176.

Patla, A. E., & Shumway-Cook, A. (1999). Dimensions of mobility: Defining the complexity and difficulty associated with community mobility. *Journal of Aging and Physical Activity*, *7*(1), 7–19.

Prohaska, T. R., Anderson, L. A., Hooker, S. P., Hughes, S. L., & Belza, B. (2011). Mobility and aging: Transference to transportation. *Journal of Aging Research*, *2011*, 392751.

Rantanen, T. (2013). Promoting mobility in older people. *Journal of Preventive Medicine and Public Health, 46*(Suppl 1), S50.

Rantanen, T., Guralnik, J. M., Ferrucci, L., Leveille, S., & Fried, L. P. (1999). Coimpairments: Strength and balance as predictors of severe walking disability. *The Journals of Gerontology Series A: Biological Sciences and Medical Sciences, 54*(4), M172–M176.

Rivera, J. A., Fried, P. L., Weiss, C. O., & Simonsick, E. M. (2008). At the tipping point: Predicting severe mobility difficulty in vulnerable older women. *Journal of the American Geriatrics Society, 56,* 147–1423.

Robson, K. (2015). Exploration of falls in Inland Australia. *Unpublished doctoral thesis.* Albury, Australia: Charles Sturt University.

Rose, D. J., Jones, J. C., & Lucchese, N. (2002). Predicting the probability of falls in community-residing older adults using the 8-foot Up-and-Go: A new measure of functional mobility. *Journal of Aging and Physical Therapy, 10*(40), 466–475.

Rubenstein, L. Z. (2006). Falls in older people: Epidemiology, risk factors and strategies for prevention. *Age and Aging, 35-S2,* ii37–ii41.

Rubenstein, L. Z., & Josephson, K. R. (2002). The epidemiology of falls and syncope. *Clinical Geriatric Medicine, 18,* 141–158.

Salzman, B. (2010). Gait and balance disorders in older adults. *American Family Physician, 82*(1), 61–68.

Satariano, W. A., Guralnik, J. M., Jackson, R. J., Marottoli, R. A., Phelan, E. A., & Prohaska, T. R. (2012). Mobility and aging: New directions for public health action. *American Journal of Public Health, 102*(8), 1508–1515.

Shumway-Cook, A., Baldwin, M., Polissar, N. L., & Gruber, W. (1997). Predicting the probability for falls in community-dwelling older adults. *Physical Therapy, 77*(8), 812–819.

Shumway-Cook, A., Patla, A., Stewart, A., Ferrucci, L., Ciol, M. A., & Guralnik, J. M. (2003). Environmental components of mobility disability in community-living older persons. *Journal of the American Geriatrics Society, 51*(3), 393–398.

Smith, R., Quine, S., Anderson, J., & Black, K. (2002). Assistive devices: Self-reported use by older people in Victoria. *Australian Health Review, 25*(4), 169–177.

Stenholm, S., Shardell, M., Bandinelli, S., Guralnik, J. M., & Ferrucci, L. (2015). Physiological factors contributing to mobility loss over 9 years of follow-up – results from the InCHIANTI Study. *Journals of Gerontology: Medical Sciences,* 591–597.

Steultjens, E. M., Dekker, J., Bouter, L. M., Jellema, S., Bakker, E. B., & Van Den Ende, C. H. (2004). Occupational therapy for community dwelling elderly people: A systematic review. *Age and Ageing, 33*(5), 453–460.

Stevens, J. A., Corso, P. S., Finkelstein, E. A., & Miller, T. R. (2006). The costs of fatal and non-fatal falls among older adults. *Injury Prevention, 12*(5), 290–295.

Tiedemann, A., Shimada, H., Sherrington, C., Murray, S., & Lord, S. (2008). The comparative ability of eight functional mobility tests for predicting falls in community dwelling older people. *Age and Aging, 37*(4), 430–435.

Thorbahn, L. D. B., & Newton, R. A. (1996). Use of the Berg Balance Test to predict falls in elderly persons. *Physical Therapy, 76*(6), 576–583.

Tinetti, M. E., & Williams, C. S. (1997). Falls, injuries due to falls, and the risk of admission to a nursing home. *New England Journal of Medicine, 337*(18), 1279–1284.

Tse, T. (2005). The environment and falls prevention: Do environmental modifications make a difference? *Australian Occupational Therapy Journal, 52,* 271–281.

Verghese, J., LeValley, A., Hall, C. B., Katz, M. J., Ambrose, A. F., & Lipton, R. B. (2006). Epidemiology of gait disorders in community-residing older adults. *Journal of the American Geriatrics Society, 54*(2), 255–261.

Watson, W. L., Clapperton, A. J., & Mitchell, R. J. (2011). The cost of fall-related injuries among older people in NSW, 2006-07. *NSW Public Health Bulletin, 22*(3-4), 55–59.

Webber, S. C., Porter, M. M., & Menec, V. H. (2010). Mobility in older adults: A comprehensive framework. *The Gerontologist, 50*(4), 433–450.

Whittle, M. W. (2002). *Gait analysis: An introduction* (3rd ed.). Oxford, UK: Butterworth Heimemann.

World Health Organization. (2007). *World Health Organization Global Report on Falls Prevention in Older Age.* Geneva: World Health Organization.

Zhang, J., Ishikawa-Takata, K., Yamazaki, H., & Ohta, T. (2004). Is a type A behavior pattern associated with falling among the community-dwelling elderly? *Archives of Gerontology and Geriatrics, 38,* 145–152.

Zecevic, A. A., Salmoni, A. W., Speechley, M., & Vandervoort, A. A. (2006). Defining a fall and reasons for falling: Comparisons among the views of seniors, health care providers, and the research literature. *The Gerontologist, 46*(3), 367–376.

47

WHEELED MOBILITY AND SEATING SYSTEMS

RACHAEL LEIGH MCDONALD

CHAPTER OUTLINE

Abstract

People who have difficulty with or are unable to walk independently often require wheeled mobility and seating system to assist with their mobility. People who have increasing impairments often need extra cushions or special cushions placed within their wheeled mobility and seating system. The prescription and evaluation of wheeled mobility and seating system and their accessories is a growing area of occupational therapy practice. The goal of providing wheeled mobility and seating system is to enable a person to engage in occupations, even though the provision itself is a technical

intervention. Traditional approaches to wheeled mobility and seating system provision have tended towards a medical model; however, occupational therapists have been uncomfortable only concentrating on the impairments of body functions and structures. It is the occupational therapist's role to address the cognitive, affective and spiritual elements of the person, along with the self-care, leisure and productivity aspects of occupation and the cultural, institutional and social aspects of the environment. The occupational therapist is able to help the person by enabling mobility, and therefore a range of occupations, in a way that is person-centred. An integral part of the provision of wheeled mobility and seating intervention is a detailed and thorough assessment, which takes into account the person's age, life stage and roles, funding considerations, environmental barriers and facilitators and social and personal factors, as well as more technical considerations, such as body biomechanics and prevention of pressure ulcers. Collaboration between the occupational therapist and the person, education and appropriate supports are essential for the wheeled mobility and seating system provision to be meaningful to the person and enable the person to perform his or her desired activities.

KEY POINTS

▪ People with restricted mobility often require wheeled mobility and seating systems to enable them to engage in the occupations that they want and need to do.

▪ Mobility is fundamental to occupational engagement. Limitations to mobility can be enhanced or replaced by wheeled mobility and seating system.

▪ People use wheeled mobility and seating system not only to increase their mobility but also as a basis for participation in life. The number of people using wheeled mobility and seating system is growing, and so it is an important technical skill for occupational therapists to develop.

▪ Seating assessment and provision depends on working through the person's mobility and life goals, considering the person's body function and structure along with the activities and occupations that he or she wants and needs to do.

▪ When providing advice on mobility, occupational therapists should consider the person's age, life stage and stage of adjustment, funding, environmental barriers and facilitators, social and personal factors, collaboration, education and support.

INTRODUCTION

People who have challenges with walking independently or walking for long periods may use a wheeled mobility and seating system for their mobility (Best, Kirby, Smith, & Macleod, 2005; Sakakibara, Miller, Routhier, Backman, & Eng, 2014). The assessment and prescription of wheeled mobility and seating systems can be an interdisciplinary intervention that can involve a number of professionals, including occupational therapists (for engagement in daily occupations), physiotherapists (for body posture), nurses and doctors (for pressure management), and rehabilitation engineers (for design). For all these professionals, the provision of wheeled mobility and seating systems can be classified as a technical intervention, in which the goal is to enable participation in daily occupations (Reid, Laliberte-Rudman, & Hebert, 2002). Traditional approaches to this technical intervention have tended towards a medical model of

providing a piece of equipment that enables the person to be transported from one place to another or that focuses on 'fixing' body functions and structures, and in so doing has not considered people's occupational needs. However, if done well, this interdisciplinary intervention enables people with restricted mobility to participate in life and undertake the things that they want and need to do.

The importance of developing skills for the effective assessment and prescription of wheeled mobility and seating systems is reinforced by the fact that at a population level, internationally, people are aging, and with age often people experience restrictions in both mobility and access to their community (Löfqvist, Pettersson, Iwarsson, & Brandt, 2012). Furthermore, those people who acquire impairments – both congenitally or through accident, disease or trauma – are living longer and often have mobility issues. Impaired mobility often leads to a lack of access to the environment and becomes a factor in reducing involvement in activities and social, economic and community participation (Mortenson, Miller, Backman, & Oliffe, 2012; Ripat, Brown, & Ethans, 2015; Torkia et al., 2015).

Occupational therapists who work with people with a mobility impairment arrange for the modification of their environments, teach them skills to deal with environmental barriers and advocate at a public policy level for universal design and access to community activities and the built environment. In addition, occupational therapists also help people with mobility impairments to investigate and trial alternative methods of mobility to enable them to participate in the occupations that they want and need to do. Wheeled mobility and seating systems are an alternative method of mobility. Occupational therapists working with people who require a wheeled mobility and seating system need to understand the technical dimensions of the wheeled mobility device itself and match that to the body function and structural needs of the person to enable the person to actively participate in daily life. Enabling a person's occupational performance is based upon a deep understanding of personal factors – including an understanding of the roles and occupations that person needs and wants to do and the personal goals the person wants to achieve.

Increasingly, the International Classification of Functioning, Disability and Health (ICF) (World Health Organization, 2001) is being used as a framework for assessment and intervention by people working in the field of wheeled mobility and seating systems (Cohen, 2007; Sprigle, 2007a, 2007b). The ICF fits with the provision of wheeled mobility and seating systems because of the individualised contextual factors of personal preference, environmental limitations and a person's activity and participation, which are given equal weight to the person's health condition or impairments in body functions and structures (McDonald, Surtees, & Wirz, 2004). The ICF resonates with occupational therapists who base their practice on occupation models as they are able to understand and relate to the concept of participation and the multiple factors that enable participation. As a result, occupational therapists can make a unique and valuable contribution to the interdisciplinary team involved in wheeled mobility and seating provision (Hjelle & Vik, 2011).

One challenge of wheeled mobility and seating provision is that these devices have a dual purpose. The first purpose is that of a medicinal product, prescribed and funded in the same manner as other aids and devices with the role of compensating for or improving impairment of body functions and structure (Sprigle, 2007b). The other role is that of performance, in which wheeled mobility and seating has the potential to enable a person without independent mobility to be independent. However, as wheeled mobility and seating has the potential to cause harm, it is important to understand the impact of inappropriate provision (Cohen, Fitzgerald, Lane, & Boninger, 2005). Effective provision of wheeled mobility and seating enables the user to have health, to enhance the user's occupational performance and to facilitate the user to engage in activities and to participate in life roles. Enabling people to have a wheeled mobility and seating system that meets their goals can positively influence other factors that promote both physical and mental health and well-being, such as community connectedness.

If the occupational therapist concentrates on providing equipment to accommodate only the physical needs and impairments of a person, then the cognitive, affective and spiritual elements of the person, along with the self-care, leisure, and productivity aspects of occupation and the cultural, institutional and social aspects of the environment, are not considered (Townsend & Polatajko, 2007). The effectiveness of wheeled mobility and seating provision is dependent on person-centred practice, using the individual's seating and positioning devices as a way of enhancing each person's participation in occupational performance and engagement (Rudman, Hebert, & Reid, 2006). The key to providing wheeled mobility and seating that addresses a person's whole needs involves setting measurable and achievable goals with the person, and the person's caregivers where appropriate, to enable an individual to participate and engage in daily occupations (Mortenson, Miller, & Miller-Pogar, 2007). This is mirrored in the philosophy of occupational therapy (Creek, 2003; Law et al., 1996; Townsend & Polatajko, 2007) and is an important reason why occupational therapists are involved in this technical area of practice. The impact of seating and positioning is complex, and an individual's underlying physical illness, injury or impairment has dominated the provision of seating and mobility devices; this dominance of body functions and structures has meant that enablement of engagement in occupation has been a secondary issue (Alexander, Hwang, & Sipski, 2001).

POPULATIONS – WHO USES WHEELED MOBILITY AND SEATING SYSTEMS?

Health conditions that cause mobility impairment or seating difficulty range from a person who needs wheeled mobility and seating system occasionally to help access the community, to someone who is unable to sit upright independently and therefore needs both a wheeled mobility device and sophisticated positioning equipment.

The total population estimated to use wheeled mobility ranges from 0.61% of people living outside institutions in the United States of America (Kaye, Kang, & Laplante, 2002) to 1.46% of the population in the United Kingdom (Audit Commission, 2000; Sanderson, Place, & Wright, 2000). The number of people who use wheeled mobility and seating systems in the United States of America may be anywhere between 1.8 to 4.4 million people, with 900,000 users in the United Kingdom, and between 125,000 to 300,000 users in Australia. The number of people who use wheeled mobility and seating systems for their daily mobility is expected to increase at a rate of between 2% and 10% per year in the coming years (Audit Commission, 2000, 2002; Cooper, Ferretti, Oyster, Kelleher, & Cooper, 2008; Jelier & Turner-Smith, 1997; Sanderson, Place, & Wright, 2000). This partly is due to the increasing older population as the proportion of people using wheeled mobility and seating systems increases with age. Currently the highest rate of both manual and electric wheelchair use is among the elderly (65 years or older), with working-age adults the next most prominent group and children and young people having the least prevalence.

Health Conditions of People Who Use Wheeled Mobility and Seating Systems

People who have neurological, musculoskeletal or cognitive conditions may have difficulty with their mobility. Often the impact of these conditions will change throughout the lifespan or with the progression of the disease. The role of the occupational therapist may change as the difficulties people have with their occupational performance and engagement change.

Conditions that are neurological or have neuromuscular implications include congenital or genetic disorders such as cerebral palsy, spina bifida or muscular dystrophy; acquired conditions such as cerebrovascular accident, traumatic brain injury or spinal cord injury; and other conditions such as multiple sclerosis, Parkinson's disease, Guillain-Barre syndrome or Huntington's chorea. The impact of the neurological impairment results in alterations of muscle tone, muscle weakness or paralysis and sensory disorders. The group of users with neurological conditions may also have difficulties secondary to their original diagnosis. For example, a large proportion of people diagnosed with cerebral palsy may have had dislocated hips when they were children (O'Connor, Boyd, & Shields, 2006) and in later life may have developed scoliosis (Majd, Muldowny, & Holt, 1997; Sadani et al., 2012), leading to extra positioning needs.

Musculoskeletal conditions may also interfere with the mobility of the person. One of the most common symptoms of these conditions is acute or chronic pain (Bearne, Coomer, & Hurley, 2007; Estes, Bochenek, & Fasler, 2000). Other symptoms of musculoskeletal disorders include painful, swollen and stiff joints, with muscle wasting around the affected joints leading to contractures (Estes et al., 2000). Other health conditions that can affect an individual's mobility are cognitive disorders, such as pervasive developmental disorders, intellectual impairments and Alzheimer's disease.

Wheeled mobility and seating systems are also commonly used by two other groups of people: those classified as frail elderly and people with chronic health conditions. Frail elderly people are the highest proportion of users of wheeled mobility and seating systems because of their reduced capacity to safely cover short and long distances, in the absence of an underlying health condition or impairment. However, this group is often poorly served in the area of wheeled mobility and seating (Barks et al., 2015; Jones & Rader, 2015; Requejo, Furumasu, & Mulroy, 2015). Factors such as a lack of resources to purchase a wheeled mobility and seating system, lack of competence in therapists assessing and prescribing wheeled mobility and seating systems, and living in residential aged care are all contributors to this (Chen, Huang, Cheng, Li, & Chang, 2015; Cohen, Fitzgerald, Lane, & Boninger, 2005; Giesbrecht, Mortenson, & Miller, 2012; Jones & Rader, 2015). This then becomes an important occupational justice issue.

The primary health condition is often the reason why the person may need a wheeled mobility and seating system. However, personal and environmental factors, along with a person's activity and participation needs, contribute significantly to the successful provision of a wheeled mobility and seating system. The individual's health condition and impairments of body function and structure in the context of his or her desired activity, ability to participate and various institutional and personal factors are illustrated in Practice Story 47.1. This practice story also illustrates how a change in one part of the process can have a major impact on a person's life.

Many people experience difficulties with their health that can also interfere with their wheeled mobility and seating system use. For example, people with a spinal cord injury will often experience other issues with functioning and health that are not part of seating and positioning but that need to be taken into account when the person is considering which wheeled mobility and seating system is best suited to their needs. The types of issues that a person with a spinal cord injury may have that can affect the prescription of a wheeled mobility and seating system include urinary tract and

---

PRACTICE STORY 47.1

Orlando: Potential Outcomes with Wheeled Mobility and Seating System (with Thanks to Dr Natasha Layton)

This comparative practice story illustrates the key role assistive technology plays in supporting body structure and function, as well as engagement in activities and participation in daily occupations. A critical path analysis enables the comparison of likely outcomes for an individual with and without an optimal wheelchair and pressure cushion and illustrates a complexity of other factors that must be considered alongside the wheelchair itself.

CRITICAL PATH 1: OPTIMAL OUTCOME

Orlando, 27, had a spinal cord injury resulting from a traffic accident, which meant that he was eligible for third party funding. He underwent rehabilitation and was discharged home with a combination of environmental adaptations, assistive technologies and a personal care plan. The environmental adaptations included a stepless shower base and accessible toilet, both able to be accessed via a padded, self-propelled over-toilet/shower chair to minimise unnecessary transfers. His manual wheelchair was ultralight (8 kg), minimising the load he had to propel, and was light enough for him to pull into the passenger seat of a car and stow during car trips. The customised seat angle and rake supported an active posture, and the wheel camber maximised his self-propulsion. A lightweight, low-rise pressure-relieving/pressure-reducing cushion was fitted concurrently. The combination of the wheelchair itself with the lightweight, pressure-relieving/pressure-reducing cushion, meant that the wheelchair was very easy for him to propel. Orlando was a 'beginner' at the time of being prescribed his wheelchair and cushion but developed high-level wheelchair skills over the next 12 to 18 months. Hence, it was important when initially prescribing the wheelchair to consider the possibility of being able to further adjust it to ensure Orlando did not 'grow out' of its capacity too soon. Orlando was actively involved in establishing his individualised package of personal care (hours and personnel); he decreased the hours he required a personal care assistant over time as he became 'hardened' to daily activities. In the future, Orlando wanted to establish full independence, work full time, play sport, drive a car with hand controls and engage in usual occupational opportunities for a person of his age.

CRITICAL PATH 2: SUBOPTIMAL OUTCOME

In this practice story, a fall from a ladder at home caused Orlando's spinal cord injury, and thus he was not compensable. He underwent the same rehabilitation process, but the environmental adaptations and assistive technologies provided were based upon public funding limits, which capped both type and cost of items regardless of an individual's need. Orlando returned to a rental property where major modifications were not permitted; thus he needed to engage in multiple daily transfers onto a bathseat and toilet and had a midcost, relatively heavy pressure-relieving/pressure-reducing cushion and a 15-kg manual wheelchair that was adjusted to fit but not customised for him. His tended to have a sacral sitting posture when sitting in the wheelchair, which resulted in him sitting in a flexed position, slightly compressing his chest cavity, and put him at a slight biomechanical disadvantage when self-propelling his wheelchair and when reaching while sitting in his wheelchair. His personal care consisted of twice weekly visits from community nurses, which limited his capacity to make appointments or leave the house on those days as they came within a 4-hour window. He had limited capacity to travel

Continued on following page

Orlando: Potential Outcomes with Wheeled Mobility and Seating System (with Thanks to Dr Natasha Layton) *(Continued)*

in vehicles as he required assistance to lift and stow the wheelchair; therefore his participation in community activities was minimal. Orlando's subsequent critical path thus included frequent readmissions with pressure areas and compromised shoulder function. Bed rest to relieve pressure ulcers led to a decrease in physical fitness, upper limb strength and independence. A powered wheelchair was eventually required to enable independent mobility when travelling a distance, costing considerably more than an optimal manual wheelchair would have. Orlando's eventual outcome was a nursing home, where care costs plus his inability to work decreased his disposable income to below pension level. He was no longer eligible for government funding for a replacement wheelchair as he was in residential care, further compounding his impoverished occupational opportunities and failure to accomplish life tasks.

CONCLUSION

The health condition is the same, but the outcomes are profoundly different. As can be seen, an appropriate wheelchair is

one essential component to ensure Orlando's critical path is on an upward trajectory. One critical difference is the resources available. Another is the professional reasoning of the prescribing occupational therapist. The occupational therapist who collaborates with the person to establish the person's occupational goals and takes a whole-of-life approach can argue for best outcomes in view of the likely life trajectory of the person, enabling the achievement of occupational potential.

When providing advice on mobility, Orlando's occupational therapist must consider the following:

- Age, life stage and stage of adjustment
- Pragmatic constraints such as funding
- Environmental barriers and facilitators
- Social and personal factors that shape the individual's situation
- Temporal aspects that affect the wheelchair and cushion throughout a day and into the future
- Collaboration, education and support

---

bowel problems, pressure ulcers, spasticity, musculoskeletal and neuropathic pain, sexual dysfunction and respiratory and cardiovascular disorders (Adriaansen et al., 2013).

PRESCRIBING WHEELED MOBILITY AND SEATING SYSTEMS

It is useful to think of people who need to use a wheeled mobility and seating system as on a continuum in terms of their physical abilities or body functions and structures, as shown in Fig. 47.1. Whatever the involvement of the occupational therapist, many individuals considering using a wheeled mobility and seating

system will find this confronting and extremely challenging as it provides evidence of the severity of their impairment (Farley et al., 2003).

For convenience, wheeled mobility and seating system prescription to enhance an individual's seated occupational performance may be divided into two areas:

1. Enablement of mobility
2. Management of posture

There is often overlap between the two, but generally on the continuum of physical difficulties, those with fewer care needs will require a less complex wheeled mobility and seating system.

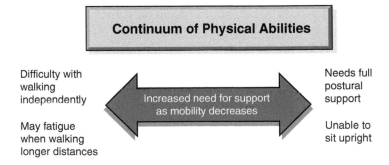

FIG. 47.1 ■ Continuum of people who use wheeled mobility and seating systems.

Enablement of Mobility

Mobility is fundamental to the independent occupational engagement of individuals. Wheeled mobility and seating systems may not need to have high-specification cushions or seating devices but when inappropriately prescribed can have a detrimental effect on the abilities and future body functions and structures of the user.

To prescribe a wheeled mobility and seating system it is important to consider what outcomes are to be achieved and how best to determine the achievement of these outcomes. Measurement of outcomes takes the form of either performance of the wheeled mobility device itself (Rushton, Kirby, & Miller, 2012), assessment of the skills of the user (Askari, Kirby, Parker, Thompson, & O'Neill, 2013), or generic assessments that cover many assistive devices (Arthanat, Bauer, Lenker, Nochajski, & Wu, 2007; Fuhrer, Jutai, Scherer, & Deruyter, 2003; Ryan et al., 2006). Some of these can also be used as predictors of the effective use of devices (Arthanat et al., 2007). Outcome measurements continue to evolve as concepts such as quality of life and participation are increasingly used to measure the effectiveness of the mobility for the person (Davin, 2015; Frank, De Souza, Frank, & Neophytou, 2012; Hutzler, Chacham-Guber, & Reiter, 2013; Liu, Cooper, Kelleher, & Cooper, 2014).

Assessment should begin with asking the person about his or her personal goals and expectations for the mobility system. However, basic physical assessment is always a requirement to ensure that the wheeled mobility and seating system fit correctly. The basic measurements that a therapist needs to take to determine the size of the wheeled mobility and seating system are illustrated in Fig. 47.2. It is important to ensure that the measurements taken are as accurate as possible to ensure that the correctly

sized wheeled mobility and seating system is provided. When a wheeled mobility and seating system is too big or too small for a person, it can negatively affect the person's sitting posture, which can result in significant postural and pressure complications. The possible effects on a person's body function and structure and on occupational performance of the size of the wheeled mobility and seating system being incorrect are listed in Table 47.1.

When deciding on the wheeled mobility device there are three main types of wheeled mobility bases to be considered: self-propelling wheelchairs or independent manual mobility

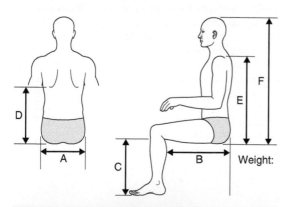

Basic seating measurements
A, Widest measure across the hips
B, Rear of the buttocks to the inside of the bent knee
C, Bottom of the heel to the inside of the bent knee
D, Seat to scapula
E, Seat to top of shoulder
F, Seat to top of head

FIG. 47.2 ■ Basic seating measurements.

TABLE 47.1

Examples of Effects of Poorly Fitting Seat on the Person Using a Wheeled Mobility and Seating System

Description of Fit of Wheeled Mobility and Seating System	Leads to Difficulties in Body Functions and Structures and Outcome	Leads to Occupational Performance Difficulties
Wheeled mobility and seating system seat too wide	Inability to reach wheels to self-propel. Encourages pelvic obliquity or unstable sitting base – hips and thighs tend to be in an abducted position.	Poor stability in seating leads to decreased upper limb and head skills, leading to difficulties in eating, using hands and other instrumental ADL skills. Decreases independence by hampering self-propulsion or independent driving. Environmental barriers are increased.
Wheeled mobility and seating system seat too narrow	Encourages pelvic obliquity, instability. Leads to discomfort. Increases risk of pressure ulcers.	Discomfort decreases ability to perform independent functional activity. Causes instability (as earlier). Pressure ulcer development reduces person's health and well-being.
Wheeled mobility and seating system seat too long	Pulls person forwards in chair, increasing pressure on sacrum, encourages slumping and instability. Compromises circulation of lower	Person is unable to use hands. Pressure ulcer development reduces person's health and well-being.

Continued on following page

TABLE 47.1		
Examples of Effects of Poorly Fitting Seat on the Person Using a Wheeled Mobility and Seating System *(Continued)*		
Description of Fit of Wheeled Mobility and Seating System	Leads to Difficulties in Body Functions and Structures and Outcome	Leads to Occupational Performance Difficulties
	limb and creates pressure area behind knees. Does not support person's spine.	
Wheeled mobility and seating system seat too short	Encourages instability by reducing base of support. Increases pressure on thigh and supporting area.	Pressure ulcer development reduces person's health and well-being. Unstable sitting base leads to decreased ability to use hands and head to perform daily activities.
Armrests too high	Elevates shoulders, resulting in discomfort, encouragement of kyphosis and hyperextension of neck. Reduces ability to use arms if relying on armrest for support.	Reduces ability to self-propel or drive. Reduces health and quality of life.
Armrests too low	Encourages slumping either forwards or to the side because of lack of support.	Possibly leads to reduction of respiration, thus increasing fatigue. Instability decreases physical ability to perform daily activities.
Footplates too high	Causes discomfort in hips and knees. Can lead to abduction of hips. Can cause adduction and internal rotation of hips, leading to increased risk of dislocation. Increases pressure on buttocks and sacrum. Reduces base of support.	Instability decreases ability to perform daily activities. Pressure ulcer development reduces person's health and well-being.

TABLE 47.1		
Examples of Effects of Poorly Fitting Seat on the Person Using a Wheeled Mobility and Seating System *(Continued)*		
Description of Fit of Wheeled Mobility and Seating System	Leads to Difficulties in Body Functions and Structures and Outcome	Leads to Occupational Performance Difficulties
Footplates too low	May hit front castors or hit pavements/curbs. Pulls pelvis forwards and encourages slumping and poor sitting stability.	Potential environmental barriers are increased. May lead to secondary deformities.

ADL, Activity of daily living.

systems, attendant-propelled wheelchairs or dependent mobility systems and powered wheeled mobility devices.

Self-propelling Wheelchairs or Independent Manual Mobility Systems

Self-propelling or independent manual wheelchairs are for people who can propel the device by themselves. The chairs have either a 'fixed frame' (Fig. 47.3) or 'folding frame' (Fig. 47.4). The chairs have big wheels at the rear and small wheels at the front to enable the user to push the chair in the most effective and efficient way. In general, fixed-frame chairs are easier to push and are more sturdy but are unable to fold, and a folding-frame chair has more apparatus and is heavier to push but is more convenient for storage. Recent studies have found that it is imperative that the configuration of the wheelchair for the individual who self-propels is correctly set up, as incorrect solutions can cause secondary problems, such as carpal tunnel or shoulder injuries (Mulroy et al., 2015; Rice, Jayaraman, Hsiao-Wecksler, & Sosnoff, 2014; Zukowski et al., 2014).

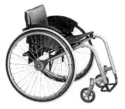

FIG. 47.3 ■ Lightweight fixed-frame wheelchair. The increased seat-to-back angle and position of the seat decrease the stability of the chair but increase the mobility for a highly skilled user.

Attendant-Propelled Wheelchairs or Dependent Mobility System

Attendant-propelled wheelchairs (Fig. 47.5) are used by people who are unable to push themselves and include buggies or push-chairs for younger users, as well as wheelchairs that are purely for someone else to push. This type of chair tends to have small wheels at the back and the front and may be an essential backup for people who use a powered wheelchair as their main form of independent mobility.

Powered Wheeled Mobility Devices

Powered wheelchairs (Fig. 47.6A) are used by people who are capable of independent mobility but unable to achieve this through pushing themselves. They are usually driven using a joystick that controls the movement, but other controls are available for people who have limited upper limb use. An alternative to powered wheelchairs for people who need some help is a mobility scooter (Fig. 47.6B), with a seat at the back and steered by handles at the front of the chair. This can be used by people who are safe to get in and out of the device.

Powered wheeled mobility devices can enable mobility and increase the occupational performance, competence, adaptability and self-esteem of people using these devices (Buning, Angelo, & Schmeler, 2001). These devices can enable users to increase their mobility within their community and their opportunities to participate in daily activities. For example, the provision of a scooter to a person who cannot walk long distances may enable this person to do grocery shopping. Some people might be reluctant to use a powered wheeled mobility device as they fear that they might lose skills, become less active or put on weight. However, recent studies have found that people who begin to use powered wheeled mobility devices do not increase their weight but do increase their participation in occupations and show improvements in measurements of their wellness and quality of life (Bottos, Bolcati, Sciuto, Ruggeri, & Feliciangeli, 2001;

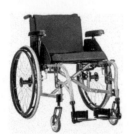

FIG. 47.4 ■ Lightweight folding chair. Often used for people who need mobility help for short distances or are pushed by someone else.

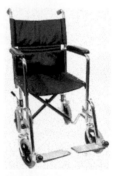

FIG. 47.5 ■ Attendant-propelled manual wheelchair, which has increased stability but no possibility for independent mobility.

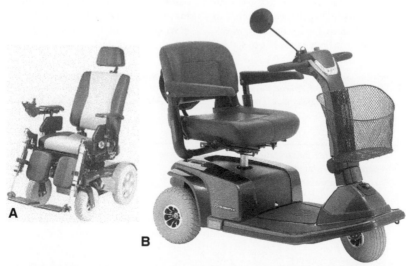

A

B

FIG. 47.6 ■ (A) Powered wheelchair, with joystick control on right-hand side. (B) Mobility scooter.

Brandt, Iwarsson, & Stahle, 2004; Davies, De Souza, & Frank, 2003; Kotsch, 2003; Yang, Wilson, Oda, & Yan, 2007).

There are different means of controlling a powered wheelchair. The most common way is to 'drive' the wheelchair using a joystick. For people who have weakness of the upper limb, the weight required to push a joystick may need to be modified, through the use of either a program in the computer system of the powered chair itself or a specially made joystick. If a person is unable to use his or her hands to operate a joystick, then alternative controls are available, such as single or multiple switches to operate a scanning interface. Alternatives to standard joystick control of a powered wheelchair can be expensive and often complex. However, providing the means for independent powered wheeled mobility for people who have an illness, injury or impairment can make an enormous difference to their quality of life and well-being.

Special Types of Mobility Systems

In addition to the three main types of wheeled mobility bases there are a number of special types of mobility systems. These include high-performance sports wheelchairs, bariatric wheelchairs, stand-up wheelchairs, elevating wheelchairs and tilt-in-space wheelchairs.

High-performance sports wheelchairs. People who are very proficient at using their wheelchairs, such as people who have a low spinal cord injury, often use high-performance wheelchairs. These can significantly enhance people's ability to participate in their daily occupations. These wheelchairs often have a fixed frame, so to transport the chair without the user in it often involves unclipping the wheels and folding the back rest. In order to gain speed and manoeuvrability, the user sacrifices some of the stability of the chair.

Bariatric wheelchairs. The term *bariatric* refers to the branch of medicine that deals with obesity. Regular wheelchairs can usually support a body weight up to 135 kg. Bariatric wheelchairs can accommodate people with body mass of up to 450 kg.

Stand-up wheelchairs. There are a number of environmental restrictions when using a wheelchair, as users are in a sitting position and hence limited in how high they can reach. To promote independence and increase access to activities, some people prefer to use a stand-up wheelchair. Stand-up wheelchairs are specialised devices, and there are a number of prerequisites for use, usually concerning safety and postural requirements. Biomechanical considerations of centre of gravity are extremely important to consider

Elevating wheelchairs. As previously mentioned, the seated wheelchair position presents an environmental barrier to many activities that require standing height. An alternative to standing wheelchairs is an elevating wheelchair – instead of the individual assuming an assisted standing device, the whole seat is able to move into an elevated position.

Tilt-in-Space wheelchairs. Some wheelchairs have reclining backs or have the option of the whole seat being able to tilt backwards. This is important for people who are unable to move their body in the wheelchair to relieve pressure or attain a more comfortable position.

Management of Posture

A thorough assessment for wheeled mobility, in addition to basic body measurements (see Fig. 47.2), should also involve activity, participation, personal and environmental considerations as well as body functions and posture. Consider the practice story of Orlando (Practice Story 47.1) and the fact that the difference between optimal and suboptimal outcomes had a great deal to do with considering all the contexts within which an individual performs. Until recently, there were very few standardised assessments, but there has been recognition of the need for outcome measures in this field, and there has been rapid development recently. A noncomprehensive list of assessments can be found in Table 47.2.

TABLE 47.2			
Outcome Measurement Tools for Wheeled Mobility and Seating Systems			
Name or Type of Assessment	What It Does	Who It Is For	Author(s)
Pressure mapping systems	Measure skin interface pressure between the seated surface and the skin of the user	All, but primarily adults	Brienza et al., 2001; Crawford, Stinson, Walsh, & Porter-Armstrong, 2005; Davin, 2013; Davin, 2015; Fradet et al., 2011; McDonald et al., 2011; Nelson, 1997; Pellow, 1999
Usability Scale for Assistive Technology	Self-reported degree of usability of assistive technology (including wheeled mobility and seating systems)	People able to self-report who use assistive technology	Arthanat et al., 2007

Name or Type of Assessment	What It Does	Who It Is For	Author(s)
Wheelchair Propulsion Test	Wheeling 10 m while timed, number of cycles and propulsion methods	Anyone able to propel a wheelchair	Askari et al., 2013
Seating and Mobility Script Concordance Test of Spinal Cord Injury	Assesses competencies in professional reasoning of therapists providing seating equipment.	Seating therapists	Cohen et al., 2005; Cohen et al., 2009
Tool for Assessing Wheelchair disComfort (TAWC)	Assessment to determine comfort within a wheelchair	Adults who use a wheeled mobility and seating system full-time and have intact sensation	Crane, Holm, Hobson, Cooper, & Reed, 2007
Seating assessment tool for community use	Guidelines for allocation of pressure cushions	Adults who use a wheeled mobility device and seating system who are at risk of compromised tissue integrity	Shipperley & Collins, 1999
Wheelchair Outcome Measure (WhOM)	Person-specific tool which identifies individual goals for seating	Adults who use a wheeled mobility device and seating system	Mortenson et al., 2007
Functioning Everyday in a Wheelchair (FEW)	Self-report questionnaire to assess everyday functioning when using a wheelchair	Adults who use a wheeled mobility device and seating system	Mills et al., 2002
Functioning Everyday in a Wheelchair Performance (FEW-P)	Observational assessment of performance to accompany FEW questionnaire	Adults who use a wheeled mobility device and seating system	Mills et al., 2002
Seated Postural Control Measure	Observational assessment divided into two parts; physical assessment and seated function	Developed for children with neurological disorders but adapted recently for adults with neurological impairments	Field & Roxborough, 2011; Fife et al., 1991; Gagnon, Noreau, & Vincent, 2005a, 2005b
Wheelchair User's Shoulder Pain Index (WUSPI)	Index of shoulder pain and discomfort	Adults who actively use a wheeled mobility device and seating system	Curtis et al., 1995a, 1995b
Obstacle Course Assessment of Wheelchair User Performance (OCAWUP)	10 items that represent environmental barriers to people using different types of wheelchairs	People who use a wheeled mobility device and seating system	Routhier et al., 2003, 2004, 2005
Seated Posture Scale (SPS)	Pen-and-paper test of wheelchair seated posture	Older adults	Barks et al., 2015
Adapted Manual Wheelchair Circuit (AMWC)	Wheelchair circuit to determine wheelchair performance	People who use a manual wheelchair	Cowan, Nash, De Groot, & Van Der Woude, 2011
Accelerometers	Measures physical activity of the person who uses a wheeled mobility and seating system	People who use a manual wheelchair	Gendle et al., 2012
Visual analogue scales and pain drawings	Define pain in seating systems	People who are nonverbal and may have issues with cognition	Gibson & Frank, 2005
Power Mobility Road Test	Virtual reality to simulate real-world driving	People being assessed for powered mobility	Mahajan, Dicianno, Cooper, & Ding, 2013
Transfer Assessment Instrument	Assesses quality of transfers the person who uses a wheeled mobility and seating system	People who use a wheeled mobility device and seating system and who can transfer	Mcclure, Boninger, Ozawa, & Koontz, 2011
Posture Assessment Software	Electronic measurement of body angles	People who need postural assessment	Metring, Gaspar, Mateus-Vasconcelos, Gomes, & De Abreu, 2012

Before assessing a person in detail, the therapist needs some basic understanding of biomechanical principles, the forces that act on the body that underpin seating and positioning. The ability to sit and be stable comes from the underlying structural stability of the musculoskeletal system in conjunction with the body's biomechanical alignment and neurological and vestibular systems. However, people with some spinal, neurological, orthopaedic or other injuries may not have the underlying structural stability to support themselves in a regular seated position. Prerequisites for stable sitting are a stable base of support through the pelvis and lower limbs, as well as stability of the trunk and upper body.

During the assessment for a wheeled mobility and seating system, the therapist must investigate, consider and make a judgement about the effects of the forces acting on the body of a person. It is important to understand that the forces acting on the body are not always obvious and that they may be internal as well as external. Consideration of biomechanics and the forces acting on the body when conducting a wheeled mobility postural assessment can be used to do the following:

- Enable somebody to attain and maintain a stable position
- Encourage occupation through comfort, stability and enabling the person to perform occupations they want and need to do
- Prevent deformity by counteracting the forces that are acting on the body as a result of muscle tone
- Prevent the development of pressure ulcers

Effect of Force on Seating

Forces can act either internally (e.g. a spastic muscle) or externally (e.g. a seating system or orthotic). Stable or balanced seating is achieved when there is a balance of forces acting on a person. These forces include compression forces, shearing forces and gravitational forces. Most people are able to hold themselves up against gravitational forces, but for people with low muscle tone, this is difficult and becomes an important consideration for seating and positioning.

A compression force is when the stress or force is perpendicular to the surface (in the case of sitting in a wheeled mobility device, the surface referred to is the skin of the buttock). In sitting, compression force refers to a force that compresses the blood vessels, muscles and skin tissue. This means oxygenation of the cells in the area being compressed is reduced. Shear force is parallel or tangential to the face of the surface (again the surface referred to in this case is the skin of the buttock). Shear forces can cause rubbing of the skin over the bone (e.g. blisters from uncomfortable shoes), and this leads to sores, which, combined with compression forces, may lead to the development of pressure ulcers.

Centre of Mass

The centre of mass or composite mass is the place where a person's weight is concentrated, in a downward way, together with gravity. When seated, the centre of mass changes – generally, it falls in front of the body, outside the trunk. For a person to be stable, the centre of mass must fall within the person's base of support; when a person is standing, the base of support is his or her two feet, and when a person is sitting in a wheeled mobility and seating system, the base of support is the wheel base of the system. The centre of mass is very important in the provision of seating, as the effect of gravity on the wheeled mobility and seating system will determine the stability of the system. For example, if the rear wheels of a wheelchair are moved forwards of the centre of mass, the wheelchair will become unsteady and will more easily tip backwards; if the width of the wheels at the front is too narrow, the wheelchair is more likely to tip sideways; and if the front wheels are too far back, the wheelchair is more likely to tip forwards. Hence, consideration of the position of the centre of mass is essential for the safety and stability of a person and for the person's ability to perform activities.

Tissue Integrity and Pressure Ulcers

There are a number of reasons why some basic understanding of the forces acting on the body is required. These reasons include understanding the impact of forces on the development of pressure ulcers and deformity that affect a person's body, and ultimately the impact that forces can have on a person's ability to engage and participate in occupation.

People who have reduced sensory and motor functions and who spend a long period in the same position may develop pressure ulcers (Arias et al., 2015). A pressure ulcer can initially be noticed by reddened skin (stage 1), which, if the pressure is not relieved, can go on to form a blister or an open sore (stage 2), and then a sore that looks like a crater (stage 3). If the pressure is not relieved at stage 3, it is possible for the pressure ulcer to become so deep that it causes damage to the muscle and bone (stage 4). The secondary effects of this include infection leading to poor health, leading to restrictions in mobility, enforced bed rest and even the need for surgery (Adriaansen et al., 2013; Brillhart, 2005; De Laat, Scholte, Reimer, & Van Achterberg, 2005).

Compression forces that cause pressure that blocks or occludes the vessels transporting blood to the tissues and the vessels that remove the metabolic waste products away from the tissues are the major factors causing pressure ulcers. As force and in turn the pressure increase, the amount of time required to develop a blockage decreases; therefore the aim of many interventions is to keep the amount of pressure to a minimum. The bones on which an individual sits – the ischial tuberosities and sacrum – are particularly at risk. Pressure (P) is equal to force (F) divided by area (a) ($P = F/a$), and as such, if weight (force) is distributed over a small area (such as the ischial tuberosities), the pressure will be more than if it is distributed over a large area (such as the whole of a person's buttocks).

Friction, caused by shearing forces, where skin is pulled sideways over bone when moving, is another cause of pressure ulcers (Aissaoui, Boucher, Bourbonnais, Lacoste, & Dansereau, 2001; Brillhart, 2005). Other factors that increase susceptibility to developing pressure ulcers include moisture (from incontinence or sweating), decreased skin elasticity as a result of aging and excess weight or malnourishment (Apatsidis, Solomonidis, & Michael, 2002; Stinson, Porter-Armstrong, & Eakin, 2003).

The Skeletal System and Deformity

The skeletal system is the scaffolding that holds the body upright, but for people who have neuromuscular difficulties such as cerebral palsy, those who have had a cerebrovascular accident, or people who have musculoskeletal difficulties, such as rheumatoid arthritis, the skeleton may not be symmetrical or straight. This is referred to as a bony or postural deformity. There are three terms commonly used to describe a bony or postural deformity: *mobile deformity, fixed deformity,* and *structural deformity.* A mobile deformity is maintained by muscle power or gravity and can be corrected passively. A fixed deformity

(or contracture) is one that cannot be corrected passively as the soft tissues (muscle, ligament, etc.) do not allow a full range of movement at a joint. Structural deformity is one that is caused by abnormal bone shape or lack of joint integrity. Trying to correct a fixed or structural deformity by positioning may cause discomfort and even stress and strain on the long bones of the person and increase the risk of pressure ulcer development.

The role of postural management is either to attempt to correct a deformity that is not fixed or accommodate a deformity that is fixed, thereby preventing the development of secondary deformity. When a person's posture is fixed in a position that is not typical, it affects the rest of that person's body. Some possible secondary difficulties that individuals may experience that are caused by inappropriate wheelchair provision, along with possible solutions to reduce or eliminate each identified difficulty, are identified in Table 47.3. These possible solutions are sometimes called 'postural management'.

TABLE 47.3

Body Positions in Wheeled Mobility and Seating Systems, Description of Movement, Effects and Possible Solutions

Description of Body Position	Description of Movement	Secondary Physical or Occupational Performance Difficulties Caused by Movement	Possible Solutions
Posterior pelvic tilt	Pelvis is rotated or slumped backwards because of spasticity in hip extensors, lack of muscle tone through the trunk.	Pain where vertebrae are pushed together. Protraction of shoulders reduce hand and upper limb activities. Chin poking or hyperextension of neck occurs, which may affect safety of swallowing.	Check that length of seat is not too long. Equipment such as pelvic belts, antithrust seats and pelvic bars can be employed.
Anterior pelvic tilt	Pelvis is rotated forwards possibly as a result of weakness of trunk musculature, hip flexion contractures or hyper tonicity of lumbar extensors.	Increased risk of hip dislocating anteriorly. Instability of arms and head as pushed forwards. Pain.	Ensure seat is flat, not hammocked. Hip belt positioned to counter the effect of the tilt.
Pelvic obliquity	Pelvis is elevated on one side, judged by feeling the anterior sacroiliac spine (ASIS), and comparing line between them to the horizontal.	Likelihood of secondary scoliosis increased. Decreased stability of sitting position as balanced on one ischial tuberosity, often compensatory side flexion of trunk.	Check the width of the seat.
Pelvic rotation	Pelvis is rotated backwards on one side and forwards on the other, due to asymmetry of muscle tone around the hip and trunk, OR seat is too long on one side.	Increases likelihood of developing secondary scoliosis. Reduced stability in sitting. Reduced ability to use hands — shoulder also rotated forwards.	Assess and accommodate for leg length discrepancy or hip abduction/adduction contracture. 45-degree bifurcate (Y-shaped) hip belt. ASIS bar, rigid bar placed immediately below the ASIS.

Continued on following page

TABLE 47.3

Body Positions in Wheeled Mobility and Seating Systems, Description of Movement, Effects and Possible Solutions (Continued)

Description of Body Position	Description of Movement	Secondary Physical or Occupational Performance Difficulties Caused by Movement	Possible Solutions
Scoliosis and kyphosis of spine	Neuromuscular or idiopathic curvature of the spine. May be internally rotated around the vertebrae.	Physical issues such as decreased respiration, increased gastrooesophageal reflux. Difficulty using one or both hands. Difficulty holding head upright.	Accommodation of fixed deformity, support of the body above and below the curve. Accommodation of spinal orthotic, if worn. May require spinal surgery.
Side flexion (postural scoliosis) of trunk	Imbalance of tone throughout trunk, low tone of trunk and slumps to preferred side, or compensation for pelvic obliquity.	Inability to use hands. Increased susceptibility to develop fixed scoliosis. Discomfort. Poor head control.	Firm seat base to reduce pelvic obliquity cause by hammocking of sling seat. Pads or moulded seat to counteract trunk position. Spinal orthotic.
Forwards flexion (kyphosis) of trunk	Possible compensation for backwards pelvic tilt. Weight of arms pulls trunk forwards with poor abdominal strength.	Poor head and neck control, may influence safety in eating. Discomfort or pain. Difficulty using hands and arms for functional movement.	Firm support of seat base and throughout the back. Use of armrests and or tray. Accommodate if has fixed kyphosis. Tilt back in space.
Hip extension	Spasticity of hip extensors, hamstring contractures.	Unstable base of support means difficulty with all movements of upper limbs and head and neck.	Firm seat and back. Wedged or contoured seat. Accommodate to fixed hamstring contractures in seat.
Hip flexion	Spasticity of hip flexors, or hip flexion contractures.	Unstable base of support means difficulty with all movements of upper limbs and head and neck.	Ensure seat length and footplate height is correct. Accommodate fixed contractures. Firm seat, trial forwards tilt.
Adduction of hips	Caused by spasticity of adductor muscles, contracture, subluxation or dislocation of hip. Could be due to footplate height.	Pain and discomfort as the hip begins to sublux. Instability, poor use of arms, hands, head and neck. Secondary issues of spine.	Firm, contoured seat to support the thighs. Use of pommel, or abduction straps. Use of kneeblock and sacral pad. Control pelvic rotation, but accommodate to fixed contracture.
Abduction of hips	Caused by spasticity of abductors, contracture or adduction of the opposite hip.	Instability and discomfort. May create environmental barriers.	Accommodate to fixed contracture. Use of hip guides or lateral supports along the thighs. Control for pelvic rotation.
Head and neck positioning	Flexion or extension of the neck, secondary to either poor positioning or lack of head control.	May effect eating and drinking, communication, eye pointing. May be unsafe.	Good firm base of support/ postural support throughout the whole body. Possible head band or neck supports. Tilt seating system in space.

Mechanical Assessment Tool Postural Assessment

A Mechanical Assessment Tool (MAT) assessment can also be referred to as a biomechanical assessment or physical examination for seating. It is commonly used by therapists to provide a thorough measurement of a person's body posture to ensure that any seating given to the person meets that person's particular combination of best body posture and reduced risk of deformity. The tool examines the person's range of motion, as well as joint flexibility, muscle length and skeletal or postural alignment. It involves looking at the person's body position in that person's current seating system, followed by measuring body angles on a firm surface in supine and in sitting. At the same time, the person's neurological issues, such as tone and spasm, are recorded, as these will also affect how that person sits. This is important because the position and posture of a person will affect that person's ability to sit comfortably and to control a powered wheelchair or push a manual wheelchair (Buck, 2009).

Adaptive Seating Systems and Pressure-Relieving/Pressure-Reducing Cushion for Postural Management

There are two main types of postural systems, used to provide postural support and reduced the risk of pressure ulcers, that can be prescribed for people using a wheeled mobility and seating system; adaptive seating and pressure-relieving/pressure-reducing cushions.

Adaptive seating systems. Adaptive seating systems are devices that seek to correct or accommodate a person's postural difficulty using mechanical forces. Adaptive seating systems provide postural management when the biomechanical forces on the body mean that the person requires extra support. Postural management equipment needs to encourage the development of skills and independence and at the same time respond to growth and changes in body shape, environment and intervention plans throughout the person's lifespan (Cox, 2003).

It is important to remember that adaptive seating systems are used for people with complex physical impairments, and the aim is to increase the person's ability to engage in occupations as well as prevent the development of secondary postural problems. A list of some of the body segments that often cause difficulties in symmetrical or individual sitting for an individual are listed in Table 47.3. Each body segment needs to be measured individually – it is an extension of the information in Table 47.1, but for individuals who have complex needs. Whatever the 'prescription', the adaptive seating system needs to be individually tailored to the individual's needs and goals. The limited research that has been done suggests that improving people's postural stability does improve their function (Costigan & Light, 2011).

Pressure-relieving/pressure-reducing cushions. As previously mentioned, a pressure ulcer is tissue necrosis caused by occlusion of the blood supply usually resulting when external pressure acts upon a bony prominence (Brienza, Karg, Geyer, Kelsey, & Trefler,

2001). In an attempt to reduce the pressure that may lead to an ulcer, pressure-relieving/pressure-reducing cushions are supplied (Brienza et al., 2001). It has been found that pressure-relieving/pressure-reducing seating surfaces are essential to the maintenance of skin integrity for a person who is at risk of developing pressure ulcers (Brienza et al., 2010). Cushions for pressure management are available; the cushions are designed based on the biomechanical principle of increasing the load-bearing area to reduce the pressure over a single surface.

The aims of a pressure cushion is to do the following:

- Distribute and decrease the pressure by increasing the area of support over a larger support surface (i.e. over the whole buttock rather than just the ischial tuberosities)
- Remove or reduce the weight, and compressive and shearing forces from the bony prominences
- Control temperature and moisture

The technology involved in pressure-relieving/pressure-reducing cushions is rapidly developing, with cushion design now including combinations of air, pressure-relieving gel and foam technologies (Brillhart, 2005). A range of cushions are shown in Fig. 47.7, which use air, memory foam and gel to increase the surface area of support and thus reduce pressure on the seated surface of the individual.

One way to manage pressure in people who use powered wheelchairs is to tilt or recline the seat to reduce the seating load away from the ischial tuberosities. However, caution must be taken to ensure that the pressure is not redistributed to other bony areas, such as the coccyx (Yanni et al., 2014). To have an impact on pressure, the seat must be tilted back at least 30 degrees, with 45 degrees having a noticeable change in pressure.

SOME CONSIDERATION WHEN PRESCRIBING WHEELED MOBILITY AND SEATING SYSTEMS

Manual Wheelchair Skills Training

Providing training in wheelchair skills is important for people to learn to use their wheelchairs safely (Rushton et al., 2012), gain competence and mastery (Sawatzky, Hers, & Macgillivray, 2015b; Taylor et al., 2015) and prevent secondary problems (Sawatzky, Digiovine, Berner, Roesler, & Katte, 2015a). Wheelchair skills are not just about learning to wheel the chair in the most efficient way, but also to learn how to maintain the chair, including things like what tyre pressure is best for the most efficient use (Booka et al., 2015).

Learning how to use a manual wheelchair is like any other skill; it takes time and practice (Zwinkels, Verschuren, Janssen, Ketelaar, & Takken, 2014). There has been an increase in training programmes to enable users to become fully competent in their wheelchair skills training (Fliess-Douer, Vanlandewijck, Lubel Manor, & Van Der Woude, 2010). Zukowski et al. (2014) demonstrated that appropriate training

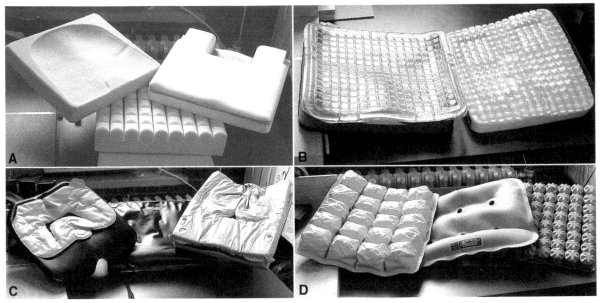

FIG. 47.7 ■ Examples of seat cushion designed to manage pressure in wheelchair seat. (A) Foam cushions. (B) Gel cushions. (C) Viscous fluid cushions. (D) Air cushions.

programmes can prevent or reduce the development of issues such as carpal tunnel syndrome. Furthermore, the setup of the chair is important – factors such as axle position, changes in tyre type and the adding of accessories can affect whether or not shoulder injuries will develop (Caspall, Seligsohn, Dao, & Sprigle, 2013), and this needs to be included in training. Furthermore, training has been demonstrated to reduce the likelihood of wheelchair-related accidents (Chen et al., 2011).

Although there are lots of different wheelchair skills training packages available, the packages available at the wheelchair skills programme housed by Dalhousie University are comprehensive for both assessment and teaching of wheelchair skills (see http://www.wheelchairskillsprogram.ca/eng/index.php).

Teaching Powered Mobility

Driving a powered mobility device does involve the risk of accidents to the person who uses a wheeled mobility and seating system and to others. One emerging way of determining whether someone has the potential for independent powered mobility use is the use of simulated environments (Hasdai, Jessel, & Weiss, 1998; Linden, Whyatt, Craig, & Kerr, 2013; Mahajan, 2012). Most recently these have involved virtual reality (Adelola, Cox, & Rahman, 2009). A virtual reality session can be used for assessment and training of skills and as an outcome measure, to determine whether someone can attain and maintain the skills necessary for driving a chair in a safe way. When using virtual reality, the training experienced by the person must be equivalent to the experience of driving a chair and can complement training programmes (Archambault, Tremblay,

Cachecho, Routhier, & Boissy, 2012). Training in simulated environments has also been found to be an effective and safe way of enhancing skills that are needed to be safe in a powered wheelchair (Wei Pin et al., 2015).

Powered Mobility and Older Adults

Often older adults do not have access to powered mobility. This is particularly true when people live in residential aged care or nursing homes (Mortenson, Hurd Clarke, & Best, 2013), even though it has been found that access to powered mobility improves and enhances engagement in occupations and increases quality of life (Auger et al., 2010). This is discriminatory, and as such, an important role for an occupational therapist is to advocate for older adults to ensure that they have access to the devices that will improve their quality of life and use them to their full potential (Mortenson et al., 2013). It appears that lack of access to powered mobility for older adults is not always because of the underlying skills or engagement of the persons themselves but is the result of an inability to access funding or the inability of professionals to accurately assess older adults' abilities.

Shoulder Pain in People Who Propel Their Own Wheelchairs

Shoulder joints are delicate, and up to 40% of people who propel their own wheelchair can develop shoulder pain (Akhigbe et al., 2015). The risk of developing shoulder pain increases with age and years after injury (Alm, Saraste, & Norrbrink, 2008) and in people who have more severe injuries (Yildirim, Comert, &

Ozengin, 2010). The development of shoulder pain can affect a person's ability to participate in daily occupations and limit a person's ability to transfer into and out of a wheelchair.

Shoulder pain can be prevented using a number of different mechanisms. Initially, this can be done by the person using a wheelchair learning to propel in the most efficient manner, the strain on joints will be reduced. Similarly, people using wheelchairs should be taught to recognise early signs of discomfort and pain and take steps to manage that pain rather than pushing through and causing joint damage. Other strategies include using different assistive technologies, such as different wheels or even powered mobility for a time to reduce strain on the joint (Alm et al., 2008; Collinger et al., 2008).

Being Physically Active

Staying healthy and well is important for people who use wheeled mobility and seating systems, as is participation in the community (Cooper, Ferretti, Oyster, Kelleher, & Cooper, 2011). Lack of exercise is a major risk factor for developing secondary physical and mental health conditions in people who use wheeled mobility and seating systems – including people who use powered devices (Barfield & Malone, 2013). It is important to encourage physical activity in people who use wheeled mobility and seating systems of all types, and there is developing evidence for the benefit of this (Conger & Bassett, 2011). It has been found, for example, that if people using a powered wheelchair can increase their physical activity and participation in the community, this will lead to an improvement in the person's quality of life (Davies, De Souza, & Frank, 2003).

Personal and Environmental Factors Related to Participation in Life When Using a Wheeled Mobility and Seating System

Despite legislation to the contrary, commonplace physical environments such as public transport remain barriers to participation in everyday life for people who use wheeled mobility and seating systems (Hoenig, Landerman, Shipp, & George, 2003; Hunt, 2005). There are wheeled mobility devices available that have special facilities to overcome environmental barriers, including wheelchairs that are elevating and those which have a standing frame as integral to the design. However, these devices are usually expensive and do not suit every individual. Furthermore, decreased access to the environment reduces an individual's ability to participate in all activities and occupations, which affects a person's self-esteem and worldview.

Whether or not a wheeled mobility and seating system is useful ultimately is due to the personal factors and acceptance by the user. Research on adherence and agreement with all assistive technologies has found that failure to consider the opinions and preferences, as well as degree of confidence in assistive technology devices, results in the abandonment and rejection of these devices (Cushman & Scherer, 1996; Demers, Weiss-Lambrou, & Ska, 1996, 2000; Hocking, 1999). White (1999) found that

there is a need for greater collaboration between therapists, carers and users of special seating systems, partly for the very reason that collaboration and communication is likely to have an effect both on compliance in using the system, as well as overall satisfaction with the service the user receives (Pain, Gore, & Mclellan, 2000; White, 1999). Collaboration in which the person who uses a wheeled mobility and seating system is engaged in the decision-making process helps to optimise the provision of the system to ensure the best outcome.

EMERGING TECHNOLOGIES

There are a number of exciting new technologies and developments with wheeled mobility and seating systems that will enhance the mobility and quality of life for people who require these systems. It is important for the occupational therapist to be aware of these new developments, together with the evidence supporting their use. A brief overview of some of them is provided:

Pushrim Activated Power Assist Wheelchairs (PAPAWs): This is a regular manual wheelchair to which motorised wheels are added to provide power to the wheelchair, turning the wheelchair into a hybrid between a manual wheelchair and a power wheelchair (Alm et al., 2008; Giesbrecht, Ripat, Cooper, & Quanbury, 2011).

Intellwheels: This is a system that enables a wheelchair to be driven by voice, for people whose motor impairment means that they cannot drive a powered wheelchair easily using a joystick or switch access system (Braga, Beng, Reis, & Moreira, 2011).

Solar battery charging pack: The use of solar power to extend the battery life of a powered wheelchair will allow people whose batteries on their powered chairs often run low to charge the battery while driving their chairs (Chi-Sheng, Tung-Yung, Tze-Yuan, Tsung-Yuan, & Tzer-Min, 2014).

Alternative drive and access systems for people with severe physical illness, injury or impairment: Different ways to drive the chair and access many of the chair's features are in development, such as the *Tongue Drive System (TDS).* This will enable people with severe physical impairments to access computers, drive powered wheelchairs and control their environments using their voluntary tongue movements (Huo, 2011). *Intelligent powered wheelchairs* that have inbuilt safety mechanisms such as anticollide mechanisms have been found to increase social participation for people with complex difficulties (Rushton et al., 2015).

CONCLUSION

In terms of occupational engagement, the person is at the core, and the occupational therapist must ensure above all that the wheeled mobility and seating system meets the personal needs of the user. Age, life stage and stage of adjustment must all be considered. Collaboration with the person, so that his or her ability to participate in occupation is enhanced and developed, is essential to the assessment and provision of a wheeled mobility and seating system. It is important to remember that 'the role of the occupational therapist in wheelchairs and seating is to enhance the user's participation in occupation through technical intervention' (Reid et al., 2002, p. 261). All occupational therapists who participate in the assessment of wheeled mobility and seating systems have a responsibility to ensure that provision is cost effective and safe for the person. Primarily, though, the wheeled mobility and seating system must enhance the user's ability to participate in purposeful and meaningful occupation.

 http://evolve.elsevier.com/Curtin/OT

REFERENCES

Adelola, I. A., Cox, S. L., & Rahman, A. (2009). Virtual environments for powered wheelchair learner drivers: Case studies. *Technology & Disability, 21*, 97–106.

Adriaansen, J. J. E., Van Asbeck, F. W. A., Lindeman, E., Van Der Woude, L. H. V., De Groot, S., & Post, M. W. M. (2013). Secondary health conditions in persons with a spinal cord injury for at least 10 years: Design of a comprehensive long-term cross-sectional study. *Disability & Rehabilitation, 35*, 1104–1110.

Aissaoui, R., Boucher, C., Bourbonnais, D., Lacoste, M., & Dansereau, J. (2001). Effect of seat cushion on dynamic stability in sitting during a reaching task in wheelchair users with paraplegia. *Archives of Physical Medicine and Rehabilitation, 82*, 274–281.

Akhigbe, T., Chin, A. S., Svircev, J. N., et al. (2015). A retrospective review of lower extremity fracture care in patients with spinal cord injury. *Journal of Spinal Cord Medicine, 38*, 2–9.

Alexander, C. J., Hwang, K., & Sipski, M. (2001). Mothers with spinal cord injuries: Impact on family division of labor, family decision making, and rearing of children. *Topics in Spinal Cord Injury Rehabilitation, 7*, 25–36.

Alm, M., Saraste, H., & Norrbrink, C. (2008). Shoulder pain in persons with thoracic spinal cord injury: prevalence and characteristics. *Journal of Rehabilitation Medicine (Stiftelsen Rehabiliteringsinformation), 40*, 277–283.

Apatsidis, D., Solomonidis, S. E., & Michael, S. M. (2002). Pressure distribution at the seating interface of custom-molded wheelchair seats: Effect of various materials. *American Academy of Physical Medicine and Rehabilitation*, 1151–1156.

Archambault, P. S., Tremblay, S., Cachecho, S., Routhier, F., & Boissy, P. (2012). Driving performance in a power wheelchair simulator. *Disability & Rehabilitation: Assistive Technology, 7*, 226–233.

Arias, S., Cardiel, E., Garay, L., et al. (2015). Effects on interface pressure and tissue oxygenation under ischial tuberosities during the application of an alternating cushion. *Journal of Tissue Viability, 24*, 91 101.

Arthanat, S., Bauer, S. M., Lenker, J. A., Nochajski, S. M., & Wu, Y. W. B. (2007). Conceptualization and measurement of assistive technology usability. *Disability and Rehabilitation Assistive Technology, 2*, 235–248.

Askari, S., Kirby, R. L., Parker, K., Thompson, K., & O'Neill, J. (2013). Wheelchair Propulsion Test: Development and measurement properties of a new test for manual wheelchair users. *Archives of Physical Medicine & Rehabilitation, 94*, 1690–1698.

Audit Commission (2000). *Fully equipped – The provision of equipment services to older or disabled people by the NHS and social services in England and Wales.* London: Audit Commission.

Audit Commission (2002). *Fully Equipped 2002 – Assisting independence.* London: Audit Commission.

Auger, C., Demers, L., Gélinas, I., Miller, W. C., Jutai, J. W., & Noreau, L. (2010). Life-space mobility of middle-aged and older adults at various stages of usage of power mobility devices. *Archives of Physical Medicine & Rehabilitation, 91*, 765–773.

Barfield, J. P., & Malone, L. A. (2013). Perceived exercise benefits and barriers among power wheelchair soccer players. *Journal of Rehabilitation Research & Development, 50*, 231–238.

Barks, L., Luther, S. L., Brown, L. M., Schulz, B., Bowen, M. E., & Powell-Cope, G. (2015). Development and initial validation of the Seated Posture Scale. *Journal of Rehabilitation Research & Development, 52*, 201–210.

Bearne, L. M., Coomer, A. F., & Hurley, M. V. (2007). Upper limb sensorimotor function and functional performance in patients with rheumatoid arthritis. *Disability & Rehabilitation, 29*, 1035–1039.

Best, K., Kirby, R. L., Smith, C., & Macleod, D. A. (2005). Wheelchair skills training for community-based manual wheelchair users: A randomized controlled trial. *Archives of Physical Medicine & Rehabilitation, 86*, 2316–2323.

Booka, M., Yoneda, I., Hashizume, T., Lee, H., Oku, H., & Fujisawa, S. (2015). Effect of tire pressure to physical workload at operating a manual wheelchair. *Studies in Health Technology & Informatics, 217*, 929–934.

Bottos, M., Bolcati, C., Sciuto, L., Ruggeri, C., & Feliciangeli, A. (2001). Powered wheelchairs and independence in young children with tetraplegia. *Developmental Medicine & Child Neurology, 43*, 769–777.

Braga, R. A. M., Beng, M. P., Reis, L. P., & Moreira, A. N. P. (2011). IntellWheels: Modular development platform for intelligent wheelchairs. *Journal of Rehabilitation Research & Development, 48*, 1061–1076.

Brandt, A., Iwarsson, S., & Stahle, A. (2004). Older people's use of powered wheelchairs for activity and participation. *Journal of Rehabilitation Medicine, 36*, 70–77.

Brienza, D. M., Karg, P. E., Geyer, M. J., Kelsey, S., & Trefler, E. (2001). The relationship between pressure ulcer incidence and buttock-seat cushion interface pressure in at-risk elderly wheelchair users. *Archives of Physical Medicine and Rehabilitation, 82*, 529–533.

Brienza, D., Kelsey, S., Karg, P., et al. (2010). A randomized clinical trial on preventing pressure ulcers with wheelchair seat cushions. *Journal of the American Geriatric Society, 58*(12), 2308–2314. http://dx.doi.org/10.1111/j.1532.2010.03168.x.

Brillhart, B. (2005). Pressure sore and skin tear prevention and treatment during a 10-month program. *Rehabilitation Nursing, 30*, 85–91.

Buck, S. (2009). *More than 4 wheels: Applying clinical practice to seating, mobility and assistive technology.* Toronto: Therapy Now.

Buning, M. E., Angelo, J. A., & Schmeler, M. R. (2001). Occupational performance and the transition to powered mobility: A pilot study. *American Journal of Occupational Therapy, 55*, 339–344.

Caspall, J. J., Seligsohn, E., Dao, P. V., & Sprigle, S. (2013). Changes in inertia and effect on turning effort across different wheelchair configurations. *Journal of Rehabilitation Research & Development, 50*, 1353–1361.

Chen, K.-M., Huang, H.-T., Cheng, Y.-Y., Li, C.-H., & Chang, Y.-H. (2015). Sleep quality and depression of nursing home older adults in wheelchairs after exercises. *Nursing Outlook, 63*, 357–365.

Chen, W.-Y., Jang, Y., Wang, J.-D., Huang, W.-N., Chang, C.-C., Mao, H.-F., & WANG, Y.-H. (2011). Wheelchair-related accidents: Relationship with wheelchair-using behavior in active community wheelchair users. *Archives of Physical Medicine & Rehabilitation, 92*, 892–898.

Chi-Sheng, C., Tung-Yung, H., Tze-Yuan, L., Tsung-Yuan, K., & Tzer-Min, L. (2014). Design and development of solar power-assisted manual/electric wheelchair. *Journal of Rehabilitation Research & Development, 51*, 1411–1425.

Cohen, L. (2007). Research priorities: Wheeled mobility. *Disability and Rehabilitation Assistive Technology, 2*, 173–180.

Cohen, L. J., Fitzgerald, S. G., Lane, S., & Boninger, M. L. (2005). Development of the seating and mobility script concordance test of spinal cord injury: Obtaining content validity evidence. *Assistive Technology, 17*, 122–132.

Cohen, L., Fitzgerald, S., Lane, S., Boninger, M., Minkel, J., & Mccue, M. (2009). Validation of the seating and mobility script concordance test. *Assistive Technology, 27*(1), 47–56. http://dx.doi.org/10.1080/10400430902945546.

Collinger, J. L., Boninger, M. L., Koontz, A. M., et al. (2008). Shoulder biomechanics during the push phase of wheelchair propulsion: A multisite study of persons with paraplegia. *Archives of Physical Medicine & Rehabilitation, 89*, 667–676.

Conger, S. A., & Bassett, J. D. R. (2011). A compendium of energy costs of physical activities for individuals who use manual wheelchairs. *Adapted Physical Activity Quarterly, 28*, 310–325.

Cooper, R. A., Cooper, R., & Boninger, M. L. (2008). Trends and issues in wheelchair technologies. *Assistive Technology, 20*, 61–72.

Cooper, R. A., Ferretti, E., Oyster, M., Kelleher, A., & Cooper, R. (2011). The relationship between wheelchair mobility patterns and community participation among individuals with spinal cord injury. *Assistive Technology, 23*, 177–183.

Costigan, F. A., & Light, J. (2011). Functional seating for school-age children with cerebral palsy: An evidence-based tutorial. *Language, Speech & Hearing Services in Schools, 42*, 223–236.

Cowan, R. E., Nash, M. S., De Groot, S., & Van Der Woude, L. H. (2011). Adapted manual wheelchair circuit: Test-retest reliability and discriminative validity in persons with spinal cord injury. *Archives of Physical Medicine & Rehabilitation, 92*, 1270–1280.

Cox, D. L. (2003). Wheelchair needs for children and young people: A review. *British Journal of Occupational Therapy, 66*, 219–223.

Crane, B. A., Holm, M. B., Hobson, D., Cooper, R. A., & Reed, M. P. (2007). Responsiveness of the TAWC tool for assessing wheelchair discomfort. *Disability and Rehabilitation Assistive Technology, 2*, 97–103.

Crawford, S. A., Stinson, M. D., Walsh, D. M., & Porter-Armstrong, A. P. (2005). Impact of sitting time on seat-interface pressure and on pressure mapping with multiple sclerosis patients. *Archives of Physical Medicine and Rehabilitation, 86*, 1221–1225.

Creek, J. (2003). *Occupational therapy defined as a complex intervention.* London: College of Occupational Therapists.

Curtis, K. A., Roach, K. E., Applegate, E. B., et al. (1995a). Development of the Wheelchair User's Shoulder Pain Index (WUSPI). *Paraplegia, 33*, 290–293.

Curtis, K. A., Roach, K. E., Applegate, E. B., et al. (1995b). Reliability and validity of the Wheelchair User's Shoulder Pain Index (WUSPI). *Paraplegia, 33*, 595–601.

Cushman, L. A., & Scherer, M. J. (1996). Measuring the relationship of assistive technology use, functional status over time, and consumer-therapist perceptions of ATs. *Assistive Technology, 8*, 103–109.

Davies, A., De Souza, L. H., & Frank, A. O. (2003). Changes in the quality of life in severely disabled people following provision of powered indoor/outdoor chairs. *Disability & Rehabilitation, 25*, 286–290.

Davin, D. K. (2015). Pressure mapping for wheelchair users. *Exceptional Parent, 45*, 32–34.

Davin, K. N. (2013). Pressure mapping reveals the complete picture for seating and positioning solutions. *Rehabilitation Management: The Interdisciplinary Journal of Rehabilitation, 26*, 8–15.

De Laat, E. H., Scholte, O. P., Reimer, W. J., & Van Achterberg, T. (2005). Pressure ulcers: Diagnostics and interventions aimed at wound-related complaints: A review of the literature. *Journal of Clinical Nursing, 14*, 464–472.

Demers, L., Weiss-Lambrou, R., & Ska, B. (1996). Development of the Quebec User Evaluation of Satisfaction with Assistive Technology (QUEST). *Assistive Technology, 8*, 3–13.

Demers, L., Weiss-Lambrou, R., & Ska, B. (2000). Item analysis of the Quebec User Evaluation of Satisfaction with Assistive Technology (QUEST). *Assistive Technology, 12*, 96–105.

Estes, J. P., Bochenek, C., & Fasler, P. (2000). Osteoarthritis of the fingers. *Journal of Hand Therapy, 13*, 108–123.

Farley, R., Clark, J., Davidson, C., et al. (2003). What is the evidence for the effectiveness of postural management?… including commentary by Roxborough L. *International Journal of Therapy & Rehabilitation, 10*, 449–455.

Field, D. A., & Roxborough, L. A. (2011). Responsiveness of the seated postural control measure and the level of sitting scale in children with neuromotor disorders. *Disability & Rehabilitation: Assistive Technology, 6*, 473–482.

Fife, S. E., Roxborough, L. A., Armstrong, R. W., Harris, S. R., Gregson, J. L., & Field, D. (1991). Development of a clinical measure of postural control for assessment of adaptive seating in children with neuromotor disabilities. *Physical Therapy, 71*, 981–993.

Fliess-Douer, O., Vanlandewijck, Y. C., Lubel Manor, G., & Van Der Woude, L. H. V. (2010). A systematic review of wheelchair skills tests for manual wheelchair users with a spinal cord injury: Towards a standardized outcome measure. *Clinical Rehabilitation, 24*, 867–886.

Fradet, L., John, T., Mcgrath, M., Murray, E., Braatz, F., & Wolf, S. I. (2011). The use of pressure mapping for seating posture characterisation in children with cerebral palsy. *Disability & Rehabilitation: Assistive Technology, 6*, 47–56.

Frank, A. O., De Souza, L. H., Frank, J. L., & Neophytou, C. (2012). The pain experiences of powered wheelchair users. *Disability & Rehabilitation, 34*, 770–778.

Fuhrer, M. J., Jutai, J. W., Scherer, M. J., & Deruyter, F. (2003). A framework for the conceptual modelling of assistive technology device outcomes. *Disability & Rehabilitation*, 25, 1243–1251.

Gagnon, B., Noreau, L., & Vincent, C. (2005a). Reliability of the seated postural control measure for adult wheelchair users. *Disability & Rehabilitation*, 27, 1479–1491.

Gagnon, B., Vincent, C., & Noreau, L. (2005b). Adaptation of a seated postural control measure for adult wheelchair users. *Disability & Rehabilitation*, 27, 951–959.

Gendle, S. C., Richardson, M., Leeper, J., Hardin, L. B., Green, J. M., & Bishop, P. A. (2012). Wheelchair-mounted accelerometers for measurement of physical activity. *Disability & Rehabilitation: Assistive Technology*, 7, 139–148.

Gibson, J., & Frank, A. (2005). Pain experienced by electric-powered chair users: A pilot exploration using pain drawings. *Physiotherapy Research International*, 10, 110–115.

Giesbrecht, E. M., Mortenson, W. B., & Miller, W. C. (2012). Prevalence and facility level correlates of need for wheelchair seating assessment among long-term care residents. *Gerontology*, 58, 378–384.

Giesbrecht, E. M., Ripat, J. D., Cooper, J. E., & Quanbury, A. O. (2011). Experiences with using a pushrim-activated power-assisted wheelchair for community-based occupations: A qualitative exploration. *Canadian Journal of Occupational Therapy*, 78, 127–136.

Hasdai, A., Jessel, A. S., & Weiss, P. L. (1998). Use of a computer simulator for training children with disabilities in the operation of a powered wheelchair. *American Journal of Occupational Therapy*, 52, 215–220.

Hjelle, K. M., & Vik, K. (2011). The ups and downs of social participation: Experiences of wheelchair users in Norway. *Disability & Rehabilitation*, 33, 2479–2489.

Hocking, C. (1999). Function or feelings: Factors in abandonment of assistive devices. *Technology and Disability*, 11.

Hoenig, H., Landerman, L. R., Shipp, K. M., & George, L. (2003). Activity restriction among wheelchair users. *Journal of the American Geriatrics Society*, 51, 1244–1251.

Hunt, P. C. (2005). *Factors associated with wheelchair use and the impact on quality of life among individuals with spinal cord injury*. Doctoral dissertation: University of Pittsburgh.

Huo, X. (2011). *Tongue drive: A wireless tongue-operated assistive technology for people with severe disabilities*. Georgia Institute of Technology: Doctoral dissertation.

Hutzler, Y., Chacham-Guber, A., & Reiter, S. (2013). Psychosocial development of participants with disabilities throughout a reverse-integrated wheelchair basketball program. *Palaestra*, 27, 33–36.

Jelier, P., & Turner-Smith, A. (1997). Review of wheelchair services in England. *British Journal of Occupational Therapy*, 60, 150–155.

Jones, D. A., & Rader, J. (2015). Seating and wheeled mobility for older adults living in nursing homes. *Topics in Geriatric Rehabilitation*, 31, 10–18.

Kaye, S., Kang, T., & Laplante, M. P. (2002). Wheelchair use in the United States. *Disability Statistics Abstract*, 23, 1–4.

Kotsch, L. (2003). Wheelchair provision to the young disabled [correspondence]. *International Journal of Therapy and Rehabilitation*, 10, 285.

Law, M., Cooper, B. A., Strong, S., Stewart, D., Rigby, P., & Letts, L. (1996). The Person-Environment-Occupational Model: A transactive approach to occupational performance. *Canadian Journal of Occupational Therapy*, 63, 9–23.

Linden, M. A., Whyatt, C., Craig, C., & Kerr, C. (2013). Efficacy of a powered wheelchair simulator for school aged children: A randomized controlled trial. *Rehabilitation Psychology*, 58, 405–411.

Liu, H.-Y., Cooper, R., Kelleher, A., & Cooper, R. A. (2014). An interview study for developing a user guide for powered seating function usage. *Disability & Rehabilitation: Assistive Technology*, 9, 499–512.

Löfqvist, C., Pettersson, C., Iwarsson, S., & Brandt, A. (2012). Mobility and mobility-related participation outcomes of powered wheelchair and scooter interventions after 4-months and 1-year use. *Disability & Rehabilitation: Assistive Technology*, 7, 211–218.

Mahajan, H. P. (2012). *Development and validation of simulators for power wheelchair driving evaluations*. Doctoral dissertation: University of Pittsburgh.

Mahajan, H. P., Dicianno, B. E., Cooper, R. A., & Ding, D. (2013). Assessment of wheelchair driving performance in a virtual reality-based simulator. *Journal of Spinal Cord Medicine*, 36, 322–332.

Majd, M. E., Muldowny, D. S., & Holt, R. T. (1997). Natural history of scoliosis in spastic cerebral palsy. *Spine*, 22, 1461–1466.

Mcclure, L. A., Boninger, M. L., Ozawa, H., & Koontz, A. (2011). Reliability and validity analysis of the transfer assessment instrument. *Archives of Physical Medicine & Rehabilitation*, 92, 499–508.

McDonald, R., Surtees, R., & Wirz, S. (2004). The International Classification of Functioning, Disability and Health provides a model for adaptive seating interventions for children with cerebral palsy. *British Journal of Occupational Therapy*, 67, 293–302.

Mcdonald, R. L., Wilson, G. N., Molloy, A., & Franck, L. S. (2011). Feasibility of three electronic instruments in studying the benefits of adaptive seating. *Disability & Rehabilitation: Assistive Technology*, 6, 483–490.

Metring, N. L., Gaspar, M. I. F. A. S., Mateus-Vasconcelos, E. C. L., Gomes, M. M., & De Abreu, D. C. C. (2012). Influence of different types of seat cushions on the static sitting posture in individuals with spinal cord injury. *Spinal Cord*, 50, 627–631.

Mills, T., Holm, M. B., Trefler, E., Schmeler, M., Fitzgerald, S., & Boninger, M. (2002). Development and consumer validation of the Functional Evaluation in a Wheelchair (FEW) instrument. *Disability and Rehabilitation*, 24, 38–46.

Mortenson, B. W., Hurd Clarke, L., & Best, K. (2013). Prescribers' experiences with powered mobility prescription among older adults. *American Journal of Occupational Therapy*, 67, 100–107.

Mortenson, W. B., Miller, W. C., Backman, C. L., & Oliffe, J. L. (2012). Association between mobility, participation, and wheelchair-related factors in long-term care residents who use wheelchairs as their primary means of mobility. *Journal of the American Geriatrics Society*, 60, 1310–1315.

Mortenson, W. B., Miller, W. C., & Miller-Pogar, J. (2007). Measuring wheelchair intervention outcomes: Development of the Wheelchair Outcome Measure. *Disability and Rehabilitation Assistive Technology*, 2, 275–285.

Mulroy, S. J., Hatchett, P., Eberly, V. J., Lighthall Haubert, L., Conners, S., & Requejo, P. S. (2015). Shoulder strength and physical activity predictors of shoulder pain in people with paraplegia from spinal injury: Prospective cohort study. *Physical Therapy, 95,* 1027–1038.

Nelson, G. G. (1997). Wheelchair seating. *Rehabilitation Management: The Interdisciplinary Journal of Rehabilitation, 10,* 34–35.

O'Connor, B., Boyd, R. N., & Shields, N. (2006). A systematic review of postural management of hip displacement in children with cerebral palsy. *Developmental Medicine & Child Neurology, 48,* 42–43.

Pain, H., Gore, S., & Mclellan, D. L. (2000). Parents' and therapists' opinion on features that make a chair useful for a young disabled child. *International Journal of Rehabilitation Research, 23,* 75–80.

Pellow, T. R. (1999). A comparison of interface pressure readings to wheelchair cushions and positioning: a pilot study. *Canadian Journal of Occupational Therapy, 66,* 140–149.

Reid, D., Laliberte-Rudman, D., & Hebert, D. (2002). Impact of wheeled seated mobility devices on adult users' and their caregivers' occupational performance: A critical literature review. *Canadian Journal of Occupational Therapy – Revue Canadienne d Ergotherapie, 69,* 261–280.

Requejo, P. S., Furumasu, J., & Mulroy, S. J. (2015). Evidence-based strategies for preserving mobility for elderly and aging manual wheelchair users. *Topics in Geriatric Rehabilitation, 31,* 26–41.

Rice, I. M., Jayaraman, C., Hsiao-Wecksler, E. T., & Sosnoff, J. J. (2014). Relationship between shoulder pain and kinetic and temporal-spatial variability in wheelchair users. *Archives of Physical Medicine & Rehabilitation, 95,* 699–704.

Ripat, J. D., Brown, C. L., & Ethans, K. D. (2015). Barriers to wheelchair use in the winter. *Archives of Physical Medicine & Rehabilitation, 96,* 1117–1122.

Routhier, F., Desrosiers, J., Vincent, C., & Nadeau, S. (2005). Reliability and construct validity studies of an obstacle course assessment of wheelchair user performance [corrected] [published erratum appears in Int J Rehabil Res 2005;28(2):185]. *International Journal of Rehabilitation Research, 28,* 49–56.

Routhier, F., Vincent, C., Desrosiers, J., & Nadeau, S. (2003). Mobility of wheelchair users: A proposed performance assessment framework. *Disability and Rehabilitation, 25,* 19–34.

Routhier, F., Vincent, C., Desrosiers, J., Nadeau, S., & Guerette, C. (2004). Development of an obstacle course assessment of wheelchair user performance (OCAWUP): A content validity study. *Technology and Disability, 16,* 19–31.

Rudman, D. L., Hebert, D., & Reid, D. (2006). Living in a restricted occupational world: The occupational experiences of stroke survivors who are wheelchair users and their caregivers. *Canadian Journal of Occupational Therapy, 73,* 141–152.

Rushton, P. W., Kairy, D., Archambault, P. S., et al. (2015). The potential impact of intelligent power wheelchair use on social participation: Perspectives of users, caregivers and clinicians. *Disability and Rehabilitation Assistive Technology, 10,* 191–197.

Rushton, P. W., Kirby, R. L., & Miller, W. C. (2012). Manual wheelchair skills: Objective testing versus subjective questionnaire. *Archives of Physical Medicine & Rehabilitation, 93,* 2313–2318.

Ryan, S., Campbell, K. A., Rigby, P., Germon, B., Chan, B., & Hubley, D. (2006). Development of the new family impact of assistive technology scale. *International Journal of Rehabilitation Research, 29,* 195–200.

Sadani, S., Jones, C., Seal, A., Bhakta, B., Hall, R., & Levesley, M. (2012). A pilot study of scoliosis assessment using radiation free surface topography in children with GMFCS IV and V cerebral palsy. *Child: Care, Health & Development, 38,* 854–862.

Sakakibara, B. M., Miller, W. C., Routhier, F., Backman, C. L., & Eng, J. J. (2014). Association between self-efficacy and participation in community-dwelling manual wheelchair users aged 50 years or older. *Physical Therapy, 94,* 664–674.

Sanderson, D., Place, M., & Wright, D. (2000). *Evaluation of the powered wheelchair and voucher scheme initiatives.* York: York Health Economics Consortium, Department of Health.

Sawatzky, B., Digivine, C., Berner, T., Roesler, T., & Katte, L. (2015a). The need for updated clinical practice guidelines for preservation of upper extremities in manual wheelchair users. *American Journal of Physical Medicine & Rehabilitation, 94,* 313–324.

Sawatzky, B., Hers, N., & Macgillivray, M. K. (2015b). Relationships between wheeling parameters and wheelchair skills in adults and children with SCI. *Spinal Cord, 53,* 561–564.

Shipperley, T. F., & Collins, F. (1999). A seating assessment tool for community use. *Journal of Wound Care, 8,* 119–120.

Sprigle, S. (2007a). Research priorities: Seating and positioning. *Disability and Rehabilitation Assistive Technology, 2,* 181–187.

Sprigle, S. (2007b). State of the science on wheeled mobility and seating measuring the health, activity and participation of wheelchair users. *Disability and Rehabilitation Assistive Technology, 2,* 133–135.

Stinson, M. D., Porter-Armstrong, A., & Eakin, P. (2003). Seat-interface pressure: A pilot study of the relationship to gender, body mass index, and seating position. *Archives of Physical Medicine and Rehabilitation, 84,* 405–409.

Taylor, S., Gassaway, J., Heisler-Varriale, L. A., et al. (2015). Patterns in wheeled mobility skills training, equipment evaluation, and utilization: Findings from the SCIRehab Project. *Assistive Technology, 27,* 59–68.

Torkia, C., Reid, D., Korner-Bitensky, N., et al. (2015). Power wheelchair driving challenges in the community: A users' perspective. *Disability and Rehabilitation Assistive Technology, 10,* 211–215.

Townsend, E., & Polatajko, H. (2007). *Enabling occupation II: Advancing an occupational therapy vision for health, well-being & justice through occupation.* Ottawa: CAOT Publications ACE.

Wei Pin, H., Chia Cheng, W., Jo Hua, H., et al. (2015). Joystick-controlled video console game practice for developing power wheelchairs users' indoor driving skills. *Journal of Physical Therapy Science, 27,* 495–498.

White, E. (1999). Wheelchair special seating: Need and provision. *British Journal of Therapy & Rehabilitation, 6,* 285–286.

World Health Organization. (2001). *International classification of functioning, disability and health.* Geneva: World Health Organization.

Yang, W., Wilson, L., Oda, I., & Yan, J. (2007). The effect of providing power mobility on body weight change. *American Journal of Physical Medicine & Rehabilitation, 86,* 746–753.

Yanni, C., Jue, W., Chi-Wen, L., Yang, T. D., Crane, B. A., & Yih-Kuen, J. (2014). Effect of tilt and recline on ischial and coccygeal interface pressures in people with spinal cord injury. *American Journal of Physical Medicine & Rehabilitation, 95,* 1019–1030.

Yildirim, N. U., Comert, E., & Ozengin, N. (2010). Shoulder pain: A comparison of wheelchair basketball players with trunk control and without trunk control. *Journal of Back & Musculoskeletal Rehabilitation, 23,* 55–61.

Zukowski, L. A., Roper, J. A., Shechtman, O., Otzel, D. M., Hovis, P. W., & Tillman, M. D. (2014). Wheelchair ergonomic hand drive mechanism use improves wrist mechanics associated with carpal tunnel syndrome. *Journal of Rehabilitation Research & Development, 51,* 1515–1523.

Zwinkels, M., Verschuren, O., Janssen, T. W. J., Ketelaar, M., & Takken, T. (2014). Exercise training programs to improve hand rim wheelchair propulsion capacity: A systematic review. *Clinical Rehabilitation, 28,* 847–861.

48

DRIVING AND COMMUNITY MOBILITY

MARILYN DI STEFANO

CHAPTER OUTLINE

Abstract

The ability to drive plays an important part in the life roles of many people in industrially developed countries, because it is often the preferred means of maintaining good community mobility. Driving-related issues can therefore be very important for occupational therapists to address, because one goal of occupational therapy is to improve the occupational engagement of the people with whom they work. Driving a motor vehicle is an activity of daily living that requires a combination of sensory, perceptual/cognitive and motor abilities, which together enable a driver to develop the skills necessary to manoeuvre and navigate a vehicle through complex, dynamic environments. Occupational therapists working in a number of areas of practice have responsibility for identifying and educating individuals about the potential impact of sensory, perceptual/cognitive and motor limitations on their driving and community mobility. Many also provide education, resources and training related to alternative community mobility. Specialised individual assessments

and interventions that are more specific to driving are usually the domain of occupational therapists who have completed recognised postgraduate training in driver assessment and rehabilitation. Such professionals are referred to in this chapter as *occupational therapy driving specialists*. Some of the main theoretical and empirically based foundations of occupational therapy practice in these areas are described in this chapter, along with an outline of the limitations most likely to affect driving and community mobility, the content and general procedures involved in driver assessments and associated rehabilitation approaches.

KEY POINTS

- Driving is a common occupation in industrially developed countries.

- The maintenance of independent driving or community mobility is important to support participation, socialisation and other forms of community engagement.

- A range of health, impairment and age-related factors may affect safe driving and mobility.

- Occupational therapists play an important role in supporting individuals to maintain independence in these domains, and they assess and provide interventions related to community mobility.

- Occupational therapists educate and inform drivers about the impact of sensory, perceptual/cognitive and motor impairment on driving.

- Occupational therapy driving specialists have a specific role in evaluating driver-related skills and devising customised rehabilitation programmes.

- There are many ways that drivers with limitations can be assisted to obtain or maintain their driving independence.

- Vehicle adaptations and modifications support drivers with physical impairment to access, sit within and safely operate motor vehicles, thus optimising driving independence.

INTRODUCTION

In many industrialised societies with sprawling urban populations and poor transport infrastructure, increasing numbers of people are dependent on the car for transportation. In regions where there are very limited public or community transport options, or where long travel distances are involved, this reliance on personal vehicular modes of transport can create major problems for those unable to drive (Chihuri et al., 2015). For these reasons driving an automobile is an important and valued occupation, especially for individuals with impairment (Norweg, Jette, Houlihan, Ni, & Boninger, 2011; Tsai, Graves, & Lai, 2014).

Research on people's driving abilities in relation to their transport needs has focused largely on older drivers, most of whom have been driving regularly throughout their adult lives and expect to continue doing so indefinitely (Oxley & Whelan, 2008). There are various reasons why people's ability to drive safely may deteriorate significantly as they age – particularly beyond 75 years of age. However, people often do not plan for the time when they may need to reduce their driving or perhaps cease driving altogether (Liddle et al., 2014). In addition, various health- and impairment-related causes of disruption to driving abilities may affect drivers across the lifespan (Charlton et al., 2010)

In this context, occupational therapists can play several important roles. They may have an educational role in explaining the impact of impairment on driving abilities and in explaining drivers' obligations within the relevant driver licensing jurisdiction. They may be required to develop remediation programmes to help people who have an illness, injury or impairment regain performance skills related to driving and

to facilitate and promote community mobility among those unable to drive. Importantly, they can refer to and explain the role of occupational therapy driving specialists and possible driver rehabilitation interventions, funding options and licence conditions. The occupational therapy driving specialists are responsible for assessing the driving-related abilities and driving performance of individual drivers as well as implementing interventions such as prescribing vehicle modifications and developing retraining programmes.

In pursuing these objectives, occupational therapists have multiple responsibilities – both to the individuals with whom they work and to the wider community. At an individual level, driving can be centrally important in maintaining a person's community mobility. At a societal level, drivers with some types of perceptual or cognitive impairments and certain health conditions can threaten both their own safety and that of others as a result of their increased risk of road accident involvement (Charlton et al., 2010; Rudin-Brown & Jamson, 2013).

DRIVING, COMMUNITY MOBILITY AND HEALTH

Community mobility refers to the extent to which people are able to travel within their community in accord with their needs and preferences. This can be accomplished by walking; by using human-powered devices such as bicycles or manual wheelchairs, or electric-powered versions of such devices; by using public or community-based transportation systems (e.g. buses, taxis, trains); or by catching a ride with family or friends. But for many people often the preferred option is to independently drive a car (Macdonald, Pellerito, & Di Stefano, 2006).

Coughlin (2001, p. v) highlighted the importance of transportation options to community mobility and the quality of people's lives:

[Community] mobility, the ability to travel from point A to point B when and how one chooses, is the means by which individuals maintain their connection to society. Transportation has been described as the 'glue' that holds together all the activities that we call life. Ready access to family, friends, social activities, health care, and goods and services are vital to full participation in daily life.

Many drivers see their ability to drive as centrally important to their well-being. Evidence supports the reality of this view in cases where loss of a driver's licence has reduced the individual's community mobility and contributed to increased incidence of illnesses, such as depression (Chihuri et al., 2015; Mann, 2011).

When people become unable to drive as a result of health problems, it might be thought that they should then start to walk rather than drive, or use other options such as public or community-based transport to travel longer distances. However, for older individuals, many of the most common chronic

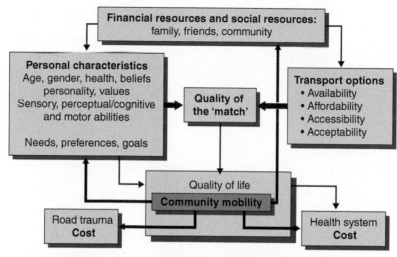

FIG. 48.1 ■ Determinants of community mobility.

deteriorating health conditions and age-related impairments may have a greater effect on *personal* mobility (i.e. their ability to walk around) than on driving performance (Whelan, Langford, Oxley, Koppel, & Charlton, 2006). This means that for many older people, driving may be the most effective and sometimes the only means by which they can participate in activities outside their own homes, whether to perform essential tasks, such as shopping and visiting doctors, or to participate in social or recreational activities.

Regardless of the particular transport mode, the primary determinant of community mobility is the quality of the match between an individual's personal characteristics and transport options. As shown in Fig. 48.1, both sides of this equation are influenced by the individual's own resources – both financial and social.* Among the personal characteristics shown here, sensory, perceptual/cognitive and motor abilities are the most directly relevant, particularly if driving is the preferred transport option, because of the increased risk of road accidents if these abilities are inadequate. Some of the other personal characteristics, particularly driver age and a range of medical conditions, have been found to influence a person's abilities (Charlton et al., 2010; Dobbs, 2005).

*Fig. 48.1 is based on the premise – drawn from the field of human factors psychology or ergonomics – that adequacy of system functioning is dependent on the 'goodness of fit' between individual characteristics (including physical, cognitive and psychomotor capacities, personal needs and preferences) and the demands and other characteristics of the activities they wish to undertake (e.g. see Oborne, 1982; Sanders & McCormick, 1993). It is also consistent with Ecological Systems Theory as formulated by Bronfenbrenner (1979, 1989); and with European research on community mobility in relation to older people's quality of life (e.g. Mollenkopf, 2003).

The potential effects of these factors on community mobility and more general quality of life, which in turn have consequences for health, for road crash risk, and for the costs associated with both, are also illustrated in Fig. 48.1. This conceptualisation is consistent with the models of human occupation or activity engagement that have been developed to guide occupational therapy professional practice, a defining characteristic of which is the person-centred approach to service delivery. Such models are helpful in promoting understanding of the wide range of factors that influence driving and mobility engagement. The Model of Human Occupation (Kielhofner, 2002), the Person–Environment–Occupation model (Law et al., 1996), the Occupational Adaptation Model (Schultz & Schkade, 2003) and the Canadian Model of Occupational Performance and Engagement (Townsend & Polatajko, 2007) all identify relationships among human, task, social and environmental factors that change over the lifespan and affect successful performance in a particular situation. The Ecology of Human Performance Framework (Dunn, McClain, Brown, & Youngstrom, 1998), which is an interdisciplinary model that shares some of the aforementioned characteristics, has also been applied to driver assessment and rehabilitation (Stav, Justiss, Belchior, & Lanford, 2006b).

Balancing Road Safety and an Individual's Mobility Needs

For occupational therapists working with drivers, a centrally important issue is the need to maintain a person's community mobility while at the same time maintaining road safety. This refers not only to the safety of the driver but also the safety of passengers, along with other drivers and users of the road traffic system, including pedestrians and cyclists.

For many people, driving a vehicle in ordinary traffic is among the most hazardous activities routinely undertaken.

The risk of death or serious injury as a result of road crashes is particularly high for drivers who are either very young or very old. The underlying reasons for these differences in crash risk are complex (e.g. see Braver & Trempel, 2004; Keall & Frith, 2004). Self-regulation is one method by which drivers of any age with insight into their limitations may reduce their driving exposure. For example, such drivers might limit driving at night, during peak traffic hours or in inclement weather. However, recent research has highlighted that self-regulation cannot necessarily be assumed. For example, although older driver self-rated driving performance is usually high (good/excellent), it is not necessarily predictive of driving safety (e.g. as measured by citations and crashes). This raises the possibility that insight and self-regulation may be limited in some drivers (Ross, Dodson, Edwards, Ackerman, & Ball, 2012), highlighting the reason why families may take extreme measures to report unfit drivers to the licensing authority (Meuser, Carr, Unger, & Ulfarsson, 2015).

Older drivers are also more likely than young ones to sustain the kind of illness-related impairments that commonly result in driving cessation. Apart from specific diagnosed illnesses, the more general aging process also leads eventually to impairments and limitations (e.g. vision decrements, slower cognitive processing) that are likely to increase crash risk substantially, as outlined later. This situation contrasts with that of *young* drivers, who are most likely to require the services of occupational therapy driving specialists because of congenital impairments or impairments resulting from accidents (including road crashes), such as acquired brain injuries or spinal injuries.

People presenting to occupational therapy driving specialists for driver evaluations may have a variety of diagnoses and comorbidities, including stroke, closed head injuries, spinal/multiple injuries, dementia and neurological conditions (Korner-Bitensky, Bitensky, Sofer, Man-Son-Hing, & Gelinas, 2006; Lovell & Russell, 2005). Across all age ranges, the following health conditions have been identified by researchers as associated with a substantial increase in crash risk: dementia, epilepsy, multiple sclerosis, psychiatric disorders (grouped into one category), sleep apnoea, alcohol abuse, and cataracts (Charlton et al., 2010).

The driving performance of people with dementia has been a particular focus of research because the condition can develop quite rapidly and affected drivers may not be able to perceive and take account of decrements in their driving performance (Bradshaw, Di Stefano, & Catchpole, 2013; Breen, Breen, Moore, Breen, & O'Neill, 2007). In light of the aging populations in many countries, such issues have been widely discussed at both national and international levels (e.g. Organisation for Economic Co-operative Development, 2001; SafetyNet, 2009; U.S. Department of Transportation, 2003, 2004).

Occupational therapists have considerable scope to help people develop and implement strategies to maintain reasonably good community mobility while reducing their exposure to mobility-related accident risks. For example, better forward planning might lead to less frequent driving trips; or trips might be better planned to avoid high-risk situations such as driving at night, or in heavy or high-speed traffic, or when visibility is poor because of the weather. Apart from driving, potential means of maintaining community mobility for those without major cognitive-perceptual or musculoskeletal difficulties may include use of public transport, motorised devices such as scooters or use of a bicycle or tricycle. The remainder of this chapter focuses predominantly on driving as the preferred community mobility option.

Reporting of Health- and Impairment-related Conditions That May Impair Driving

In some jurisdictions, health professionals, including doctors and occupational therapists, have legal obligations to report some types of health- and impairment-related conditions, including, for example, dementia, major visual field loss and cognitive/perceptual impairments.* It is therefore important for both generalist occupational therapists and those with specialist training in driver assessment to familiarise themselves with the licensing and medicolegal frameworks within which they practice. Guidelines for medical and health professionals are readily available on the Internet – see, for example, those produced by the American, Australian, British and Canadian transport or medical/health associations (American Medical Association & National Highway Traffic Safety Administration, 2010; Austroads, 2016; Canadian Medical Association, 2012; Department of Transport, U.K., 2014).

Although these documents provide some guidance, their usefulness is limited by wide variability in the type and severity of impairments that are associated with many medical diagnoses. Consequently, such guidelines are necessarily worded in quite general terms, and diagnosis of a specific medical condition, per se, is in reality likely to be a weak indicator of the quality of an individual's current driving performance (Di Stefano & Macdonald, 2003a). To support the effective identification of those individuals whose driving is likely to present a substantial road crash risk, it is therefore very important for occupational therapists to be able to assess the quality of the match between each individual's sensory, perceptual/cognitive and motor abilities and the safe accessibility of driving as a transport option for that individual (see Fig. 48.1).

Driving as an Information Processing Task

The safe accessibility of driving is determined by the demands that drivers have to cope with as they perform the task of driving a vehicle within the road traffic system. Driving requires some physical abilities, such as adequate strength and range of motion of limbs required to move operational controls. However, it is sensory, perceptual and cognitive functioning that are most important in enabling drivers to predict and manage

---

*Apart from the reporting obligations of professionals, drivers may have self-reporting obligations.

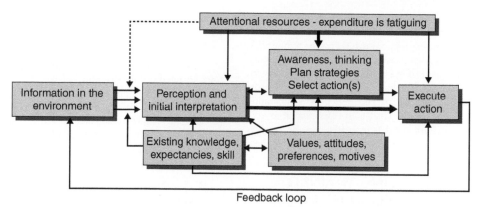

FIG. 48.2 ■ A generic depiction of how people 'process' information during activities such as driving. *(From Macdonald, W. (2004). Human error: Causes and countermeasures. In Proceedings of the Safety in Action Conference 2004. Safety Institute of Australia, Victorian Division.)*

safety-critical demands. To understand more about perceptual and cognitive abilities, it is helpful to view driving as an 'information processing' task, as shown in Fig. 48.2. The relationships between human information processing capacities and limitations with interacting system characteristics have been well documented in the literature (e.g. see seminal references like Proctor & Van Zandt, 1994; and Wickens & Hollands, 2000).

Fig. 48.2 shows information from the environment (on the left) impinging on the driver's sensory organs, with some of this being registered in sensory stores, where it is very briefly retained. In the case of driving, *visual* information is clearly the most important type of sensory input, which means that effective visual sensory functioning is an important requirement for competent driving performance. It should be noted that *dynamic* visual acuity may be more important than the *static* acuity that is more routinely tested. Only a subset of the information registered in sensory stores progresses further into the system to be 'perceived'. Perception is the point where some initial interpretation occurs, based on the driver's preexisting knowledge and skills, and influenced also by attitudes and motivational factors. This perceptual stage is critical for road safety because it both sustains the driver's awareness of road and traffic conditions and provides the basis for cognitive predictions of the immediate future road traffic situations to enable appropriate vehicle control actions and more general 'situation awareness' (Bolstad & Hess, 2000).

Only a subset of *perceived* information goes on to the central, *cognitive* stage of processing, which is when the driver becomes fully aware or conscious of it. Processing of information at this stage requires the allocation of attentional resources, and because these resources are in limited supply, this is where humans' information processing capacity is at its most limited. Associated with this, there is a maximum rate at which humans can process information. This limitation can result in drivers sometimes being at risk of information overload. It also makes

it important that drivers allocate their available attentional resources optimally across different aspects of the task.

Some aspects of cognitive performance typically decline with old age: attentional limitations have been identified as particularly important (Riddle, 2007). Also, suboptimal *allocation* of available attentional resources becomes an increasingly common problem among the oldest drivers (Brayne et al., 1999, 2000). As noted earlier, research has found that it is perceptual and cognitive impairments rather than purely physical ones that are significantly linked to higher crash risk (Charlton et al., 2010). Attentional issues may also be of concern with younger individuals who are cognitively compromised (e.g. those with congenital brain impairment, rapidly progressive neurological conditions or acquired brain injury).

Older people usually have the advantage of being highly experienced drivers. This means that when they are driving in familiar surroundings, a substantial part of the incoming information can be processed in an automatic, or partially automatic, fashion, indicated by the large arrow in Fig. 48.2 connecting 'Perception and Initial Interpretation' directly to 'Execute Action'. Importantly, this arrow bypasses conscious awareness, which is the stage most demanding of attentional resources. Very experienced drivers are therefore able to cope with completely routine aspects of the driving task within highly familiar road environments without there being heavy demands on their attentional resources – for example, to undertake steering, accelerator and brake operations, smooth speed control and appropriate vehicle lane positioning.

Regardless of age, the process of learning to drive (for young, cognitively compromised individuals) or relearning to drive (for more experienced drivers after a major injury or illness) may place high demands on available attentional resources, because some of the required actions or performance strategies may not have been encountered or will probably be different from those previously learned. Also, it is important to remember that even in very familiar environments there is always the possibility of unexpected events to which drivers need to be able to respond quickly. Even the most experienced drivers can be temporarily overloaded by very sudden increases in driving task demands.

Furthermore, aspects of the information processing system can be affected by diseases, symptoms of conditions or treatments (e.g. medication side effects, persistent pain or fluctuating arousal levels) (Lococo & Staplin, 2006). Therefore it is very important that a person's status is evaluated and the person's 'readiness' for driver assessment and rehabilitation is established.

ROLE OF NONDRIVING TRAINED OCCUPATIONAL THERAPIST IN RELATION TO DRIVING

All occupational therapists, whether they are generalists or specialist driver assessors, need to have a good understanding of the issues outlined earlier. For generalists, this is necessary because they routinely address a wide variety of issues with people and their families, including self-care, education, work, leisure and social participation (Redepenning, 2006). In many of these contexts, driving and community mobility issues may be important considerations.

The usual starting point for both generalist and specialist occupational therapists is to identify those people who may present an unacceptable crash risk as a driver and, independent of effects on crash risk, to identify whether they are likely to experience difficulties when driving. This is a complex process, and as yet there is no single battery of validated assessments or tests suitable for all health conditions to support definitive decision making, which could replace on-road assessments. Researchers continue to explore alternatives to on-road testing such as computer-based simulators (Classen & Brooks, 2014). However, current evaluation protocols for specific diagnostic groups (e.g. stroke, dementia) are based on literature reviews or are opinion-based, such as consensus statements (e.g. Iverson et al., 2010; Molnar, Byszewski, Marshall, & Man-Son-Hing, 2005).

The use of impairment-related 'red flags' is emerging as a potentially useful screening approach. One simple tool that has acceptable face validity based on a literature review (its empirical validity requires investigation) is the SAFEDRIVE checklist (Wiseman & Souder, 1996). This tool is used by medical and allied health personnel to identify whether an individual's history or presenting signs and symptoms are indicative of the need to investigate driving-related abilities. The acronym refers to the following assessment cues:

S – safety record and history of crashes
A – attention deficits and skills
F – family report a history of driving-related problems
E – history of ethanol use
D – drug and/or medication use
R – reaction time–related limitations associated with neurological or musculoskeletal problems

I – intellectual impairment
V – vision-related problems
E– executive cognition limitations or concerns

Factors affecting driving or community mobility may be identified in referral documentation or emerge from occupational therapy assessment procedures that are routinely conducted when working with a range of individuals. Concerns may also be raised by family or significant others. Various assessment checklists, including the SAFEDRIVE mentioned earlier, may trigger the need for further investigations. In such cases, the generalist occupational therapist's role may encompass the following:

■ Identification of individuals who may not meet driver medical/licensing guidelines and who may require referral for medical assessment and specialist occupational therapy or mobility centre driver evaluation.
■ Occupational profile analysis to highlight the significance of independent driving and mobility in relation to life roles and goals.
■ Occupational performance evaluation to identify specific gaps in performance abilities that also affect driving performance.
■ Remediation or compensation-related interventions aimed at improving abilities to enable driver or mobility rehabilitation.
■ Education interventions for individuals and significant others regarding driving and community mobility.
■ Advocacy interventions such as seeking funding for driver/mobility assessment and rehabilitation, vehicle modifications or mobility aides.

In addition, there is a more general need to assess the level of driver insight. Individuals demonstrating a lack of insight into major decrements may be a risk to their own or the public's safety when driving, especially in relicensing systems that place the onus only on the individual to report their health or impairment status.

OCCUPATIONAL THERAPY DRIVING SPECIALIST: ASSESSMENT AND INTERVENTION

The Practice Context

Occupational therapists specialising in driver assessment and rehabilitation rarely work *only* in this field. Typically, they also provide services for a range of other people, depending on the context of their practice. Such practice contexts include private practice, rehabilitation units (e.g. for people who have had a stroke, spinal cord or acquired brain injury), geriatric assessment facilities, mental health units, and community health centres or within 'mobility centres' that specialise in driver assessment and community mobility (Brooks & Hawley, 2005).

In these various contexts, they are often part of teams (Stav, Justiss, Belchior, & Lanford, 2006b). Team members usually include family members or caregivers, medical practitioners, other treating health practitioners (including generalist occupational therapists, physiotherapists, optometrists, orthotists), case managers, driving instructors and vehicle modifiers (Pellerito & Blanc, 2006). The size of the team will depend on the range and extent of issues faced by individual drivers. In some driver licensing jurisdictions, specialist occupational therapists may be required to register with the driver licensing authority, after having completed their specialist training, in order to offer their services (Di Stefano & Macdonald, 2006b).

Referral Systems for Specialist Mobility and Driver Assessment Services

Individuals might be referred to occupational therapy driver specialists by personnel of medical, rehabilitation, educational, vocational training or other centres; by family members; and in some driver licensing jurisdictions, by the driver licensing authority. For individuals, the first part of the referral process often involves a specific medical assessment, with the doctor completing an official report (e.g. see VicRoads, 2008).

As part of this process, people might need to complete an Informed Consent form, because privacy legislation in some jurisdictions limits the type of information about an individual that can be obtained or disseminated. Permission from the person might be required for the occupational therapist to contact the person's family members, medical practitioner, the referrer or the driver licensing authority.

Characteristics of Individuals Referred for Driver Assessment

Occupational therapy driver assessments are commonly provided for individuals with a wide range of health, impairment and aging issues that may affect their driving performance and activity participation (Table 48.1). Referrals commonly fall into the following broad categories:

1. Learners: young adults with a congenital or acquired impairment who want to know if they have the capacity to drive (e.g. those with conditions such as spina bifida and cerebral palsy or on the higher functioning end of the intellectual impairment or autism spectrum disorders)
2. Individuals who are adapting to, or *recovering* from, physical, neurological or psychosocial conditions that often indicate a need to evaluate their driving performance (e.g. those with spinal cord injury, acquired brain impairment, long-term mental health problems)
3. Individuals with a *deteriorating* chronic illness (e.g. neurological conditions such as multiple sclerosis, muscular dystrophy, dementia, Parkinson's disease)
4. *Older* members of the community whose capacity has deteriorated as a result of the aging process or a combination of other factors identified earlier.

Driving-related Assessments

There are a number of published articles or booklets describing occupational therapy–related driver assessment practices (see e.g. Di Stefano and Macdonald, 2010; Korner-Bitensky, Bitensky, Sofer, Man-Son-Hing, & Gelinas, 2006; Redepenning, 2006; Stav, 2004). The evidence base for the application of specific assessments and interventions used in occupational therapy driver assessment is increasing. At times the interpretation and general application of research findings is problematic because of heterogeneous diagnoses and the unknown baseline functional status of participants, different research methodologies, and variable outcome measures used in the studies (e.g. Kua, Korner-Bitensky, Desrosiers, Man-Son-Hing, & Marshall, 2007). A wide range of screening and assessment procedures are currently used in the assessment of older drivers specifically (see e.g. Dobbs, 2005; Kua et al., 2007; Molnar, Byszewski, Marshall, & Man-Son-Hing, 2006; Redepenning, 2006; Stav, Hunt, & Arbesman, 2006a).

The Occupational Therapy Driver Off-Road Assessment, developed by Unsworth et al. (2012), is a one off-road screening battery that can be used with people with a wide range of diagnoses. The battery includes a range of standardised assessments, has been empirically developed and has demonstrated preliminary content and predictive validity versus on-road assessment outcomes.

The point at which people present for driving evaluation during the course of their deteriorating chronic condition (e.g. Parkinson's disease, dementia) or rehabilitation after a health event (e.g. stroke, acquired brain injury) can significantly affect intervention outcomes. A general overview of the timing of referral and both components of the driver evaluation procedure is presented here.

The timing of driver assessments within the overall habilitation or rehabilitation process is determined by a number of factors, including requirements of medical fitness-to-drive guidelines; the nature and extent of a person's injuries; the acute, chronic or progressive nature of a person's medical condition; rehabilitation team concerns; and individual factors, such as age, medication intake and medication compliance, driving experience, financial status and more general motivation and behavioural issues. For example, it would be inappropriate to assess someone who has experienced a major stroke within weeks of the event if the person is likely to obtain the greatest extent of sensory, perceptual/cognitive and motor return within 3 to 6 months. Undertaking the assessment *after* the person has had sufficient time for recovery is more likely to reflect his or her longer-term abilities, an important consideration if the driver is considering expensive vehicle modifications.

In most cases, the specialist occupational therapy driver assessment procedure consists of two components: off-road screening and on-road in-car evaluation. Usually a core set of tests is used in the off-road screening to provide a consistent set of baseline measures across all individuals seen within the service (Lovell & Di Stefano, 2007). For this purpose it is preferable to use tests that are standardised and are known to have

		TABLE 48.1		
Health or Impairment Issues and How They Might Influence Driver-Related Performance				
Health/Impairment Issue: Abilities Still Compliant with Requirements of Relevant Medical Guidelines*		DRIVING PERFORMANCE		
	Planning of Driving Trip: Timing and/or Route	Contextual Factors/ Vehicle Control (e.g. Steering, Use of Accelerator or Brake Pedal)	Interacting with Traffic and Other Road Users	Participation/Life Roles, Goals and Skills for Living
Reduced upper limb movement (e.g. incoordination, pain or weakness)	Performance may be influenced by diurnal fluctuations in pain/ function. Trip length may need to be extended to cope with need for more frequent rest breaks.	Difficulties with ignition, use of steering wheel, indicators and secondary controls, slower movement time.	May experience restricted ability to steer vehicle around objects quickly or respond to situations requiring skilful, quick manoeuvring.	Difficulties with driving independence may affect ability to retain previous or attempt new paid worker roles.
Reduced or absent lower limb movement (e.g. amputation, weakness)		Difficulties with ingress/ egress, use of foot-operated pedals, seating balance.	Sustained or quick acceleration or braking may be difficult.	Reliance on aides for mobility may increase need to depend on vehicular-related mobility independence.
Minor reduction in visual acuity, visuoperceptual and/or cognitive abilities	May experience difficulties driving at night or in adverse weather or peak hour conditions. Complex or new routes may create additional undesirable mental workload over and above reserves required to compensate for impairments.	May not see, interpret or respond to important aspects of the road environment accurately; may not scan sufficiently to compensate; slower reaction time.	May not be able to attend to environmental stimuli or recall appropriate strategies fast enough to cope with driving in complex conditions with many fast-moving, unpredictable road users. Reacting to unexpected movements/actions of vehicles or road users may be difficult or inconsistent.	Difficulty with performance demands other than associated with routine daytime driving may affect life roles as parent, carer or worker. May reduce occupational engagement with leisure, family, religious or community pursuits.

*Note: Medical guidelines applicable to different countries/jurisdictions normally need to be met before drivers are eligible for licensure. Modified from Hatakka et al. (1999) and World Health Organization (2001) and assessed by occupational therapy driving specialists – see, for example, Austroads (2016); American Medical Association & National Highway Traffic Safety Administration (2010); Canadian Medical Association (2012); and Department of Transport, U.K. (2014).

good validity and reliability. Additional specific tests might be added to the battery, depending on an individual's presenting problems.

Off-road Screening

Off-road screening typically comprises the following elements:

- Review of the contents of medical or allied health reports
- Interview to obtain information regarding driving history, occupational profile, level of insight into the impact

of impairments upon driving performance, types of vehicles driven and licences held
- Recording of medication taken and any side effects
- Assessment of the following:
    - Vision (includes acuity, eye movement and coordination, visual fields, possibly contrast sensitivity)
    - Hearing
    - Other sensory abilities relevant to driving task demands (e.g. superficial sensation, proprioception, kinaesthesia)

- Physical abilities relevant to driving task demands (e.g. muscle strength, range of motion, coordination, sitting balance, mobility and transfer abilities)
- Pain, physical and mental endurance
- Knowledge about road law and driving procedures (e.g. via a written or computer-based test)
- Simple and choice reaction times (e.g. by use of a brake reaction machine of some kind)
- Some perceptual/cognitive abilities by using tests such as the Mini-Mental State Examination (Folstein, Folstein, & McHugh, 1975), Trail Making Tests (Reitan, 1985), Useful Field of View (UFOV) (Owsley et al., 1998), or other such tests as deemed appropriate
  - Observations throughout the session, to assess more general perceptual/cognitive abilities or dysfunction (e.g. aspects of memory, attention, perception, visuoperceptual, problem-solving), which may be of concern in relation to driving task demands

Off-road screening also offers the opportunity to observe and discuss the following, as appropriate:

- A person's insight into his or her limitations
- A person's emotional status and contact with reality
- Likely impact of the impairments on driving performance
- Possible vehicle adaptations that may be needed
- Nature of the on-road driving assessment
- Driving requirements in relation to work, study, family, leisure, etc.
- Impact of likely licence conditions on independence/life roles

As a result of findings from this screening procedure, the occupational therapy driving specialist may sometimes require further information about a particular area of sensory, perceptual/cognitive or motor abilities – for example, more detailed visual assessment by an ophthalmologist or an evaluation by a neuropsychologist. At times it may be appropriate for the people being assessed to await further recovery or undertake targeted rehabilitation in order to maximise his or her potential. Of particular importance is the need to ensure that the prospective driver meets minimum medical guidelines for fitness for driving, such as minimum vision requirements

(Austroads, 2016). So that evaluation is efficient and interpretations of on-road behaviour are accurate, it is important that individuals perform while at their optimum (e.g. with vision corrected reflecting current status and having achieved maximum motor and sensory recovery after illness or trauma).

At the conclusion of the off-road screening, the occupational therapist will have clarified issues, such as the following:

- Type of vehicle required (e.g. automatic transmission or manual)
- Adaptive devices that may be required (e.g. hand controls, modified seating)
- Type and duration of the on-road assessment route to be used
- Special requirements of the driving instructor
- Requirement for an interpreter
- The likely impact of presenting impairments on the person's ability to manage the various tasks associated with driving
- Any specific cognitive-perceptual or other abilities to be tested during the drive

Such information assists the occupational therapy driving specialist in the professional reasoning required to identify and interpret issues emerging during the on-road assessment, where an important focus is on identifying possibilities for interventions. The off-road screen is thus a very important component of the overall occupational therapy driver evaluation.

On-road Assessment

Many occupational therapy assessments include a component in which the occupational therapist observes the individual while he or she attempts to complete a task; the on-road driver evaluation involves just this in relation to driving. The assessment usually takes place in a vehicle with dual controls, with a driving instructor seated in the front passenger seat to provide navigational instructions and take responsibility for maintaining safety. The occupational therapist sits in the rear seat on the opposite side from the driver, usually directs the assessment process and takes detailed notes using a checklist. Some examples of driver performance routinely evaluated are shown in Table 48.2.

TABLE 48.2

Examples of Behavioural and Performance Aspects Assessed During On-Road Evaluation

Person: Impact of Impairment on Driving Skill Components	Performance Components	Road Law Application to the Following	Road Craft
Cognitive-perceptual function	Maintaining lane position	Speed limits	Vehicle position at intersections
Pain levels	Right and left turns at various intersections	Intersection give way laws	Application of indicators
Endurance			
Use of limbs to manage vehicle adaptations	Observations	Other road users (e.g. pedestrians)	Use of gears, accelerator and brake
Visual abilities	Slow-speed manoeuvres	Merging and lane changing	Manoeuvring in tight spaces

To optimise safety, the driving course usually starts off in a low-demand situation such as a quiet car park or segment of road with little or no traffic. It is graded in this way so that the driver can have some time to become familiar with the vehicle by attempting basic operational tasks before venturing out into situations that are more complex, requiring interacting with multiple road users under more demanding conditions. The road test can last up to 60 minutes, depending on the goals of the assessment and driver anxiety, fatigue and other considerations.

On-road tests used in the evaluation of impaired drivers reported in the literature vary considerably. In some cases, licensing authority tests are used, with or without slight modification (e.g. Kantor, Mauger, Richardson, & Tschantz-Unroe, 2004). In other cases, specific tests have been developed for particular populations (e.g. Dobbs, Heller, & Schopflocker, 1998; Hunt et al., 1997).

To ensure reliability and validity of any on-road assessment, adequate numbers and types of different test items should be included. This is to ensure that adequate behavioural sampling occurs, providing drivers with sufficient opportunities to demonstrate their skills under a range of conditions. Assessment items include manoeuvres such as pulling to the curb, parking, completing turns at various intersections, and interacting with other traffic and road users, including merging into streams of traffic or overtaking. In addition, the checklists used during on-road assessment should have route details and prespecification of particular points along the route at which observations are to be made, as well as documenting the specific behavioural items to be assessed (Di Stefano & Macdonald, 2006b). Most occupational therapists have one or more standard routes for their on-road assessments, including those with sufficient item complexity and difficulty that would be consistent with the provision of an 'open area' license (allowing the driver to drive where they choose). This is to distinguish these routes from those used for a 'local area' test.

If a local area licence is being considered, a route around the person's home may be used, following familiar travel paths to most frequent destinations, such as to shops, medical and recreational facilities. Commonly resultant licenses are used as either an interim measure for drivers who may be continuing to make improvements but are still not able to deal with new or unpredictable driving situations, or as a step towards maintaining some degree of community mobility while gradually reducing driving privileges if the driver has a deteriorating condition. Depending on the occupational therapy service delivery model, personnel other than occupational therapy driver specialists may take responsibility for some aspects of the on-road assessment (Stav, Hunt, & Arbesman, 2006a). Australian occupational therapy driving specialists support measures required to optimise the reliability and validity of on-road test procedures to improve service delivery and equity. This is particularly important as many jurisdictions in Australia accept the occupational therapy driving specialist's on-road assessment in lieu of a formal driver licencing authority test (Di Stefano & Macdonald, 2010).

Possible Driver Evaluation Outcomes

At the conclusion of the on-road driver assessment, the individual, driving instructor and occupational therapy driving specialist discuss the findings. A decision has to made about whether the person has passed, passed with provisions, needs further interventions before being reassessed or has failed. Feedback about driving behaviours is offered as well as advice about vehicle choice, adaptations, planning and organising driving activities to accommodate functional limitations, transfer aids and seating considerations. Recommendations could include the following:

- Await further recovery from illness or injury and/or undergo a period of remediation to optimise abilities before considering reassessment and/or the continuation of driver rehabilitation.
- Undertake driving lessons, for the purpose of developing or improving general driving or other skills related to use of compensatory strategies and/or modified vehicle controls.
- Drive under restricted licence conditions, such as with a supervising driver, only within a local area limit, or only in a vehicle of a certain type or fitted with specific devices (e.g. hand controls, left external mirrors, or automatic transmission).
- Undertake further health reassessments/reviews after specified amounts of time to track either improvement or deterioration in abilities.

Some examples of impairment issues and possible interventions and licensing considerations are presented in Table 48.3.

Modifying vehicles or using aids to support access, egress, seated posture and safe operation of primary and secondary controls are commonly applied interventions. Modifications can range from simple and inexpensive (e.g. gloves, steering wheel covers, back support cushions, transfer boards) to complex and expensive (e.g. lowering/raising vehicle floor/roof, customised computerised primary and secondary controls, automatic wheelchair lock-down systems, hoists and seats). For these latter options, the occupational therapy driving specialist may need to carefully consider a range of complex individual health, ergonomics and lifestyle issues. Liaising with vehicle modifiers and engineers and funding bodies and licensing authorities may be required to ensure vehicle changes prescribed are completed in accord with required product standards criteria and approval or legislative processes (Di Stefano & Stuckey, 2015).

If the person fails the on-road assessment, the occupational therapist must decide what driving options, if any, are available to the driver. Professional reasoning, informed by referral and medical information and results of the off-road screening and on-road test, is used to evaluate available options. The occupational therapist must decide if there is any likelihood of further recovery or if the driver might benefit from driver rehabilitation. If individuals have advanced neurological conditions (e.g. dementia, Parkinson's disease or multiple sclerosis) or if there is a significant lack of insight into major limitations,

TABLE 48.3

Examples of Different Impairments and Possible Occupational Therapy Interventions Involving the Person, Vehicle, Training and Broader System (License) Issues

Health or Impairment Issue: Abilities Still Compliant with Requirements of Relevant Medical Guidelines*	Person	Vehicle Options/ Modifications	Training/Task/Road conditions	Licence Conditions/ Restrictions (These May Apply to Any of the Impairments in First Column)
Reduced upper limb movement (e.g. incoordination, pain or weakness)	Received remediation to improve movement related to range of motion, movement and strength required for upper limb. Review pain management strategies.	Use automatic vehicle with power steering and steering aid. Apply steering wheel cover to improve hand grip.	Receive lessons for training related to use of vehicle modifications. Grade exposure to driving tasks to evaluate stamina and improve endurance.	Driving only a certain type of car (e.g. automatic transmission) and/or with certain vehicle adaptations; requires a licence condition.

Check regulations regarding use of mirrors – may require a licence condition. |
| Reduced or absent lower limb movement (e.g. amputation, weakness) | Receive remediation to optimise residual abilities. If feasible, retrain left foot to operate accelerator/brake. | Use automatic vehicle with either left foot accelerator or hand controls to replace foot-operated pedals. | Initially avoid city or other driving environments requiring a lot of deceleration/ acceleration, turns or difficult parking manoeuvres. | Licence restriction to drive only in familiar areas may be required to reduce likelihood of encountering unfamiliar and demanding driving situations.

Drivers with chronic and/or deteriorating conditions may be required to undertake periodic medical and/or license testing reviews. |
| Minor reduction in visual acuity, visuoperceptual and/or cognitive abilities | Receive remediation to improve abilities. Develop compensatory strategies to optimise performance. Ensure optimal driver seating position and access/use of all controls. | Use automatic vehicle to simplify driving task. Ensure optimal view out of all windows and size, number and placement of mirrors. Additional mirrors may be installed to facilitate use of compensatory strategies. | Receive lessons for training related to in-car compensatory strategies and use of mirrors or other aids. Grade exposure to increasingly complex driving tasks to evaluate application of techniques and performance consistency over time. Assess problem-solving skills when faced with both common and unusual or more complex road scenarios. | |

*Note: Medical guidelines applicable to different countries/jurisdictions normally need to be met before drivers are eligible for licensure and assessed by occupational therapy driving specialists – see, for example, Austroads (2016); American Medical Association & National Highway Traffic Safety Administration (2010); Canadian Medical Association (2012); Department of Transport, U.K. (2014).

driver, passenger and community safety may be at risk if the person continues to drive. In such cases the occupational therapist and driving instructor may recommend that a driver ceases driving altogether. Such recommendations are always based on

sound, objective documented evidence and are usually forwarded to the licensing authority for further action.

Decisions to recommend license suspension or cancellation are not undertaken lightly as this may impose significant practical transportation difficulties and lifestyle restrictions for the former driver. The research to date examining the effects of licence cancellation on older people has highlighted the detrimental effect this can have on psychosocial health and occupational roles (Chihuri et al., 2015; Fonda, Wallace & Herzog, 2001; Marottoli et al., 1997; Marotolli, et al., 2000). The family, carers and other health personnel involved should always be advised of this outcome. A referral for counselling may be warranted. In addition, information about relevant funding schemes and community mobility alternatives, including walking, motorised devices (e.g. scooters), public and community-based transport services and taxi services, are provided.

Practice Story 48.1, involving Sue, who sustained an acquired brain injury, highlights some of the driving-related issues that can be associated with multiple system impairments. Although Sue did not require vehicle modifications, she was tested, retrained and eventually passed her second assessment, in a vehicle with automatic transmission. Driving an automatic car helps reduce the amount of both mental and physical workload associated with driving. Sue's progress through various types of health services also reinforces the importance of addressing driving-related issues very early in the rehabilitation process and depicts the collaborative and integrated efforts made by the three occupational therapists involved in her care.

OCCUPATIONAL THERAPY DRIVER ASSESSMENT AND REHABILITATION: EMERGING ISSUES

With increasing longevity and expectations that a high quality of life should be sustainable into old age, there will be increasing demands for occupational therapy community mobility and driver specialist services that maintain personal and driving independence, despite impairment and advancing age (Di Stefano, Stuckey, & Lovell, 2012). Concurrent with this, occupational therapy driver specialists will face the need to address a number of factors that, in future, are likely to affect practice and mobility/driver independence. For example:

- In-vehicle technologies that may provide additional distractions or mental workload on individuals with compromised abilities, such as personal mobile communication, in-vehicle entertainment and navigation devices (Di Stefano & Macdonald, 2003b)
- In-vehicle technologies that support driving independence, such as crash avoidance systems and parking aids (Di Stefano & Macdonald, 2006a)
- Emerging types of individual mobility options, such as motorised push bikes and Segway Personal Tranporters (Segway, 2008)
- Computer- or simulator-based methods of evaluating mobility and driver prerequisite skills
- The need to evaluate and use validated on-road and driver skill rehabilitation interventions (Unsworth & Baker, 2014)

CONCLUSION

Occupational therapists have a vital role to play in assisting people with sensory, perceptual/cognitive or motor limitations to maximise their independence by means of driving, or by whatever other means are most appropriate to achieve and sustain good community mobility. From a road safety viewpoint it is commonly a person's cognitive and perceptual limitations that are most important, but physical limitations also need to be addressed. In addition to directly supporting individuals to explore community mobility options, occupational therapists have an important role in educating and helping to optimise the abilities of the people they refer for specialist occupational therapy driver evaluations. Occupational therapists with specialist training in driver assessment and rehabilitation typically work in a team context in achieving driving-related objectives with individuals. Centrally important to the task of these occupational therapists is the careful evaluation of each driver's skills in relation to the requirements for consistently safe driving performance. To maximise the quality of the match between a person's characteristics and driving task demands, occupational therapists may use adaptive equipment, modified vehicle controls, remediation strategies, retraining or restricted licence conditions, with the aim of providing individuals with sensory, perceptual/cognitive and motor limitations opportunities to commence or resume safe driving.

PRACTICE STORY 48.1

Sue

DRIVER PROFILE AND RELEVANT OCCUPATIONAL HISTORY

Sue was a 21-year-old university student when she sustained an acquired brain injury and multiple fractures (pelvis, left humerus and right clavicle) as a result of a motor vehicle accident. After spending several months in an acute care setting, Sue was transferred to a rehabilitation facility. A further 3 months passed before Sue was fit enough to be discharged.

She was making a good recovery, having regained full sensorimotor function, although she still experienced mild upper limb coordination difficulties and a neuropsychological assessment confirmed that she was still displaying some mild residual cognitive deficits, which affected her executive skills (information processing rate, divided attention, planning and problem solving). Sue was subsequently discharged to live at home with her family as she was independent with minimal support

PRACTICE STORY 48.1

Sue (Continued)

(e.g. adaptive devices, memory aids). After discharge she attended a community-based rehabilitation programme three mornings per week.

At the time of referral for occupational therapy driver assessment, some 9 months after her accident, Sue expressed a desire to remain living at home while resuming her university studies, hopefully the following year. She indicated that she wanted to return to driving to help her travel to university (she lived 30 km from the campus) and assist her to lead a more independent lifestyle.

Before the accident, Sue had been living in a university hall of residence and had 3 years of driving experience in a manual car.

GENERALIST OCCUPATIONAL THERAPY INTERVENTION: REHABILITATION PHASES

Rehabilitation Facility

During the rehabilitation phase of her recovery, the occupational therapist initially discussed driving and considered this in relation to Sue's self-care, study and recreational pursuits. Driving was included in the rehabilitation plan goals and discussed at team and family meetings. The occupational therapist incorporated some computer-based driving-related games and education tools into Sue's programme, as well as relating some of the activities in the general rehabilitation programme to driving goals. For example, Sue was encouraged to play table soccer and use a sewing machine under supervision to test her memory, eye–hand coordination and visuospatial and reaction time abilities.

Community-based Setting

Upon transfer to the service, the community-based occupational therapist reviewed the referral documentation and used the SAFEDRIVE checklist (Wiseman & Souder, 1996) to confirm if attention deficits and skills, coordination, reaction time and executive cognitive limitations might affect Sue's driving abilities. Consequently, the occupational therapist also considered driving-related goals in the intervention plan, recommending that Sue do the following:

- Revise the content of the road rule handbook
- Undertake a programme aimed at physical reconditioning (swimming and water aerobics)
- Resume cycling in a graded programme (off-road initially, then low-demand open road environment)
- Play computer-based driving games

These were implemented with the intention of improving coordination, hazard perception and road awareness skills before considering driver assessment. In addition, a cognitive-perceptual programme (developed in conjunction with a neuropsychologist) was also commenced to improve skills in this activity domain.

OCCUPATIONAL THERAPY DRIVING SPECIALIST INTERVENTION

The community-based occupational therapist initially discussed referral with the occupational therapy driver specialist. Sue was reviewed by her rehabilitation medical specialist for the purpose of completing the specific jurisdiction's medical assessment for drivers form. This was a legal requirement and had to be completed before attempting the driver evaluation with the occupational therapy driver specialist.

Off-road Screen

The off-road interview and assessment highlighted that Sue was very motivated to resume driving and her family were supportive. The screening tests and referral information revealed that Sue still experienced mild problems in relation to executive cognitive abilities and a slight reduction in her reaction time, although she had adequate upper limb coordination, excellent insight, self-regulated her activities to avoid potential overload situations and was rigorously following her rehabilitation programme. No concerns were raised regarding road law knowledge and application.

On-road Test and Subsequent Driver Rehabilitation

The on-road test was undertaken in a car with automatic transmission to simplify the driving task. Sue did not require any other vehicle modifications. Only one half of the usual on-road assessment route was completed because of anxiety levels and errors. Sue agreed not to resume sole independent driving until a further assessment was completed and in the interim to undertake a programme of staged driver rehabilitation involving a series of graded lessons with a specialist driving instructor. In addition, home-based rehabilitation activities were prescribed using opportunities Sue had to practice driving from the passenger's seat. For example, 'commentary driving' was recommended, which involved Sue's mother driving and Sue providing a verbal commentary of the driving task, noting key elements and events requiring driver responses. Over this period the occupational therapy driving specialist liaised with Sue, her mother and the driving instructor to monitor progress.

Reassessment Post–driver Rehabilitation

After 3 months, and a total of 12 formal lessons in addition to regular sessions with her mother, Sue was reassessed by the occupational therapy driver specialist. This time the full on-road route was completed successfully and Sue was subsequently granted a licence to drive independently in an automatic car. A medical review to track her progress was recommended after 12 months, with further occupational therapy assessment dependent on medical referral, if required.

http://evolve.elsevier.com/Curtin/OT

REFERENCES

American Medical Association & National Highway Traffic Safety Administration (2010). *Physician's Guide to Assessing and Counselling Older Drivers*. Retrieved from, http://geriatricscareonline.org/ProductAbstract/physicians-guide-to-assessing-and-counseling-older-drivers/B013.

Austroads. (2016). *Assessing fitness to drive: For commercial and private vehicle drivers: Medical Standards for licensing and clinical management guidelines* (4th ed.). Sydney: Austroads Incorporated.

Bolstad, C. A., & Hess, T. M. (2000). Situation awareness and aging. In M. R. Endsley, & D. J. Garland (Eds.), *Situation awareness, analysis and measurement* (pp. 277–301). Mahwah, NJ: Lawrence Erlbaum Associates.

Bradshaw, C., Di Stefano, M., & Catchpole, J. (2013). *Dementia and driving: Report for the RACV, Research Report 13/1*. Retrieved from, https://vic.fightdementia.org.au/sites/default/files/VIC/documents/RACV-Dementia-and-Driving-2013.pdf.

Braver, E. R., & Trempel, R. E. (2004). Are older drivers actually at higher risk of involvement in collisions resulting in deaths or non-fatal injuries among their passengers and other road users? *Injury Prevention, 10,* 27–32.

Brayne, C., Dufouil, C., Ahmed, A., et al. (2000). Very old drivers: Findings from a population cohort of people aged 84 and over. *International Journal of Epidemiology, 29,* 704–707.

Brayne, C., Spiegelhalter, D. J., Dufouil, C., et al. (1999). Estimating the true extent of cognitive decline in the old. *Journal of the American Geriatrics Society, 47,* 1283–1288.

Breen, D. A., Breen, D. P., Moore, J. W., Breen, P. A., & O'Neill, D. (2007). Driving and dementia. *British Medical Journal, 334,* 1365–1369.

Bronfenbrenner, U. (1979). *The ecology of human development.* Cambridge, MA: Harvard University Press.

Bronfenbrenner, U. (1989). Ecological systems theory. In R. Vasta (Ed.), *Annals of child development* (6th ed., pp. 187–251). Greenwich, CT: JAI.

Brooks, N., & Hawley, C. A. (2005). Return to driving after traumatic brain injury: A British perspective. *Brain Injury, 19*(3), 165–175.

Canadian Medical Association. (2012). *Determining medical fitness to operate motor vehicles* (8th ed.). Retrieved from, http://viewer.zmags.com/publication/b948d3f8#/b948d3f8/2.

Charlton, J., Koppel, S., Oldell, M., et al. (2010). Influence of chronic illness on crash involvement of motor vehicle drivers. (Literature review No. 300)In (2nd ed.). Melbourne: Monash University Accident Research Centre. Retrieved from, http://www.monash.edu.au/miri/research/reports/muarc300.pdf.

Chihuri, S., Mielenz, T. J., DiMaggio, C. J., et al. (2015). *Driving cessation and health outcomes in older adults: A longROAD study.* Washington, DC: AAA Foundation for Road Safety. Retrieved from, https://www.aaafoundation.org/driving-cessation-and-health-outcomes-older-adults-longroad-study.

Classen, S., & Brooks, J. (2014). Driving simulators for occupational therapy screening, assessment and intervention. *Occupational Therapy in Healthcare, 28*(2), 154–162.

Coughlin, J. F. (2001). *Transportation and older persons: Perceptions and preferences.* A report on focus groups. Retrieved from, http://www.aarp.org/research/searchResults.html?search_keyword=coughlin&x=20&y=8.

Department of Transport, U.K (2014). *Current medical guidelines: DVLA guidance for professionals, transport regulations and safety and transport.* Retrieved from, https://www.gov.uk/current-medical-guidelines-dvla-guidance-for-professionals-conditions-a-to-c.

Di Stefano, M., & Macdonald, W. (2003a). Assessment of older drivers: Relationships among on-road errors, medical conditions and test outcome. *Journal of Safety Research, 34*(5), 415–429.

Di Stefano, M., & Macdonald, W. (2003b). Intelligent transport systems and occupational therapy practice. *Occupational Therapy International, 10*(1), 56–74.

Di Stefano, M., & Macdonald, W. (2006a). *In-vehicle intelligent transport systems.* St Louis: Mosby Elsevier.

Di Stefano, M., & Macdonald, W. (2006b). On-the-road evaluation of driving performance. In J. Pellerito (Ed.), *Driver rehabilitation and community mobility: Principles and practice* (pp. 255–274). St. Louis: Mosby Elsevier.

Di Stefano, M., & Macdonald, W. (2010). Australian occupational therapy driver assessors' opinions on improving on-road driver assessment procedures. *American Journal of Occupational Therapy, 64*(2), 325–335.

Di Stefano, M., & Stuckey, R. (2015). Ergonomic considerations for vehicle driver-cabin configurations: Optimising the fit between drivers with a disability and motor vehicles. In I. Soderback (Ed.), *International handbook of occupational therapy interventions* (2nd ed.). Basel: Springer.

Di Stefano, M., Stuckey, R., & Lovell, R. (2012). Promotion of safe community mobility: Challenges and opportunities for occupational therapy practice. *Australian Occupational Therapy Journal, 59,* 98–102.

Dobbs, A., Heller, R., & Schopflocker, D. (1998). A comparative approach to identify unsafe older drivers. *Accident Analysis and Prevention, 30*(3), 363–370.

Dobbs, B. (2005). *Medical conditions and driving: A review of the literature 1960-2000.* (Technical Report No. DOT HS 809 690). Washington, DC: US Department of Transportation. Retrieved from, http://www.nhtsa.dot.gov/people/injury/research/Medical_Condition_Driving/pages/Sec1-Intro.htm.

Dunn, W., McClain, L. H., Brown, C., & Youngstrom, M. J. (1998). The ecology of human performance. In M. E. Neistadt, & E. B. Crepeau (Eds.), *Willard and Spackman's occupational therapy* (9th ed., pp. 525–535). Philadelphia: Lippincott, Williams & Wilkins.

Folstein, M. F., Folstein, S. E., & McHugh, P. R. (1975). Mini Mental State – a practical method for grading the cognitive state of patients for the clinician. *Journal of Psychiatric Research, 12,* 189 198.

Fonda, S. J., Wallace, R. B., & Herzog, A. R. (2001). Changes in driving patterns and worsening depressive symptoms among older adults. *The Journals of Gerontology Series B: Psychological Sciences and Social Sciences, 56,* S343–S351.

Hatakka, M., Keskinen, E., Gregersen, N. P., & Glad, A. (1999). Theories and aims of educational and training measures. In S. E. Siegrist (Ed.), *Driver training, testing and licensing – towards theory-based management of young drivers' injury risk in road traffic* (pp. 13–44). Berne, Switzerland: Human Research Department, Swiss Council for Accident Prevention (BFU).

Hunt, L. A., Murphy, C., Carr, D. B., Duchek, J., Buckles, V., & Morris, J. (1997). Reliability of the Washington University Road Test: A performance-based assessment for drivers with dementia of the Alzheimer type. *Archives of Neurology, 54*, 707–712.

Iverson, D., Gronseth, G., Reger, M., Classen, S., Dubinsky, R., & Rizzo, M. (2010). Practice Parameter update: Evaluation and management of driving risk in dementia – Report of the Quality Standards Subcommittee of the American Academy of Neurology. *Neurology, 17*(16), 1316–1324.

Kantor, B., Mauger, L., Richardson, V. E., & Tschantz-Unroe, K. (2004). An analysis of an Older Driver Evaluation Program. *Journal of the American Geriatrics Society, 52*(8), 1326–1330.

Keall, M. D., & Frith, W. J. (2004). Older driver crash rates in relation to type and quantity of travel. *Traffic Injury Prevention, 5*, 26–36.

Kielhofner, G. (2002). *A model of human occupation: Theory and application* (3rd ed.). Baltimore: Williams & Wilkins.

Korner-Bitensky, N., Bitensky, J., Sofer, S., Man-Son-Hing, M., & Gelinas, I. (2006). Driving evaluation practices of clinicians working in the United States and Canada. *The American Journal of Occupational Therapy, 60*(4), 428–434.

Kua, A., Korner-Bitensky, N., Desrosiers, J., Man-Son-Hing, M., & Marshall, S. (2007). Older driver retraining: A systematic review of evidence of effectiveness. *Journal of Safety Research, 38*, 81–90.

Law, M., Cooper, B. A., Strong, S., Stewart, C., Rigby, P., & Letts, L. (1996). The person-environment-occupation model: A transactive approach to occupational performance. *Canadian Journal of Occupational Therapy, 63*, 9–23.

Liddle, J., Haynes, M., Pachana, N. A., Mitchell, G., Mckenna, K., & Gustafsson, L. (2014). Effect of a group intervention to promote older adults' adjustment to driving cessation on community mobility: A randomized controlled trial. *The Gerontologist, 54* (3), 409–422.

Lococo, K. H., & Staplin, L. (2006). *Literature review of polypharmacy and older drivers: Identifying strategies to study drug usage and driving functioning among older drivers*. Retrieved from, http://www.nhtsa.dot.gov/people/injury/olddrive/DrugUse_OlderDriver/pages/content.htm.

Lovell, R., & Di Stefano, M. (2007). *Driver education and rehabilitation course manual for Occupational Therapists*. Melbourne: School of Occupational Therapy, La Trobe University.

Lovell, R., & Russell, K. (2005). Developing referral and reassessment criteria for drivers with dementia. *Australian Occupational Therapy Journal, 52*, 26–33.

Macdonald, W. (2004). Human Error: Causes and countermeasures. In: *Paper presented at the Proceedings of the Safety in Action Conference 2004*. Melbourne: Australia.

Macdonald, W., Pellerito, J., & Di Stefano, M. (2006). Introduction to driver rehabilitation and community mobility. In J. Pellerito (Ed.), *Driver rehabilitation and community mobility: Principles and practice* (pp. 5–35). Philadelphia: Elsevier.

Mann, W. (Ed.). (2011). *Community mobility: Driving and transportation alternatives for older persons*. New York: Taylor & Francis.

Marottoli, R. A., Mendes de Leon, C., Glass, T., et al. (1997). Driving cessation and increased depressive symptoms: Prospective evidence from the New Haven EPESE. *Journal of the American Geriatric Society, 45*, 202–206.

Marottoli, R. A., Mendes de Leon, C. F., Glass, T. A., Williams, C. S., Cooney, L. M., & Berkman, L. F. (2000). Consequences of driving cessation: Decreased out-of-home activity levels. *Journal of Gerontology and Social Sciences, 55B*(6), S334–S340.

Meuser, T. M., Carr, D. B., Unger, E. A., & Ulfarsson, G. F. (2015). Family reports of medically impaired drivers in Missouri: Cognitive concerns and licensing outcomes. *Accident Analysis and Prevention, 74*, 17–23.

Molnar, F. J., Byszewski, A. M., Marshall, S. C., & Man-Son-Hing, M. (2005). In-office evaluation of medical fitness to drive: Practical approaches for assessing older people. *Canadian Family Physician, 51*(March), 372–379.

Molnar, F. J., Patel, A., Marshall, S., Man-Son-Hing, M., & Wilson, K. G. (2006). Clinical utility of office-based cognitive predictors of fitness to drive in persons with dementia: A systematic review. *Journal of the American Geriatric Society, 54*, 1809–1824.

Mollenkopf, H. (2003). *Mobility in later life – the European view. Position paper presented at the Second Meeting of STELLA Focus Group 3: Society, Behavior, and Private/Public Transport*. Arlington, Virginia, USA: U.S. National Science Foundation. 13 January – 14 January.

Norweg, A., Jette, A. M., Houlihan, B., Ni, P., & Boninger, M. L. (2011). Patterns, predictors, and associated benefits of driving a modified vehicle after spinal cord injury: Findings from the National Spinal Cord Injury Model Systems. *Archives of Physical Medicine & Rehabilitation, 92*(3), 477–483.

Oborne, D. J. (1982). *Ergonomics at work*. New York: John Wiley. &. Sons.

Organisation for Economic Co-operative Development. (2001). *Aging and transport: Mobility needs and transport issues; OECD Report*. Retrieved from, Geneva, Switzerland: Organisation for Economic Co-operative Development. http://www.ocs.polito.it/biblioteca/mobilita/OECDAgeing.pdf.

Owsley, C., Ball, K., McGwin, G., et al. (1998). Visual processing impairment and risk of motor vehicle crash among older adults. *Journal of the American Medical Association, 279*(14), 1083–1088.

Oxley, J., & Whelan, M. (2008). It cannot be all about safety: The benefits of prolonged mobility. *Traffic Injury Prevention, 9*(4), 367–378.

Pellerito, J., & Blanc, C. A. (2006). The driver rehabilitation team. In J. Pellerito (Ed.), *Driver rehabilitation and community mobility: Principles and practice* (pp. 53–68). St. Louis: Mosby Elsevier.

Proctor, R. W., & Van Zandt, T. (1994). *Human factors in simple and complex systems*. Boston: Allyn and Bacon.

Redepenning, S. (2006). *Driver rehabilitation across age and disability: An occupational therapy guide*. Bethesda, MD: American Occupational Therapy Association.

Reitan, R. M. (1985). *The Halstead-Reitan neuropsychology battery: Theory and clinical practice*. Tucson: Neuropsychology Press.

Riddle, D. R. (Ed.). (2007). *Brain aging: Models, methods and mechanisms*. Boca Raton, FL: Taylor & Francis.

Ross, L., Dodson, J., Edwards, J., Ackerman, M., & Ball, K. (2012). Self-rated driving and driving safety in older adults. *Accident Analysis and Prevention, 48*, 523–527.

Rudin-Brown, C., & Jamson, S. (2013). *Behavioural adaptation and road safety: Theory, evidence and action*. Boca Raton, FL: CRC Press, Taylor & Francis.

SafetyNet (2009). *Older drivers: Report for the European Commission, Directorate-General Transport and Energy*. Retrieved from, http://ec.europa.eu/transport/road_safety/specialist/knowledge/pdf/olderdrivers.pdf.

Sanders, J. S., & McCormick, E. J. (1993). *Human factors in engineering and design* (7th ed.). New York: McGraw Hill.

Schultz, S., & Schkade, J. K. (2003). Occupational adaptation. In E. B. Crepeau, E. S. Cohn, & B. A. Boyt Schell (Eds.), *Willard and Spackman's occupational therapy* (pp. 220–227). Philadelphia: Lippincott Williams & Wilkins.

Segway. (2008). *About Segway: Dedicated to moving you*. Retrieved from, http://www.segway.com.

Stav, W. B. (2004). *Driving rehabilitation: A guide for assessment and intervention*. San Antonio: PsychCorp.

Stav, W. B., Hunt, L. A., & Arbesman, M. (2006a). *Occupational therapy practice guidelines for driving and community mobility for older adults*. Bethesda, MD: American Occupational Therapy Association.

Stav, W. B., Justiss, M. D., Belchior, P., & Lanford, D. N. (2006b). Clinical practice in driving rehabilitation. *Topics in Geriatric Rehabilitation, 22*(2), 153–161.

Townsend, E. A., & Polatajko, H. J. (2007). *Enabling occupation II: Advancing an occupational therapy vision for health, well-being, & justice through occupation*. Ottawa: CAOT Publications ACE.

Tsai, I. H., Graves, D. E., & Lai, C. H. (2014). The association of assistive mobility devices and social participation in people with spinal cord injuries. *Spinal Cord, 52*(3), 209–215.

Unsworth, C. A., Baker, A., Taitz, C., et al. (2012). Development of a standardised occupational therapy—driver off-road assessment battery to assess older and/or functionally impaired drivers. *Australian Occupational Therapy Journal, 59*(1), 23–36.

Unsworth, C. A., & Baker, A. (2014). Driver rehabilitation: A systematic review of the types and effectiveness of interventions used by occupational therapists to improve on-road fitness-to-drive. *Accident Analysis and Prevention, 71*, 106–114.

U.S. Department of Transportation. (2003). *Safe mobility for a maturing society: Challenges and opportunities*. Retrieved from, http://www.crag.uab.edu/safemobility/SafeMobility.pdf.

U.S. Department of Transportation (2004). *Quantifying the relationships: Aging, driving cessation, health and costs*. Retrieved from, http://www.volpe.dot.gov/hf/docs/memo012804.doc.

VicRoads. (2008). *Resources and guidelines for OT driving assessors* (2nd ed.). Melbourne: Roads Corporation. Retrieved from, https://www.google.com.au/url?url=https://www.vicroads.vic.gov.au/~/media/files/formsandpublications/licences/guidelines_for_occupational_therapy_ot_driver_assessors.pdf.

Whelan, M., Langford, J., Oxley, J., Koppel, S., & Charlton, J. (2006). *The elderly and mobility: A review of the literature*. Retrieved from, http://www.monash.edu.au/muarc/reports/muarc255.html.

Wickens, C. D., & Hollands, J. G. (2000). *Engineering psychology and human performance* (3rd ed.). Upper Saddle River, NJ: Prentice Hall.

Wiseman, E. J., & Souder, E. (1996). The older driver: A handy tool to assess competence behind the wheel. *Geriatrics, 51*(7), 36–38. 41-42, 45.

World Health Organization. (2001). *International classification of functioning, disability and health: ICF*. Geneva: World Health Organization.

MOVING AND HANDLING

TESS WHITEHEAD

Abstract

The handling of people is a particular risk factor because of the unpredictable nature of the task. People vary in size, shape and physical/cognitive abilities, and the adult human form is difficult to hold because of an uneven distribution of weight. The potential for uncooperative or aggressive behaviour increases the risk of injury for therapists and carers. Additionally, the psychosocial impact of organisational and other work issues, such as high levels of demand, low levels of support or lack of control over workload, have been found to increase stress in employees, exacerbating symptoms of existing musculoskeletal disorder or heightening awareness of musculoskeletal pain. Occupational therapists involved in moving and handling risk assessments need an understanding of the biomechanics and ergonomic principles of safe handling and the equipment options available. Balanced decision making is essential to provide people with every opportunity to facilitate assisted or independent movement and maximise occupational engagement.

KEY POINTS

- Understanding of biomechanics and normal human movement is essential in the analysis and safe facilitation of moving and handling people.

- Moving and handling practice and policy must be underpinned by legislation and risk assessment.

- Therapists and all who assist people to move need to have an awareness of personal joint and back care and mechanisms of injury.

- Independence in movement should be encouraged when possible, using rehabilitation or compensatory approaches or a combination of both.
- Care handling and therapeutic handling can be used together.
- Active participation of individuals can be encouraged by the appropriate use of equipment; this also reduces the risk of injury to all involved.
- Balanced decision making in risk assessment must take account of the needs and protection of everyone involved in the moving and handling task.

INTRODUCTION

Moving and handling is much more than simply ensuring legal obligations are met. It is also concerned with how health professionals promote a balanced, proportionate approach to handling tasks, ensuring that every opportunity is available for the people receiving health services to participate and be as involved as is possible within the challenges of their illness, injury or impairment.

Independent normal movement is taken for granted by most people. People do not think about how they are going to turn in bed or stand up, as all these movement patterns are learned at the preverbal stage of development in infancy. When mobility is restricted by illness, injury or impairment, the occupational therapist plays a key role in analysing the demands of daily occupations, assessing the abilities of individuals and identifying the physical, social, cultural, attitudinal and legislative factors that may enable or disable each person in their daily routines and then modifying the activity or the environment to better support their occupational engagement (World Health Organization, 2012). Moving and handling is an intrinsic part of this process and includes direct handling of an individual and guidance and instruction to carers (College of Occupational Therapists, 2006). Understanding of normal movement and biomechanics is crucial when developing the most appropriate and safe interventions. When considering moving and handling interventions with an individual, a balance must be maintained between the needs and human rights of that individual and the safety of those assisting the person to move (Mandelstam, 2011).

Moving and handling, in this chapter, refers to any activity involving transporting, supporting, lifting, putting down, pushing, pulling, carrying or moving a person or load (Health and Safety Executive (HSE), 2004, 2012). Such activities may be carried out by hand or using body force, or in conjunction with handling equipment. It encompasses all aspects of assisting people to move any part of their body; therefore activities ranging from supporting a limb while splinting, through to hoisting a person from the floor, all require knowledge and skill to maintain safety for the therapist and individual concerned. Application of safe moving and handling principles is essential if therapists are to protect themselves and those with whom they are working. This application of safe moving and handling principles will be illustrated throughout all the practice stories presented in this chapter, starting with Practice Story 49.1.

An overview of moving and handling principles is the focus of this chapter. It is not within the remit of this chapter to discuss the wide variety of methods and equipment available for safer moving and handling. This is dealt with comprehensively in other texts, such as *The Guide to the Handling of People* (6th ed.) (Smith, 2011) and *Manual Handling of Children* (Alexander & Johnson, 2011).

IMPACT OF MOVING AND HANDLING ON THE BODY – RISKS TO THE OCCUPATIONAL THERAPIST

Musculoskeletal disorders (MSDs) are a group of painful disorders of muscles, tendons, joints and nerves. All parts of the body can be affected, although the upper limbs and back are the most common areas affected. MSDs arise from movements such as bending, straightening, gripping, holding, twisting, clenching, squatting, kneeling and reaching. These movements are not particularly hazardous in themselves; it is the continued repetition, static loading, speed of the movements and lack of time for recovery between them that contribute to the development of MSDs (European Agency for Safety and Health at Work, 2015).

Students and newly qualified therapists can be particularly at risk of MSDs. Passier and McPhail (2011) carried out the first preliminary empirical study of work-related musculoskeletal disorders (WRMDs) specific to occupational therapists. Sixty-three percent of respondents experienced one or more WRMDs within the previous 12 months and 80.4% over the course of their career. The physically demanding nature of work tasks and practice demands of delivering hands-on interventions, the physical handling of loads and a culture of underreporting are believed to contribute to this high incidence of WRMDs among therapists.

With improved training programmes, policies and procedures, therapists are much better informed regarding best practice to avoid hazardous handling and improve safe handling techniques and strategies for risk reduction musculoskeletal injury (HSE, 2014b; MacGregor, 2016). Possible sources of back pain that can affect therapists can be found in Box 49.1.

Not all stressful tasks involve straightforward direct lifts of people; awkward and static body postures, holding loads away from the body and repetitive movements increase the risk of musculoskeletal injury. Repositioning a person in a chair or bed, feeding a person or assisting with personal care are typical examples of activities that can cause muscular overload of ligaments and tendons. Occupational therapists must be aware of the risk exposure when undertaking these activities, especially when teaching family members or carers (Practice Story 49.2).

The combination of a high injury prevalence associated with handling people and the large estimates of biomechanical stress

PRACTICE STORY 49.1

Introducing Caroline

Caroline is 54 years old. She is in hospital after a fall. She has multiple sclerosis, is intermittently ambulant, no longer able to work and lives in a two-bedroom house with her husband, who works long hours from Monday to Friday. The occupational therapist involved with Caroline is responsible for ensuring her safe discharge and continuing care in the community. Safe mobility and assistance with moving are key areas of concern for Caroline as she is on her own for periods during the day and her husband is often physically and mentally exhausted when he finishes work at the end of each day. Her interests are gardening and painting and she wishes to continue engaging in these occupations for as long as possible.

Caroline's diagnosis and prognosis are important considerations when shaping any interventions. Using the medical model to consider the future effects of the disease process signposts her potential medical needs; however, occupational therapists are also concerned with any psychosocial and environmental effects on Caroline's occupational performance and engagement. Using the International Classification of Functioning, Disability and Health (ICF) (World Health Organization, 2002), social and environmental aspects of her lifestyle and surroundings need to be assessed to establish what factors may enable or disable her in the immediate and longer term. With this in mind, the potential need for equipment or adaptation must be considered, taking into account environmental and social issues, in order to facilitate safe mobility for as long as possible for the sake of Caroline, her husband and any other carers.

Occupational analysis will be central to the interventions used with Caroline and her family. Issues of mobility and assistance with moving will have a significant impact on the way she manages her daily life and carries out her chosen occupations. To facilitate optimum conditions for Caroline's mobility and handling needs and to protect those who assist her, the occupational therapist needs to have knowledge of the following:

- Normal movement for each task or activity she wishes to carry out
- Changes in her abilities which may affect the way in which she carries out these tasks
- Compensatory approaches used to enable her to carry out chosen tasks
- Her priorities for task completion
- Structure, components and order of the tasks she carries out
- The ability of her husband, and other carers, to assist her
- Equipment and resources available for her mobility and activity needs
- Skill levels required to assist her to move or those required to use equipment

---

BOX 49.1
POSSIBLE SOURCES OF BACK PAIN IN THE WORKPLACE

Examples of known sources of back pain (for therapists) in the workplace:
- Heavy manual labour (e.g. lifting equipment into the back of a car, lifting or transferring heavy people)
- Manual handling in awkward places (e.g. bathrooms or toilets)
- Repetitive tasks (e.g. carrying out exercises with a person)
- Working in the same position for long periods (e.g. sitting at a workstation for a long time if the workstation is not correctly arranged or adjusted to fit the person)
- Driving long distances, particularly if the seat is not properly adjusted
- Inadequate training in injury prevention
- Treating a large number of people in one day
- Difficulty in performing safe handling techniques because of a person's condition, size or shape

Examples of physical activities that can aggravate back pain:
- Continuing to work when injured or hurt
- Stooping, bending over or crouching, including poor posture when working with computers
- Lifting objects that are heavy or bulky, carrying objects awkwardly
- Pushing, pulling or dragging excessive loads
- Working beyond or at normal ability limits and when physically overtired
- Using poor lifting techniques (where compromised because of other risk factors)
- Stretching, twisting and reaching
- Spending prolonged periods in one position, leading to postural strain
- Understaffing, which leads to psychosocial risk stressors

Adapted from Health and Safety Executive (2007) and Glover et al. (2005).

PRACTICE STORY 49.2

Beginning to Identify Risks

For the safety of Caroline and her carers, the occupational therapist needs to be aware of mechanisms of injury and how the daily activities for Caroline and her husband may potentially increase risk of injury to either Caroline or any of her carers. By listing Caroline's essential and chosen daily activities, when these occur and how they are prioritised, the therapist can begin to identify where risks may be higher; for example, Caroline needing physical assistance to move into bed at night. Manual handling activities such as this may place her husband at increased risk of musculoskeletal disorders as he is often exhausted from work at the end of the day. Her husband therefore risks injury through trying to work beyond his physical capability at that time.

The therapist needs to help the couple prioritise where formal care or careful use of equipment (such as transfer board or, at a later stage, a ceiling track hoist) is needed in order to protect both Caroline and her husband from injury and to facilitate maximum participation and independence for Caroline. Once activities have been identified and prioritised, the therapist needs to look at Caroline's performance and the fluctuations in her ability. Application of normal movement and biomechanical principles will help identify areas of risk for her and her carers during mobility tasks. From this, a more detailed risk assessment can be carried out to develop a personal handling profile.

---

associated with moving and handling techniques in these situations have led to the use of risk assessment tools such as the Rapid Entire Body Assessment, Rapid Upper Limb Assessment, and Borg Rating of Perceived Exertion to analyse the biomechanics of handling techniques. At the same time safer handling techniques have been developed and specialist equipment designed to facilitate independence and minimise risk to the therapist doing the moving and handling.

PRINCIPLES OF MOVEMENT

It is not the remit of this chapter to discuss the neurophysiological principles of movement, but to make decisions related to moving or handling people, it is necessary to understand how a person moves in the absence of physical limitations. In the context of moving and handling a person, this is called *normal movement*. Put simply, it is the way that a person would normally move: the voluntary and automatic movements produced by the nerve pathways and action of muscles on bones and joints, which then achieve a movement task in an energy-efficient, coordinated way. Patterns of movement are sequences of movement for the achievement of a motor goal. Normal movement requires combinations of movement patterns.

If a whole year group of occupational therapy students were lying supine on a floor, arms by their sides, legs straight, and on a given cue turned on to their right sides, there would many common components to their methods of completing the task. Movement generally starts with the head – looking to the right in this instance. The left shoulder girdle will follow the rotation of the cervical spine, and the left arm reaches across the chest. In order for the body mass to move, it is likely that the left knee will bend, the foot will be placed on the floor, and the 'reach' with the arm and the 'push' with the foot will cause the body to roll onto

its side. Figs. 49.1A to D illustrate this sequence of 'normal' movement for turning to the side from supine.

Variations will of course occur – because of previous injury, body shape, age, medical condition and so on – but because the human form is generally made up of the same component parts, movement patterns are somewhat predictable. If therapists are going to ask a person to move, and perhaps give the person instructions to do so, it is important that the therapist first understands how a person would normally achieve the task and then consider the most effective and efficient way for the person.

The objective of the therapist is usually to enable people to do as much for themselves as possible. Placing a person in an optimum starting position, making use of biomechanical advantage and giving opportunity for recruitment of muscles and joints may be sufficient to enable the person to complete a moving task or help the therapist to identify the missing components or which compensatory movements the person is using. To meet this objective, therapists need to have a sound knowledge of anatomy and basic principles of biomechanics.

BIOMECHANICAL PRINCIPLES

Stability

The stability of an object is its ability to withstand external and internal forces and remain in its current position or shape. Stability in the human body is dependent on a number of factors, such as the size of the base of support (BOS), location of the body (or body segment), centre of gravity (COG) and, as a consequence, where the line of gravity (LOG) falls within the BOS (McMillan & Carin-Levy, 2013). Stability is also affected to a degree by friction and internal and external forces acting on the body.

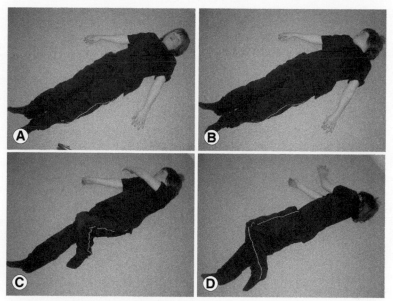

FIG. 49.1 ■ Normal movement sequence for turning onto the side in supine lying. (A) Supine lying. (B) Turning the head in the direction of the move. (C) Bending the knee and placing foot flat on the floor while reaching across the chest with the arm. Reaching with the arm and pushing with the foot to turn onto the side.

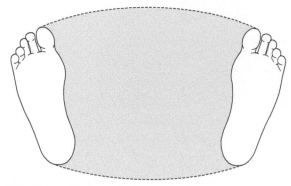

FIG. 49.2 ■ Base of support.

Base of Support

The BOS is denoted by the contact points of an object or person with the ground and all the area inside those contact points, as illustrated in Fig. 49.2. A large BOS provides greater stability (Fig. 49.3). A small BOS means that the person is less stable (Fig. 49.4).

Stability is also linked to the position of the COG and LOG relative to the BOS.

Centre of Gravity and Line of Gravity

The point at which gravity is thought to act on an object is described as its COG. In the adult human body, while standing

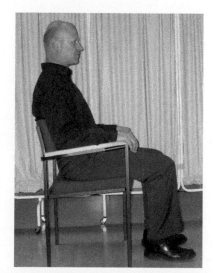

FIG. 49.3 ■ Large base of support (BOS) from back legs of chair to front of person's feet.

or lying in the anatomical position, the COG of the whole body is estimated to be anterior to the second sacral vertebrae (Norkin & Levangie, 2011). The precise location of the COG changes constantly with every new position of the body and limbs. The body proportions of the individual also affect the location of the COG. Each segment in the human body has its own COG;

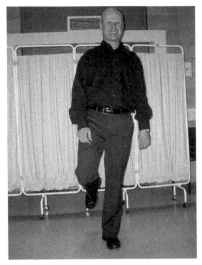

FIG. 49.4 ■ Small base of support (BOS) denoted by one foot in contact with the ground.

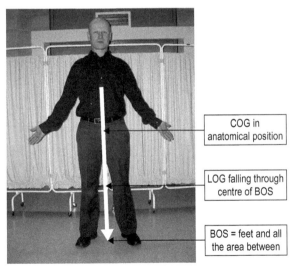

FIG. 49.5 ■ Centre of gravity (COG) in anatomical position and line of gravity (LOG) falling within centre of the BOS.

COG in anatomical position

LOG falling through centre of BOS

BOS = feet and all the area between

however, within the remit of moving and handling, it is usual to refer to the COG of the whole body. The LOG is an imaginary line drawn vertically from the COG to the ground and helps to estimate, at any time, where the COG is relative to the BOS. Knowing this helps to estimate the stability of a person. The more central the COG and LOG are, within the BOS, the greater a person's stability (Fig. 49.5). A low COG increases a person's stability; therefore when people are lying in prone or supine they are at their most stable (Fig. 49.6).

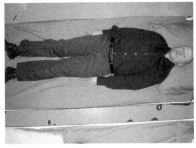

FIG. 49.6 ■ Large base of support (BOS) with low centre of gravity (COG) leads to maximum stability.

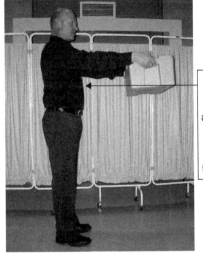

Due to rearrangement of body segments and addition of weight on the arms, the COG moves up and forward decreasing the person's stability

FIG. 49.7 ■ Position of decreased stability due to higher centre of gravity (COG).

Conversely, raising the COG (Fig. 49.7) decreases stability. In addition, as people rearrange the segments of their bodies, the COG of the whole body moves. It can move in any direction and can be outside the physical body (Norkin & Levangie, 2011). If this movement results in the LOG moving towards the edge of or outside the BOS, the person becomes unstable, as in Fig. 49.8.

In summary, when a person has a small BOS (see Fig. 49.2) it will take very little movement of the body for the COG to fall towards or outside the edge of the BOS, thus causing that person to experience postural instability. Equally changing the weight distribution of the body may raise the COG, which will also reduce stability. Although a high degree of stability is necessary for safety, when, for example, a person is supporting a load, reduced stability is necessary for movement to occur. If a person was to keep his COG and LOG centrally within a wide BOS all

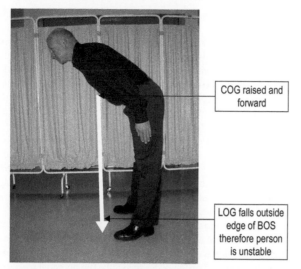

FIG. 49.8 ■ Position of line of gravity (LOG) outside base of support (BOS) creates instability.

COG raised and forward

LOG falls outside edge of BOS therefore person is unstable

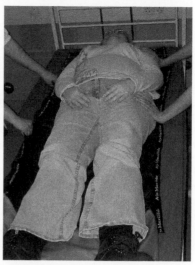

FIG. 49.9 ■ Reducing dynamic friction using slide sheets to make movement easier.

the time (see Fig. 49.3), the person would find it very difficult to change position.

In rehabilitation, interventions generally begin with the person in a position of maximum stability. Having a low COG and large BOS requires the least amount of energy consumption and muscle tone (e.g. in supine lying; see Fig. 49.6). The objective may be to progress to movement in a position of less stability in order to retrain muscle tone, balance reactions and so on. An example of this would be the person ultimately being able to stand on tip-toe with arms raised to lift an object into a high cupboard. This position is one of reduced stability as the COG is raised (because of reorganisation of body segments and added weight through the arms), and the BOS is small. Any shift in position of the COG now will more easily result in the LOG falling outside the BOS, thus destabilising the person. To maintain balance in this position of reduced stability, the person is dependent on recruitment of appropriate muscle groups, vestibular and visual function and intact proprioception.

Friction

Another factor potentially affecting a person's ability to move, the effort required and the quality of movement is friction. Where two objects are in contact with each other, friction will occur to a greater or lesser extent, depending on the type of surfaces in contact and the pressure between them. It is important to understand the effects of friction coefficients in different materials and their effects on movement. A surface with a high friction coefficient will resist movement across it – for example, a deep-pile wool carpet. Alternatively a surface with a low friction coefficient will enable movement to occur more easily and reduce the degree of shearing forces on the moving object – for example, a slide sheet (Norkin & Levangie, 2011).

Two types of friction exist: static and dynamic. Static friction resists movement. Therefore when a person sits still in a chair (see Fig. 49.3), static friction between the thighs/buttocks and the chair seat prevents the person from slipping out of the chair. To overcome this static friction a person must create movement through internal or external forces. Once movement begins, dynamic friction occurs between the surfaces in contact with each other. For the therapist and person, this can be either beneficial or a hindrance. If the person in Fig. 49.3 wishes to stand out of the chair, the high friction coefficient and his body weight will necessitate greater internal and external forces to enable him to move. Therefore a high friction coefficient will be beneficial in enabling him to stay in the chair but will make moving out of the chair more difficult. This is often the case when people are in bed (see Fig. 49.6). Static friction between the person's body and the bed means that the person is very stable; however, when the person needs to move, the dynamic friction between the two surfaces increases the risk of shearing forces on a person's skin. The therapist also has to exert much larger external forces to initiate movement, increasing his or her risk of musculoskeletal injury. Using slide sheets, which have a very low friction coefficient, reduces the impact of shearing forces and requires less external force to create movement. This principle applies equally where people are able to sit up and move themselves on a bed. Using small slide sheets between themselves and the bed reduces shearing forces and minimises the amount of effort required to move (Fig. 49.9).

Levers and Forces

To understand how people move, it is important to understand levers. A lever system comprises an axis, an effort force and a resistance force. In the human body the axis is commonly a joint. The effort force is denoted by the direction of movement of the body or body segment, and the resistance force opposes the movement. The process of standing from sitting neatly illustrates all these aspects and enables an analysis of why this activity can sometimes be difficult and how to make it easier. In order for this movement to be easy, the distance of the effort force from the axis should be equal to or greater than the distance of the resistance force, as the larger the distance of a force from an axis, the greater its mechanical advantage. The effort force in this case is the quadriceps muscles, which extend the knee. The axis is the knee joint and the resistance force is the body weight, the central point of which is the COG. Figs. 49.10A and B show that the distance of the resistance force from the axis is greater than the distance of the effort force, which is common, as muscle attachments cannot move and therefore are generally close to a joint.

When sitting upright in a chair, a person has a large BOS with the LOG falling through the centre of this support. The person is therefore very stable. In order to stand up, the person needs to destabilise the body. Figs. 49.10A and B illustrate the biomechanical differences between static upright sitting and preparation for standing and explains how changing the position of the body's COG facilitates easier standing.

To make standing even easier, therapists can ask or assist the person to move hips forward in the chair to bring the LOG closer to the edge of the BOS, thus destabilising the person further. Additionally, by using chair raisers to increase the overall height of the chair, the angle at the hips and knees when sitting is decreased and the body's COG (resistance force) is automatically closer to the knees (axis). Its mechanical advantage is therefore decreased even further in relation to the quadriceps muscles (effort force).

Having an understanding of biomechanics and normal patterns of movement in an able-bodied adult of average body mass provides a working baseline from which it is possible to understand the impact of changes in tone (increased or decreased), body mass (increased or decreased, as in pregnancy or amputation) or joint function (pain, etc.) on movement. Application of this understanding of biomechanics and normal patterns of movement is illustrated in Practice Story 49.3.

For the most part there is no single 'correct' way of moving a person to achieve a task. Most importantly, having a sound knowledge of biomechanics and human movement enables an accurate assessment of risk to achieve completion of tasks while promoting maximum ability and facilitating occupational engagement.

RISK ASSESSMENT

Moving a person has to take into consideration a multitude of factors, such as weight distribution, asymmetrical body mass, unpredictable behaviour, and medical and sensory issues, such as muscle spasms, loss of spatial awareness, visual impairment and so on. The amount of assistance that the individual can offer at any point may also vary, so each time the task is performed the risks may be different. Added to this are environmental considerations such as confined spaces and other factors of attitude, knowledge base and frequency of the task.

Avoidance of injury through manual handling should be a primary concern for employers and staff alike. Under health and safety legislation, employers must take measures to eliminate handling tasks which put staff at risk of injury. Where this is not possible, risks must be assessed and reduced to the lowest level that is reasonably practicable. This must be regularly reviewed. A useful acronym for this is AARR: Avoid Assess Reduce and Review (HSE, 2012).

People live in a world full of hazards; it is unrealistic to expect that a person can always eliminate all risks, and this is particularly true in the work environment. Therefore risk assessments need to be carried out in order to reduce the potential for accidents and injury, particularly in the case of handling people. When carrying out risk assessments therapists need to strike a balance between the potential benefits to the person being moved against the risk of injury to the handler (Johnson, 2011).

For the occupational therapist, personal risks will be high where active rehabilitation (therapeutic handling) is taking place. In this situation the therapist will be testing the boundaries of the person's abilities in order to optimise occupational performance. Professional reasoning and expertise will enable the therapist to decide what is reasonable in terms of risk and balance this with the potential benefit to each individual.

In care handling situations the therapist may be making detailed risk assessments of the everyday handling needs of each individual to ensure safest practice for carers. These differing approaches form the basis of the care–therapy handling continuum, which is illustrated in Table 49.1.

Risk assessment involves identifying hazards within a given situation and deciding whether these hazards pose a risk of injury to those carrying out associated tasks. Risk assessment should be undertaken where any handling task is considered to present a health risk to those involved (HSE, 2015). Risk assessments may be *generic* or *individual*.

Generic risk assessments cover all common tasks carried out within an area, including people and inanimate load handling. They seek to identify and highlight key hazards and control measures associated with general locations, events or activites. For example, in a residential setting, profiling beds may be recommended to replace manually adjustable beds. Increasing a resident's independent movement on the bed reduces the need for manual assistance from staff for activities such as sitting up in bed. This results in reduced risk of musculoskeletal injury to both staff and residents (Fergusson Burt, 2007) while encouraging residents to be more independent, improving self-esteem and encouraging occupational engagement. As can be seen from this example, *generic risk assessments* are important tools for managers and their teams, as they can provide the basis for

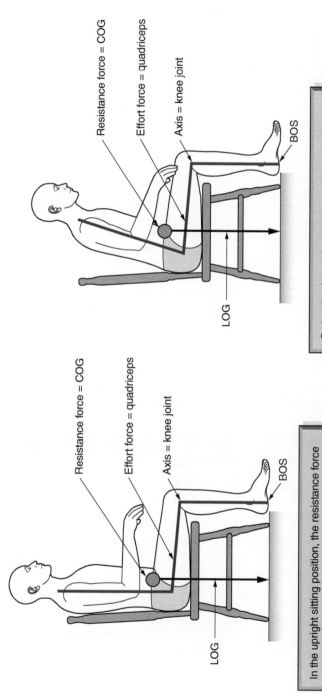

Resistance force = COG

Effort force = quadriceps

Axis = knee joint

BOS

LOG

By leaning forward, the resistance force (COG) is bought closer to the axis (knee), reducing its mechanical advantage relative to the effort force (quadriceps). The LOG now falls closer to the edge of the BOS, therefore stability is decreased. This results in reduced effort for standing.

B

Resistance force = COG

Effort force = quadriceps

Axis = knee joint

BOS

LOG

In the upright sitting position, the resistance force (COG) is much further from the axis (knee) than the effort force (from quadriceps). The resistance force therefore has greater mechanical advantage and more effort is required to overcome gravity in order to stand. The line of gravity also falls from the COG near to the centre of the BOS therefore stability is high.

A

FIG. 49.10 ■ Biomechanical principles related to upright sitting and preparation for standing.

PRACTICE STORY 49.3

Considering Principles of Normal Movement and Biomechanics

Caroline's condition may necessitate greater assistance to help her move at the end of the day because of fatigue. By understanding the principles of normal movement and biomechanics, the occupational therapist can reduce the potential for injury for both Caroline and her carers. Should Caroline wish to transfer from a chair or wheelchair to the bed, her husband might typically adopt a controversial technique known as the 'bear hug' to help her to stand. As is common in these situations, he may not be aware of his own body postures. By standing in front of her and grasping her round the waist he reduces Caroline's ability to use normal movement by blocking her potential to lean forward. He becomes the effort force. Caroline's centre of gravity (COG; resistance force) is a significant distance from her knees (axis). As a result, he will need to use extra effort to bring her COG towards the edge of her base of support, thus destabilising her enough to move. Through careful task analysis, the occupational therapist should be able to offer training in alternatives, such as those described here:

- Use chair raisers to raise the height of the chair. Caroline to utilise normal movement as described earlier to position herself ready to stand. Her husband can then position himself at her side and provide minimal assistance to enable her to lean forward and stand to transfer.
- Suggest the use of a handling belt.
- Reduce the risk of falls through fatigue by training the couple in the safe use of a transfer board. This enables

Caroline to continue using normal movement to transfer from chair or wheelchair into bed in the evenings.

In terms of assisting a person to move, a distinction is made between 'therapeutic handling' and 'care handling'. The differences are listed in Table 49.1. By Health and Safety Executive (2004) definition, handling of a person involves the application of human effort using the hands or any other part of the body, either directly or indirectly, to transport, support, move, steady or position a load. For therapists this includes guiding, facilitating, manipulating or providing resistance (Chartered Society of Physiotherapy, 2003). So in fact *all* physical contact with a person, wherever that takes place, will potentially involve manual handling − including work with rehabilitation equipment.

NB: When defining an intervention programme which involves specific methods of moving and handling with the person, the therapist is responsible for carrying out those handling techniques. A therapist must not expect other professionals or untrained staff to carry out therapeutic handling techniques with a person unless the therapist has specifically trained and assessed the competence of individuals in methods specific to that person (College of Occupational Therapists, 2006). It is also important to remember that the code of professional conduct empowers therapists to say 'no' to performing a task if they are not competent to complete it safely, and this also applies to moving and handling tasks (College of Occupational Therapists, 2015).

TABLE 49.1
Types of Person Handling

Therapeutic Handling	Care Handling
Takes place within a structured setting or therapy session, usually by a therapist in a department, hospital ward or within a person's home.	Takes place in wards, residential settings, a person's home, a school or other day facility.
Is of short duration and may include active/passive moving, use of equipment or positioning with a specific goal in mind.	Is potentially carried out a number of times throughout a 24-hour period and may include active/passive moving, use of equipment or positioning of the person.
Requires cooperation from the individual.	Although cooperation is encouraged, care handling of necessity may not involve active participation from the person because of limitations in physical or cognitive ability.
Improves or maintains performance.	Maintains performance, with or without the use of equipment, and may help improve overall mobility and quality of life. Can involve compensatory approaches.
Involves highly trained qualified staff.	Involves formal/informal carers, family members, school assistants, etc., who have received training from an occupational therapist or moving and handling advisor.
Involves calculated risks in order to improve performance. Requires professional reasoning and expertise and completion of risk assessment documentation to support this. Needs to take account of required performance in a variety of environments.	Involves completion of detailed risk assessments and handling management plan to assist with essential activities of daily living.

prioritising funds for additional resources. The stages of generic risk assessment are summarised in Box 49.2.

Individual risk assessments are carried out where individuals have specific handling and/or complex needs which fall outside generic protocols. From these, handling management plans are developed, providing more specific detail about processes, equipment, numbers and skill base of handlers and type of assistance required for each given handling task. Handling management plans should take into account the individual's wishes and needs (Madelstam, 2011; Human Rights Act, 1998), their fluctuating ability, plus the physical and psychosocial influences on all those involved in the tasks (HSE, 2013).

To help employers determine when risk assessment of inanimate handling tasks that cannot be avoided is required, the Health and Safety Executive published Lifting and Lowering Guidelines. However, these apply to objects, not people, and the guideline weights are for infrequent operations – up to about 30 operations per hour – where the pace of work is not forced, adequate pauses to rest or use different muscles are possible, and the load is not supported by the handler for any length of time. However, it is a useful tool that can be used to indicate whether further detailed risk assessment of each identified task is necessary. The individual risk assessment process is summarised in Box 49.3.

TILE(O) is a simple and easily applied acronym to identify the main components of a moving and handling assessment (HSE, 2004), standing for: Task, Individual capacity, Load, Environment and Other factors (Box 49.4). An ergonomic approach to risk assessment requires analysis of all these components. The reader is referred *The Guide to the Handling of People* (6th ed.) (Smith, 2011) for a more detailed description of the individual elements of a TILEO risk assessment.

In addition to these considerations, therapists need to consider potential *triggers* for adverse behaviour particularly when handling people with complex needs or challenging behaviour. Fear of equipment or experiences of pain from poor handling procedures or use of equipment may trigger physiological responses, such as muscle spasm, or behavioural responses, such as aggression. These all increase the risk of injury to individuals and their handlers.

When considering risk assessment, the law does not identify a maximum weight limit. The Manual Handling Operations Regulations guidance gives basic guideline figures for lifting and lowering which indicate when a more detailed risk assessment should be carried out. It places duties on employers to manage or control risk; measures to take to meet this duty will vary depending on the circumstances of the task. Things to be considered include the individual carrying out the handling operation (e.g. strength, fitness, underlying medical conditions), the weight to be lifted and distance to be carried, the nature of the load and the postures to be adopted or the availability of equipment to facilitate the lift.

Having completed the risk assessment, all risks identified must be reduced to the lowest level reasonably practicable and clearly recorded in the risk reduction steps in a Handling Management Plan or Safe System of Work. These must be dated and signed and must also indicate a timescale for review or be reviewed whenever there is significant change in a person's or carer's circumstances (HSE, 2015; Johnson, 2011).

It is not always appropriate to use only one risk assessment tool where there are complex handling situations. A risk assessment filter is initially required to establish the need for formal risk assessment. The choice of assessment tool will then depend on the activity and the circumstances in which it is being used. A range of possible assessments are listed in Box 49.5. Additional qualitative and quantitative assessment tools are described in the *Guide to the Handling of People* (6th ed.).

BOX 49.4

TILEO ASSESSMENT TOOL HANDLING OF PEOPLE

Task	What is the task? (Object): e.g. lifting a box of slings (Person): e.g. personal care, standing transfers Does it need to be done? What does it entail (twisting, stooping, reaching, pushing, pulling, carrying long distances, sudden movements, prolonged effort, insufficient recovery periods)? Are there inherent risks to the handler or others from carrying it out?
Individual	*This refers to the handler(s).* Do they have correct/sufficient skills and training? Are they in an at risk group for injury? Are they wearing the correct clothing and footwear?
Load	Is this inanimate or a person? What is the weight of the load and the distribution of this weight? Is it bulky, difficult to grasp, unstable? What is the ability/diagnosis of the person? Are there factors of unpredictability? What clothing is the person wearing? What are the effects of present condition; of the medication, etc? Is the person cooperative? Is the person able to weight bear? How much assistance is needed? Is the person able to communicate? What is the viability of the person's tissue? Are there able behavioural concerns? Are there any cultural issues? Does the person use/wear any splints, catheters, and/or orthoses?
Environment	What are the levels of lighting, ambient temperature and humidity and do these enable safe handling? Are there any slip or trip hazards; inanimate or otherwise? Is the floor or ground surface safe for moving on? What are the space contraints on posture?
Other	Is movement or posture hindered by clothing or personal protective equipment?

BOX 49.4

TILEO ASSESSMENT TOOL HANDLING OF PEOPLE *(Continued)*

Is there an absence of the correct/suitable Personal Protective Equipment being worn?
Are there personal factors between the client and handler?
What equipment is available/in place?
Is it well maintained, serviced, fit for purpose, appropriate for the task?
Is equipment accessible?
Have handlers been trained to use it?

From Smith (2011)

BOX 49.5

EXAMPLES OF QUALITATIVE AND QUANTITATIVE RISK ASSESSMENTS

- Rapid Entire Body Assessment (REBA) (Hignet & McAtamney, 2000)
- Finnish Work Ability Index (Ilmarinen, 1998)
- Ergonomic Workplace Analysis (Ahonen et al.,1989)
- Benner Scale (Benner, 1984)
- Functional Independence Measure (FIM) (Granger et al., 1993)
- Manual Tasks Risk Assessment Tool (ManTRA) (Straker et al., 2004)
- Rapid Upper Limb Assessment (RULA) (McAtamney & Corlett, 1993)
- NIOSH equation for lifting tasks (NIOSH, 1991)
- Manual Handling Assessment Chart (MAC) (Health and Safety Executive, 2003)
- Ovako Working Posture System (OWAS, 2007)

The risk assessment process as applied to Caroline is illustrated in Practice Story 49.4.

Reviewing Risk Assessments

The Heath and Safety Executive do not set a frequency for carrying out a review of a risk assessment. Instead, therapists are advised to review if it is no longer valid or if there has been a significant change; this can include, but is not limited to changes in a person's condition, the general environment, the tasks being performed, and the care worker's situation.

EQUIPMENT PROVISION AND USE

The provision of specialist equipment for moving and handling is a commonly used intervention. Appropriate equipment

PRACTICE STORY 49.4

Detailed Risk Assessment

Regular assessment of Caroline's performance and needs will be required as her ability will potentially fluctuate, as well as deteriorate. It is not appropriate to introduce equipment too early, as she will want to retain as much independence as possible, for both her and her husband's sake. Interprofessional collaboration will be key to enabling her to retain her abilities and the occupational therapist will possibly be the coordinating professional, ensuring contact with statutory and voluntary bodies to provide support. Task analysis will enable us to identify elements of daily activities in which Caroline may be independent, partially dependent or totally dependent. Maintenance of mobility through analysis of normal movement and application of biomechanical principles to tasks will enable Caroline to focus her energy on activities that are most important to her.

Having established Caroline's priorities for activities and identified those which may present a risk of injury to her or her carers, application of the risk assessment filter will help the therapist decide which activities present risk significant enough to apply formal risk assessment. From here the therapist must select the most appropriate tools to use. Generally the TILEO assessment is used initially to establish the presence of significant risk; however, in Caroline's case, it may also be useful to use the Dreyfus model of skill acquisition to indicate the skill level required for those assisting her and to direct the therapist to potential training and equipment needs.

After performing manual handling risk assessments for all activities where assistance is required and where there may be risk of injury to Caroline, her carers or therapists working to maintain her mobility will be in a position to produce a handling management plan. This should detail how and when Caroline needs assistance with mobility, methods to be used and equipment required. The plan should give a clear indication of how and when equipment is to be used, what the criteria are for these and who is able to use it. It will be important to gain consent from Caroline for both manual assistance and introduction of equipment to aid mobility. Environmental issues such as access, circulation space for equipment, aesthetics and potential hazards must all be assessed, particularly with regards to any mobility aids used by Caroline. The occupational therapist must consider alternative approaches to be used at different times of the day and night to facilitate safest practice for anyone assisting Caroline with mobility. There must also be a clear indication of any specific treatment handling which takes place, when this happens and with whom.

The therapist must provide or source appropriate training and assessment of competence for all carers in both techniques and equipment use in order to reduce risk of musculoskeletal injury. Although the Manual Handling Operations Regulations 1992 (amended 2004; Health and Safety Executive, 2004) serve to protect the formal carers, the Human Rights Act (1998) must be considered, particularly when recommending formal care or equipment. Balanced decision making (Mandelstam, 2011) is important in order to enable Caroline to feel an active participant rather than a passive recipient. This will help minimise risk of triggers such as anxiety-induced muscle spasm or emotional rejection of recommendations which may affect both Caroline's and her carer's safety. Most importantly, the handling management plan and risk assessment must be regularly reviewed, adapted and signed, to account for changes in Caroline's or her carer's functional ability or needs.

TILEO, **T**ask, **I**ndividual capacity, **L**oad, **E**nvironment and **O**ther factors.

---

solutions can improve productivity, enhance comfort, reduce costs and increase a person's independence (Sturman-Floyd, 2011). Although equipment may be essential, the therapist should first address mobility issues using detailed task analysis and risk assessment. It is important to establish those elements of the task that are problematic and those that the individual can carry out with minimal or no assistance, always encouraging as much active participation as possible.

Having completed a baseline task analysis for an activity, identified normal movement requirements and any physical, cognitive, and sensory limitations and risks associated with task completion for the person and carers, there is a need to identify equipment that either the person can use without assistance or that can be used by carers to safely move the person. Careful assessment of motor, sensory and cognitive ability is essential before the provision of equipment. The therapist must be confident that the person operating the equipment can follow instructions and understand safety principles to ensure its safe and appropriate use. The therapist must ensure the equipment and environment are compatible with the target activity and be clear about the rationale and potential risks related to the use of such equipment and that any equipment selected meets safety criteria as set out by the Medical and Health Care Products Regulations Agency (2008).

Moving and handling equipment, legislation, organisational polices and best practice exist in an effort to protect people and and those assisting them. Therapists who routinely move, handle, reposition and transfer a person without technology or assistive aids, are inherently at greater risk of sustaining a musculoskeletal injury even when proper body mechanics are used (Frost & Barkley, 2012). However, despite the availability of safer systems of work, opinion exists among therapists within rehabilitation settings that the use of handling equipment may impede a person's recovery (Waters & Rockefeller, 2010). In contrast, Arnold, Radawiec, Campo, & Wright, (2011) and Darragh et al. (2013) found that therapists using equipment during intervention increased their options for therapeutic activites, allowing them to mobilise people earlier and decreasing the length of hospital stay.

Examples of equipment that may be used either by the person to assist movement or by carers, when the person is more dependent, are listed in Table 49.2.

Transfer/Handling Belts

Most transfer belts are made of fabric or cushioned material and have multiple loops or handholds. Carers should hold on to the handles from the outside and never put their thumbs inside or through the loops in case the person falls and the carer is unable to disengage his or her hands. Transfer belts are secured around person's waists and adjusted until firm but not tight. Transfer belts are used to assist the development of mobility and rehabilitation for people who are minimally dependent, have weight-bearing capacity and are cooperative. They can also assist with people who might be difficult to hold, either because of size or discomfort or because the person is uncomfortable with being assisted. Transfer slings are often used for bed-to-chair, chair-to-chair, and chair-to-car transfers, repositioning a person in a chair and supporting a person while walking. Transfer belts should never be used to lift a person.

TABLE 49.2	
Examples of Equipment Used to Facilitate Independent or Assisted Movement	
Hand blocks	Lightweight plastic body with nonslip pads on the base designed to help a person move himself or herself in bed by 'lengthening' his or her arms. Can be used singly or in pairs or in conjunction with sliding sheets.
Transfer belt (handling belt, gait belt, walking belt)	A belt placed around a person's waist during several types of transfer and for assisted walking for rehabilitation.
Leg lifters or handling slings	Enable the person or carer to lift legs into baths, onto beds or wheelchair footplates, reducing the risk of bruising through finger pressure on the legs and limiting the risk of back pain for carers through stooping to reach person's feet.
Slide sheet	A sheet made of low-friction material and used under a person to allow easy repositioning in bed and lateral transfers.
One-way glide cushion (glide and lock sheet)	Nonslip is a tubular cushion with a nonslip outer material that grips to any surface. Allows sliding easily in one direction while resisting sliding in the other direction. Suitable for users who slides forward when sitting.
Swivel cushion (rota cushion, swivelling seat)	Low-friction swivel cushion that allows the user to slide and turn into the desired position in a car seat or chair.
Turning disc (transfer disc, turning aid, transfer turntable)	To support moving feet during seated transfer, such as transfer between bed, wheelchair, chair, shower chair, toilet and commode.
Transfer board (slide board, banana board)	Length of board made from wood or plastic, used to bridge gaps for person to transfer from one surface to another, such as from a stretcher or wheelchair to a bed
Person turner (transfer disc, transfer platform)	Aluminium platform and frame with handholds for sit to stand transfers by pushing or pulling up. Smooth rotational movement operated by carer. Some versions have small casters to facilitate movement across small distances.
In-bed management systems (two-way glide, four-way glide)	Draw sheet and base slide sheet that can be left underneath a person to enable easier turning and repositioning in bed. Base slide sheet can be used independently; two-way sheet allows sideways movement; four-way allows multidirectional movement.
Inflatable lifting cushion	Air-filled cushion designed to lift a person from the floor. Effective in small confined spaces such as the bedroom or bathroom where alternative person lifter devices may not be suitable.
Standing hoist (sit-to-stand hoist, standing lift, stand aid hoist)	A specific type of mobile hoist designed to assist people between sitting and standing positions. Standing hoists are designed to fit under and around chairs.
Mobile hoist (floor hoist, floor lift, mechanical lift, portable hoist)	A hoist on casters that can be moved along the floor, used for transferring a person using a compatible sling.
Ceiling hoist (overhead hoist, ceiling lift, H frame, XY system)	A hoist attached to permanently mounted ceiling track that moves a person inside a sling.
Gantry hoists (free-standing gantry, two-post hoist/system)	Floor-standing frames that can be used with a mains-powered hoist unit or a battery-powered portable hoist unit. Usually installed over a bed.

Slide Sheets

Slide sheets are one of the most popular and versatile pieces of moving and handling equipment. They are inexpensive, come in a range of sizes and are relatively straightforward to use; despite this, training is necessary in the correct application to avoid injury. Slide sheets are made from lightweight fabric and have low friction surfaces when placed together to allow for multidirectional moves. Procedures such as turning in bed, moving higher up or lower in bed or readjusting a person who is in a prone position become easier to achieve with a slide sheet, even with a heavier or passive user. For a person who has fallen into a confined space, slide sheets can be used to move the person along the floor to a location where a hoist can be used.

Hoists

There are three general categories of hoist: standing hoists, mobile floor hoists and ceiling track hoists (sometimes called overhead hoists, H frames and XY systems). All hoists use slings to support the person during the transfer. Hoists and slings should be clearly labelled with their safe working loads (SWL). Before transferring any person the therapist must carry out precautionary safety checks before each use. These include, but are not limited to, the following:

- Read and follow the handling/hoisting plan.
- Conduct an 'on the spot' risk assessment to check there is no significant change from the handling/hoisting plan and do a visual check of all equipment before using it. These visual check would include the following:
  - Ensuring (in relation to the hoist):
    - □ the safe working load SWL of the hoist is adequate for the person and that the SWL is clearly displayed;
    - □ hoist is fully charged, the battery and leads are fitted and connected correctly and the emergency stop button is correctly set;
    - □ there are no obvious signs of damage, fluid leaks, the lifting tape is intact and not frayed (applies to ceiling track, certain mobile hoists), castors move freely (i.e. free from carpet fibres/fluff, etc.), base adjustment of mobile and standing hoists move freely and the raise/lowering mechanism works; and
    - □ Lifting Operations and Lifting Equipment Regulations (LOLER) checks are in date.
  - Ensuring (in relation to the sling):
    - □ sling has been assessed for the individual, fit for purpose and is compatible with the person and the hoist;
    - □ all labels are legible and show SWL and unique identifier;
    - □ there are no signs of fraying or tears or worn areas, and all stitching is intact;
    - □ Velcro (if applicable) is clean and free of fibres/fluff;
    - □ the buckle (if applicable) and/or loops or clips have no obvious signs of damage;
    - □ sling is clean, especially if shared, to prevent spread of infection; and
    - □ LOLER checks are in date.
  - Ensuring (in relation to the environment):
    - □ there is sufficient space to use the hoist safely;
    - □ the floor is clear of obstacles;
    - □ there is sufficient access around and under furniture;
    - □ there is a suitable and safe area to store and charge (if applicable) the hoist; and
    - □ the environment is prepared for the task.

If a fault is identified with either the hoist or sling, it should be immediately withdrawn from use and organisational reporting procedures followed.

Mobile Hoists

Where weight bearing and trunk stability are very limited or absent, it may be necessary to use a mobile hoist for some or all transfers. Mobile hoists (sometimes called floor hoists) can be very cost effective and often can be procured more quickly than overhead hoist systems. For this reason, they are often included in the 'standard' Community Equipment Store range and are readily available for both hospital and community therapists to prescribe. They offer versatility in terms of being moved to different locations within a single setting and used for a variety of tasks. There are factors that need to be taken into consideration, such as the space constraints where the hoist is to be used and whether the legs of the hoist will fit under or around any furniture, such as bed, bath or chair. Carers may also need a lot of strength to move the equipment, particularly in areas with carpet (especially if a hoist has small wheels). Depending on the sling type being used, not all mobile hoists have sufficient lifting height to clear the sides of the transfer surface (e.g. bed, wheelchair) if a standing/jacket harness is being used. The abililty to pick up a person from floor level in an emergency also needs to be checked as not all hoists are capable of this.

Ceiling Hoists

Ceiling track hoists (CTH) run along tracks permanently fixed to ceiling joists or wall-mounted brackets. Thought needs to be given to structural considerations: ceiling joists may need to be reinforced and doorways altered to accommodate the track. There are different tracking solutions available:

- A single track system transfers a person from one defined pickup point to another; a major limitation of this is that it only allows transfers to take place in a straight line. Coverage can be increased by adding turntables and 90-degree bends for a number of pickup points in different rooms.
- The most versatile are H or XY systems. These involve two straight sections of track being fixed adjacent to each other on each side of the room with another track joining

the two. The track slides along the two parallel tracks, providing whole room coverage of any given room allowing total flexibility in terms of transfer positions.

CTH can usually lift over a greater height range from floor to ceiling. They do not take up valuable floor space and can therefore be used safely in confined or restricted ennvironments where it would not be possible to use a mobile hoist. They require little physical exertion as the transfer of the person takes place without the friction of castors on the floor. CTHs are generally powered by mains electricity, with either a powered or manual raising and lowering mechanism; a fully powered hoist can be operated by a person independently, something which is not possible with any floor-standing system. The constant availability means it is more likely to be used by carers than a mobile hoist, which may not be to hand immediately when required.

CTHs are generally more expensive than other type of hoisting equipment. However, they can often be used by a single carer as the person can be easily raised, lowered, turned and traversed with no physical effort. Statutory service reviews conducted over the past 5 years have evidenced how care costs have been dramatically reduced with the right equipment provision and well-trained care staff (Phillips, Mellson, & Richardson, 2014).

Hoists and Specialist Walking Harnesses

Although hoists are traditionally perceived as the equipment of choice for transferring more dependent people, there has been an increase in the use of hoists with specialist walking harnesses to facilitate therapeutic intervention. Skilled use of a hoist with a walking or standing harness enables the therapist to test and improve trunk stability and mobility in standing. In addition, it reduces the risk of the therapist obtaining a musculoskeletal injury as there is no need to manually support a person during standing activities (Darragh et al., 2013). Walking harnesses have gained in popularity with the paediatric population. A standing or walking harness can be viewed as more acceptable than a fully supportive sling, as the children are still given the opportunity to take weight through their lower limbs, and can be used as part of a therapy programme and make transferring into a standing frame much easier.

The Number of Handlers Required When Using a Hoist

There are many publications providing advice on the supply and use of hoisting equipment; however, there is no authoritative guidance on the number of people required to safely operate such equipment. Historically, there has been a misinterpretation of the National Minimum Standards Regulations for Domiciliary Care, (Department of Health, 2003), which indicates that two people fully trained in current safe handling techniques and the equipment to be used are always involved in the provision of care when the need is identified from the manual handling risk assessment. The Standards clearly require that an individual risk assessment is carried out to determine the appropriate level of service provision, not a blanket policy applied regardless of the circumstances.

Phillips et al. (2014) found in their research that insufficient knowledge of specialist equipment and an often outdated and inflexible approach have led to too much generalisation regarding the perceived need for two carers as opposed to one.

Standing Equipment

For those people unable to achieve independent part or entire movement using small equipment, the therapist may consider a greater degree of manual intervention, to include larger handling equipment. Even at this stage, hoists are not the immediate answer for those with limited mobility. People are often able to stand for short periods if provided with a biomechanical advantage for sitting to standing. However, maintenance of standing or walking may be unreliable because of an underlying pathological condition, environmental risks or anxiety as a result of previous falls. Where standing and walking are unreliable but some weight bearing is possible, standing aids may be considered for certain transfers.

A mobile standing hoist (also called a stand aid, sit-to-stand lift, or standing and raising aid) is a specific type of mobile hoist used to move a person from one seated surface to another such as from a chair to a bed or a toilet. The hoist has a platform or footrest on which the person stands. The person is supported by a unique stand aid sling or vest fitted around the trunk and knee blocks to secure the legs in place. Standing hoists are only suitable for people who are partially weight bearing and those who can support most of their own weight while standing. Standing hoists are useful as they allow more access to person's clothing compared with a full hoist and have therapeutic benefit by providing an opportunity to increase weight-bearing tolerance. These hoists should only be used for transporting people for short distances, such as within a room or to an adjacent bathroom, and not for longer distances such as corridors.

It is important to remember that stand aids generally do not encourage normal movement patterns during the sit to stand movement; therefore thorough needs analysis is required to direct the use of these, either as an alternative to normal movement or as part of a rehabilitation programme. However, stand-assist devices may be preferable to incorrectly performed manual transfers.

Thorough assessment of the person's physical and cognitive ability is essential to ensure safety for all when using this equipment. The person must have active extension in the knees, be able to weight bear through feet and ankles and be able to sustain that activity. He or she must not have uncontrolled movements or variable spasms.

The therapist must understand the functions and purpose of the chosen equipment to prevent misuse and risk of injury; a stand aid must never be used for convenience as a means of saving time or in the absence of or as an alternative to a full hoisting system. Incorrect use can result in soft tissue damage caused by pressure on the knee pads and under the axilla if the sling rides up as a result of inadequate lower limb strength. The shoulder joint is particularly susceptible to injuries because of its great mobility and inherent instability.

Standing aids may be manual or electric. Manual stand aids require an individual to pull himself or herself into standing on a platform, to be transferred from one seated position to another. Electric stand aids pull the individual into a semistand or standing position by the use of specifically designed slings.

Competency to Use Equipment

Occupational therapists should only provide services and use techniques and equipment for which they are qualified by education, training or experience and are within their professional competence (College of Occupational Therapists, 2006). This is particularly true of moving and handling equipment, as professional qualification alone does not automatically imply expertise in this area. If occupational therapists are in any doubt or lack the expertise in assessing for and providing manual handling equipment, they should seek expert advice.

Providing Instruction to Others

Occupational therapists may often be perceived as the experts in the provision and use of equipment. However, professional status does not necessarily imply expertise in this area and training and delegation of tasks to others must be carefully considered within the realms of personal skills and knowledge. Where there is doubt about personal levels of experience or expertise in this area, the occupational therapist should not engage in training others or delegation of tasks related to moving and handling or use of equipment. Principles of delegation and guidance to others in moving and handling are discussed in *Manual Handling Guidance 3* (College of Occupational Therapists, 2006) and in the *Code of Ethics and Professional Conduct* (College of Occupational Therapists, 2015).

Providing instructions and information on the safe use of the equipment is crucial in establishing safe working systems and is a legal responsibility. Failure to provide instructions has resulted in liability – for example, *Colclough v Staffordshire County Council*, 1998, cited in Mandelstam (2009).

To help avoid confusion when using the equipment, especially hoists and slings, written instructions are often supported with photographs or drawings to incorporate into the handling management plan for reference by anyone providing care to the person. The therapist must also be aware of communication barriers and provide the information in alternative formats for the handlers and support workers, such as another language or large print. Pictorial instructions are particularly beneficial for those who are educationally disadvantaged. The College of Occupational Therapists (2006) recommends that any written instructions should:

- be clearly and simply phrased and formatted, without unnecessary jargon or detail;
- be accompanied by pictures or photographs if appropriate;
- include the contact details of the organisation of the prescribing occupational therapist;
- provide contact details in connection with broken or faulty equipment;
- indicate points of safe use and basic maintenance arrangements; and
- include the manufacturer's instructions.

TRAINING

Employers have a legal responsibility to provide a safe system of work and to provide adequate information, instruction, training and supervison to meet the health and safety requirements of their employees (HSE, 2012).

Management of Health and Safety at Work Regulations 1999 (Regulation 13(2) and (3)) require employers to provide health and safety training:

1. On recruitment
2. When risks change
3. To be repeated periodically as appropriate
4. To be adapted to take account of any changes required
5. To take place during working hours

Although there is no single institute or body that accredits moving and handling training courses, the National Back Exchange has produced professional standards and guidelines to ensure compliance with the law, meet requirements of best practice, meet continuing professional development (CPD) requirements and promote national consistency (National Back Exchange, 2010).

Training in principles of safe handling, techniques and equipment provision are all essential elements to ensure a safe system of work for both therapists and the people receiving therapy services. There is, however, evidence to show that educational moving and handling training in isolation is largely ineffective in changing working practises and reducing back pain and back injury, and often the principles learned during training are not applied in the working environment (Clemes, Haslam, & Haslam, 2010). Strategies found to be effective include making training more relevant to workers using task-specific examples and observation and reinforcement of training in the workplace (Clemes et al., 2010; College of Occupational Therapists, 2006; HSE, 2014a; National Back Exchange, 2010; Rose, 2011). Many organisations have recognised the need and adopted specific moving and handling practical training supplemented with the theory of safe handling. Effective training always needs to work alongside appropriate levels of workplace supervision. This will ensure that staff can be identified as competent and compliant to instruction and that this is being maintained throughout their undertaking of people-handling activities in the workplace (Phillips et al., 2014).

The Health and Safety Executive does not publish prescriptive guidance on what 'good' manual handling training courses should include or how long formal training should last, simply that training should be suitable for the individual, the tasks and the environment involved and should last long enough to cover all relevant information. The need to update training on a regular basis is strongly advised (National Back Exchange, 2010).

PRINCIPLES OF SAFER HANDLING

There is no single correct way to move a person or load (HSE, 2014a). Each situation will demand a different approach. Therefore basic principles are important to ensure optimum safety for handlers and the people being moved. A balanced approach to handling tasks, ensuring the rights of the person as well as the safety of handlers, encourages cooperation, reducing the risk of adverse reactions and the subsequent risk of injury (College of Occupational Therapists, 2006). These issues are illustrated in Practice Story 49.5.

LEGISLATION

The UK legislation regarding the moving and handling of people has two main objectives: to protect those doing the handling and those being handled. The Manual Handling Operations Regulations (HSE, 1992) within the United Kingdom sits under the umbrella of the Health and Safety at Work Act (1974), which is part of criminal law (College of Occupational Therapists, 2006). The Manual Handling Operations Regulations (HSE, 1992) were developed as a result of a European Union directive in Health and Safety for member states, established in 1990. For a long time specific sections of the legal framework for manual handling that pertained to the handling of inanimate objects in the workplace were taken and applied to the handling of people. Applied out of context, these regulations and directives were interpreted by some organisations in such a way as to make any manual handling too risky and this led to blanket no-lifting policies. People have been failed in terms of their rehabilitation and occupational potential because of the restrictions placed on employees; these policies have therefore been subject to scrutiny in the United Kingdom because of their perceived inflexible nature and lack of consideration for the human rights of the individual concerned.

The Manual Handling Operations Regulations 1992 (as amended) do not prohibit individual types of manual handling or endorse no-lifting policies. However, manual handling should be limited to those times when it cannot be avoided and only where the risk has been assessed and minimised. Employers cannot simply pass on the risk to employees, and a balanced approach to risk is advocated to ensure that workers are not required to perform tasks that put them at unreasonable risk.

A judicial review conducted in East Sussex in England reenforced the importance of an individual moving and handling assessment. Lord Chief Justice Mumby stated that 'the assessment must be focussed on the particular circumstances of the individual case. Just as context is everything so the individual assessment is all' (Mandelstam, 2011, p. 4). The court went on to state that blanket no-lifting policies would be highly likely to be unlawful. This is because such policies would prejudge the outcome of a moving and handling risk assessment (Mandelstam, 2011).

There are now many recent acts and rights that address this imbalance, and a much more realistic and holistic approach to moving and handling people now prevails. When handling people or enabling them to move themselves, an ergonomic assessment based on a range of relevant factors should be used to determine the risk and so point the way to how the risk can be reduced. Legislation such as The Care Act 2014, The Human Rights Act (1998), The National Health Service and Community Care Act (1990) and the Chronically Sick and Disabled Person's Act (1970) need to be considered in order to make suitable assessment of manual handling needs in the home, at work, in education institutions and when engaged in leisure pursuits. Application of these acts, alongside other key legislation relevant to manual handling in the United Kingdom outlined in Table 49.3, allows for balanced decision

---

PRACTICE STORY 49.5

Applying Principles of Safer Handling

Consent, cultural awareness and clear communication are paramount if changes to Caroline's environment and routine are implemented or equipment or alternative practices are introduced to ensure safer handling. The environment must be safe for carers to work in and they must be sufficiently trained to enable them to apply safe handling principles when working with Caroline. There needs to be a clear distinction between when therapy handling and care handling approaches are to be used. In addition, given her deteriorating condition, a falls management strategy may need to be considered. Careful introduction and use of equipment will reduce the risk of negative physiological or psychological responses during handling tasks. If after careful consideration of the situation, it is necessary to assist Caroline to move, either manually or with the use of equipment, the principles outlined in Fig. 49.11 should be applied to ensure best practice and safety during and after the manoeuvre.

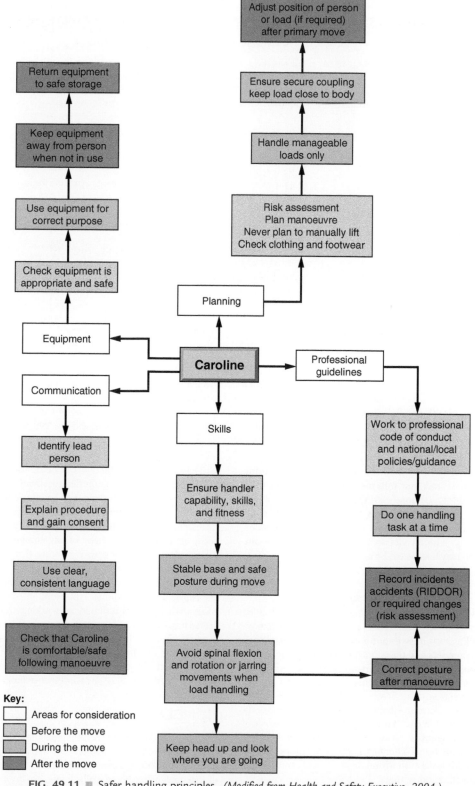

FIG. 49.11 ■ Safer handling principles. *(Modified from Health and Safety Executive, 2004.)*

TABLE 49.3	
Summary of UK Legislation Relevant to Moving and Handling	
Health and Safety at Work Act (HSWA), 1974	The employer is to ensure, so far as is reasonably practicable, the health, safety and welfare of all employees. Employees must also take reasonable care for the health and safety of themselves and others while at work.
Manual Handling Operations Regulations (MHOR), 1992	Employers must ensure that employees do the following: ■ Avoid hazardous manual handling ■ Assess that which cannot be avoided ■ Take action to reduce the risk to the lowest level reasonably practicable ■ Review risks regularly
Provision and Use of Work Equipment Regulations (PUWER), 1992	Employers must ensure that all work equipment is suitable for its intended use and is regularly serviced.
Workplace Health Safety and Welfare Regulations (W(HSW)R), 1992	Employers must ensure a suitable environment for employees to work in, including appropriate light, temperature, ventilation, flooring and suitable workstations (which may include treatment plinths, etc.)
Lifting Operations and Lifting Equipment Regulations (LOLER), 1998	Requires employers to ensure that lifting equipment: ■ is adequate for the tasks required; ■ is positioned/installed safely; ■ displays safe working load; ■ is in good working order when installed; and ■ is examined by a competent person every 6 months.
Human Rights Act (HRA), 1998	Most relevant to health and personal injury are the following: ■ Article 2 – right to life ■ Article 3 – prohibition of torture, inhumane or degrading treatment or punishment ■ Article 8 – right to respect for private and family life
Management of Health and Safety at Work Regulations (MHSWR), 1999	Requires employers to make suitable and sufficient assessment of all risks to the health and safety of employees while at work and provide training where appropriate.

making, when considering the needs of both the people being moved and those carrying out moving and handling tasks (Mandelstam, 2011). Dimond (2011) suggests it would be very difficult for occupational therapists to eliminate risk of injury through manual handling without an unacceptable reduction in person choice. Within civil law therapists have a duty of care to anyone who may be affected by a therapist's actions or omissions. Therefore therapists should aim to reduce risk of injury to the lowest level reasonably practicable (HSE, 2011), taking into account the needs and rights of the person.

It is not within the remit of this chapter to provide detailed descriptions and application of all legislation pertaining to moving and handling. It is important for occupational therapists to investigate and understand the context of national, regional and local legislation to protect themselves, carers and individuals under their care, when assessing handling risks and recommending intervention.

The reader is directed to Chapters 1 and 2 of the *Guide to the Handling of People* (6th ed.) (Smith, 2011) and to the College of Occupational Therapists' *Manual Handling Guidance 3*, (College of Occupational Therapists, 2006) for more detailed application of this legislation within the context of general treatment and rehabilitation settings.

The occupational therapist should also understand the importance of reporting injuries sustained at work, in order for safety and risk management to be improved. In the United Kingdom, the Reporting of Injuries Diseases and Dangerous Occurrences Regulations (1995 Reg. 3) requires employers to notify an enforcing authority of any employee injuries or illnesses originating at or caused by work that has an impact of longer than 3 days' duration.

To ensure best practice when dealing with the handling needs of people, interprofessional collaboration is essential and the occupational therapist should be working closely with other professionals, such as physiotherapists, back care/manual handling advisers and tissue viability nurses, to assess risks to people and staff and develop realistic and safe handling protocols. The consideration of legislation in relation to the moving and handling of a person is illustrated in Practice Story 49.6.

CONCLUSION

The issue of moving and handling people, ranging from facilitating independent movement to maximising occupational engagement, through assisted movement to enable completion of essential activities of daily living, to the use of specialist

PRACTICE STORY 49.6

Consideration of Relevant Legislation

The therapist will need to balance the wishes and needs of Caroline with the safety of the therapist, Caroline's husband and others involved in her care, taking account of relevant legislation. Central to this is adherence to the *Code of Ethics and Professional Conduct* (College of Occupational Therapists, 2015) in order to ensure the safety and dignity of Caroline and the safety of her carers. In addition, local policies and procedures related to moving and handling and equipment provision must be available and applied in all moving and handling situations. This applies to both general care handling and, more specifically, to therapeutic handling protocols.

Underpinning the occupational therapists safe practice will be up-to-date training in person handling, either through local service provision or attendance at a nationally recognised course. It is imperative that the therapist has experience and expertise in assessing for and recommending appropriate equipment and handling techniques if this is to be part of the intervention plan for Caroline. Along with this is the therapist's responsibility to ensure adequate training, assessment of competence and documentation in the safe use of any equipment and specific handling techniques recommended for carers.

---

techniques and equipment to move the more dependent person, has been addressed in this chapter. Introduction of the Manual Handling Operations Regulations and other guidance from 1992 onward focused assessment on reducing risks to professionals and carers who manually assist people to move. Since then, the introduction of the Human Rights Act (1998) has encouraged more balanced decision making (Mandelstam, 2011) in terms of the rights of both professionals and carers and the people who require their services and has encouraged a more collaborative approach between professionals and those receiving therapy or care. To provide therapists with a 'toolbox' of principles with which to analyse moving and handling tasks and establish appropriate levels of intervention across the continuum from care handling to treatment and therapeutic handling, the principles of risk assessment, legislation and safe handling along with principles of normal movement and biomechanics have been covered. Therapists are reminded that there is no one correct way to move or handle a person and because of this moving and handling should be guided by sound principles, to establish safe approaches within the boundaries of professional practice and expertise. Task and activity analysis forms the basis of occupational therapy practice, and this should always be applied in the field of people handling to guide decision making and enable the best outcome for both individuals and therapists and carers.

 http://evolve.elsevier.com/Curtin/OT

REFERENCES

Ahonen, M., Launis, M., & Kuorinka, T. (1989). *Ergonomic workplace analysis.* Transl. by Georgianna Oja. Helsinki, Finland: Ergonomics Section Finnish Institute of Occupational Health: (p. 33). Cited in Ramadan, P.A. & Ferreira, M. (2006). Risk Factors Associated with the Reporting of Musculoskeletal Symptoms in Workers at a Laboratory of Clinical Pathology. *Annals of Occupational Hygiene 50*(3), 297–303.

Alexander, P., & Johnson, C. (2011). *Manual handling of children.* Middlesex: BackCare.

Arnold, M., Radawiec, S., Campo, M., & Wright, L. R. (2011). Changes in functional independence measure ratings associated with a safe patient handling and movement program. *Rehabilitation Nursing, 36,* 138–144.

Benner, P. (1984). From Novice to Expert: Excellence and Power in Clinical Nursing Practice. Menlo-Park: Addison-Wesley. Cited by Crumpton E and Johnson C. In J Smith (Ed.), (2005) *The Guide to the Handling of People (5th ed) Middlesex.* BackCare and Royal College of Nursing.

Care Act (2014). Retrieved from, http://www.legislation.gov.uk/ukpga/2014/23/contents/enacted.

College of Occupational Therapists. (2006). *Manual handling guidance 3.* London: College of Occupational Therapists.

College of Occupational Therapists. (2015). *Code of ethics and professional conduct.* London: College of Occupational Therapists.

Clemes, S. A., Haslam, C. O., & Haslam, R. A. (2010). What constitutes effective manual handling training? A systematic review. *Occupational Medicine, 60,* 101–107.

Chartered Society of Physiotherapy (2003). *Guidance in Manual Handling for Physiotherapists.* London: Chartered Society of Physiotherapy.

Chronically Sick and Disabled Persons Act (1970). Retrieved from http://www.opsi.gov.uk/RevisedStatutes/Acts/ukpga/1970/cukpga_19700044_en_1.

Darragh, A. R., Campo, M. A., Frost, L., Miller, M., Pentico, M., & Argulis, H. (2013). Safe-patient handling equipment in therapy practice: Implications for rehabilitation. *American Journal of Occupational Therapy, 67,* 45–53.

Department of Health (2003). *Domiciliary Care National Minimum Standards.* Retrieved from http://www.housingcare.org/downloads/kbase/2553.pdf.

Dimond, B. (2011). *Legal aspects of occupational therapy.* London: Wiley-Blackwell.

European Agency for Safety and Health at Work, (2015). *Risk factors for musculoskeletal disorders in manual handling of loads.*

Retrieved from (2015). https://oshwiki.eu/wiki/Risk_factors_for_musculoskeletal_disorders_in_manual_handling_of_loads.

Fergusson Burt, L. (2007). The potential benefits of the introduction of electric profiling beds in preference to manually height-adjustable Kings Fund beds within the NHS: A literature review. Column, 19(2), 12–15.

Frost, L., & Barkley, W. M. (2012). Patient handling methods taught in occupational therapy curricula. American Journal of Occupational Therapy, 66, 463–470.

Glover, W., Sullivan, C., & Hague, J. (2005). Work related musculoskeletal disorders affecting members of the Chartered Society of Physiotherapy. London: Chartered Society of Physiotherapy.

Granger, C. V., Hamilton, B. B., Linacre, J. M., Heinemann, A. W., & Wright, B. D. (1993). Performance profiles of the functional independence measure. American Journal of Phys Med Rehabil, Vol. 72, p 84–89. Cited by Crumpton E and Johnson C. In: Smith J (Ed.) (2005). The Guide to the Handling of People (5th ed) Middlesex. BackCare and Royal College of Nursing.

Health and Safety Executive (1974). Health and Safety at Work Act. Retrieved from http://www.healthandsafety.co.uk/haswa.htm.

Health and Safety Executive (1992). Workplace (health safety and welfare) regulations. A short guide for managers. Retrieved from http://www.hse.gov.uk/pubns/indg244.pdf.

Health and Safety Executive (2003). Manual Handling Assessment Charts (MAC). London. HSE.

Health and Safety Executive (2004). Manual handling operations regulations 1992 (as amended): Guidance on regulations. L23. Norwich: HMSO.

Health and Safety Executive (2007). What can lead to back pain in the workplace. Retrieved from http://www.hse.gov.uk/msd/backpain/wkp.htm.

Health and Safety Executive (2008). Risk Management. Available from http://www.hse.gov.uk/risk/fivesteps.htm.

Health and Safety Executive (2012). Manual handling at work: A brief guide. Retrieved from http://www.hse.gov.uk/pubns/indg143.htm.

Health and Safety Executive (2013). Ergonomics and human factors at work: A brief guide. Retrieved from http://www.hse.gov.uk/pubns/indg90.htm.

Health and Safety Executive (2014a). FAQs – Manual handling and labelling loads. Retrieved from http://www.hse.gov.uk/msd/faq-manhand.htm.

Health and Safety Executive (2014b). Health and safety in care homes. Retrieved from www.hse.gov.uk/pUbns/priced/hsg220.pdf.

Health and Safety Executive (2015). What you need to do – Moving and handling. Retrieved from http://www.hse.gov.uk/healthservices/moving-handling-do.htm.

Hignet, S., & McAtamney, L. (2000). Rapid Entire Body Assessment. Applied Ergonomics, 31, 201–205.

Human Rights Act (1998). Retrieved from http://www.opsi.gov.uk/ACTS/acts1998/19980042.htm.

Ilmarinen, J. (1998). Work Ability Index. Finland: Finnish Institute of Occupational Health.

Johnson, C. (2011). Manual handling risk management. In J. Smith (Ed.), The guide to the handling of people (6th ed.). Middlesex: BackCare.

MacGregor, H. (2016). Moving and handling patients at a glance. Hoboken, NJ: Wiley-Blackwell.

Mandelstam, M. (2009). Community care practice and the law (4th ed.). London: Jessica Kingsley.

Mandelstam, M. (2011). Manual handling: Legal framework and balanced decision making. In J. Smith (Ed.), The guide to the handling of people (6th ed.). Middlesex: BackCare.

McAtamney, L., & Corlett, E. N. (1993). RULA: a survey method for the investigation of work-related upper limb disorders. Applied Ergonomics, 24, 91–99.

McMillan, I., & Carin-Levy, G. (2013). Tyldesley and Grieve's muscles, nerves and movement in human occupation (4th ed.). Oxford, UK: Blackwell Science.

National Back Exchange (2010). Standards in manual handling: Taining guidelines. Retrieved from http://www.nationalbackexchange.org/files/training_guidelines/training_guidelines.pdf.

NIOSH (1991). National Institute for Occupational Safety and Health: Safe Patient Handling and Movement (SPHM). http://www.cdc.gov/niosh/index.htm.

Norkin, C. C., & Levangie, P. K. (2011). Joint structure and function: A comprehensive analysis (5th ed.). Philadelphia: FA Davis.

OWAS (WinOWAS) (2007). A computerized system for the analysis of work postures. Available at; http://turva1.mc.tut.fi/owas/index.html.

Passier, L., & McPhail, S. (2011). Work-related injuries amongst occupational therapists: A preliminary investigation. British Journal of Occupational Therapy, 74(3), 143–147.

Phillips, J., Mellson, J., & Richardson, N. (2014). It takes two? Exploring the manual handling myth. Wakefield, West Yorkshire: Prism Medical UK. Retrieved from, https://prismmedical.co.uk/wp-content/uploads/.../Does-it-Take-Two.pdf.

Rose, P. (2011). Manual handling risk management. In J. Smith (Ed.), The guide to the handling of people (6th ed.). Middlesex: BackCare.

Smith, J. (Ed.). (2011). The guide to the handling of people (6th ed.). Middlesex: BackCare/Royal College of Nursing.

Straker, L., Burgess-Limerick, R., Pollock, C., & Egeskov, R. (2004). A randomized and controlled trial of a participative ergonomics intervention to reduce injuries associated with manual tasks: physical risk and legislative compliance. Ergonomics, 47(2), 166–188.

Sturman-Floyd, M. (2011). Reducing the incidence and risk of pressure sores, manual handling loading and carer costs using 'In-bed systems'. Retrieved from, (2011). http://www.communityequipment.org.uk/wp-content/uploads/SturmanFloyd-paper-2011-Complete-final-paper.pdf.

Waters, T. R., & Rockefeller, K. (2010). Safe patient handling for rehabilitation professionals. Rehabilitation Nursing, 35, 216–222.

World Health Organization (2002). International Classification of Functioning, Disability and Health. Retrieved from http://www.who.int/classifications/icf/icfbeginnersguide.pdf.

World Health Organization (2012). International classification of functioning, disability and health. Retrieved from http://www.who.int/classifications/icf/en.

ENABLING SKILLS AND STRATEGIES - EXCERPTS FROM BONUS PRACTICE STORIES

ⓔ [Read the full practice stories on Evolve at http://evolve.elsevier.com/Curtin/OT]

ⓔ ## MRS TREMBLAY: A PRACTICE STORY OF A PERSON EXPERIENCING REHABILITATION FOLLOWING A STROKE - ENABLING SKILLS AND STRATEGIES

DOROTHY KESSLER, KATRINE SAUVÉ-SHENK, & VALERIE METCALFE

Part 1: Acute Care

Implement the plan

1. Bed Positioning: I provided Mrs Tremblay with a positioning aid to be used when in bed to support her left arm and shoulder in a neutral position ...

ⓔ **To read the full Practice Story and complete a reflective exercise please visit Evolve at http://evolve.elsevier.com/Curtin/OT**

ⓔ ## KARIN: A PRACTICE STORY OF A PERSON EXPERIENCING RHEUMATOID ARTHRITIS - ENABLING SKILLS AND STRATEGIES

MATHILDA BJÖRK & INGRID THYBERG

Part 1: Initial Diagnosis

Implement the plan. I provided Karin with a wrist support bandage to her right wrist. The bandage was easy for Karin to put on herself. She stated that she really liked the black colour since it looked sporty and gave a more active impression than the skin coloured. I recommended that she use the wrist bandage when performing heavy activities at home or at work ...

ⓔ **To read the full Practice Story and complete a reflective exercise please visit Evolve at http://evolve.elsevier.com/Curtin/OT**

ⓔ ## ANGELA: A PRACTICE STORY OF A PERSON EXPERIENCING PALLIATIVE CARE - ENABLING SKILLS AND STRATEGIES

DEIDRE MORGAN & CELIA MARSTON

Implement the plan. The aim of the intervention strategies were to restore physical components of Angela's function based upon motor learning theory. I encouraged Angela to participate as much as she was able with her self-care, in particular to eat and dressing herself with minimal or no assistance ...

ⓔ **To read the full Practice Story and complete a reflective exercise please visit Evolve at http://evolve.elsevier.com/Curtin/OT**

Section 7

REFLECTING ON PRACTICE

50 REFLECTING ON PRACTICE

GENEVIÈVE PÉPIN

Abstract

Reflective practice is one of the distinguishing features between a technician and a professional. It helps to make the link among theory, evidence, and practice, supporting therapeutic decision making. It is essential to competent occupational therapy practice. In doing so, reflective practice can support practitioners in implementing the last two action points of the Canadian Practice Process Framework (CPPF), evaluating the outcomes of the therapeutic process and concluding or pursuing the interventions.

How reflective practice supports professional decision making associated with these two action points of the CPPF will be illustrated in this chapter. First, reflective practice is described. This is followed by identifying the underpinnings of reflective practice and importance of critical reflection and intuition to competent occupational therapy practice. Then the different levels of reflection are presented, described and illustrated, along with strategies to develop and apply reflection in practice. A model of reflection is presented and applied to a practice story illustrating the journey of Joel, an occupational therapist, in evaluating occupational therapy intervention and deciding to conclude the intervention.

KEY POINTS

- Reflective practice is an essential characteristic of a competent therapist.

- Reflective practice requires therapists to critically think about their actions and to identify new strategies to further enhance their practice.

- Reflective practice can be abstract, less tangible and more difficult to understand but it can be learned, improved and developed.

- Reflective practice can guide and frame the therapeutic process.

- There are different levels of reflective practice, and therapists should work towards developing critical reflection.

- Gibbs' model of reflection is a tool that enables students and therapists to become reflective practitioners.

INTRODUCTION

The last two action points of the Canadian Practice Process Framework (CPPF) are about evaluating the outcomes of the therapeutic process and concluding or pursuing the interventions. When evaluating the outcomes, the therapist, collaboratively with the person receiving therapy services, determines whether the goals have been met or if new goals must be considered and new interventions developed and implemented. In the next action point the therapist and person decide together either to continue the therapeutic process or terminate it. In this chapter, Joel, an occupational therapist practising in palliative care, has been working with Janet for a few months and together they have decided to end the occupational therapy intervention. Principles of reflective practice will be linked to the evaluation of the therapeutic process and integrated in Joel's practice story. Finally, strategies to apply reflective practice will be identified.

REFLECTIVE PRACTICE

To determine whether the therapy process should cease or continue and assess the quality and relevance of the interventions put into place, it is essential to take the time to review the intervention plan and think back on therapeutic goals, as well as how therapy unfolded. Reflective practice is the process through which this is achieved.

Developing a reflective approach is an essential component of occupational therapy practice to ensure therapists remain lifelong learners and continue to develop and consolidate their competencies (Larkin & Pépin, 2013). There are several other reasons why reflective practice is important:

■ It has been identified as a necessary characteristic of competent professional practice (Johnson & Bird, 2006; Wald & Reis, 2010).
■ It contributes significantly to developing professionalism (Mann, Gordon & MacLeod, 2009; Schaub-de Jong, Schönrock-Adema, Dekker, Verkerk, & Cohen-Schotanus, 2011).
■ It improves practice skills, strengthens problem solving (Aukes, Geertsma, Cohen-Schotanus, Zwierstra, & Slaets, 2007), and supports flexible thinking and lifelong learning (Epstein, 2008; Mamede & Schmidt, 2004; Mann et al., 2009; Sandars, 2009).
■ It enables therapists, and students, to evaluate their strengths and limitations, and identify relevant learning needs (Mann et al., 2009), and in doing so promotes an individualised professional development planning (Fitzgerald, Moores, Coleman, & Fleming, 2015).
■ It improves self-awareness (Hays & Gay, 2011) and as a result anchors person-centred practice.

In practice settings, reflective practice is used to appraise and critique therapeutic interventions and processes. When reflecting, therapists think critically and ask themselves questions such as *what* (went well, did not go well, happened throughout therapy, is really going on in therapy), *why* (did things unfold in a specific way, were actions chosen) and *how* (can things improve, be done differently to reach better outcomes for the person). However, reflective practice can be hard to define and understand; it can be an abstract concept. Yet it is expected that occupational therapy students will begin developing reflective practice from the start of their occupational therapy degree.

Practice Story 50.1 illustrates the application of reflective practice within an occupational therapy context. In this practice

---

PRACTICE STORY 50.1

Joel and Janet

As Joel was completing his notes about Janet, he thought back on the intervention plan and the occupational therapy process. He initially thought of the referral he received and when he first met Janet:

> Joel had been working with Janet, a 79-year-old woman who lived in a single terrace house with Paul, her husband of 57 years, in an inner city suburb. Janet and Paul had a daughter and a son living close by and who were very involved and supportive of their parents. They had three grandchildren and a close circle of friends who they met regularly for dinner or coffee.
>
> Janet had ongoing heart problems and was diagnosed with slow-progressing carcinoid cancer with tumours along her small intestine. The first course of action after the diagnosis of this cancer would usually have been surgery to remove the tumours; however, Janet's general health was too precarious and her oncologist advised against

> it. Therefore Janet was undertaking a course of radiation therapy and was monitored closely by the medical team. The radiation was making Janet very tired and weak. She was quite concerned about the long-term side effects of the radiation and the impact that not having the tumours removed would have on her overall prognosis. Joel met Janet and her husband after he received a referral for home modifications and equipment provision to help Janet complete her activities of daily living (ADL) and other occupations. During the first visit, Joel took the time to explain his role and why he was visiting Janet and Paul in their home. They took Joel around the house and showed him each room. Their main concerns at this stage were the separate toilet room, and the small size of the shower. Joel was able to observe Janet and how she moved around the house. He noted that Janet had difficulty transitioning from a sitting to standing position and going up and down stairs; this included the four steps at the front and the back of the house. He also noticed

PRACTICE STORY 50.1

Joel and Janet (Continued)

that Janet held on to benches or leaned against walls when she was in a standing position for several minutes. After assessing Janet's occupational performance and her environment, Joel and Janet agreed on the following therapeutic goals:

- To increase Janet's independence in performing her ADL
- To improve Janet's engagement in meaningful occupations

Joel then remembered his next home visit, where he had a plan to propose to Janet and Paul.

He suggested that Janet would benefit from the installation of hand rails to help her move up and down the steps at the front and back of the house. He also suggested some equipment and structural changes to the toilet and bathroom to help Janet more safely use the toilet and to have a shower. He advised Janet to use a walking frame as this could reduce the fatigue she experienced when standing for long periods. Joel also thought that if Janet used the walking frame, she and Paul would be able to walk to the shops, which were just around the corner from their house. Janet agreed to have the rails installed, try the equipment and for the structural changes to be done to the bathroom and toilet.

In the following weeks, the equipment was provided and trialled. Joel did some teaching and training on how to use the equipment and he made sure he involved Paul so he could help Janet when needed. In Joel's opinion, there were ups and downs throughout the intervention process where the equipment was not used or was used inappropriately. At times, he felt there might be a lack of motivation or perhaps a lack of understanding; so he provided further education about the appropriate and safe use of the equipment to Janet and Paul. He also provided Janet further information, even, in his enthusiasm, copies of journal articles he had read that described the effectiveness and the impact of using adequate equipment on function and independence in doing every day activities. On reflection, he was not sure that providing the journal articles was the most effective way of providing education to Janet and Paul.

When the home modification started, Janet and Paul were very excited. While the construction took place, Janet and Paul stayed at their friends' house who happened to be travelling overseas. Staying in their friends' house was convenient as Janet and Paul's children and grandchildren could visit them, and Janet and Paul were able to walk around the neighbourhood and meet their friends. It also allowed Janet to rest and deal with the effects of the radiotherapy. Her oncologist was relatively pleased with the results, but he decided a second course of radiation was needed. He kept monitoring Janet's condition closely. Interestingly, none of the equipment provided by Joel was taken to the house and used. Janet told Joel she could not bring anything with her as there was not enough space in their friends' house.

While Janet and Paul stayed at their friends' house, the home modifications were completed. They were both satisfied with the changes made to the toilet room and the shower. The bathroom and toilet room were made larger so that there was more space to move around. Hand rails were installed on both the front and back steps. Janet also had a walking frame, which she could use when she felt she needed more support.

Joel then began to reflect on his final home visit:

During this visit, Joel, Janet and Paul discussed the reasons for the occupational therapy referral, which were: home modifications and equipment provision to help Janet complete her ADL and other meaningful occupations. Joel mentioned that when he first met Janet and Paul, Janet's access to the toilet and the shower were the main problems that they wanted addressed. The changes made to the house combined with the equipment provided enabled Janet to complete her ADL, including toileting and showering, and participate in other important occupations, such as running errands, seeing their family and socialising with friends. Janet admitted that it had taken her some time to get used to the idea that she had reached a stage in her life where she needed to have those modifications done to her home. Intellectually she understood how to use the equipment and its value, but emotionally she did not want to be that person who needed special equipment yet. Together, as the treatment goals were met, Janet and Joel decided to end the occupational therapy intervention.

As Joel was reflecting on the intervention he provided Janet and Paul while he wrote his discharge summary, key moments in the therapeutic process stood out. For example, he remembered feeling a bit disappointed and surprised that Janet did not use the equipment he provided. His first reaction was to wonder what he could do differently to make sure Janet used the equipment he provided her. Joel realised he had matured as a therapist. Instead of thinking that the problem was with Janet because she was not using the equipment, he thought of other actions he could implement to encourage her to use the equipment. Previously, he would have tried to fix the situation, do something about it as the therapist and expert in occupational performance and therapy. Joel still saw himself as a doer and as a person who listened to his instincts when deciding on a course of action. However, he often felt that listening to his instinct was at odds with the need to support occupational therapy practice with evidence and research. As he gained more experience, he learned to combine his instincts and feelings with recent and relevant evidence to support his decision-making process. Remembering his last conversation with Janet, Joel realised he spent too much time listening to his own instincts and not enough listening to Janet's feelings. This realisation left Joel feeling a bit uncomfortable.

story, Joel was an occupational therapist who worked in palliative care. He just returned from his last home visit for Janet and Paul, a couple to whom he was providing services, and he was writing his discharge summary.

Intuition

What Joel meant by listening to his instinct when making a decision can be referred to as intuition. Witteman, Spaanjaars, & Aarts (2012) have defined intuition as a process that occurs without a person's awareness and that is akin to feelings or emotions. For example, in Joel's story, when he found out Janet was not using the equipment, he *felt* something was not working and that there might be a lack of motivation or understanding and this *feeling* guided his interventions. Intuition, or the feeling or sense that something is going on or that things are not what they appear to be, does not rely on evidence or on a structured and organised critique or analysis of a practice situation. As such, intuition has been criticised by some researchers (English, 1993; Gaudiano, Brown, & Miller, 2011) as lacking rigour and not relying on current evidence, whereas others have acknowledged its value (Welsh & Lyons, 2001; Witteman et al., 2012), especially when combined with experience and a more structured reflective practice (Schön, 1995). Interestingly, intuition has been associated to reflecting in action, which can be considered as the basis of reflective practice (Welsh & Lyons, 2001).

Critically and Consciously Thinking

Reflective practice involves the process of thinking critically and consciously about a series of actions, or in Joel's case, his occupational therapy practice and interventions. Thinking critically means that a therapist or a student takes the time to think about what happened in therapy, questions a course of action and interventions and considers alternative actions and their impacts on the person receiving therapy services and on the outcome of therapy. Nolan and Sim (2011) have summarised reflective practice as being able to

> Identify one's own values, beliefs and assumptions, consider other perspectives or alternative ways of viewing the world; being able to identify what perspectives are missing from one's account; identify how one's own views can have a particular bias that privileges one view over another; perceive contradictions and inconsistencies in one's own account of events; and imagine other possibilities. (p. 123)

When Joel realised Janet was not using the equipment he provided her with, he identified his own values, beliefs and assumptions. As he mentioned, earlier in his career he might have *assumed* that the problem was with Janet, that perhaps she was not motivated enough. Joel appears to *value* Janet's independence. He seems to *believe* in empowering Janet and supporting her to engage in important occupations. Joel also *considered* other perspectives and wondered what was missing, what Janet needed from him to be motivated to use the equipment safely.

As a result, he provided further information and training about the equipment and also gave Janet some literature about what she was using and why they were useful tools to help her reengage with the occupations that were important to her.

The application of Nolan and Sim's (2011) approach to reflective practice can help identify other questions Joel could have asked himself. For example, what was missing from the situation? What were Janet's perspectives and views? What were those of her husband and close relatives and friends? Although Joel reflected on a specific situation within the therapeutic process, a critique of his reflective practice could suggest Joel takes the time to talk to Janet and find out her views to understand how she felt about having rails added to the front and back of her house. How did she feel about going out using a walking frame? Also, have Joel's own views influenced the interventions, narrowing the opportunities to consider other possibilities? We could also recommend Joel explore Paul's perspectives and explore if there were discrepancies between Janet's and Paul's views of the intervention plan and equipment provided.

Four Levels of Reflection

As mentioned earlier, reflective practice can be an abstract concept that might be hard to grapple with. The ability to critically reflect on occupational therapy practice can be difficult to acquire and, although some people are naturally reflective, others might find it more challenging (Larkin & Pepin, 2013). Thankfully it is possible to learn and develop reflective thinking (Kek & Huijser, 2011). Kember, McKay, Sinclair, & Wong, (2008) have described the following four levels of reflection.

Habitual action/nonreflection
Understanding
Reflection
Critical reflection

Habitual Action/Nonreflection

At the level of *nonreflection,* there can be very detailed descriptions of a situation or circumstances related to a particular experience. In providing a detailed description only, there is no opportunity for deeper thinking and no thoughts are given to imagine the other possibilities mentioned by Nolan and Kim (2011). The example in Practice Story 50.2 illustrates Joel's reflective thinking at a *nonreflection* level.

Understanding

At the level of *understanding* there is the emergence of an attempt to try and understand what the situation truly is, including further characteristics, perspectives and opinions. In Practice Story 50.3 there is an example of Joel's reflective thinking at a level of *understanding.*

Reflection

The level of actual *reflection* is when knowledge and information are integrated with a real-life circumstance (or a practice situation) and personal experiences. This is when 'personal insights that go beyond book theory' are demonstrated (Kember et al., 2008, p. 374). Joel demonstrated this level of *reflection* when thinking back about a home visit; this is presented in Practice Story 50.4.

Critical Reflection

The last level of reflective thinking is *critical reflection,* and it happens when there is a 'transformation of perspective' (Kember et al., 2008, p. 374). In other words, *critical reflection* occurs when there is evidence of a change in thinking and perspective. It also implies that personal values, beliefs and assumptions are brought to a conscious level and addressed to lead to the transformation identified by Kember et al. In Practice Story 50.5 there is an example of Joel's *critical reflection.*

PRACTICE STORY 50.2

Joel's Reflective Thinking at Habitual Action/Nonreflection Level

Today I went to Janet's and Paul's house to verify how Janet was doing and how the new equipment I provided – the walking frame and the hand rails at the front and the back of the house, the shower stool and the rails in the shower – was helping her. When I asked Janet about the equipment, Paul answered. He said she was not really using the walker and was not getting out that much. I asked Janet why she was not using the equipment and she said she was a bit tired with the radiation therapy and was not really strong enough to go out. Paul was very enthusiastic about the walking frame and the hand rails, demonstrating to me and to Janet how easy it was to move around and go up and down the steps. I agreed with Paul and reminded Janet about the goals that we identified on our first visit.

PRACTICE STORY 50.3

Joel's Reflective Thinking at a Level of Understanding

After the home visit, I wrote my progress notes and realised that I did not gather as much information as I could have. It felt like Janet and I did not go into enough depth. I think I probably asked too many questions and provided too many reasons why she should use the equipment. I probably did not let Janet think for herself and tell me her views and opinions. I know the equipment provided will help her engage in important occupations and that she will not get as tired as when she does not use the equipment. I tried to convince her, with the help of her husband, instead of giving her time to think and respond.

PRACTICE STORY 50.4

Joel's Reflective Thinking at a Level of Reflection

I don't think I was being person-centred today during the home visit. I don't think I was being a good occupational therapist. I realise now that I actually felt uncomfortable in this situation. I am a doer, I thrive on action, and I found it hard to slow down and take the time to talk to Janet and reconsider the plan. Especially when I knew what I had prescribed was the best equipment for her. I let myself get carried away by Paul's enthusiasm and probably pressured Janet into using the equipment. Although providing information and more education about the equipment is a good strategy, I should have been more person-centred and focused on Janet's point of view.

PRACTICE STORY 50.5

Joel's Reflective Thinking at a Level of Critical Reflection

After my last home visit, I know that in the future I need to change the way I go about encouraging the people I work with to use the equipment I prescribe them. I need to change what I do and mostly how I do it to ensure they are engaging in therapy with me – that we work collaboratively. First of all I need to put aside my own ideas and beliefs and put myself in their shoes. I need to show more empathy. This means putting my occupational therapy knowledge aside and taking the time to involve them in the changes I am introducing. I have to realise that having changes made to people's homes or to their way of maintaining their independence might be difficult to accept for a variety of reasons. It was only during our last therapy session that Janet told me how she felt. I was shocked. I had not once taken the time to ask or let Janet tell me how she felt. I must stop myself from trying to 'fix' things. I provided Janet with more training and journal articles to read to highlight my point when what she needed was time to adjust – both strategies, which, on reflection, were not appropriate for Janet and where she was at. I found some interesting articles and textbooks about person-centred practice and how to empower people in decision-making processes, and on therapeutic use of self. I found out about the Intentional Relationship model (Taylor, 2008) and tools to identify preferred therapeutic modes and how to adapt these modes to each person to facilitate a more collaborative relationship. This new knowledge will be useful for me.

Transformation of Perspectives

Knowing and gaining a better understanding of how to think critically and reflect in practice using the four levels of reflection described by Kember et al. (2008) provides clearer information about how to develop a reflective practice. Therapists and students should strive to achieve the level of *critical reflection* and aim for the transformation mentioned by Kember et al. (2008) even if this transformation is at times uncomfortable. This is illustrated in Joel's story when he realised he had not used a person-centred approach and had failed to discuss the impact of the changes he was making to Janet's home and life with her. In Joel's case the transformation of perspectives implied learning about a new model that would strengthen his therapeutic use of self.

GIBBS' MODEL OF REFLECTION

Once therapists and students develop and further enhance their reflective abilities, it is important to put them in to practice and apply them to the therapeutic process. In doing so it becomes possible to evaluate the outcomes of the therapeutic process and to determine whether it is appropriate to conclude or pursue interventions.

There are different models of reflective practice in the literature. Graham Gibbs (1988) developed a model of reflection (Fig. 50.1) based on an iterative approach. It includes six steps, and each step informs the next. Gibbs' model was a precursor to others' work and claims that reflective practice should challenge assumptions and explore new ideas, that it encourages the

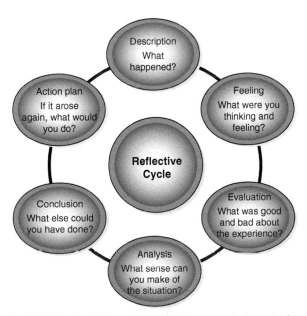

FIG. 50.1 ■ Gibbs' model of reflection (1988). *(From Larkin & Pépin, 2013, p. 39.)*

identification of strengths and limitations as well as the identification and implementation of actions to keep improving practice. By integrating essential elements of reflection and reflective thinking, Gibbs' model provides a framework to apply reflective practice to specific circumstances.

Gibbs' model rests on the evolution of levels of reflection mentioned earlier in this chapter. First, it starts with the description of an experience. Then the practitioner has to identify and explore the feelings and thoughts associated with the detailed experience. In completing this second step of the model, the practitioner starts to question what happens and why it happened in a specific way. It is the first step of challenging assumptions.

The third step is when the combination of factual information and emotional content is evaluated to determine the strengths and limitations of the overall experience. There needs to be some reflection on the experience to identify what went well and what did not go well. The fourth step consists of analysing the experience. This is when the practitioner tries to make sense of the experience. It means further reflection is done to identify reasons to explain what has happened. Why were there successes and why were there challenges? It is about trying to find true and honest justifications.

Once the analysis of the experience has been completed, it is time to answer the question: *What else could have been done?* This refers to the ability to imagine new perspectives and possibilities identified earlier by Nolan and Sim (2011). This is also where the transformation of perspectives discussed by Kember et al. (2008) in the description of *critical reflection* emerges. Finally, and to confirm and crystallise the transformation, an *action plan* is developed and made ready to be implemented. The integration of 'new knowledge, behaviours and skills learnt from the experience' translates in to clear strategies and actions that will enable the practitioner to 'approach a similar experience in the future from a different perspective' (Larkin & Pépin, 2013, p. 38).

Gibbs' model of reflective practice can be used when reflecting about a specific therapeutic event or when reflecting about an entire occupational therapy process. As such it is possible to make interesting links between Gibbs' model and the eight action points of the CPPF, especially when evaluating the outcome of the therapy (Action Point 7) and deciding whether or not to conclude the therapy (Action Point 8). Using Joel's example, Gibbs' model will be used in conjunction with the CPPF to help decide if the therapeutic process should be concluded or if it should continue to evaluate the outcome of therapy (Practice Story 50.6).

CONCLUSION

Reflective practice is an essential characteristic of a competent occupational therapist. Being a reflective practitioner means that a therapist or a student is able to use intuition, knowledge, evidence and expertise and critical thinking and transform their perspectives to guide and inform practice to reach the best outcomes possible for a person. Reflective practice enables occupational therapists and occupational therapy students to provide strong justifications for their choices and actions confidently and be accountable for their interventions to the people receiving their services and to their colleagues.

Reflective practice, although it can be an abstract concept that is difficult to gasp, can be learned and developed. Some of the definitions, examples and models presented in this chapter are intended to provide further information and clarity as well as strategies to integrate reflective practice in to the implementation and evaluation of the therapeutic process.

PRACTICE STORY 50.6

Combining the CPPF and Gibbs' Model of Reflection

As Joel and Janet engaged in the occupational therapy process, Joel collected relevant information about Janet, her occupations and environment as well as her conditions and their effects on her occupational performance (Action Point 1: Enter/initiate and Action Point 2: Set the stage). Assessments were completed to determine goals and interventions strategies. The main goals and reason why Janet was referred to Joel were to provide equipment and determine the home modifications that would enable Janet to do her ADL and other meaningful occupations without assistance (Action Point 3: Assess/evaluate). The environment needed to be assessed and a home visit was necessary for Joel to fully understand and consider Janet's environment and how it influenced her occupational performance (Action Point 3: Assess/evaluate). An action plan was then developed, presented to Janet and her husband, considering the implication of the home modifications for both of them (Action Point 4: Agree on objectives, plan), and implemented (Action Point 5: Implement plan). During the home visits, Joel was able to monitor Janet's progress towards her goals. Further education and information was provided about the safe use of equipment when Joel found out Janet did not use the walking frame, shower stools and hand rails (Action Point 6: Monitor/modify). As Janet started to use the equipment provided safely and could complete her ADL and reengage in meaningful occupations, the home modifications were completed, further enabling her occupational performance. When goals were met and previous occupational issues had been resolved through the implementation of the plan and there were no further occupational issues to address, the therapeutic process was concluded (Action Point 7: Evaluate outcome and Action Point 8: Conclude/exit).

Throughout the implementation of the different action points, Joel, as a reflective practitioner, could continuously collect information to be able to provide a detailed description of the therapeutic process and interventions (*Description*). He could take the time to identify and explore his feeling as therapy unfolded (*Feeling*). This ensured Joel's own views and assumptions did not overly influence the therapeutic process. The *Evaluation* of the therapeutic process was an opportunity

for Joel to reflect on the entire intervention with Janet. This was where he was able to identify the strengths and limitations of the therapeutic process. Including Janet's husband early on in the therapeutic process was positive because he was able to better support his wife. Joel's knowledge of equipment provision and use of evidence to support his decision were strengths of the therapeutic process. Other strengths of the therapeutic process were Joel's expertise and his ability to assess Janet's level of function to determine that the goals had been met.

By reflecting further on the therapeutic process, Joel was able to identify some limitations and things that did not go as well as they could have. He realised that he did not spend enough time setting the stage with Janet (Action Point 2). He did not take enough time to ask Janet's opinions and views of her occupational story. He did not know what she really perceived as being her occupational issues. He realised also that he did not structure his intervention plan around a specific occupational therapy model or framework.

The next step for Joel was to make sense of what happened and provide reasons and justifications for what occurred (or did not occur) in the therapeutic process (*Analysis*). Was he too focused on fixing what he saw as problems? Did he have sufficient knowledge of occupational therapy theories and models? Did he have the level of communication skills required to find out Janet's perspectives and true opinions about her occupational issues and about the interventions that were going to be implemented? In the *Conclusion* step of Gibbs' model, Joel identified what could have been done differently to improve the therapy outcomes. He could identify skills that he needed to further develop and the resources and strategies that he needed. Finally, Joel had put an *action plan* together for him to ensure he had the skills and knowledge to set the stage better in the future. He knew there were strengths in his approach to therapy and he knew how to ensure he maintained and upgraded these strengths. He also knew what he needed to improve and had identified a course of action to implement the improvements. He had transformed his perspectives and gained new knowledge and skills, which he would use in the future.

ADL, Activity of daily living; *CPPF,* Canadian Practice Process Framework.

ACKNOWLEDGEMENT

I acknowledge the input of my colleague Helen Larkin, who willingly discussed, and assisted with the development of, this chapter.

 http://evolve.elsevier.com/Curtin/OT

REFERENCES

Aukes, L. C., Geertsma, J., Cohen-Schotanus, J., Zwierstra, R. P., & Slaets, J. P. (2007). The development of a scale to measure personal reflection in medical practice and education. *Medical Teacher, 29*, 77–82.

English, I. (1993). Intuition as a function of the expert nurse: A critique of Benner's novice to expert model. *Journal of Advanced Nursing, 18*, 387–393.

Epstein, R. M. (2008). Reflection, perception and the acquisition of wisdom. *Medical Education, 2008*(42), 1048–1050.

Fitzgerald, C., Moores, A., Coleman, A., & Fleming, J. (2015). Supporting new graduate professional development: A clinical learning framework. *Australian Occupational Therapy Journal, 62*, 13–20.

Gaudiano, B. A., Brown, L. A., & Miller, W. M. (2011). Let your intuition be your guide? Individual differences in the evidence-based practice attitudes of psychotherapists. *Journal of Evaluation in Clinical Practice, 17*, 628–634.

Gibbs, G. (1988). *Learning by doing: A guide to teaching and learning methods.* Oxford, UK: Further Education Unit, Oxford Brookes University.

Hays, R., & Gay, S. (2011). Reflection or 'pre-reflection': What are we actually measuring in reflective practice? *Medical Education, 45*, 116–118.

Johnson, C., & Bird, J. (2006). How to …: Teach reflective practice. *Education for Primary Care, 17*, 640–642.

Kek, M., & Huijser, H. (2011). The power of problem-based learning in developing critical thinking skills: Preparing students for tomorrow's digital futures in today's classrooms. *Higher Education Research & Development, 30*(3), 329–341.

Kember, D., McKay, J., Sinclair, K., & Wong, F. K. Y. (2008). A four-category scheme for coding and assessing the level of reflection in written work. *Assessment & Evaluation in Higher Education, 33*(4), 369–379.

Larkin, H., & Pépin, G. (2013). Becoming a reflective practitioner. In K. Stagnitti, A. Schoo, & D. Welch (Eds.), *Clinical and fieldwork placement in the health professions* (2nd ed., pp. 31–42). Melbourne: Oxford University Press.

Mamede, S., & Schmidt, H. G. (2004). The structure of reflective practice in medicine. *Medical Education, 38*, 1302–1308.

Mann, K., Gordon, J., & MacLeod, A. (2009). Reflection and reflective practice in health professions education: A systematic review. *Advances in Health Sciences Education, 14*, 595–621.

Nolan, A., & Sim, J. (2011). Exploring and evaluating levels of reflection in pre-service early childhood teachers. *Australasian Journal of Early Childhood, 36*(3), 122–130.

Sandars, J. (2009). The use of reflection in medical education: AMEE Guide No. 44. *Medical Teacher, 31*, 685–695.

Schaub-de Jong, M. A., Schönrock-Adema, J., Dekker, H., Verkerk, M., & Cohen-Schotanus, J. (2011). Development of a student rating scale to evaluate teachers' competencies for facilitating reflective learning. *Medical Education, 45*, 155–165.

Schön, D. D. A. (1995). *Reflective practitioner: How professionals think in action.* Aldershot: Arena.

Taylor, R. (2008). The Intentional Relationship Model: occupational therapy and use of self. Philadelphia: F.A.: Davis Co.

Wald, H. S., & Reis, S. P. (2010). Beyond the margins: Reflective writing and development of reflective capacity in medical education. *Journal of General Internal Medicine, 25*, 746–749.

Welsh, I., & Lyons, C. M. (2001). Evidence-based care and the case for intuition and tacit knowledge in clinical assessment and decision making in mental health nursing practice: An empirical contribution to the debate. *Journal of Psychiatric and Mental Health Nursing, 8*, 299–305.

Witteman, C., Spaanjaars, N., & Aarts (2012). Clinical intuition in mental health care: A discussion and focus groups. *Counselling Psychology Quarterly, 25*(1), 19–29.

REFLECTING ON PRACTICE - EXCERPTS FROM BONUS PRACTICE STORIES

 [Read the full practice stories on Evolve at http://evolve.elsevier.com/Curtin/OT]

MRS TREMBLAY: A PRACTICE STORY OF A PERSON EXPERIENCING REHABILITATION FOLLOWING A STROKE - REFLECTING ON PRACTICE

DOROTHY KESSLER, KATRINE SAUVÉ-SHENK, & VALERIE METCALFE

Part 1: Acute Care

Conclude/exit. Mrs Tremblay was discharged from the acute care unit and transferred to inpatient stroke rehabilitation at another facility. Mrs Tremblay was pleased with the proposed transfer and the progress she had made in acute care. I completed all documentation and discharged her from my caseload ...

To read the full Practice Story and complete a reflective exercise please visit Evolve at http://evolve.elsevier.com/Curtin/OT

KARIN: A PRACTICE STORY OF A PERSON EXPERIENCING RHEUMATOID ARTHRITIS - REFLECTING ON PRACTICE

MATHILDA BJÖRK & INGRID THYBERG

Part 1: Initial Diagnosis

Conclude/exit. As Karin only wanted to focus on reducing the pain and swelling of her right wrist and she responded positively to the intervention it was decided that she had successfully obtained her goals. Karin indicated that she was feeling positive, full of energy and empowered ...

To read the full Practice Story and complete a reflective exercise please visit Evolve at http://evolve.elsevier.com/Curtin/OT

ANGELA: A PRACTICE STORY OF A PERSON EXPERIENCING PALLIATIVE CARE - REFLECTING ON PRACTICE

DEIDRE MORGAN & CELIA MARSTON

Conclude/exit. The occupational therapist's role in terminal care varies from setting to setting. It may entail provision of assistive equipment like a hospital bed or air mattress to enable a person to die at home. It is possible to support a person's occupational preferences even at this time. For example, if a person prefers to be amongst the activity of family everyday life, the person's hospital bed could be situated in a family living area ...

To read the full Practice Story and complete a reflective exercise please visit Evolve at http://evolve.elsevier.com/Curtin/OT

INDEX

Note: Page numbers followed by *f* indicate figures, *t* indicate tables and *b* indicate boxes.